POCKET VERSION

drug facts and comparisons®

Drug Facts and Comparisons® Pocket Version, Second Edition, 1998

Adapted from *Drug Facts and Comparisons®* loose-leaf drug information service. Previous copyrights 1947-1997 by Facts and Comparisons.

ISBN 1-57439-032-5

Printed in the United States of America

Published by
Facts and Comparisons®
111 West Port Plaza, Suite 300
St. Louis, Missouri 63146-3098
314/878-2515

FACTS AND COMPARISONS® PUBLISHING GROUP

Vincent J. Parker
President

Denise S. Threlkeld
Coordinating Editor

Paul S. Heirendt
Director, Marketing and Sales

Rachel C. Hagemann, RPh
Technical Editor

Renée M. Short
Assistant Editor

Steven K. Hebel, RPh
Director, Editorial/Production

Bernie R. Olin, PharmD
Director, Drug Information

Renée Rivard, PharmD
Drug Information Specialist

Sara L. Schweain
Assistant Editor

Jennifer K. Walsh
Composition Specialist

DRUG FACTS AND COMPARISONS® POCKET VERSION REVIEWERS

Daniel L. Brown, PharmD
Director of Pharmacy Services
Merced Community Medical Center
Merced, California

Dennis J. Cada, PharmD
Publisher, Health Systems
Facts and Comparisons
St. Louis, Missouri

Kate Farthing, PharmD
Drug Information Coordinator
Oregon Health Sciences University
Drug Information Service

Steven K. Hebel, RPh
Director, Editorial/Production
Facts and Comparisons
St. Louis, Missouri

Joyce A. Generali, RPh, MS
Director, Drug Information Center
Clinical Associate Professor
University of Kansas Medical Center
Kansas City, Kansas

Mary J. Ferrill, PharmD
Assistant Professor
Drug Information Specialist
University of the Pacific
School of Pharmacy
Stockton, California

Mary Beth Shirk, PharmD
Clinical Pharmacy Specialist, Pain Management
The Ohio State University Medical Center
Columbus, Ohio

Burgunda V. Sweet, PharmD
Chief, Drug Information Services
The University of Michigan Hospitals
Ann Arbor, Michigan

FACTS AND COMPARISONS® EDITORIAL ADVISORY PANEL

CONTRIBUTING REVIEW PANEL

Siret D. Jaanus, PhD
Acting Chairman
Department of Biomedical Sciences
State University of New York
State College of Optometry
New York, New York

Robert E. Kates, PharmD, PhD
President
Analytical Solutions, Inc.
Sunnyvale, California

Julio R. Lopez, PharmD
Assistant Professor, School of Pharmacy, University of the Pacific
Assistant Clinical Professor, School of Pharmacy, University of California, San Francisco
Director, Drug Information Center, VA Medical Center
Martinez, California

Susan O'Donoghue, MD
Associate Director, Cardiac Arrhythmia Center
Washington Hospital Center
Washington, DC

Richard M. Oksas, PharmD, MPh
Pharmaceutical Consultant
Medication Information Service
Torrance, California

Edward V. Platia, MD
Director, Cardiac Arrhythmia Center
Washington Hospital Center
Professor of Medicine
George Washington University School of Medicine

Michael T. Reed, PharmD
Associate Professor of Clinical Pharmacy
Arnold and Marie Schwartz College of Pharmacy and Health Sciences of Long Island University
Brooklyn, New York
The Mount Sinai Medical Center
New York, New York

J. James Rowsey, MD
Professor and Chairman
Department of Ophthalmology
University of South Florida College of Medicine
Tampa, Florida

Frederick L. Ruben, MD
Infectious Disease Division
Montefiore University Hospital
University of Pittsburgh
Pittsburgh, Pennsylvania

Mary Beth Shirk, PharmD
Clinical Pharmacy Specialist, Pain Management
The Ohio State University Medical Center
Columbus, Ohio

Burgunda V. Sweet, PharmD
Clinical Pharmacist, Home Medication Infusion Service
The University of Michigan Hospitals
Ann Arbor, Michigan

Udho Thadani, MBBS, FRCP(C), FACC
Professor of Medicine
Vice Chief of Cardiology and Director of Clinical Research
University of Oklahoma Health Sciences Center
Oklahoma City, Oklahoma

Robert A. Wild, MD
Chief, Section of Research & Education in Women's Health
Department of Obstetrics and Gynecology
University of Oklahoma Health Sciences Center
Oklahoma City, Oklahoma

Thom J. Zimmerman, MD, PhD
Chairman of Department of Ophthalmology and Visual Sciences
Professor of Pharmacology & Toxicology
University of Louisville

Table of Contents

HOW TO USE

Drug monographs in *Drug Facts and Comparisons®, Pocket Version* are arranged by use. Drugs with similar therapeutic or pharmacologic characteristics have been grouped together to allow the healthcare provider to compare these drugs easily and determine the most appropriate drug therapy. Standard sections within the monographs occur in a consistent format. Once the user is familiar with the organization of the data, the desired information can be located quickly.

Monograph Organization

1. *Therapeutic class:* Drugs that share the same therapeutic class will share a common title that appears on the left-hand pages. If there is no shared class, the monograph title will repeat.
2. *Drug name:* Generic names and any common synonyms appear in a horizontal bar which introduces a new monograph. Synonyms follow the generic name in parentheses and are separated by semicolons.
3. *Product table:* Doseforms and strengths of generic drugs are listed in the left column with their schedules (eg, *Rx*, *otc*, *c-II*). If more than one generic entity is included in the monograph (eg, beta blockers), the drugs appear in all caps with specific information below. The more common trade names, with their specific manufacturers/distributors, are listed in the righthand column. If the drug is available generically, the word "Various" appears at the beginning of the trade name listing.
4. *Warning box:* Potentially life-threatening reactions specified in the product labeling will appear in a box. *Not included in sample.*
5. *Actions:* A brief discussion of significant pharmacologic and pharmacokinetic information.
6. *Indications:* All FDA-approved indications are included. In addition, off-label uses with substantial documentation may appear under the term "Unlabeled uses".
7. *Contraindications:* All known contraindications are included.
8. *Warnings:* A brief description of major warnings associated with the drug. Standard sections (eg, Pregnancy, Lactation, Children) appear at the end of this section. The Pregnancy section generally only lists the Standard Pregnancy Category (A, B, C, D or X). A description of these categories can be found in the Appendix.
9. *Precautions:* Potential conditions for which the patient should be cautioned (eg, photosensitivity) are included, as well as other significant situations where caution is warranted.
10. *Drug Interactions:* Drugs that may interact (affect or be affected by the interacting agent) are listed. Lab test and drug/food interactions are also included.
11. *Adverse Reactions:* Where possible, reactions that occur in 3% or more of patients have been listed. When percentages were not available, significant reactions not discussed in Warnings or Precautions are included.
12. *Administration and Dosage:* Appropriate dosage, dosage range, etc is included. When available, specific information for administration in situations such as renal impairment, elderly patients, etc. is included.

1

112 **DANAZOL**

2 **DANAZOL**

Capsules: 50, 100 and 200 mg (*Rx*) Various, *Danocrine* (Sanofi Winthrop) 3

4

Actions:

5 *Pharmacology:* A synthetic androgen derived from ethisterone, danazol suppresses the pituitary-ovarian axis by inhibiting the output of pituitary gonadotropins. Danazol depresses the output of both follicle-stimulating hormone (FSH) and luteinizing hormone (LH). Danazol acts by direct enzymatic inhibition of sex steroid synthesis and competitively inhibits binding of steroids to their cytoplasmic receptors in target tissues.

In endometriosis, danazol alters the normal and ectopic endometrial tissue so that it becomes inactive and atrophic.

Pharmacokinetics: Blood levels of danazol do not increase proportionately with increases in dose. When the dose is doubled, plasma levels increase only about 35% to 40%.

6 **Indications:**

Endometriosis: For the treatment of endometriosis amenable to hormonal management.

Fibrocystic breast disease: Danazol is usually effective in decreasing nodularity, pain and tenderness, but it alters hormone levels; recurrence of symptoms is very common after cessation of therapy.

Hereditary angioedema: For the prevention of attacks of angioedema in males and females.

Unlabeled uses: Danazol has been used to treat precocious puberty, gynecomastia and menorrhagia. It has also been studied in the treatment of idiopathic immune thrombocytopenia, lupus-associated thrombocytopenia and autoimmune hemolytic anemia.

7 **Contraindications:**

Undiagnosed abnormal genital bleeding; markedly impaired hepatic, renal or cardiac function; pregnancy and lactation.

8 **Warnings:**

Carcinoma of the breast should be excluded before initiating therapy for fibrocystic breast disease.

Long-term experience with danazol is limited. Long-term therapy with other steroids alkylated at the 17 position has been associated with serious toxicity (cholestatic jaundice, peliosis hepatis). Similar toxicity may develop after long-term danazol.

Androgenic effects may not be reversible even when the drug is discontinued. Watch patients closely for signs of virilization.

Pregnancy: Use a nonhormonal method of contraception. If a patient becomes pregnant during treatment, discontinue use. Continuing treatment may result in androgenic effects in the fetus.

9 **Precautions:**

Fluid retention: Conditions influenced by edema require careful observation.

Hepatic dysfunction has been reported; perform periodic liver function tests.

Semen should be checked for volume, viscosity, sperm count and motility every 3 to 4 months, especially in adolescents.

10 **Drug Interactions:**

Drugs that may interact with danazol include insulin and warfarin.

11 **Adverse Reactions:**

Significant adverse reactions include: Edema; vaginitis; nervousness; emotional lability; hepatic dysfunction; elevated blood pressure; pelvic pain; carpal tunnel syndrome; sleep disorders; fatigue; tremor; visual disturbances; anxiety; depression; gastroenteritis.

12 **Administration and Dosage:**

Endometriosis: Begin therapy during menstruation or make sure the patient is not pregnant. Administer 800 mg/day in 2 divided doses to best achieve amenorrhea and rapid response to painful symptoms. Downward titration to a dose sufficient to main-

PREFACE

The Pocket Version of *Drug Facts and Comparisons®* (*DFC*) is an abridged version of the full *DFC* publication designed for quick reference by the health-care professional. The purpose of *DFC Pocket Version* is to provide an easy-to-use, concise, portable version that can be utilized in daily practice. It is not intended to replace the complete information found in *DFC*; however, it provides the same reliable source of drug information.

In addition to the extensive review panel for *DFC*, a separate panel of drug information specialists and hospital pharmacists was established to determine which drug monographs would be most valuable to you along with the data for each drug you need most. The book is arranged therapeutically in 12 chapters in a consistent format. Single-agent monographs have been pared down to provide the essential information that a healthcare provider needs to aid in drug therapy decisions. Product tables, which list trade names, doseforms, strengths and manufacturers, are included at the beginning of each monograph. Group monographs contain product information and dosing instructions for each of the drugs in a specific class (eg, beta blockers). Actions, indications, contraindications, warnings, drug interactions and significant adverse reactions (those occurring in ≥ 3% of patients) are also included for all monographs. Most important, the useful tables that are so common to *DFC* have, for the most part, been retained in the Pocket Version.

Appendix material (eg, Management of Overdosage, FDA Pregnancy Categories) is also available for reference. A comprehensive index will help you reach the desired information quickly and easily.

Facts and Comparisons® hopes you find *Drug Facts and Comparisons® Pocket Version* a valuable tool in daily practice. As always, your comments and suggestions are appreciated.

Steven K. Hebel, RPh
Director, Editorial/Production

Chapter 1
NUTRITIONALS

RECOMMENDED DIETARY ALLOWANCES OF VITAMINS AND MINERALS

Recommended Dietary Allowances (RDA) are published by the Food and Nutrition Board, National Research Council-National Academy of Sciences, as a guide for nutritional problems and to provide standards of good nutrition for different age groups. They are revised periodically.

The RDA values are *not requirements*;they are *recommended* daily intakes of certain essential nutrients. Based on available scientific knowledge, they are believed to be adequate for known nutritional needs for most *healthy* persons under usual environmental stresses. The recommended allowances vary for age and sex, with extra allowances for women during pregnancy and lactation. The most commonly used RDA values (the "reference male" and "reference female") are those of adults 23 to 50 years of age. With the exception of energy (kilocalories), the RDA provide for individual requirement variations and prevent symptoms of clinical deficiency of 97% of the population.

RDA have been established for many essential nutrients; however, present knowledge of human nutritional needs of pantothenic acid and biotin is incomplete. Therefore, to ensure adequate nutrient intake, obtain the recommended allowances from as varied a selection of foods as possible. Nutritionists suggest that dietary planning include regular intake of each of the four basic food groups:

1.) Milk, cheese, dairy products — Minimum 2 servings/day.
2.) 2. Meat, poultry, fish, beans — Minimum 2 servings/day.
3.) 3. Vegetables, fruit — Minimum 4 servings/day.
4.) 4. Bread, cereal (whole-grain and enriched or fortified) — Minimum 4 servings/day.

Such a balance, in sufficient quantities, will provide about 1200 kcal enough protein, and most of the vitamins and minerals required daily. A person may increase nutrient and energy intake by consuming larger quantities (or more servings/day) of the four basic food groups. Nutrient and energy intake may also be increased by selecting food from the fifth group, fats-sweets-alcohol, which mainly provides energy.

RDA quantities apply only to healthy persons and are not intended to cover therapeutic nutritional requirements in disease or other abnormal states (ie, metabolic disorders, weight reduction, chronic disease, drug therapy). Although certain single nutrients in larger quantities may have pharmacologic actions, these are unrelated to nutritional functions. There is no convincing evidence that consuming excessive quantities of single nutrients will cure or prevent nonnutritional diseases.

The "official" listings of United States Recommended Daily Allowances (US-RDAs) should not be confused with the RDA values. US-RDA are derived from the 1968 RDA and serve as legal standards for nutritional labeling of food and dietary food and dietary supplement products controlled by the Food and Drug Administration. Generally, they represent the higher value of the male or female RDA and are grouped into only three age brackets plus one category for pregnant or lactating women. Prior to 1972, these allowances were erroneously listed as minimum daily requirements (MDR). A second fallacy perpetuated by US-RDA labeling of foods is the implication that a food is defective if it does not contain all the officially established nutrients in their full US-RDA quantities. No individual food is nutritionally complete, but several foods together should complement each other to provide maximal nutrient balance and to minimize naturally occurring toxic principles consumed from any individual foodstuff.

The Recommended Dietary Allowances (RDA) for adult males and adult females are included in each individual vitamin monograph. The table on the following page presents the listing of vitamin and mineral RDA values for all age groups as published in Recommended Dietary Allowances, 10th Edition, National Academy of Sciences, Washington, D.C., 1989.

RECOMMENDED DIETARY ALLOWANCES[1]

Patient Parameters						Fat-Soluble Vitamins				Water-Soluble Vitamins							Minerals						
Age (years) or Condition	Weight[2] (kg)	Weight[2] (lb)	Height[2] (cm)	Height[2] (in)	Protein g	Vitamin A μg RE[3]	Vitamin D IU[4]	Vitamin E IU[5]	Vitamin K μg	Ascorbic Acid (C) mg	Thiamine (B_1) mg	Riboflavin (B_2) mg	Niacin (B_3) mg	Pyridoxine (B_6) mg	Folate μg	Cyanocobalamin (B_{12}) μg	Calcium mg	Phosphorus mg	Magnesium mg	Iron mg	Zinc mg	Iodine μg	Selenium μg
Infants																							
0.0-0.5	6	13	60	24	13	375	300	4	5	30	0.3	0.4	5	0.3	25	0.3	400	300	40	6	5	40	10
0.5-1	9	20	71	28	14	375	400	6	10	35	0.4	0.5	6	0.6	35	0.5	600	500	60	10	5	50	15
Children																							
1-3	13	29	90	35	16	400	400	9	15	40	0.7	0.8	9	1	50	0.7	800	800	80	10	10	70	20
4-6	20	44	112	44	24	500	400	10	20	45	0.9	1.1	12	1.1	75	1	800	800	120	10	10	90	20
7-10	28	62	132	52	28	700	400	10	30	45	1	1.2	13	1.4	100	1.4	800	800	170	10	10	120	30
Males																							
11-14	45	99	157	62	45	1000	400	15	45	50	1.3	1.5	17	1.7	150	2	1200	1200	270	12	15	150	40
15-18	66	145	176	69	59	1000	400	15	65	60	1.5	1.8	20	2	200	2	1200	1200	400	12	15	150	50
19-24	72	160	177	70	58	1000	400	15	70	60	1.5	1.7	19	2	200	2	1200	1200	350	10	15	150	70
25-50	79	174	176	70	63	1000	200	15	80	60	1.5	1.7	19	2	200	2	800	800	350	10	15	150	70
51 +	77	170	173	68	63	1000	200	15	80	60	1.2	1.4	15	2	200	2	800	800	350	10	15	150	70
Females																							
11-14	46	101	157	62	46	800	400	12	45	50	1.1	1.3	15	1.4	150	2	1200	1200	280	15	12	150	45
15-18	55	120	163	64	44	800	400	12	55	60	1.1	1.3	15	1.5	180	2	1200	1200	300	15	12	150	50
19-24	58	128	164	65	46	800	400	12	60	60	1.1	1.3	15	1.6	180	2	1200	1200	280	15	12	150	55
25-50	63	138	163	64	50	800	200	12	65	60	1.1	1.3	15	1.6	180	2	800	800	280	15	12	150	55
51 +	65	143	160	63	50	800	200	12	65	60	1	1.2	13	1.6	180	2	800	800	280	10	12	150	55
Pregnant					60	800	400	15	65	70	1.5	1.6	17	2.2	400	2.2	1200	1200	320	30	15	175	65
Lactating – 1st 6 mo.					65	1300	400	18	65	95	1.6	1.8	20	2.1	280	2.6	1200	1200	355	15	19	200	75
2nd 6 mo.					62	1200	400	16	65	90	1.6	1.7	20	2.1	260	2.6	1200	1200	340	15	16	200	75

Reproduced from: *Recommended Dietary Allowances,* 10th edition, 1989, National Academy of Sciences, National Academy Press, Washington, DC.

[1] The allowances, expressed as average daily intakes over time, are intended to provide for individual variations among most normal persons as they live in the US under usual environmental stresses. Diets should be based on a variety of common foods in order to provide other nutrients for which human requirements have been less well defined.

[2] Weights and heights of Reference Adults are actual medians for the US population of the designated age, as reported by NHANES II. The median weights and heights of those under 19 years of age were taken from Hamill PV et al. *Am J Clin Nutr* 1979;32:607-29. The use of these figures does not imply that the height-to-weight ratios are ideal.

[3] Retinol equivalents. 1 retinol equivalent = 1 μg retinol or 6 μg β-carotene.

[4] As cholecalciferol. 10 μg cholecalciferol = 400 IU of vitamin D.

[5] α-Tocopherol equivalents. 1 mg d-α-tocopherol = α-TE = 1.49 IU.

PYRIDOXINE HCl (B_6)

Tablets: 25, 50 and 100 mg (*otc*)	Various, *Nestrex* (Fielding)
Tablets, timed release: 100 mg (*otc*)	*Vitamin* B_6 (Mission)
Injection: 100 mg per ml	Various

Actions:

Pharmacology: Vitamin B_6 activity in natural substances, pyridoxine in plants, and pyridoxal or pyridoxamine in animals, are converted to physiologically active forms of vitamin B_6, pyridoxal phosphate (codecarboxylase) and pyridoxamine phosphate.

Vitamin B_6, a water-soluble vitamin, acts as a coenzyme in the metabolism of protein, carbohydrates and fat. In protein metabolism, it participates in the decarboxylation of amino acids; conversion of tryptophan to niacin or serotonin (5-hydroxytryptamine); and deamination, transamination and transulfuration of amino acids. In carbohydrate metabolism, it is responsible for the breakdown of glycogen to glucose-1-phosphate.

Pharmacokinetics: Pyridoxine is readily absorbed from the GI tract. Its biologic half-life is 15 to 20 days. Vitamin B_6 is degraded to 4–pyridoxic acid in the liver. This metabolite is excreted in the urine.

Indications:

Oral: Pyridoxine deficiency, including: Inadequate diet; drug-induced deficiency (eg, isoniazid, hydralazine, oral contraceptives); inborn errors of metabolism (eg, B_6-dependent seizures or B_6-responsive anemia).

Parenteral: The parenteral route is indicated when oral use is not feasible.

Unlabeled uses:

Hydrazine poisoning. Although experience is limited, reversal of neurologic symptoms and CNS depression have been reported.

Premenstrual syndrome (PMS) has been treated with pyridoxine 40 to 500 mg/day, but with conflicting results.

Hyperoxaluria type I (and oxalate kidney stones) has been treated with pyridoxine in low doses (25 to 300 mg/day).

Nausea and vomiting in pregnancy is sometimes treated with pyridoxine.

Contraindications:

Sensitivity to pyridoxine.

Warnings:

Pregnancy: Category A. Pyridoxine requirements are increased during pregnancy and lactation.

Lactation: Pyridoxine may inhibit lactation by prolactin suppression.

Children: Safety and efficacy have not been established for use in children.

Precautions:

Pyridoxine deficiency alone is rare; multiple vitamin deficiencies can be expected in any inadequate diet. Some drugs may result in increased pyridoxine requirements, including: Cycloserine, hydralazine, isoniazid, oral contraceptives and penicillamine.

Drug abuse and dependence: Noted in adults withdrawn from 200 mg/day.

Drug Interactions:

Drugs that may interact include levodopa, phenobarbital and phenytoin.

Adverse Reactions:

Sensory neuropathic syndromes; unstable gait; numb feet; awkwardness of hands; perioral numbness; decreased sensation to touch, temperature and vibration; paresthesia; somnolence; low serum folic acid levels.

Administration and Dosage:

Recommended Dietary Allowances (RDAs): Adult males, 1.7 to 2 mg; adult females, 1.4 to 1.6 mg. Requirements are greater in persons having certain genetic defects or those receiving INH or oral contraceptives. For a complete listing of RDAs by age, sex and condition, see the Recommended Dietary Allowances table.

Dietary deficiency: 10 to 20 mg/day for 3 weeks. Follow-up is recommended daily for several weeks with an oral therapeutic multivitamin containing 2 to 5 mg pyridoxine. Correct poor dietary habits and encourage a well balanced diet.

Vitamin B_6 dependency syndrome: May require a therapeutic dosage of as much as 600 mg/day and 30 mg/day for life.

Deficiencies due to isoniazid: Some advocate pyridoxine prophylaxis for all isoniazid patients; others advocate prophylaxis only for those predisposed to neuropathy. Recommended prophylactic doses range from 6 to 100 mg daily, but the lower doses appear more common. Treatment of established neuropathy requires 50 to 200 mg daily.

INH poisoning (> 10 g), given an equal amount of pyridoxine: 4 g IV followed by 1 g IM every 30 minutes. Pyridoxine can be toxic, but doses of 70 to 357 mg/kg have been administered without incident.

VITAMIN C (Ascorbic Acid)

ASCORBIC ACID	
Tablets: 25, 50, 100, 250, 500 and 1000 mg (*otc*)	Various, *One A Day Extras Vitamin* C (Miles)
Tablets, chewable: 60, 100, 250 and 500 mg (*otc*)	Various, *Flavorcee* (Hudson)
Tablets and caplets, timed release: 500, 1000 and 1500 mg (*otc*)	Various
Caplets: 500 mg (*otc*)	*SunKist Vitamin* C (Ciba)
Capsules, timed release: 500 mg (*otc*)	Various, *Ascorbicap* (ICN), *Cebid Timecelles* (Hauck), *Cevi-Bid* (Geriatric)
Lozenges: 60 mg (*otc*)	*N'ice Vitamin C Drops* (SmithKline Beecham Consumer)
Crystals: 4 g per teaspoonful (*otc*)	*Vita*-C (Freeda)
Powder: 4 g per teaspoonful (*otc*)	*Dull*-C (Freeda)
Liquid: 35 mg per 0.6 ml (*otc*)	*Ce-Vi-Sol* (Mead Johnson Nutritional)
Solution: 100 mg per ml (*otc*)	*Cecon* (Abbott)
Syrup: 500 mg per 5 ml (*otc*)	Various
Injection: 250 and 500 mg per ml	Various
SODIUM ASCORBATE	
Tablets: 585 mg (equiv. to 500 mg ascorbic acid) (*otc*)	Various
Crystals: 1020 mg (equiv. to 900 mg ascorbic acid) per ¼ tspful (*otc*)	Various
Injection: 250 mg/ml (equiv. to 222 mg/ml ascorbic acid) (*Rx*)	Various
562.5 mg per ml (equiv. to 500 mg/ml ascorbic acid) (*Rx*)	*Cenolate* (Abbott), *Cevalin* (Lilly)
CALCIUM ASCORBATE	
Tablets: 610 mg (equiv. to 500 mg ascorb. acid)	Various
Powder: 1 g (equiv. to 826 mg ascorb. acid) per ¼ tspful	Various

Actions:

Pharmacology: Vitamin C, a water-soluble vitamin, is an essential vitamin in man; however, its exact biological functions are not fully understood. It is essential for the formation and the maintenance of intercellular ground substance and collagen, for catecholamine biosynthesis, for synthesis of carnitine and steroids, for conversion of folic acid to folinic acid and for tyrosine metabolism.

The deficiency state *scurvy* is characterized by degenerative changes in the capillaries, bone and connective tissues. Mild vitamin C deficiency symptoms may include faulty bone and tooth development, gingivitis, bleeding gums and loosened teeth. Febrile states, chronic illness and infection increase the need for ascorbic acid. Premature and immature infants require relatively large amounts of the vitamin. Hemovascular disorders, burns and delayed fracture and wound healing are indications for an increase in daily intake.

Absorption of dietary ascorbate from the intestines is nearly complete. Vitamin C is readily available in citrus fruit, tomatoes, potatoes and leafy vegetables.

Indications:

Prevention and treatment of scurvy. Parenteral administration is desirable in an acute deficiency or when absorption of oral ascorbic acid is uncertain.

Unlabeled uses: Vitamin C in high doses has been advocated for prevention of the common cold, for treatment of asthma, atherosclerosis, wounds, schizophrenia and for treatment of cancer; however, clinical data do not justify these uses.

Vitamin C (≥ 2 g/day) may be used as a urinary acidifier in conjunction with methenamine therapy. Data regarding the efficacy of ascorbic acid for this purpose are conflicting. Failure of vitamin C to significantly lower urine pH may be attributed to inadequate dosage (< 2 g/day).

Vitamin C in doses of at least 150 mg has been used to control idiopathic methemoglobinemia (less effective than methylene blue).

Warnings:

Excessive vitamin C doses: Diabetics, patients prone to recurrent renal calculi, those undergoing stool occult blood tests and those on sodium restricted diets or anticoagulant therapy should not take excessive doses of vit. C over an extended time period.

Pregnancy: Category C. Do not administer ascorbic acid to pregnant women in excess of the amount needed for treatment. The possibility of the fetus adapting to high levels of the vitamin could result in a scorbutic condition after birth when the intake drops to normal levels. This action is controversial.

Lactation: Ascorbic acid is excreted in breast milk, but does not necessarily increase in response to increasing doses.

Drug Interactions:

Contraceptives (oral) and estrogens: Ascorbic acid increases serum levels of estrogen and estrogen contained in oral contraceptives, possibly resulting in adverse reactions.

Warfarin: The anticoagulant action of warfarin may be reduced.

Drug/Lab test interactions: Large doses (> 500 mg) of vitamin C may cause false-negative urine **glucose determinations.**

No exogenous vitamin C should be ingested for 48 to 72 hours before amine-dependent stool **occult blood** tests are conducted because possible false-negative results may occur.

Adverse Reactions:

Large doses may cause diarrhea and precipitation of cystine, oxalate or urate renal stones if the urine becomes acidic during therapy.

Transient mild soreness may occur at the site of IM or SC injection. Too rapid IV administration may cause temporary faintness or dizziness.

Administration and Dosage:

Recommended Dietary Allowances (RDAs): Adults, 60 mg. For a complete listing of RDAs by age, sex and condition, refer to the Recommended Dietary Allowances table.

Parenteral: Administer IV, IM or SC. Avoid too rapid IV injection. Absorption and utilization are somewhat more efficient with the IM route, which is usually preferred.

Infants: Average daily protective requirement is 30 mg. The usual curative dose is 100 to 300 mg daily, continued as long as clinical symptoms persist or until saturation, as indicated by excretion tests, has been attained.

Premature infants: May require 75 to 100 mg/day.

Adults: The average protective dose is 70 to 150 mg daily. For scurvy, 300 mg to 1 g daily is recommended. However, up to 6 g/day has been administered parenterally to normal adults without evidence of toxicity.

Enhanced wound healing – Doses of 300 to 500 mg daily for 7 to 10 days both preoperatively and postoperatively are adequate, although considerably larger amounts have been recommended.

Burns – For severe burns, daily doses of 1 to 2 g are recommended.

In other conditions in which the need for vitamin C is increased, 3 to 5 times the daily optimum allowances appears adequate.

CALCIUM

CALCIUM ACETATE	
Tablets: 667 mg (169 mg calcium) (*Rx*)	*Calphron* (Nepro-Tech), *PhosLo* (Braintree)
CALCIUM CARBONATE	
Tablets: 650 and 667 mg, and 1.25 and 1.5 g (260 mg calcium) (*otc*)	Various, *Cal-Plus* (Geriatric Pharm.), *Caltrate 600* (Lederle), *Os-Cal 500* (SmithKline Beecham), *Oyster Shell Calcium-500* (Vangard)
Tablets, chewable: 750 mg and 1.25 g (*otc*)	*Calci-Chew* (R & D), *Caltrate, Jr.* (Lederle), *Os-Cal 500*, *Tums 500* (SmithKline Beecham)
Capsules: 125 mg (50 mg calcium) (*otc*)	*Cal-Guard Softgels* (Rugby)
1250 mg powdered calcium carbonate (500 mg calcium) (*otc*)	*Calci-Mix* (R & D)
Oral Suspension: 1.25 g (500 mg calcium) per 5 ml (*otc*)	Various
Powder: 6.5 g (2400 mg calcium) per packet (*otc*)	*Cal Carb-HD* (Konsyl Pharm.)
CALCIUM CITRATE	
Tablets: 950 mg (200 mg calcium) (*otc*)	*Citracal* (Mission)
Tablets, effervescent: 2376 mg (500 mg calcium) (*otc*)	*Citracal Liquitab* (Mission)
CALCIUM GLUBIONATE	
Syrup: 1.8 mg calcium glubionate (115 mg calcium) per 5 ml (*otc*)	*Neo-Calglucon* (Sandoz)
CALCIUM GLUCONATE	
Tablets: 500 mg (45 mg calcium), 650 mg (58.5 mg calcium), 975 mg (87.75 mg calcium), 1 g (90 mg calcium) (*otc*)	Various
Injection: 10% (*Rx*)	Various
CALCIUM GLUCEPTATE	
Injection: 1.1 g per 5 ml (*Rx*)	Various
CALCIUM LACTATE	
Tablets: 325 mg (42.25 mg calcium), 650 mg (84.5 mg calcium) (*otc*)	Various
CALCIUM CHLORIDE	
Injection: 10% (*Rx*)	Various
CALCIUM SALT COMBINATIONS	
Injection: 50 mg calcium glycerophosphate and 50 mg calcium lactate per 10 ml in sodium chloride solution (0.08 mEq Ca/ml) (*Rx*)	*Calphosan* (Glenwood)
TRICALCIUM PHOSPHATE	
Tablets: 1565.2 mg (600 mg calcium) (*otc*)	*Posture* (Whitehall)

Actions:

Pharmacology: Calcium is essential for the functional integrity of the nervous and muscular systems, for normal cardiac contractility and the coagulation of blood. It also functions as an enzyme cofactor and affects the secretory activity of endocrine and exocrine glands. Normal levels are 8.5 to 10.5 mg/dl.

Hypocalcemia –

Symptoms: Tetany; paresthesias; laryngospasm; muscle spasms; seizures (usually grand mal); irritability; depression; psychosis; prolonged QT interval; intestinal cramps and malabsorption; respiratory arrest. Prolonged hypocalcemia may be associated with ectodermal defects including the nails, skin and teeth.

Pharmacokinetics: Calcium acetate, when taken with meals, combines with dietary phosphate to form insoluble calcium phosphate which is excreted in the feces.

Elemental Calcium Content of Calcium Salts

Calcium salt	% Calcium	mEq Ca^{++}/g
Calcium glubionate	6.5	3.3
Calcium gluconate	9.3	4.6
Calcium lactate	13	9.2
Calcium citrate	21	12
Calcium acetate	25	12.6
Tricalcium phosphate	39	19.3

Elemental Calcium Content of Calcium Salts		
Calcium salt	% Calcium	mEq Ca^{++}/g
Calcium carbonate	40	20
Calcium chloride	27.3	13.6
Calcium gluceptate	8.2	4.1

Differences in absorption and bioavailability between various calcium salts appear to exist, as well as between different preparations of the same salt.

Approximately 80% of body calcium is excreted in the feces as insoluble salts; urinary excretion accounts for the remaining 20%.

Indications:

Oral: As a dietary supplement when calcium intake may be inadequate.

In the treatment of calcium deficiency states which may occur in diseases such as: Tetany of newborn; end stage renal disease, mild to moderate renal insufficiency; renal osteodystrophy; acute and chronic hypoparathyroidism; pseudohypoparathyroidism; postmenopausal and senile osteoporosis; rickets and osteomalacia. Some studies have suggested that the use of calcium citrate is more effective than calcium carbonate in the treatment of postmenopausal osteoporosis.

Calcium acetate (PhosLo) – Control of hyperphosphatemia in end stage renal failure; does not promote aluminum absorption.

Parenteral:

Hypocalcemia – For a prompt increase in plasma calcium levels (eg, neonatal tetany and tetany due to parathyroid deficiency, vitamin D deficiency, alkalosis); prevention of hypocalcemia during exchange transfusions; conditions associated with intestinal malabsorption.

Calcium chloride and gluconate – Adjunctive therapy in the treatment of insect bites or stings, such as Black Widow spider bites to relieve muscle cramping; sensitivity reactions, particularly when characterized by urticaria; depression due to overdosage of magnesium sulfate; acute symptoms of lead colic; rickets; osteomalacia.

Calcium chloride – To combat the deleterious effects of severe hyperkalemia as measured by ECG, pending correction of increased potassium in the extracellular fluid.

Cardiac resuscitation: Particularly after open heart surgery, when epinephrine fails to improve weak or ineffective myocardial contractions.

Calcium gluconate – To decrease capillary permeability in allergic conditions, nonthrombocytopenic purpura and exudative dermatoses such as dermatitis herpetiformis; for pruritus of eruptions caused by certain drugs; in hyperkalemia, calcium gluconate may aid in antagonizing the cardiac toxicity, provided the patient is not receiving digitalis therapy.

Unlabeled uses:

Oral – Calcium supplementation may lower blood pressure in some hypertensive patients with indices suggesting calcium "deficiency." However, other hypertensives may experience a pressor response.

In one study, calcium administration significantly reduced premenstrual symptoms of fluid retention, pain and negative affect.

Parenteral – Calcium salts have been used to treat verapamil overdose, treat acute hypotension from verapamil and prevent initial hypotension in patients requiring verapamil for whom decreases in blood pressure could be detrimental.

Contraindications:

Oral: Renal calculi; hypophosphatemia; hypercalcemia.

Parenteral: Hypercalcemia; ventricular fibrillation; digitalized patients.

Warnings:

Extravasation: **Calcium chloride** and **gluconate** can cause severe necrosis, sloughing and abscess formation with IM or SC administration. Take great care to avoid extravasation or accidental injection into perivascular tissues.

PhosLo: End stage renal failure patients may develop hypercalcemia when given calcium with meals. Do not give other calcium supplements concurrently with *PhosLo*.

Chronic hypercalcemia may lead to vascular and other soft tissue calcification. Monitor serum calcium levels twice weekly during the early dose adjustment period. Do not allow serum calcium times phosphate product to exceed 66.

Pregnancy: Category C. (*PhosLo* and parenteral).

Precautions:

Oral:

Hypercalcemia/hypercalciuria may result when therapeutic amounts are given for prolonged periods; it is most likely to occur in hypoparathyroid patients receiving high doses of vitamin D. Avoid by frequent monitoring of plasma and urine calcium levels.

Calcium citrate –

Renal function impairment: Avoid concurrent aluminum- containing antacids.

Parenteral:

Cardiovascular effects – It is particularly important to prevent a high concentration of calcium from reaching the heart because of the danger of cardiac syncope.

Drug Interactions:

Drugs that may affect calcium include thiazide diuretics.

Drugs that may be affected by calcium include atenolol, sodium polystyrene sulfonate, tetracyclines and verapamil. *Oral only:* Iron salts, quinolones; *parenteral only:* Digitalis glycosides.

Drug/Lab test interactions: Transient elevations of plasma 11-hydroxy-cortico- steroid levels (Glenn-Nelson technique) may occur when IV calcium is administered, but levels return to control values after 1 hour. In addition, IV calcium gluconate can produce false-negative values for serum and urinary magnesium.

Drug/Food interactions: Diets high in dietary fiber have been shown to decrease absorption of calcium due to decreased transit time in the GI tract and complexing of fiber with the calcium.

Adverse Reactions:

Oral: GI disturbances are rare. Mild hypercalcemia (Ca^{++} > 10.5 mg/dl) may be asymptomatic or manifest itself as: Anorexia; nausea; vomiting; constipation; abdominal pain; dry mouth; thirst; polyuria. More severe hypercalcemia (Ca^{++} 12 mg/dl) is associated with confusion, delirium, stupor and coma.

The risk of hypercalcemia with calcium acetate may be less than that of calcium carbonate and calcium citrate.

IM administration: Mild local reactions may occur (calcium gluceptate). Local necrosis and abscess formation may occur with **calcium gluconate,** and severe necrosis and sloughing may occur with IM or SC administration of **calcium chloride.**

IV administration: Rapid IV administration may cause bradycardia, sense of oppression, tingling, metallic, calcium or chalky taste or "heat waves". Rapid IV **calcium gluconate** may cause vasodilation, decreased blood pressure, cardiac arrhythmias, syncope and cardiac arrest. **Calcium chloride** injections cause peripheral vasodilation and a local burning sensation; blood pressure may fall moderately.

Administration and Dosage:

Oral: Calcium must be in a soluble, ionized form to be absorbed. Solubility (except calcium lactate) is increased by acidic pH. Give with meals to maximize acidity and solubility.

Recommended Dietary Allowances (RDAs) – Adults (25 to > 51 years of age), 800 mg. For a complete listing of RDAs by age, sex and condition, refer to the RDA table in the Nutritionals chapter.

Dietary supplement – The usual daily dose is 500 mg to 2 g, 2 to 4 times daily.

An NIH Consensus Development conference recommends a calcium intake for adults of 1000 to 1500 mg/day to reduce bone loss associated with aging.

PhosLo – 2 tablets with each meal. The dosage may be increased to bring the serum phosphate value < 6 mg/dl, as long as hypercalcemia does not develop. Most patients require 3 to 4 tablets with each meal.

Parenteral: Calcium gluconate is generally preferred over calcium chloride as it is less irritating.

IV – Warm solutions to body temperature and give slowly (0.5 to 2 ml/min); stop if patient complains of discomfort. Resume when symptoms disappear. Following injection, patient should remain recumbent for a short time. Repeated injections may be needed because of the rapid calcium excretion. Inject **calcium chloride** and **gluconate** through a small needle into a large vein to minimize venous irritation.

IM administration of **calcium gluceptate** and **gluconate** may be tolerated; however, reserve this route for emergencies when technical difficulty makes IV injection impossible. Administer **calcium gluconate** only by the IV route and **calcium chloride** by the IV or intraventricular route.

CALCIUM GLUCONATE – For IV use only, either directly or by infusion; SC or IM injection may cause severe necrosis and sloughing. Do not exceed a rate of 0.5 to 2 ml/minute. Calcium gluconate may also be administered by intermittent infusion at a rate not exceeding 200 mg/min, or by continuous infusion. Discontinue injection if the patient complains of discomfort. Do not use IM, as abscess formation and local necrosis may occur.

Adults: 2.3 to 9.3 mEq (5 to 20 ml) as required. Dosage range is 4.65 to 70 mEq/day.

Children: 2.3 mEq/kg/day or 56 mEq/m ^{2}/day, well diluted; give slowly in divided doses.

Infants: Not more than 0.93 mEq (2 ml).

Emergency elevation of serum calcium:

Adults – 7 to 14 mEq (15 to 30.1 ml) IV.

Children – 1 to 7 mEq (2.2 to 15 ml).

Infants – < 1 mEq (2.2 ml). Depending on patient response, these doses can be repeated every 1 to 3 days.

Hypocalcemic tetany:

Adults – 4.5 to 16 mEq of calcium (9.7 to 34.4 ml) may be given IM until therapeutic response occurs.

Children – 0.5 to 0.7 ,mEq/kg (1.1 to 1.5 ml/kg) IV 3 or 4 times daily or until tetany is controlled.

Neonates – 2.4 mEq/kg/day (5.2 ml/kg/day) in divided doses.

Hyperkalemia with secondary cardiac toxicity: Administer IV to provide 2.25 to 14 mEq (4.8 to 30.1 ml) while monitoring ECG. If necessary, repeat doses after 1 to 2 min.

Magnesium intoxication:

Adults – Initial dose is 4.5 to 9 mEq (9.7 to 19.4 ml) IV. Adjust subsequent doses to patient response. If IV use is not possible, give 2 to 5 mEq (4.3 to 10.8 ml) IM.

Exchange transfusion:

Adults – Approximately 1.35 mEq (2.9 ml) IV concurrent with each 100 ml of citrated blood.

Neonates – Administer IV at a dosage of 0.45 mEq (1 ml)/100 ml of exchanged citrated blood.

Admixture incompatibilities: Calcium salts should not generally be mixed with **carbonates, phosphates, sulfates** or **tartrates** in parenteral admixtures; they are conditionally compatible with potassium phosphates, depending on concentration. Calcium ions will chelate **tetracycline.**

CALCIUM GLUCEPTATE –

IM: 2 to 5 ml (0.44 to 1.1 g). Inject 5 ml (1.1 g) doses in the gluteal region or, in infants, in the lateral thigh.

IV: 5 to 20 ml (1.1 to 4.4 g). Warm solution to body temperature and administer slowly (≤ 2 ml/min).

Exchange transfusions in newborns: 0.5 ml (0.11 g) after every 100 ml of blood exchanged.

CALCIUM CHLORIDE –

For IV use only. Injection is irritating to veins and must not be injected into tissues, since severe necrosis and sloughing may occur. Avoid extravasation. Administer slowly (not to exceed 0.5 to 1 ml/minute).

Intraventricular administration – In cardiac resuscitation, injection may be made into the ventricular cavity; do not inject into the myocardium. Intraventricular injection may be administered by personnel who are well trained in the technique and familiar with possible complications. Break off the IV needle supplied with the syringe and replace with a suitable intracardiac needle by affixing it firmly to the Luer taper provided on the syringe. After the injection has been completed, remove the needle/syringe assembly from the injection site by grasping the needle at the Luer fitting.

The intraventricular dose usually ranges from 200 to 800 mg (2 to 8 ml).

Hypocalcemic disorders:

Adults – 500 mg to 1 g at intervals of 1 to 3 days, depending on response of patient or serum calcium determinations. Repeated injections may be required.

Children – 0.2 ml/kg up to 1 to 10 ml/day.

Magnesium intoxication: Give 500 mg promptly; observe patient for signs of recovery before further doses are given.

Hyperkalemic ECG disturbances of cardiac function: Adjust dosage by constant monitoring of ECG changes during administration.

Cardiac resuscitation:

Adults – Dose ranges from 500 mg to 1 g IV or 200 to 800 mg injected into the ventricular cavity.

Children – 0.2 ml/kg

PHOSPHORUS REPLACEMENT PRODUCTS

Tablets: 250 mg phosphorus, 49.4 mg potassium, 250.5 mg sodium (*Rx*)	*Uro-KP-Neutral* (Star)
250 mg phosphorus, 45 mg potassium, 298 mg sodium (*Rx*)	*K-Phos Neutral* (Beach)
Powder: 250 mg phosphorus, 278 mg potassium, 164 mg sodium (*otc*)	*Neutra-Phos* (Willen)
250 mg phosphorus, 556 mg potassium (*otc*)	*Neutra-Phos-K* (Willen)

Actions:

Pharmacology: Phosphorus functions intracellularly for 1) Energy transport and production in the form of ATP and ADP; 2) phospholipids in cell membranes responsible for nutrient transport; 3) part of nucleic acids (RNA, DNA); 4) buffering systems and calcium transport.

Phosphate administration lowers urinary calcium levels and increases urinary phosphate levels and urinary pyrophosphate inhibitor. Orthophosphates appear to decrease the aggregation and number of oxalate crystals in the urine of calculous patients.

Indications:

Dietary supplements of phosphorus, particularly if the diet is restricted or if needs are increased.

Contraindications:

Addison's disease; hyperkalemia; acidification of urine in urinary stone disease; patients with infected urolithiasis or struvite stone formation; severely impaired renal function; presence of hyperphosphatemia.

Warnings:

Pregnancy: Category C.

Precautions:

Monitoring: The following determinations are important in patient monitoring (other tests may be warranted in some patients): Renal function; serum calcium; serum phosphorus; serum potassium; serum sodium. Monitor at periodic intervals during therapy.

Sodium/Potassium restriction: Use with caution if patient is on sodium or potassium restricted diet. These products provide significant amounts of sodium or potassium.

Special risk patients: Use with caution when the following medical problems exist: Cardiac disease (particularly in digitalized patients); acute dehydration; renal function impairment or chronic renal disease; extensive tissue breakdown; myotonia congenita; cardiac failure; cirrhosis of the liver or severe hepatic disease; peripheral and pulmonary edema; hypernatremia; hypertension; preeclampsia; hypoparathyroidism; osteomalacia; acute pancreatitis; rickets (rickets may benefit from phosphate therapy; however, use caution).

Kidney stones: Warn patients with kidney stones of the possibility of passing old stones when phosphate therapy is started.

Drug Interactions:

Drugs that may affect phosphorus include antacids, calcium, vitamin D, potassium-containing agents and potassium-sparing agents.

Adverse Reactions:

Individuals may experience a mild laxative effect for the first few days. If this persists, reduce the daily intake until this effect subsides, or, if necessary, discontinue use.

GI upset (eg, diarrhea, nausea, stomach pain, vomiting) may occur with phosphate therapy.

Administration and Dosage:

Recommended dietary allowances (RDAs): Adults, 800 to 1200 mg. For a complete listing of RDAs by age, sex and condition, refer to the RDA table.

Capsules must be reconstituted. Do *not* swallow capsules. Refer to manufacturers' labeling for reconstitution of capsules and powder.

MAGNESIUM

Tablets: 400 mg magnesium (oxide) (*otc*)	*Mag-200* (Optimox)
400 mg magnesium oxide (241.3 mg mangesium) (*otc*)	*Mag-Ox 400* (Blaine)
500 mg magnesium gluconate (27 mg magnesium) (*otc*)	*Almora* (Forest), *Magonate* (Fleming)
500 mg magnesium gluconate (29 mg magnesium) (*otc*)	*Magtrate* (Mission)
500 mg magnesium amino acids chelate (100 mg mangesium) (*otc*)	*Chelated Magnesium* (Freeda)
Tablets, sustained release: 535 mg magnesium chloride hexahydrate (64 mg magnesium) (*otc*)	*Slow-Mag* (Searle)
Caplets, sustained release: 84 mg magnesium (as lactate) (*otc*)	*Mag-Tab SR* (Niche)
Capsules: 140 mg magnesium oxide (84.5 mg magnesium) (*otc*)	*Uro-Mag* (Blaine)
Liquid: 54 mg/5 ml magnesium (as gluconate) (*otc*)	*Magonate* (Fleming)
Injection: 20% magnesium chloride (1.97 mEq/ml) (*Rx*)	Various
Injection: Magnesium sulfate. 10% (0.8 mEq/ml), 12.5% (1 mEq/ml) and 50% (4 mEq/ml) (*Rx*)	Various

Actions:

Pharmacology: Magnesium is an electrolyte which is necessary in a number of enzyme systems, phosphate transfer, muscular contraction and nerve conduction. Magnesium deficiency may occur in: Malabsorption syndromes; prolonged diarrhea or steatorrhea; vomiting; pancreatitis; aldosteronism; renal tubular damage; chronic alcoholism; prolonged IV therapy with magnesium-free solutions; diuretic therapy; during hemodialysis; renal tubular damage; disorders associated with hypokalemia and hypocalcemia; in patients on digitalis therapy. While there are large stores of magnesium present intracellularly and in bone in adults, these stores often are not mobilized sufficiently to maintain plasma levels; therefore serum levels may not reflect total magnesium stores.

Indications:

As a dietary supplement.

Unlabeled uses: A pyridoxine/magnesium oxide combination has been used to prevent recurrence of calcium oxalate kidney stones.

Oral magnesium gluconate may be a cost-effective and clinically effective alternative to oral ritodrine as a tocolytic for continued inhibition of contractions following parenteral magnesium sulfate.

Warnings:

Pregnancy: There is weak evidence that magnesium supplementation reduces the risk of poor perinatal outcome. However, since magnesium deficiency is rare, there appears to be no need for routine supplementation during pregnancy.

Precautions:

Renal disease: Do not use without physician supervision due to potential accumulation.

Excessive dosage may cause diarrhea and GI irritation.

Drug Interactions:

Drugs that may be affected by magnesium salts include aminoquinolines, digoxin, nitrofurantoin, penicillamine and tetracyclines.

Administration and Dosage:

1 g Mg = 83.3 mEq (41.1 mmol).

Dietary supplement: 54 to 483 mg/day in divided doses. Refer to product labeling.

Recommended dietary allowances (RDAs):

Adult – Males, 350 to 400 mg; females, 280 to 300 mg. For a complete listing of RDAs by age, sex and condition, refer to the RDA table.

Magnesium-containing antacids may also be used.

POTASSIUM REPLACEMENT PRODUCTS

Tablets, controlled release: 6.7 mEq (500 mg) potassium chloride in a wax matrix (*Rx*)	*Kaon-Cl* (Adria)
8 and 10 mEq (600 and 750 mg) potassium chloride in a wax matrix (*Rx*)	Various, *Klor-Con 8* (Upsher-Smith), *Slow-K* (Summit), *Kaon Cl-10* (Adria), *Klor-Con 10* (Upsher-Smith), *Klotrix* (Bristol), *K-Tab* (Abbott)
Tablets, extended release: 750 mg potassium chloride equivalent to 10 mEq potassium in a wax matrix (*Rx*)	Various
Tablets, controlled release: 750 mg microencapsulated potassium chloride equivalent to 10 mEq potassium (*Rx*)	*K-Dur 10* (Key), *Ten-K* (Summit)
1500 mg microencapsulated potassium chloride equivalent to 20 mEq potassium (*Rx*)	*K-Dur 20* (Key)
Tablets: 500 mg potassium gluconate (83.45 mg potassium) (*Rx*)	Various
595 mg potassium gluconate (99 mg potassium) (*Rx*)	Various
Tablets, effervescent: 20 mEq potassium (from potassium bicarbonate) (*Rx*)	*K + Care ET* (Alra)
20 mEq potassium (from potassium chloride and bicarbonate and lysine hydrochloride) (*Rx*)	*Klorvess* (Sandoz)
25 mEq potassium (from potassium chloride and bicarbonate and lysine hydrochloride) (*Rx*)	*K•Lyte/Cl* (Bristol)
50 mEq potassium (from potassium Cl and bicarbonate, l-lysine monohydrochloride and citric acid) (*Rx*)	*K•Lyte/Cl 50* (Bristol)
25 mEq potassium (from potassium bicarbonate) (*Rx*)	*K + Care ET* (Alra)
25 mEq potassium (as bicarbonate and citrate) (*Rx*)	Various, *Effer-K* (Nomax), *Klor-Con/EF* (Upsher-Smith), *K•Lyte* (Bristol)
50 mEq potassium (from potassium bicarbonate and citrate and citric acid) (*Rx*)	*K•Lyte DS* (Bristol)

Capsules, controlled release: 600 mg potassium chloride equivalent to 8 mEq potassium. Microencapuslated particles (*Rx*)	*Micro-K Extencaps* (Robins)
10 mEq (750 mg) potassium chloride. Microencapsulated particles (*Rx*)	Various, *K-Lease* (Adria), *K-Norm* (Fisons), *Micro-K 10 Extencaps* (Robins)
Liquid: 20 mEq/15 ml potassium and chloride (10% KCl) (*Rx*)	Various, *Cena-K* (Century), *Kaochlor 10% and S-F* (Adria), *Kay Ciel* (Forest), *Klorvess* (Sandoz)
30 mEq/15 ml potassium and chloiride (15% KCl) (*Rx*)	*Rum-K* (Fleming)
40 mEq/15 ml potassium and chloride (20% KCl) (*Rx*)	Various, *Cena-K* (Century), *Kaon-Cl 20%* (Adria)
20 mEq/15 ml potassium (as potassium gluconate) (*Rx*)	Various, *Kaon* (Adria), *K-G Elixir* (Geneva)
45 mEq/15 ml potassium (from potassium acetate, potassium bicarbonate and potassium citrate) (*Rx*)	*Tri-K* (Century)
20 mEq/15 ml potassium (as potassium gluconate & potassium citrate) (*Rx*)	*Twin-K* (Boots)
20 mEq potassium and 3.4 mEq chloride/15 ml (from potassium gluconate and potassium chloride (*Rx*)	*Kolyum* (Fisons)
Powder: 15 mEq potassium chloride per packet (*Rx*)	*K + Care* (Alra)
20 mEq potassium chloride per packet (*Rx*)	Various, *Gen-K* (Goldline), *Kay Ciel* (Forest), *K + Care* (Alta), *K-Lor* (Abbott), *Klor-Con* (Upsher-Smith), *Micro-K LS* (Robins)
25 mEq potassium chloride per dose (*Rx*)	*K•Lyte/Cl* (Mead-J)
20 mEq each potassium & chloride (potassium chloride, bicarbonate and citrate & lysine hydrochloride)/packet (*Rx*)	*Klorvess Effervescent Granules* (Sandoz)

Actions:

Pharmacology: Potassium participates in a number of essential physiological processes, such as maintenance of intracellular tonicity and a proper relationship with sodium across cell membranes, cellular metabolism, transmission of nerve impulses, contraction of cardiac, skeletal and smooth muscle, acid-base balance and maintenance of normal renal function. Normal potassium serum levels range from 3.5 to 5 mEq/L.

mEq/g of Various Potassium Salts	
Potassium salt	mEq/g
Potassium gluconate	4.3
Potassium citrate	9.8
Potassium bicarbonate	10
Potassium acetate	10.2
Potassium chloride	13.4

Hypokalemia – Potassium depletion is usually a consequence of prolonged therapy with oral diuretics, primary or secondary hyperaldosteronism, diabetic ketoacidosis, severe diarrhea (especially if associated with vomiting) or inadequate replacement during prolonged parenteral nutrition. Potassium depletion due to these causes is usually accompanied by a concomitant deficiency of chloride and is manifested by hypokalemia and metabolic alkalosis.

The use of potassium salts in patients receiving diuretics for uncomplicated essential hypertension is often unnecessary when such patients have a normal diet. However, if hypokalemia occurs, dietary supplementation with potassium-containing foods may be adequate. In more severe cases, potassium salt supplementation may be indicated.

Symptoms: Weakness; fatigue; ileus; tetany; polydipsia; flaccid paralysis or impaired ability to concentrate urine (in advanced cases). ECG may reveal atrial and ventricular ectopy, prolongation of QT interval, ST segment depression, conduction defects, broad or flat T waves or appearance of U waves.

Indications:

Treatment of hypokalemia in the following conditions: With or without metabolic alkalosis; digitalis intoxication; familial periodic paralysis; diabetic acidosis; diarrhea and vomiting; surgical conditions accompanied by nitrogen loss, vomiting, suction drainage, diarrhea and increased urinary excretion of potassium; certain cases of uremia; hyperadrenalism; starvation and debilitation; corticosteroid or diuretic therapy.

Prevention of potassium depletion when dietary intake is inadequate in the following conditions: Patients receiving digitalis and diuretics for CHF; significant cardiac arrhythmias; hepatic cirrhosis with ascites; states of aldosterone excess with normal renal function; potassium-losing nephropathy; certain diarrheal states.

When hypokalemia is associated with alkalosis, use potassium chloride. When acidosis is present, use the bicarbonate, citrate, acetate or gluconate potassium salts.

Unlabeled uses: In patients with mild hypertension, the use of potassium supplements appears to result in a long-term reduction of blood pressure.

Contraindications:

Severe renal impairment with oliguria or azotemia; untreated Addison's disease; hyperkalemia from any cause; adynamia episodica hereditaria; acute dehydration; heat cramps; patients receiving potassium-sparing diuretics or aldosterone-inhibiting agents.

Warnings:

Hyperkalemia: In patients with impaired potassium excretion, potassium salts can produce hyperkalemia or cardiac arrest. This occurs most commonly in patients given IV potassium, but may also occur in patients given oral potassium. Potentially fatal hyperkalemia can develop rapidly and may be asymptomatic.

Hyperkalemia may be manifested only by an increased serum potassium concentration and characteristic ECG changes. However, the following may also occur: Paresthesias; heaviness, muscle weakness and flaccid paralysis of the extremities; listlessness; mental confusion; decreased blood pressure; shock; cardiac arrhythmias; heart block.

GI lesions: Potassium chloride tablets have produced stenotic or ulcerative lesions of the small bowel and death. These lesions are caused by a concentration of potassium ion in the region of a rapidly dissolving tablet, which injures the bowel wall and produces obstruction, hemorrhage or perforation. The reported frequency of small bowel lesions is much less with wax matrix tablets and microencapsulated tablets than with enteric coated tablets. Discontinue either type of tablet immediately and consider the possibility of bowel obstruction or perforation if severe vomiting, abdominal pain or distention or GI bleeding occurs.

Patients at greatest risk for developing potassium chloride-induced GI lesions include: The elderly, the immobile and those with scleroderma, diabetes mellitus, mitral valve replacement, cardiomegaly or esophageal stricture/compression.

Metabolic acidosis and hyperchloremia: In some patients (eg, those with renal tubular acidosis), potassium depletion is rarely associated with metabolic acidosis and hyperchloremia. Replace with potassium bicarbonate, citrate, acetate or gluconate.

Renal function impairment requires careful monitoring of the serum potassium concentration and appropriate dosage adjustment.

Pregnancy: Category C.

Children: Safety and efficacy for use in children have not been established.

Drug Interactions:

Drugs that may interact include ACE inhibitors, potassium-sparing diuretics and digitalis.

Adverse Reactions:

Adverse reactions may include nausea, vomiting, diarrhea, flatulence and abdominal discomfort due to GI irritation. They are best managed by diluting the preparation further, by taking with meals or by dose reduction. Severe reactions may include hyperkalemia; GI obstruction, bleeding, ulceration or perforation.

Administration and Dosage:

The usual dietary intake of potassium ranges between 40 to 150 mEq/day.

Individualize dosage. Usual range is 16 to 24 mEq/day for the prevention of hypokalemia to 40 to 100 mEq/day or more for the treatment of potassium depletion.

Reserve slow release potassium chloride preparations for patients who cannot tolerate liquids or effervescent potassium preparations, or for patients in whom there is a problem of compliance with these preparations.

Some studies suggest the "microencapsulated" preparations are less likely to cause GI damage; however, evidence conflicts and a specific recommendation of one solid oral product over another cannot be made. Avoid enteric coated products.

Potassium intoxication may result from any therapeutic dosage.

SODIUM CHLORIDE

Tablets: 650 mg, 1 and 2.25 g (*otc*)	Various
Tablets, slow release: 410 mg sodium chloride and 150 mg potassium chloride in wax matrix (*otc*)	*Slo-Salt-K* (Mission)

Indications:

Prevention or treatment of extracellular volume depletion, dehydration or sodium depletion; aid in the prevention of heat prostration.

Warnings:

Acclimatization: Inappropriate salt administration in an effort to acclimatize to a hot environment can be dangerous. Balanced electrolytes and adequate hydration are essential.

Salt tablets may pass through the GI tract undigested. Avoid their use in treating heat cramps since they may cause vomiting, pooling of oral fluids and potassium depletion. Use oral salt solutions instead.

Pregnancy/Lactation: Seek professional advice before using these products while pregnant or breastfeeding.

Precautions:

Supplementation: Individuals with adequate dietary sodium intake and normal renal function should not require sodium chloride supplementation. Balanced electrolyte supplements may be preferred to prevent hypokalemia.

Use with caution in the presence of CHF, kidney dysfunction, peripheral or pulmonary edema or preeclampsia.

Administration and Dosage:

Refer to specific product labeling for dosage guidelines.

SODIUM CHLORIDE

Solution: 0.45% (77 mEq/L sodium, 77 mEq/L chloride) (*Rx*)	Various
0.9% (154 mEq/L sodium, 154 mEq/L chloride) (*Rx*)	Various
3% (513 mEq/L sodium, 513 mEq/L chloride) (*Rx*)	Various
5% (855 mEq/L sodium, 855 mEq/L chloride) (*Rx*)	Various
Solution: 0.9% sodium chloride (as Bacteriostatic Sodium Chloride Inj) (*Rx*)	Various
Concentrated Solution: 14.6% and 23.4% sodium chloride (*Rx*)	Various

Actions:

Pharmacology: Normal osmolarity of the extracellular fluid ranges between 280 to 300 mOsm/L; it is primarily a function of sodium and its accompanying ions, chloride and bicarbonate. Sodium chloride is the principal salt involved in maintenance of plasma tonicity. One g of sodium chloride provides 17.1 mEq sodium and 17.1 mEq chloride.

Hyponatremia (< 135 mEq/L) – Symptoms may include weakness, nausea, disorientation, lethargy and headache; severe cases may progress to seizures and coma.

Indications:

Hyponatremia: For parenteral restoration of sodium ion in patients with restricted oral intake. Sodium replacement is specifically indicated in patients with hyponatremia or low salt syndrome. Sodium Chloride may also be added to compatible carbohydrate solutions such as Dextrose in Water to provide electrolytes.

Diluents: Sodium Chloride Injections are also indicated as pharmaceutic aids and diluents for the infusion of compatible drug additives.

0.9% Sodium Chloride (Normal Saline), which is isotonic, restores both water and sodium chloride losses. Other indications for parenteral 0.9% saline include: Diluting or dissolving drugs for IV, IM or SC injection; flushing of IV catheters; extracellular fluid replacement; treatment of metabolic alkalosis in the presence of fluid loss and mild sodium depletion; as a priming solution in hemodialysis procedures and to initiate and terminate blood transfusions without hemolyzing red blood cells.

0.45% Sodium Chloride (Hypotonic) is primarily a hydrating solution and may be used to assess the status of the kidneys, since more water is provided than is required for salt excretion. It may also be used in the treatment of hyperosmolar diabetes where the use of dextrose is inadvisable and there is a need for large amounts of fluid without an excess of sodium ions.

3% or 5% Sodium Chloride (Hypertonic) is used in hyponatremia and hypochloremia due to electrolyte and fluid loss replaced with sodium-free fluids; drastic dilution of body water following excessive water intake; emergency treatment of severe salt depletion.

Bacteriostatic Sodium Chloride: Only for diluting or dissolving drugs for IV, IM or SC injection.

Concentrated Sodium Chloride: As an additive in parenteral fluid therapy for use in patients who have special problems of sodium electrolyte intake or excretion. It is intended to meet the specific requirements of the patient with unusual fluid and electrolyte needs. After available clinical and laboratory information is considered and correlated, determine the appropriate number of milliequivalents of Concentrated Sodium Chloride Injection, USP and dilute for use.

Contraindications:

Hypernatremia; fluid retention; when the administration of sodium or chloride could be clinically detrimental.

3% and 5% sodium chloride solutions: Elevated, normal or only slightly decreased plasma sodium and chloride concentrations.

Bacteriostatic sodium chloride: Newborns; for fluid or sodium chloride replacement.

Warnings:

Fluid/solute overload: Excessive amounts of sodium chloride by any route may cause hypokalemia and acidosis. Administration of IV solutions can cause fluid or solute overload resulting in dilution of serum electrolyte concentrations, CHF, overhydration, congested states or acute pulmonary edema, especially in patients with cardiovascular disease and in patients receiving corticosteroids or corticotropin or drugs that may give rise to sodium retention. The risk of dilutional states is inversely proportional to the electrolyte concentration. The risk of solute overload causing congested states with peripheral and pulmonary edema is directly proportional to the electrolyte concentration.

Infusion of > 1 L of isotonic (0.9%) sodium chloride may supply more sodium and chloride than normally found in serum, resulting in hypernatremia; this may cause a loss of bicarbonate ions, resulting in an acidifying effect. Infusion during or immediately after surgery may result in excessive sodium retention.

Bacteriostatic Sodium Chloride: Do not use in newborns. Benzyl alcohol as a preservative in Bacteriostatic Sodium Chloride Injection has been associated with toxicity in newborns. This toxicity may result from both high cumulative amounts (mg/kg) of benzyl alcohol and the limited detoxification capacity of the neonate liver. These solutions have not been reported to cause problems in older infants, children and adults. It is estimated that a 30 ml IV dose may be given to adults without toxic effects. Use preservative-free Sodium Chloride Injection for flushing intravascular catheters. Where a sodium chloride solution is required for preparing or diluting medications for use in newborns, use only preservative-free 0.9% Sodium Chloride.

Concentrated Sodium Chloride Injection is hypertonic and must be diluted before use. Inadvertent direct injection or absorption of concentrated Sodium Chloride Injection may give rise to sudden hypernatremia and such complications as cardiovascular shock, CNS disorders, extensive hemolysis, cortical necrosis of the kidneys and severe local tissue necrosis (if administered extravascularly). Do not use unless solution is clear. When administered peripherally, slowly infuse through a small bore needle placed well within the lumen of a large vein to minimize venous irritation. Carefully avoid infiltration.

Surgical patients should seldom receive salt-containing solutions immediately following surgery unless factors producing salt depletion are present. Because of renal retention of salt during surgery, additional electrolyte given IV may result in fluid retention, edema and overloading of the circulation.

Renal function impairment: Infusions of sodium ions may result in excessive sodium retention; administer with care.

Pregnancy: Category C.

Children: Safety and efficacy have not been established.

Precautions:

Monitoring: Clinical evaluation and periodic laboratory determinations are necessary to monitor changes in fluid balance, electrolyte concentrations and acid-base balance during prolonged parenteral therapy or whenever the condition of the patient warrants such evaluation. Significant deviations from normal concentrations may require tailoring of the electrolyte pattern.

Extraordinary electrolyte losses may necessitate additional electrolyte supplementation. Supply additional essential electrolytes, minerals and vitamins as needed.

Hypokalemia may result from excessive administration of potassium-free solutions.

Special risk patients: Administer cautiously to patients with decompensated cardiovascular, cirrhotic and nephrotic disease, circulatory insufficiency, hypoproteinemia, hypervolemia, urinary tract obstruction, CHF and to patients with concurrent edema and sodium retention, those receiving corticosteroids or corticotropin and those retaining salt.

Elderly or postoperative patients: Exercise care in administering sodium-containing solutions in renal or cardiovascular insufficiency, with or without CHF.

3% and 5% sodium chloride solutions: Infuse very slowly and use with caution to avoid pulmonary edema; observe patients constantly.

Administration and Dosage:

In the average adult, daily requirements of sodium and chloride are met by the infusion of 1 L of 0.9% sodium chloride (154 mEq each of sodium and chloride). Base fluid administration on calculated maintenance or replacement fluid requirements.

IV catheters: Prior to and after administration of the medication, entirely flush the catheter with 0.9% Sodium Chloride for Injection. Use in accord with any warnings or precautions appropriate to the medication being administered.

Calculation of sodium deficit: To calculate the amount of sodium that must be administered to raise serum sodium to the desired level, use the following equation (TBW = total body water): Na deficit (mEq) = TBW (desired – observed plasma Na).

Base the repletion rate on the degree of urgency in the patient. Use of hypertonic saline (eg, 3% or 5%) will correct the deficit more rapidly.

Concentrated Sodium Chloride: Not for direct infusion. *Must* be diluted before use.

The dosage as an additive in parenteral fluid therapy is predicated on specific requirements of the patient. The appropriate volume is then withdrawn for proper dilution. Having determined the mEq of sodium chloride to be added, divide by four to calculate the number of ml to be used. Withdraw this volume and transfer into appropriate IV solutions such as 5% Dextrose Injection. The properly diluted solution may be given IV.

Admixture incompatibilities: Some additives may be incompatible. Consult a pharmacist.

To minimize the risk of possible incompatibilities arising from mixing this solution with other additives that may be prescribed, inspect the final infusate for cloudiness or precipitation immediately after mixing, prior to administration and periodically during administration. Do not store.

POTASSIUM SALTS

POTASSIUM ACETATE	
Injection: 2 and 4 mEq/ml (*Rx*)	Various
POTASSIUM CHLORIDE CONCENTRATE	
Injection: 2 mEq/ml and 10, 20, 30, 40, 60 and 90 mEq (*Rx*)	Various

Actions:

Pharmacology: The principal intracellular cation, potassium is essential for maintenance of intracellular tonicity; transmission of nerve impulses; contraction of cardiac, skeletal and smooth muscle; and maintenance of normal renal function. Potassium participates in carbohydrate utilization and protein synthesis and is critical in regulating nerve conduction and muscle contraction, particularly in the heart.

Hypokalemia – Gradual potassium depletion occurs via renal excretion, through GI loss or because of inadequate intake (excretion > intake). Depletion usually results from diuretic therapy, primary or secondary hyperaldosteronism, diabetic ketoacidosis, severe diarrhea (especially if associated with vomiting) or inadequate replacement during prolonged parenteral nutrition.

Potassium depletion sufficient to cause 1 mEq/L drop in serum potassium requires a loss of about 100 to 200 mEq of potassium from the total body store.

Symptoms: Weakness; fatigue; ileus; polydipsia; flaccid paralysis or impaired ability to concentrate urine (in advanced cases).

ECG may reveal premature atrial and ventricular contractions, prolongation of QT interval, ST segment depression, broad and flat T waves or appearance of U waves. Severe cases may lead to muscular weakness, paralysis, respiratory failure.

Pharmacokinetics: Normally about 80% to 90% of potassium intake is excreted in urine with the remainder voided in stool and, to a small extent, in perspiration. Kidneys do not conserve potassium well; during fasting or in patients on a potassium-free diet, potassium loss from the body continues, resulting in potassium depletion. A deficiency of either potassium or chloride will lead to a deficit of the other.

Indications:

Prevention and treatment of moderate or severe potassium deficit when oral replacement therapy is not feasible.

Potassium acetate is useful as an additive for preparing specific IV fluid formulas when patient needs cannot be met by standard electrolyte or nutrient solutions.

Also indicated for marked loss of GI secretions by vomiting, diarrhea, GI intubation or fistulas; prolonged diuresis; prolonged parenteral use of potassium-free fluids; diabetic acidosis, especially during vigorous insulin and dextrose treatment; metabolic alkalosis; attacks of hereditary or familial periodic paralysis; hyperadrenocorticism; primary aldosteronism; overmedication with adrenocortical steroids, testosterone or corticotropin; healing phase of scalds or burns; cardiac arrhythmias, especially due to digitalis glycosides.

Contraindications:

Diseases where high potassium levels may be encountered; hyperkalemia; renal failure and conditions in which potassium retention is present; oliguria or azotemia; anuria; crush syndrome; severe hemolytic reactions; adrenocortical insufficiency (untreated Addison's disease); adynamica episodica hereditaria; acute dehydration; heat cramps; hyperkalemia from any cause; early postoperative oliguria except during GI drainage.

Warnings:

Potassium intoxication: Do not infuse rapidly. High plasma concentrations of potassium may cause death through cardiac depression, arrhythmias or arrest. Monitor potassium replacement therapy whenever possible by continuous or serial ECG. In addition to ECG effects, local pain and phlebitis may result when a > 40 mEq/L concentration is infused.

Renal impairment or adrenal insufficiency may cause potassium intoxication. Potassium salts can produce hyperkalemia and cardiac arrest. Potentially fatal hyperkalemia can develop rapidly and be asymptomatic. Use with great caution, if at all.

Concentrated potassium solutions are for IV admixtures only; do not use undiluted. Direct injection may be instantaneously fatal.

Metabolic alkalosis: Potassium depletion is usually accompanied by an obligatory loss of chloride resulting in hypochloremic metabolic alkalosis. Treat the underlying cause of potassium depletion and administer IV potassium chloride.

Use solutions containing acetate ion carefully in metabolic or respiratory alkalosis, and when there is an increased level or impairment of utilization of this ion.

Metabolic acidosis: Treat associated hypokalemia with an alkalinizing potassium salt.

Musculoskeletal/Cardiac effects: When serum sodium or calcium concentration is reduced, moderate elevation of serum potassium may cause toxic effects on the heart and skeletal muscle. Weakness and later paralysis of voluntary muscles, with consequent respiratory distress and dysphagia, are generally late signs, sometimes significantly preceding dangerous or fatal cardiac toxicity.

Renal function impairment: Normal kidney function permits safe potassium therapy. Although temporary elevation of serum potassium level due to renal insufficiency secondary to dehydration or shock may mask an intracellular potassium deficit, do not replenish potassium until renal function is reestablished by overcoming dehydration and shock. Discontinue potassium-containing solutions if signs of renal insufficiency develop during infusions.

Pregnancy: Category C.

Precautions:

Monitoring: Close medical supervision with frequent ECGs and serum potassium determinations. Plasma levels are not necessarily indicative of tissue levels.

Special risk patients: Use with caution in the presence of cardiac disease, particularly in digitalized patients or in the presence of renal disease, metabolic acidosis, Addison's disease, acute dehydration, prolonged or severe diarrhea, familial periodic paralysis, hypoadrenalism, hyperkalemia, hyponatremia and myotonia congenita.

Fluid/Solute overload: IV administration can cause fluid or solute overloading resulting in dilution of serum electrolyte concentrations, overhydration, congested states or pulmonary edema.

Drug Interactions:

Drugs that may interact include ACE inhibitors, potassium-sparing diuretics, potassium-containing salt substitutes and digitalis.

Adverse Reactions:

Hyperkalemia: Adverse reactions involve the possibility of potassium intoxication. Signs and symptoms include: Paresthesias of extremities; flaccid paralysis; muscle or respiratory paralysis; areflexia; weakness; listlessness; mental confusion; weakness and heaviness of legs; hypotension; cardiac arrhythmias; heart block; ECG abnormalities such as disappearance of P waves, spreading and slurring of the QRS complex with development of a biphasic curve and cardiac arrest.

GI: Nausea; vomiting; abdominal pain; diarrhea.

Administration and Dosage:

mEq/g of Various Potassium Salts

Potassium salt	mEq/g
Potassium acetate	10.2
Potassium chloride	13.4
Dibasic potassium phosphate[1]	11.5
Monobasic potassium phosphate[1]	7.3

[1] Commercial preparations of potassium phosphate injection contain a mixture of both mono- and dibasic salts.

Do not administer undiluted potassium. Potassium preparations must be diluted with suitable large volume parenteral solutions, mixed well and given by slow IV infusion.

Too rapid infusion of hypertonic solutions may cause local pain and, rarely, vein irritation. Adjust rate of administration according to tolerance. Use of the largest peripheral vein and a small bore needle is recommended.

The usual additive dilution of potassium chloride is 40 mEq/L of IV fluid. The maximum desirable concentration is 80 mEq/L, although extreme emergencies may dictate greater concentrations.

In critical states, potassium chloride may be administered in saline (unless saline is contraindicated) since dextrose may lower serum potassium levels by producing an intracellular shift.

Avoid "layering" of potassium by proper agitation of the prepared IV solution. Do not add potassium to an IV bottle in the hanging position.

Individualize dosage. Guide dosage and rate of infusion by ECG and serum electrolyte determinations. The following may be used as a guide:

Potassium Dosage/Rate of Infusion Guidelines

Serum K+	Maximum infusion rate	Maximum concentration	Maximum 24 hour dose
> 2.5 mEq/L	10 mEq/hr	40 mEq/L	200 mEq
< 2 mEq/L	40 mEq/hr	80 mEq/L	400 mEq

Add electrolytes to the mixed solutions only after considering electrolytes already present and potential incompatibilities such as calcium and phosphate or sulfate.

Children: IV infusion up to 3 mEq/kg or 40 mEq/m^2/day. Adjust volume of administered fluids to body size.

MAGNESIUM

MAGNESIUM CHLORIDE	
Injection: 20% (1.97 mEq/ml) (*Rx*)	Various
MAGNESIUM SULFATE	
Injection: 10% (0.8 mEq/ml), 12.5% (1 mEq/ml), 50% (4 mEq/ml) (*Rx*)	Various

Actions:

Pharmacology: Magnesium is a cofactor in a number of enzyme systems, and is involved in neurochemical transmission and muscular excitability. As a nutritional adjunct in hyperalimentation, the precise mechanism of action is uncertain.

Magnesium deficiency is rare in well nourished individuals, except in malabsorption syndromes. Magnesium deficiency may occur in malabsorption syndromes, chronic alcoholism, malnutrition, intestinal bypass surgery, diuretic therapy, severe diarrhea, prolonged nasogastric suction, steatorrhea, during hemodialysis, diabetes mellitus, pancreatitis, primary aldosteronism and renal tubular damage. Early symptoms of hypomagnesemia (< 1.5 mEq/L) may develop as early as 3 to 4 days or within weeks. Predominant deficiency effects are neurological. Hypocalcemia and hypokalemia often follow low serum levels of magnesium. While large stores of magnesium are found intracellularly and in bone in adults, they often are not mobilized sufficiently to maintain plasma levels. Parenteral magnesium therapy repairs the plasma deficit and causes deficiency signs and symptoms to cease. The normal adult body contains 20 to 30 g (2000 mEq) magnesium.

Magnesium prevents or controls convulsions by blocking neuromuscular transmission and decreasing the amount of acetylcholine liberated at the end plate by the motor nerve impulse. Magnesium is said to have a depressant effect on the CNS, but it does not adversely affect the mother, fetus or neonate when used as directed in eclampsia or preeclampsia. Normal plasma magnesium levels range from 1.5 to 2.5 mEq.

Magnesium acts peripherally to produce vasodilation. With low doses, only flushing and sweating occur; larger doses cause a lowering of blood pressure and CNS depression. The central and peripheral effects of magnesium poisoning are antagonized by IV administration of calcium.

One g of magnesium sulfate provides 8.12 mEq of magnesium.

Hypermagnesemia – As plasma magnesium rises above 4 mEq/L, the deep tendon reflexes are first decreased and then disappear as the plasma level approaches 10 mEq/L. At this level respiratory paralysis may occur. Heart block also may occur at this or lower plasma levels of magnesium. Serum magnesium concentrations in excess of 12 mEq may be fatal.

Pharmacokinetics: IM injection results in therapeutic plasma levels within 60 minutes and persists for 3 to 4 hours. IV doses provide immediate effects that last for 30 minutes. Effective anticonvulsant serum levels range from 2.5 to 7.5 mEq/L. Magnesium is excreted by the kidneys at a rate proportional to the plasma concentration and glomerular filtration.

Indications:

Hypomagnesemia: Magnesium sulfate is used as replacement therapy in magnesium deficiency especially in acute hypomagnesemia accompanied by signs of tetany similar to those observed in hypocalcemia. In such cases, the serum magnesium (Mg;) level is usually below the lower limit of normal (1.5 to 2.5 or 3 mEq/L) and the serum calcium (Ca++) level is normal (4.3 to 5.3 mEq/L) or elevated.

Total parenteral nutrition patients may develop hypomagnesemia (<1.5 mEq/L) without supplementation. Magnesium is added to correct or prevent hypomagnesemia.

Preeclampsia/eclampsia/nephritis (magnesium sulfate): Prevention and control of convulsions of severe preeclampsia and eclampsia and for control of hypertension, encephalopathy and convulsions associated with acute nephritis in children.

Unlabeled uses: Inhibition of premature labor (tocolytic); however, it is not a first-line agent.

In suspected acute myocardial infarction patients immediately after admission to counteract post-infarctional hypomagnesemia and subsequent arrhythmias.

Magnesium IV is effective as a bronchodilator and, therefore, may be useful in some asthmatic patients.

Since magnesium deficiency may play a role in chronic fatigue syndrome, it has been suggested that magnesium administration may be beneficial in this condition; however, there are conflicting reports and further study is needed.

Contraindications:

Magnesium sulfate: Heart block or myocardial damage; IV magnesium to patients with preeclampsia during the 2 hours preceding delivery.

Magnesium chloride: Renal impairment; marked myocardial disease; coma.

Warnings:

Renal function impairment: Because magnesium is excreted by the kidneys, use with caution. Parenteral use in the presence of renal insufficiency may lead to magnesium intoxication.

Elderly: Geriatric patients often require reduced dosage because of impaired renal function. In patients with severe impairment, dosage should not exceed 20 g in 48 hours. Monitor serum magnesium in such patients.

Pregnancy: Category A.

When administered by continuous IV infusion (especially for > 24 hours preceding delivery) to control convulsions in toxemic mothers, the newborn may show signs of magnesium toxicity, including neuromuscular or respiratory depression.

Lactation: Magnesium is distributed into milk during parenteral magnesium sulfate administration.

Children: Safety and efficacy in children have not been established.

Precautions:

Monitoring: Maintain urine output at a level of ≥ 100 ml every 4 hours. Monitor serum magnesium levels and clinical status to avoid overdosage in preeclampsia.

Clinical indications of safe dosage regimen include presence of the patellar reflex (knee jerk) and absence of respiratory depression. Serum magnesium levels usually sufficient to control convulsions range from 3 to 6 mg/dl (2.5 to 5 mEq/L). Strength of deep tendon reflexes begins to diminish when magnesium levels exceed 4 mEq/L. Reflexes may be absent at 10 mEq/L, where respiratory paralysis is possible. Keep an injectable calcium salt immediately available to counteract potential hazards of magnesium intoxication in eclampsia.

Flushing/Sweating: Administer with caution if flushing or sweating occurs.

Drug Interactions:

Effects of nondepolarizing neuromuscular blocking agents may be increased by concurrent magnesium sulfate.

Adverse Reactions:

Adverse effects are usually the result of magnesium intoxication and include: Flushing; sweating; hypotension; stupor; depressed reflexes; flaccid paralysis; hypothermia; circulatory collapse; cardiac and CNS depression proceeding to respiratory paralysis (the most life-threatening effect).

Hypocalcemia with signs of tetany secondary to magnesium sulfate therapy for eclampsia has occurred.

Administration and Dosage:

IV administration: Do not exceed 1.5 ml/min of a 10% concentration (or its equivalent), except in cases of severe eclampsia with seizures. Dilute IV infusion solutions to a concentration of ≤ 20% prior to IV administration. The most commonly used diluents are 5% Dextrose Injection and 0.9% Sodium Chloride Injection.

IM administration: Deep IM injection of the undiluted (50%) solution is appropriate for adults, but dilute to ≤ 20% concentration prior to IM injection in children.

Admixture incompatibilities: Magnesium sulfate in solution may result in a precipitate formation when mixed with solutions containing: Alcohol (in high concentrations);

alkali carbonates and bicarbonates; alkali hydroxides; arsenates; barium; calcium; clindamycin phosphate; heavy metals; hydrocortisone sodium succinate; phosphates; polymyxin B sulfate; procaine HCl; salicylates; strontium; tartrates.

Hyperalimentation: Maintenance requirements are not precisely known. Maintenance dose range:

Adults – 8 to 24 mEq/day.

Infants – 2 to 10 mEq/day.

Mild magnesium deficiency:

Adults – 1 g (8.12 mEq; 2 ml of 50% solution) IM every 6 hours for 4 doses (total of 32.5 mEq/24 hours).

Severe hypomagnesemia:

IM – As much as 2 mEq/kg (0.5 ml of 50% solution) within 4 hours if necessary.

IV – 5 g (≈ 40 mEq)/L of 5% Dextrose Injection or 0.9% Sodium Chloride solution, infused over 3 hours. In treatment of deficiency states, observe caution to prevent exceeding renal excretory capacity.

Seizures associated with preeclampsia/eclampsia/nephritis: Refer to Anticonvulsants, Miscellaneous for complete dosing information.

SODIUM BICARBONATE

Injection: 4.2% (0.5 mEq/ml), 5% (0.6 mEq/ml), 7.5% (0.9 mEq/ml), 8.4% (1 mEq/ml) (*Rx*)	Various
Neutralizing Additive Solution: 4% (0.48 mEq/ml) (*Rx*)	*Neut* (Abbott)
4.2%(0.5 mEq/ml) (*Rx*)	Various

Actions:

Pharmacology: Increases plasma bicarbonate; buffers excess hydrogen ion concentration; raises blood pH; reverses the clinical manifestations of acidosis.

One g sodium bicarbonate provides 11.9 mEq each of sodium and bicarbonate.

Pharmacokinetics: Sodium bicarbonate in water dissociates to provide sodium and bicarbonate ions. Sodium is the principal cation of extracellular fluid. Bicarbonate is a normal constituent of body fluids and normal plasma level ranges from 24 to 31 mEq/L. Plasma concentration is regulated by the kidney. Bicarbonate anion is considered "labile" since, at a proper concentration of hydrogen ion, it may be converted to carbonic acid, then to its volatile form, carbon dioxide, excreted by lungs. Normally, a ratio of 1:20 (carbonic acid: bicarbonate) is present in extracellular fluid. In a healthy adult with normal kidney function, almost all the glomerular filtered bicarbonate ion is reabsorbed; < 1% is excreted in urine.

Indications:

Metabolic acidosis: In severe renal disease, uncontrolled diabetes, circulatory insufficiency due to shock, anoxia or severe dehydration, extracorporeal circulation of blood, cardiac arrest and severe primary lactic acidosis where a rapid increase in plasma total CO_2 content is crucial. Treat metabolic acidosis in addition to measures designed to control the cause of the acidosis. Since an appreciable time interval may elapse before all ancillary effects occur, bicarbonate therapy is indicated to minimize risks inherent to acidosis itself.

At one time it was suggested to administer bicarbonate during cardiopulmonary resuscitation following cardiac arrest; however, recent evidence suggests that little benefit is provided and its use may be detrimental. For treatment of acidosis in this clinical situation, concentrate efforts on restoring ventilation and blood flow. According to the American Heart Association guidelines, use as a last resort after other standard measures have been utilized.

Urinary alkalinization: In the treatment of certain drug intoxications (eg, salicylates, lithium) and in hemolytic reactions requiring alkalinization of the urine to diminish nephrotoxicity of blood pigments.

Severe diarrhea which is often accompanied by a significant loss of bicarbonate.

Neutralizing additive solution: To reduce the incidence of chemical phlebitis and patient discomfort due to vein irritation at or near the infusion site by raising the pH of IV acid solutions.

Contraindications:

Losing chloride by vomiting or from continuous GI suction; receiving diuretics known to produce a hypochloremic alkalosis; metabolic and respiratory alkalosis; hypocalcemia in which alkalosis may produce tetany, hypertension, convulsions or congestive heart failure (CHF); when sodium use could be clinically detrimental.

Neutralizing additive solution: Do not use as a systemic alkalinizer.

Warnings:

Cardiac effects:

Cardiac arrest – The risk of rapid infusion must be weighed against the potential for fatality due to acidosis.

CHF – Since sodium accompanies bicarbonate, use cautiously in patients with CHF or other edematous or sodium-retaining states.

Fluid/Solute overload: IV administration can cause fluid or solute overloading resulting in dilution of serum electrolyte concentrations, overhydration, congested states or pulmonary edema. The risk of dilutional states is inversely proportional to the electrolyte concentrations of administered parenteral solutions. The risk of solute overload causing congested states with peripheral and acute pulmonary edema is directly proportional to the electrolyte concentrations of such solutions. Rapid or excessive administration of Sodium Bicarbonate Injection may produce tetany due to a decrease in ionized calcium and hypokalemia as potassium reenters the cells. Hypertonic solutions may cause vein damage. Avoid extravasation.

Extravasation of IV hypertonic solutions of sodium bicarbonate may cause chemical cellulitis (because of their alkalinity), with tissue necrosis, ulceration or sloughing at the site of infiltration. Prompt elevation of the part, warmth and local injection of lidocaine or hyaluronidase are recommended to prevent sloughing.

Too rapid infusion of hypertonic solutions may cause local pain and venous irritation. Adjust the rate of administration according to tolerance. Use of the largest peripheral vein and a well placed small bore needle is recommended.

Too rapid or excessive administration may result in hypernatremia and alkalosis accompanied by hyperirritability or tetany. Hypernatremia may be associated with edema and exacerbation of CHF due to the retention of water, resulting in an expanded extracellular fluid volume.

Renal function impairment: Administration of solutions containing sodium ions may result in sodium retention. Use with caution. Also use cautiously in oliguria or anuria.

Elderly: Exercise particular care when administering sodium-containing solutions to elderly or postoperative patients with renal or cardiovascular insuffiency, with or without CHF.

Pregnancy: *Category* C.

Children:

Neonates and children (< 2 years old) – Rapid injection (10 ml/min) of hypertonic sodium bicarbonate solutions may produce hypernatremia, a decrease in cerebrospinal fluid pressure and possible intracranial hemorrhage. Do not administer > 8mEq/kg/day. A 4.2% solution is preferred for such slow administration.

Precautions:

Monitoring: Adverse reactions may result from an excess or deficit of one or more of the ions in the solution; frequent monitoring of electrolyte levels is essential.

Avoid overdosage and alkalosis by giving repeated small doses and periodic monitoring by appropriate laboratory tests.

Potassium depletion may predispose to metabolic alkalosis, and coexistent hypocalcemia may be associated with carpopedal spasm as the plasma pH rises. Minimize by treating electrolyte imbalances prior to or concomitantly with bicarbonate.

Chloride loss: Patients losing chloride by vomiting or GI intubation are more susceptible to developing severe alkalosis if given alkalinizing agents.

Neutralizing additive solution: Administer this solution promptly. When introducing additives, mix thoroughly and do not store. Raising pH of IV fluids with neutralizing additive solution will only reduce incidence of chemical irritation caused by infusate; it will not diminish any foreign body effects caused by needle or catheter.

Extraordinary electrolyte losses such as may occur during protracted nasogastric suction, vomiting, diarrhea or GI fistula drainage may necessitate additional electrolyte supplementation.

Drug Interactions:

Drugs that may interact include chlorpropamide, lithium, methotrexate, salicylates, tetracyclines, anorexiants, flecainide, mecamylamide, quinidine and sympathomimetics.

Adverse Reactions:

Extravasation; local pain; venous irritation; hypernatremia; alkalosis.

Administration and Dosage:

Cardiac arrest: Bicarbonate administration in this situation may be detrimental. Administer according to results of arterial blood pH and $PaCO_2$ and calculation of base deficit. Flush IV lines before and after use.

Adults – A rapid IV dose of 200 to 300 mEq of bicarbonate, given as a 7.5% or 8.4% solution.

Infants (≤ 2 years of age) – 4.2% solution for IV administration at a rate not to exceed 8 mEq/kg/day to guard against the possibility of producing hypernatremia, decreasing CSF pressure and inducing intracranial hemorrhage.

Initial dose – 1 to 2 mEq/kg/min given over 1 to 2 minutes followed by 1 mEq/kg every 10 minutes of arrest. If base deficit is known, give calculated dose of 0.3 × kg × base deficit. If only 7.5% or 8.4% sodium bicarbonate is available, dilute 1:1 with 5% Dextrose in Water before administration.

Severe metabolic acidosis – Administer 90 to 180 mEq/L (≈ 7.5 to 15 g) at a rate of 1 to 1.5 L during the first hour. Adjust to patient's needs for further management.

Less urgent forms of metabolic acidosis – Sodium Bicarbonate Injection may be added to other IV fluids. The amount of bicarbonate to be given to older children and adults over a 4 to 8 hour period is approximately 2 to 5 mEq/kg, depending on the severity of the acidosis as judged by the lowering of total CO_2 content, blood pH and clinical condition. Initially, an infusion of 2 to 5 mEq/kg over 4 to 8 hours will produce improvement in the acid-base status of the blood.

Alternatively, estimates of the initial dose of sodium bicarbonate may be based on the following equation:

$$0.5\ (\text{L/kg}) \times \text{body weight (kg)} \times \text{desired increase in serum } HCO_3^- \ (\text{mEq/L}) = \text{bicarbonate dose (mEq)}$$

or

$$0.5\ (\text{L/kg}) \times \text{body weight (kg)} \times \text{base deficit (mEq/L)} = \text{bicarbonate dose (mEq)}.$$

The next step of therapy is dependent on the clinical response of the patient. If severe symptoms have abated, reduce frequency of administration and dose.

If the CO_2 plasma content is unknown, a safe average dose of sodium bicarbonate is 5 mEq (420 mg)/kg.

It is unwise to attempt full correction of a low total CO_2 content during the first 24 hours, since this may accompany an unrecognized alkalosis due to delayed readjustment of ventilation to normal. Thus, achieving total CO_2 content of about 20 mEq/L at the end of the first day will usually be associated with a normal blood pH.

Neutralizing additive solution – One vial of neutralizing additive solution added to 1 L of any of the commonly used parenteral solutions including Dextrose, Sodium Chloride, Ringer's, etc, will increase the pH to a more physiologic range (specific pH may vary slightly).

Note – Some products such as amino acid solutions and multiple electrolyte solutions containing dextrose will not be brought to near physiologic pH by the addition of sodium bicarbonate neutralizing additive solution. This is due to the relatively high buffer capacity of these fluids.

Admixture incompatibilities – Avoid adding sodium bicarbonate to parenteral solutions containing **calcium**, except where compatibility is established; precipitation or haze may result. **Norepinephrine, dopamine** and **dobutamine** are incompatible.

Chapter 2

BLOOD MODIFIERS

IRON-CONTAINING PRODUCTS, ORAL

FERROUS SULFATE	
Tablets: 195, 300 and 324 mg	Various, *Feratab* (Upsher-Smith), *Mol-Iron* (Schering-Plough)
Tablets, timed release: 525 mg	*Fero-Gradumet Filmtab* (Abbott)
Capsules: 250 mg	Various (Geneva, Parmed, Rugby)
Syrup: 90 mg	*Fer-In-Sol* (Mead Johnson Nutritionals)
Elixir: 220 mg	Various, *Feosol* (SmithKline-Beecham)
Drops: 75 mg	Various, *Fer-In-Sol* (Mead Johnson Nutritionals)
FERROUS SULFATE EXSICCATED	
Tablets: 200 mg	*Feosol* (SmithKline-Beecham)
Tablets, slow release: 160 mg	*Slow FE* (Ciba Consumer)
Capsules: 190 mg	*Fer-In-Sol* (Mead Johnson Nutritionals)
Capsules, timed release: 159 mg	*Feosol* (SmithKline-Beecham)
250 mg dried ferrous sulfate equivalent	Various (Parmed)
FERROUS GLUCONATE	
Tablets: 300, 320 and 325 mg	Various, *Fergon* (Sterling Health), *Ferralet* (Mission)
Tablets, sustained release: 320 mg	*Ferralet Slow Release* (Mission)
Capsules, soft gelatin: 86 mg	*Simron* (SmithKline-Beecham)
Elixir: 300 mg	*Fergon* (Sterling Health)
FERROUS FUMARATE	
Tablets: 63, 195, 200, 324, 325 and 350 mg	Various, *Femiron* (Menley & James), *Ferretts* (Pharmics), *Fumerin* (Laser), *Hemocyte* (U.S. Pharm.), *Fumasorb* (MiLance), *Ircon* (Kenwood)
Capsules, controlled release: 325 mg	*Span-FF* (Lexis)
Tablets, chewable: 100 mg	*Feostat* (Forest)
Suspension: 100 mg	*Feostat* (Forest)
Drops: 45 mg	*Feostat* (Forest)
POLYSACCHARIDE-IRON COMPLEX	
Tablets: 50 mg	*Niferex* (Central)
Capsules: 150 mg	*Hytinic* (Hyrex), *Niferex-150* (Central), *Nu-Iron 150* (Mayrand)
Elixir: 100 mg iron per 5 ml	*Niferex* (Central), *Nu-Iron* (Mayrand)

Actions:

Pharmacology: Iron, an essential mineral, is a component of hemoglobin, myoglobin and a number of enzymes. The total body content of iron is approximately 50 mg/kg in men and 35 mg/kg in women. Approximately two-thirds of total body iron is in the circulating red blood cell mass in hemoglobin, the major factor in oxygen transport.

Pharmacokinetics:

Absorption/Distribution The average dietary intake of iron is 18 to 20 mg/day; however, only about 10% of this iron is absorbed (1 to 2 mg/day) in individuals with adequate iron stores. Absorption is enhanced (20% to 30%) when storage iron is depleted or when erythropoiesis occurs at an increased rate. Sustained release or enteric coated preparations reduce the amount of available iron; absorption from these doseforms is reduced because iron is transported beyond the duodenum. Dose also influences the amount of iron absorbed. The amount of iron absorbed increases progressively with larger doses; however, the percentage decreases. Food can decrease the absorption of iron by 40% to 66%; however, gastric intolerance may often necessitate administering the drug with food.

Elemental Iron Content of Iron Salts	
Iron salt	% Iron
Ferrous sulfate	≈ 20
Ferrous sulfate, exsiccated	≈ 30
Ferrous gluconate	≈ 12
Ferrous fumarate	≈ 33

Indications:

For the prevention and treatment of iron deficiency anemias.

Unlabeled uses: Iron supplementation may be required by most patients receiving epoetin therapy. Failure to administer iron supplements (oral or IV) during epoetin therapy can impair the hematologic response to epoetin.

Contraindications:

Hemochromatosis; hemosiderosis; hemolytic anemias.

Warnings:

Chronic iron intake: Individuals with normal iron balance should not take iron chronically.

Precautions:

GI effects: Occasional GI discomfort, such as nausea, may be minimized by taking with meals and by slowly increasing to the recommended dosage.

Drug Interactions:

Iron salts may be affected by the following agents: Antacids, ascorbic acid, chloramphenicol, cimetidine and tetracyclines.

Agents that may be affected by iron salts include: Levodopa, methyldopa, penicillamine, quinolones and tetracyclines.

Drug/Food interactions: Eggs and milk inhibit iron absorption. Coffee and tea consumed with a meal or 1 hour after a meal may significantly inhibit the absorption of dietary iron; clinical significance has not been determined. Administration of calcium and iron supplements with food can reduce ferrous sulfate absorption by one-third. If combined iron and calcium supplementation is required, iron absorption is not decreased if calcium carbonate is used and the supplements are taken between meals.

Adverse Reactions:

GI irritation; anorexia; nausea; vomiting; constipation; diarrhea. Stools may appear darker in color. Iron-containing liquids may cause temporary staining of the teeth.

Administration and Dosage:

Recommended Dietary Allowances (RDAs): Adult males (≥ 19 years old) – 10 mg; adult females (11 to 50 years old) – 15 mg, (≥ 51 years old) – 10 mg; pregnancy – 30 mg; lactation – 15 mg.

For a complete listing of RDAs by age and sex, refer to the RDA table in the Nutritionals chapter.

Iron replacement therapy in deficiency states:

Adults – 100 to 200 mg (2 to 3 mg/kg) elemental iron daily in three divided doses is the usual therapeutic dose.

Children (2 to 12 years) – 3 mg/kg/day in 3 to 4 divided doses; *(6 months to 2 years)* – up to 6 mg/kg/day in 3 to 4 divided doses.

Infants – 10 to 25 mg daily in 3 to 4 divided doses.

The length of iron therapy depends upon the cause and severity of the iron deficiency. In general, approximately 4 to 6 months of oral iron therapy is required to reverse uncomplicated iron deficiency anemias.

Iron supplementation: Consider only in individuals with documented risk factors for iron deficiency.

Pregnancy – 30 mg elemental iron daily (not taken with meals) should be adequate to meet the daily requirement of the last 2 trimesters.

IRON DEXTRAN

Injection: 50 mg iron per ml (as dextran) (*Rx*) — *InFeD* (Schein)

Warning:

The parenteral use of complexes of iron and carbohydrates has resulted in fatal anaphylactic-type reactions. Deaths associated with such administration have been reported; therefore, use iron dextran injection only in those patients in whom the indications have been clearly established and laboratory investigations confirm an iron deficient state not amenable to oral iron therapy.

Actions:

Pharmacology: Iron dextran, a hematinic agent, is a complex of ferric hydroxide and dextran for IM or IV use. The iron dextran complex is dissociated by the reticuloendothelial system, and the ferric iron is transported by transferrin and incorporated into hemoglobin and storage sites.

Indications:

For treatment of patients with documented iron deficiency in whom oral administration is unsatisfactory or impossible.

Unlabeled uses: Iron supplementation may be required by most patients receiving epoetin therapy. Failure to administer iron supplements (oral or IV) during epoetin therapy can impair the hematologic response to epoetin.

Contraindications:

Hypersensitivity to the product.

Warnings:

Hepatic function impairment: Use this preparation with extreme caution in the presence of serious impairment of liver function.

Pregnancy: Do not use in pregnancy or in women of child-bearing potential unless potential benefits outweigh possible hazards.

Precautions:

Iron overload: Unwarranted therapy with parenteral iron will cause excess storage of iron with the consequent possibility of exogenous hemosiderosis.

Allergies/Asthma: Use with caution in patients with history of significant allergies/asthma.

Arthritis: Patients with iron deficiency anemia and rheumatoid arthritis may have an acute exacerbation of joint pain and swelling following IV administration.

Adverse Reactions:

Anaphylactic reactions including fatal anaphylaxis; other hypersensitivity reactions including dyspnea, urticaria, other rashes, itching, arthralgia, myalgia and febrile episodes; variable degree of soreness and inflammation at or near injection site, including sterile abscesses (IM); brown skin discoloration at injection site (IM); peripheral vascular flushing with overly rapid IV administration; hypotensive reaction.

The following pattern of signs/symptoms has been reported as a delayed (1 to 2 days) reaction at recommended doses: Modest-high fever; chills; backache; headache; myalgia; malaise; nausea; vomiting; dizziness. These reactions have been reported in an unexpectedly high incidence with certain batches.

Administration and Dosage:

Maximum dose: 2 ml of undiluted iron dextran daily.

Iron deficiency anemia:

Dosage – Use periodic hematologic determinations as a guide in therapy. Recognize that iron storage may lag behind the appearance of normal blood morphology. This total iron requirement reflects the amount of iron needed to restore hemoglobin to normal or near normal levels plus an additional 50% allowance to provide adequate replenishment of iron stores in most individuals with moderately or severely reduced levels of hemoglobin.

Note: The table is applicable for dosage determinations only in patients with iron deficiency anemia.

Total Amount of Iron Dextran Required (to the nearest ml) for Restoration of Hemoglobin and Replacement of Depleted Iron Stores, Based on Observed Hemoglobin and Body Weight					
Patient weight		Amount required (ml) based on observed hemoglobin			
lb	kg	4 g/dl	6 g/dl	8 g/dl	10 g/dl
10	4.5	3	3	2	2
20	9.1	7	6	4	3
30	13.6	10	8	7	5
40	18.1	18	14	11	8
50	22.7	22	18	14	10
60	27.2	26	21	17	12
70	31.8	31	25	19	14
80	36.3	35	28	22	16
90	40.8	39	32	25	18
100	45.4	44	35	28	20
110	49.9	48	39	30	21
120	54.4	53	42	33	23
130	59	57	46	36	25
140	63.5	61	50	39	27
150	68.1	66	53	41	29
160	72.6	70	57	44	31
170	77.1	74	60	47	33
180	81.7	79	64	50	35

Iron deficiency anemia: The total amount of iron dextran required for the treatment of iron deficiency anemia is determined from the preceding table.

Test dose – Prior to administering the first therapeutic dose, give all patients a test dose of 0.5 ml. It is recommended that a period of ≥ 1 hour elapse before the remainder of the initial therapeutic dose is given.

IV injection – Individual doses of ≤ 2 ml may be given on a daily basis until the calculated total amount required has been reached.

Give undiluted and slowly (≤ 1 ml/min).

IM injection – If no adverse reactions are observed, the injection can be given according to the following schedule until the calculated total amount required has been reached. Each day's dose should ordinarily not exceed 0.5 ml (25 mg iron) for infants < 10 lb, 1 ml (50 mg iron) for children < 20 lb and 2 ml (100 mg iron) for other patients.

Inject only into the muscle mass of the upper outer quadrant of the buttock (never into the arm or other exposed areas) and inject deeply with a 2 or 3 inch 19 or 20 gauge needle. If the patient is standing, have them bear their weight on the leg opposite the injection site, or if in bed, have them in a lateral position with injection site uppermost. To avoid injection or leakage into the subcutaneous tissue, a Z-track technique (displacement of the skin laterally prior to injection) is recommended.

Iron replacement for blood loss – Direct iron therapy in these patients toward replacement of the equivalent amount of iron represented in the blood loss. The table and formula described under *Iron deficiency anemia* are not applicable for simple iron replacement values.

The following formula is based on the approximation that 1 ml of normocytic, normochromic red cells contains 1 mg elemental iron:

Replacement iron (in mg) = Blood loss (in ml) x hematocrit

FOLIC ACID (Folacin; Pteroylglutamic Acid; Folate)

Tablets: 0.4 mg, 0.8 mg, 1 mg (*Rx*[1])	Various
Injection: 5 mg/ml (*Rx*)	Various, *Folvite* (Lederle)

[1] Although most folic acid products carry the *Rx* legend, products which provide 0.4 mg or less (or 0.8 mg for pregnant or lactating women) may be *otc* items.

Actions:

Pharmacology: Exogenous folate is required for nucleoprotein synthesis and maintenance of normal erythropoiesis. Folic acid stimulates production of red and white blood cells and platelets in certain megaloblastic anemias.

Pharmacokinetics: Dietary folic acid is present in foods (eg, liver, dried beans, peas, lentils, oranges, whole-wheat products, vegetables such as asparagus, beets, broccoli, brussels sprouts and spinach), primarily as reduced folate polyglutamate. It must undergo hydrolysis, reduction and methylation in the GI tract before it is absorbed. Oral synthetic folic acid is a monoglutamate and is completely absorbed following administration, even in the presence of malabsorption syndromes.

Folic acid appears in the plasma ≈ 15 to 30 minutes after an oral dose; peak levels are generally reached within 1 hour. After IV administration, the drug is rapidly cleared from the plasma. Folic acid is metabolized in the liver. Normal serum levels of total folate have been reported to be 5 to 15 ng/ml; normal CSF levels are ≈ 16 to 21 ng/ml. In general, folate serum levels < 5 ng/ml indicate folate deficiency, and levels < 2 ng/ml usually result in megaloblastic anemia. A majority of the metabolic products appeared in the urine after 6 hours; excretion was generally complete within 24 hours.

Indications:

Megaloblastic anemia: Treatment of megaloblastic anemias due to a deficiency of folic acid as seen in tropical or nontropical sprue, anemias of nutritional origin, pregnancy, infancy or childhood.

Contraindications:

Treatment of pernicious anemia and other megaloblastic anemias where vitamin B_{12} is deficient (not effective).

Warnings:

Pernicious anemia: Folic acid in doses > 0.1 mg daily may obscure pernicious anemia in that hematologic remission can occur while neurologic manifestations remain progressive.

Except during pregnancy and lactation, folic acid should not be given in therapeutic doses > 0.4 mg daily until pernicious anemia has been ruled out. Daily doses exceeding the Recommended Dietary Allowance should not be included in multivitamin preparations; if therapeutic amounts are necessary, folic acid should be given separately.

Elderly: It may be prudent to consider the status of folate in persons > 65 years of age.

Pregnancy: Category A. Pregnant women are more prone to develop folate deficiency as reflected in larger dosage recommendations. Folate-deficient mothers may be more prone to complications of pregnancy and fetal abnormalities, including fetal anomalies, placental abruption, toxemia, abortions, placenta previa, low-birth-weight and premature delivery. The Recommended Dietary Allowance of folate during pregnancy is 0.4 mg/day.

Lactation: Folic acid is excreted in breast milk.

Drug Interactions:

Drugs that may interact with folic acid include aminosalicylic acid, oral contraceptives, dihydrofolate reductase inhibitors (eg, methotrexate, trimethoprim), sulfasalazine, hydantoins.

Adverse Reactions:

Adverse reactions may include erythema, skin rash, nausea, abdominal distention, altered sleep patterns, irritability, mental depression, confusion and impaired judgement.

Administration and Dosage:

Give orally, except in severe intestinal malabsorption. Although most patients with malabsorption cannot absorb food folates, they are able to absorb folic acid given orally.

Parenteral administration is not advocated but may be necessary in some individuals (eg, patients receiving parenteral or enteral alimentation). Give IM, IV or SC if disease is very severe or GI absorption is very severely impaired. Doses > 0.1 mg should not be used unless anemia due to vitamin B_{12} deficiency has been ruled out or is being adequately treated with cobalamin.

Usual therapeutic dosage: Up to 1 mg daily. Resistant cases may require larger doses.

Maintenance: When clinical symptoms have subsided and the blood picture has normalized, use the dosage below. Never give < 0.1 mg/day. Keep patients under close supervision and adjust maintenance dose if relapse appears imminent. In the presence of alcoholism, hemolytic anemia, anticonvulsant therapy or chronic infection, the maintenance level may need to be increased.

Infants – 0.1 mg/day.
Children (< 4 years of age) – Up to 0.3 mg/day.
Adults and children (> 4 years of age) – 0.4 mg/day.
Pregnant and lactating women – 0.8 mg/day.

Recommended Dietary Allowances (RDAs): Adult males, 0.15 to 0.2 mg/day; females, 0.15 to 0.18 mg/day.

For a complete listing of RDAs by age and sex, refer to the RDA table in the Nutritionals chapter.

LEUCOVORIN CALCIUM (Folinic Acid; Citrovorum Factor)

Tablets: 5 mg (*Rx*)	Various, *Wellcovorin* (Burroughs Wellcome)
15 mg (*Rx*)	Various
25 mg (*Rx*)	Various, *Wellcovorin*(Burroughs Wellcome)
Injection: 3 mg/ml (*Rx*)	Various
Powder for Injection: 50, 100 and 350 mg/vial (*Rx*)	Various, *Wellcovorin* (Burroughs Wellcome)

Actions:

Pharmacology: Leucovorin is one of several active, chemically reduced derivatives of folic acid. It is useful as an antidote to drugs which act as folic acid antagonists. Administration of leucovorin can counteract the therapeutic and toxic effects of folic acid antagonists such as methotrexate (MTX), which act by inhibiting dihydrofolate reductase.

Pharmacokinetics:

Leucovorin Pharmacokinetics[1]

Parameter	IV	IM	Oral
Total reduced folates:			
Mean peak conc. (ng/ml)	1259 (range, 897-1625)	436 (range, 240 to 725)	393 (range, 160 to 550)
Mean time to peak	10 min	52 min	2.3 hrs
Terminal half-life	6.2 hrs	6.2 hrs	5.7 hrs
5-Methyl-THF[2]			
Mean peak conc. (ng/ml)	258	226	367
Mean time to peak	1.3 hrs	2.8 hrs	2.4 hrs
5-Formyl-THF[3]			
Mean peak conc. (ng/ml)	1206	360	51
Mean time to peak	10 min	28 min	1.2 hrs

[1] Following administration of a 25 mg dose.
[2] The major metabolite to which leucovorin is primarily converted in the intestinal mucosa and which becomes the predominant circulating form of the drug.
[3] The parent compound.

Following oral administration leucovorin is rapidly absorbed and expands the serum pool of reduced folates. Oral absorption of leucovorin is saturable at doses > 25 mg. The apparent bioavailability of leucovorin was 97% for 25 mg, 75% for 50 mg and 37% for 100 mg.

Indications:

Oral and parenteral: Leucovorin "rescue" after high-dose methotrexate therapy in osteosarcoma.

Parenteral: Treatment of megaloblastic anemias due to folic acid deficiency when oral therapy is not feasible.

In combination with 5-fluorouracil to prolong survival in the palliative treatment of patients with advanced colorectal cancer.

Contraindications:

Pernicious anemia and other megaloblastic anemias secondary to the lack of vitamin B_{12}.

Warnings:

Anemias: Leucovorin is improper therapy for pernicious anemia and other megaloblastic anemias secondary to the lack of vitamin B_{12}.

5-Fluorouracil dosage/toxicity: Leucovorin enhances the toxicity of 5-FU.

Therapy with leucovorin/5-FU must not be initiated or continued in patients who have symptoms of GI toxicity of any severity, until those symptoms have completely resolved. Patients with diarrhea must be monitored with particular care until the diarrhea has resolved, as rapid clinical deterioration leading to death can occur.

Methotrexate concentrations: Monitoring of the serum MTX concentration is essential in determining the optimal dose and duration of treatment with leucovorin. Delayed MTX excretion may be caused by a third space fluid accumulation, renal insufficiency or inadequate hydration. Under such circumstances, higher doses of leucovorin or prolonged administration may be indicated. Doses higher than those recommended for oral use must be given IV.

Calcium content: Because of the calcium content of the leucovorin solution, inject no more than 160 mg/min IV.

Folic acid antagonist overdosage: In the treatment of accidental overdosages of folic acid antagonists, administer leucovorin as promptly as possible. As the time interval between antifolate administration (eg, MTX) and leucovorin rescue increases, leucovorin's effectiveness in counteracting toxicity decreases.

Elderly: Take particular care in the treatment of elderly or debilitated colorectal cancer patients, as these patients may be at increased risk of severe toxicity.

Pregnancy: Category C.

Lactation: It is not known whether this drug is excreted in breast milk.

Drug Interactions:

Drugs that may be affected by leucovorin include anticonvulsants.

Adverse Reactions:

Allergic sensitization, including anaphylactoid reactions and urticaria, following administration of both oral and parenteral leucovorin.

The following adverse events occurred when leucovorin was administered at both high (200 mg/m^2) and low (20 mg/m^2) doses in combination with 5–FU: Leukopenia, thrombocytopenia, infection, nausea, vomiting, diarrhea, stomatitis, constipation, lethargy/malaise/fatigue, alopecia, dermatitis, anorexia.

Administration and Dosage:

Oral administration of doses > 25 mg is not recommended.

Advanced colorectal cancer: Either of the following two regimens is recommended:

1) Leucovorin 200 mg/m^2 by slow IV injection over a minimum of 3 minutes, followed by 5-FU 370 mg/m^2 by IV injection.

2) Leucovorin 20 mg/m^2 by IV injection followed by 5-FU 425 mg/m^2 by IV injection.

Treatment is repeated daily for 5 days. This 5 day treatment course may be repeated at 4 week (28 day) intervals for 2 courses and then repeated at 4 to 5 week (28 to 35 day) intervals provided that the patient has completely recovered from the toxic effects of the prior treatment course.

Institute dosage modifications of 5-FU as follows, based on the most severe toxicities: If diarrhea or stomatitis are moderate, WBC/mm^3 nadir is 1000–1900 or platelets/mm^3 are 25,000 to 75,000, reduce the 5–FU dose by 20%; if diarrhea or stomatitis are severe, WBC/mm^3 nadir is < 1000, or platelets/mm^3 are < 25,000, reduce the 5–FU dose by 30%.

If no toxicity occurs, the 5-FU dose may increase 10%.

Defer treatment until WBCs are 4000/mm^3 and platelets are 130,000/mm^3. If blood counts do not reach these levels within 2 weeks, discontinue treatment.

Leucovorin rescue after high-dose MTX therapy: The recommendations for leucovorin rescue are based on an MTX dose of 12 to 15 g/m^2 administered by IV infusion over 4 hours. Leucovorin rescue at a dose of 15 mg ($\approx$ 10 mg/m^2) every 6 hours for 10 doses starts 24 hours after the beginning of the MTX infusion. In the presence of GI toxicity, nausea or vomiting, administer leucovorin parenterally.

Determine serum creatinine and MTX levels at least once daily. Continue leucovorin administration, hydration and urinary alkalinization (pH of $\geq$ 7) until the MTX level is $< 5 \times 10^{-8}$M (0.05 micromolar).

If significant clinical toxicity is observed, extend leucovorin rescue for an additional 24 hours (total of 14 doses over 84 hours) in subsequent courses of therapy.

Impaired MTX elimination or inadvertent overdosage: Begin leucovorin rescue as soon as possible after an inadvertent overdosage and within 24 hours of MTX administration when there is delayed excretion (see Warnings). Administer leucovorin 10 mg/m^2 IV, IM or orally every 6 hours until the serum MTX level is $< 10^{-8}$M. In the presence of GI toxicity, nausea or vomiting, administer leucovorin parenterally.

Determine serum creatinine and MTX levels at 24 hour intervals. If the 24 hour serum creatinine has increased 50% over baseline or if the 24 or 48 hour MTX level is $> 5 \times 10^{-6}$M or $> 9 \times 10^{-7}$M, respectively, increase the dose of leucovorin to 100 mg/m^2 IV every 3 hours until the MTX level is $< 10^{-8}$M.

Megaloblastic anemia due to folic acid deficiency: $\leq$ 1 mg leucovorin/day. There is no evidence that doses > 1 mg/day have greater efficacy than 1 mg doses.

VITAMIN B_{12}

HYDROXOCOBALAMIN	
Injection: 1000 mcg/ml (*Rx*)	Various, *LA-12* (Hyrex), *Hydro-Crysti-12* (Roberts Hauck)
CYANOCOBALAMIN	
Tablets: 500 and 1000 mcg (*otc*)	Various
Injection: 100 and 1000 mcg per ml (*Rx*)	Various, *Crysti 1000* (Roberts Hauck), *Cyanoject* (Mayrand)

Actions:

Pharmacology: Vitamin B_{12} is essential to growth, cell reproduction, hematopoiesis and nucleoprotein and myelin synthesis. Its physiologic role is associated with methylation, participating in nucleic acid and protein synthesis. Cyanocobalamin participates in red blood cell formation through activation of folic acid coenzymes. Cyanocobalamin has hematopoietic activity apparently identical to that of the antianemia factor in purified liver extract. Hydroxocobalamin (vitamin B_{12a}) functions the same as cyanocobalamin.

The normal range of plasma B_{12} is 200 to 750 pg/ml, which represents ≈ 0.1% of the total body content. The total daily loss ranges from 2 to 5 mcg. Because of its slow rate of utilization and considerable body stores, vitamin B_{12} deficiency may take many months to appear. The average diet supplies about 5 to 15 mcg/day of vitamin B_{12}.

Pharmacokinetics: Absorption of vitamin B_{12} depends on the presence of sufficient intrinsic factor and calcium. In general, absorption of oral B_{12} is inadequate in malabsorptive states and in pernicious anemia (unless intrinsic factor is simultaneously administered).

Cyanocobalamin is rapidly absorbed from IM and SC injection sites; the plasma level peaks within 1 hour. Once absorbed, it is bound to plasma proteins, stored mainly in the liver and is slowly released when needed to carry out normal cellular metabolic functions. Within 48 hours after injection of 100 to 1000 mcg of vitamin B_{12}, 50% to 98% of the dose appears in the urine. The major portion is excreted within the first 8 hours. More rapid excretion occurs with IV administration; there is little opportunity for liver storage.

Hydroxocobalamin (vitamin B_{12a}) is more highly protein bound and is retained in the body longer than cyanocobalamin. However, it has no advantage over cyanocobalamin.

Indications:

Vitamin B_{12} deficiency: due to malabsorption syndrome as seen in pernicious anemia; GI pathology, dysfunction or surgery; fish tapeworm infestation; malignancy of pancreas or bowel; gluten enteropathy; sprue; small bowel bacterial overgrowth; total or partial gastrectomy; accompanying folic acid deficiency.

Increased vitamin B_{12} requirements: associated with pregnancy, thyrotoxicosis, hemolytic anemia, hemorrhage, malignancy and hepatic and renal disease.

Vitamin B_{12} absorption test (Schilling test).

Unlabeled uses: Hydroxocobalamin has been used to prevent and to treat cyanide toxicity associated with sodium nitroprusside. It lowers red blood cell and plasma cyanide concentrations by combining with cyanide to form cyanocobalamin, which is nontoxic and excreted in the urine.

Contraindications:

Hypersensitivity to cobalt, vitamin B_{12} or any component of these products.

Warnings:

Inadequate response: A blunted or impeded therapeutic response may be due to infection, uremia, bone marrow suppressant drugs, concurrent iron or folic acid deficiency or misdiagnosis.

Vitamin B_{12} deficiency allowed to progress for > 3 months may produce permanent degenerative lesions of the spinal cord.

Optic nerve atrophy: Patients with early Leber's disease (hereditary optic nerve atrophy) treated with cyanocobalamin suffer severe and swift optic atrophy.

Hypokalemia: and sudden death may occur in severe megaloblastic anemia which is treated intensely.

Pregnancy: Category C (parenteral). B_{12} is an essential vitamin and needs are increased during pregnancy. The National Academy of Sciences has recommended that 2.2 mcg/day should be consumed during pregnancy.

Lactation: Vitamin B_{12} is excreted in breast milk in concentrations that approximate the mother's vitamin B_{12} blood level. Amounts of B_{12} recommended by the Food and Nutrition Board, National Academy of Sciences-National Research Council (2.6 mcg daily) should be consumed during lactation.

Children: The Food and Nutrition Board, National Academy of Sciences-National Research Council recommends a daily intake of 0.3 to 0.5 mcg/day for infants < 1 year of age and 0.7 to 1.4 mcg/day for children 1 to 10 years of age.

Precautions:

Monitoring: During treatment of severe megaloblastic anemia, monitor serum potassium levels closely for the first 48 hours and replace potassium if necessary. Obtain reticulocyte counts, hematocrit and vitamin B_{12}, iron and folic acid plasma levels prior to treatment and between the fifth and seventh days of therapy, and then frequently until the hematocrit is normal. If folate levels are low, also administer folic acid.

Test dose: Anaphylactic shock and death have occurred after parenteral vitamin B_{12} administration. Give an intradermal test dose in patients sensitive to the cobalamins.

Folate: Doses > 10 mcg daily may produce hematologic response in patients with folate deficiency. Indiscriminate use may mask the true diagnosis of pernicious anemia.

Doses of folic acid > 0.1 mg/day may result in hematologic remission in patients with vitamin B_{12} deficiency. Neurologic manifestations will not be prevented with folic acid, and if not treated with vitamin B_{12}, irreversible damage will result.

Polycythemia vera: Vitamin B_{12} deficiency may suppress the signs of polycythemia vera.

Vegetarian diets containing no animal products (including milk products or eggs) do not supply any vitamin B_{12}.

Immunodeficient patients: Vitamin B_{12} malabsorption may occur in patients with AIDS or HIV infection. Consider monitoring levels.

Drug Interactions:

Drugs that may affect vitamin B_{12} include: Aminosalicylic acid, chloramphenicol, colchicine and alcohol.

Drug/Lab test interactions: Methotrexate, pyrimethamine and most antibiotics invalidate folic acid and vitamin B_{12} diagnostic microbiological blood assays.

Adverse Reactions:

The following reactions are associated with parenteral vitamin B_{12}: Anaphylactic shock, death, pulmonary edema, congestive heart failure early in treatment, severe and swift optic nerve atrophy.

Administration and Dosage:

HYROXYCOBALAMIN, CRYSTALLINE: Administer IM only. The recommended dosage is 30 mcg/day for 5 to 10 days, followed by 100 to 200 mcg monthly. Children may be given a total of 1 to 5 mg over 2 or more weeks in doses of 100 mcg, then 30 to 50 mcg every 4 weeks for maintenance. Institute concurrent folic acid therapy at the beginning of treatment if needed.

CYANOCOBALAMIN, CRYSTALLINE:

Addisonian pernicious anemia – Parenteral therapy is required for life; oral therapy is not dependable. Administer 100 mcg daily for 6 or 7 days by IM or deep SC injection. If there is clinical improvement and a reticulocyte response, give the same amount on alternate days for 7 doses, then every 3 to 4 days for another 2 to 3 weeks. By this time, hematologic values should have become normal. Follow this regimen with 100 mcg monthly for life. Administer folic acid concomitantly if needed.

Other patients with vitamin B_{12} deficiency – In seriously ill patients, administer both vitamin B_{12} and folic acid. It is not necessary to withhold therapy until the precise cause of B_{12} deficiency is established. For hematologic signs, children may be given 10 to 50 mcg/day for 5 to 10 days followed by 100 to 250 mcg/dose every 2 to 4 weeks; for neurologic signs, 100 mcg/day for 10 to 15 days, then once or twice weekly for several months, possibly tapering to 250 to 1000 mcg monthly by 1 year.

Oral – Up to 1000 mcg/day. Oral vitamin B_{12} therapy is not usually recommended for vitamin B_{12} deficiency. The maximum amount of vitamin B_{12} that can be absorbed from a single oral dose is 1 to 5 mcg. The percent absorbed decreases with increasing doses.

IM or SC – 30 mcg daily for 5 to 10 days followed by 100 to 200 mcg monthly. Larger doses (eg, 1000 mcg) have been recommended, even though a larger amount is lost through excretion. However, it is possible that a greater amount is retained, allowing for fewer injections.

Schilling test: The flushing dose is 1000 mcg IM.

PHYTONADIONE (K_1, Phylloquinone, Methylphytyl Napthoquinone)

Tablets: 5 mg (*Rx*)	*Mephyton* (Merck)
Injection (aqueous colloidal solution): 2 mg per ml (*Rx*)	Various, *AquaMEPHYTON* (Merck), *Konakion* (Roche)
Injection (aqueous dispersion): 10 mg per ml (*Rx*)	*AquaMEPHYTON* (Merck), *Konakion* (Roche)

Warning:

IV use: Severe reactions, including fatalities, have occurred during and immediately after IV injection, even with precautions to dilute the injection and to avoid rapid infusion. These severe reactions resemble hypersensitivity or anaphylaxis, including shock and cardiac or respiratory arrest. Some patients exhibit these severe reactions on receiving vitamin K for the first time. Therefore, restrict the IV route to those situations where other routes are not feasible and the serious risk involved is justified.

Actions:

Pharmacology: Vitamin K promotes the hepatic synthesis of active prothrombin (factor II), proconvertin (factor VII), plasma thromboplastin component (factor IX) and Stuart factor (factor X). The mechanism by which vitamin K promotes formation of these clotting factors involves the hepatic post-translational carboxylation of specific glutamate residues to gamma-carboxylglutamate residues in proteins involved in coagulation, thus leading to their activation.

Phytonadione (vitamin K_1) is a lipid-soluble synthetic analog of vitamin K. Phytonadione possesses essentially the same type and degree of activity as the naturally occurring vitamin K.

Pharmacokinetics: Phytonadione is only absorbed from the GI tract via intestinal lymphatics in the presence of bile salts. Although initially concentrated in the liver, vitamin K is rapidly metabolized and very little tissue accumulation occurs.

Parenteral phytonadione is generally detectable within 1 to 2 hours. Phytonadione usually controls hemorrhage within 3 to 6 hours. A normal prothrombin level may be obtained in 12 to 14 hours. Oral phytonadione exerts its effect in 6 to 10 hours.

The US daily allowances for vitamin K have not been officially established, but have been estimated to be 10 to 20 mcg for infants, 15 to 100 mcg for children and adolescents and 70 to 140 mcg for adults. Usually, dietary vitamin K will satisfy these requirements, except during the first 5 to 8 days of the neonatal period.

Recommended Dietary Allowances as published by the National Academy of Sciences are as follows: Adult males, 45 to 80 mcg/day; adult females, 45 to 65 mcg/day.

Indications:

Coagulation disorders due to faulty formation of factors II, VII, IX and X when caused by vitamin K deficiency or interference with vitamin K activity.

Oral: Anticoagulant-induced prothrombin deficiency (see Warnings); hypoprothrombinemia secondary to salicylates or antibacterial therapy; hypoprothrombinemia secondary to obstructive jaundice and biliary fistulas, but only if bile salts are administered concomitantly with phytonadione.

Parenteral: Anticoagulant-induced prothrombin deficiency; hypoprothrombinemia secondary to conditions limiting absorption or synthesis of vitamin K (eg, obstructive jaundice, biliary fistula, sprue, ulcerative colitis, celiac disease, intestinal resection, cystic fibrosis of the pancreas, regional enteritis); drug-induced hypoprothrombinemias due to interference with vitamin K metabolism (eg, antibiotics, salicylates); prophylaxis and therapy of hemorrhagic disease of the newborn.

Contraindications:

Hypersensitivity to any component of the product.

Warnings:

Oral anticoagulant-induced hypoprothrombinemia: Vitamin K will not counteract the anticoagulant action of heparin.

Immediate coagulant effect should not be expected. It takes a minimum of 1 to 2 hours for a measurable improvement in the prothrombin time (PT).

The prothrombin test is sensitive to the levels of factors II, VII and X. Fresh plasma or blood transfusions may be required for severe blood loss or lack of response to vitamin K.

With phytonadione use and anticoagulant therapy indicated, the patient is faced with the same clotting hazards prior to starting anticoagulant therapy. Phytonadione is not a clotting agent, but overzealous therapy may restore original thromboembolic phenomena conditions. Keep dosage as low as possible and check PT regularly.

Hepatic function impairment: Hypoprothrombinemia due to hepatocellular damage is not corrected by administration of vitamin K. Repeated large doses of vitamin K are not warranted in liver disease if the initial response is unsatisfactory (Koller test). Failure to respond to vitamin K may indicate a coagulation defect or a condition unresponsive to vitamin K. In hepatic disease, large doses may further depress liver function.

Paradoxically, giving excessive doses of vitamin K or its analogs in an attempt to correct hypoprothrombinemia associated with severe hepatitis or cirrhosis may actually result in further depression of the prothrombin concentration.

Pregnancy: Category C.

Lactation: Vitamin K is excreted in breast milk.

Children: Safety and efficacy in children have not been established. Hemolysis, jaundice and hyperbilirubinemia in newborns, particularly in premature infants, have been reported with vitamin K. These effects may be dose-related. Therefore, do not exceed recommended dose.

Drug Interactions:

Drugs that may interact include anticoagulants and mineral oil.

Adverse Reactions:

Adverse reactions from parenteral administration may include transient "flushing sensations" and "peculiar" sensations of taste. Deaths have occurred after IV administration. Hyperbilirubinemia has been observed in the newborn following administration of phytonadione. Anaphylactoid reactions may occur with either doseform.

Administration and Dosage:

If possible, discontinue or reduce the dosage of drugs interfering with coagulation mechanisms (eg, salicylates, antibiotics) as an alternative to phytonadione. The severity of the coagulation disorder should determine whether the immediate administration of phytonadione is required in addition to discontinuation or reduction of interfering drugs.

Inject SC or IM when possible. In older children and adults, inject IM in the upper outer quadrant of the buttocks. In infants and young children, the anterolateral aspect of the thigh or the deltoid region is preferred. When IV administration is unavoidable, inject very slowly, not exceeding 1mg/min.

Anticoagulant-induced prothrombin deficiency in adults: 2.5 to 10 mg or up to 25 mg (rarely, 50 mg) initially. Determine subsequent doses by PT response or clinical condition. If in 6 to 8 hours after parenteral administration (or 12 to 48 hours after oral administration), the PT has not been shortened satisfactorily, repeat dose. If shock or excessive blood loss occurs, transfusion of blood or fresh frozen plasma may be required.

Hemorrhagic disease of the newborn:

Prophylaxis – Single IM dose of 0.5 to 1 mg within 1 hour after birth. This may be repeated after 2 to 3 weeks if the mother has received anticoagulant, anticonvulsant, antituberculous or recent antibiotic therapy during her pregnancy. Twelve to 24 hours before delivery, 1 to 5 mg may be given to the mother.

Oral doses of 2 mg have been shown to be adequate for prophylaxis.

Treatment – 1 mg SC or IM. Higher doses may be necessary if the mother has been receiving oral anticoagulants. Empiric administration of vitamin K_1 should not replace proper laboratory evaluation. A prompt response (shortening of the PT in 2 to 4 hours) is usually diagnostic of hemorrhagic disease of the newborn; failure to respond indicates another diagnosis or coagulation disorder. Give blood or blood products such as fresh frozen plasma if bleeding is excessive. This therapy, however, does not correct the underlying disorder; give phytonadione concurrently.

Hypoprothrombinemia due to other causes in adults: 2.5 to 25 mg (rarely, up to 50 mg); amount and route of administration depends on severity of condition and response obtained. Avoid oral route when clinical disorder would prevent proper absorption. Give bile salts with tablets when endogenous supply of bile to GI tract is deficient.

EPOETIN ALFA (Erythropoietin; EPO)

Injection: 2000, 3000, 4000 and 10,000 units per ml (*Rx*) *Epogen* (Amgen), *Procrit* (Ortho Biotech)

Actions:

Pharmacology: Erythropoietin is a glycoprotein which stimulates red blood cell production. It is produced in the kidney and stimulates the division and differentiation of erythroid progenitors in bone marrow. Epoetin alfa, a 165 amino acid glycoprotein manufactured by recombinant DNA technology, has the same biological effects as endogenous erythropoietin.

Endogenous production of erythropoietin is regulated by the level of tissue oxygenation. Hypoxia and anemia generally increase the production of erythropoietin, which in turn stimulates erythropoiesis. In normal subjects, plasma erythropoietin levels range from 0.01 to 0.03 U/ml and increase up to 100- to 1000-fold during hypoxia or anemia. In patients with chronic renal failure (CRF), erythropoietin production is impaired; this deficiency is the primary cause of their anemia.

Epoetin alfa stimulates erythropoiesis in anemic patients on dialysis and those who do not require regular dialysis. The first evidence of a response to epoetin alfa administration is an increase in the reticulocyte count within 10 days, followed by increases in the red cell count, hemoglobin and hematocrit, usually within 2 to 6 weeks. Once the hematocrit reaches the suggested target range (30% to 36%), that level can be sustained by epoetin alfa therapy in the absence of iron deficiency and concurrent illnesses.

The rate of hematocrit increase varies between patients and is dependent upon the dose of epoetin alfa within a therapeutic range of ≈ 50 to 300 U/kg 3 times weekly; a greater biologic response is not observed at doses > 300 U/kg 3 times weekly. Other factors affecting rate and extent of response include availability of iron stores, baseline hematocrit and concurrent medical problems.

Pharmacokinetics: Epoetin alfa IV is eliminated via first-order kinetics with a circulating half-life of 4 to 13 hours in patients with CRF. Within the therapeutic dosage range, detectable levels of plasma erythropoietin are maintained for at least 24 hours. After SC administration of epoetin alfa to patients with CRF, peak serum levels are achieved within 5 to 24 hours after administration and decline slowly thereafter. The half-life in healthy volunteers is ≈ 20% shorter than in CRF patients.

Indications:

Treatment of anemia associated with CRF, including patients on dialysis (end-stage renal disease) and patients not on dialysis, to elevate or maintain the red blood cell level (as manifested by the hematocrit or hemoglobin determinations) and to decrease the need for transfusions.

Treatment of anemia related to zidovudine therapy in HIV-infected patients: To elevate or maintain the red blood cell level (as manifested by the hematocrit or hemoglobin determinations) and to decrease the need for transfusions in these patients when the endogenous erythropoietin level is ≤ 500 mU/ml and the dose of zidovudine is ≤ 4200 mg/week.

Not indicated for the treatment of anemia in HIV-infected patients due to other factors such as iron or folate deficiencies, hemolysis or GI bleeding which should be managed appropriately.

Treatment of anemia in cancer patients on chemotherapy: Treatment of anemia in patients with non-myeloid malignancies where anemia is due to the effect of concomitantly administered chemotherapy. It is intended to decrease the need for transfusions in patients who will be receiving chemotherapy for a minimum of 2 months.

Unlabeled uses: Epoetin alfa is effective in increasing the procurement of autologous blood in patients about to undergo elective surgery.

Contraindications:

Uncontrolled hypertension; hypersensitivity to mammalian cell-derived products or to human albumin.

Warnings:

Anemia: Not intended for CRF patients who require correction of severe anemia; epoetin alfa may obviate the need for maintenance transfusions but is not a substitute for emergency transfusion. Not indicated for treatment of anemia in HIV-infected patients or cancer patients due to other factors such as iron or folate deficiencies, hemolysis or GI bleeding which should be managed appropriately.

Hypertension: Up to 80% of patients with CRF have a history of hypertension. Do not treat patients with uncontrolled hypertension; monitor blood pressure adequately before initiation of therapy. Although there does not appear to be any direct pressor effects of epoetin, blood pressure may rise during therapy. During the early phase of treatment when the hematocrit is increasing, ≈ 25% of patients on dialysis may require initiation of, or increases in, antihypertensive therapy. Hypertensive encephalopathy and seizures have occurred in patients with CRF treated with epoetin.

Take special care to closely monitor and aggressively control blood pressure in epoetin-treated patients. If blood pressure is difficult to control by initiation of appropriate measures, the hematocrit may be reduced by decreasing or withholding the epoetin dose. A clinically significant decrease in hematocrit may not be observed for several weeks. It is recommended that the epoetin dose be decreased if the hematocrit increase exceeds 4 points in any 2 week period because of the possible association of excessive rate of rise of hematocrit with an exacerbation of hypertension.

Seizures: The relationship to seizures is uncertain. The baseline incidence of seizures in the untreated dialysis population appears to be 5% to 10% per patient-year. In patients on dialysis, there appeared to be a higher incidence of seizures during the first 90 days of therapy when compared to subsequent 90 day periods. Monitor the presence of premonitory neurologic symptoms closely.

Since the relationship between seizures and the rate of rise of hematocrit is uncertain, decrease the dose of epoetin alfa if the hematocrit increase exceeds 4 points in any 2 week period.

Thrombotic events: During hemodialysis, patients treated with epoetin alfa may require increased anticoagulation with heparin to prevent clotting of the artificial kidney.

Overall, for patients with CRF (whether on dialysis or not), other thrombotic events have occurred at an annualized rate of < 0.04 events per patient-year of epoetin alfa. Monitor patients with pre-existing vascular disease closely.

Allergic reactions: Skin rashes and urticaria are rare, mild and transient. There is no evidence of antibody development to erythropoietin, including those receiving epoetin alfa for > 4 years. Nevertheless, if an anaphylactoid reaction occurs, immediately discontinue the drug and initiate appropriate therapy. Refer to Management of Acute Hypersensitivity Reactions.

Pregnancy: Category C.

Lactation: It is not known whether epoetin alfa is excreted in breast milk.

Children: Safety and efficacy have not been established.

Precautions:

Monitoring:

Patients with CRF not requiring dialysis – Monitor blood pressure and hematocrit no less frequently than for patients maintained on dialysis. Closely monitor renal function and fluid and electrolyte balance, as an improved sense of well-being may obscure the need to initiate dialysis in some patients.

Determine the hematocrit twice a week until it has stabilized in the target range and the maintenance dose has been established. After any dose adjustment, determine the hematocrit twice weekly for at least 2 to 6 weeks until the hematocrit has stabilized; then monitor at regular intervals.

Perform complete blood count with differential and platelet counts regularly. Modest increases have occurred in platelets and white blood cell counts, but values remained within normal ranges.

Monitor serum chemistry values (including blood urea nitrogen [BUN], uric acid, creatinine, phosphorus and potassium) regularly. In patients on dialysis, modest increases occurred in BUN, creatinine, phosphorus and potassium. In some patients, modest increases in serum uric acid and phosphorus were observed. The values remained within the ranges normally seen in patients with CRF.

Zidovudine-treated, HIV-infected patients – Measure hematocrit once a week until it is stabilized; measure periodically thereafter.

Iron evaluation – During therapy, absolute or functional iron deficiency may develop. Functional iron deficiency, with normal ferritin levels but low transferrin saturation, is presumably due to the inability to mobilize iron stores rapidly enough to support increased erythropoiesis. Transferrin saturation should be at least 20%, and ferritin should be at least 100 ng/ml. Prior to and during therapy, evaluate the patient's iron status, including transferrin saturation (serum iron divided by iron binding capacity) and serum ferritin. Virtually all patients will eventually require supplemental iron to increase or maintain transferrin saturation to levels that will adequately support epoetin alfa-stimulated erythropoiesis.

Hematology: The elevated bleeding time characteristic of CRF decreases toward normal after correction of anemia in epoetin alfa-treated patients. Reduction of bleeding time also occurs after correction of anemia by transfusion.

Allow sufficient time to determine a patient's responsiveness before adjusting the dose. Because of the time required for erythropoiesis and the red cell half-life, an interval of 2 to 6 weeks may occur between the time of a dose adjustment (initiation, increase, decrease or discontinuation) and a significant change in hematocrit.

Porphyria exacerbation has been observed rarely in epoetin alfa-treated patients with CRF. Use with caution in patients with known porphyria.

Bone marrow fibrosis is a complication of CRF and may be related to secondary hyperparathyroidism or unknown factors.

Delayed or diminished response: If the patient fails to respond or to maintain a response to doses within the recommended range, consider and evaluate the following etiologies:

1.) Functional iron deficiency may develop with normal ferritin levels but low transferrin saturation (< 20%), presumably due to the inability to mobilize iron stores rapidly enough to support increased erythropoiesis. Virtually all patients will eventually require supplemental iron therapy.
2.) Underlying infectious, inflammatory or malignant processes.
3.) Occult blood loss.
4.) Underlying hematologic diseases (eg, thalassemia, refractory anemia or other myelodysplastic disorders).
5.) Vitamin deficiencies: Folic acid or vitamin B_{12}.
6.) Hemolysis.
7.) Aluminum intoxication.
8.) Osteitis fibrosa cystica.
9.) Increase in zidovudine dosage.

Diet: As the hematocrit increases and patients experience an improved sense of well-being, reinforce the importance of compliance with dietary guidelines and frequency of dialysis.

Hyperkalemia is not uncommon in patients with CRF.

Dialysis management: Therapy with epoetin alfa results in an increase in hematocrit and a decrease in plasma volume that could affect dialysis efficiency. This has not adversely affected dialyzer function or the efficiency of high-flux hemodialysis.

Adverse Reactions:

CRF patients: Epoetin alfa is generally well tolerated. The following adverse reactions are frequent (> 3%) sequelae of CRF and are not necessarily due to epoetin alfa therapy: Hypertension, headache, arthralgia, nausea, edema, fatigue, diarrhea, vomiting, chest pain, asthenia, dizziness and clotted vascular access.

Zidovudine-treated HIV-infected patients: Adverse experiences > 3% were consistent with the progression of HIV infection: Pyrexia, fatigue, headache, cough, diarrhea, rahs, nausea, respiratory congestion, shortness of breath, asthenia and dizziness.

Cancer patients in chemotherapy: Adverse reactions > 3% were consistent with the underlying disease state: Pyrexia, diarrhea, nausea, vomiting, edema, asthenia, fatigue, shortness of breath, paresthesia, upper respiratory infection, dizziness and trunk pain.

Administration and Dosage:

CRF patients:

Epoetin Alfa: General Therapeutic Guidelines in CRF Patients	
Starting dose	50 to 100 U/kg 3 times weekly IV or SC
Reduce dose when:	1) Hematocrit approaches 36% or 2) Hematocrit increases > 4 points in any 2 week period.
Increase dose if:	Hematocrit does not increase by 5 to 6 points after 8 weeks of therapy, and hematocrit is below suggested target range.
Maintenance dose	Individualize.
Suggested target hematocrit range	30% to 36%

Starting doses over the range of 50 to 100 U/kg 3 times weekly are safe and effective in increasing hematocrit and eliminating transfusion dependency in patients with CRF. Reduce the dose as the hematocrit approaches 36% or increases by > 4 points in any 2 week period. Individualize the dosage to maintain the hematocrit within the suggested target range. At the physician's discretion, the suggested target hematocrit range may be expanded to achieve maximal patient benefit.

Epoetin alfa may be given either as an IV or SC injection. In patients on hemodialysis, epoetin alfa usually has been administered as an IV bolus 3 times/week. While the administration is independent of the dialysis procedure, epoetin alfa may be administered into the venous line at the end of the dialysis procedure to obviate the need for additional venous access.

Dose adjustment – Following therapy, a period of time is required for erythroid progenitors to mature and be released into circulation resulting in an eventual increase in hematocrit. Additionally, red blood cell survival time affects hematocrit and may vary due the uremia. As a result the time required to elicit a clinically significant change in hematocrit (increase or decrease) following any dose adjustment may be 2 to 6 weeks.

Dose adjustment should not be made more frequently than once a month, unless clinically indicated. After any dose adjustment, determine the hematocrit twice weekly for at least 2 to 6 weeks.

- If the hematocrit is increasing and approaching 36%, reduce the dose to maintain the suggested target hematocrit range. If the reduced dose does not stop the rise in hematocrit and it exceeds 36%, temporarily withhold doses until the hematocrit begins to decrease, then reinitiate at a lower dose.
- At any time, if the hematocrit increases by > 4 points in a 2 week period, immediately decrease the dose. After the dose reduction, monitor the hematocrit twice weekly for 2 to 6 weeks and make further dose adjustments as outlined in the maintenance dose section.
- If a hematocrit increase of 5 to 6 points is not achieved after an 8 week period and iron stores are adequate, the dose may be incrementally increased. Further increases may be made at 4 to 6 week intervals until the desired response is attained.

Maintenance – Individualize dosage.

Dialysis patients: Median dose is 75 U/kg 3 times weekly (range, 12.5 to 525 U/kg 3 times weekly).

Nondialysis CRF patients: Dose of 75 to 150 U/kg *per week* has maintained hematocrits of 36% to 38% for up to 6 months.

Delayed or diminished response – Over 95% of patients with CRF responded with clinically significant increases in hematocrit, and virtually all patients were transfusion-independent within approximately 2 months of initiation of therapy.

If a patient fails to respond or maintain a response, consider other etiologies and evaluate as clinically indicated.

Zidovudine-treated, HIV-infected patients: Prior to beginning therapy, determine the endogenous serum erythropoietin level prior to transfusion. Available evidence suggests that patients receiving zidovudine with endogenous serum erythropoietin levels > 500 mU/ml are unlikely to respond to therapy.

Initial dose – For patients with serum erythropoietin levels ≤ 500 mU/ml who are receiving a dose of zidovudine ≤ 4200 mg/week, the recommended starting dose is 100 U/kg as an IV or SC injection 3 times weekly for 8 weeks.

If the response is not satisfactory in terms of reducing transfusion requirements or increasing hematocrit after 8 weeks of therapy, the dose can be increased by 50 to 100 U/kg 3 times weekly. Evaluate response every 4 to 8 weeks thereafter and adjust the dose accordingly by 50 to 100 U/kg increments 3 times weekly. If patients have not responded satisfactorily to a 300 U/kg dose 3 times weekly, it is unlikely that they will respond to higher doses.

Maintenance dose – When the desired response is attained, titrate the dose to maintain the response based on factors such as variations in zidovudine dose and the presence of intercurrent infectious or inflammatory episodes. If the hematocrit exceeds 40%, stop the dose until the hematocrit drops to 36%. When resuming treatment, reduce the dose by 25%, then titrate to maintain the desired hematocrit.

Cancer patients on chemotherapy:

Starting dose – 150 units/kg SC 3 times weekly. In general, patients with lower baseline serum erythropoietin levels responded more vigorously to epoetin alfa. Treatment of patients with grossly elevated erythropoietin levels (eg, > 200 mU/ml) is not recommended. Monitor hematocrit on a weekly basis until hematocrit becomes stable.

Dose adjustment – If response is not satisfactory in terms of reducing transfusion requirement or increasing hematocrit after 8 weeks of therapy, the dose may be increased up to 300 units/kg 3 times weekly. If patients do not respond, it is unlikely that they will respond to higher doses. If hematocrit exceeds 40%, hold the dose until it falls to 36%. Reduce dose by 25% when treatment is resumed and titrate to maintain desired hematocrit. If initial dose includes a very rapid hematocrit response (eg, increase of > 4 percentage points in any 2 week period), reduce the dose.

FILGRASTIM (Granulocyte Colony Stimulating Factor; G-CSF)

Injection: 300 mcg/ml (*Rx*)	*Neupogen* (Amgen)

Actions:

Pharmacology: Filgrastim is a human granulocyte colony stimulating factor (G-CSF), produced by recombinant DNA technology. Filgrastim is produced by *Escherichia coli* bacteria inserted with the human G-CSF gene. G-CSF regulates the production of neutrophils within the bone marrow; endogenous G-CSF is a glycoprotein produced by monocytes, fibroblasts and endothelial cells. It has minimal direct in vivo or in vitro effects on the production of other hematopoietic cell types.

Pharmacokinetics: Absorption and clearance follow first-order pharmacokinetics without apparent concentration dependence. A positive linear correlation occurs between the parenteral dose and both the serum concentration and area under the concentration-time curves. Continuous IV infusion of 20 mcg/kg filgrastim over 24 hours resulted in mean and median serum concentrations of ≈ 48 and 56 ng/ml, respectively. SC administration of 3.45 and 11.5 mcg/kg resulted in maximum serum concentrations of 4 and 49 ng/ml, respectively, within 2 to 8 hours. The volume of distribution averaged 150 ml/kg in both healthy subjects and cancer patients. The elimination half-life in both healthy subjects and cancer patients was ≈ 3.5 hours. Clearance rates were ≈ 0.5 to 0.7 ml/min/kg. Continuous 24 hour IV infusions at 20 mcg/kg over an 11 to 20 day period produced steady-state serum concentrations of filgrastim with no evidence of drug accumulation over the time period investigated.

Indications:

Cancer patients:

Myelosuppressive chemotherapy – To decrease the incidence of infection, as manifested by febrile neutropenia, in patients with non-myeloid malignancies receiving myelosuppressive anti-cancer drugs associated with a significant incidence of severe neutropenia with fever.

Bone marrow transplant (BMT) – To reduce the duration of neutropenia and neutropenia-related clinical sequelae (eg, febrile neutropenia) in patients with non-myeloid malignancies undergoing myeloablative chemotherapy followed by marrow transplantation.

Peripheral Blood Progenitor Cell (PBPC) Collection – For the mobilization of hematopoietic progenitor cells into the peripheral blood for leukapheresis collection.

Severe chronic neutropenia (SCN): Chronic administration to reduce the incidence and duration of sequelae of neutropenia (eg, fever, infections, oropharyngeal ulcers) in symptomatic patients with congenital, cyclic or idiopathic neutropenia.

Unlabeled uses: Although further studies are needed, filgrastim may be beneficial in AIDS, aplastic anemia, hairy cell leukemia, myelodysplasia, drug-induced and congenital agranulocytosis, alloimmune neonatal neutropenia and congenital, acquired or cyclic neutropenia.

Contraindications:

Hypersensitivity to *E coli*-derived proteins, filgrastim or any product components.

Warnings:

Hypersensitivity: Allergic-type reactions have occurred on initial or subsequent treatment in < 1 in 4000 patients treated with filgrastim. These have generally been characterized by systemic symptoms involving at least two body systems, most often skin (rash, urticaria, facial edema), respiratory (wheezing, dyspnea) and cardiovascular (hypotension, tachycardia). Reactions tended to occur within the first 30 minutes after administration and appeared to occur more frequently in patients receiving IV filgrastim. Rapid resolution of symptoms occurred in most cases after administartion of antihistamines, steroids, bronchodilators or epinephrine. Symptoms recurred in > 50% of patients who were rechallenged. Refer also to Management of Acute Hypersensitivity Reactions.

Pregnancy: Category C.

Lactation: It is not known whether filgrastim is excreted in breast milk.

Children: Safety data indicates that filgrastim does not exhibit any greater toxicity in children than in adults. Filgrastim has been used to treat 128 pediatric severe chronic neutropenia patients (3 months to 18 years of age); doses used were 0.6 to 120 mcg/kg/day for up to 3 years. Such doses were well tolerated, and the overall pattern of adverse events in children and adults appeared to be similar.

Precautions:

Monitoring:

Myelosuppressive chemotherapy – Obtain CBC and platelet counts prior to chemotherapy, and at regular intervals (twice per week) during therapy to avoid leukocytosis and to monitor the neutrophil count. Following cytotoxic chemotherapy, the neutrophil nadir occurred earlier during cycles when filgrastim was administered and WBC differentials demonstrated a left shift, including the appearance of promyelocytes and myeloblasts. In addition, the duration of severe neutropenia was reduced and was followed by an accelerated recovery in the neutrophil counts. Therefore, regular monitoring of WBC counts, particularly at the time of the recovery from the post-chemotherapy nadir, is recommended in order to avoid excessive leukocytosis.

BMT – Obtain CBC and platelet counts at a minimum of 3 times per week following marrow infusion to monitor the recovery of marrow reconstitution.

Simultaneous use with chemotherapy and radiation: Because of the potential sensitivity of rapidly dividing myeloid cells to cytotoxic chemotherapy, do not use filgrastim 24 hours before to 24 hours after the administration of cytotoxic chemotherapy.

Safety and efficacy have not been evaluated in patients receiving concurrent radiation therapy. Avoid simultaneous use of filgrastim.

Growth factor potential: Filgrastim is a growth factor that primarily stimulates neutrophils. However, the possibility that filgrastim can act as a growth factor for any tumor type, particularly myeloid malignancies, cannot be excluded. Therefore, exercise caution in using this drug in any malignancy with myeloid characteristics.

Leukocytosis: White blood cell counts of $\geq$ 100,000/mm^3 were observed in $\approx$ 2% of patients receiving doses > 5 mcg/kg/day. In order to avoid potential complications of excessive leukocytosis, a complete blood count (CBC) is recommended twice per week during therapy.

Premature discontinuation of therapy: A transient increase in neutrophil counts is typically seen 1 to 2 days after therapy initiation. However, for a sustained therapeutic response, continue therapy until the post nadir ANC reaches 10,000/mm^3. Therefore, premature discontinuation of therapy prior to recovery from the expected neutrophil nadir is generally not recommended.

Chronic administration: The safety and efficacy of chronic administration of filgrastim have not been established. Subclinical splenomegaly was the most frequently observed adverse effect, occurring in approximately 33% of patients receiving chronic administration of filgrastim; 3% of patients were noted to have clinical splenomegaly.

Hematologic effects: Because of the potential of receiving higher doses of chemotherapy, the patient may be at greater risk of thrombocytopenia, anemia and non-hematologic consequences of increased chemotherapy doses. Regular monitoring of the hematocrit and platelet count is recommended. Furthermore, exercise care in the use of filgrastim in conjunction with other drugs known to lower the platelet count. In septic patients, be alert to the possibility of adult respiratory distress syndrome, due to the possible influx of neutrophils at the inflammation site.

Cardiac events (eg, myocardial infarctions, arrhythmias) have occurred in 11 of 375 cancer patients receiving filgrastim; the relationship to filgrastim therapy is unknown. However, closely monitor patients with preexisting cardiac conditions.

Medullary bone pain occurred in 24% of patients. This bone pain was generally of mild to moderate severity, and could be controlled in most patients with non-narcotic analgesics; infrequently, bone pain was severe enough to require narcotic analgesics. Bone pain occurred more frequently in patients treated with higher doses administered IV, and less frequently in patients treated with lower SC doses.

Cutaneous vasculitis: There have been rare reports of cutaneous vasculitis in patients receiving filgrastim. In most cases the severity was moderate or severe. Most reports involved patients with severe chronic neutropenia receiving long-term therapy. Symptoms of vasculitis generally developed simultaneously with an increase in the ANC and abated when the ANC decreased. Many patients were able to continue therapy at a reduced dose.

Drug Interactions:

Drugs which may potentiate the release of neutrophils, such as lithium, should be used with caution.

Adverse Reactions:

Myelosuppressive chemotherapy: Medullary bone pain, nausea/vomting, skeletal pain, alopecia, diarrhea, neutropeinic fever, mucositis, fever, fatigue, anorexia, dyspnea, headache, cough, skin rash, chest pain, generalized weakness, sore throat, stomatitis, constipation.

Bone marrow transplant: Nausea, vomiting, hypertension and rash. Generally, adverse reactions occurred in a minority of patients and were of mild-to-moderate severity.

PBPC Collection: Decreased platelet counts (97%); anemia (65%); mild to moderate musculoskeletal symptoms (44%); medullary bone pain (33%); headache (7%); increases in alkaline phosphatase (21%); increases in neutrophil counts.

Administration and Dosage:

Myelosuppressive chemotherapy: Recommended starting dose is 5 mcg/kg/day, given as a single daily injection by SC bolus injection, by short IV infusion (15 to 30 minutes) or by continuous SC or IV infusion. Obtain CBC and platelet count before instituting therapy; monitor twice weekly during therapy. Doses may be increased in increments of 5 mcg/kg for each chemotherapy cycle according to duration and severity of the ANC nadir.

Administer no earlier than 24 hours after cytotoxic chemotherapy and not in the 24 hours before administration of chemotherapy. Give daily for up to 2 weeks until ANC has reached 10,000/mm^3 following the expected chemotherapy-induced neutrophil nadir. Duration of therapy needed to attenuate chemotherapy-induced neutropenia may depend on the myelosuppressive potential of the chemotherapy regimen employed. Discontinue therapy if the ANC surpasses 10,000/mm^3 after the expected chemotherapy-induced neutrophil nadir. In clinical trials, efficacy was observed at doses of 4 to 8 mcg/kg/day.

Bone marrow transplant: Recommended dose following BMT is 10 mcg/kg/day given as an IV infusion of 4 or 24 hours or as a continuous 24 hour SC infusion. For patients receiving BMT, administer the first dose of filgrastim at least 24 hours after cytotoxic chemotherapy and at least 24 hours after bone marrow infusion.

During the period of neutrophil recovery, titrate the daily dose against the neutrophil response as follows:

Filgrastim Dose Based on Neutrophil Response	
Absolute neutrophil count	Filgrastim dose adjustment
When ANC > 1000/mm^3 for 3 consecutive days	Reduce to 5 mcg/kg/day[1]
If ANC remains > 1000/mm^3 for 3 more consecutive days	Discontinue filgrastim
If ANC decreases to < 1000/mm^3	Resume at 5 mcg/kg/day

[1] If ANC decreases to < 1000/mm^3 at any time during the 5 mcg/kg/day administration, increase filgrastim to 10 mcg/kg/day and follow the steps in the table.

PBPC collection: 10 mcg/kg/day SC, either as a bolus or a continuous infusion. It is recommended that filgrastim be given for at least 4 days before the first leukapheresis procedure and continued until the last leukapheresis. Administration of filgrastim for 6 to 7 days with leukaphereses on days 5, 6 and 7 was found to be safe and effective.

SARGRAMOSTIM (Granulocyte Macrophage Colony Stimulating Factor; GM-CSF)

Powder for Injection, lyophilized: 250 and 500 mcg (*Rx*) *Leukine* (Immunex)

Actions:

Pharmacology: Sargramostim is a recombinant human granulocyte-macrophage colony stimulating factor produced by recombinant DNA technology in a yeast (*S. cerevisiae*) expression system. GM-CSF is a hematopoietic growth factor which stimulates proliferation and differentiation of hematopoietic progenitor cells.

Pharmacokinetics: In eight patients receiving 250 mcg/m^2 of sargramostim by 2 hour IV infusion, serum concentration ranged from 120 to 1500 pg/ml at the termination of the infusion. Then the serum levels decreased with a mean initial half-life and terminal half-life of ≈ 11 minutes and 1.6 hours, respectively, while the mean area under the plasma concentration-time curve (AUC) was 5.35 mcg/ml/hr. When the same patients were treated with 250 mcg/m^2 sargramostim SC, serum levels peaked at 3 hours and ranged between 100 and 1500 pg/ml. The serum levels decreased with a mean terminal half-life and terminal half-life of ≈ 2.6 hours, while the mean AUC was 4.65 mcg/ml/hr. The mean serum levels remained >100 pg/ml for 12 hours after the SC injection and 6 hours after the 2 hour infusion.

Indications:

Acceleration of myeloid recovery in patients with non-Hodgkin's lymphoma (NHL), acute lymphoblastic leukemia (ALL) and Hodgkin's disease undergoing autologous bone marrow transplantation (BMT).

Bone marrow transplantation (BMT) failure or engraftment delay: For patients who have undergone allogeneic or autologous BMT in whom engraftment is delayed or has failed.

Inducation chemotherapy in acute myelogenous leukemia (AML): For use following induction chemotherapy in older patients with AML to shorten neutrophil recovery time and reduce severe and life-threatening infections resulting in death. Safety and efficacy have not been established in AML patients < 55 years of age.

Mobilization and following transplantation of autologous PBPC: For mobilization of hematopoletic progenitor cells into peripheral blood collection by leukapheresis. Mobilization allows collection of increased progenitor cells capable of engraftment compared with collection without mobilization.

Myeloid reconstitution after allogeneic BMT: For acceleration of myeloid recovery in patients undergoing allogeneic BMT from human lymphocyte antigen (HLA)-matched related donors. Safety and efficacy have been established in accelerating myeloid engraftment, reducing the incidence of bacteremia and other culture positive infections and shortening the median duration of hospitilization.

Unlabeled uses: GM-CSF has been used in the following conditions:

To increase WBC counts in patients with myelodysplastic syndromes and in AIDS patients receiving zidovudine.

To decrease nadir of leukopenia secondary to myelosuppressive chemotherapy and decrease myelosuppression in preleukemic patients.

To correct neutropenia in aplastic anemia patients.

To decrease transplantation-associated organ system damage, particularly in the liver and kidney (consistent with the observation that the duration of neutropenia correlates with organ system injury).

Contraindications:

Excessive leukemic myeloid blasts in the bone marrow or peripheral blood (≥ 10%); known hypersensitivity to GM-CSF, yeast-derived products or any component of the product; simultaneous administration with cytotoxic chemotherapy or radiotherapy, or administration 24 hours preceding or following chemotherapy or radiotherapy.

Warnings:

Cardiovascular symptoms: Occasional transient supraventricular arrhythmia has occurred during administration, particularly in patients with a previous history of cardiac arrhythmia. However, these arrhythmias have been reversible after discontinuation of sargramostim.

Respiratory symptoms: Sequestration of granulocytes in the pulmonary circulation has occurred following sargramostim infusion, occasionally with dyspnea. Give special attention to respiratory symptoms during or immediately following infusion, especially in patients with preexisting lung disease.

Fluid retention: Peripheral edema, pleural or pericardial effusion have occurred in patients after administration. In patients with preexisting pleural and pericardial effusions, administration of sargramostim may aggravate fluid retention. Use with caution in preexisting fluid retention, pulmonary infiltrates or congestive heart failure.

Hypersensitivity: Use appropriate precautions during parenteral administration of recombinant proteins in case an allergic or untoward reaction occurs. Transient rashes and local injection site reactions have occasionally been observed. Serious allergic or anaphylactic reactions have been reported rarely. If any anaphylactoid reaction occurs, immediately discontinue and initiate appropriate therapy. Refer to Management of Acute Hypersensitivity Reactions.

Renal/Hepatic function impairment: In some patients with preexisting renal or hepatic dysfunction in uncontrolled clinical trials, sargramostim has induced elevation of serum creatinine or bilirubin and hepatic enzymes. Biweekly monitoring of renal and hepatic function in patients with renal or hepatic dysfunction prior to treatment is recommended during administration.

Pregnancy: Category C.

Lactation: It is not known whether sargramostim is excreted in breast milk.

Children: Safety and efficacy in children have not been established; however, available data indicate that sargramostim does not exhibit any greater toxicity in children than adults.

Precautions:

Monitoring: Sargramostim can induce variable increases in WBC or platelet counts. To avoid potential complications of excessive leukocytosis (WBC > 50,000 cells/mm^3; ANC > 20,000 cells/mm^3), perform a CBC twice per week during therapy. Biweekly monitoring of renal and hepatic function in patients with renal or hepatic dysfunction prior to initiation of treatment is recommended during administration.

Growth factor potential: Sargramostim is a growth factor that primarily stimulates normal myeloid precursors. However, the possibility that sargramostim can act as a growth factor for any tumor type, particularly myeloid malignancies, cannot be excluded.

Use in patients with AML or MDS is not recommended due to possible proliferative effects on abnormal myeloid cells.

First dose effects: Respiratory distress, hypoxia, tachycardia, hypotension with flushing and syncope has occurred rarely following the first use. These signs have resolved with symptomatic treatment and have not recurred with subsequent doses in the same cycle of treatment.

Rapid increase in peripheral blood counts: Stimulation of marrow precursors with sargramostim may result in a rapid rise in white blood cell (WBC) count. If the ANC exceeds 20,000 cells/mm^3 or if the platelet count exceeds 500,000/mm^3, interrupt administration or reduce the dose by half. Base the decision to reduce the dose or interrupt treatment on the clinical condition of the patient. Excessive blood counts have returned to normal or baseline levels within 3 to 7 days following cessation of therapy. Perform biweekly monitoring of CBC with differential (including examination for the presence of blast cells) to preclude development of excessive counts.

Patients receiving purged bone marrow: Sargramostim is effective in accelerating myeloid recovery in patients receiving bone marrow purged by monoclonal antibodies. If in vitro marrow purging with chemical agents causes a significant decrease in the number of responsive hematopoietic progenitors the patient may not respond to sargramostim.

When the bone marrow purging process preserves a sufficient number of progenitors, a beneficial effect of sargramostim on myeloid engraftment has occurred.

Previous exposure to intensive chemotherapy/radiotherapy: In patients who before autologous BMT have received extensive radiotherapy to hematopoietic sites for the treatment of primary disease in the abdomen or chest, or have been exposed to multiple myelotoxic agents, the effect of sargramostim on myeloid reconstitution may be limited.

Concomitant use with chemotherapy and radiotherapy: Because of potential sensitivity of rapidly dividing hematopoietic progenitor cells to cytotoxic chemotherapeutic or radiologic therapies, sargramostim should not be administered within 24 hours preceding or following chemotherapy, or within 12 hours preceding or following radiotherapy.

Drug Interactions:

Drugs which may potentiate the myeloproliferative effects of sargramostim, such as lithium and corticosteroids, should be used with caution.

Adverse Reactions:

The most frequent adverse events were fever, asthenia, headache, bone pain, chills and myalgia. Other reports include arrhythmia, eosinophilia, hypotension, injection site reactions, pain (including abdominal, back, chest and joint pain) tachycardia, thrombosis and transient liver function abnormalities.

Administration and Dosage:

Myeloid reconstitution after autologous bone marrow transplantation: 250 mcg/m^2/day for 21 days as a 2 hour IV infusion beginning 2 to 4 hours after the autologous bone marrow infusion, and not less than 24 hours after the last dose of chemotherapy and 12 hours after the last dose of radiotherapy. If a severe adverse reaction occurs, reduce or temporarily discontinue the dose until the reaction abates. If blast cells appear or progression of the underlying disease occurs, discontinue the treatment. Interrupt or reduce dose by half if the ANC > 20,000 cells/mm^3. Patients should not receive sargramostim until the post-marrow infusion ANC is < 500 cells/mm^3.

Neutrophil recovery following chemotherapy in AML: 250 mcg/m^2/day IV over a 4 hour period starting ≈ day 11 or 4 days following the completion of induction chemotherapy, if the day 10 bone marrow is hypoplastic with < 5% blasts. If a second cycle of induction chemotherapy is necessary, administer ≈ 4 days after the completion of chemotherapy if the bone marrow is hypoplastic with < 5% blasts. Continue sargramostim until an ANC > 1500/mm^3 for 3 consecutive days or a maximum of 42 days. Discontinue immediately if leukemic regrowth occurs. If a severe adverse reaction occurs, reduce the dose by 50% or temporarily discontinue the dose until the reaction abates.

Mobilization of PBPC: 250 mcg/m^2/day IV over 24 hours or SC once daily. Continue at the same dose through the period of PBPC collection. The optimal schedule for PBPC collection has not been established. In clinical studies, collection of PBPC was usually begun by day 5 and performed daily until protocol specified targets were achieved. If WBC > 50,000 cells/mm^3, reduce the dose by 50%. If adequate numbers of progenitor cells are not collected, other metabolization therapy should be considered.

Post peripheral blood progenitor cell transplantation: 250 mcg/m^2/day IV over 24 hours or SC once daily beginning immediately following infusion of progenitor cells and continuing until an ANC > 1500 for 3 consecutive days is attained.

Bone marrow transplantation failure or engraftment delay: 250 mcg/m^2/day for 14 days as a 2 hour IV infusion. The dose can be repeated after 7 days off therapy if engraftment has not occurred. If engraftment still has not occurred, a third course of 500 mcg/m^2/day for 14 days may be tried after another 7 days off therapy. If there is still no improvement, it is unlikely that further dose escalation will be beneficial. If a severe adverse reaction occurs, the dose can be reduced or temporarily discontinued until the reaction abates. If blast cells appear or disease progression occurs, discontinue the treatment.

DIPYRIDAMOLE

Tablets: 25, 50 and 75 mg (*Rx*) — Various, *Persantine* (Boehringer Ingelheim)

Actions:

Pharmacology: Dipyridamole lengthens abnormally shortened platelet survival time in a dose-dependent manner.

Dipyridamole is a platelet adhesion inhibitor, although the mechanism of action has not been fully elucidated. The mechanism may relate to: 1) Inhibition of red blood cell uptake of adenosine, itself an inhibitor of platelet reactivity, 2) phosphodiesterase inhibition leading to increased cyclic-3', 5'-adenosine monophosphate within platelets and 3) inhibition of thromboxane A_2 formation which is a potent stimulator of platelet activation.

Pharmacokinetics:

Metabolism – Following an oral dose of dipyridamole, the average time to peak concentration is about 75 minutes. The decline in plasma concentration fits a two-compartment model. The α half-life (the initial decline following peak concentration) is ≈ 40 minutes. The β half-life (the terminal decline in plasma concentration) is ≈ 10 hours. Dipyridamole is highly bound to plasma proteins. It is metabolized in the liver where it is conjugated as a glucuronide and excreted with the bile.

Indications:

Thromboembolic complications: Adjunct to coumarin anticoagulants in the prevention of postoperative thromboembolic complications of cardiac valve replacement.

Unlabeled uses: At one time, dipyridamole was indicated as a "possibly effective" long term therapy for chronic angina pectoris. The FDA, however, has withdrawn approval for this indication.

Dipyridamole in combination with aspirin has been commonly used in the prevention of myocardial reinfarction and reduction of mortality post MI. However, combination therapy appears to be no more beneficial than the use of aspirin alone.

Warnings:

Fertility impairment: A significant reduction in number of corpora lutea with consequent reduction in implantations and live fetuses was observed at 155 times the maximum recommended human dose.

Pregnancy: Category B.

Lactation: Dipyridamole is excreted in breast milk.

Children: Safety and efficacy in children < 12 years of age have not been established.

Precautions:

Hypotension: Use with caution in patients with hypotension since it can produce peripheral vasodilation.

Adverse Reactions:

Adverse reactions at therapeutic doses are usually minimal and transient. With long-term use, initial side effects usually disappear. The following reactions were reported in two heart valve replacement trials comparing dipyridamole and warfarin therapy to either warfarin alone or warfarin and placebo: Dizziness, abdominal distress, headache and rash.

On those uncommon occasions when adverse reactions have been persistent or intolerable, they have ceased on withdrawal of the medication.

Administration and Dosage:

Adjunctive use in prophylaxis of thromboembolism after cardiac valve replacement: The recommended dose is 75 to 100 mg, 4 times daily as an adjunct to the usual warfarin therapy.

TICLOPIDINE HCl

Tablets: 250 mg (*Rx*) *Ticlid* (Syntex)

Warning:

Neutropenia defined as an absolute neutrophil count (ANC) < 1200 neutrophils/mm^3 occurred in 50 of 2048 (2.4%) stroke patients who received ticlopidine in clinical trials. Neutropenia is calculated as follows: ANC = WBC x % neutrophils.

Severe neutropenia (< 450 neutrophils/mm^3) or agranulocytosis occurred in 17 patients (0.8%) who received ticlopidine. When the drug was discontinued, the neutrophil counts returned to normal (> 1200 neutrophils/mm^3) within 1 to 3 weeks.

Mild to moderate neutropenia (451 to 1200 neutrophils/mm^3) occurred in 33 patients (1.6%) who received ticlopidine. Eleven of the patients discontinued treatment and recovered within a few days. In the remaining 22 patients, the neutropenia was transient and did not require discontinuation of therapy.

The onset of severe neutropenia occurred 3 weeks to 3 months after the start of therapy with no documented cases of severe neutropenia beyond that time. The bone marrow typically showed a reduction in myeloid precursors. It is therefore essential that CBCs and white cell differentials be performed every 2 weeks starting from the second week to the end of the third month of therapy, but more frequent monitoring is necessary for patients whose absolute neutrophil counts have been consistently declining or are 30% less than the baseline count.

If clinical evaluation and repeat laboratory testing confirm the presence of neutropenia, discontinue the drug. In clinical trials, when therapy was discontinued immediately upon detection of neutropenia, the neutrophil counts returned to normal within 1 to 3 weeks.

After the first 3 months of therapy, CBCs need to be obtained only for patients with signs or symptoms suggestive of infection.

Actions:

Pharmacology: Ticlopidine is a platelet aggregation inhibitor. When taken orally, ticlopidine causes a time and dose-dependent inhibition of both platelet aggregation and release of platelet granule constituents, as well as a prolongation of bleeding time. Ticlopidine interferes with platelet membrane function by inhibiting ADP-induced platelet-fibrinogen binding and subsequent platelet-platelet interactions. The effect on platelet function is irreversible for the life of the platelet.

After discontinuation of ticlopidine, bleeding time and other platelet function tests return to normal within 2 weeks in the majority of patients. At the recommended therapeutic dose (250 mg twice daily), ticlopidine has no known significant pharmacological actions in man other than inhibition of platelet function and prolongation of the bleeding time.

Pharmacokinetics: Ticlopidine is rapidly absorbed (> 80%), with peak plasma levels occurring at ≈ 2 hours after dosing, and is extensively metabolized. Administration after meals results in a 20% increase in the area under the plasma concentration-time curve (AUC). Ticlopidine displays non-linear pharmacokinetics and clearance decreases markedly on repeated dosing. in older volunteers, the apparent half-life after a single 250 mg dose is about 12.6 hours; with repeat dosing at 250 mg twice daily, the terminal elimination half-life rises to 4 to 5 days and steady-state levels of ticlopidine in plasma are obtained after ≈ 14 to 21 days.

Ticlopidine binds reversibly (98%) to plasma proteins, mainly to serum albumin and lipoproteins. The binding to albumin and lipoproteins is nonsaturable over a wide concentration range. Ticlopidine also binds to alpha-1 acid glycoprotein; at concentrations attained with the recommended dose, ≤ 15% in plasma is bound to this protein.

Ticlopidine is metabolized extensively by the liver; only trace amounts of intact drug are detected in the urine. Following an oral dose, 60% is recovered in the urine and 23% in the feces. Approximately, one-third of the dose excreted in the feces is intact ticlopidine, possibly excreted in the bile. Approximately 40% to 50% of the metabolites circulating in plasma are covalently bound to plasma proteins, probably by acylation. Although analysis of urine and plasma indicates at least twenty metabolites, no metabolite which accounts for the activity of ticlopidine has been isolated.

Indications:

Thrombotic stroke: To reduce the risk of thrombotic stroke (fatal or nonfatal) in patients who have experienced stroke precursors, and in patients who have had a completed thrombotic stroke.

Because ticlopidine is associated with a risk of neutropenia/agranulocytosis, which may be life-threatening, reserve for patients who are intolerant to aspirin therapy where indicated to prevent stroke.

Unlabeled uses: Ticlopidine has also been utilized in various other conditions; further study is needed:Intermittent claudication; chronic arterial occlusion; subarachnoid hemorrhage; uremic patients with AV shunts or fistulas; open heart surgery; coronary artery bypass grafts; primary glomerulonephritis; sickle cell disease.

Contraindications:

Hypersensitivity to the drug; presence of hematopoietic disorders such as neutropenia and thrombocytopenia; presence of a hemostatic disorder or active pathological bleeding; severe liver impairment.

Warnings:

Thrombocytopenia: Rarely, thrombocytopenia may occur in isolation or together with neutropenia. If clinical evaluation and repeat laboratory testing confirm the presence of thrombocytopenia, discontinue the drug.

Cholesterol elevation: Ticlopidine therapy causes increased serum cholesterol and triglycerides. Serum total cholesterol levels are increased 8% to 10% within 1 month of therapy and persist at that level. The ratios of lipoprotein subfractions are unchanged.

Hematological effects: Rare cases of pancytopenia and thrombotic thrombocytopenia purpura, some of which have been fatal, have occurred.

Anticoagulant drugs: If a patient is switched from an anticoagulant or fibrinolytic drug to ticlopidine, discontinue the former drug prior to ticlopidine administration.

Renal function impairment: Patients with mildly or moderately impaired renal function were compared to healthy subjects. AUC values of ticlopidine increased by 28% and 60% in mild and moderately impaired patients, respectively, and plasma clearance decreased by 37% and 52%, respectively, but there were no statistically significant differences in ADP-induced platelet aggregation. Bleeding times showed significant prolongation only in the moderately impaired patients. Nevertheless, for renally impaired patients it may be necessary to reduce ticlopidine dosage or discontinue it altogether if hemorrhagic or hematopoietic problems are encountered.

Hepatic function impairment: The average plasma concentration in patients with advanced cirrhosis was slightly higher than that seen in older subjects. Because of limited experience in patients with severe hepatic disease, who may have bleeding diatheses, the use of ticlopidine is not recommended.

Elderly: Clearance of ticlopidine is somewhat lower in elderly patients and trough levels are increased. No overall differences in safety or efficacy were observed between elderly patients and younger patients, but greater sensitivity of some older individuals cannot be ruled out.

Pregnancy: Category B.

Lactation: It is not known whether this drug is excreted in human breast milk.

Children: Safety and efficacy in patients < 18 years of age have not been established.

Precautions:

Increased bleeding risk: Use with caution in patients who may be at risk of increased bleeding from trauma, surgery or pathological conditions. If it is desired to eliminate the antiplatelet effects of ticlopidine prior to elective surgery, discontinue the drug 10 to 14 days prior to surgery. Increased surgical blood loss has occurred in patients undergoing surgery during treatment with ticlopidine. In TASS and CATS it was recommended that patients have ticlopidine discontinued prior to elective surgery. Several hundred patients underwent surgery during the trials, and no excessive surgical bleeding was reported.

Prolonged bleeding time is normalized within 2 hours after administration of 20 mg methylprednisolone IV. Platelet transfusions may also be used to reverse the effect of ticlopidine on bleeding.

GI bleeding: Ticlopidine prolongs template bleeding time. Use with caution in patients who have lesions with a propensity to bleed (such as ulcers). Use drugs that might induce such lesions with caution in patients on ticlopidine.

Drug Interactions:

The dose of drugs metabolized by hepatic microsomal enzymes with low therapeutic ratios, or being given to patients with hepatic impairment, may require adjustment to maintain optimal therapeutic blood levels when starting or stopping concomitant therapy with ticlopidine.

Drugs that may interact include antacids, cimetidine, aspirin, digoxin and theophylline.

Drug/Food interactions: The oral bioavailability of ticlopidine is increased by 20% when taken after a meal. Administration with food is recommended to maximize GI tolerance.

Adverse Reactions:

Adverse reactions were relatively frequent, with > 50% of patients reporting at least one. Most involved the GI tract. Most adverse effects are mild, but 21% of patients discontinued therapy because of an adverse event, principally diarrhea, rash, nausea, vomiting, GI pain and neutropenia. Most adverse effects occur early in the course of treatment, but a new onset of adverse effects can occur after several months. Ticlopidine has been associated with a number of bleeding complications such as ecchymosis, epistaxis, hematuria, conjunctival hemorrhage, GI bleeding and perioperative bleeding. The incidence of elevated alkaline phosphatase (> 2 times upper limit of normal) was 7.6% in ticlopidine patients.The incidence of elevated AST (> 2 times upper limit of normal) was 3.1% in ticlopidine patients.

Administration and Dosage:

Recomended dose: 250 mg twice daily taken with food.

ABCIXIMAB

Injection: 2 mg/ml (*Rx*)	*ReoPro* (Lilly)

Actions:

Pharmacology: Abciximab is the Fab fragment of the chimeric human-murine monoclonal antibody 7E3. Abciximab binds to the intact glycoprotein IIb/IIIa (GPIIb/IIIa) receptor of human platelets, which is a member of the integrin family of adhesion receptors and the major platelet surface receptor involved in platelet aggregation. The drug inhibits platelet aggregation by preventing the binding of fibrinogen, von Willebrand factor and other adhesive molecules to GPIIb/IIIa receptor sites on activated platelets. Low levels of GPIIb/IIIa receptor blockade are present for up to 10 days following cessation of the infusion.

Pharmacokinetics: Following IV bolus administration, free plasma concentrations of abciximab decrease rapidly with an initial half-life of < 10 minutes and a second phase half-life of about 30 minutes, probably related to rapid binding to the platelet receptors. Platelet function generally recovers over the course of 48 hours, although abciximab remains in the circulation for up to 10 days in a platelet-bound state. IV administration of a 0.25 mg/kg bolus dose of abciximab followed by continuous infusion of 10 mcg/min produces almost constant free plasma concentrations throughout the infusion. At the termination of the infusion period, free plasma concentrations fall rapidly for about 6 hours and then decline at a slower rate.

Indications:

Platelet aggregation inhibition: Adjunct to percutaneous transluminal coronary angioplasty or atherectomy (PTCA) for the prevention of acute cardiac ischemic complications in patients at high risk for abrupt closure of the treated coronary vessel.

Abciximab is intended for use with aspirin and heparin.

Contraindications:

Because abciximab increases the risks of bleeding, it is contraindicated in the following clinical situations: Active internal bleeding; recent (within 6 weeks) GI or GU bleeding of clinical significance; history of cerebrovascular accident (CVA) within 2 years or CVA with a significant residual neurological deficit; bleeding diathesis; administration of oral anticoagulants within 7 days unless prothrombin time is < 1.2 times control; thrombocytopenia; recent (within 6 weeks) major surgery or trauma; intracranial neoplasm, arteriovenous malformation or aneurysm; severe uncontrolled hypertension; presumed or documented history of vasculitis; use of IV dextran before PTCA or intent to use it during PTCA; hypersensitivity to any component of this product or to murine proteins.

Warnings:

Bleeding: Abciximab is associated with an increased frequency of major bleeding complications including retroperitoneal bleeding, spontaneous GI and GU bleeding and bleeding at the arterial access site. In the following conditions, clinical data suggest that the risks of major bleeds due to therapy may be increased and should be weighed against the anticipated benefits: Patients who weigh < 75 kg; patients > 65 years old; history of prior GI disease; patients receiving thrombolytics; heparin anticoagulation.

The following conditions are also associated with an increased risk of bleeding in the angioplasty setting which may be additive to that of abciximab: PTCA within 12 hours of the onset of symptoms for acute MI; prolonged PTCA (lasting > 70 minutes); failed PTCA.

Should serious bleeding occur that is not controllable with pressure, stop the infusion of abciximab and any concomitant heparin.

Bleeding sites – Therapy with abciximab requires careful attention to all potential bleeding sites (including catheter insertion, arterial and venous puncture, cutdown, needle puncture, GI, GU and retroperitoneal sites).

Femoral artery access site: Abciximab is associated with an increase in bleeding rate particularly at the site of arterial access for femoral sheath placement. Use care when attempting vascular access so that only the anterior wall of the femoral artery is punctured, avoiding a Seldinger technique for obtaining sheath access. Avoid femoral vein sheath placement unless needed. While the vascular sheath is in place, maintain patients on complete bed rest with the head of the bed ≤ 30° and restrain the affected limb in a straight position.

Discontinue heparin at least 4 hours prior to arterial sheath removal. Following sheath removal, apply pressure to the femoral artery for at least 30 minutes using either manual compression or a mechanical device for hemostasis. Apply a pressure dressing following hemostasis. Maintain the patient on bed rest for 6 to 8 hours following sheath removal or discontinuation of abciximab, whichever is later.

Frequently check the sheath insertion site and distal pulses of affected leg(s) while the femoral artery sheath is in place, and for 6 hours after femoral artery sheath removal. Measure any hematoma and monitor for enlargement.

General nursing care: Arterial and venous punctures, IM injections and use of urinary catheters, nasotracheal intubation, nasogastric tubes and automatic blood pressure cuffs should be minimized. When obtaining IV access, avoid non-compressible sites (eg, subclavian or jugular veins). Consider saline or heparin locks for blood drawing. Document and monitor vascular puncture sites. Provide gentle care when removing dressings.

High-risk patients: Patients at high risk for abrupt closure include those undergoing PTCA with at least one of the following conditions: Unstable angina or a non-Q-wave MI; an acute Q-wave MI within 12 hours of the onset of symptoms.

Other high-risk clinical or morphologic characteristics include: Two type B lesions in the artery to be dilated; one type B lesion in the artery to be dilated in a woman of at least 65 years of age; one type B lesion in the artery to be dilated in a patient with diabetes mellitus; one type C lesion in the artery to be dilated; angioplasty of an infarct-related lesion within 7 days of MI.

Hypersensitivity: Administration of abciximab may result in human anti-chimeric antibody (HACA) formation that can cause allergic or hypersensitivity reactions, thrombocytopenia or diminished benefit upon readministration of abciximab. Patients with HACA titers may have allergic or hypersensitivity reactions when treated with other diagnostic or therapeutic monoclonal antibodies. Anaphylaxis may occur at any time during administration. If it does, immediately stop administration of abciximab and initiate standard appropriate resuscitative measures.

Pregnancy: Category C.

Lactation: It is not known whether this drug is excreted in breast milk or absorbed systemically after ingestion.

Children: Safety and efficacy in children have not been established.

Precautions:

Monitoring: Before infusion of abciximab, measure platelet count, prothrombin time and APTT to identify pre-existing hemostatic abnormalities. During and after treatment, closely monitor platelet counts and extent of heparin anticoagulation, as assessed by activated clotting time or APTT.

Concomitant therapy: In a clinical trial, abciximab was used concomitantly with heparin and aspirin. Because abciximab inhibits platelet aggregation, use caution when it is used with other drugs that affect hemostasis, including thrombolytics, oral anticoagulants, nonsteroidal anti-inflammatory drugs, dipyridamole and ticlopidine.

Low molecular weight dextran and oral anticoagulants were usually given for the deployment of a coronary stent. In the 11 patients who received low molecular weight dextran with abciximab, 5 had major bleeding events and 4 had minor bleeding events.

Thrombocytopenia: Monitor platelet counts prior to treatment, 2 to 4 hours following the bolus dose of abciximab and at 24 hours or before discharge, whichever is first. If a patient experiences an acute platelet decrease (eg, decrease to < 100,000 cells/mcl or a decrease of at least 25% from pretreatment value), determine additional platelet counts. If true thrombocytopenia is verified, immediately discontinue abciximab and appropriately monitor and treat the condition.

Restoration of platelet function: In the event of serious uncontrolled bleeding or the need for surgery (especially major procedures within 48 to 72 hours of treatment with abciximab), determine a bleeding time. Preliminary evidence suggests that platelet function may be restored, at least in part, with platelet transfusions.

Adverse Reactions:

The most common complication of abciximab therapy is bleeding (see Warnings). Adverse reactions occurring in > 3% of abciximab patients include: Hypotension, bradycardia, nausea, vomiting, thrombocytopenia, atrial fibrillation/flutter and miscellaneous pain.

Administration and Dosage:

Abciximab is intended for use in patients undergoing PTCA. The safety and efficacy of abciximab have only been investigated with concomitant administration of heparin and aspirin.

Failed PTCAs: In patients with failed PTCAs, stop the continuous infusion of abciximab because there is no evidence for abciximab efficacy in that setting.

Serious bleeding: In the event of serious bleeding that cannot be controlled by compression, discontinue abciximab and heparin.

The recommended dosage is an IV bolus of 0.25 mg/kg administered 10 to 60 minutes before the start of PTCA, followed by a continuous IV infusion of 10 mcg/min for 12 hours.

Administration instructions:

1.) Do NOT use preparations of abciximab containing visibly opaque particles.
2.) Anticipate hypersensitivity reactions whenever protein solutions such as abciximab are administered. Epinephrine, dopamine, theophylline, antihistamines and corticosteroids should be available for immediate use. If symptoms of an allergic reaction or anaphylaxis appear, stop the infusion and give appropriate treatment.
3.) Withdraw the necessary amount of abciximab (2 mg/ml) for bolus injection through a sterile, non-pyrogenic, low protein-binding 0.2 or 0.22 micron filter into a syringe. Administer the bolus 10 to 60 minutes before the procedure.
4.) Withdraw 4.5 ml of abciximab for the continuous infusion through a sterile, non-pyrogenic, low protein-binding 0.2 or 0.22 micron filter into a syringe. Inject into 250 ml of sterile 0.9% saline or 5% dextrose and infuse at a rate of 17 ml/hr (10 mcg/min) for 12 hours via a continuous infusion pump equipped with an in-line sterile, non-pyrogenic, low protein-binding 0.2 or 0.22 micron filter. Discard the unused portion at the end of the 12-hour infusion.

ANTICOAGULANTS

Blood coagulation resulting in the formation of a stable fibrin clot involves a cascade of proteolytic reactions involving the interaction of clotting factors, platelets and tissue materials. Clotting factors (see table) exist in the blood in inactive form and must be converted to an enzymatic or activated form before the next step in the clotting mechanism can be stimulated. Each factor is stimulated in turn until an insoluble fibrin clot is formed.

Two separate pathways, intrinsic and extrinsic, lead to the formation of a fibrin clot. Both pathways must function for hemostasis.

Intrinsic pathway: All the protein factors necessary for coagulation are present in circulating blood. Clot formation may take several minutes and is initiated by activation of factor XII.

Extrinsic pathway: Coagulation is activated by release of tissue thromboplastin, a factor not found in circulating blood. Clotting occurs in seconds because factor III bypasses the early reactions.

Refer to the next page for the complete coagulation pathway.

Anticoagulants used therapeutically include heparin, warfarin (a coumarin derivative) and anisindione (an indandione derivative).

Blood Clotting Factors

Factor	Synonym	Vitamin K-dependent
I	Fibrinogen	no
II	Prothrombin	yes
III	Tissue thromboplastin, tissue factor	no
IV	Calcium	no
V	Labile factor, proaccelerin	no
VII	Proconvertin	yes
VIII	Antihemophilic factor, AHF	no
IX	Christmas factor, plasma thromboplastin component, PTC	yes
X	Stuart factor, Stuart-Prower factor	yes
XI	Plasma thromboplastin antecedent, PTA	no
XII	Hageman factor	no
XIII	Fibrin stabilizing factor, FSF	no
HMW-K	High molecular weight Kininogen, Fitzgerald factor	no
PL	Platelets or phospholipids	no
PK	Prekallikrein, Fletcher factor	no
Protein C[1]		yes
Protein S[2]		yes

[1] Partially responsible for inhibition of the extrinsic pathway. Inactivates factors V and VIII and promotes fibrinolysis. Activity declines following warfarin administration.

[2] A cofactor to accelerate the anticoagulant activity of protein C. Decreased levels occur following warfarin administration.

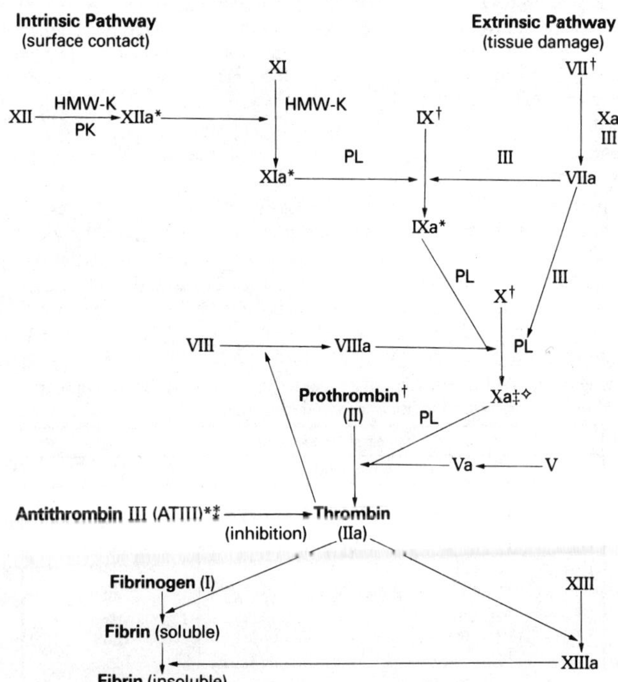

* Major site of activity for unfractionated heparin
† Site of activity for warfarin and anisindione
‡ Major site of activity for fractionated heparin
⁑ Minor site of activity for fractionated heparin
✧ Minor site of activity for fractionated heparin

ENOXAPARIN SODIUM

Injection: 30 mg/0.3 ml (*Rx*)	*Lovenox* (Rhone-Poulenc Rorer)

Actions:

Pharmacology: Enoxaparin is a low molecular weight heparin obtained by depolymerization of unfractionated porcine heparin. It has antithrombotic properties characterized by a higher ratio of anti-Factor Xa to anti-Factor IIa activity than unfractionated heparin and has relatively less lipase release activity.

Pharmacokinetics: Maximum anti-Factor Xa and antithrombin (anti-Factor IIa) activities occur 3 to 5 hours after SC injection of enoxaparin. Mean absolute bioavailability based on anti-Factor Xa activity is 92% in healthy volunteers. The volume of distribution of anti-Factor Xa activity is about 6 L. Following IV dosing, the total body clearance is 25 ml/min. Elimination half-life based on anti-Factor Xa activity was about 4.5 hours after SC administration. Following a 40 mg dose significant anti-Factor Xa activity persists in plasma for about 12 hours. Following IV dosing, 8% to 20% of anti-Factor Xa activity was recovered in urine in 24 hours.

Indications:

Prevention of deep vein thrombosis, which may lead to pulmonary embolism, following hip replacement surgery.

Unlabeled uses: Enoxaparin is currently being investigated for use following knee replacement.

Contraindications:

Active major bleeding; thrombocytopenia associated with a positive in vitro test for anti-platelet antibody in the presence of enoxaparin; hypersensitivity to enoxaparin, heparin or pork products.

Warnings:

Interchangeability with heparin: Enoxaparin cannot be used interchangeably (unit for unit) with unfractionated heparin or other low molecular weight heparins.

Hemorrhage: Like other anticoagulants, use with extreme caution in conditions with increased risk of hemorrhage. Bleeding can occur at any site during therapy with enoxaparin.

Thrombocytopenia: Moderate thrombocytopenia occurred at a rate of about 2% in patients given enoxaparin, 3% in patients given heparin, and 0% in patients receiving placebo in clinical trials. Closely monitor thrombocytopenia of any degree.

Heparin-induced thrombocytopenia: Use with extreme caution in patients with a history of this condition.

Renal function impairment: Delayed elimination of enoxaparin may occur.

Elderly: An increase of 25% in the area under anti-Factor Xa activity vs time curve was observed following once-daily dosing in healthy elderly subjects for 10 days. Delayed elimination of enoxaparin may occur.

Pregnancy: Category B.

Lactation: It is not known whether this drug is excreted in breast milk.

Children: Safety and efficacy in children have not been established.

Precautions:

Monitoring: Periodic complete blood counts, including platelet count, and stool occult blood tests are recommended during the course of treatment with enoxaparin.

Special risk patients: Use with care in patients with a bleeding diathesis, uncontrolled arterial hypertension or a history of recent GI ulceration and hemorrhage.

Thromboembolic events: If thromboembolic events occur despite enoxaparin prophylaxis, discontinue and initiate appropriate therapy.

Drug Interactions:

Anticoagulants and platelet inhibitors: Use enoxaparin with care.

Drug/Lab test interactions: Asymptomatic increases in transaminase levels (AST and ALT) > 3 times the upper limit of normal of the laboratory reference range have been reported in two of 10 healthy subjects and in up to 5% of patients during treatment with enoxaparin. Such elevations are fully reversible and are rarely associated with increases in bilirubin. Since transaminase determinations are important in the differential diagnosis of myocardial infarction, liver disease and pulmonary emboli, interpret elevations that might be caused by drugs like enoxaparin with caution.

Adverse Reactions:

Adverse reactions associated with enoxaparin include: Hemorrhage, thrombocytopenia, local irritation following SC administration, fever, nausea, edema, peripheral edema and hyochromic anemia.

Administration and Dosage:

Adults: In patients undergoing hip replacement, the recommended dose is 30 mg twice daily administered by SC injection with the initial dose given as soon as possible after surgery, but not more than 24 hours postoperatively. Continue treatment throughout the period of postoperative care until the risk of deep vein thrombosis has diminished. Up to 14 days administration has been well tolerated in controlled clinical trials. The average duration of administration is 7 to 10 days.

Screen all patients prior to prophylactic administration of enoxaparin to rule out a bleeding disorder. There is usually no need for daily monitoring of the effect of enoxaparin in patients with normal presurgical coagulation parameters.

Administration: Administer by SC injection. Do not administer by IM injection.

SC injection technique: Patients should be lying down; administer by deep SC injection. Alternate administration between the left and right anterolateral and left and right posterolateral abdominal wall. Introduce the whole length of the needle into a skin fold held between the thumb and forefinger; hold the skin fold throughout the injection.

DALTEPARIN SODIUM

Solution: 2500 anti-Factor Xa/0.2 ml (*Rx*) *Fragmin* (Pharmacia)

Actions:

Pharmacology: Dalteparin is a low molecular weight heparin for injection with antithrombotic properties. It acts by enhancing the inhibition of Factor Xa and thrombin by antithrombin. Dalteparin potentiates preferentially the inhibition of coagulation factor Xa, while only slightly affecting clotting time (eg, activated partial thromboplastin time [APTT]).

Pharmacokinetics:

Absorption/Distribution – Mean peak levels of plasma anti-Factor Xa activity following single SC doses of 2500, 5000 and 10,000 IU were 0.19, 0.41 and 0.82 IU/ml, respectively, and were attained in about 4 hours in most subjects. Absolute bioavailability in healthy volunteers, measured as the anti-Factor Xa activity, was 87%. Increasing the dose from 2500 to 10,000 IU resulted in an overall increase in anti-Factor Xa AUC that was greater than proportional by ≈ 33%. Peak anti-Factor Xa activity increased more or less linearly with dose.

The volume of distribution for dalteparin anti-Factor Xa activity was 40 to 60 ml/kg. The mean plasma clearances of dalteparin anti-Factor Xa activity in healthy volunteers following single IV bolus doses of 30 and 120 anti-Factor Xa IU/kg were 24.6 and 15.6 ml/hr/kg, respectively. Their corresponding mean disposition half-lives are 1.47 and 2.5 hrs.

Following IV doses of 40 and 60 IU/kg, mean terminal half-lives were 2.1 and 2.3 hrs, respectively. Longer apparent terminal half-lives (3 to 5 hrs) are observed following SC dosing, possibly due to delayed absorption.

Indications:

Deep vein thrombosis: Prophylaxis against DVT. Patients at risk include patients who are > 40 years of age, obese, undergoing surgery under general anesthesia lasting > 30 minutes or who have additional risk factors such as malignancy or a history of DVT or pulmonary embolism.

Contraindications:

Hypersensitivity to the dalteparin, heparin or pork products; active major bleeding; thrombocytopenia associated with positive in vitro tests for antiplatelet antibody in the presence of dalteparin.

Warnings:

Product interchangeability: Dalteparin cannot be used interchangeably (unit for unit) with unfractionated heparin or other low molecular weight heparins.

Hemorrhage: Use dalteparin, like other anticoagulants, with extreme caution in patients who have an increased risk of hemorrhage. Bleeding can occur at any site during therapy with dalteparin. An unexpected drop in hematocrit or blood pressure should lead to a search for a bleeding site.

Thrombocytopenia: Closely monitor thrombocytopenia of any degree. Heparin-induced thrombocytopenia can occur with administration of dalteparin. Use with extreme caution in patients with history of heparin-induced thrombocytopenia.

Renal/Hepatic function impairment: Use with caution in patients with severe liver or kidney insufficiency. In patients with chronic renal insufficiency requiring hemodialysis, the mean terminal half-life of anti-Factor Xa activity following a single IV dose of 5000 IU was 5.7 hrs (considerably longer than values observed in healthy volunteers), therefore greater accumulation can be expected in these patients.

Pregnancy: Category B.

Lactation: It is not known whether dalteparin is excreted in breast milk.

Children: Safety and efficacy in children have not been established.

Precautions:

Monitoring: Periodic routine complete blood counts, including platelet count and stool occult blood tests are recommended during the course of treatment.

Retinopathy: Use with caution in patients with hypertensive or diabetic retinopathy.

Thromboembolic event: If a thromboembolic event should occur despite dalteparin prophylaxis, discontinue the drug and initiate appropriate therapy.

Laboratory tests: Asymptomatic increases in transaminase levels (AST and ALT) > 3 times the upper limit of normal of the laboratory reference range have been reported.

Drug Interactions:

Use dalteparin with care in patients receiving oral anticoagulants or platelet inhibitors because of increased risk of bleeding.

Adverse Reactions:

Adverse reactions may include hematoma at the injection site; thrombocytopenia; wound hematoma.

Administration and Dosage:

Route of administration: Dalteparin is administered by SC injection. It must not be administered by IM injection.

Dosage: In patients undergoing abdominal surgery with a risk of thromboembolic complications, administer 2500 IU each day, SC only, starting 1 to 2 hours prior to surgery and repeated once daily for 5 to 10 days postoperatively. Dosage adjustment and routine monitoring of coagulation parameters are not required if these dosage and administration recommendations are followed.

HEPARIN

HEPARIN SODIUM	
Injection: 1000, 5000, 10,000 and 20,000 units/ml (multiple dose vials) (*Rx*)	Various, *Liquaemin Sodium* (Organon)
Injection: 1000, 5000, 10,000 and 20,000 units/ml (single dose amps and vials) (*Rx*)	Various, *Liquaemin Sodium Preservative Free* (Organon)
Injection: 1000, 2500, 5000, 7500, 10,000 and 20,000 units/ml (unit dose vials) (*Rx*)	Various
HEPARIN SODIUM AND SODIUM CHLORIDE	
Injection: 1000 and 2000 units (*Rx*)	*Heparin Sodium and 0.9% Sodium Chloride* (Clintec)
Injection: 12,500 and 25,000 units (*Rx*)	*Heparin Sodium and 0.45% Sodium Chloride* (Abbott)
HEPARIN SODIUM LOCK FLUSH	
Injection: 10 and 100 units/ml (*Rx*)	Various, *Hep-Lock* (Elkins-Sinn)

Actions:

Pharmacology: The major rate-limiting step in the coagulation cascade is the activation of factor X, which is involved in both intrinsic and extrinsic pathways. Small amounts of heparin in combination with antithrombin III (heparin cofactor) inhibit thrombosis by inactivating factor Xa and inhibiting the conversion of prothrombin to thrombin. Once active thrombosis has developed, larger amounts of heparin can inhibit further coagulation by inactivating thrombin and preventing the conversion of fibrinogen to fibrin. In combination with antithrombin III, heparin inactivates factors IX, X, Xa, XI, XII and thrombin, inhibiting conversion of fibrinogen to fibrin. The heparin-antithrombin III complex is 100 to 1000 times more potent as an anticoagulant than antithrombin III alone. Heparin also prevents the formation of a stable fibrin clot by inhibiting the activation of factor XIII (the fibrin stabilizing factor). Other effects include the inhibition of thrombin-induced activation of factors V and VIII.

Commercial products contain both low and high molecular weight heparin fractions. Low molecular weight heparin has a greater inhibitory effect on factor Xa, and less antithrombin activity than the high molecular weight fraction.

Heparin inhibits reactions that lead to clotting, but does not significantly alter the concentration of the normal clotting factors of blood. Although clotting time is prolonged by full therapeutic doses, in most cases it is not measurably affected by low doses of heparin. Bleeding time is usually unaffected.

Heparin also enhances lipoprotein lipase release, (which clears plasma of circulating lipids), increases circulating free fatty acids and reduces lipoprotein levels.

Pharmacokinetics:

Absorption/Distribution – Heparin is not adsorbed from the GI tract. An IV bolus results in immediate anticoagulant effects. The duration of action is dose-dependent. Peak plasma levels of heparin are achieved 2 to 4 hours following SC use. Once absorbed, heparin is distributed in plasma and is extensively protein bound.

Metabolism/Excretion – Following administration, heparin demonstrates a biphasic elimination curve. The lack of relationship between plasma and pharmacologic half-lives may reflect factors such as protein binding. Heparin is rapidly cleared from plasma with an average half-life of 30 to 180 minutes. Half-life is dose-dependent and may be significantly prolonged at higher doses. Heparin is partially metabolized by liver heparinase and the reticuloendothelial system. There may be a secondary site of metabolism in the kidneys. Apparent volume of distribution is 40 to 60 ml/kg. In patients with deep venous thrombosis, plasma clearance is more rapid and half-life is shorter than in patients with pulmonary embolism. Heparin is excreted in urine as unchanged drug (up to 50%) particularly after large doses. Some urinary degradation products have anticoagulant activity.

Indications:

Prophylaxis and treatment of venous thrombosis and its extension; pulmonary embolism; peripheral arterial embolism; atrial fibrillation with embolization.

Diagnosis and treatment of acute and chronic consumption coagulopathies (disseminated intravascular coagulation [DIC]).

Postoperative: Low dose regimen for prevention of postoperative deep venous thrombosis (DVT) and pulmonary embolism in patients undergoing major abdominothoracic surgery or patients who are at risk of developing thromboembolic disease.

According to National Institutes of Health Consensus Development Conference, low-dose heparin is treatment of choice as prophylaxis for DVT and pulmonary embolism in urology patients > 40 years old; pregnant patients with prior thromboembolism; stroke patients; those with heart failure, acute MI or pulmonary infection; also recommended as suggested prophylaxis in high-risk surgery patients, moderate and high-risk gynecologic patients without malignancy, neurology patients with extracranial problems and patients with severe musculoskeletal trauma.

Prevention of clotting in arterial and heart surgery, blood transfusions, extracorporeal circulation, dialysis procedures and blood samples for laboratory purposes.

Unlabeled uses: Prophylaxis of left ventricular thrombi and cerebrovascular accidents post-MI.

Continuous infusion for treatment of myocardial ischemia in unstable angina refractory to conventional treatment. Heparin decreases the number of anginal attacks and silent ischemic episodes and reduces the daily duration of ischemia. Intermittent heparin is not as effective.

Prevention of cerebral thrombosis in the evolving stroke.

As an adjunct in treatment of coronary occlusion with acute myocardial infarction (MI). Although there is some controversy regarding the efficacy of heparin therapy with concurrent antiplatelet therapy (eg, aspirin) in the prevention of rethrombosis/reocclusion after primary thrombolysis with thrombolytics during acute MI, it is recommended by the American College of Cardiology and the American Heart Association. Generally, administer heparin IV immediately after thrombolytic therapy, usually within 2 to 8 hours (depending on the thrombolytic used), and maintain the infusion for at least 24 hours. Begin aspirin therapy immediately as soon as the patient is admitted, and continue its administration.

Contraindications:

Hypersensitivity to heparin; severe thrombocytopenia; uncontrolled bleeding (except when it is due to DIC); any patient for whom suitable blood coagulation tests cannot be performed at the appropriate intervals (there is usually no need to monitor coagulation parameters in patients receiving low-dose heparin).

Warnings:

Hemorrhage can occur at virtually any site in patients receiving heparin. An unexplained fall in hematocrit, fall in blood pressure or any other unexplained symptom should lead to serious consideration of a hemorrhagic event. An overly prolonged coagulation test or bleeding can usually be controlled by withdrawing the drug. Signs and symptoms will vary according to the location and extent of bleeding and may present as paralysis, headache, chest, abdomen, joint or other pain, shortness of breath, difficulty breathing or swallowing, unexplained swelling or unexplained shock. GI or urinary tract bleeding may indicate an underlying occult lesion. Certain hemorrhagic complications may be difficult to detect.

Use heparin with extreme caution in disease states in which there is increased danger of hemorrhage. These include:

Cardiovascular – Subacute bacterial endocarditis; arterial sclerosis; dissecting aneurysm; increased capillary permeability; severe hypertension.

CNS – During and immediately following spinal tap, spinal anesthesia or major surgery, especially of the brain, spinal cord or eye.

Hematologic – Hemophilia; some vascular purpuras; thrombocytopenia.

GI – Ulcerative lesions, diverticulitis or ulcerative colitis; continuous tube drainage of the stomach or small intestine.

Obstetric – Threatened abortion; menstruation.

Other – Liver disease with impaired hemostasis; severe renal disease.

Hyperlipidemia: Heparin may increase free fatty acid serum levels by induction of lipoprotein lipase. The catabolism of serum lipoproteins by this enzyme produces lipid fragments which are rapidly processed by the liver. Patients with dysbetalipoproteinemia (type III) are unable to catabolize the lipid fragments, resulting in hyperlipidemia.

Resistance: Increased resistance to the drug is frequently encountered in fever, thrombosis, thrombophlebitis, infections with thrombosing tendencies, MI, cancer and postoperative states.

Thrombocytopenia has occurred in patients receiving heparin. The incidence of heparin-associated thrombocytopenia is higher with bovine than with porcine heparin. The severity also appears to be related to heparin dose.

Early thrombocytopenia (Type I) develops 2 to 3 days after starting heparin, tends to be mild and is due to a direct action of heparin on platelets.

Delayed thrombocytopenia (Type II) develops 7 to 12 days after either low-dose or full-dose heparin, can have serious consequences and may reflect the presence of an immunoglobulin that induces platelet aggregation.

Mild thrombocytopenia may remain stable or reverse even if heparin is continued. However, closely monitor thrombocytopenia of any degree. If a count falls below $100,000/mm^3$ or if recurrent thrombosis develops, discontinue heparin. If continued heparin therapy is essential, administration of heparin from a different organ source can be reinstituted with caution.

White clot syndrome – Rarely, patients may develop new thrombus formation in association with thrombocytopenia resulting from irreversible aggregation of platelets induced by heparin, the so-called "white clot syndrome." The process may lead to severe thromboembolic complications. Monitor platelet counts before and during therapy. If significant thrombocytopenia occurs, immediately terminate heparin and institute other therapeutic measures.

Hypersensitivity: Heparin is derived from animal tissue; use with caution in patients with a history of allergy. Before a therapeutic dose is given, a trial dose may be advisable. Have epinephrine 1:1000 immediately available.

Vasospastic reactions may develop 6 to 10 days after starting therapy and last 4 to 6 hours. The affected limb is painful, ischemic and cyanotic. An artery to this limb may have been recently catheterized. After repeated injections, the reaction may gradually increase to generalized vasospasm with cyanosis, tachypnea, feeling of oppression and headache. Itching and burning, especially on the plantar side of the feet, is possibly based on a similar allergic vasospastic reaction. Chest pain, elevated blood pressure, arthralgias or headache have also been reported in the absence of definite peripheral vasospasm.

Hepatic function impairment: Heparin half-life may be prolonged in liver disease.

Elderly: A higher incidence of bleeding has occurred in women > 60 years of age.

Pregnancy: *Category* C. Safety for use during pregnancy has not been established. Heparin does not cross the placenta. However, its use during pregnancy has been associated with 13% to 22% unfavorable outcomes, including stillbirths and prematurity. This contrasts with a 31% incidence with coumarin derivatives. Heparin is probably the preferred anticoagulant during pregnancy, but it is not risk free.

Lactation: Heparin is not excreted in breast milk.

Children: Safety and efficacy have not been determined in newborns; germinal matrix intraventricular hemorrhage occurs more often in low-birth-weight infants receiving heparin.

Use heparin lock flush solution with caution in infants with disease states in which there is an increased danger of hemorrhage. The use of the 100 unit/ml concentration is not advised because of bleeding risk, especially in low-birth-weight infants.

Precautions:

Monitoring: The most common test used to monitor heparin's effect is APTT. Other tests used include Activated Coagulation Time (ACT) and Lee White-Whole Blood Clotting Time (WBCT). If the coagulation test is unduly prolonged or if hemorrhage occurs, discontinue the drug promptly. Perform periodic platelet counts, hematocrit and tests for occult blood in stool during the entire course of therapy, regardless of route of administration.

Hyperkalemia may develop, probably due to induced hypoaldosteronism. Use with caution in patients with diabetes or renal insufficiency. Monitor patient closely.

Drug Interactions:

Drugs that may interact include cephalosporins, nitroglycerin, penicillins and salicylates.

Drug/Lab test interactions: Significant elevations of **aminotransferase** (AST and ALT) levels have occurred in a high percentage of patients. Cautiously interpret aminotransferase increases that might be caused by heparin.

If heparin comprises ≥ 10% of the total volume of a sample for blood gas analysis, errors in measurements of **carbon dioxide pressure, bicarbonate concentration** and **base excess** may occur.

Adverse Reactions:

Adverse reactions associated with heparin include hemorrhage, chills, fever, urticaria and thrombocytopenia.

Administration and Dosage:

Give by intermittent IV injection, continuous IV infusion or deep SC (ie, above the iliac crest of abdominal fat layer) injection. Continuous IV infusion is generally preferable due to the higher incidence of bleeding complications with other routes. Avoid IM injection because of the danger of hematoma formation.

Adjust dosage according to coagulation test results prior to each injection. Dosage is adequate when WBCT is ≈ 2.5 to 3 times control value, or when APTT is 1.5 to 2 times normal.

When given by continuous IV infusion, perform coagulation tests every 4 hours in the early stages. When administered by intermittent IV infusion, perform coagulation tests before each dose during early stages and at appropriate intervals thereafter. After deep SC injection, perform tests 4 to 6 hours after the injections.

General heparin dosage guidelines: Although dosage must be individualized, the following may be used as guidelines:

Heparin Dosage Guidelines		
Method of administration	Frequency	Recommended dose[1]
Subcutaneous[2]	Initial dose	10,000 – 20,000 units[3]
	Every 8 hours	8000 – 10,000 units
	Every 12 hours	15,000 – 20,000 units
Intermittent IV	Initial dose	10,000 units[4]
	Every 4 to 6 hours	5000 – 10,000 units[4]
IV Infusion	Continuous	20,000 – 40,000 units/day[3]

[1] Based on a 68 kg (150 lb) patient.
[2] Use a concentrated solution.
[3] Immediately preceded by IV loading dose of 5,000 units.
[4] Administer undiluted or in 50 to 100 ml 0.9% NaCl.

Children: In general, the following dosage schedule may be used as a guideline:

Initial dose – 50 units/kg IV bolus.

Maintenance dose – 100 units/kg/dose IV drip every 4 hours, or 20,000 units/m^2/24 hours continuous IV infusion.

Low-dose prophylaxis of postoperative thromboembolism: Low-dose heparin prophylaxis, prior to and after surgery, will reduce the incidence of postoperative DVT in the legs and clinical pulmonary embolism. Give 5000 units SC 2 hours before surgery and 5000 units every 8 to 12 hours thereafter for 7 days or until the patient is fully ambulatory, whichever is longer. Administer by deep SC injection above the iliac crest or abdominal fat layer, arm or thigh using a concentrated solution. Use a fine guage needle (25 to 26 guage) to minimize tissue trauma. Reserve such prophylaxis for patients > 40 years of age undergoing major surgery. Exclude patients on oral anticoagulants or drugs that affect platelet function or in patients with bleeding disorders, brain or spinal cord injuries, spinal anesthesia, eye surgery or potentially sanguineous operations.

If bleeding occurs during or after surgery, discontinue heparin and neutralize with protamine sulfate. If clinical evidence of thromboembolism develops despite low-dose prophylaxis, give full therapeutic doses of anticoagulants until contraindicated. Prior to heparinization, rule out bleeding disorders; perform appropriate coagulation tests just prior to surgery. Coagulation test values should be normal or only slightly elevated at these times.

Surgery of the heart and blood vessels: Give an initial dose of not less than 150 units/kg to patients undergoing total body perfusion for open heart surgery. Often, 300 units/kg is used for procedures < 60 minutes and 400 units/kg is used for procedures > 60 minutes.

Extracorporeal dialysis: Follow equipment manufacturers' operating directions.

Laboratory samples: Add 70 to 150 units per 10 to 20 ml sample of whole blood to prevent coagulation of sample.

Clearing intermittent infusion (heparin lock) sets: To prevent clot formation in a heparin lock set, inject dilute heparin solution (Heparin Lock Flush Solution, USP; or a 10 to 100 units/ml heparin solution) via the injection hub in a quantity sufficient to fill the entire set to the needle tip. Replace this solution each time the heparin lock is used. If the administered drug is incompatible with heparin, flush the entire heparin lock set with sterile water or normal saline before and after the medication is administered; following the second flush, the dilute heparin solution may be reinstilled into the set. Consult the set manufacturer's instructions.

Converting to oral anticoagulant therapy: Perform baseline coagulation tests to determine prothrombin activity when heparin activity is too low to affect PT or INR. When the results of the initial prothrombin determinations are known, initiate the oral anticoagulant in the usual amount. Thereafter, perform coagulation tests and prothrombin activity at appropriate intervals. When the prothrombin activity reaches the desired therapeutic range, discontinue heparin and continue oral anticoagulants.

COUMARIN AND INDANDIONE DERIVATIVES

WARFARIN SODIUM	
Tablets: 1, 2, 2.5, 4, 5, 7.5 and 10 mg (*Rx*)	*Coumadin* (DuPont)
ANISINDIONE	
Tablets: 50 mg (*Rx*)	*Miradon* (Schering)
DICUMAROL	
Tablets: 25 mg (*Rx*)	*Dicumarol* (Abbott)

Actions:

Pharmacology: Coumarins (dicumarol and warfarin) and indandiones (anisindione) interfere with the hepatic synthesis of vitamin K-dependent clotting factors which results in an in vivo depletion of clotting factors VII, IX, X and II (prothrombin). Anticoagulant effects are dependent on the half-lives of these clotting factors, which are 6, 24, 36 and 50 hours, respectively. Hence, the reduction in the rate of synthesis of the clotting factors determines the clinical response. Although factor VII is quickly depleted and an initial prolongation of the prothrombin time (PT) is seen in 8 to 12 hours, maximum anticoagulation (thus, antithrombotic effects) is not approached for 3 to 5 days as the other factors are depleted and the drug achieves steady-state.

Oral anticoagulants have no direct effect on an established thrombus, nor do they reverse ischemic tissue damage. However, once thrombosis has occurred, anticoagulant treatment may prevent further extension of the formed clot and prevent secondary thromboembolic complications which may result in serious and possibly fatal sequelae.

Warfarin is available as a racemic mixture containing the R(+) and S(–) enantiomers in equal proportions; however, the S-isomer is 3 to 6 times more potent as an anticoagulant than the R-isomer.

Pharmacokinetics:

Absorption – The oral anticoagulants are generally rapidly and completely absorbed.

Distribution – Oral anticoagulants are highly bound to plasma proteins (97% to > 99%), primarily albumin.

Metabolism/Excretion – These agents are metabolized by hepatic microsomal enzymes and are excreted primarily in the urine and feces as inactive metabolites.

Various Pharmacokinetic Parameters of Oral Anticoagulants			
Oral anticoagulant	Half-life (days)	Peak activity (days)	Duration[1] (days)
Coumarin derivatives			
Dicumarol	1-2	1.5-2	5-6
Warfarin	1-2.5[2]	1.5-3	2-5
Indandione derivative			
Anisindione	3-5	2-3	1-3

[1] Following drug discontinuation
[2] S-isomer ≈ 2 days; R-isomer ≈ 1.33 days

Indications:

Warfarin/Anisindione/Dicumarol: Prophylaxis and treatment of venous thrombosis and its extension; treatment of atrial fibrillation with embolization; prophylaxis and treatment of pulmonary embolism.

Warfarin: Prophylaxis of atrial fibrillation with embolism. As an adjunct in the prophylaxis of systemic embolism after myocardial infarction (MI).

Anisindione/Dicumarol: As an adjunct in the treatment of coronary occlusion. Warfarin is generally the drug of choice.

Unlabeled uses: Oral anticoagulants have been used to prevent recurrent transient ischemic attacks and to reduce the risk of recurrent MI, but data conflict. Warfarin has shown potential benefit as an adjunct in the treatment of small cell carcinoma of the lung, given concomitantly with chemotherapy and radiation.

Contraindications:

Pregnancy (see Warnings); hemorrhagic tendencies; hemophilia; thrombocytopenic purpura; leukemia; recent or contemplated surgery of the eye or CNS, major regional lumbar block anesthesia, or surgery resulting in large, open surfaces; patients bleeding from the GI, respiratory or GU tract; threatened abortion; aneurysm (cerebral, dissecting aortic); ascorbic acid deficiency; history of bleeding diathesis; prostatectomy; continuous tube drainage of the small intestine; polyarthritis; diverticulitis; emaciation; malnutrition; cerebrovascular hemorrhage; eclampsia and pre-eclampsia; blood dyscrasias; severe uncontrolled or malignant hypertension; severe renal or hepatic disease; pericarditis and pericardial effusion; subacute bacterial endocarditis; visceral carcinoma; following spinal puncture and other diagnostic or therapeutic procedures (ie, IUD insertion) with potential for uncontrollable bleeding; unsupervised senility; alcoholism; psychosis; open wounds; history of warfarin-induced necrosis.

Warnings:

Monitoring:

PT – Treatment is highly individualized. Control dosage by periodic determination of PT or other suitable coagulation tests (eg, INR). Monitor PT daily during the initiation of therapy and whenever any other drug is added to or discontinued from therapy which may alter the patient's response. Concurrent heparin therapy will elevate the PT 10% to 20%; if target PT levels are not increased by the same percentage during concurrent therapy, the patient could be inadequately anticoagulated when the heparin therapy is discontinued. Once stabilized, monitor PT every 4 to 6 weeks.

INR –

INR is based on the determination of an International Normalized Ratio which provides a common basis for PT results and interpretations of therapeutic ranges. For a discussion of the relationship between PT and INR in clinical practice, refer to Administration and Dosage.

Hemorrhage/Necrosis: The most serious risks associated with anticoagulant therapy are hemorrhage in any tissue or organ and, less frequently, necrosis or gangrene of skin and other tissues; this has resulted in death or permanent disability. The risk of hemorrhage is related to the level of intensity and duration of therapy. Discontinue therapy when anticoagulants are the suspected cause of developing necrosis; consider heparin therapy.

Hemorrhagic tendency may be manifested by hematuria, skin petechiae, hemorrhage into or from a wound or ulcerating lesion or petechial and purpuric hemorrhages throughout the body.

Bleeding during anticoagulant therapy does not always correlate with prothrombin activity. Bleeding that occurs when the PT or INR is within the therapeutic range warrants investigation since it may unmask a previously unsuspected lesion (eg, tumor, ulcer).

Independent risk factors that may provide a basis for predicting major bleeding with anticoagulants include: ≥ 65 years of age; history of stroke; history of GI bleeding; serious comorbid condition (eg, recent MI, renal insufficiency, severe anemia); atrial fibrillation.

"Purple toe syndrome" – Anticoagulant therapy may enhance the release of atheromatous plaque emboli thereby increasing the risk of complications from systemic cholesterol microembolization including the "purple toe syndrome."

Excessive uterine bleeding may occur, but menstrual flow is usually normal. Women may be at risk of developing ovarian hemorrhage at the time of ovulation.

Oral anticoagulants should not be used in the treatment of acute completed strokes due to the risk of fatal cerebral hemorrhage.

Adrenal hemorrhage with resultant acute adrenal insufficiency has occurred.

Special risk patients: There is an increased risk with use of anticoagulants in the following conditions: Trauma; infection (concomitant antibiotic therapy may alter intestinal flora); renal insufficiency; prolonged dietary insufficiencies (eg, sprue, vitamin K deficiency); severe to moderate hypertension; polycythemia vera; vasculitis; severe allergic disorders; anaphylactic disorders; indwelling catheters; severe diabetes; surgery or trauma resulting in large exposed raw surfaces.

Use with caution in patients with active tuberculosis, severe diabetes, history of ulcerative disease of the GI tract and during menstruation and the postpartum period.

Protein C deficiency: Known or suspected hereditary, familial or clinical deficiency in protein C has been associated with necrosis following warfarin therapy.

Agranulocytosis and hepatitis have been associated with anisindione use.

Rebound hypercoagulability was thought to occur upon sudden anticoagulant withdrawal, but has not been reproducible. Also there is no evidence that thrombosis will recur following abrupt withdrawal. Therefore, tapering the dose to discontinuation appears unnecessary, although tapering the dose gradually over 3 to 4 weeks is recommended if possible.

CHF: Patients with CHF may become more sensitive to dicumarol.

Hypersensitivity: Delayed reactions are rare and occur within 1 to 3 months following the start of anisindione; 10% of cases are fatal. Discontinue the medication at the first sign of hypersensitivity reactions.

Renal/Hepatic function impairment: Use with caution.

Elderly: May be more sensitive to these agents.

Pregnancy: *Category X.*

If oral anticoagulants are used in pregnant women, do not administer during the first trimester, and discontinue prior to labor and delivery.

Some clinicians suggest the replacement of oral anticoagulants with heparin therapy before term. After 5 to 7 days, therapy with oral anticoagulants may be resumed if indicated.

Lactation: Warfarin appears in breast milk in an inactive form. Infants nursed by warfarin-treated mothers had no change in PT.

Anisindione and dicumarol or their metabolites may be excreted in breast milk in amounts sufficient to cause a prothrombopenic state and bleeding in the newborn.

Children: Safety and efficacy in children < 18 years old have not been established. Oral anticoagulants may be beneficial in children with rare thromboembolic disorder secondary to other disease states such as the nephrotic syndrome or congenital heart lesions. Heparin is probably the initial anticoagulant of choice because of its immediate onset of action.

Precautions:

Enhanced anticoagulant effects: Several endogenous factors that may result in an increased response to the oral anticoagulants or an increased PT or INR include: Carcinoma; hepatic disorders including hepatitis or obstructive jaundice; biliary fistula; febrile states; preparatory bowel sterilization; recent surgery; x-ray therapy; vitamin K deficiency; steatorrhea; CHF; diarrhea; poor nutritional state or collagen disease; renal insufficiency; hyperthyroidism; elevated temperature. Also, female and elderly patients are more sensitive to these agents.

Decreased anticoagulant effects: Endogenous factors that may reduce the response to the oral anticoagulants or decrease the PT or INR include: Edema; hyperlipidemia; diabetes mellitus; hypothyroidism; hereditary resistance to oral anticoagulants.

Drug Interactions:

The oral anticoagulants have a great potential for clinically significant drug interactions. Warn all patients about potential hazards and instruct against taking **any** drug, including nonprescription products, without the advice of a physician or pharmacist.

Careful monitoring and appropriate dosage adjustments usually will permit safe administration of combined therapy. Critical times during therapy occur when an interacting drug is added to or discontinued from a patient stabilized on anticoagulants.

Coumarin and indandione derivatives are affected by many drugs. Those that may significantly affect coumarin and indandione derivatives include amiodarone, 17–alkyl androgens, barbiturates, clofibrate, dextrothyroxine, erythromycin, histamine H_2 antagonists, metronidazole, miconazole, phenylbutazones, quinine derivatives, salicylates, sulfinpyrazone, sulfonamides, thioamines, thyroid hormones and vitamin E.

Drug/Lab test interactions: Oral anticoagulants may cause red-orange discoloration of alkaline urine; this may interfere with some lab tests.

Adverse Reactions:

Hemorrhage is the principal adverse effect of oral anticoagulants.

Other adverse reactions include: Nausea; diarrhea; pyrexia; dermatitis; exfoliative dermatitis; urticaria; alopecia; sore mouth; mouth ulcers; fever; abdominal cramping; leukopenia; red-orange urine; priapism (causal relationship not established); paralytic ileus and intestinal obstruction from submucosal or intramural hemorrhage.

Administration and Dosage:

Dosage: Individualize dosage.

Available clinical evidence indicates that prolongation of the PT to 1.2 to 1.5 times control, when measuring with the less sensitive thromboplastin reagents, is sufficient for prophylaxis and treatment of venous thromboembolism and minimizes the risk of hemorrhage associated with more prolonged PT values. In cases where the risk of thromboembolism is great, such as in patients with recurrent systemic embolism, maintain a PT of 1.5 to 2 times control. A ratio of > 2 appears to provide no additional therapeutic benefit in most patients and is associated with a higher risk of bleeding.

For the three commercial rabbit brain thromboplastins currently used in North America, a PT ratio of 1.3 to 2 is equivalent to an INR of 2 to 4. For other thromboplastins, the INR can be calculated as:

$$\text{INR} = (\text{observed PT ratio})^{\text{ISI}}$$

where the ISI (International Sensitivity Index) is the calibration factor and is available from the manufacturers of the thromboplastin reagent and observed PT ratio is:

$$\frac{\text{PT observed}}{\text{PT control}}$$

Following are the recommended therapeutic ranges for oral anticoagulant therapy from the American College of Chest Physicians (ACCP) and the National Heart, Lung and Blood Institute (NHLBI):

ACCP/NHLBI Recommended Therapuetic Range for Oral Anticogulant Therapy		
Condition	PT Ratio[1]	INR
Acute MI[2]	1.3 to 1.5	2 to 3
Atrial fibrillation[2]	1.3 to 1.5	2 to 3
Mechanical prosthetic valves	1.5 to 2	3 to 4.5
Pulmonary embolism, treatment	1.3 to 1.5	2 to 3
Systemic embolism		
Prevention	1.3 to 1.5	2 to 3
Recurrent	1.5 to 2	3 to 4.5
Tissue heart valves[2]	1.3 to 1.5	2 to 3
Valvular heart disease[2]	1.3 to 1.5	2 to 3
Venous thrombosis		
Prophylaxis (high-risk surgery)	1.3 to 1.5	2 to 3
Treatment	1.3 to 1.5	2 to 3

[1] ISI of 2.4
[2] To prevent systemic embolism

Transfer from heparin therapy: To provide continuous adequate anticoagulation in a patient on heparin, switch to oral anticoagulation. Since there is a delayed onset of oral anticoagulant effects, give heparin and warfarin simultaneously from the first day, or alternatively, start warfarin on the third to sixth day of heparin therapy. Use concurrent therapy until a therapeutic PT or INR is achieved.

Elderly: Lower dosages are recommended.

Duration of therapy: In the determination of the duration of long-term anticoagulant therapy, consider history of recurrent thromboembolism, underlying diseases, reason for anticoagulant therapy (eg, atrial fibrillation) and risks of adverse effects.

WARFARIN:

Induction – Initiate with 10 mg/day for 2 to 4 days; adjust daily dosage according to PT or INR determinations. Use of a large loading dose (eg, 30 mg) may increase the incidence of hemorrhagic and other complications, does not offer more rapid protection against thrombi formation and is not recommended.

Maintenance – 2 to 10 mg daily, based on PT or INR.

Bioequivalence problems have been documented for warfarin sodium products marketed by different manufacturers. Brand interchange is not recommended.

Treatment during dentistry and surgery – In patients who must be anticoagulated prior to, during or immediately following dental or surgical procedures, adjusting the dosage to maintain the PT at the low end of the therapeutic range (or maintain the corresponding INR value) may safely allow for continued anticoagulation. Limit the operative site to permit effective use of local measures for hemostasis. Under these conditions, dental and surgical procedures may be performed without undue risk of hemorrhage.

Minidose warfarin may be beneficial as prophylaxis against venous thrombosis after major surgery. In one study, 1 mg daily given before surgery (mean 20 days) significantly lowered the incidence of DVT compared to controls; there was no difference between the 1 mg/day and the full-dose anticoagulation group. APTT and PT were not prolonged beyond normal on the day of surgery using the minidose therapy.

ANISINDIONE: 300 mg the first day, 200 mg the second day, 100 mg the third day and 25 to 250 mg daily for maintenance.

DICUMAROL: 200 to 300 mg the first day, 25 to 200 mg on subsequent days.

Treatment during dentistry and surgery – If it is elected to administer anticoagulants prior to, during or immediately following dental or surgical procedures, it is recommended that the dosage of dicumarol be adjusted to maintain the prothrombin time at ≈ 1½ to 2½ times the control level.

Chapter 3
HORMONES

ESTROGENS

Product	Manufacturer
ESTRONE AQUEOUS	
Injection: 2 and 5 mg per ml (*Rx*)	Various, *Aquest* (Dunhall), *Estrone 5* (Keene), *Kestrone 5* (Hyrex)
ESTROGENIC SUBSTANCE OR ESTROGENS (MAINLY ESTRONE) AQUEOUS SUSPENSION	
Injection: 2 mg per ml estrogenic substance or estrogens (mainly estrone) (*Rx*)	Various
ESTRADIOL TRANSDERMAL SYSTEM	
Transdermal Patch: 0.0375 mg, 0.05 mg, 0.075 mg and 0.1 mg per 24 hours (*Rx*)	*Estraderm* (Ciba), *Climara* (Berlex), *Vivelle* (Ciba)
ESTRADIOL, ORAL	
Tablets: 0.5, 1 and 2 mg micronized estradiol (*Rx*)	*Estrace* (Bristol-Myers Squibb)
ESTRADIOL VALERATE in oil	
Injection: 10, 20 and 40 mg per ml (*Rx*)	Various, *Delestrogen* (Mead Johnson), *Dioval* (Keene), *Estra-L* (Pasadena), *Gynogen L.A.* (Forest), *Valergan* (Hyrex),
CONJUGATED ESTROGENS, ORAL	
Tablets: 0.3, 0.625, 0.9, 1.25 and 2.5 mg (*Rx*)	*Premarin* (Wyeth-Ayerst)
CONJUGATED ESTROGENS, PARENTERAL	
Injection: 25 mg conjugated estrogens (*Rx*)	*Premarin Intravenous* (Wyeth-Ayerst)
ESTERIFIED ESTROGENS	
Tablets: 0.3, 0.625, 1.25 mg, 2.5 mg (*Rx*)	*Estratab* (Solvay Pharm.), *Menest* (SK-Beecham)
ESTROPIPATE	
Tablets: 0.75, 1.5 and 3 mg estropipate (*Rx*)	Various, *Ogen* (Abbott), *Ortho-Est* (Ortho)
QUINESTROL	
Tablets: 100 mcg (*Rx*)	*Estrovis* (Parke-Davis)
ETHINYL ESTRADIOL	
Tablets: 0.02, 0.05, 0.5 mg (*Rx*)	*Estinyl* (Schering)
DIETHYLSTILBESTROL (DES)	
Tablets: 1 and 5 mg (*Rx*)	Various
CHLOROTRIANISENE	
Capsules: 12 and 25 mg (*Rx*)	*Tace* (Marion Merrell Dow)
ESTRADIOL CYPIONATE IN OIL	
Injection: 5 mg per ml (*Rx*)	Various, *depGynogen* (Forest), *Depo-Estradiol Cypionate* (Upjohn), *Depogen* (Hyrex), *Estro-Cyp* (Keene)

Warning:

Estrogens have been reported to increase the risk of endometrial carcinoma.

When estrogens are used for the treatment of menopausal symptoms, use the lowest dose and discontinue medication as soon as possible. When prolonged treatment is indicated, reassess the patient at least semiannually to determine the need for continued therapy. Cyclic administration of low doses of estrogen may carry less risk than continuous administration.

Do not use estrogens during pregnancy.

The use of female sex hormones (both estrogens and progestins) during early pregnancy may seriously damage the offspring.

If estrogens are used during pregnancy, or if the patient becomes pregnant while taking estrogens, inform her of the potential risks to the fetus.

Actions:

Pharmacology: Although six different natural estrogens have been isolated from the human female, only three are present in significant quantities: Estradiol, estrone and estriol. The most potent and major secretory product of the ovary, estradiol, is rapidly oxidized to estrone. Hydration of estrone produces the much weaker estriol. The estrogenic potency of estradiol is 12 times estrone's and 80 times estriol's.

Estrogens, important in developing and maintaining female reproductive system and secondary sex characteristics, promote growth and development of vagina, uterus, fallopian tubes and breasts. They affect release of pituitary gonadotropins; cause capillary dilatation, fluid retention, protein anabolism and thin cervical mucus; inhibit or facilitate ovulation; prevent postpartum breast discomfort. Indirectly, they contribute to: Shaping the skeleton (conserving calcium and phosphorus and encouraging bone formation); maintenance of tone and elasticity of urogenital structures; changes in epiphyses of long bones that allow for pubertal growth spurt and its termination; growth of axillary and pubic hair; pigmentation of nipples and genitals.

Menstruation – Decline of estrogenic activity at the end of the menstrual cycle can induce menstruation, although cessation of progesterone secretion does the same to an estrogen-primed endometrium. However, in the preovulatory or nonovulatory cycle, estrogen withdrawal is the primary determinant of the onset of menstruation.

Menopause – The beginning of menopause is marked by hot flushes, decreasing frequency and quality of ovulation, associated with skips and delays of menses or variable periods of amenorrhea and later by decreasing estrogen secretion. Estrogen production, first to appear at menarche, is last to decline at menopause. The declining estrogen secretion is accompanied by signs and symptoms of hormone deficits in the estrogen-dependent organs, including pituitary, uterus, cervix, vagina and breasts. Pituitary gonadotropin secretion rises, reflected by increased quantities of gonadotropin in blood and urine. The endometrium becomes atrophic, myometrial mass decreases and the vaginal epithelium becomes thin as, deficient in glycogen, it fails to become keratinized. The ovarian stroma producing androgens persist at variable amounts of time.

Pharmacokinetics:

Absorption/Distribution – Absorption of most natural estrogens and their derivatives from the GI tract is complete. The limited oral effectiveness of natural estrogens and their esters is due to their metabolism. About 80% of estradiol is bound to sex hormone binding globulin; most of the rest is loosely bound to albumin and about 2% is unbound. Estrone is highly bound to protein as it circulates in the blood, primarily as a conjugate with sulfate.

Transdermal system: In contrast to oral estradiol, the skin metabolizes estradiol via the transdermal system only to a small extent. Therefore, transdermal use produces therapeutic serum levels of estradiol with lower circulating levels of estrone and estrone conjugates, and requires smaller total doses. Transdermal use produces mean serum estradiol concentrations comparable to those produced by daily oral administration at about 20 times the daily transdermal dose.

Metabolism/Excretion – Metabolism and inactivation occur primarily in the liver. During cyclic passage through the liver, estrogens are degraded to less active estrogenic compounds conjugated with sulfuric and glucuronic acids.

Indications:

Moderate to severe vasomotor symptoms associated with menopause: The primary indication is to treat hot flushes. Sleep deprivation associated with this can aggravate depression. Estrogens are not the drug of choice for treating depression.

Atrophic vaginitis; kraurosis vulvae.

Female hypogonadism; female castration; primary ovarian failure.

Breast cancer: Palliation only in selected women and men or those with metastatic disease.

Prostatic carcinoma: Palliative therapy of advanced disease.

Osteoporosis: **Conjugated estrogens** are indicated in postmenopausal women, with evidence of loss or deficiency of bone mass, to retard further bone loss and estrogen-deficiency-induced osteoporosis. Use with other important measures such as diet, calcium and physiotherapy. A more favorable benefit/risk ratio exists if women have had a hysterectomy; there is no risk of endometrial carcinoma.

The FDA has also approved the use of the other oral short-acting estrogens (DES, esterified estrogens, estradiol, ethinyl estradiol and estropipate) in the treatment of osteoporosis.

Abnormal uterine bleeding due to hormonal imbalance in the absence of organic pathology (**conjugated estrogens, parenteral**).

Unlabeled uses: Oral DES is an effective postcoital contraceptive when given in doses of 25 mg twice daily for 5 days if therapy is started no later than 72 hours after intercourse. Ethinyl estradiol, conjugated estrogens and other estrogens have also been evaluated for postcoital contraception.

Ethinyl estradiol – A 5 mcg tablet is being investigated for use in the treatment of Turner's syndrome.

Contraindications:

Breast cancer, except in appropriately selected patients being treated for metastatic disease; estrogen-dependent neoplasia; undiagnosed abnormal genital bleeding; active thrombophlebitis or thromboembolic disorders; history of thrombophlebitis, thrombosis or thromboembolic disorders associated with previous estrogen use (except when used in treatment of breast or prostatic malignancy); known or suspected pregnancy.

Warnings:

Induction of malignant neoplasms: Estrogens may increase the risk of endometrial carcinoma.

Gallbladder disease: There is a 2– to 3–fold increase in risk of gallbladder disease in women receiving postmenopausal estrogens. This may be related to large doses.

Effects similar to those caused by estrogen-progestin oral contraceptives (OCs): Consider the following effects noted in OC users as potential risks of estrogen use:

Elevated blood pressure is common, but is less frequent with estrogen replacement therapy than with OC use.

Thromboembolic disease – OC users have an increased risk of thromboembolic and thrombotic vascular diseases, including thrombophlebitis, pulmonary embolism, stroke and myocardial infarction. Cases of retinal thrombosis, mesenteric thrombosis and optic neuritis have been reported. The risk of several of these adverse reactions is dose-related. An increased risk of postsurgical thromboembolic complications has also been reported.

Do not use in persons with active thrombophlebitis or thromboembolic disorders or in persons with a history of such disorders associated with estrogen use (except in treatment of malignancy).

Large doses (conjugated estrogens 5 mg/day), comparable to those used to treat prostate and breast cancer, have increased risk of nonfatal MI, pulmonary embolism and thrombophlebitis in men. When such estrogen doses are used, the thromboembolic and thrombotic adverse effects associated with OC use are a clear risk.

Hypercalcemia: Estrogens may lead to severe hypercalcemia in patients with breast cancer and bone metastases. If this occurs, discontinue the drug and take appropriate measures to reduce the serum calcium level.

Glucose tolerance: Usual replacement doses of estrogen improve insulin sensitivity.

Hepatic function impairment: Patients with a history of jaundice during pregnancy have an increased risk of recurrence while on estrogen-containing OCs. If jaundice develops in any patient on estrogen, discontinue medication and investigate the cause. Estrogens may be poorly metabolized in impaired liver function; use with caution.

Pregnancy: Category X (See Warning Box).

Lactation: Estrogens have been shown to decrease the quantity and quality of breast milk and may be excreted in breast milk. Administer only when clearly needed.

Children: Safety and efficacy are not established. Because of effects on epiphyseal closure, use judiciously in young patients in whom bone growth is incomplete.

Precautions:

History/Physical exam: Before initiating estrogens, take complete medical and family history. Pretreatment and periodic history and physical exams every 6 to 12 months should include blood pressure, breasts, abdomen, pelvic organs and a Papanicolaou smear. Generally, do not prescribe for > 1 year between physical examinations.

Excessive estrogenic stimulation: Certain patients may develop undesirable manifestations of excessive estrogenic stimulation (eg, abnormal or excessive uterine bleeding, mastodynia). Advise the pathologist of estrogen therapy when relevant specimens are submitted.

Fluid retention: Estrogens may cause some degree of fluid retention; conditions which might be influenced by this factor (eg, asthma, epilepsy, migraine and cardiac or renal dysfunction) require careful observation.

Calcium and phosphorus metabolism is influenced by estrogens; use caution in patients with metabolic bone diseases associated with hypercalcemia or in renal insufficiency.

Prolonged unopposed estrogen therapy may increase risk of endometrial hyperplasia.

Acute intermittent porphyria may be precipitated by estrogens.

Benzyl alcohol, contained in some of these products as a preservative, has been associated with a fatal "gasping syndrom" in premature infants.

Photosensitivity: Photosensitization may occur; therefore, caution patients to take protective measures (ie, sunscreens, protective clothing) against exposure to ultraviolet light or sunlight until tolerance is determined.

Tartrazine sensitivity: Some of these products contain tartrazine which may cause allergic-type reactions (including bronchial asthma) in susceptible individuals. Although the incidence of sensitivity is low, it is frequently seen in patients who also have aspirin hypersensitivity.

Drug Interactions:

Drugs that may be affected by estrogens include oral anticoagulants, tricyclic antidepressants, dantrolene, hydantoins and corticosteroids.

Drugs that may affect estrogens include barbiturates, rifampin and hydantoins.

Drug/Lab test interactions: Certain endocrine and liver function tests may be affected by estrogen-containing OCs. Expect these similar changes with larger doses:

Increased **sulfobromophthalein retention.**

Increased **prothrombin** and **factors** VII, VIII, IX and X; decreased **antithrombin** III; increased norepinephrine-induced **platelet aggregability.**

Increased **thyroid binding globulin (TBG)** leading to increased circulating total thyroid hormone, as measured by **PBI,** T_4 by column or T_4 by radioimmunoassay. **Free T_3 resin uptake** is decreased, reflecting the elevated TBG; **free T_4** concentration is unaltered.

Impaired **glucose tolerance**; decreased **pregnanediol excretion**; reduced response to **metyrapone test**; reduced **serum folate** concentration; increased **serum triglyceride** and **phospholipid** concentration.

Adverse Reactions:

Significant adverse reactions include breakthrough bleeding; spotting; change in menstrual flow; dysmenorrhea; premenstrual-like syndrome; amenorrhea during and after treatment; nausea; vomiting; abdominal cramps; bloating; cholestatic jaundice; chloasma or melasma (may persist when drug is discontinued); erythema nodosum/multiforme; hemorrhagic eruption; urticaria; dermatitis; steepening of corneal curvature; intolerance to contact lenses; headache; migraine; dizziness; mental depression; convulsions; pain at injection site; sterile abscess; postinjection flare; redness and irritation at application site with the estradiol transdermal system (17%); aggravation of porphyria; edema; changes in libido; breast tenderness, enlargement or secretion.

Administration and Dosage:

Concomitant progestin therapy: Addition of a progestin for 7 or more days of a cycle of estrogen has lowered the incidence of endometrial hyperplasia. Morphological and biochemical studies of endometrium suggest that 10 to 13 days of progestin are needed to provide maximal maturation of the endometrium and to eliminate any hyperplastic changes.

ESTRONE: Administer IM only. Shake vial and syringe well prior to withdrawal and injection (using a 21 to 23 gauge needle) to properly suspend medication.

Cyclically –

Replacement therapy of estrogen deficiency associated conditions (eg, hypogonadism, female castration, primary ovarian failure): Initial relief of symptoms may be achieved through the administration of 0.1 to 1 mg of estrone weekly in single or divided doses. Some patients may require 0.5 to 2 mg weekly.

Senile vaginitis and kraurosis vulvae: Generally, 0.1 to 0.5 mg 2 or 3 times/week.

Abnormal uterine bleeding due to hormone imbalance: May respond to brief courses of intensive therapy. Usual dose range is 2 to 5 mg daily for several days.

Chronically –

Inoperable progressing prostatic cancer: For palliation in prostatic cancer, use estrone at 2 to 4 mg, 2 or 3 times/week. If a response to therapy is going to occur, it should be apparent within 3 months of beginning therapy. If a response does occur, continue the hormone until the disease is again progressive.

Inoperable progressing breast cancer in appropriately selected men and postmenopausal women: 5 mg ≥ 3 times/week according to severity of pain.

ESTRADIOL TRANSDERMAL SYSTEM:

Initiation of therapy –

Treatment of menopausal symptoms: Start with the 0.05 mg system applied to the skin twice weekly. Adjust dose as necessary to control symptoms. Use the lowest dosage necessary to control symptoms, especially in women with an intact uterus. Make attempts to taper or discontinue the drug at 3 to 6 month intervals.

Prophylaxis to prevent postmenopausal bone loss: Initiate with 0.05 mg/day as soon as possible after menopause. Adjust dosage if necessary to control concurrent menopausal symptoms. Discontinuation may reestablish natural rate of bone loss.

In women who are not taking oral estrogens, start treatment immediately. In women who are currently taking oral estrogens, start treatment 1 week after withdrawal of oral therapy or sooner if symptoms reappear in < 1 week.

Therapeutic regimen – Therapy may be given continuously in patients who do not have an intact uterus. In patients with an intact uterus, therapy may be given on a cyclic schedule (eg, 3 weeks therapy followed by 1 week off).

Estraderm and *Vivelle* are applied twice a week; the *Climara* patch lasts for 7 days.

Application of system – Place adhesive side of the system on a clean, dry area on the trunk of the body (including the buttocks and abdomen). Do not apply to breasts. Rotate application site with an interval of at least 1 week between applications to a particular site. The area should not be oily, damaged or irritated. Avoid the waistline, since tight clothing may rub the system off. Apply the system immediately after opening pouch and removing protective liner. Press firmly in place with the palm for ≈10 seconds. Make sure there is good contact, especially around the edges. In the unlikely event that a system should fall off, the same system may be reapplied. If necessary, apply a new system. In either case, continue the original treatment schedule.

ESTRADIOL, ORAL:

Moderate to severe vasomotor symptoms, vulva/vaginal atrophy associated with menopause, female hypogonadism, female castration, primary ovarian failure – Initiate treatment with 1 or 2 mg/day; adjust to control presenting symptoms. Titrate to determine the minimal effective dose for maintenance therapy.

Prostatic cancer (androgen-dependent, inoperable, progressing) – Administer 1 to 2 mg 3 times daily. Judge the effectiveness of therapy by phosphatase determinations and by symptomatic improvement of the patient.

Breast cancer (inoperable, progressing) – Given chronically in appropriately selected men and women, the usual dose is 10 mg 3 times daily for at least 3 months.

Osteoporosis prevention – Administer cyclically (eg, 23 weeks on, 5 days off) 0.5 mg/day as soon as possible after menopause. Adjust dosage if necessary to control concurrent menopause symptoms. Discontinuation may reestablish natural rate of bone loss.

ESTRADIOL VALERATE IN OIL: Provides 2 to 3 weeks of estrogenic effect from a single IM injection.

For IM injection only.

Moderate to severe vasomotor symptoms, atrophic vaginitis or kraurosis vulvae associated with menopause, female hypogonadism, female castration or primary ovarian failure – 10 to 20 mg every 4 weeks.

Prostatic carcinoma – 30 mg or more every 1 or 2 weeks.

CONJUGATED ESTROGENS, ORAL: Administer cyclically (3 weeks of daily estrogen and 1 week off) for all indications except selected cases of carcinoma.

Moderate to severe vasomotor symptoms associated with menopause – 1.25 mg/day. If the patient has not menstruated in 2 months or more, administration is started arbitrarily. If the patient is menstruating, begin administration on day 5 of bleeding.

Atrophic vaginitis and kraurosis vulvae associated with menopause – 0.3 to 1.25 mg or more daily, depending on tissue response of the patient.

Female hypogonadism – 2.5 to 7.5 mg daily, in divided doses for 20 days, followed by a rest period of 10 days. If bleeding does not occur by the end of this period, repeat dosage schedule. The number of courses of estrogen therapy necessary to produce bleeding may vary, depending on the responsiveness of the endometrium.

If bleeding occurs before the end of the 10 day period, begin a 20 day estrogen-progestin cyclic regimen with estrogen, 2.5 to 7.5 mg daily in divided doses. During the last 5 days of estrogen therapy, give an oral progestin. If bleeding occurs before this regimen is concluded, discontinue therapy and resume on the fifth day of bleeding.

Female castration and primary ovarian failure – 1.25 mg/day. Adjust according to severity of symptoms and patient response. For maintenance, adjust to lowest effective level.

Osteoporosis – 0.625 mg/day, cyclically.

Mammary carcinoma (for palliation) – 10 mg 3 times daily for at least 3 months.

Prostatic carcinoma (for palliation) – 1.25 to 2.5 mg 3 times daily. Effectiveness can be judged by phosphatase determinations as well as by symptomatic improvement.

CONJUGATED ESTROGENS, PARENTERAL: Treatment of abnormal uterine bleeding due to hormonal imbalance in the absence of organic pathology. Administration IV produces a more rapid response and is preferred. Usual dose is one 25 mg injection IV or IM. Repeat in 6 to 12 hours if necessary. Inject slowly to obviate the occurrence of flushes.

Compatibility – Infusion of conjugated estrogens with other agents is not recommended. In emergencies, however, when an infusion has already been started, make the injection into the tubing just distal to the infusion needle. Solution is compatible with normal saline, dextrose and invert sugar solutions. It is not compatible with protein hydrolysate, ascorbic acid or any solution with an acid pH.

ESTERIFIED ESTROGENS:

Moderate to severe vasomotor symptoms, atrophic vaginitis or kraurosis vulvae associated with menopause – Cyclic therapy for short-term use. Average dose is 0.3 to 1.25 mg daily. Adjust dosage to the lowest effective level and discontinue as soon as possible.

Female hypogonadism – Administer 2.5 to 7.5 mg daily in divided doses for 20 days followed by a 10 day rest period. If bleeding does not occur by the end of this period, repeat the same dosage schedule. The number of courses of estrogen therapy necessary to produce bleeding varies, depending on endometrial responsiveness.

If bleeding occurs before the end of the 10 day period, begin a 20 day estrogen-progestin cyclic regimen of 2.5 to 7.5 mg daily in divided doses for 20 days. During the last 5 days of estrogen therapy, give an oral progestin. If bleeding occurs before this regimen is concluded, discontinue therapy; resume on the fifth day of bleeding.

Female castration and primary ovarian failure – Give 1.25 mg daily, cyclically.

Prostatic carcinoma (inoperable, progressing) – 1.25 to 2.5 mg 3 times a day. Judge the effectiveness of therapy by symptomatic response and phosphatase determinations.

Breast cancer (inoperable, progressing) – In appropriately selected men and postmenopausal women, give 10 mg 3 times a day for at least 3 months.

QUINESTROL:

Moderate to severe vasomotor symptoms associated with menopause, atrophic vaginitis, kraurosis vulvae, female hypogonadism, female castration and primary ovarian failure – Initially, 100 mcg daily for 7 days; follow with 100 mcg once weekly for maintenance starting 2 weeks after treatment begins. Increase dosage to 200 mcg per week if the therapeutic response is not desirable or optimal.

ESTROPIPATE (Piperazine Estrone Sulfate):

Moderate to severe vasomotor symptoms, atrophic vaginitis or kraurosis vulvae associated with menopause – Give cyclically for short-term use. The lowest dose and regimen that will control symptoms should be chosen. Usual dosage range is 0.625 to 5 mg/day.

Female hypogonadism, female castration or primary ovarian failure – Administer cyclically, 1.25 to 7.5 mg/day for the first 3 weeks, followed by a rest period of 8 to 10 days. Repeat if bleeding does not occur by the end of the rest period. The duration of therapy necessary to produce withdrawal bleeding will vary according to the responsiveness of the endometrium. If satisfactory withdrawal bleeding does not occur, give an oral progestin in addition to estrogen during the third week of the cycle.

Osteoporosis prevention – 0.625 mg daily for 25 days of a 31 day cycle per month.

ETHINYL ESTRADIOL:

Moderate to severe vasomotor symptoms associated with menopause – Usual dosage range is 0.02 to 0.5 mg/day. The effective dose may be as low as 0.02 mg every other day. Dosage schedule for early menopause, while spontaneous menstruation continues, is 0.05 mg once/day for 21 days followed by a 7 day rest period. May add a progestational agent during the latter part of the cycle.

For initial treatment of late menopause, the same regimen is indicated with 0.02 mg for the first few cycles, after which the 0.05 mg dosage may be substituted. In more severe cases, such as those due to surgical and roentgenologic castration, give 0.05 mg 3 times daily at the start of treatment. With adequate clinical improvement, usually obtainable in a few weeks, dosage may be reduced to 0.05 mg/day. A progestational agent may be added during the latter part of a planned cycle.

Female hypogonadism – 0.05 mg 1 to 3 times daily during the first 2 weeks of a theoretical menstrual cycle. Follow with a progestin during the last half of the arbitrary cycle. Continue for 3 to 6 months. The patient is then untreated for 2 months. Prescribe additional therapy if the cycle cannot be maintained without hormonal therapy.

Cancer of the female breast (inoperable, progressing) – In appropriately selected postmenopausal women, 1 mg 3 times daily given chronically for palliation.

Prostatic carcinoma (inoperable, progressing) – 0.15 to 2 mg/day given chronically for palliation.

DIETHYLSTILBESTROL (DES):

Prostatic carcinoma (inoperable, progressing) – Given chronically, the usual dosage is 1 to 3 mg/day initially, increased in advanced cases; dosage may later be reduced to an average of 1 mg/day.

Breast cancer (inoperable, progressing) – Given chronically in appropriately selected men and postmenopausal women, the usual dosage is 15 mg/day.

CHLOROTRIANISENE:

Moderate to severe vasomotor symptoms associated with menopause – 12 to 25 mg/day given cyclically for 30 days; one or more courses may be prescribed.

Atrophic vaginitis and kraurosis vulvae – 12 to 25 mg/day cyclically for 30 to 60 days.

Female hypogonadism – 12 to 25 mg/day given cyclically for 21 days. May be followed immediately by 100 mg progesterone IM or by an oral progestin during the last 5 days of therapy. Next course may begin on the fifth day of induced uterine bleeding.

Prostatic carcinoma (inoperable, progressing) – Given chronically, the usual dose is 12 to 25 mg/day.

ESTRADIOL CYPIONATE IN OIL:

Moderate to severe vasomotor symptoms associated with menopause – Usual dosage range is 1 to 5 mg IM, every 3 to 4 weeks.

Female hypogonadism – 1.5 to 2 mg IM at monthly intervals.

MISCELLANEOUS ESTROGENS, VAGINAL

Cream: 1.5 mg estropipate/g (Rx)	*Ogen* (Upjohn)
Cream: 0.1 mg estradiol/g (Rx)	*Estrace* (Bristol-Myers Squibb)
Cream: 0.625 mg conjugated estrogens/g (Rx)	*Premarin* (Wyeth-Ayerst)
Cream: 0.01% dienestrol (Rx)	*Ortho Dienestrol* (Ortho Pharm)

Actions:

Pharmacology: The signs and symptoms of vulvovaginal epithelial atrophy (atrophic vaginitis) may be alleviated by the topical application of an estrogenic hormone.

Indications:

Treatment of atrophic vaginitis and kraurosis vulvae associated with the menopause.

Warnings:

Vaginal bleeding: Since there is a possibility of absorption through the vaginal mucosa, uterine bleeding might be provoked by excessive administration in menopausal women. Cytologic study, endometrial assessment/sampling or D and C may be required to differentiate this uterine bleeding from carcinoma. Breast tenderness and vaginal discharge due to mucus hypersecretion may result from excessive estrogenic stimulation; endometrial withdrawal bleeding may occur if use is suddenly discontinued.

Administration and Dosage:

Treatment of atrophic vaginitis, kraurosis vulvae associated with menopause: Choose the lower dose that will control symptoms and discontinue medication as promptly as possible. Make attempts to discontinue or taper medication at 3 to 6 month intervals.

Estropipate and conjugated estrogens – Administer cyclically; 3 weeks on and 1 week off. Give ½ to 2 g daily of conjugated estrogens and 2 to 4 g daily of estropipate intravaginally depending on severity of condition.

Estradiol – 2 to 4 g daily for 2 weeks. Gradually reduce to one-half initial dosage for a similar period. A maintenance dose of 1 g 1 to 3 times a week may be used after restoration of the vaginal mucosa has been achieved.

Dienestrol – Usual dosage is 1 applicatorful once or twice daily for 1 or 2 weeks, then reduce to initial dosage for a similar period. A maintenance dosage of 1 applicatorful 1 to 3 times a week may be used after restoration of vaginal mucosa has been achieved.

PROGESTINS

HYDROXYPROGESTERONE IN OIL	
Injection: 125 and 250 mg/ml (Rx)	Various, *Hylutin* (Hyrex), *Hyprogest 250* (Keene)
MEDROXYPROGESTERONE	
Tablets: 2.5 mg, 5 mg (Rx)	*Cycrin* (ESI Pharma), *Provera* (Upjohn)
Tablets: 10 mg (Rx)	Various, *Amen* (Carnrick), *Curretab* (Solvay), *Provera* (Upjohn)
MEGESTROL ACETATE	
Suspension: 40 mg/ml (Rx)	*Megace* (Mead Johnson Oncology)
NORETHINDRONE ACETATE	
Tablets: 5 mg (Rx)	*Aygestin* (Wyeth-Ayerst)
PROGESTERONE IN OIL	
Injection: 50 mg/ml (Rx)	Various
PROGESTERONE POWDER	
Powder (Rx)	Various

Warning:

Pregnancy: Progestins have been used beginning with the first trimester of pregnancy to prevent habitual abortion or treat threatened abortion; however, there is no adequate evidence that such use is effective. There is evidence of potential harm to the fetus when given during the first 4 months of pregnancy. Therefore, the use of such drugs during the first 4 months of pregnancy is not recommended.

The cause of abortion is generally a defective ovum, which progestational agents could not be expected to influence. In addition, progestational agents have uterine relaxant properties that may cause a delay in spontaneous abortion when given to patients with fertilized defective ova.

Actions:

Pharmacology: Progesterone, a principle of corpus luteum, is the primary endogenous progestational substance. Progestins (progesterone and derivatives) transform proliferative endometrium into secretory endometrium. They inhibit (at the usual dose range) the secretion of pituitary gonadotropins, which in turn prevents follicular maturation and ovulation. They also inhibit spontaneous uterine contraction. Progestins may demonstrate some estrogenic, anabolic or androgenic activity. The precise mechanism by which megestrol produces effects in anorexia and cachexia is unknown.

Pharmacokinetics: Absorption of oral tablets and parenteral oily solutions of progestins is rapid; however, the hormone undergoes prompt hepatic transformation.

Indications:

Amenorrhea; abnormal uterine bleeding; endometriosis.

Megestrol: Treatment of anorexia, cachexia or an unexplained significant weight loss in patients with a diagnosis of acquired immunodeficiency syndrome (AIDS).

Palliative treatment of advanced carcinoma of the breast or endometrium.

Unlabeled uses: Medroxyprogesterone acetate (10 mg/day) has been used in the treatment of menopausal symptoms and to stimulate respiration in obstructive sleep apnea and other forms of chronic hypoventilation.

Adding progestin for ≥ 7 days of a cycle of estrogen replacement for menopause has lowered incidence of endometrial hyperplasia.

Progesterone suppositories (rectal or vaginal, 200 to 400 mg twice daily) have been used in premenstrual syndrome (PMS).

Progesterone has been used successfully in premature labor in late stages of pregnancy. Progesterone suppositories have been used during the luteal phase to the end of the first trimester to decrease spontaneous abortions in previous aborters and in ovulatory women receiving clomiphene citrate or human menopausal gonadotropins, and in luteal phase defects to improve fertility. However, see Warning Box.

Norethindrone (5 mg/day) appears to be effective in the treatment of hyperparathyroidism associated with mild hypercalcemia in postmenopausal women.

Contraindications:

Hypersensitivity to progestins; thrombophlebitis, thromboembolic disorders, cerebral hemorrhage or patients with a history of these conditions; impaired liver function or disease; carcinoma of the breast; undiagnosed vaginal bleeding; missed abortion; as a diagnostic test for pregnancy; known or suspected pregnancy; prophylactic use to avoid weight loss (megestrol).

Warnings:

Ophthalmologic effects: Discontinue medication pending examination if there is a sudden partial or complete loss of vision, or if there is sudden onset of proptosis, diplopia or migraine. If papilledema or retinal vascular lesions are present, discontinue use.

Thrombotic disorders (thrombophlebitis, cerebrovascular disorders, retinal thrombosis, pulmonary embolism) occasionally occur in patients taking progestins.

Pregnancy: Use is not recommended. See Warning Box.

Lactation: Detectable amounts of progestins enter the milk of mothers receiving these agents. The effect on the nursing infant has not been determined.

Medroxyprogesterone does not adversely affect lactation and may increase milk production and duration of lactation if given in the puerperium.

Precautions:

Causes of weight loss: Institute therapy with megestrol for weight loss only after treatable causes of weight loss are sought and addressed.

Respiratory infections: Long-term treatment may increase the risk of respiratory infections.

Pretreatment physical examination should include breasts and pelvic organs, as well as Papanicolaou smear.

Fluid retention may occur; therefore, conditions influenced by this factor (epilepsy, migraine, asthma, cardiac or renal dysfunction) require careful observation.

Depression: Observe patients who have a history of psychic depression and discontinue the drug if the depression recurs to a serious degree.

Menopause: The age of the patient constitutes no absolute limiting factor, although treatment with progestins may mask the onset of the climacteric.

Photosensitivity: Photosensitization (photoallergy or phototoxicity) may occur.

Drug Interactions:

Drugs that may interact with progestins include aminoglutethimide and rifampin.

Drug/Lab test interactions: Laboratory test results of **hepatic function**, coagulation tests (increase in prothrombin, Factors VII, VIII, IX and X), thyroid, metyrapone test and **endocrine functions**, may be affected by progestins or estrogens. A decrease in **glucose tolerance** has been observed in a small percentage of patients on estrogen-progestin combination drugs. **Pregnanediol** determination may be altered by the use of progestins.

Adverse Reactions:

Adverse reactions that may occur include breakthrough bleeding, spotting, change in menstrual flow, amenorrhea, changes in cervical erosion and cervical secretions; breast changes (tenderness), masculinization of the female fetus, edema, changes in weight (increase or decrease), cholestatic jaundice, rash (allergic) with and without pruritus, acne, melasma or chloasma, mental depression; alopecia, hirsutism, thromboembolic phenomena including thrombophlebitis and pulmonary embolism, sensitivity reactions ranging from pruritus and urticaria to generalized rash (medroxyprogesterone acetate).

For information concerning adverse reactions associated with combined estrogen-progestin therapy, refer to the Oral Contraceptives monograph.

Megestrol: Adverse reactions occuring in ≥ 3% of patients include: diarrhea; impotence; rash; flatulence; hypertenison; asthenia; insomnia; nausea; anemia; fever; libido decreased; hyperglycemia; headache.

Administration and Dosage:

HYDROXYPROGESTERONE IN OIL: For IM use.

Amenorrhea (primary and secondary); dysfunctional uterine bleeding; metrorrhagia – Usual adult dose: 375 mg.

Production of secretory endometrium and desquamation – Test for continuous endogenous estrogen production (Medical D and C). Usual adult dose 125 to 250 mg given on tenth day of cycle; repeat every 7 days until suppression is no longer desired.

MEDROXYPROGESTERONE ACETATE: For information on parenteral medroxyprogesterone acetate, refer to monograph in Antineoplastic section.

The duration of action of medroxyprogesterone is prolonged and variable.

Secondary amenorrhea – 5 to 10 mg daily for 5 to 10 days. A dose for inducing an optimum secretory transformation of an endometrium that has been adequately primed with either endogenous or exogenous estrogen is 10 mg daily for 10 days. Start therapy any time. Withdrawal bleeding usually occurs 3 to 7 days after therapy ends.

Abnormal uterine bleeding due to hormonal imbalance in the absence of organic pathology – 5 to 10 mg daily for 5 to 10 days, beginning on the 16th or 21st day of the menstrual cycle. To produce an optimum secretory transformation of an endometrium that has been adequately primed with either endogenous or exogenous estrogen, give 10 mg daily for 10 days, beginning on the 16th day of the cycle. Withdrawal bleeding usually occurs 3 to 7 days after discontinuing therapy. Patients with recurrent episodes of abnormal uterine bleeding may benefit from planned menstrual cycling with medroxyprogesterone acetate.

MEGESTROL ACETATE: Initial dose is 800 mg/day (20 ml/day); daily doses of 400 and 800 mg/day were found to be clinically effective. Shake container well before using.

NORETHINDRONE ACETATE: Norethindrone acetate differs from norethindrone only in potency; the acetate is approximately twice as potent.

Amenorrhea; abnormal uterine bleeding due to hormonal imbalance in the absence of organic pathology – 2.5 to 10 mg starting with day 5 of the menstrual cycle and ending on the 25th day.

Endometriosis –

Initial dose: 5 mg/day for 2 weeks; increase in increments of 2.5 mg/day every 2 weeks until 15 mg/day is reached. Therapy may be held at this level for 6 to 9 months or until breakthrough bleeding demands temporary termination.

PROGESTERONE: For IM use. The drug is irritating at the injection site.

Amenorrhea – Administer 5 to 10 mg daily for 6 to 8 consecutive days. If ovarian activity has produced a proliferative endometrium, expect withdrawal bleeding 48 to 72 hours after the last injection. Spontaneous normal cycles may follow.

Functional uterine bleeding – Administer 5 to 10 mg daily for 6 doses. Bleeding should cease within 6 days. When estrogen is also given, begin progesterone after 2 weeks of estrogen therapy. Discontinue injections when menstrual flow begins.

Progesterone is available as a micronized powder for prescription compounding.

ORAL CONTRACEPTIVES

MONOPHASIC ORAL CONTRACEPTIVES	
Tablets: Estrogens (ethinyl estradiol, mestranol), progestins (desogestrel, ethynodiol diacetate, levonorgestrel, norethindrone, norethindrone acetate, norgestimate, norgestrel) (*Rx*)	*Brevicon* (Syntex), *Demulen* (Searle), *Desogen* (Organon), *Genora* (Rugby), *Levlen* (Berlex), *Loestrin* (Parke-Davis), *Lo/Ovral* (Wyeth Ayerst), *Modicon* (Ortho), *Nelova* (Warner Chilcott), *Nordette* (Wyeth-Ayerst), *Norethin* (Roberts), *Norinyl* (Syntex), *Ortho-Cept*, *Ortho-Cyclen*, *Ortho-Novum* (Ortho), *Ovcon* (Mead Johnson), *Zovia* (Watson)
BIPHASIC ORAL CONTRACEPIVES	
Tablets: Estrogen (ethinyl estradiol), progestin (norethindrone) (*Rx*)	*Jenest-28* (Organon), *Nelova 10/11* (Warner Chilcott), *Ortho-Novum 10/11* (Ortho)
TRIPHASIC ORAL CONTRACEPTIVES	
Tablets: Estrogen (ethinyl estradiol), progestin (levonorgestrel, norethindrone, norgestimate) (*Rx*)	*Ortho-Novum 777*, *Ortho Tri-Cyclen* (Ortho), *Tri-Levlen* (Berlex), *Tri-Norinyl* (Syntex), *Triphasil* (Wyeth-Ayerst)
PROGESTIN-ONLY PRODUCTS	
Tablets: Norethindrone 0.35 mg (*Rx*)	*Micronor* (Ortho), *Nor-Q.D.* (Syntex)
Tablets: Norgestrel 0.075 mg (*Rx*)	*Ovrette* (Wyeth-Ayerst)

Actions:

Pharmacology: Oral contraceptives (OCs) include estrogen-progestin combos and progestin-only products.

Progestin-only – The mechanism by which progestin-only contraceptives prevent conception is not completely known, but they alter the cervical mucus, exert a progestational effect on the endometrium, apparently producing cellular changes that renders the endometrium hostile to implantation by a fertilized ovum (egg) and, in some patients, suppress ovulation.

Combination OCs inhibit ovulation by suppressing the gonadotropins, follicle-stimulating hormone (FSH) and luteinizing hormone (LH). Additionally, alterations in the genital tract, including cervical mucus (which inhibits sperm penetration) and the endometrium (which reduces the likelihood of implantation), may contribute to contraceptive effectiveness.

Contraceptive efficacy –

Pregnancy Rates for Various Means of Contraception (%)[1]

Method of contraception	Lowest expected[2]	Typical[3]
Oral Contraceptives		3
Combined	0.1	nd
Progestin-only	0.5	nd
Mechanical/Chemical		
Levonorgestrel implant	0.2	0.2
Medroxyprogesterone injection	0.3	0.3
IUD		
Progesterone	2	nd
Copper T 380A	0.8	nd
Condom		
Without spermicide	2	12
With spermicide[4]	1.8	4-6
Spermicide alone	3	21
Diaphragm (with spermicidal cream or gel)	6	18
Vaginal sponge		
Nulliparous	6	18
Multiparous	9	28
Female condom	2-4	12-25
Periodic abstinence (ie, rhythm; all methods)	1-9	20

Pregnancy Rates for Various Means of Contraception (%)[1]		
Method of contraception	Lowest expected[2]	Typical[3]
Sterility		
Vasectomy	0.1	0.15
Tubal ligation	0.2	0.4
No contraception	85	85

[1] nd = No data.During first year of continuous use.
[2] Best guess of percentage expected to experience an accidental pregnancy among couples who initiate a method and use it consistently and correctly.
[3] A "typical" couple who initiate a method and experience an accidental pregnancy.
[4] Used as a separate product (not in condom package).

There are three types of combination OCs: Monophasic, biphasic and triphasic. The biphasic and triphasic OCs are intended to deliver hormones in a fashion similar to physiologic processes.

Monophasic – Fixed dosage of estrogen to progestin throughout the cycle.

Biphasic – Amount of estrogen remains the same for the first 21 days of the cycle. Decreased progestin:estrogen ratio in first half of cycle allows endometrial proliferation. Increased ratio in second half provides adequate secretory development.

Triphasic – Estrogen amount remains the same or varies throughout cycle. Progestin amount varies.

Pharmacokinetics:

Estrogens – Ethinyl estradiol is rapidly absorbed with peak concentrations attained in 1 to 2 hours. It undergoes considerable first-pass elimination. Mestranol is demethylated to ethinyl estradiol. Ethinyl estradiol is approximately 98% bound to plasma albumin. Half-life varies from 6 to 20 hours. It is excreted in bile and urine as conjugates, and undergoes some enterohepatic recirculation.

Progestins – Peak concentrations of norethindrone occur 0.5 to 4 hours after oral administration; it undergoes first-pass metabolism with an overall bioavailability around 65%. Levonorgestrel reaches peak concentrations between 0.5 to 2 hours, does not undergo a first-pass effect and is completely bioavailable. Desogestrel is rapidly and completely absorbed and converted into 3–keto-desogestrel, the biologically active metabolite. Relative bioavailability is ≈ 84%. Maximum concentrations of the metabolite are reached at 1.4 ± 0.8 hours. Norgestimate is well absorbed; peak serum concentrations are observed within 2 hours followed by a rapid decline to levels generally below assay within 5 hours. However, a major metabolite, 17–deacetyl norgestimate, appears rapidly in serum with concentrations greatly exceeding that of the parent. Both norethynodrel and ethynodiol diacetate are converted to norethindrone. Terminal half-life of the progestins are as follows: Norethindrone, 5 to 14 hours; levonorgestrel, 11 to 45 hours; desogestrel (metabolite), 38 ± 20 hours; norgestimate (metabolite), 12 to 30 hours.

Indications:

Contraceptive: For the prevention of pregnancy. Start new patients on preparations containing ≤ 35 mcg estrogen.

Unlabeled uses: Ovral (50 mcg ethinyl estradiol and 0.5 mg norgestrel) in high doses has been used successfully as a postcoital contraceptive or "morning after" pill. Patients are given 2 tablets within 72 hours of unprotected intercourse at the initial visit and 2 tablets 12 hours later.

Contraindications:

Thrombophlebitis; thromboembolic disorders; history of deep-vein thrombophlebitis; cerebral vascular disease; myocardial infarction; coronary artery disease; known or suspected breast carcinoma or estrogen-dependent neoplasia; carcinoma of endometrium or other; hepatic adenomas/carcinomas; past or present angina pectoris; undiagnosed abnormal genital bleeding; known or suspected pregnancy; cholestatic jaundice of pregnancy/jaundice with prior pill use.

Warnings:

> *Cigarette smoking* increases the risk of cardiovascular side effects from OCs. This risk increases with age and with heavy smoking (≥ 15 cigarettes per day) and is quite marked in women > 35 years of age. Women who use OCs should not smoke.

Risks of OC use: The use of OCs is associated with increased risk of thromboembolism, stroke, MI, hepatic neoplasia and gallbladder disease, although risk of serious morbidity or mortality is very small in healthy women without underlying risk factors.

Mortality associated with all methods of birth control is low and below that associated with childbirth, with the exception of OC use in women ≥ 35 who smoke and ≥ 40 who do not smoke. However, the Fertility and Maternal Health Drugs Advisory Committee recommended that the benefits of low-dose OC use by healthy nonsmoking women > 40 years of age may outweigh the possible risks.

Thromboembolic and cardiovascular problems: Risk of thromboembolism, including coronary thrombosis, appears to be directly related to estrogen dose used; however, estrogen quantity may not be the sole factor involved.

Myocardial infarction (MI) risk associated with OC use is increased. The highest risk group includes women 40 to 49 years old who used OCs for ≥ 5 years.

Smoking – OC users who also smoke have about a fivefold increased risk of fatal infarction compared to nonsmoking users, but a 10- to 12-fold increased risk compared to nonusers who do not smoke.

Cerebrovascular diseases – OCs increase the risks of cerebrovascular events (thrombotic and hemorrhagic strokes), although, in general, the risk is greatest in hypertensive women > 35 years of age who also smoke.

Vascular disease – A positive association is observed between the amount of estrogen and progestin in OCs and the risk of vascular disease. A decline in serum high density lipoproteins (HDL) has occurred with progestins. Because estrogens increase HDL cholesterol, the net effect depends on a balance achieved between doses of estrogen and progestin and the androgenic activity of the progestin.

Age – The risk of cerebrovascular and circulatory disease in OC users is substantially increased in women ≥ 35 years of age with other risk factors (eg, smoking, uncontrolled hypertension, hypercholesterolemia [LDL 190], obesity, diabetes).

Postsurgical thromboembolism risk is increased 2– to 4-fold. If possible, discontinue OCs at least 2 to 4 weeks before and 2 weeks after surgery as OCs are associated with an increased risk of thromboembolism.

Subarachnoid hemorrhage has been increased by OC use.

Persistence of risk – An increased risk may persist for at least 6 years after discontinuation of OC use for cerebrovascular disease and at least 9 years for MI in users 40 to 49 years of age who had used OCs ≥ 5 years.

Ocular lesions such as optic neuritis or retinal thrombosis have been associated with the use of OCs.

Carcinoma: While there are conflicting reports, the overall evidence in the literature suggests that use of OCs is not associated with an increase in the risk of developing any cancer, regardless of age and parity of first use.

Hepatic lesions (adenomas, focal nodular hyperplasia, hepatocellular carcinoma, etc): Benign and malignant hepatic adenomas have been associated with the use of OCs. Severe abdominal pain, shock or death may be due to rupture and hemorrhage of a liver tumor.

Pregnancy test: Do not administer progestin-only products or progestin-estrogen combinations to induce withdrawal bleeding as a test for pregnancy.

Carbohydrate metabolism: Glucose tolerance may decrease, which is directly related to estrogen dose.

Lipid profile: Triglycerides may increase. Some progestins decrease HDL, while some estrogens increase HDL.

Elevated blood pressure and hypertension may occur within a few months of beginning use.

Headaches: Onset or exacerbation of migraine or development of headache of a new pattern which is recurrent, persistent or severe, requires OC discontinuation and evaluation.

Bleeding irregularities: Breakthrough bleeding (BTB), spotting and amenorrhea are frequent reasons for discontinuing OCs. Progestin-only products are more likely to cause an alteration in menstrual patterns.

Menopause: Treatment with OCs may mask the onset of the climacteric.

Fertility impairment may occur in women discontinuing OCs; however, impairment diminishes with time.

Pregnancy: Category X. Rule out pregnancy before initiating or continuing the OCs, and always consider it if withdrawal bleeding does not occur.

Lactation: Oral contraceptives may interfere with lactation, decreasing both the quantity and the quality of breast milk. Furthermore, a small fraction of the hormones in OCs are excreted in breast milk. A few adverse effects on the nursing infant have been reported, including jaundice and breast enlargement.

Precautions:

Monitoring: Pretreatment and periodic exams should include blood pressure, breasts, abdomen and pelvic organs, including Papanicolaou smear.

Uterine fibroids: Preexisting uterine leiomyomata (uterine fibroids) may increase in size. However, there is no evidence of this with low-dose OCs.

Pyridoxine deficiency: OC users may have relative pyridoxine deficiency.

Depression: The incidence of depression in OC users ranges from < 5% to 30%. Pyridoxine deficiency may be a factor in the depression.

Fluid retention: OCs may cause fluid retention.

Hepatic function: Patients with a history of jaundice during pregnancy have an increased risk of recurrence of jaundice.

Serum folate levels may be depressed by therapy.

Acute intermittent porphyria: Estrogens have been reported to precipitate attacks of acute intermittent porphyria.

Vomiting/Diarrhea: Several cases of OC failure have been reported in association with vomiting or diarrhea. If significant GI disturbance occurs, a back-up method of contraception for the remainder of the cycle is recommended.

Sexually transmitted diseases (STDs): Advise patients that OCs do not protect against HIV infection and other STDs.

Photosensitivity: Photosensitization (photoallergy or phototoxicity) may occur.

Drug Interactions:

Drugs that may affect oral contraceptives include antibiotics, barbiturates, hydantoins and rifampin. Drugs that may be affected by oral contraceptives include acetaminophen, anticoagulants, benzodiazepines, beta blockers, caffeine, clofibrate, corticosteroids, salicylates, theophyllines and tricyclic antidepressants.

Drug/Lab test interactions: Estrogen-containing OCs may cause the following alterations in serum, plasma or blood, unless specified otherwise.

Increased – Sulfobromophthalein retention; factors I (prothrombin), VII, VIII, IX, X; decreased tissue plasminogen, fibrinogen; norepinephrine-induced platelet aggregation; thyroid binding globulin (TBG), leading to increased total thyroid hormone (as measured by protein bound iodine or T_4 by column or radioimmunoassay); transcortin; corticosteroid levels; triglycerides and phospholipids; ceruloplasmin; aldosterone; amylase; gamma-glutamyltranspeptidase; iron binding capacity; transferrin; prolactin; renin activity; vitamin A.

Decreased – Antithrombin III; free T_3 resin uptake; response to metyrapone test; folate; glucose tolerance; albumin; cholinesterase; haptoglobin; zinc; vitamin B_{12}.

Adverse Reactions:

Serious adverse reactions that may occur include: Thrombophlebitis and venous thrombosis with or without embolism; pulmonary embolism; coronary thrombosis; MI; cerebral thrombosis; arterial thromboembolism; cerebral hemorrhage; hypertension; gallbladder disease; hepatic adenomas or benign liver tumors; hepatocellular carcinoma; mesenteric thrombosis; Budd-Chiari syndrome. Other adverse reactions that may occur include: Nausea and vomiting (10% to 30% of patients during the first cycle, less common with low doses, and majority resolve in 3 months); abdominal cramps; bloating; breakthrough bleeding (majority, > 80%, resolve in 3 months); spotting; change in menstrual flow; amenorrhea during and after treatment; change in cervical erosion and cervical secretions; vaginal candidiasis; breast changes; melasma; rash (allergic); migraine; mental depression; contact lens intolerance; edema; weight change (increase or decrease).

Administration and Dosage:

Product choice: Only low-dose pills should be routinely used now; there is rarely a need for 50 mcg estrogen component tablets.

Sunday-Start packaging: If the instructions recommend starting the regimen on Sunday, take the first tablet on the first Sunday after menstruation begins. If menstruation begins on Sunday, take the first tablet on that day.

21-Day regimen: Day 1 of the cycle is the first day of menstrual bleeding. Take 1 tablet daily for 21 days, beginning on day 5 of cycle. No tablets are taken for 7 days; whether bleeding has stopped or not, start a new course of 21 days.

28-Day regimen: To eliminate the need to count the days between cycles, some products contain 7 inert or iron-containing tablets to permit continuous daily dosage during the entire 28-day cycle. Take the 7 tablets on the last 7 days of the cycle.

Biphasic and triphasic OCs: Follow instructions on the dispensers or packs. As with the monophasic OCs, 1 tablet is taken each day; however, as the color of the tablet changes, the strength of the tablet also changes (ie, the estrogen/progestin ratio varies).

Missed dose:

One tablet – Take it as soon as remembered, or take 2 tablets the next day; alternatively take 1 tablet, discard the other missed tablet, continue as scheduled and use another form of contraception for the 7 days after the pills missed, preferably for the remainder of the cycle..

Two consecutive tablets – Take 2 tablets as soon as remembered with the next pill at the usual time, or take 2 tablets daily for the next 2 days, then resume the regular schedule. Use an additional form of contraception for the 7 days after pills are missed, preferably for the remainder of the cycle.

Three consecutive tablets – Begin a new compact of tablets, starting on day one of the cycle after the last pill was taken or starting 7 days after the last tablet was taken.

Postpartum administration in non-nursing mothers may begin at the first postpartum examination (4 to 6 weeks), regardless of whether spontaneous menstruation has occurred. Also, start no earlier than 4 to 6 weeks after a midtrimester pregnancy termination.

Dosage adjustments:

Achieving Proper Hormonal Balance In An Oral Contraceptive			
Estrogen		Progestin	
Excess	Deficiency	Excess	Deficiency
Nausea, bloating Cervical mucorrhea, polyposis Melasma Hypertension Migraine headache Breast fullness or tenderness Edema	Early or midcycle breakthrough bleeding Increased spotting Hypomenorrhea	Increased appetite Weight gain Tiredness, fatigue Hypomenorrhea Acne, oily scalp[1] Hair loss, hirsutism[1] Depression Monilial vaginitis Breast regression	Late breakthrough bleeding Amenorrhea Hypermenorrhea

[1] Result of androgenic activity of progestins.

Pharmacological Effects of Progestins Used in Oral Contraceptives[1]				
	Progestin	Estrogen	Antiestrogen	Androgen
Norgestrel/levonorgestrel	+++	0	++	+++
Desogestrel	+++	0/+	+++	0/+
Norgestimate	+++	0	+++	0
Ethynodiol diacetate	++	+[2]	+[2]	++
Norethindrone acetate	+	+	+++	++
Norethindrone	+	+[2]	+[2]	++
Norethynodrel	+	+++	0	0

[1] *Symbol Key:* *+++ pronounced effect* *++ moderate effect* *+ slight effect* *0 no effect*
[2] Has estrogenic effect at low doses; may have antiestrogenic effect at higher doses.

Progestin-only products: Administer daily, starting on the first day of menstruation. Take one tablet at the same time each day, every day of the year.

Postpartum administration – May be initiated no earlier than 4 weeks postpartum.

Missed dose –

One tablet: Because of the slightly higher failure rate of the progestin-only products, a more conservative approach is to discontinue the regimen if only 1 tablet is missed and use other nonhormonal contraceptive methods until menses occurs or pregnancy is ruled out.

Two consecutive tablets: Do not take the missed tablets; discard and take the next tablet at the regular time (*Micronor* and *Nor-Q.D.*), or take 1 of the missed tablets, discard the other and take daily tablet at usual time (*Ovrette*).

Three consecutive tablets: Discontinue immediately.

LEVONORGESTREL IMPLANTS

Kit: 6 capsules (each contains 36 mg levonorgestrel) (*Rx*) — *Norplant System* (Wyeth-Ayerst)

Actions:

Pharmacology: Diffusion of levonorgestrel through the wall of each capsule provides a continuous low dose of the progestin. Because of the range of variability in blood levels and variation in individual response, blood levels alone are not predictive of the risk of pregnancy in an individual woman.

Pharmacokinetics: Levonorgestrel concentrations among women show considerable variation. They reach a maximum, or near maximum, within 24 hours after placement with mean values of 1600 pg/ml. Levels decline rapidly over the first month partially due to a circulating protein, SHBG, that binds levonorgestrel and is depressed by the presence of levonorgestrel. Mean levels decline to values of around 400 pg/ml at 3 months to 258 pg/ml at 60 months.

Concentrations decreased with increasing body weight by a mean of 3.3 pg/ml/kg. After capsule removal, mean concentrations drop to < 100 pg/ml by 96 hours and to below assay sensitivity (50 pg/ml) by 5 to 14 days. Fertility rates return to levels comparable to those seen in the general population of women using no method of contraception. Circulating concentrations can be used to forecast the risk of pregnancy only in a general statistical sense. Mean concentrations associated with pregnancy have been 210 ± 60 pg/ml.

Contraceptive efficacy – Lowest expected failure rate during the first year of use is < 1.

Indications:

Prevention of pregnancy: The implant system is a long-term (up to 5 years) reversible contraceptive system. Remove the capsules by the end of the 5th year; new capsules may be inserted at that time if continuing contraceptive protection is desired.

Contraindications:

Active thrombophlebitis or thromboembolic disorders; undiagnosed abnormal genital bleeding; known or suspected pregnancy; acute liver disease; benign or malignant liver tumors; known or suspected carcinoma of the breast.

Warnings:

Bleeding irregularities: Most women can expect some variation in menstrual bleeding patterns. Irregular menstrual bleeding, intermenstrual spotting, prolonged episodes of bleeding and spotting, and amenorrhea occur in some women. Overall, these irregularities diminish with continuing use. Since some users experience periods of amenorrhea, missed menstrual periods cannot serve as the only means of identifying early pregnancy. Perform pregnancy tests whenever a pregnancy is suspected. After a pattern of regular menses, ≥ 6 weeks of amenorrhea may signal pregnancy. If pregnancy occurs, the capsules must be removed.

Delayed follicular atresia: If follicular development occurs, atresia of the follicle is sometimes delayed and the follicle may continue to grow beyond the size it would attain in a normal cycle. These enlarged follicles cannot be distinguished clinically from ovarian cysts. In the majority of women, enlarged follicles will spontaneously disappear and should not require surgery. Rarely, they may twist or rupture, sometimes causing abdominal pain; surgical intervention may be required.

Ectopic pregnancies have occurred among levonorgestrel implant users. The risk of ectopic pregnancy may increase with the duration of use and, possibly, with increased weight of the user. Any patient who presents with lower abdominal pain must be evaluated to rule out ectopic pregnancy.

Ocular lesions: Although it is believed that this reaction is related to the estrogen component of oral contraceptives, remove capsules if there is unexplained partial or complete vision loss, onset of proptosis or diplopia, papilledema or retinal vascular lesions. Undertake appropriate diagnostic and therapeutic measures immediately.

Foreign body carcinogenesis: Rarely, cancers have occurred at the site of foreign body intrusions or old scars. Because of the resistance of human beings to these cancers and because of the small size of the capsules, the risk to users is judged to be minimal.

Thromboembolic disorders: Patients who develop active thrombophlebitis or thromboembolic disease should have the levonorgestrel capsules removed. Also consider removal in women who will be immobilized for a prolonged period due to surgery or other illnesses.

Lactation: Levonorgestrel has been identified in breast milk. No significant effects were observed on growth or health of infants whose mothers used implants beginning 6 weeks after parturition compared with mothers using IUDs or barrier methods.

Precautions:

Physical examination and follow-up: Take a complete medical history and physical examination prior to the implantation or re-implantation of levonorestrel implants and at least annually during its use. Carefully monitor women with a strong family history of breast cancer or who have breast nodules.

Carbohydrate and lipid metabolism: Effects of implants on carbohydrate metabolism appear to be minimal. Carefully observe diabetic and prediabetic patients.

Closely follow women who are being treated for hyperlipidemias.

Liver function: If jaundice develops consider removing the capsules.

Fluid retention: Prescribe with caution, and only with careful monitoring, in patients with conditions which might be aggravated by fluid retention.

Emotional disorders: Consider removing the capsules in women who become significantly depressed since the symptom may be drug-related. Carefully observe women with a history of depression and consider removal if depression recurs to a serious degree.

Contact lens wearers who develop changes in vision or in lens tolerance should be assessed by an ophthalmologist.

Insertion and removal: To be sure that the woman is not pregnant at the time of capsule placement and to assure contraceptive efficacy during the first cycle of use, insert capsules during the first 7 days of the cycle or immediately after an abortion. Insertion is not recommended before 6 weeks postpartum in breastfeeding women.

Expulsion of capsules is uncommon. It occurs more frequently when placement of the capsules is extremely shallow, too close to the incision, or when infection is present. Replacement of an expelled capsule must be accomplished using a new sterile capsule. If infection is present, treat and cure before replacement. Contraceptive efficacy may be inadequate with < 6 capsules.

Provisions for removal: Advise women that the capsules will be removed at any time for any reason. The removal should be done on such request or at the end of 5 years of usage by personnel instructed in the removal technique.

Drug Interactions:

Carbamazepine and phenytoin: Reduced efficacy (pregnancy) has occurred. Warn users of the possibility of decreased efficacy with use of any related drugs.

Drug/Lab test interactions: Certain endocrine tests may be affected by levonorgestrel implants: Sex hormone binding globulin concentrations are decreased; thyroxine concentrations may be slightly decreased and triiodothyronine uptake increased.

Adverse Reactions:

Adverse reactions occuring in ≥ 3% of patients include prolonged bleeding; spotting; amenorrhea; irregular bleeding; frequent bleeding onsets; removal difficulties affecting patients; scanty bleeding; breast discharge; cervicitis; musculoskeletal pain; abdominal discomfort; leukorrhea; vaginitis; pain or itching near implant site.

Administration and Dosage:

Levonorgestrel implants consist of six *Silastic* capsules; each capsule is 2.4 mm in diameter and 34 mm in length and contains 36 mg levonorgestrel. Total administered (implanted) dose is 216 mg. Perform implantation of all six capsules during the first 7 days of menses onset. The initial dose is ≈ 85 mcg/day, followed by a decline to ≈ 50 mcg/day by 9 months, and to ≈ 35 mcg/day by 18 months, with a further decline thereafter to ≈ 30 mcg/day. Insertion is subdermal in the mid-portion of the upper arm (see literature included with the product.)

MEDROXYPROGESTERONE ACETATE

Injection (Rx)	*Depo-Provera* (Upjohn)

Actions:

Pharmacology: Medroxyprogesterone, when administered IM at the recommended dose to women every 3 months, inhibits the secretion of gonadotropins which, in turn, prevents follicular maturation and ovulation and results in endometrial thinning. These actions produce its contraceptive effect.

Pharmacokinetics: Following a single 150 mg IM dose, medroxyprogesterone concentrations increase for ≈ 3 weeks to reach peak plasma concentrations of 1 to 7 ng/ml. The levels then decrease exponentially until they become undetectable (< 100 pg/ml) between 120 to 200 days following injection. The apparent half-life following IM administration is ≈ 50 days.

Indications:

Prevention of pregnancy. It is a long-term injectable contraceptive in women when administered at 3 month intervals.

Contraindications:

Known or suspected pregnancy or as a diagnostic test for pregnancy; undiagnosed vaginal bleeding; known or suspected malignancy of breast; active thrombophlebitis, or current or past history of thromboembolic disorders, or cerebral vascular disease; liver dysfunction or disease; hypersensitivity to medroxyprogesterone or any of its other ingredients.

Warnings:

Bleeding irregularities: Most women using medroxyprogesterone experience disruption of menstrual bleeding patterns. If abnormal bleeding persists or is severe, institute appropriate investigation to rule out the possibility of organic pathology, and institute appropriate treatment when necessary.

As women continue using medroxyprogesterone, fewer experience intermenstrual bleeding and more experience amenorrhea.

Bone mineral density changes: Use of medroxyprogesterone may be considered among the risk factors for development of osteoporosis. The rate of bone loss is greatest in the early years of use and then subsequently approaches the normal rate of age-related fall.

Thromboembolic disorders: Be alert to the earliest manifestations of thrombotic disorders. If any of these occur or are suspected, do not readminister the drug.

Ocular disorders: Do not readminister pending examination if there is a sudden partial or complete loss of vision or if there is a sudden onset of proptosis, diplopia or migraine. If examination reveals papilledema or retinal vascular lesions, do not readminister.

Carcinogenesis: Long-term case-controlled surveillance of users found slight or no increased overall risk of breast cancer and no overall increased risk of ovarian, liver or cervical cancer and a prolonged, protective effect of reducing the risk of endometrial cancer in the population of users.

Pregnancy: Category X.

Lactation: Detectable amounts of the drug have been identified in the milk of mothers receiving medroxyprogesterone. In nursing mothers treated with medroxyprogesterone, milk composition, quality and amount are not adversely affected. Infants exposed to medroxyprogesterone via breast milk have been studied for developmental and behavioral effects through puberty; no adverse effects have been noted.

Precautions:

Physical examination: The pretreatment and annual history and physical examination should include special reference to breast and pelvic organs, as well as a Papanicolaou smear.

Fluid retention: Because progestational drugs may cause some degree of fluid retention, conditions that might be influenced by this condition require careful observation.

Weight changes: There is a tendency for women to gain weight while on medroxyprogesterone therapy.

Return of fertility: Medroxyprogesterone has a prolonged contraceptive effect. It is expected that 68% of women who do become pregnant may conceive within 12 months, 83% may conceive within 15 months and 93% may conceive within 18 months from the last injection.

CNS disorders and convulsions: Carefully observe patients who have a history of psychic depression; do not readminister if the depression recurs.

There have been a few reported cases of convulsions. Association with drug use or preexisting conditions is not clear.

Carbohydrate metabolism: A decrease in glucose tolerance has been observed in some patients. Carefully observe diabetic patients during therapy.

Liver function: If jaundice develops, consider not readministering the drug.

Drug Interactions:

Drugs that may interact with medroxyprogesterone include aminoglutethimide.

Drug/Lab test interactions: The following laboratory tests may be affected by medroxyprogesterone: Plasma and urinary steroid levels are decreased; gonadotropin levels are decreased; sex-hormone binding globulin concentrations are decreased; protein bound iodine and butanol extractable protein bound iodine may increase; T_3 uptake values may decrease; coagulation test values for prothrombin (Factor II), and Factors VII, VIII, IX, and X may increase. Sulfobromophthalein and other liver function test values may be increased; the effects of medroxyprogesterone acetate on lipid metabolism are inconsistent. Both increases and decreases in total cholesterol, triglycerides, low-density lipoprotein (LDL) cholesterol, and high-density lipoprotein (HDL) cholesterol have been observed.

Adverse Reactions:

Common (> 3%) adverse reactions include: Menstrual irregularities; weight changes; headache; nervousness; abdominal pain; discomfort; asthenia; dizziness.

Administration and Dosage:

Shake the vial vigorously just before use to ensure that the dose being administered represents a uniform suspension.

The recommended dose is 150 mg every 3 months administered by deep IM injection in the gluteal or deltoid muscle. To increase assurance that the patient is not pregnant at the time of the first administration, give this injection only during the first 5 days after the onset of a normal menstrual period; within 5 days postpartum if not breastfeeding; or, if breastfeeding, at 6 weeks postpartum. If the period between injections is > 14 weeks, determine that the patient is not pregnant before administering the drug.

ANDROGENS

FLUOXYMESTERONE	
Tablets: 2 mg, 5 mg (*c-iii*)	*Halotestin 1* ,(Upjohn)
Tablets: 10 mg (*c-iii*)	Various, *Halotestin* (Upjohn)
METHYLTESTOSTERONE	
Tablets: 10 mg (*c-iii*)	Various, *Android-10* (ICN), *Oreton Methyl* (Schering)
Tablets: 25 mg (*c-iii*)	Various, *Android-25* (ICN)
Tablets (Buccal): 10 mg (*c-iii*)	Various, *Oreton Methyl* (Schering)
Capsules: 10 mg (*c-iii*)	*Testred* (ICN), *Virilon* (Star)
TESTOSTERONE, SHORT-ACTING	
TESTOSTERONE (IN AQUEOUS SUSPENSION)	
Injection: 25 mg/ml, 50 mg/ml (*c-iii*)	Various
Injection: 100 mg/ml (*c-iii*)	Various, *Histerone 100* (Roberts Hauck), *Tesamone* (Dunhall)
TESTOSTERONE PROPIONATE (IN OIL)	
Injection: 100 mg/ml (*c-iii*)	Various
TESTOSTERONE, LONG-ACTING	
TESTOSTERONE ENANTHATE (IN OIL)	
Injection: 100 mg/ml (*c-iii*)	Various
Injection: 200 mg/ml (*c-iii*)	Various, *Andro L.A. 200* (Forest), *Andropository-200* (Rugby), *Delatestryl* (Bio-Technology General), *Durathate-200* (Roberts Hauck)
TESTOSTERONE CYPIONATE (IN OIL)	
Injection: 100 mg/ml, 200 mg/ml (*c-iii*)	Various, *depAndro* (Forest), *Depotest* (Hyrex) *Depo-Testosterone* (Upjohn), *Duratest* (Roberts Hauck)
TESTOSTERONE TRANSDERMAL SYSTEM	
Patch: 10, 15 mg testosterone (*c-iii*)	*Testoderm* (Alza)
Patch: 12.2 mg testosterone (*c-iii*)	*Androderm* (SmithKline Beecham)
TESTOSTERONE SUBCUTANEOUS	
Pellets: 75 mg testosterone (*c-iii*)	*Testopel* (Bartor Pharmacal)

Effective February 27, 1991, these agents were switched to a *c-iii* status by the DEA because of their abuse potential.

Actions:

Pharmacology: Testosterone, produced by the Leydig cells of the testis, is the primary natural androgen. In women, small amounts are synthesized by the ovary and adrenal cortex. Fluoxymesterone and methyltestosterone are synthetic derivatives of testosterone which have predominant anabolic and minor androgenic activity. Esterification (enanthate and propionate) prolongs the duration of action as the esters are hydrolyzed in vivo to free testosterone. Alkylation (methyltestosterone and fluoxymesterone) and halogenation at position 9 (fluoxymesterone) increase the pharmacologic activity per unit weight compared to oral testosterone.

Endogenous androgens are responsible for the normal growth and development of the male sex organs and for maintenance of secondary sex characteristics. Androgens are responsible for the growth spurt of adolescence and for the termination of linear growth by fusion of the epiphyseal growth centers. During administration of exogenous androgens, endogenous testosterone release is inhibited through feedback inhibition of pituitary luteinizing hormone (LH). Large doses of exogenous androgens may suppress spermatogenesis through feedback inhibition of pituitary follicle stimulating hormone (FSH).

Pharmacokinetics:

Absorption –

Oral: Testosterone is metabolized by the gut and 44% is cleared by the liver in the first pass. The synthetic androgens are less extensively metabolized by the liver and have longer half-lives and are more suitable than testosterone for oral administration. Buccal administration permits methyltestosterone to be absorbed directly into the systemic venous return so that the unmetabolized hormone is carried directly into the tissues. The buccal tablets have approximately twice the potency of oral methyltestosterone.

IM: Testosterone esters are less polar than free testosterone. Testosterone esters in oil injected IM are absorbed slowly from the lipid phase; thus, testosterone cypionate and enanthate can be given at intervals of 2 to 4 weeks.

Transdermal:

Testoderm – Following placement of *Testoderm* on scrotal skin, the serum testosterone concentration rises to a maximum at 2 to 4 hours and returns toward baseline within ≈ 2 hours after system removal. Serum levels reach a plateau at 3 to 4 weeks.

Androderm – Following application to non-scrotal skin, testosterone is continuously absorbed during the 24–hour dosing period. Daily application of 2 systems at ≈ 10:00 p.m. results in a serum testosterone concentration profile that mimics the normal circadian variation observed in healthy young men. Maximum concentrations occur in the early morning hours with minimum concentrations in the evening.

Distribution – Testosterone in plasma is about 98% bound to a specific testosterone-estradiol binding globulin. There are considerable variations in the reported half-life of testosterone, ranging from 10 to 100 minutes. The half-life of testosterone cypionate IM is approximately 8 days; for oral fluoxymesterone, it is ≈ 9.2 hours; and for methyltestosterone it is 2.5 to 3 hours.

Metabolism/Excretion – Inactivation of testosterone occurs primarily in the liver. About 90% of a testosterone dose is excreted in the urine as conjugates of testosterone and its metabolites; about 6% of a dose is excreted in the feces.

Indications:

Males:

Replacement therapy in hypogonadism associated with a deficiency or absence of endogenous testosterone. Prior to puberty, androgen replacement therapy is needed for development of secondary sexual characteristics. Prolonged treatment is required to maintain sexual characteristics in these and other males who develop testosterone deficiency after puberty. Appropriate adrenal cortical and thyroid hormone replacement therapy are still necessary, however, and are of primary importance.

Primary hypogonadism (congenital or acquired): Testicular failure due to cryptorchidism, bilateral torsion, orchitis, vanishing testis syndrome or orchidectomy.

Hypogonadotropic hypogonadism (congenital or acquired): Idiopathic gonadotropin or luteinizing hormone releasing hormone (LHRH) deficiency or pituitary-hypothalamic injury from tumors, trauma or radiation.

Delayed puberty: To stimulate puberty in carefully selected males with clearly delayed puberty. Brief treatment with conservative doses may be justified if these patients do not respond to psychological support.

Impotence and male climacteric symptoms (methyltestosterone): For treatment when conditions are secondary to androgen deficiency.

Transdermal system –

Replacement therapy in males for conditions associated with a deficiency or absence of endogenous testosterone.

Primary hypogonadism (congenital or acquired) – Testicular failure due to cryptorchidism, bilateral torsion, orchitis, vanishing testis syndrome, orchidectomy, Klinefelter's syndrome, chemotherapy or toxic damage from alcohol or heavy metals.

Secondary Hypogonadotropic hypogonadism (congenital or acquired) – Idiopathic gonadotropin or LHRH deficiency or pituitary-hypothalamic injury from tumors, trauma or radiation. These men have low testosterone serum levels but have gonadotropins in the normal or low range.

Appropriate adrenal cortical and thyroid hormone replacement therapy may be necessary in patients with multiple pituitary or hypothalamic abnormalities.

Females:

Metastatic cancer – May be used secondarily in women with advancing inoperable metastatic (skeletal) breast cancer who are 1 to 5 years postmenopausal. Primary goals of therapy include ablation of the ovaries. This treatment has been used in premenopausal women with breast cancer who have benefited from oophorectomy and have a hormone-responsive tumor.

Postpartum breast pain/engorgement – Androgens (methyltestosterone, fluoxymesterone and testosterone propionate) have been used for the management of postpartum breast pain and engorgement, but there is no satisfactory evidence that they prevent or suppress lactation.

Unlabeled uses: In one study, weekly injections of testosterone enanthate 200 mg maintained safe, stable, effective and reversible contraception for at least 12 months in healthy fertile men rendered azoospermic.

Contraindications:

Patients with serious cardiac, hepatic or renal diseases; hypersensitivity to the drug; in men with carcinomas of the breast or prostate; pregnancy (see Warnings); sensitivity/allergy to mercury compounds (Histerone).

Warnings:

Athletic performance: Although the anabolic steroids are generally the agents that are abused for enhancement of athletic performance, these agents have also been used for such purposes. However, these drugs are not safe and effective for this use and have a potential risk of serious side effects.

Product interchange: Do not use testosterone cypionate interchangeably with testosterone propionate because of differences in duration of action.

Breast cancer and immobilized patients: Androgen therapy may cause hypercalcemia by stimulating osteolysis.

Hepatotoxicity: Prolonged use of high doses of androgens has been associated with the development of potentially life-threatening peliosis hepatis, hepatic neoplasms and hepatocellular carcinoma. Cholestatic hepatitis and jaundice occur with fluoxymesterone and methyltestosterone at relatively low doses. Drug-induced jaundice is reversible when the medication is discontinued.

Oligospermia and reduced ejaculatory volume may occur after prolonged administration or excessive dosage.

Edema, with or without congestive heart failure, may be a serious complication in patients with preexisting cardiac, renal or hepatic disease.

Gynecomastia frequently develops and occasionally persists in patients being treated for hypogonadism.

Bone maturation: Use cautiously in healthy males with delayed puberty. Monitor bone maturation by assessing bone age of the wrist and hand every 6 months.

Carcinogenesis: There are rare reports of hepatocellular carcinoma in patients receiving long-term therapy with androgens in high doses.

Elderly males treated with androgens may be at an increased risk of developing prostatic hypertrophy and prostatic carcinoma. Marked increase in libido may occur.

Pregnancy: Category X. Androgens cause virilization of the external genitalia of the female fetus. The degree of masculinization is related to the amount of drug given and the age of the fetus. Masculinization is most likely to occur in the female fetus when androgens are given in the first trimester.

Lactation: It is not known whether androgens are excreted in breast milk.

Children: Use androgens very cautiously in children; the drugs should only be given by specialists who are aware of the adverse effects on bone maturation. Androgens may accelerate bone maturation without producing compensatory gain in linear growth. This adverse effect may result in compromised adult stature. The younger the child, the greater the risk of compromising final mature height.

Precautions:

Monitoring: Frequently determine urine and serum calcium levels during the course of therapy in women with disseminated breast carcinoma. Periodically perform liver function tests. Make periodic (every 6 months) x-ray examinations of bone age during treatment of prepubertal males to determine the rate of bone maturation and the effects of the androgen therapy on the epiphyseal centers. Check hemoglobin and hematocrit periodically for polycythemia in patients who are receiving high doses of androgens.

Virilization: Observe women for signs of virilization (deepening voice, hirsutism, acne, clitoromegaly and menstrual irregularities). Discontinue therapy at the time of evidence of mild virilism to prevent irreversible virilization.

Benign prostatic hypertrophy: Patients with benign prostatic hypertrophy may develop acute urethral obstruction. Priapism or excessive sexual stimulation may develop. Oligospermia may occur after prolonged administration or excessive dosage.

Acute intermittent porphyria: Androgens have precipitated attacks of acute intermittent porphyria.

Hypercholesterolemia: Serum cholesterol may be altered during therapy.

Drug Interactions:

Drugs that may interact with testosterone include anticoagulants and imipramine.

Drug/Lab test interactions:

Thyroid function tests – Decreased levels of thyroxine-binding globulin, resulting in decreased total T_4 serum levels and increased resin uptake of T_3 and T_4. Free thyroid hormone levels remain unchanged, and there is no clinical evidence of thyroid dysfunction.

Adverse Reactions:

Females: Amenorrhea and other menstrual irregularities; inhibition of gonadotropin secretion and virilization, including deepening voice and clitoral enlargement.

Males: Gynecomastia; excessive frequency and duration of penile erections; decreased ejaculatory volume; oligospermia (high dosages).

Males and females: Hirsutism; male pattern baldness; acne; seborrhea; hypercalcemia (particularly in immobile patients and in those patients with metastatic breast carcinoma); nausea; cholestatic jaundice; alterations in liver function tests; increased or decreased libido; headache; anxiety; depression; generalized paresthesia; sleep apnea syndrome; rash.

Administration and Dosage:

FLUOXYMESTERONE:

Males –

Hypogonadism: 5 to 20 mg daily.

Females –

Inoperable breast carcinoma: 10 to 40 mg daily in divided doses. Continue for 1 month for a subjective response and 2 to 3 months for an objective response.

Prevention of postpartum breast pain and engorgement: 2.5 mg shortly after delivery. Then administer 5 to 10 mg daily in divided doses for 4 to 5 days.

METHYLTESTOSTERONE: Absorption through buccal mucosa into systemic circulation provides twice the androgenic activity of oral tablets.

Males –

Hypogonadism, male climacteric and impotence: 10 to 40 mg/day orally.

Androgen deficiency: 10 to 50 mg/day orally (5 to 25 mg buccal).

Postpubertal cryptorchidism: 30 mg/day orally.

Females –

Postpartum breast pain and engorgement: 80 mg/day orally for 3 to 5 days.

Breast cancer: 50 to 200 mg/day orally (25 to 100 mg buccal).

TESTOSTERONE, SHORT-ACTING: For IM use only. Administer deep in the gluteal muscle. Do not inject IV. Shake well.

Suggested dosage for androgens varies depending on age, sex and diagnosis of the patient. Adjust dosage according to response and appearance of adverse reactions.

Androgen replacement therapy – The guideline dose is 25 to 50 mg 2 to 3 times weekly.

Delayed puberty – Dosages are generally in the lower ranges and for a limited duration (eg, 4 to 6 months). Various regimens have been used to induce pubertal changes in hypogonadal males. Some experts advocate lower initial doses, gradually increasing the dose as puberty progresses, with or without a decrease to maintenance levels. Other experts emphasize that higher dosages are needed to induce pubertal changes and lower dosages can be used for maintenance after puberty. Consider the chronological and skeletal ages when determining initial dose and adjusting dose.

Other suggested doses are as follows (injection in oil) –

Growth stimulation in Turner syndrome or constitutional delay of puberty: 40 to 50 mg/m²/dose monthly for 6 months.

Male hypogonadism: Initiation of pubertal growth, 40 to 50 mg/m²/dose monthly until the growth rate falls to prepubertal levels (approximately 5 cm/year); during terminal growth phase, 100 mg/m²/dose monthly until growth ceases; maintenance virilizing dose, 100 mg/m²/dose twice monthly or 50 to 400 mg/dose every 2 to 4 weeks.

Palliation of mammary cancer: Usual dose is 50 to 100 mg 3 times a week. Follow women with metastatic breast carcinoma closely because androgen therapy occasionally appears to accelerate the disease. Thus, many experts prefer to use the shorter-acting androgen preparations rather than those with prolonged activity for treating breast carcinoma, particularly during the early stages of androgen therapy.

Postpartum breast engorgement (testosterone propionate): 25 to 50 mg for 3 to 4 days, starting at the time of delivery

TESTOSTERONE, LONG-ACTING: For IM use only. Individualize dosage. In general, > 400 mg/month is not required because of the prolonged action of the preparation.

Male hypogonadism –

Replacement therapy (eunuchism): 50 to 400 mg every 2 to 4 weeks.

Males with delayed puberty – 50 to 200 mg every 2 to 4 weeks for a limited duration.

Palliation of inoperable breast cancer in women – 200 to 400 mg every 2 to 4 weeks. Androgen therapy occasionally appears to accelerate metastatic breast carcinoma.

TESTOSTERONE TRANSDERMAL SYSTEM:

Testoderm – Patients should start therapy with a 6 mg/day system applied daily; if scrotal area is inadequate, use a 4 mg/day system. Place the patch on clean, dry, scrotal skin. Dry-shave scrotal hair for optimal skin contact. Do not use chemical depilatories. The testosterone transdermal system should be worn 22 to 24 hours.

After 3 to 4 weeks of daily system use, blood should be drawn 2 to 4 hours after system application for determination of serum total testosterone. Because of variability in analytical values among diagnostic laboratories, this laboratory work and later analyses for assessing the effect of the transdermal testosterone therapy should be performed at the same laboratory.

If patients have not achieved desired results by the end of 6 to 8 weeks of use, consider another form of testosterone replacement therapy.

Androderm – The usual starting dose is 2 systems applied nightly for 24 hours, providing a total dose of 5 mg/day.

Apply the adhesive side of the system to a clean, dry area of the skin on the back, abdomen, upper arms or thighs. Avoid bony prominences, such as the shoulder and hip areas. Do NOT apply to the scrotum. Rotate the sites of application, with an interval of 7 days between applications to the same site. The area selected should not be oily, damaged or irritated.

Apply the system immediately after opening the pouch and removing the protective release liner. Press the system firmly in place, making sure there is good contact with the skin, especially around the edges.

To ensure proper dosing, the morning serum testosterone concentration may be measured following system application the previous evening. If the serum concentration is outside the normal range, repeat sampling with assurance of proper system adhesion as well as appropriate application time. Confirmed serum concentrations outside the normal range may require increasing the dosage regimen to 3 systems, or decreasing the regimen to 1 system, maintaining nightly application. Because of variability in analytical values among diagnostic laboratories, this laboratory work and any later analysis for assessing the effect of therapy should be performed at the same laboratory so results can be more easily compared.

Non-virilized patient – Dosing may be initiated with 1 system nightly.

Storage – Do not store outside the pouch provided. Damaged systems should not be used. The drug reservoir may be burst by excessive pressure or heat. Discard systems in household trash in a manner that prevents accidental application or ingestion by children, pets or others.

FINASTERIDE

Tablets: 5 mg finasteride (*Rx*)	*Proscar* (Merck)

Actions:

Pharmacology: Finasteride, a synthetic 4-azasteroid compound, is a competitive and specific inhibitor of steroid 5α-reductase, an intracellular enzyme that converts testosterone into the potent androgen 5α-dihydrotestosterone (DHT). It has no affinity for the androgen receptor. The 5α-reduced steroid metabolites in blood and urine are decreased after administration of finasteride.

The development of the prostate gland is dependent on the potent androgen DHT. The enzyme 5α-reductase metabolizes testosterone to DHT in the prostate gland, liver and skin.

Pharmacokinetics: Finasteride is well absorbed after oral administration, with absolute bioavailability in humans of 63% (range, 34% to 108%). The half-life of finasteride is 4.7 to 7.1 hours.

Finasteride undergoes extensive hepatic metabolism through oxidative pathways to inactive compounds that are eliminated primarily through the bile; the mean urinary recovery of the parent drug within 24 hours of a dose was only 0.04%.

The bioavailability of finasteride is not affected by food. Approximately 90% is bound to plasma proteins. Finasteride crosses the blood-brain barrier.

Indications:

Treatment of symptomatic benign prostatic hyperplasia (BPH). Approximately 60% of patients experience an increase in urinary flow and > 30% experience improvement in symptoms of BPH.

Unlabeled uses: Finasteride is being investigated as adjuvant monotherapy following radical prostatectomy. Other potential uses include prevention of the progression of first-stage prostate cancer, treatment of male pattern baldness, acne and hirsutism.

Contraindications:

Hypersensitivity to finasteride or any component of this product; pregnancy, lactation, children.

Warnings:

Duration of therapy: A minimum of 6 months of treatment may be necessary to determine whether an individual will respond to finasteride. It is not possible to identify prospectively those patients who will respond.

Hepatic function impairment: Use caution in those patients with liver function abnormalities since finasteride is metabolized extensively in the liver.

Elderly: The elimination rate of finasteride is decreased in the elderly, but no dosage adjustment is necessary. The mean terminal half-life in subjects ≥ 70 years of age was ≈ 8 hours (range, 6 to 15 hours) compared to 6 hours (range, 4 to 12 hours) in subjects 45 to 60 years of age. As a result, mean AUC (0 to 24 hr) after 17 days of dosing was 15% higher in subjects ≥ 70 years of age.

Pregnancy: Category X.

Lactation: It is not known whether finasteride is excreted in breast milk; however, finasteride is not indicated for use in women.

Children: Safety and efficacy in children have not been established; however, finasteride is not indicated for use in children.

Precautions:

Prostate cancer evaluation: Perform digital rectal examinations, as well as other evaluations for prostate cancer, on patients with BPH prior to initiating therapy and periodically thereafter.

Finasteride causes a decrease in serum prostate specific antigen (PSA) levels in patients with BPH even in the presence of prostate cancer. Consider this reduction of PSA levels when evaluating PSA laboratory data; it does not suggest a beneficial effect of finasteride on prostate cancer.

Carefully evaluate any sustained increases in PSA levels while on finasteride, including consideration of non-compliance to therapy.

Obstructive uropathy: Since not all patients demonstrate a response to finasteride, carefully monitor patients with a large residual urinary volume or severely diminished urinary flow for obstructive uropathy. These patients may not be candidates for this therapy.

Drug Interactions:

Drug/Lab test interactions: When PSA laboratory determinations are evaluated, give consideration to the fact that PSA levels are decreased in patients treated with finasteride.

Adverse Reactions:

Adverse reactons occuring in ≥ 3 % of patients include: Impotence; decreased libido.

Administration and Dosage:

The recommended dose is 5 mg once a day, with or without meals.

Although early improvement may be seen, at least 6 to 12 months of therapy may be necessary in some patients to assess whether a beneficial response has been achieved. Perform periodic follow-up evaluations to determine whether a clinical response has occurred.

DANAZOL

Capsules: 50, 100 and 200 mg (*Rx*) — Various, *Danocrine* (Sanofi Winthrop)

Actions:

Pharmacology: A synthetic androgen derived from ethisterone, danazol suppresses the pituitary-ovarian axis by inhibiting the output of pituitary gonadotropins. Danazol depresses the output of both follicle-stimulating hormone (FSH) and luteinizing hormone (LH). Danazol acts by direct enzymatic inhibition of sex steroid synthesis and competitively inhibits binding of steroids to their cytoplasmic receptors in target tissues.

In endometriosis danazol alters the normal and ectopic endometrial tissue so that it becomes inactive and atrophic.

Pharmacokinetics: Blood levels of danazol do not increase proportionately with increases in dose. When the dose is doubled, plasma levels increase only about 35% to 40%.

Indications:

Endometriosis: For the treatment of endometriosis amenable to hormonal management.

Fibrocystic breast disease: Danazol is usually effective in decreasing nodularity, pain and tenderness, but it alters hormone levels; recurrence of symptoms is very common after cessation of therapy.

Hereditary angioedema: For the prevention of attacks of angioedema in males and females.

Unlabeled uses: Danazol has been used to treat precocious puberty, gynecomastia and menorrhagia. It has also been studied in the treatment of iodiopathic immune thrombocytopenia, lupus-associated thrombocytopenia and autoimmune hemolytic anemia.

Contraindications:

Undiagnosed abnormal genital bleeding; markedly impaired hepatic, renal or cardiac function; pregnancy and lactation.

Warnings:

Carcinoma of the breast should be excluded before initiating therapy for fibrocystic breast disease.

Long-term experience with danazol is limited. Long-term therapy with other steroids alkylated at the 17 position has been associated with serious toxicity (cholestatic jaundice, peliosis hepatitis). Similar toxicity may develop after long-term danazol.

Androgenic effects may not be reversible even when the drug is discontinued. Watch patients closely for signs of virilization.

Pregnancy: Use a nonhormonal method of contraception. If a patient becomes pregnant during treatment, discontinue use. Continuing treatment may result in androgenic effects in the fetus.

Precautions:

Fluid retention: Conditions influenced by edema require careful observation.

Hepatic dysfunction has been reported; perform periodic liver function tests.

Semen should be checked for volume, viscosity, sperm count and motility every 3 to 4 months, especially in adolescents.

Drug Interactions:

Drugs that may interact with danazol include insulin and warfarin.

Adverse Reactions:

Significant adverse reactions include: Edema; vaginitis; nervousness; emotional lability; hepatic dysfunction; elevated blood pressure; pelvic pain; carpal tunnel syndrome; sleep disorders; fatigue; tremor; visual disturbances; anxiety; depression; gastroenteritis.

Administration and Dosage:

Endometriosis: Begin therapy during menstruation or make sure the patient is not pregnant. Administer 800 mg/day in 2 divided doses to best achieve amenorrhea and rapid response to painful symptoms. Downward titration to a dose sufficient to maintain amenorrhea may be considered depending upon response. Initially, for mild cases, give 200 to 400 mg in 2 divided doses.

Fibrocystic breast disease: Begin therapy during menstruation or make sure patient is not pregnant. Dosage ranges from 100 to 400 mg/day in 2 divided doses.

Hereditary angioedema: Recommended starting dose is 200 mg 2 or 3 times a day. After a favorable initial response, determine continuing dosage by decreasing the dosage by 50% or less at intervals of 1 to 3 months or longer if frequency of attacks prior to treatment dictates. If an attack occurs, increase dosage by up to 200 mg/day.

GLUCOCORTICOIDS

BETAMETHASONE	
BETAMETHASONE, ORAL	
Tablets: 0.6 mg (*Rx*)	*Celestone* (Schering)
Syrup: 0.6 mg per 5 ml (*Rx*)	
BETAMETHASONE SODIUM PHOSPHATE	
Injection: 4 mg/ml (*Rx*)	Various, *Celestone Phosphate* (Schering)
BETAMETHASONE SODIUM PHOSPHATE AND ACETATE	
Injection: 3 mg acetate and 3 mg sodium phosphate per ml (*Rx*)	Various, *Celestone Soluspan* (Schering)
CORTISONE	
Tablets: 5, 10 and 25 mg (*Rx*)	Various, *Cortisone Acetate* (Merck)
Injection: 50 mg/ml (*Rx*)	*Cortone Acetate* (Merck)
DEXAMETHASONE	
DEXAMETHASONE, ORAL	
Tablets: 0.25, 0.5, 0.75, 1, 1.5, 2, 4 and 6 mg (*Rx*)	Various, *Decadron* (Merck), *Dexone* (Solvay), *Hexadrol* (Organon)
Elixir: 0.5 mg/5 ml (*Rx*)	Various, *Decadron* (Merck), *Hexadrol* (Organon)
Oral Solution: 0.5 mg/5 ml (*Rx*)	Various
DEXAMETHASONE ACETATE	
Injection: 8 and 16 mg/ml (*Rx*)	Various, *Dalalone L.A.* (Forest), *Dalalone D.P.* (Forest) *Decadron-LA* (Merck)
DEXAMETHASONE SODIUM PHOSPHATE	
Injection: 4, 10, 20, and 24 mg/ml (*Rx*)	Various, *Dalalone* (Forest), *Decadron Phosphate* (Merck), *Hexadrol Phosphate* (Organon)
HYDROCORTISONE (CORTISOL)	
HYDROCORTISONE	
Tablets: 5, 10 and 20 mg (*Rx*)	Various, *Cortef* (Upjohn), *Hydrocortone* (Merck)
HYDROCORTISONE CYPIONATE	
Oral Suspension: 10 mg/5 ml (*Rx*)	*Cortef* (Upjohn)
HYDROCORTISONE SODIUM PHOSPHATE	
Injection: 50 mg/ml (*Rx*)	*Hydrocortone Phosphate* (Merck)
HYDROCORTISONE SODIUM SUCCINATE	
Injection: 100, 250, 500 and 1000 mg per vial (*Rx*)	*A-Hydrocort* (Abbott), *Solu-Cortef* (Upjohn)
HYDROCORTISONE ACETATE	
Injection: 25 and 50 mg/ml (*Rx*)	Various, *Hydrocortone Acetate* (Merck)
METHYLPREDNISOLONE	
METHYLPREDNISOLONE, ORAL	
Tablets: 2, 4, 8, 16, 24 and 32 mg (*Rx*)	Various, *Medrol* (Upjohn)
METHYLPREDNISOLONE SODIUM SUCCINATE	
Powder for Injection: 40, 125 and 500 mg and 1 and 2 g per vial (*Rx*)	Various, *A-Methapred* (Abbott), *Solu-Medrol* (Upjohn)
METHYLPREDNISOLONE ACETATE	
Injection: 20, 40 and 80 mg/ml (*Rx*)	Various, *Depo-Medrol* (Upjohn), *depMedalone* (Forest), *Adlone* (UAD)
PREDNISOLONE	
PREDNISOLONE, ORAL	
Tablets: 5 mg (*Rx*)	Various, *Delta-Cortef* (Upjohn)
Syrup: 15 mg/5 ml (*Rx*)	*Prelone* (Muro)
PREDNISOLONE ACETATE	
Injection: 25 and 50 mg/ml (*Rx*)	Various, *Key-Pred 25* (Hyrex), *Key-Pred 50* (Hyrex)
PREDNISOLONE TEBUTATE	
Injection: 20 mg/ml (*Rx*)	Various, *Hydeltra-T.B.A.* (Merck)
PREDNISOLONE SODIUM PHOSPHATE	
Injection: 20 mg/ml (*Rx*)	*Hydeltrasol* (Merck)
Oral Liquid: 5 mg/5 ml (*Rx*)	*Pediapred* (Fisons)
PREDNISONE	
Tablets: 1, 2.5, 5, 10, 20 and 50 mg (*Rx*)	Various, *Meticorten* (Schering), *Orasone* (Solvay), *Deltasone* (Upjohn)

Oral Solution: 5 mg/5 ml (*Rx*)	Various
Syrup: 5 mg/5 ml (*Rx*)	*Liquid Pred* (Muro)
TRIAMCINOLONE	
TRIAMCINOLONE, ORAL	
Tablets: 1, 2, 4 and 8 mg (*Rx*)	Various, *Aristocort* (Fujisawa), *Kenacort* (Apothecon)
Syrup: 4 mg/5 ml (*Rx*)	*Kenacort* (Apothecon)
TRIAMCINOLONE DIACETATE	
Injection: 25 and 40 mg/ml (*Rx*)	Various, *Aristocort Intralesional* (Fujisawa), *Aristocort Forte* (Fujisawa), *Triamolone 40* (Forest)
TRIAMCINOLONE HEXACETONIDE	
Injection: 5 mg/ml (*Rx*)	*Aristospan Intralesional* (Fujisawa)
Injection: 20 mg/ml (*Rx*)	*Aristospan Intra-articular* (Fujisawa)
TRIAMCINOLONE ACETONIDE	
Injection: 3, 10 and 40 mg/ml (*Rx*)	Various, *Tac-3* (Herbert), *Kenalog-10* (Westwood-Squibb), *Kenalog-40* (Westwood-Squibb), *Triamonide 40* (Forest)

Actions:

Pharmacology: The naturally occurring adrenal cortical steroids have both anti- inflammatory (glucocorticoid) and salt-retaining (mineralocorticoid) properties. Glucocorticoids cause profound and varied metabolic effects. In addition, they modify the body's immune responses to diverse stimuli. These compounds are used as replacement therapy in adrenocortical deficiency states and may be used for their anti-inflammatory effects.

Pharmacokinetics: Hydrocortisone and most of its congeners are readily absorbed from the GI tract; greatly altered onsets and durations are usually achieved with injections of suspensions and esters. Hydrocortisone is metabolized by the liver, which is the rate-limiting step in its clearance. The metabolism and excretion of the synthetic glucocorticoids generally parallel hydrocortisone. Induction of hepatic enzymes will increase the metabolic clearance of hydrocortisone and the synthetic glucocorticoids.

The half-life values refer to the intrinsic activity of each agent; insoluble salts of these drugs are used as repository injections and have sustained effects due to delayed absorption from the injection site.

Glucocorticoid Equivalencies, Potencies and Half-Life

Glucocorticoid	Approximate equivalent dose (mg)	Relative anti-inflammatory (glucocorticoid) potency	Relative mineralocorticoid potency	Plasma (min)	Biologic (hrs)
Short-acting					
Cortisone	25	0.8	2	30	8-12
Hydrocortisone	20	1	2	80-118	8-12
Intermediate-acting					
Prednisone	5	4	1	60	18-36
Prednisolone	5	4	1	115-212	18-36
Triamcinolone	4	5	0	200+	18-36
Methylprednisolone	4	5	0	78-188	18-36
Long-acting					
Dexamethasone	0.75	20-30	0	110-210	36-54
Betamethasone	0.6-0.75	20-30	0	300+	36-54

Indications:

Endocrine disorders: Primary or secondary adrenal cortical insufficiency (hydrocortisone or cortisone is the drug of choice; synthetic analogs may be used in conjunction with mineralocorticoids; in infancy, mineralocorticoid supplementation is important); congenital adrenal hyperplasia; nonsuppurative thyroiditis; hypercalcemia associated with cancer.

Parenteral – Acute adrenal cortical insufficiency (hydrocortisone or cortisone is drug of choice); preoperatively or in serious trauma or illness with known adrenal insufficiency or when adrenal cortical reserve is doubtful; shock unresponsive to conventional therapy if adrenal cortical insufficiency exists or is suspected.

Various rheumatic disorders.

Collagen diseases.

Dermatologic diseases.

Allergic states: Control of severe or incapacitating allergic conditions intractable to conventional treatment in serum sickness and drug hypersensitivity reactions. Parenteral therapy is indicated for urticarial transfusion reactions and acute noninfectious laryngeal edema (epinephrine is the drug of first choice).

Ophthalmic: Severe acute and chronic allergic and inflammatory processes involving the eye and its adnexa.

Respiratory diseases.

Hematologic disorders.

Neoplastic diseases.

Edematous states: To induce diuresis or remission of proteinuria in the nephrotic syndrome (without uremia) of the idiopathic type or that due to lupus erythematosus.

GI diseases: Crohn's disease and intractable sprue.

Multiple Sclerosis

Miscellaneous: Tuberculous meningitis with subarachnoid block or impending block when accompanied by appropriate antituberculous chemotherapy; in trichinosis with neurologic or myocardial involvement.

Intralesional administration: Keloids; localized hypertrophic, infiltrated, inflammatory lesions of lichen planus, psoriatic plaques, granuloma annulare, lichen simplex chronicus (neurodermatitis); discoid lupus erythematosus; necrobiosis lipoidica diabeticorum; alopecia areata. May be useful in cystic tumors of an aponeurosis or tendon (ganglia).

Triamcinolone: Treatment of pulmonary emphysema where bronchospasm or bronchial edema plays a significant role, and diffuse interstitial pulmonary fibrosis (Hamman-Rich syndrome); in conjunction with diuretic agents to induce a diuresis in refractory CHF and in cirrhosis of the liver with refractory ascites; and for postoperative dental inflammatory reactions.

Unlabeled uses:

Glucocorticoid Unlabeled Uses

Use	Drug/Comment
Acute mountain sickness	Dexamethasone 4 mg q 6 h; prevention or treatment
Antiemetic	Dexamethasone most common, 16 to 20 mg
Bacterial meningitis	Dexamethasone 0.15 mg/kg q 6 h; to decrease incidence of hearing loss
Bronchopulmonary dysplasia in preterm infants	Dexamethasone 0.5 mg/kg, then taper.
COPD	Prednisone 30 to 60 mg/day for 1 to 2 weeks, then taper
Depression, diagnosis of	Dexamethasone 1 mg
Duchenne's muscular dystrophy	Prednisone 0.75 to 1.5 mg/kg/day; to improve strength and function
Graves ophthalmopathy	Prednisone 60 mg/day, taper to 20 mg/day
Hepatitis, severe alcoholic	Methylprednisolone 32 mg/day
Hirsutism	Dexamethasone 0.5 to 1 mg/day

Glucocorticoid Unlabeled Uses	
Use	Drug/Comment
Respiratory distress syndrome	Prevention in premature neonates (betamethasone most common); adults, methylprednisolone 30 mg/kg (controversial)
Septic shock	Methylprednisolone 30 mg/kg IV most common (very controversial)
Spinal cord injury, acute	Methylprednisolone IV within 8 hrs of injury; to improve neurologic function
Tuberculous pleurisy	Prednisolone 0.75 mg/kg/day, then taper; concurrently w/antituberculous therapy

Contraindications:

Systemic fungal infections; hypersensitivity to the drug; IM use in idiopathic thrombocytopenic purpura; administration of live virus vaccines (eg, smallpox) in patients receiving immunosuppressive corticosteroid doses (see Warnings).

Warnings:

Infections: Corticosteroids may mask signs of infection, and new infections may appear during their use. There may be decreased resistance and inability of the host defense mechanisms to prevent dissemination of the infection. Restrict use in active tuberculosis to cases of fulminating or disseminated disease in which the corticosteroid is used for disease management with appropriate chemotherapy. Corticosteroids may exacerbate systemic fungal infections and may activate latent amebiasis.

Hepatitis: Although corticosteroids have been advocated for use in chronic active hepatitis, they may be harmful in chronic active hepatitis positive for hepatitis B surface antigen.

Ocular effects: Prolonged use may produce posterior subcapsular cataracts, glaucoma with possible damage to the optic nerves, and may enhance the establishment of secondary ocular infections due to fungi or viruses.

Fluid and electrolyte balance: Average and large doses of hydrocortisone or cortisone can cause elevation of blood pressure, salt and water retention and increased excretion of potassium. These effects are less likely to occur with the synthetic derivatives except when used in large doses.

Immunosuppression: During therapy, do not use live virus vaccines (eg, smallpox). Do not immunize patients who are receiving corticosteroids, especially high doses, because of possible hazards of neurological complications and a lack of antibody response. This does not apply to patients receiving corticosteroids as replacement therapy.

Adrenal suppression: Prolonged therapy of pharmacologic doses may lead to hypothalamic-pituitary-adrenal suppression. The degree of adrenal suppression varies with the dosage, relative glucocorticoid activity, biological half-life and duration of glucocorticoid therapy within each individual. Adrenal suppression may be minimized by the use of intermediate-acting glucocorticoids (prednisone, prednisolone, methylpred-nisolone) on an alternate day schedule.

Stress: In patients receiving or recently withdrawn from corticosteroid therapy subjected to unusual stress, increased dosage of rapidly acting corticosteroids is indicated before, during and after stressful situations, except in patients on high-dose therapy.

Cardiovascular: Reports suggest an apparent association between corticosteroid use and left ventricular free wall rupture after a recent MI.

Hypersensitivity: Anaphylactoid reactions have occurred rarely with corticosteroid therapy.

Renal function impairment: Edema may occur in the presence of renal disease with a fixed or decreased glomerular filtration rate.

Elderly: Consider the risk/benefit factors of steroid use. Consider lower doses because of body changes caused by aging (ie, diminution of muscle mass and plasma volume).

Pregnancy: Corticosteroids cross the placenta (prednisone has the poorest transport). Chronic maternal ingestion during the first trimester has shown a 1% incidence of cleft palate in humans. Hypoadrenalism has occurred.

Lactation: Corticosteroids appear in breast milk and could suppress growth, interfere with endogenous corticosteroid production or cause other unwanted effects in the nursing infant. However, large doses for short periods may not harm the infant. Alternatives to consider include waiting 3 to 4 hours after the dose before breastfeeding and using prednisolone rather than prednisone.

Children: Carefully observe growth and development of infants and children on prolonged corticosteroid therapy.

Precautions:

Monitoring: Observe patients for weight increase, edema, hypertension, and excessive potassium excretion, as well as for less obvious signs of adrenocortical steroid-induced untoward effects. Monitor for a negative nitrogen balance due to protein catabolism. Evaluate blood pressure and body weight, and do routine laboratory studies, including 2 hour postprandial blood glucose and serum potassium and a chest x-ray at regular intervals during prolonged therapy. Upper GI x-rays are desirable in patients with known or suspected peptic ulcer disease or significant dyspepsia or in patients complaining of gastric distress.

Use the lowest possible dose: Make a benefit/risk decision in each individual case as to the size of the dose, duration of treatment and the use of daily or intermittent therapy, since complications of treatment are dependent on these factors.

Special risk patients: Use with caution in the following situations: Nonspecific ulcerative colitis if there is a probability of impending perforation, abscess or other pyogenic infection; diverticulitis; fresh intestinal anastomoses; hypertension; CHF; thromboembolitic tendencies; thrombophlebitis; osteoporosis; exanthema; Cushing's syndrome; antibiotic-resistant infections; convulsive disorders; metastatic carcinoma; myasthenia gravis; vaccinia; varicella; diabetes mellitus.; hypothyroidism, cirrhosis (enhanced effect of corticosteroids).

Steroid psychosis: Steroid psychosis is characterized by a delirious or toxic psychosis with clouded sensorium. Other symptoms may include euphoria, insomnia, mood swings, personality changes and severe depression. The onset of symptoms usually occurs within 15 to 30 days. Predisposing factors include doses > 40 mg prednisone equivalent, female predominance, and, possibly, a family history of psychiatric illness.

Multiple sclerosis: Although corticosteroids are effective in speeding the resolution of acute exacerbations of multiple sclerosis, they do not affect the ultimate outcome or natural history of the disease.

Repository injections: To minimize the likelihood and severity of atrophy, do not inject SC, avoid injection into the deltoid and avoid repeated IM injections into the same site, if possible. Repository injections are not recommended as initial therapy in acute situations.

Local injections: Intra-articular injection may produce systemic and local effects. A marked increase in pain accompanied by local swelling, further restriction of joint motion, fever and malaise is suggestive of septic arthritis. Frequent intra-articular injection may damage joint tissues.

Drug Interactions:

Drugs that may be affected by glucocorticoids include anticholinesterases, anticoagulants, cyclosporine, digitalis glycosides, isoniazid, nondepolarizing neuromuscular blockers, potassium-depleting agents (eg, diuretics), salicylates, somatrem and theophyllines. Drugs that may affect corticosteroids include aminoglutethimide, barbiturates, cholestyramine, oral contraceptives, ephedrine, estrogens, hydantoins, ketoconazole, macrolide antibiotics and rifampin.

Drug/Lab test interactions: Urine glucose and serum cholesterol levels may increase. Decreased serum levels of potassium, triiodothyronine (T_3), and a minimal decrease of thyroxine (T_4) may occur. Thyroid I^{131} uptake may be decreased. False-negative results with the nitroblue-tetrazolium test for bacterial infection. Dexamethasone, given for cerebral edema, may alter the results of a brain scan (decreased uptake of radioactive material).

Adverse Reactions:

Adverse reactions that may occur include: Hypertension, myocardial rupture following recent MI, anaphylactoid/hypersensitivity reactions; sodium and fluid retention; hypokalemia; metabolic alkalosis; hypocalcemia; hypotension or shock-like reactions; muscle weakness; muscle mass loss; tendon rupture; osteoporosis; spontaneous fractures; thromboembolism or fat embolism; thrombophlebitis; cardiac arrhythmias or ECG changes due to potassium deficiency; syncopal episodes; pancreatitis; abdominal distension; ulcerative esophagitis; nausea; vomiting; increased appetite and weight gain; impaired wound healing; thin fragile skin; petechiae/ecchymoses; erythema; purpura; hirsutism; acneiform eruptions; allergic dermatitis; urticaria; convulsions; vertigo; headache; neuritis/paresthesias; aggravation of preexisting psychiatric conditions; steroid psychoses; menstrual irregularities; development of Cushingoid state (eg, moonface, buffalo hump, supraclavicular fat pad enlargement, central obesity); suppression of growth in children; increased sweating; hyperglycemia; glycosuria; increased IOP; glaucoma; malaise; fatigue; insomnia.

Administration and Dosage:

The maximal activity of the adrenal cortex is between 2 and 8 am, and it is minimal between 4 pm and midnight. Exogenous corticosteroids suppress adrenocortical activity the least when given at the time of maximal activity (am). Therefore, administer glucocorticoids in the morning prior to 9 am.

Initiation of therapy: The initial dosage depends on the specific disease entity being treated. Maintain or adjust the initial dosage until a satisfactory response is noted. If after a reasonable period of time there is a lack of satisfactory clinical response, discontinue the drug and transfer the patient to other appropriate therapy. For infants and children, the recommended dosage should be governed by the same considerations rather than by strict adherence to the ratio indicated by age or body weight. It should be emphasized that dosage requirements are variable and must be individualized.

Maintenance therapy: After a favorable response is observed, determine the maintenance dosage by decreasing the initial dosage in small amounts at intervals until the lowest dosage that will maintain an adequate clinical response is reached.

Withdrawal of therapy: If, after long-term therapy, the drug is to be stopped, it must be withdrawn gradually. If spontaneous remission occurs in a chronic condition, discontinue treatment gradually.

Alternate day therapy is a dosing regimen in which twice the usual daily dose is administered every other morning. The purpose is to provide the patient requiring long-term treatment with the beneficial effects of corticosteroids while minimizing pituitary-adrenal suppression, the cushingoid state, withdrawal symptoms and growth suppression in children. The benefits of alternate day therapy are only achieved by using the intermediate-acting agents.

Intra-articular injection: Dose depends on the joint size and varies with the severity of the condition. In chronic cases, injections may be repeated at intervals of 1 to 5 or more weeks depending upon the degree of relief obtained from the initial injection. Injection must be made into the synovial space.

Miscellaneous (tendinitis, epicondylitis, ganglion): In the treatment of conditions such as tendinitis or tenosynovitis, inject into the tendon sheath rather than into the substance of the tendon. When treating conditions such as epicondylitis, outline the area of greatest tenderness and infiltrate the drug into the area.

Injections for local effect in dermatologic conditions: Avoid injection of sufficient material to cause blanching, since this may be followed by a small slough. One to four injections are usually employed.

BETAMETHASONE:

Betamethasone, oral –

Initial dosage: 0.6 to 7.2 mg/day.

Betamethasone sodium phosphate –

Systemic and local: The initial dosage may vary up to 9 mg/day.

Betamethasone sodium phosphate and acetate – Betamethasone sodium phosphate provides prompt activity, while betamethasone acetate is only slightly soluble and affords sustained activity.

Systemic: Not for IV use.

Initial dose – 0.5 to 9 mg/day. Dosage ranges are ⅓ to ½ the oral dose given every 12 hours. In certain acute, life-threatening situations, dosages exceeding the usual may be justified and may be in multiples of oral dosages.

Intrabursal, intra-articular, intradermal and intralesional: 0.5 to 2 ml.

Dermatologic conditions: 0.2 ml/cm^2 intradermally. *Maximum dose* - 1 ml/week.

Foot disorders: 0.5 to 1 ml.

CORTISONE:

Initial dosage – 25 to 300 mg/day. In less severe diseases, lower doses may suffice.

DEXAMETHASONE:

Dexamethasone, oral –

Initial dosage: 0.75 to 9 mg/day.

In acute, self-limited allergic disorders or acute exacerbations of chronic allergic disorders, the following dosage schedule combining parenteral (dexamethasone sodium phosphate injection, 4 mg/ml) and oral therapy (0.75 mg tablets) is suggested: First day, 1 or 2 ml IM; second day, 4 tablets in 2 divided doses; third day, 4 tablets in 2 divided doses; fourth day, 2 tablets in 2 divided doses; fifth day, 1 tablet; sixth day, 1 tablet; seventh day, no treatment; eighth day, follow-up visit.

Suppression tests: For Cushing's syndrome – Give 1 mg at 11 pm. Draw blood for plasma cortisol determination the following day at 8 am. For greater accuracy, give 0.5 mg every 6 hours for 48 hours. Collect 24 hour urine to determine 17-hydroxycorticosteroid excretion.

Test to distinguish Cushing's syndrome due to pituitary ACTH excess from Cushing's syndrome due to other causes – Give 2 mg every 6 hours for 48 hours. Collect 24 hour urine to determine 17-hydroxycorticosteroid excretion.

Dexamethasone acetate – Not for IV use. *Systemic:* 8 to 16 mg IM, may repeat in 1 to 3 weeks. *Intralesional:* 0.8 to 1.6 mg. *Intra-articular and soft tissue:* 4 to 16 mg; may repeat at 1 to 3 week intervals.

Dexamethasone sodium phosphate –

Systemic:

Initial dosage – 0.5 to 9 mg daily. Usual dose ranges are ⅓ to ½ the oral dose given every 12 hours. However, in certain acute, life-threatening situations, dosages exceeding the usual may be justified and may be in multiples of the oral dosages.

Cerebral edema: In adults, administer an initial IV dose of 10 mg, followed by 4 mg IM every 6 hours until maximum response has been noted. Response is usually noted within 12 to 24 hours. Dosage may be reduced after 2 to 4 days and gradually discontinued over 5 to 7 days. For palliative management of patients with recurrent or inoperable brain tumors, maintenance therapy with either the injection or tablets in a dosage of 2 mg 2 or 3 times daily may be effective.

Unresponsive shock – Reported regimens range from 1 to 6 mg/kg as a single IV injection, to 40 mg initially followed by repeated IV injections every 2 to 6 hours while shock persists.

HYDROCORTISONE (Cortisol):

Hydrocortisone, oral –

Initial dosage: 20 to 240 mg/day.

Hydrocortisone sodium phosphate – Administer by IV, IM or SC injection. Initial dose is 15 to 240 mg/day. Usually, ⅓ to ½ the oral dose every 12 hours. For acute diseases, doses > 240 mg may be required.

Hydrocortisone sodium succinate – May be administered IV or IM. The initial dose is 100 to 500 mg, and may be repeated at 2, 4 or 6 hour intervals depending on patient response and clinical condition.

Hydrocortisone acetate – For intralesional, intra-articular or soft tissue injection only. Not for IV use. Dosage range is 5 to 37.5 mg. If desired, a local anesthetic may be injected before hydrocortisone acetate or mixed in a syringe and given simultaneously.

METHYLPREDNISOLONE:

Methylprednisolone, oral –

Initial dose: 4 to 48 mg/day; adjust until a satisfactory response is noted. Determine maintenance dose by decreasing initial dose in small decrements at appropriate intervals until reaching the lowest effective dose.

Dosepak 21 therapy: Follow manufacturer's directions.

Methylprednisolone sodium succinate –

Initial dose: 10 to 40 mg IV, administered over 1 to several minutes. Give subsequent doses IV or IM.

Infants and children: Not less than 0.5mg/kg/24 hours.

For high dose therapy, give 30 mg/kg IV, infused over 10 to 20 minutes. May repeat every 4 to 6 hours, not beyond 48 to 72 hours.

Methylprednisolone acetate – Not for IV use. As a temporary substitute for oral therapy, administer the total daily dose as a single IM injection. For prolonged effect, give a single weekly dose.

Adrenogenital syndrome: A single 40 mg injection IM every 2 weeks.

Rheumatoid arthritis: Weekly IM maintenance dose varies from 40 to 120 mg.

Dermatologic lesions: 40 to 120 mg IM weekly for 1 to 4 weeks. In severe dermatitis (eg, poison ivy), relief may result within 8 to 12 hours of a single dose of 80 to 120 mg IM. In chronic contact dermatitis, repeated injections every 5 to 10 days may be necessary. In seborrheic dermatitis, a weekly dose of 80 mg IM may be adequate.

Asthma and allergic rhinitis: 80 to 120 mg IM.

Intra-articular and soft tissue: 4 to 80 mg.

Intralesional: 20 to 60 mg.

PREDNISOLONE:

Prednisolone –

Initial dosage: 5 to 60 mg/day.

Multiple sclerosis: In treatment of acute exacerbations of multiple sclerosis, 200 mg daily for a week followed by 80 mg every other day for 1 month.

Prednisolone acetate – Not for IV use.

Initial dosage: 4 to 60 mg/day, IM.

Intralesional, intra-articular or soft tissue injection: 4 mg, up to 100 mg.

Multiple sclerosis: 200 mg daily for a week, followed by 80 mg every other day or 4 to 8 mg dexamethasone every other day for 1 month.

Prednisolone tebutate –

Intra-articular, intralesional or soft tissue administration: 8 to 30 mg. Doses > 40 mg are not recommended.

Prednisolone sodium phosphate –

Parenteral: For IV or IM use.

Initial dosage – 4 to 60 mg/day.

Intra-articular, intralesional or soft tissue administration: 2 to 30 mg.

Oral: Initial dosage - 5 to 60 ml (5 to 60 mg base) per day.

Multiple sclerosis (acute exacerbations) – 200 mg daily for a week, followed by 80 mg every other day or 4 to 8 mg dexamethasone every other day for 1 month.

PREDNISONE: Initial dosage varies from 5 to 60 mg/day. Prednisone is inactive and must be metabolized to prednisolone. This may be impaired in patients with liver disease.

TRIAMCINOLONE:

Triamcinolone, oral –

Adrenocortical insufficiency: 4 to 12 mg, in addition to mineralocorticoid therapy.

Rheumatic and dermatological disorders and bronchial asthma: 8 to 16 mg.

Allergic states: 8 to 12 mg.

Ophthalmological diseases: 12 to 40 mg.

Respiratory diseases: 16 to 48 mg.

Hematologic disorders: 16 to 60 mg.

Tuberculous meningitis: 32 to 48 mg.

Acute rheumatic carditis: 20 to 60 mg.

Acute leukemia and lymphoma (adults): 16 to 40 mg. It may be necessary to give as much as 100 mg/day in leukemia; *acute leukemia (children)* — 1 to 2 mg/kg.

Edematous states: 16 to 20 mg (up to 48 mg) until diuresis occurs.

Systemic lupus erythematosus: 20 to 32 mg.

Triamcinolone diacetate –

Systemic: Not for IV use. May be administered IM for initial therapy; however, most clinicians prefer to adjust the dose orally until adequate control is attained. The average dose is 40 mg IM per week. In general, a single parenteral dose 4 to 7 times the oral daily dose controls the patient from 4 to 7 days, up to 3 to 4 weeks.

Intra-articular and intrasynovial: 5 to 40 mg.

Intralesional or sublesional: 5 to 48 mg. Do not use more than 12.5 mg per injection site. The usual average dose is 25 mg per lesion.

Triamcinolone hexacetonide – Not for IV use.

Intra-articular: 2 to 20 mg average.

Intralesional or sublesional: Up to 0.5 mg per square inch of affected area.

Triamcinolone acetonide –

Systemic:

Initial IM dose – 2.5 to 60 mg/day. Not for IV use.

Intra-articular or intrabursal administration and for injection into tendon sheaths:

Initial dose – 2.5 to 5 mg for smaller joints and 5 to 15 mg for larger joints. For adults, doses up to 10 mg for smaller areas and up to 40 mg for larger areas are usually sufficient.

Intradermal: Use only 3 or 10 mg/ml. Initial dose varies; limit to 1 mg per site.

ACARBOSE

Tablets: 50 and 100 mg (*Rx*)	*Precose* (Bayer)

Actions:

Pharmacology: Acarbose is an oral alpha-glucosidase inhibitor for use in the management of Type II (non-insulin-dependent) diabetes mellitus (NIDDM). Acarbose is a complex oligosaccharide that delays the digestion of ingested carbohydrates, thereby resulting in a smaller rise in blood glucose concentration following meals. As a consequence of plasma glucose reduction, acarbose reduces levels of glycosylated hemoglobin in patients with NIDDM.

Because its mechanism of action is different, the effect of acarbose to enhance glycemic control is additive to that of sulfonylureas when used in combination. In addition, acarbose diminishes the insulinotropic and weight-increasing effects of sulfonylureas.

Pharmacokinetics:

Absorption – Following oral dosing of healthy volunteers with 14C-labeled acarbose, peak plasma concentrations of radioactivity were attained 14 to 24 hours after dosing, while peak plasma concentrations of active drug were attained at ≈ 1 hour.

Metabolism – Acarbose is metabolized exclusively within the GI tract, principally by intestinal bacteria, but also by digestive enzymes. A fraction of these metabolites (≈ 34% of the dose) was absorbed and subsequently excreted in the urine.

Excretion – The fraction of acarbose that is absorbed as intact drug is almost completely excreted by the kidneys. When acarbose was given IV, 89% of the dose was recovered in the urine as active drug within 48 hours. In contrast, < 2% of an oral dose was recovered in the urine as active (ie, parent compound and active metabolite) drug. The plasma elimination half-life of acarbose activity is ≈ 2 hours in healthy volunteers. Consequently, drug accumulation does not occur with three times a day dosing.

Indications:

Hyperglycemia: As monotherapy as an adjunct to diet to lower blood glucose in patients with NIDDM whose hyperglycemia cannot be managed on diet alone.

Acarbose may also be used with a sulfonylurea when diet plus either acarbose or a sulfonylurea do not result in adequate glycemic control.

Contraindications:

Hypersensitivity to the drug; diabetic ketoacidosis or cirrhosis; inflammatory bowel disease; colonic ulceration; partial intestinal obstruction or predisposition to intestinal obstruction; chronic intestinal diseases associated with marked disorders of digestion or absorption; conditions that may deteriorate as a result of increased gas formation in the intestine.

Warnings:

Renal function impairment: Patients with severe renal impairment (creatinine clearance [Ccr] < 25 ml/min/1.73 m^2) attained ≈ 5 times higher peak plasma concentrations of acarbose and 6 times larger AUCs than volunteers with normal renal function. Plasma concentrations of acarbose in renally impaired volunteers were proportionally increased relative to the degree of renal dysfunction. Long-term clinical trials in diabetic patients with significant renal dysfunction (serum creatinine > 2 mg/dl) have not been conducted. Therefore, treatment of these patients with acarbose is not recommended.

Pregnancy: Category B.

Lactation: It is not known whether this drug is excreted in human breast milk. Do not administer to a nursing woman.

Children: Safety and efficacy have not been established.

Precautions:

Monitoring: Monitor therapeutic response to acarbose by periodic blood glucose tests. Measurement of glycosylated hemoglobin levels is recommended for the monitoring of long-term glycemic control.

Acarbose, particularly at doses in excess of 50 mg tid, may give rise to elevations of serum transaminases and, in rare instances, hyperbilirubinemia. It is recommended that serum transaminase levels be checked every 3 months during the first year of the treatment with acarbose and periodically thereafter. If elevated transaminases are observed, a reduction in dosage or withdrawal of therapy may be indicated, particularly if the elevations persist.

Hypoglycemia: Because of its mechanism of action, acarbose alone should not cause hypoglycemia in the fasted or postprandial state. Because acarbose given in combination with a sulfonylurea will cause a further lowering of blood glucose, it may increase the hypoglycemic potential of the sulfonylurea. Use oral glucose (dextrose), with which absorption is not inhibited by acarbose, instead of sucrose (cane sugar) in the treatment of mild to moderate hypoglycemia. Severe hypoglycemia may require the use of either IV glucose infusion or glucagon injection.

Loss of blood glucose control: When diabetic patients are exposed to stress such as fever, trauma, infection or surgery, a temporary loss of control of blood glucose may occur. At such times, timporary insulin therapy may be necessary.

Drug Interactions:

Drugs that may interact with acarbose include digestive enzymes and intestinal adsorbents (eg, charcoal).

Certain drugs tend to product hyperglycemia and may lead to loss of blood glucose control. These drugs include the thiazides and other diuretics, corticosteroids, phenothiazines, thyroid products, estrogens, oral contraceptives, phenytoin, nicotinic acid, sympathomimetics, calcium channel blocking drugs and isoniazid. When such drugs are administered to a patient receiving acarbose, closely observe the patient for loss or blood glucose control. When such drugs are withdrawn from a patient receiving acarbose in combination with sulfonylureas or insulin, closely observe patients for any evidence of hypoglycemia.

Adverse Reactions:

GI symptoms are the most common reaction to acarbose and include abdominal pain, diarrhea and flatulence.

Administration and Dosage:

There is no fixed dosage regimen for the management of diabetes mellitus with acarbose or any other pharmacologic agent. Dosage of acarbose must be individualized on the basis of both effectiveness and tolerance while not exceeding the maximum recommended dose of 100 mg 3 times daily. Start at a low dose, with gradual dose escalation as described below, to both reduce GI side effects and permit identification of the minimum dose required for adequate glycemic control of the patient.

During treatment initiation and dose titration (see below), use 1–hour postprandial plasma glucose to determine the therapeutic response to acarbose and identify the minimum effective dose for the patient. Thereafter, measure glycosylated hemoglobin at intervals of ≈ 3 months. The therapeutic goal should be to decrease both postprandial plasma glucose and glycosylated hemoglobin levels to normal or near normal by using the lowest effective dose of acarbose, either as monotherapy or in combination with sulfonylureas.

Initial dosage: The recommended starting dosage is 25 mg (half of a 50 mg tablet) given orally 3 times daily at the start (with the first bite) of each main meal.

Maintenance dosage: Adjust dosage at 4 to 8 week intervals based on 1-hour postprandial glucose levels and on tolerance. After the initial dosage of 25 mg tid, the dosage can be increased to 50 mg tid. Some patients may benefit from further increasing the dosage to 100 mg tid. The maintenance dose ranges form 50 to 100 mg tid. However, because patients with low body weight may be at increased risk for elevated serum transaminases, consider only patients with body weight > 60 kg for dose titration above 50 mg tid. If no further reduction in postprandial glucose or glycosylated hemoglobin levels is observed with titration to 100 mg tid, consider lowering the dose. Once an effective and tolerated dosage has been established, it should be maintained.

INSULIN

INSULIN INJECTION	
Injection: 100 units/ml (beef and pork) (*otc*)	*Regular Iletin* I (Lilly)
Injection: 100 units/ml (pork) (*otc*)	*Regular Insulin* (Novo Nordisk)
Injection: 100 units/ml (purified pork) (*otc*)	*Pork Regular Iletin* II (Lilly), *Regular Purified Pork Insulin* (Novo Nordisk)
Injection: 100 units per ml (human insulin [rDNA]) (*otc*)	*Humulin R* (Lilly), *Novolin R* (Novo Nordisk)
Injection: 100 units/ml (human insulin [semisynthetic]) (*otc*)	*Velosulin Human* (Novo Nordisk)
Cartridges: 100 units/ml (human insulin [rDNA]). For use with *NovoPen* (*otc*)	*Novolin R PenFill* (Novo Nordisk)
ISOPHANE INSULIN SUSPENSION (NPH; insulin combined with protamine and zinc)	
Injection: 100 units/ml (beef and pork) (*otc*)	*NPH Iletin I* (Lilly)
Injection: 100 units/ml (beef) (*otc*)	*NPH Insulin* (Novo Nordisk)
Injection: 100 units/ml (purified pork) (*otc*)	*NPH-N* (Novo Nordisk)
Injection: 100 units/ml (human insulin [rDNA]) (*otc*)	*Humulin N* (Lilly), *Novolin N* (Novo Nordisk), *Novolin N PenFill* (Novo Nordisk)
ISOPHANE INSULIN SUSPENSION AND INSULIN INJECTION	
70% isophane insulin and 30% insulin injection	
Injection: 100 units/ml (human insulin [rDNA]) (*otc*)	*Humulin 70/30* (Lilly), *Novolin 70/30* (Novo Nordisk), *Novolin 70/30 PenFill* (Novo Nordisk)
50% isophane insulin and 50% insulin injection	
Injection: 100 units/ml (human insulin [rDNA]) (*otc*)	*Humulin 50/50* (Lilly)
INSULIN ZINC SUSPENSION (LENTE; 70% crystalline and 30% amorphous insulin suspension)	
Injection: 100 units/ml (beef and pork) (*otc*)	*Lente Iletin I* (Lilly)
Injection: 100 units/ml (beef) (*otc*)	*Lente Insulin* (Novo Nordisk)
Injection: 100 units/ml (purified pork) (*otc*)	*Lente Iletin II* (Lilly), *Lente L* (Novo Nordisk)
Injection: 100 units/ml (human insulin [rDNA]) (*otc*)	*Humulin L* (Lilly), *Novolin L* (Novo Nordisk)
INSULIN ZINC SUSPENSION, EXTENDED (ULTRALENTE)	
Injection: 100 units/ml (beef) (*otc*)	*Ultralente U* (Novo Nordisk)
Injection: 100 units/ml (human insulin [rDNA]) (*otc*)	*Humulin U Ultralente* (Lilly)

Actions:

Pharmacology: Insulin, secreted by the beta cells of the pancreas, is the principal hormone required for proper glucose use in normal metabolic processes.

The bioavailability of the insulins is identical when given SC. The human insulins are slightly less antigenic than either pork or beef insulins. Human insulin is the insulin of choice for patients with insulin allergy, insulin resistance, all pregnant patients with diabetes and any patient who uses insulin intermittently.

Individual response to insulin varies and is affected by diet, exercise, concomitant drug therapy and other factors.

Pharmacokinetics and Compatibility of Various Insulins

	Insulin Preparations	Onset (hrs)	Peak (hrs)	Duration (hrs)	Compatible mixed with
Rapid-Acting	Insulin Injection (Regular)	½to 1½	2½ to 5	6 to 8	All
Intermediate-Acting	Isophane Insulin Suspension (NPH)	1 to 1½	4 to 12	24	Regular
	Insulin Zinc Suspension (Lente)	1 to 2½	7 to 15	24	Regular
Long-Acting	Protamine Zinc Insulin Suspension (PZI)	4 to 8½	14 to 24	36	Regular
	Extended Insulin Zinc Suspension (Ultralente)	4 to 8½	10 to 30	> 36	Regular

Indications:

Diabetes mellitus type I (insulin-dependent).

Diabetes mellitus type II (non-insulin-dependent) that cannot be properly controlled by diet, exercise and weight reduction.

In hyperkalemia, infusion of glucose and insulin produces a shift of potassium into cells and lowers serum potassium levels.

Insulin injection (regular insulin) may be given IV or IM for rapid effect in severe ketoacidosis or diabetic coma.

Highly purified (single component) and human insulins: Local insulin allergy, immunologic insulin resistance, injection site lipodystrophy; temporary insulin use (ie, surgery, acute stress type II diabetes, gestational diabetes); newly diagnosed diabetics.

Warnings:

Change insulins cautiously and under medical supervision. Changes in purity, strength, brand, type or species source may require dosage adjustment.

Pregnancy: Pregnancy may make diabetes management more difficult. Insulin is the drug of choice for diabetes control in pregnancy.

Lactation: Insulin does not pass into breast milk. Breastfeeding may decrease insulin requirements despite the increase in necessary caloric intake.

Precautions:

Insulin resistance occurs rarely. Insulin resistant patients require > 200 units of insulin/day for > 2 days in the absence of ketoacidosis or acute infection.

Hypoglycemia may result from excessive insulin dose or may be due to: Increased work or exercise without eating; food not being absorbed in the usual manner because of postponement or omission of a meal or in illness with vomiting, fever or diarrhea; when insulin requirements decline.

Diabetic ketoacidosis, a potentially life-threatening condition, requires prompt diagnosis and treatment. Hyperglucagonemia, hyperglycemia and ketoacidosis may result. Diabetic ketoacidosis may result from stress, illness or insulin omission, or may develop slowly after a long period of insulin control.

Symptoms of Hypoglycemia vs Ketoacidosis

Reaction	Onset	Urine glucose/ acetone	Symptoms				
			CNS	Respiration	Mouth/GI	Skin	Miscellaneous
Hypoglycemic reaction (insulin reaction)	sudden	0/0	fatigue, weakness, nervousness, confusion, headache, diplopia, convulsions, psychoses, dizziness, unconsciousness	rapid, shallow	numb, tingling, hunger, nausea	pallor, moist, shallow, or dry	normal or noncharacteristic pulse, eyeballs normal
Ketoacidosis (diabetic coma)	gradual (hours or days)	+/+	drowsiness, dim vision	air hunger	thirst, acetone breath, nausea, vomiting, abdominal pain, loss of appetite	dry, flushed	rapid pulse, soft eyeballs

Insulin allergy:

Local – Occasionally, redness, swelling and itching at the injection site may develop. This occurs if the injection is not properly made, if the skin is sensitive to the cleansing solution or if the patient is allergic to insulin or insulin additives (ie, preservatives).

Systemic reactions, less common, may present as a rash, shortness of breath, fast pulse, sweating, a drop in blood pressure, anaphylaxis or angioedema and may be life-threatening.

Lipodystrophy:

Lipoatrophy is the breakdown of adipose tissue at the insulin injection site causing a depression in the skin.

Lipohypertrophy is the result of repeated insulin injection into the same site. This condition may be avoided by rotating the injection site.

Diet: Patients must follow a prescribed diet and exercise regularly. Determine the time, number and amount of individual doses and distribution of food among the meals of the day. Do not change this regimen unless prescribed otherwise.

Drug Interactions:

Decrease Hypoglycemic Effect of Insulin		Increase Hypoglycemic Effect of Insulin	
Contraceptives, oral	Epinephrine	Alcohol	MAO inhibitors
Corticosteroids	Smoking	Anabolic steroids	Phenylbutazone
Dextrothyroxine	Thiazide diuretics	Beta-blockers[1]	Salicylates
Diltiazem	Thyroid hormone	Clofibrate	Sulfinpyrazone
Dobutamine		Fenfluramine	Tetracyclines
		Guanethidine	

[1] Nonselective beta blockers may delay recovery from hypoglycemic episodes and mask their signs/symptoms. Cardioselective agents may be alternatives.

Administration and Dosage:

The number and size of daily doses, time of administration and diet and exercise require continuous medical supervision. Dosage adjustment may be necessary when changing types of insulin, particularly when changing from single-peak to the more purified animal or human insulins.

Administer maintenance doses SC. Rotate administration sites to prevent lipodystrophy. A general rule is to not administer within 1 inch of the same site for 1 month. The rate of absorption is more rapid when the injection is in the abdomen (possibly > 50% faster), followed by the upper arm, thigh and buttocks. Therefore, it may be best to rotate sites within an area rather than rotating areas.

Dosage guidelines:

Children and adults – 0.5 to 1 U/kg/day.

Adolescents (during growth spurt) – 0.8 to 1.2 U/kg/day.

Adjust doses to achieve premeal and bedtime blood glucose levels of 80 to 140 mg/dl (children < 5 years of age, 100 to 200 mg/dl).

INSULIN INJECTION CONCENTRATED

Injection: 500 units per ml purified pork (*Rx*)	*Regular (Concentrated) Iletin II U-500* (Lilly)

Actions:

Pharmacology:

Insulin resistance – Diabetes can usually be controlled with daily insulin doses ≤ 40 to 60 units; however, an occasional patient develops such resistance or becomes so unresponsive to the effect of insulin that daily doses of several hundred or even several thousand units are required. Patients who require doses in excess of 300 to 500 units daily usually have impaired insulin receptor function.

Pharmacokinetics: Concentrated insulin injection. It frequently has a duration similar to repository insulin; a single dose demonstrates activity for 24 hours.

Indications:

Treatment of diabetic patients with marked insulin resistance (requirements > 200 units/day). A large dose may be administered SC in a reasonable volume.

Contraindications:

Patients with a history of systemic allergic reactions to pork or mixed beef/pork insulin should not receive the product unless they have been successfully desensitized.

Warnings:

Dosage adjustments: Most patients will show a "tolerance" to insulin, so that minor dosage variations will not cause untoward symptoms of insulin shock. It is not possible to identify which patients will require a dosage reduction to avoid hypoglycemia.

Insulin shock: Observe extreme caution in the measurement of dosage; inadvertent overdose may result in irreversible insulin shock.

Hypersensitivity: Less common than local allergic reactions, but potentially more serious, is systemic insulin allergy, which may cause generalized urticaria, dyspnea or wheezing and may, on continued use, progress to anaphylaxis.

Precautions:

Monitoring: Monitor blood glucose closely and often until dosage is established. Some may require only one dose daily, others may require two or three injections per day.

Insulin resistance: Patients with immunologic insulin resistance to beef insulin (this diagnosis is usually confirmed by the finding of increased serum antibody titers) may require an immediate dosage reduction of 20% to 50% when treated with pork or human insulin.

Adverse Reactions:

Significant adverse reactions include: Hypoglycemic (secondary hypoglycemic reactions may develop 18 to 24 hours after injection), erythema, swelling, pruritus.

Administration and Dosage:

Administer SC or IM. Do not inject IV (allergic or anaphylactoid reactions may develop).

Use a tuberculin syringe for dosage measurement. Dosage variations are frequent in the insulin-resistant patient, since the individual is unresponsive to the pharmacologic effect of the insulin.

SULFONYLUREAS

ACETOHEXAMIDE	
Tablets: 250 and 500 mg (*Rx*)	Various, *Dymelor* (Lilly)
CHLORPROPAMIDE	
Tablets: 100 and 250 mg (*Rx*)	Various, *Diabinese* (Pfizer)
GLIMEPIRIDE	
Tablets: 1, 2 and 4 mg (*Rx*)	*Amaryl* (Hoechst-Roussel)
GLIPIZIDE	
Tablets: 5 and 10 mg (*Rx*)	Various, *Glucotrol* (Roerig)
Tablets, extended release: 5 and 10 mg (*Rx*)	*Glucotrol XL* (Pfizer)
GLYBURIDE	
Tablets: 1.25, 2.5 and 5 mg (*Rx*)	Various, *DiaBeta* (Hoechst-Roussel), *Micronase* (Upjohn)
Tablets, micronized: 1.5, 3 and 6 mg (*Rx*)	*Glynase PresTab* (Upjohn)
TOLAZAMIDE	
Tablets: 100, 250 and 500 mg (*Rx*)	Various, *Tolinase* (Upjohn)
TOLBUTAMIDE	
Tablets: 500 mg (*Rx*)	Various, *Orinase* (Upjohn)

Actions:

Pharmacology: The sulfonylurea hypoglycemic agents are sulfonamide derivatives, but are devoid of antibacterial activity. They are used as adjuncts to diet and exercise in the treatment of non-insulin-dependent diabetes mellitus (NIDDM). NIDDM is characterized by insulin resistance and defects in insulin secretion. The sulfonylurea hypoglycemic agents appear to lower blood glucose by stimulating insulin release from beta cells in the pancreatic islets possibly due to increased intracellular cAMP. These agents are only effective in patients with some capacity for endogenous insulin production. They may improve the binding between insulin and insulin receptors or increase the number of insulin receptors.

Guidelines for oral hypoglycemic therapy in NIDDM patients may include:

- Onset of diabetes at ≥ 40 years of age
- Obese or normal body weight
- Duration of diabetes < 5 years
- Absence of ketoacidosis
- Fasting serum glucose ≤ 200 mg/dl
- Insulin requirement < 40 units/day
- Absence of renal or hepatic dysfunction

Pharmacokinetics: All sulfonylureas are strongly bound to plasma proteins, primarily albumin.

Major Pharmacokinetic Parameters of the Sulfonylureas

Sulfonylureas	Equivalent doses (mg)	Doses/ day	Serum t½ (hrs)	Onset (hrs)	Duration (hrs)	Metabolism
First generation						
Acetohexamide	500	1-2	6-8 (parent drug = metabolite)	1	12-24	Reduced in liver to potent active metabolite
Chlorpropamide	250	1	36	1	Up to 60	80% metabolized in liver; metabolite activity unknown
Tolazamide	250	1	7	4-6	12-24	Several mildly active metabolites
Tolbutamide	1000	2-3	4.5-6.5	1	6-12	Oxidized in liver to inactive metabolites
Second generation						
Glipizide	10	1-2	2-4	1-1.5	10-16	Liver metabolism to inactive metabolites
Glyburide Nonmicronized	5	1-2	10	2-4	24	Liver metabolism to weakly active metabolites
Micronized	3	1-2	≈ 4	1	24	

Indications:

As an adjunct to diet to lower the blood glucose in patients with non-insulin-dependent diabetes mellitus (Type II) whose hyperglycemia cannot be controlled by diet alone.

Unlabeled uses: Chlorpropamide has been used in the treatment of neurogenic diabetes insipidus.

Sulfonylureas have been used as temporary adjuncts to insulin therapy in selected NIDDM patients to improve diabetic control.

Contraindications:

Hypersensitivity to sulfonylureas; diabetes complicated by ketoacidosis, with or without coma; sole therapy of insulin-dependent (Type I) diabetes mellitus; diabetes when complicated by pregnancy.

Warnings:

The administration of oral hypoglycemic drugs has been associated with increased cardiovascular mortality as compared to treatment with diet alone or diet plus insulin.

Patients treated for 5 to 8 years with diet plus tolbutamide (1.5 g/day) had a rate of cardiovascular mortality approximately 2.5 times that of patients treated with diet alone. A significant increase in total mortality was not observed. Consider this for other sulfonylureas as well.

Bioavailability: Micronized glyburide 3 mg tablets provide serum concentrations that are *not* bioequivalent to those from the conventional formulation (nonmicronized) 5 mg tablets.

Renal/Hepatic function impairment: Hepatic impairment may result in inadequate release of glucose in response to hypoglycemia. Renal impairment may cause decreased elimination of sulfonylureas leading to accumulation producing hypoglycemia.

Elderly: Elderly and debilitated patients are particularly susceptible to the hypoglycemic action of the sulfonylureas. Hypoglycemia may be difficult to recognize in the elderly.

Pregnancy: *Category C; Category B (glyburide).*

Because abnormal blood glucose levels during pregnancy may be associated with a higher incidence of congenital abnormalities, insulin is recommended to maintain blood glucose levels as close to normal as possible. If used during pregnancy, discontinue at least 2 days to 4 weeks before expected delivery date.

Lactation: Chlorpropamide and tolbutamide are excreted in breast milk. It is not known if other sulfonylureas are excreted in breast milk.

Children: Safety and efficacy in children have not been established.

Precautions:

Monitoring: During the transitional period, test the urine for glucose and acetone at least 3 times daily and have the results reviewed by a physician frequently. Measurement of glycosylated hemoglobin is also useful. It is important that patients be taught to correctly and frequently self-monitor blood glucose.

Hypoglycemia: All sulfonylureas may produce severe hypoglycemia. Proper patient selection, dosage and instructions are important to avoid hypoglycemic episodes.

Asymptomatic patients: Controlling blood glucose in NIDDM with sulfonylureas has not been definitely established to be effective in preventing the long-term cardiovascular or neural complications of diabetes.

Loss of blood glucose control: When a patient stabilized on any diabetic regimen is exposed to stress such as fever, trauma, infection or surgery, a loss of control may occur. At such times, it may be necessary to discontinue drug and give insulin.

The effectiveness of any oral hypoglycemic in lowering blood glucose to a desired level decreases in many patients over time (secondary failure). Primary failure occurs when the drug is ineffective in a patient when first given. Certain patients who demonstrate an inadequate response or true primary or secondary failure to one sulfonylurea may benefit from a transfer to another sulfonylurea.

Disulfiram-like syndrome: A sulfonylurea-induced facial flushing or breathlessness reaction may occur when some sulfonylureas are administered with alcohol.

Syndrome of inappropriate secretion of antidiuretic hormone (SIADH): Water retention and dilutional hyponatremia have occurred after administration of sulfonylureas to NIDDM patients, especially those with congestive heart failure or hepatic cirrhosis.

Drug Interactions:

Drugs that may affect sulfonylureas include androgens, anticoagulants, beta blockers, charcoal, chloramphenicol, cholestyramine, clofibrate, diazoxide, ethanol, fenfluramine, fluconazole, gemfibrozil, histamine H_2 antagonists, hydantoins, magnesium salts, methyldopa, MAO inhibitors, probenecid, rifampin, salicylates, sulfinpyrazone, sulfonamides, thiazide diuretics, tricyclic antidepressants, urinary acidifiers and urinary alkalinizers. Drugs that may be affected by sulfonylureas include digitalis glycosides.

Drug/Lab test interactions: A metabolite of tolbutamide in the urine may give a false-positive reaction for **albumin** if measured by the acidification-after-boiling test, which causes the metabolite to precipitate. There is no interference with the sulfosalicylic acid test.

Drug/Food interactions: Absorption of glipizide is delayed by about 40 minutes when taken with food; the drug is more effective when given approximately 30 minutes before a meal. The other sulfonylureas may be taken with food.

Adverse Reactions:

GI disturbances (eg, nausea, epigastric fullness, heartburn) are the most common reactions. Other adverse reactions may include: Hypoglycemia, disulfiram-like reactions; allergic skin reactions; eczema; pruritus; erythema; urticaria; photosensitivity reactions; leukopenia; thrombocytopenia; aplastic anemia; agranulocytosis; hemolytic anemia; pancytopenia; weakness; paresthesia; tinnitus; fatigue; dizziness; vertigo; malaise; elevated liver function tests.

Administration and Dosage:

Short-term administration of sulfonylureas may be sufficient during periods of transient loss of control in patients usually well controlled on diet.

Transfer from other hypoglycemic agents:

Sulfonylureas – When transferring patients from one oral hypoglycemic agent to another, no transitional period and no initial or priming dose is necessary. However, when transferring patients from chlorpropamide, exercise particular care during the first 2 weeks because the prolonged retention of chlorpropamide in the body and subsequent overlapping drug effects may provoke hypoglycemia.

Insulin – During insulin withdrawal period, test blood for glucose and urine for ketones 3 times daily and report results to physician daily.

Insulin Requirement When Instituting Sulfonylurea Therapy

Insulin dose	Insulin requirement
< 20 units	Start directly on oral agent and discontinue insulin abruptly.
20-40 units	Initiate oral therapy with concurrent 25% to 50% reduction in insulin dose. Further reduce insulin as response is observed. With glyburide, insulin may be discontinued immediately.
> 40 units	Initiate oral therapy with concurrent 20% to 50% reduction in insulin dose. Further reduce insulin as response is observed.

Elderly patients may be particularly sensitive to these agents; therefore, start with a lower initial dose before breakfast, and check blood and urine glucose during the first 24 hours of therapy.

Acute complications: During the course of intercurrent complications (eg, ketoacidosis, severe trauma, major surgery, infections, severe diarrhea, nausea, vomiting), supportive therapy with insulin may be necessary.

Combination insulin therapy: Concurrent administration of insulin and an oral sulfonylurea (generally glipizide or glyburide) has been used with some success in Type II diabetic patients who are difficult to control with diet and sulfonylurea therapy alone.

ACETOHEXAMIDE:

Initial dose – 250 mg to 1.5 g/day. Patients on ≤ 1 g daily can be controlled with once daily dosage. Those receiving 1.5 g/day usually benefit from twice daily dosage before morning and evening meals. Doses > 1.5 g/day are not recommended.

CHLORPROPAMIDE:

Initial dose – 250 mg/day in the mild to moderately severe, middle-aged, stable diabetic patient; use 100 to 125 mg/day in older patients.

Maintenance therapy – ≤ 100 to 250 mg/day. Severe diabetics may require 500 mg/day. Avoid doses > 750 mg/day.

GLIMEPIRIDE:

Initial dose – 1 to 2 mg once daily, given with breakfast or the first main meal. Patients sensitive to hypoglycemic drugs should begin at 1 mg once daily; titrate carefully.

Maximum starting dose is ≤ 2 mg.

Maintenance dose – 1 to 4 mg once daily. The maximum recommended dose is 8 mg once daily. After a dose of 2 mg is reached, increase dose at increments of ≤ 2 mg at 1 to 2 week intervals based on the patient's blood glucose response.

Combination insulin therapy – The recommended dose is 8 mg once daily with the first main meal with low-dose insulin.

Transfer from other hypoglycemic agents –

Sulfonylureas: When transferring patients to glimepiride, no transition period is necessary.

GLIPIZIDE: Give approximately 30 minutes before a meal to achieve the greatest reduction in postprandial hyperglycemia.

Initial dose – 5 mg, given ≈ 30 minutes before breakfast. Geriatric patients or those with liver disease may be started on 2.5 mg.

Adjust dosage in 2.5 to 5 mg increments, as determined by blood glucose response. Several days should elapse between titration steps. If response to a single dose is not satisfactory, dividing that dose may prove effective. The maximum recommended once daily dose is 15 mg. The maximum recommended total daily dose is 40 mg.

Maintenance dose – Some patients may be controlled on a once-a-day regimen, while others show better response with divided dosing. Divide total daily doses > 15 mg and give before meals of adequate caloric content. Total daily doses > 30 mg have been safely given on a twice daily basis to long-term patients.

GLYBURIDE (Glibenclamide):

DiaBeta/Micronase –

Initial dose: 2.5 to 5 mg daily, administered with breakfast or the first main meal. For patients who may be more sensitive to hypoglycemic drugs, start at 1.25 mg daily.

Maintenance dose: 1.25 to 20 mg daily. Give as a single dose or in divided doses. Increase in increments of no more than 2.5 mg at weekly intervals based on the patient's blood glucose response. Daily doses > 20 mg are not recommended.

Glynase –

Initial dose: 1.5 to 3 mg/day, administered with breakfast or the first main meal. For patients who may be more sensitive to hypoglycemic drugs, start at 0.75 mg/day.

Maintenance dose: 0.75 to 12 mg/day. Give as a single dose or in divided doses; some patients, particularly those receiving > 6 mg/day, may have a more satisfactory response with twice-daily dosing. Increase in increments of no more than 1.5 mg at weekly intervals based on the patient's blood glucose response. Daily doses > 12 mg are not recommended.

TOLAZAMIDE:

Initial dose – 100 to 250 mg/day with breakfast or the first main meal. If fasting blood sugar (FBS) is < 200 mg/dl, use 100 mg/day, or 250 mg/day if FBS is > 200 mg/dl. If patients are malnourished, underweight, elderly or not eating properly, use 100 mg once a day. Adjust dose to response. If > 500 mg/day is required, give in divided doses twice daily. Doses > 1 g/day are not likely to improve control.

TOLBUTAMIDE:

Initial dose – 1 to 2 g/day (range, 0.25 to 3 g). A maintenance dose > 2 g/day is seldom required. Total dose may be taken in the morning, but divided doses may allow increased GI tolerance.

METFORMIN HCl

Tablets: 500 and 850 mg (*Rx*)	*Glucophage* (Bristol-Myers Squibb)

Actions:

Pharmacology: Metformin is an oral antihyperglycemic drug used in the management of non-insulin-dependent diabetes mellitus (NIDDM). It is not chemically or pharmacologically related to the oral sulfonylureas. Metformin improves glucose tolerance in NIDDM subjects, lowering both basal and postprandial plasma glucose. Metformin decreases hepatic glucose production, decreases intestinal absorption of glucose and improves insulin sensitivity (increases peripheral glucose uptake and utilization).

Pharmacokinetics:

Absorption/Distribution The absolute bioavailability of 500 mg metformin given under fasting conditions is ≈ 50% to 60%. Studies using single oral doses of 500 and

1500 mg, and 850 to 2550 mg, indicate that there is a lack of dose proportionality with increasing doses, which is due to decreased absorption rather than an alteration in elimination.

The apparent volume of distribution following single oral doses of 850 mg averaged 654 ± 358 L. Metformin is negligibly bound to plasma proteins in contrast to sulfonylureas, which are > 90% protein bound. At usual clinical doses and dosing schedules, steady-state plasma concentrations are reached within 24 to 48 hours and are generally < 1 mcg/ml.

Metabolism/Excretion Metformin is excreted unchanged in the urine and does not undergo hepatic metabolism (no metabolites have been identified in humans) nor biliary excretion. Renal clearance is ≈ 3.5 times greater than creatinine clearance (Ccr) which indicates that tubular secretion is the major route of elimination. Following oral administration, ≈ 90% of the absorbed drug is eliminated via the renal route within the first 24 hours, with a plasma elimination half-life of ≈ 6.2 hours. In blood, the elimination half-life is ≈ 17.6 hours, suggesting that the erythrocyte mass may be a compartment of distribution.

Indications:

Hyperglycemia: As monotherapy, as an adjunct to diet to lower blood glucose in patients with NIDDM whose hyperglycemia cannot be satisfactorily managed on diet alone.

Metformin may be used concomitantly with a sulfonylurea when diet and metformin or a sulfonylurea alone do not result in adequate glycemic control.

Contraindications:

Renal disease or dysfunction (eg, as suggested by serum creatinine levels > 1.5 mg/dl [males], > 1.4 mg/dl [females] or abnormal Ccr) which may also result from conditions such as cardiovascular collapse (shock), acute MI and septicemia.

Temporarily withhold metformin in patients undergoing radiologic studies involving parenteral administration of iodinated contrast materials, because use of such products may result in acute alteration of renal function.

Hypersensitivity to metformin.

Acute or chronic metabolic acidosis, including diabetic ketoacidosis, with or without coma. Treat diabetic ketoacidosis with insulin.

Warnings:

Lactic acidosis: Lactic acidosis is a rare, but serious, metabolic complication that can occur due to metformin accumulation during treatment; when it occurs, it is fatal in ≈ 50% of cases. Lactic acidosis may also occur in association with a number of pathophysiologic conditions, including diabetes mellitus and whenever there is significant tissue hypoperfusion and hypoxemia. Lactic acidosis is characterized by elevated blood lactate levels (> 5 mmol/L), decreased blood pH, electrolyte disturbances with an increased anion gap and an increased lactate/pyruvate ratio. Reported cases have occurred primarily in diabetic patients with significant renal insufficiency, including both intrinsic renal disease and renal hypoperfusion, often in the setting of multiple concomitant medical/surgical problems and multiple concomitant medications.

Promptly withhold metformin in the presence of any condition associated with hypoxemia or dehydration. Because impaired hepatic function may significantly limit the ability to clear lactate, generally avoid metformin in patients with evidence of hepatic disease. Caution patients against excessive alcohol intake (acute or chronic) since alcohol potentiates the effects of metformin on lactate metabolism. In addition, temporarily discontinue metformin prior to any intravascular radiocontrast study and for any surgical procedure. Once a patient is stabilized on any dose level of metformin, GI symptoms, which are common during initiation of therapy, are unlikely to be drug related. Later occurrence of GI symptoms could be due to lactic acidosis or other serious disease. Suspect lactic acidosis in any diabetic patient with metabolic acidosis lacking evidence of ketoacidosis (ketonuria and ketonemia).

Lactic acidosis is a medical emergency that must be treated in a hospital setting. In a patient with lactic acidosis who is taking metformin, discontinue the drug immediately and promptly institute general supportive measures. Because metformin is dialyzable (with a clearance of up to 170 ml/min under good hemodynamic conditions), prompt hemodialysis is recommended to correct the acidosis and remove the accumulated metformin. Such management often results in prompt reversal of symptoms and recovery.

Glucose control: If, after a suitable trial of such treatments, glucose control still has not been achieved, give consideration to the use of insulin.

Increased risk of cardiovascular mortality: The administration of oral antidiabetic drugs has been reported to be associated with increased cardiovascular mortality as compared to treatment with diet alone or diet plus insulin.

Renal/Hepatic function impairment: In subjects with decreased renal function (based on measured Ccr), the plasma and blood half-life of metformin is prolonged and the renal clearance is decreased in proportion to the decrease in Ccr.

Since impaired hepatic function has been associated with some cases of lactic acidosis, generally avoid metformin in patients with clinical or laboratory evidence of hepatic disease.

Pregnancy: Category B.

Lactation: Decide whether to discontinue nursing or to discontinue the drug, taking into account the importance of the drug to the mother.

Children: Safety and efficacy in children have not been established. Studies in maturity-onset diabetes of the young (MODY) have not been conducted.

Precautions:

Monitoring: Before initiation of therapy and at least annually thereafter, assess renal function and verify as normal. In patients in whom development of renal dysfunction is anticipated, assess renal function more frequently and discontinue the drug if evidence of renal impairment is present.

Evaluate a diabetic patient previously well controlled on metformin who develops laboratory abnormalities or clinical illness (especially vague and poorly defined illness) for evidence of ketoacidosis or lactic acidosis. Evaluation should include serum electrolytes and ketones, blood glucose and, if indicated, blood pH, lactate, pyruvate and metformin levels. If acidosis of either form occurs, metformin must be stopped immediately and other appropriate corrective measures initiated.

Monitor response to all diabetic therapies by periodic measurements of fasting blood glucose and glycosylated hemoglobin levels, with a goal of decreasing these levels toward the normal range. During initial dose titration, fasting glucose can be used to determine the therapeutic response. Thereafter, monitor both glucose and glycosylated hemoglobin.

Perform initial and periodic monitoring of hematologic parameters (eg, hemoglobin/hematocrit, red blood cell indices) and renal function (serum creatinine) at least on an annual basis. While megaloblastic anemia has rarely been seen with metformin therapy, if this is suspected, exclude vitamin B_{12} deficiency.

Hypoxic states: Cardiovascular collapse (shock), acute CHF, acute MI and other conditions characterized by hypoxemia have been associated with lactic acidosis and may also cause prerenal azotemia. If such events occur, discontinue metformin.

Surgical procedures: Temporarily suspend metformin for surgical procedures (unless minor and not associated with restricted intake of food and fluids). Do not restart until the patient's oral intake has resumed and renal function is normal.

Vitamin B_{12} levels: A decrease to subnormal levels of previously normal serum vitamin B_{12} levels, without clinical manifestations, is observed in ≈ 7% of patients receiving metformin in controlled clinical trials of 29 weeks duration. Annual measurement of hematologic parameters is advised in patients on metformin and any apparent abnormalities should be appropriately investigated and managed.

Certain individuals with inadequate vitamin B_{12} or calcium intake or absorption appear to be predisposed to developing subnormal vitamin B_{12} levels. In these patients, routine serum vitamin B_{12} measurements at 2 to 3 year intervals may be useful.

Hypoglycemia: Hypoglycemia does not occur in patients receiving metformin alone under usual circumstances, but could occur with deficient caloric intake, strenuous exercise not compensated by caloric supplementation, or during concomitant use with other glucose lowering agents (such as sulfonylureas) or ethanol.

Elderly, debilitated or malnourished patients, and those with adrenal or pituitary insufficiency or alcohol intoxication are particularly susceptible to hypoglycemic effects. Hypoglycemia may be difficult to recognize in the elderly and in people who are taking beta-adrenergic blocking drugs.

Loss of control of blood glucose: When a patient stabilized on any diabetic regimen is exposed to stress such as fever, trauma, infection or surgery, a temporary loss of glycemic control may occur. At such times, it may be necessary to withhold metformin and temporarily administer insulin. Metformin may be reinstituted after the acute episode is resolved.

Drug Interactions:

Drugs that may affect metformin include alcohol, cationic drugs, cimetidine, furosemide, iodinated contrast material and nifedipine.

Drugs that may be affected by metformin include glyburide and furosemide.

Certain drugs tend to produce hyperglycemia and may lead to loss of glycemic control. These drugs include thiazide and other diuretics, corticosteroids, phenothiazines, thyroid products, estrogens, oral contraceptives, phenytoin, nicotinic acid, sympathomimetics, calcium channel blocking drugs and isoniazid. When such drugs are administered to a patient receiving metformin, closely observe the patient to maintain adequate glycemic control.

Drug/Food interactions: Food decreases the extent and slightly delays the absorption of a single 850 mg dose of metformin as shown by an ≈ 40% lower peak concentration and 25% lower AUC in plasma and a 35 minute prolongation of time to peak plasma concentration compared to the same strength administered under fasting conditions. The clinical relevance of these decreases is unknown.

Adverse Reactions:

Adverse reactions occurring in ≥ 3% of patients include diarrhea; nausea; vomiting; abdominal bloating; flatulence; anorexia; an unpleasant metallic taste; asymptomatic subnormal serum vitamin B_{12} levels.

Administration and Dosage:

There is no fixed dosage regimen for the management of hyperglycemia in diabetes mellitus with metformin or any other pharmacologic agent. Dosage must be individualized on the basis of both effectiveness and tolerance, while not exceeding the maximum recommended daily dose of 2550 mg. Give in divided doses with meals and start at a low dose, with gradual dose escalation as described below, both to reduce GI side effects and to permit identification of the minimum dose required for adequate glycemic control of the patient.

Short-term administration may be sufficient during periods of transient loss of control in patients usually well controlled on diet alone.

Usual starting dose: In general, clinically significant responses are not seen at doses < 1500 mg/day. However, a lower recommended starting dose and gradually increased dosage is advised to minimize GI symptoms.

Metformin 500 mg: The usual starting dose is one 500 mg tablet twice daily, given with the morning and evening meals. Make dosage increases in increments of 500 mg every week, given in divided doses, up to a maximum of 2500 mg/day. Metformin can be administered twice a day up to 2000 mg/day (eg, 1000 mg twice daily with morning and evening meals). If a 2500 mg daily dose is required, it may be better tolerated given 3 times daily with meals.

Metformin 850 mg: The usual starting dose is one 850 mg tablet daily, given with the morning meal. Make dosage increases in increments of 850 mg every *other* week, given in divided doses, up to a maximum of 2550 mg/day. The usual maintenance dose is 850 mg twice daily with the morning and evening meals. When necessary, patients may be given 850 mg 3 times daily with meals.

Transfer from other antidiabetic therapy: When transferring patients from standard oral hypoglycemic agents other than chlorpropamide to metformin, generally no transition period is necessary. When transferring patients from chlorpropamide, exercise care during the first 2 weeks because of the prolonged retention of chlorpropamide leading to overlapping drug effects and possible hypoglycemia.

Concomitant metformin and oral sulfonylurea therapy: If patients have not responded to 4 weeks of the maximum dose of metformin monotherapy, consider gradual addition of an oral sulfonylurea while continuing metformin at the maximum dose, even if prior primary or secondary failure to a sulfonylurea has occurred. Clinical and pharmacokinetic drug-drug interaction data are available only for metformin plus glyburide. Published clinical information exists for the use of metformin with either chlorpropamide, tolbutamide or glipizide. No published clinical information exists regarding concomitant use of metformin with acetohexamide or tolazamide.

With concomitant metformin and sulfonylurea therapy, the desired control of blood glucose may be obtained by adjusting the dose of each drug. However, make attempts to identify the minimum effective dose of each drug. With concomitant metformin and sulfonylurea therapy, risk of hypoglycemia associated with sulfonylurea therapy continues and may be increased. Take appropriate precautions.

If patients have not satisfactorily responded to 1 to 3 months of concomitant therapy with the maximum doses of metformin and an oral sulfonylurea, consider institution of insulin therapy and discontinuation of these oral agents.

Elderly/Debilitated: Initial and maintenance dosing should be conservative in patients with advanced age due to the potential for decreased renal function in this population. Base any dosage adjustment on a careful assessment of renal function. Generally, elderly patients should not be titrated to the maximum dose.

In debilitated or malnourished patients, the dosing should also be conservative and based on a careful assessment of renal function.

TROGLITAZONE

Tablets: 200 and 400 mg (Rx) — *Rezulin* (Parke-Davis)

Actions:

Pharmacology: Troglitazone is a thiazolidinedione antidiabetic agent that lowers blood glucose by improving target cell response to insulin, without increasing pancreatic insulin secretion. It decreases insulin resistance. It has a unique mechanism of action that is dependent on the presence of insulin for activity. Troglitazone decreases hepatic glucose output and increases insulin-dependent glucose disposal in skeletal muscle and possibly liver and adipose tissue.

Pharmacokinetics:

Absorption – Following daily drug administration, steady-state plasma concentrations of troglitazone are reached within 3 to 5 days.

Troglitazone is absorbed rapidly following oral administration; the time for maximum plasma concentration (T_{max}) occurs within 2 to 3 hours. Food increases the extent of absorption by 30% to 85%.

Distribution – Mean apparent volume of distribution of troglitazone following multiple-dose administration ranges from 10.5 to 26.5 L/kg of body weight. Troglitazone is extensively bound (> 99%) to serum albumin.

Metabolism – After 14 days of treatment with 400 mg troglitazone, the major metabolites found in the plasma were the sulfate conjugate, followed by the quinone metabolite. Only 3.1% of the dose was detected in the urine; this was primarily in the form of the glucuronide conjugate, which is present in negligible amounts in the plasma.

Excretion – Following oral administration of troglitazone, ≈ 85% is recovered in feces and 3% in urine. Unchanged troglitazone is not recovered in urine following oral administration. Mean plasma elimination half-life of troglitazone ranges from 16 to 34 hours.

Indications:

Type II diabetes: For use in patients with type II diabetes currently on insulin therapy whose hyperglycemia is inadequately controlled (HBA_{1c} > 8.5%) despite insulin therapy of > 30 units/day given as multiple injections.

Unlabeled uses: A study showed troglitazone may be beneficial in the productive and metabolic consequences of polycystic ovary syndrome and less essential hypertension with NIDDM.

Contraindications:

Known hypersensitivity or allergy to troglitazone or any of its components.

Warnings:

Heart failure: No increased incidence of adverse events potentially related to volume expansion (eg, congestive heart failure) have been observed during controlled clinical trials. Caution is advised during the administration of troglitazone to patients with NYHA Class III or IV cardiac status.

Hepatic function impairment: Troglitazone and its metabolites plasma concentrations in patients with chronic liver disease were increased compared with those in healthy subjects without hepatic dysfunction. Use troglitazone with caution in patients with hepatic disease.

Elderly: No differences in efficacy and safety were observed between ≥ 65 year-old patients and younger patients.

Pregnancy: Category B.

Lactation: It is not known whether troglitazone is secreted in breast milk. Do not administer to breastfeeding women.

Children: Safety and efficacy in pediatric patients have not been established.

Precautions:

Type I diabetes: Because of its mechanism of action, troglitazone is active only in the presence of insulin. Therefore, do not use in type I diabetes or for the treatment of diabetic keto-acidosis.

Hypoglycemia: Patients receiving troglitazone in combination with insulin may be at risk for hypoglycemia, and a reduction in the dose of insulin may be necessary. Hypoglycemia has not been observed during the administration of troglitazone as monotherapy and would not be expected based on the mechanism of action.

Drug Interactions:

Troglitazone may induce drug metabolism by CYP3A4. Consider this when prescribing other CYP3A4 substrates such as cyclosporine, tacrolimus and some HMG-CoA reductase inhibitors.

Drugs that may affect troglitazone include cholestyramine.

Drugs that may be affected by troglitazone include acetaminophen, oral contraceptives, sulfonylureas, terfenadine and warfarin.

Drug/Lab test interactions:

Hematologic – Small decreases in hemoglobin, hematocrit, and neutrophil counts (within the normal range) may be related to increased plasma volume observed with troglitazone treatment.

Lipids – Small changes in serum lipids have been observed.

Serum transaminase levels – 2.2& of troglitazone-treated patients had reversible elevations in AST or ALT > 3 times the upper limit of normal.

Drug/Food interactions: Food increases the extent of troglitazone absorption by 30% to 85%, therefore take with food.

Adverse Reactions:

Adverse reactions that were reported in ≥ 3% of patients include: Infection; headache; pain; accidental injury; asthenia; dizziness; back pain; nausea; rhinitis; diarrhea; urinary tract infection; peripheral edema; pharyngitis.

Administration and Dosage:

Continue the current insulin dose upon initiation of troglitazone therapy. Initiate therapy at 200 mg once daily in patients on insulin therapy. For patients not responding adequately, increase the dose after ≈ 2 to 4 weeks. The usual dose is 400 mg/day. The maximum recommended dose is 600 mg/day. It is recommended that the insulin dose be decreased by 10% to 25% when fasing plasma glucose concentrations decrease to < 120 mg/dl in patients receiving concomitant insulin and troglitazone. Individualize further adjustments based on glucose-lowering response. Take with a meal.

THYROID HORMONES

THYROID DESSICATED (60 mg = 1 grain)	
Tablets: 15, 30, 60, 90, 120, 180, 240 and 300 mg (*Rx*)	*Thyroid USP* (Various), *Armour Thyroid* (Rhone-Poulenc Rorer), *Thyrar* (Rhone-Poulenc Rorer), *Thyroid Strong* (Jones Medical)
Capsules: 60, 120, 180 and 300 mg (pork thyroid suspended in soybean oil) (*Rx*)	*S-P-T* (Fleming)
LEVOTHYROXINE SODIUM	
Tablets: 0.025, 0.05, 0.075, 0.088, 0.1, 0.112, 0.125, 0.137, 0.15, 0.175, 0.2 and 3 mg (*Rx*)	Various, *Eltroxin* (Roberts), *Levo-T* (Lederle), *Levothroid* (Forest), *Levoxyl* (Daniels), *Synthroid* (Knoll)
Powder for injection, lyophilized: 200 and 500 mcg per vial (*Rx*)	Various, *Levothroid* (Forest), *Levoxine* (Daniels), *Synthroid* (Knoll)
LIOTHYRONINE SODIUM	
Tablets: 5, 25 and 50 mcg (*Rx*)	Various, *Cytomel* (SK-Beecham)
Injection: 10 mcg/ml	*Triostat* (SK-Beecham)
LIOTRIX (60 mg = 1 grain)	
Tablets: ¼, ½, 1, 2 and 3 grains (T_4:T_3 content in a 4:1 ratio) (*Rx*)	*Thyrolar* (Forest)

Actions:

Pharmacology:

Preparations – Thyroid hormones include both natural and synthetic derivatives. The natural product, desiccated thyroid, is derived from beef or pork. Although this preparation is most economical, standardization by iodine content or bioassay is inexact; synthetic derivatives are generally preferred because of more uniform standardization of potency.

Physiological effects – The mechanisms by which thyroid hormones exert their physiologic action are not well understood. It is believed that most of their effects are exerted through control of DNA transcription and protein synthesis. Their principal effect is to increase metabolic rate of body tissues noted by increases in: Oxygen consumption; respiratory rate; body temperature; cardiac output; heart rate; blood volume; rate of fat, protein and carbohydrate metabolism; enzyme system activity; growth and maturation. Thyroid hormones exert a profound influence on every organ system and are particularly important in CNS development. Thyroid hormones are also concerned with growth and differentiation of tissues.

Regulation of thyroid secretion: Endogenous thyroid hormone secretion is suppressed when exogenous thyroid hormones are given to euthyroid individuals in excess of the normal gland's secretion. Thyroid administration increases basal metabolic rate. The primary effect of the thyroid hormones is the result of T_3 activity.

Pharmacokinetics:

Absorption – Absorption of T_4 from the GI tract varies from 48% to 79% of the dose administered. In 4 hours, T_3 is 95% absorbed.

Various Pharmacokinetic Parameters of Thyroid Hormones

Hormone	Ratio released from thyroid gland	Biologic potency	Half-life (days)	Protein binding (%)[2]
Levothyroxine (T_4)	20	1	6-7[1]	99+
Liothyronine (T_3)	1	4	≤ 2	99+

[1] 3 to 4 days in hyperthyroidism, 9 to 10 days in myxedema.
[2] Includes TBg, TBPA and TBa.

Indications:

Hypothyroidism: As replacement or supplemental therapy in hypothyroidism of any etiology, except transient hypothyroidism during the recovery phase of subacute thyroiditis.

Pituitary TSH suppressants: In the treatment or prevention of various types of euthyroid goiters, including thyroid nodules, subacute or chronic lymphocytic thyroiditis (Hashimoto's), multinodular goiter and in the management of thyroid cancer.

Thyrotoxicosis: May be used with antithyroid drugs to treat thyrotoxicosis, to prevent goitrogenesis and hypothyroidism and thyrotoxicosis during pregnancy.

Diagnostic use in suppression tests to differentiate suspected hyperthyroidism from euthyroidism.

Contraindications:

Acute myocardial infarction and thyrotoxicosis uncomplicated by hypothyroidism; where hypothyroidism and hypoadrenalism (Addison's disease) coexist, unless treatment of hypoadrenalism with adrenocortical steroids precedes the initiation of thyroid therapy; hypersensitivity to active or extraneous constituents.

Warnings:

> *Obesity* has been treated with thyroid hormones. In euthyroid patients, hormonal replacement doses are ineffective for weight reduction. Larger doses may produce serious or even life-threatening toxicity, particularly when given with sympathomimetic amines such as anorexiants.

Cardiovascular disease: Use caution when the integrity of the cardiovascular system, particularly the coronary arteries, is suspect. This includes patients with angina or the elderly, in whom there is a greater likelihood of occult cardiac disease.

Observe patients with coronary artery disease during surgery, since the possibility of precipitating cardiac arrhythmias may be greater in those treated with thyroid hormones.

Endocrine disorders: Thyroid hormone therapy in patients with concomitant diabetes mellitus or insipidus or adrenal insufficiency (Addison's disease) exacerbates the intensity of their symptoms. Correct adrenal insufficiency with corticosteroids before administering thyroid hormones.

Morphologic hypogonadism and nephrosis – Rule out prior to initiating therapy.

Myxedema – Patients with myxedema are particularly sensitive to thyroid preparations. Begin treatment with small doses and gradual increments.

Hyperthyroid effects – In rare instances the administration of thyroid hormone may precipitate a hyperthyroid state or may aggravate existing hyperthyroidism.

Pregnancy: Category A.

Lactation: Minimal amounts of thyroid hormones are excreted in breast milk. Thyroid is not associated with serious adverse reactions.

Children: Congenital hypothyroidism – Pregnant women provide little or no thyroid hormone to the fetus. Routine determinations of serum T_4 or TSH are strongly advised in neonates in view of the deleterious effects of thyroid deficiency on growth and development. In infants, excessive doses of thyroid hormone preparations may produce craniosynostosis. In children, partial loss of hair may be experienced in the first few months of thyroid therapy; this is usually a transient phenomenon that results in later recovery.

Precautions:

Monitoring: Treatment of patients with thyroid hormones requires the periodic assessment of thyroid status by means of appropriate laboratory tests. The TSH suppression test can be used to test the effectiveness of any thyroid preparation. Serum T_4 levels can be used to test the effectiveness of all thyroid medications except T_3. When the total serum T_4 is low but TSH is normal, a test specific to assess unbound (free) T_4 levels is warranted.

Decreased bone density: Long-term levothyroxine therapy has been associated with decreased bone density in the hip and spine in pre- and postmenopausal women.

Drug Interactions:

Drugs that may affect thyroid hormones include cholestyramine, colestipol and estrogens. Drugs that may be affected by thyroid hormones include anticoagulants, beta blockers, digitalis glycosides and theophyllines.

Drug/Lab test interactions: Consider changes in TBg concentration when interpreting T_4 and T_3 values. In such cases, measure the unbound (free) hormone.

Effects of Drugs on Thyroid Function Tests

Blank space signifies no data ↑ Increased ⇧ Slightly increased ↓ Decreased ⇩ Slightly decreased 0 No effect	Free T_4	Serum T_4	T_3 uptake resin	Free thyroxine index (FTI)	Serum T_3	Serum TSH
p-aminosalicylic acid		↓		↓		
Aminoglutethimide		↓				↑
Amiodarone	0/↑	↑		↑	↓	↑
Anabolic steroids/androgens	0	↓	↑	0	↓	0
Antithyroid (PTU, methimazole)	0	0	↓	0	↓	0
Asparaginase		↓	↑	0	↓	0
Barbiturates	0	↓	0/⇧	↓	0	0
Carbamazepine	0/↓	↓	0/↑	↓	0/↑	0/↑
Chloral hydrate		↓	0/⇧	0	⇩	0
Cholestiramine	0	↓		↓	0/↑	0
Clofibrate	0	↑	↓	0	↑	0
Colestipol	0	↓		↓	0/↑	0/↑
Contraceptives, oral	0	↑	↓	0	↓	0
Corticosteroids	0	↓	↑	0	↓	0/↓
Danazol	0	↓	↑	0	↓	0
Diazepam		↓		⇩		
Estrogens	0	↑	↓	0/⇧	↑	0
Ethionamide		↓				
Fluorouracil		↓	0/⇧	0	↓	0
Heparin (IV)		↓	0/↑	↑	0	
Insulin		↑				
Lithium carbonate		0/↓	0/↓	0/↓	0/↓	0/↑
Methadone		↑	↓	0	↑	0
Mitotane		↓	0/⇧	0	↓	0
Nitroprusside		↓				
Oxyphenbutazone/phenylbutazone		↓	0/⇧	0	↓	0
Perphenazine		↑	↓	↓	↑	
Phenytoin	0/↓	↓	0/⇧	↓	0/↑	0/↑
Propranolol	0	0/↓	0/↑	0/↓	0/↓	0
Resorcinol (excessive topical use)		↓	↓	↓	↓	↑
Salicylates (large doses)	0	↓	0/⇧	0	↓	0
Sulfonylureas		↓	0	0		
Thiazides		0			↑	

Drug/Food interactions: Fasting increases the absorption of T_4 from the GI tract.

Adverse Reactions:

Adverse reactions other than those indicating hyperthyroidism due to therapeutic overdosage, either initially or during the maintenance period, are rare. Symptoms of overdosage include: Palpitations; tachycardia; arrhythmias; angina pectoris; cardiac arrest; tremors; headache; nervousness; insomnia; diarrhea; vomiting; weight loss; menstrual irregularities; sweating; heat intolerance; fever.

Administration and Dosage:

Generally, institute thyroid therapy at relatively low doses and slowly increase in small increments until the desired response is obtained. Administer thyroid as a single daily dose, preferably before breakfast.

Treatment of choice for hypothyroidism is T_4 under most circumstances because of its consistent potency, restoration of normal constant serum levels of T_4 and T_3 and its prolonged duration of action. However, it has a slow onset of action and its effects are cumulative over several weeks.

Dosage equivalents of thyroid products: In changing from one thyroid product to another, the following dosage equivalents may be used. However, each patient may still require fine dosage adjustments because these equivalents are only estimates.

Dosage Equivalents of Thyroid Products

Preparation	Composition ratio T_4	Composition ratio T_3	Dosage equivalents
Crude hormone			
Thyroid USP	2 to 5	1	60 mg (1 grain)
Thyroglobulin	2.5	1	60 mg
Thyroid Strong	3.1	1	45 mg
Synthetic hormone			
Levothyroxine	1	0	0.05 to 0.06 mg[1]
Liothyronine	0	1	15 to 37.5 mcg
Liotrix	4	1	50 to 60 mcg T_4 and 12.5 to 15 mcg T_3

[1] Previously considered to be 0.1 mg.

THYROID DESICCATED:

Hypothyroidism –

Initial dosage: Usual starting dose is 30 mg, with increments of 15 mg every 2 to 3 weeks. Use 15 mg/day in patients with long-standing mxyedema, particularly if cardiovascular impairment is suspected.

Maintenance dosage: 60 to 120 mg/day; failure to respond to 180 mg doses suggests lack of compliance or malabsorption.

Thyroid cancer – Larger amounts of thyroid hormone than those used for replacement therapy are required.

Children – In infants with congenital hypothyroidism, institute therapy with full doses as soon as diagnosis is made.

Recommended Pediatric Dosage of Dessicated Thyroid for Congenital Hypothyroidism

Age	Dose per day (mg)	Daily dose per kg (mg)
0 to 6 mos	15 to 30	4.8 to 6
6 to 12 mos	30 to 45	3.6 to 4.8
1 to 5 yrs	45 to 60	3 to 3.6
6 to 12 yrs	60 to 90	2.4 to 3
> 12 yrs	> 90	1.2 to 1.8

LEVOTHYROXINE SODIUM (T_4; L-thyroxine):

Hypothyroidism –

Initial dosage: Usual starting dose is 0.05 mg, with increments of 0.025 mg every 2 to 3 weeks. Use ≤ 0.025 mg/day in patients with long-standing hypothyroidism, particularly if cardiovascular impairment is suspected.

Maintenance dosage: Most patients require no more than 0.2 mg/day; failure to respond to 0.3 mg doses suggests lack of compliance or malabsorption.

IV or IM injection can be substituted for the oral dosage form when oral ingestion is precluded for long periods of time. The initial parenteral dosage should be ≈ ½ of the previously established oral dosage.

Myxedema coma – Consider a medical emergency. Levothyroxine may be administered via nasogastric tube, but the IV route is preferred. A starting dose of 0.4 mg given rapidly is usually well tolerated, even in elderly.

The initial dose is followed by daily supplements of 0.1 to 0.2 mg IV. Normal T_4 levels are achieved in 24 hours followed in 3 days by threefold elevation of T_3. Maintain continued daily IV administration of lesser amounts until the patient is fully capable of accepting a daily oral dose.

A daily maintenace dose of 0.05 to 0.1 mg parenterally should suffice to maintain the euthyroid state, once established. Resume oral therapy as soon as the clinical situation has been stabilized and the patient is able to take oral medication.

TSH suppression in thyroid cancer, nodules and euthyroid goiters – Larger amounts of thyroid hormone than those used for replacement therapy are required. This therapy is also used in treating nontoxic solitary nodules and multi-nodular goiters, and to prevent thyroid enlargement in chronic (Hashimoto's) thyroiditis.

Thyroid suppression therapy – 2.6 mcg/kg/day for 7 to 10 days. These doses usually yield normal serum T_4 and T_3 levels and lack of response to TSH.

Children – Follow the recommendations in the following table. In infants with congenital hypothyroidism, institute therapy with full doses as soon as diagnosis is made.

Levothyroxine tablets may be given to infants and children who cannot swallow intact tablets. Crush the proper dose tablet and suspend in a small amount of formula or water. The suspension can be given by spoon or dropper. Do NOT store the suspension for any period of time. The crushed tablet may also be sprinkled over a small amount of food such as cooked cereal or applesauce.

Recommended Pediatric Dosage for Congenital Hypothyroidism

Age	Dose per day (mcg)	Daily dose per kg (mcg)
0 to 6 months	25 to 50	8 to 10
6 to 12 months	50 to 75	6 to 8
1 to 5 years	75 to 100	5 to 6
6 to 12 years	100 to 150	4 to 5
> 12 years	> 150	2 to 3

Alternative suggested doses include: 0 to 1 year, 8 to 10 mcg/kg/day; 1 to 5 years, 4 to 6 mcg/kg/day; > 5 years to adolescence, 3 to 4 mcg/kg/day.

LIOTHYRONINE SODIUM (T_3):

Mild hypothyroidism – Starting dose is 25 mcg/day. Daily dosage may then be increased by 12.5 or 25 mcg every 1 or 2 weeks. Usual maintenance dose is 25 to 75 mcg/day. Smaller doses may be fully effective in some patients, while dosages of 100 mcg/day may be required in others.

Congenital hypothyroidism – Starting dose is 5 mcg/day, with a 5 mcg increment every 3 to 4 days until the desired response is achieved. Infants a few months old may require only 20 mcg/day for maintenance. At 1 year of age, 50 mcg/day may be required. Above 3 years, full adult dosage may be necessary.

Simple (nontoxic) goiter – Starting dose is 5 mcg/day. Dosage may be increased every 1 to 2 weeks by 5 or 10 mcg. When 25 mcg/day is reached, dosage may be increased every 1 to 2 weeks by 12.5 or 25 mcg. Usual maintenance dosage is 75 mcg/day.

T_3 suppression test – 75 to 100 mcg daily for 7 days, then repeat I^{131} Thyroid Uptake test.

Myxedema – Starting dose is 5 mcg/day. This may be increased by 5 to 10 mcg/day every 1 to 2 weeks. When 25 mcg/day is reached, dosage may be increased by 12.5 or 25 mcg every 1 or 2 weeks. Usual maintenance dose is 50 to 100 mcg/day.

Myxedema coma/precoma (injection only) – Liothyronine injection is for IV use only; do not give IM or SC. Proper administration of an adequate dose is important in determining clinical outcome. Give ≥ 4 hours, and ≤ 12 hours, apart. Giving ≥ 65 mcg/day initially is associated with lower mortality. There is limited experience with > 100 mg/day.

An initial IV dose ranging from 25 to 50 mcg is recommended in the emergency treatment of myxedema complications in adults. In patients with known or suspected cardiovascular disease, an initial dose of 10 to 20 mcg is suggested.

Switching to oral therapy: Resume oral therapy as soon as the clinical situation has been stabilized and the patient is able to take oral medication.

Elderly or children – Start therapy with 5 mcg/day; increase only by 5 mcg increments at the recommended intervals.

LIOTRIX:

Hypothyroidism –

Initial dosage: Usual starting dose is 30 mg with 15 mg increments every 2 to 3 weeks. Use 15 mg/day in patients with long-standing hypothyroidism, particularly if cardiovascular impairment is suspected.

Maintenance dosage: Most patients require 60 to 120 mg/day; failure to respond to 180 mg doses suggests lack of compliance or malabsorption.

Thyroid cancer: Larger amounts of thyroid hormone than those used for replacement therapy are required.

Children – In infants with congenital hypothyroidism, institute therapy with full doses as soon as diagnosis is made.

Recommended Pediatric Dosage for Congenital Hypothyroidism		
	Tetraiodothyronine (T_4, levothyroxine) sodium	
Age	Dose per day	Daily dose per kg of body weight
0-6 mos	25-50 mcg	8-10 mcg
6-12 mos	50-75 mcg	6-8 mcg
1-5 yrs	75-100 mcg	5-6 mcg
6-12 yrs	100-150 mcg	4-5 mcg
over 12 yrs	over 150 mcg	2-3 mcg

ANTITHYROID AGENTS

PROPYLTHIOURACIL	
Tablets: 50 mg (*Rx*)	Various
METHIMAZOLE	
Tablets: 5 and 10 mg (*Rx*)	*Tapazole* (Lilly)

Actions:

Pharmacology: Propylthiouracil (PTU) and methimazole inhibit the synthesis of thyroid hormones and, thus, are effective in the treatment of hyperthyroidism. They do not inactivate existing thyroxine (T_4) and triiodothyronine (T_3) nor do they interfere with the effectiveness of exogenous thyroid hormones. PTU partially inhibits the peripheral conversion of T_4 to T_3.

Pharmacokinetics:

Various Pharmacokinetic Parameters of Antithyroid Agents						
Antithyroid agent	Bioavailability (%)	Protein binding (%)	Transplacental passage	Breast milk levels (M:P)[1]	Half-life(hrs)	Excreted in urine (%)
Propylthiouracil	80-95	75-80	Low	Low (0.1)	1-2	< 35
Methimazole	80-95	0	High	High (1)	6-13	< 10

[1] Approximate milk:plasma ratio.

Indications:

Hyperthyroidism: Long-term therapy may lead to disease remission. Also used to ameliorate hyperthyroidism in preparation for subtotal thyroidectomy or radioactive iodine therapy.

PTU is also used when thyroidectomy is contraindicated or not advisable.

Unlabeled uses: PTU may help reduce the mortality due to alcoholic liver disease by reducing the hepatic hypermetabolic state induced by alcohol.

Contraindications:

Hypersensitivity to antithyroid drugs; lactation.

Warnings:

Agranulocytosis is potentially the most serious side effect of therapy. Leukopenia, thrombocytopenia and aplastic anemia (pancytopenia) may also occur.

Pregnancy: Category D. These agents, used judiciously, are effective drugs in hyperthyroidism complicated by pregnancy. Because they readily cross the placenta and can induce goiter and even cretinism in the developing fetus, it is important that a sufficient, but not excessive, dose be given. If an antithyroid agent is needed, PTU is preferred because it is less likely than methimazole to cross the placenta and induce fetal/neonatal complications.

Lactation: Postpartum patients receiving antithyroid preparations should not nurse their babies. However, if necessary, the preferred drug is PTU.

Children: In several case reports, PTU hepatotoxicity has occurred in pediatric patients.

Precautions:

Monitoring: Monitor thyroid function tests periodically during therapy.

Hemorrhagic effects: Because PTU may cause hypoprothrombinemia and bleeding, monitor prothrombin time during therapy, especially before surgical procedures.

Drug Interactions:

Drugs that may interact with antithyroid agents include anticoagulants.

Adverse Reactions:

Agranulocytosis is the most serious effect.

Administration and Dosage:

PROPYLTHIOURACIL (PTU): Usually given in 3 equal doses at ≈ 8 hour intervals.

Adults –

Initial: 300 mg/day. In patients with severe hyperthyroidism, very large goiters, or both, the initial dosage is usually 400 mg/day; an occasional patient will require 600 to 900 mg/day initially.

Maintenance: Usually, 100 to 150 mg daily.

Children –

6 to 10 years: Initial dose is 50 to 150 mg/day.

≥ 10 years: Initial dose is 150 to 300 mg/day.

Maintenance: Determined by patient response.

Another suggested dosage for children is as follows:

Initial: 5 to 7 mg/kg/day or 150 to 200 mg/m^2/day in divided doses q8h.

Maintenance: ⅓ to ⅔ the intial dose beginning when the patient is euthyroid.

METHIMAZOLE: Usually given in 3 equal doses at ≈ 8 hour intervals.

Adults –

Initial: 15 mg daily for mild hyperthyroidism, 30 to 40 mg/day for moderately severe hyperthyroidism and 60 mg/day for severe hyperthyroidism.

Maintenance: 5 to 15 mg/day.

Children –

Initial: 0.4 mg/kg daily.

Maintenance: ≈ ½ the initial dose.

Another suggested dosage for children is as follows:

Initial: 0.5 to 0.7 mg/kg/day or 15 to 20 mg/m^2/day in 3 divided doses.

Maintenance: ⅓ to ⅔ of intial dose beginning when the patient is euthyroid.

Maximum: 30 mg/24 hours.

BISPHOSPHONATES

ALENDRONATE	
Tablets: 10 and 40 mg (*Rx*)	*Fosamax* (Merck)
ETIDRONATE DISODIUM (ORAL)	
Tablets: 200 and 400 mg (*Rx*)	*Didronel* (Procter & Gamble Pharm.)
ETIDRONATE DISODIUM (PARENTERAL)	
Injection: 300 mg per amp (*Rx*)	*Didronel IV* ,(MGI Pharma)
PAMIDRONATE DISODIUM	
Powder for Injection, lyophilized: 30, 60 and 90 mg (*Rx*)	*Aredia* (Ciba)

Actions:

Pharmacology: Etidronate disodium (EHDP) and pamidronate disodium (APD) are bisphosphonates that act primarily on bone. Their major pharmacologic action is the inhibition of normal and abnormal bone resorption. The exact mechanism(s) is not fully understood, but may be related to inhibition of hydroxyapatite crystal dissolution or its action on bone resorbing cells. Secondarily, etidronate reduces bone formation since formation is coupled to resorption; pamidronate inhibits bone resorption apparently without inhibiting bone formation and mineralization. Alendronate, a highly selective inhibitor of resoprtion, is a 100- to 500-fold more potent inhibitor of bone resorption. Reduction of abnormal bone resorption is responsible for therapeutic benefit in hypercalcemia.

Pharmacokinetics:

Alendronate – There is no evidence that alendronate is metabolized. Relative to an IV reference dose, mean oral bioavailability in women was 0.7%. Oral bioavailability of the 10 mg tablet in men (0.59%) was similar to that in women (0.78%). Mean steady-state volume of distribution (exclusive of bone) is ≥ 28 L. Protein binding in plasma is ≈ 78%. After a single IV dose, ≈ 50% was excreted in the urine with little or none recovered in the feces. Plasma levels fell by > 95% within 6 hours after IV administration. The terminal half-life is estimated to exceed 10 years, probably reflecting alendronate release from the skeleton.

Etidronate is not metabolized. Absorption averages about 1% of an oral dose of 5 mg/kg/day, increasing to about 2.5% at 10 mg/kg/day and 6% at 20 mg/kg/day. Most absorbed drug is cleared from blood in 6 hours. Within 24 hours, about half the absorbed dose is excreted in urine. The remainder is chemically adsorbed to bone and is slowly eliminated. Unabsorbed drug is excreted intact in feces.

A large fraction of the infused dose is excreted rapidly and unchanged in the urine. The mean volume of distribution at steady state in healthy subjects is 1370 ± 203 ml/kg while the plasma half-life is 6 ± 0.7 hours. In these same subjects, nonrenal clearance from the exchangeable pool amounts to 30% to 50% of the infused dose. This nonrenal clearance is due to uptake by bone; subsequently, the drug is slowly eliminated through bone turnover. The half-life on bone is > 90 days.

Pamidronate – In cancer patients who were given a 60 mg IV infusion over 4 or 24 hours, a mean of 51% (32% to 80%) was excreted unchanged in urine within 72 hours. Body retention during this period was calculated to be a mean of 49% (range, 20% to 68%) of the dose. Urinary excretion rate profile after 60 mg over 4 hours exhibited biphasic disposition characteristics with an alpha half-life of 1.6 hours and a beta half-life of 27.2 hours.

Indications:

Alendronate: Osteoporosis in postmenopausal women.

Paget's disease of the bone.

Etidronate:

Paget's disease of bone, symptomatic (oral) –

Heterotopic ossification (oral) – Prevention and treatment following total hip replacement or due to spinal injury.

Hypercalcemia of malignancy inadequately managed by dietary modification or oral hydration (parenteral).

Hypercalcemia of malignancy which persists after adequate hydration has been restored (parenteral).

Pamidronate: *Paget's disease of bone.*
Hypercalcemia of malignancy

Unlabeled uses:
Etidronate has been used to treat postmenopausal osteoporosis.
Pamidronate may be useful in treating the following conditions: Postmenopausal osteoporosis; bone metastases from breast cancer to prevent further tumor-related hypercalcemia and reduce incidence of pathological fractures and severe bone pain; hyperparathyroidism; to prevent glucocorticoid-induced osteoporosis; to reduce bone pain in patients with prostatic carcinoma and multiple myeloma osteolytic lesions; immobilization-related hypercalcemia.

Contraindications:
Hypersensitivity to bisphosphonates or any component of the products; hypocalcemia (alendronate); Class Dc and higher renal impairment (serum creatinine > 5 mg/dl; etidronate only).

Warnings:
Osteoporosis (alendronate): Consider causes other than estrogen deficiency and aging.

Paget's disease (etidronate): Response may be slow and may continue for months after treatment discontinuation. Do not increase dosage prematurely or resume treatment before there is evidence of reactivation of disease process.

Renal function impairment: It is likely that alendronate elimination via the kidney will be reduced in impaired renal function. Therefore, somewhat greateraccumulation of alendronate in bone might be expected in impaired renal function. No dosage adjustment is necessary in mild-to-moderate renal insufficiency. Alendronate use is not recommended in more severe renal insufficiency. Occasional mild to moderate renal function abnormalities (elevated BUN or serum creatinine) have occurred when etidronate was given to patients with hypercalcemia of malignancy. Reduction of the etidronate dose, if used at all, may be advisable in Class Cc renal functional impairment. In patients with Class Dc and higher renal functional impairment, withhold etidronate. Patients with hypercalcemia who receive an IV infusion of pamidronate should have periodic lab and clinical evaluations of renal function.

Pregnancy: *Category B (oral etidronate); Category C (alendronate, parenteral etidronate and pamidronate).*

Lactation: It is not known whether these drugs are excreted in breast milk. Do not give alendronate to a nursing mother.

Children: Safety and efficacy for use in children have not been established. Children have been treated with etidronate at doses recommended for adults, to prevent heterotopic ossifications or soft tissue calcifications.

Precautions:
Monitoring: Carefully monitor standard hypercalcemia-related metabolic parameters, such as serum levels of calcium, phosphate, magnesium and potassium following pamidronate initiation. Asymptomatic hypophosphatemia (16%), hypokalemia (7% to 9%), hypomagnesemia (11% to 12%) and hypocalcemia (5% to 12%) have occurred. Also, closely monitor electrolytes, creatinine as well as CBC, differential and hematocrit/hemoglobin. Carefully monitor patients who have pre-existing anemia, leukopenia or thrombocytopenia in the first 2 weeks following treatment.

Nutrition: Patients should maintain adequate nutrition, particularly an adequate intake of calcium and vitamin D.

GI disorders: Use caution when using bisphosphonates in patients with active upper GI problems. Etidronate therapy has been withheld from patients with enterocolitis because diarrhea is seen in some patients, particularly at higher doses.

Osteoid: Etidronate suppresses bone turnover and may retard mineralization of osteoid laid down during the bone accretion process.

Fracture: In Paget's patients, treatment regimens of etidronate exceeding the recommended daily maximum dose of 20 mg/kg or continuous administration for periods > 6 months may be associated with an increased risk of fracture.

Hormone replacement therapy: Concomitant use with alendronate for osteoporosis in postmenopausal women is not recommended.

Hypocalcemia: In one trial, 33 of 185 patients (18%) treated one or more times with etidronate had serum calcium values below lower limits of normal.

Hypocalcemia (5% to 12%) has occurred with pamidronate therapy.

Hypocalcemia must be corrected before therapy initiation with alendronate. Presumably due to the effects of alendronate on increasing bone mineral, small asymptomatic decreases in serum calcium and phosphate may occur, especially in patients with Paget's disease, in whom the pretreatment rate of bone turnover may be greatly elevated.

Drug Interactions:

Drugs that may interact with alendronate include ranitidine, calcium supplements, antacids and aspirin. The patient should wait ≥ 30 minutes after taking alendronate before taking any other drug.

Drug/Food interactions: Absorption of etidronate, complete in 2 hours, may be reduced by foods or other preparations containing divalent cations.

Adverse Reactions:

Alendronate: Musculoskeletal pain (4% to 6%); asymptomatic, mild and transient decreases in serum calcium and phosphate (≈ 18% and 10%, respectively).

Etidronate: GI complaints (≈ 6.7%). At 10 to 20 mg/kg/day, this may increase to 20% or 30%. Increased or recurrent bone pain at pagetic sites, or the onset of pain at previously asymptomatic sites has occurred. At 5 mg/kg/day, ≈ 10% report these phenomena. At higher doses, the incidence rises to ≈ 20%. In ≈ 10% of patients, occasional mild to moderate abnormalities in renal function (increases of > 0.5 mg/dl serum creatinine) were observed during or immediately after treatment. A metallic, altered or loss of taste, which usually disappeared within hours, occurred in 5% of patients.

Pamidronate: Transient mild elevation of temperature by at least 1°C was noted 24 to 48 hours after administration (21% to 34%). Drug-related local soft tissue symptoms (redness, swelling or induration and pain on palpation) at the site of catheter insertion were most common (18%) in patients treated with 90 mg. When all on-therapy events are considered, that rate rises to 41%. Adverse reactions in at least 15% of patients include: Fluid overload; generalized pain; hypertension; abdominal pain; anorexia; constipation; nausea; vomiting; urinary tract infection; bone pain; anemia; hypokalemia; hypomagnesemia; hypophosphatemia. Other adverse reactions include: Hypertension, arthrosis, bone pain, headache (10%); fever, nausea, back pain (5%).

Bisphosphonate Adverse Reactions (%)[1]

	Pamidronate			Etidronate (n = 35)	Alendronate (n = 196)[2]
Adverse reaction	60 mg over 4 hr (n = 23)	60 mg over 24 hr (n = 17)	90 mg over 24 hr (n = 17)	7.5 mg/kg x 3 days	10 mg/day
General					
Fever	26	19	18	9	0
Infusion site reaction	0	4	18	0	0
Fatigue	0	0	12	0	0
Moniliasis	0	0	6	0	0
Fluid overload	0	0	0	6	0
Respiratory					
Rales/Rhinitis	0	0	6	0	0
URI	0	3	0	0	0
Dyspnea	0	0	0	3	0
Cardiovascular					
Atrial fibrillation	0	0	6	0	0
Hypertension	0	0	6	0	0
Syncope	0	0	6	0	0
Tachycardia	0	0	6	0	0

Bisphosphonate Adverse Reactions (%)[1]					
	Pamidronate			Etidronate (n = 35)	Alendronate (n = 196)[2]
Adverse reaction	60 mg over 4 hr (n = 23)	60 mg over 24 hr (n = 17)	90 mg over 24 hr (n = 17)	7.5 mg/kg x 3 days	10 mg/day
GI					
Nausea	4	0	18	6	3.6
Anorexia	4	1	12	0	0
Constipation	4	0	6	3	3.1
GI hemorrhage	0	0	6	0	0
Abdominal pain	0	1	0	0	6.6
Stomatitis	0	1	0	3	0
Diarrhea	0	1	0	0	3.1
Dyspepsia	4	0	0	0	3.6
Vomiting	4	0	0	0	1
CNS					
Somnolence	0	1	6	0	0
Psychosis	4	0	0	0	0
Convulsions	0	0	0	3	0
Hemic/Lymphatic					
Anemia	0	0	6	0	0
Leukopenia	4	0	0	0	0
Lab abnormalities					
Hypophosphatemia	0	9	18	3	0
Hypokalemia	4	4	18	0	0
Hypomagnesemia	4	10	12	3	0
Hypocalcemia	0	1	12	0	0
Abnormal hepatic function	0	0	0	3	0
Other					
Hypothyroidism	0	0	6	0	0
Uremia	4	0	0	0	0
Taste perversion	0	0	0	3	0.5

[1] Data are pooled from separate studies and are not necessarily comparable.
[2] Alendronate was used for osteoporosis in postmenopausal women in this study.

Administration and Dosage:

ETIDRONATE DISODIUM (ORAL): Administer as a single dose. However, if GI discomfort occurs, divide the dose.

Paget's disease –

Initial treatment: 5 to 10 mg/kg/day (not to exceed 6 months) or 11 to 20 mg/kg/day (not to exceed 3 months). Reserve doses > 10 mg/kg/day for use when lower doses are ineffective, when there is an overriding requirement for suppression of increased bone turnover or when prompt reduction of elevated cardiac output is required. Doses > 20 mg/kg/day are not recommended.

Retreatment: Initiate only after an etidronate-free period of at least 90 days and if there is biochemical, symptomatic or other evidence of active disease process. Retreatment regimens are the same as for initial treatment. For most patients, the original dose will be adequate for retreatment.

Heterotopic ossification –

Due to spinal cord injury: 20 mg/kg/day for 2 weeks, followed by 10 mg/kg/day for 10 weeks; total treatment period is 12 weeks. Institute as soon as feasible following the injury, preferably prior to evidence of heterotopic ossification.

Complicating total hip replacement: 20 mg/kg/day for 1 month preoperatively, then 20 mg/kg/day for 3 months postoperatively; total treatment period is 4 months.

ETIDRONATE DISODIUM (PARENTERAL):

Recommended dose is 7.5 mg/kg/day for 3 successive days.

Infusion time – Administer the diluted dose IV over a period of at least 2 hours. Slow infusion is important. The usual course of treatment is one infusion of 7.5 mg/kg/day on each of 3 consecutive days, but some patients have been treated for up to 7 days.

Retreatment may be appropriate if hypercalcemia recurs. There should be at least a 7 day interval between courses of treatment. The dose and manner of retreatment is the same as that for initial treatment. With renal impairment, dose reduction may be advisable.

Oral editronate may be started on the day after the last infusion. The recommended oral dose for patients who have had hypercalcemia is 20 mg/kg/day for 30 days. If serum calcium levels remain normal or clinically acceptable, treatment may be extended. Use for > 90 days is not adequately studied and is not recommended.

PAMIDRONATE DISODIUM:

Hypercalcemia of malignancy –

Moderate hypercalcemia: The recommended dose in moderate hypercalcemia is 60 to 90 mg. The 60 mg dose is given as an initial, *single-dose*, IV infusion over at least 4 hours. The 90 mg dose must be given by an initial, *single-dose*, IV infusion over 24 hours.

Severe hypercalcemia: Recommended dose (corrected serum calcium > 13.5 mg/dl) is 90 mg, which must be given by initial *single-dose*, IV infusion over 24 hrs.

Retreatment: Retreatment, in patients who show complete or partial response initially, may be carried out if serum calcium does not return to normal or remain normal after initial treatment. Allow a minimum of 7 days to elapse before retreatment to allow for full response to the initial dose. The dose and manner of retreatment are identical to that of the initial therapy.

Paget's disease – The recommended dose in patients with moderate to severe Paget's disease of bone is 30 mg daily, given as a 4 hour infusion on 3 consecutive days for a total dose of 90 mg.

Retreatment: When clinically indicated, retreat at the dose of initial therapy.

ALENDRONATE: Alendronate must be taken at least 30 minutes before the first food, beverage or medication of the day with plain water only. Other beverages (including mineral water), food and some medications are likely to reduce the absorption of alendronate. Waiting > 30 minutes or taking the drug with food, berverages (other than plain water) or other medications will lessen the effect of the drug by decreasing its absoprtion. To facilitate delivery to the stomach, take with a full glass of water (6 to 8 oz.) and avoid lying down for at least 30 minutes thereafter.

Osteoporosis in postmenopausal women – 10 mg once a day. Safety of treatment for > 4 years has not been studied (extension studies are ongoing).

Paget's disease of bone – 40 mg once a day for 6 months.

Retreatment: Relapses during the 12 months following therapy occurred in 9% of patients who responded to treatment. Retreatment with alendronate may be considered, following a 6 month posttreatment evaluation period, in patients who have relapsed based on increases in serum alkaline phosphatase.

Chapter 4

CARDIOVASCULARS

THIAZIDES AND RELATED DIURETICS

BENDROFLUMETHIAZIDE	
Tablets: 5 and 10 mg (*Rx*)	*Naturetin* (Princeton)
BENZTHIAZIDE	
Tablets: 50 mg (*Rx*)	*Exna* (Robins)
CHLOROTHIAZIDE	
Tablets: 250 and 500 mg (*Rx*)	Various, *Diuril* (Merck), *Diurigen* (Goldline)
Suspension: 250 mg/5 ml (*Rx*)	*Diuril* (Merck)
Powder for injection, lyophylized:500 mg (as sodium) (*Rx*)	*Sodium Diuril* (Merck)
CHLORTHALIDONE	
Tablets: 15, 25, 50 and 100 mg (*Rx*)	Various, *Hygroton* (Rhone-Poulenc Rorer), *Thalitone* (Horus Therapeutics)
HYDROCHLOROTHIAZIDE	
Tablets: 25, 50 and 100 mg (*Rx*)	Various, *Esidrix* (Ciba), *Ezide* (Econo Med), *Hydro-DIURIL* (Merck), *Hydro-Par* (Parmed), *Oretic* (Abbott)
Solution: 50 mg per 5 ml (*Rx*)	*Hydrochlorothiazide* (Roxane)
HYDROFLUMETHIAZIDE	
Tablets: 50 mg (*Rx*)	Various, *Diucardin* (Wyeth-Ayerst), *Saluron* (Apothecon)
INDAPAMIDE	
Tablets: 1.25 and 2.5 mg (*Rx*)	Various, *Lozol* (Rhone-Poulenc Rorer)
METHYCLOTHIAZIDE	
Tablets: 2.5 and 5 mg (*Rx*)	Various, *Aquatensen* (Wallace), *Enduron* (Abbott)
METOLAZONE	
Tablets: 2.5, 5 and 10 mg (*Rx*)	*Zaroxolyn* (Fisons)
0.5 mg (*Rx*)	*Mykrox* (Fisons)
POLYTHIAZIDE	
Tablets: 1, 2 and 3 mg (*Rx*)	*Renese* (Pfizer)
QUINETHAZONE	
Tablets: 50 mg (*Rx*)	*Hydromox* (Lederle)
TRICHLORMETHIAZIDE	
Tablets: 2 and 4 mg	Various, *Diurese* (American Urologicals), *Metahydrin* (Marion Merrell Dow), *Naqua* (Schering)

Actions:

Pharmacology: Thiazide diuretics increase the urinary excretion of sodium and chloride in approximately equivalent amounts. They inhibit reabsorption of sodium and chloride in the cortical thick ascending limb of the loop of Henle and the early distal tubules. Other common actions include: Increased potassium and bicarbonate excretion, decreased calcium excretion and uric acid retention. At maximal therapeutic dosages all thiazides are approximately equal in diuretic efficacy.

The antihypertensive action requires several days to produce effects. Administration for up to 2 to 4 weeks is usually required for optimal therapeutic effect. The duration of the antihypertensive effect of the thiazides is sufficiently long to adequately control blood pressure with a single daily dose.

Pharmacokinetics:

Pharmacokinetics of Thiazides and Related Diuretics

Diuretic	Onset (hours)	Peak (hours)	Duration (hours)	Equivalent dose (mg)	Percent absorbed	Half-life (hours)
Bendroflumethiazide	2	4	16 to 12	5	≈ 100	3 to 3.9
Benzthiazide	2	4 to 6	16 to 18	50	nd[1]	nd[1]
Chlorothiazide	2[2]	4[2]	16 to 12	500	10 to 21[3]	0.75 to 2
Chlorthalidone	2 to 3	2 to 6	24 to 72	50	64[3]	40
Hydrochlorothiazide	2	4 to 6	16 to 12	50	65 to 75	5.6 to 14.8
Hydroflumethiazide	2	4	16 to 12	50	50	≈ 17

Pharmacokinetics of Thiazides and Related Diuretics						
Diuretic	Onset (hours)	Peak (hours)	Duration (hours)	Equivalent dose (mg)	Percent absorbed	Half-life (hours)
Indapamide	1 to 2	within 2	up to 36	2.5	93	≈ 14
Methyclothiazide	2	6	24	5	nd[1]	nd[1]
Metolazone[4]	1	2	12 to 24	5	65	nd[1]
Polythiazide	2	6	24 to 48	2	nd[1]	25.7
Quinethazone	2	6	18 to 24	50	nd[1]	nd[1]
Trichlormethiazide	2	6	24	2	nd[1]	2.3 to 7.3

[1] nd = No data.
[2] Following IV use, onset of action is 15 minutes; peak occurs in 30 minutes.
[3] Bioavailability may be dose-dependent.
[4] *Mykrox only:* Peak plasma concentrations reached in 2 to 4 hrs, t½ ≈ 14 hrs.

Indications:

Edema: Adjunctive therapy in edema associated with congestive heart failure (CHF), hepatic cirrhosis and corticosteroid and estrogen therapy. Useful in edema due to renal dysfunction (ie, nephrotic syndrome, acute glomerulonephritis, chronic renal failure).

Indapamide alone is indicated for edema associated with CHF.

Metolazone, rapidly acting (Mykrox) has not been evaluated for the treatment of CHF or fluid retention due to renal or hepatic disease, and the correct dosage for these conditions and other edematous states has not been established.

Hypertension: As the sole therapeutic agent or to enhance other antihypertensive drugs in more severe forms of hypertension.

Unlabeled uses:

Calcium nephrolithiasis – Thiazide diuretics have been used alone and in combination with amiloride or allopurinol to prevent formation and recurrence of calcium nephrolithiasis in hypercalciuric and normal calciuric patients.

Osteoporosis – Thiazide diuretics may be useful in reducing the incidence of osteoporosis in postmenopausal women, either alone or in combination with calcium or estrogen.

Diabetes insipidus – Thiazide diuretics reduce urine volume by 30% to 50%. They constitute the mainstay of therapy for nephrogenic diabetes insipidus.

Contraindications:

Anuria; renal decompensation; hypersensitivity to thiazides or related diuretics or sulfonamide-derived drugs; hepatic coma or precoma (metolazone).

Warnings:

Parenteral use: Use IV **chlorothiazide** only when patients are unable to take oral medication or in an emergency. In infants and children, IV use is not recommended.

Lupus erythematosus exacerbation or activation has occurred.

Hypersensitivity: Hypersensitivity reactions may occur in patients with or without a history of allergy or bronchial asthma; cross-sensitivity with sulfonamides may also occur. Refer to Management of Acute Hypersensitivity Reactions.

Renal function impairment: Use with caution in severe renal disease since these agents may precipitate azotemia. Cumulative effects of the drug may develop in patients with impaired renal function. Monitor renal function periodically.**Metolazone** is the only thiazide-like diuretic that may produce diuresis in patients with GFR < 20 ml/min. Indapamide may also be useful in patients with impaired renal function.

Pregnancy: Category B *(chlorothiazide, chlorthalidone, hydrochlorothiazide, indapamide, metolazone)*; Category C *(bendroflumethiazide, benzthiazide, hydroflumethiazide, methyclothiazide, trichlormethiazide)*. Routine use during normal pregnancy is inappropriate.

Lactation: Thiazides may appear in breast milk. Discontinue nursing or the drug.

Children: Bendroflumethiazide, benzthiazide, chlorthalidone, hydrochlorothiazide, methyclothiazide, metolazone, hydroflumethiazide, trichlormethiazide – Safety and efficacy have not been established. Metolazone is not recommended for use in children. In infants and children, IV use of chlorothiazide has been limited and is generally not recommended.

Precautions:

Fluid/electrolyte balance: Perform initial and periodic determinations of serum electrolytes, BUN, uric acid and glucose. Observe patients for clinical signs of fluid or electrolyte imbalance (eg, hyponatremia, hypochloremic alkalosis, hypokalemia, changes in serum and urinary calcium).

Hypokalemia may develop during concomitant corticosteroids, ACTH and especially with brisk diuresis, with severe liver disease or cirrhosis, vomiting or diarrhea, or after prolonged therapy.

Hyponatremia/Hypochloremia – A chloride deficit is generally mild and usually does not require specific treatment, except in extraordinary circumstances (as in liver or renal disease). Thiazide-induced hyponatremia has been associated with death and neurologic damage in elderly patients.

Hypomagnesemia – Thiazide diuretics have been shown to increase urinary excretion of magnesium, resulting in hypomagnesemia.

Hypercalcemia – Calcium excretion may be decreased by thiazide diuretics.

Hyperuricemia may occur or acute gout may be precipitated in certain patients receiving thiazides, even in those patients without a history of gouty attacks.

Glucose tolerance – Hyperglycemia may occur with thiazide diuretics.

Lipids: Thiazides may cause increased concentrations of total serum cholesterol, total triglycerides and LDL (but not HDL) in some patients, although these appear to return to pretreatment levels with long-term therapy.

Photosensitivity: Photosensitization may occur.

Drug Interactions:

Drugs that may be affected by thiazides include: Allopurinol; anesthetics; anticoagulants; antigout agents; antineoplastics; calcium salts; diazoxide; digitalis glycosides; insulin; lithium; loop diuretics; methyldopa; nondepolarizing muscle relaxants; sulfonylureas; vitamin D. Drugs that may affect thiazides include: Amphotericin B; anticholinergics; bile acid sequestrants; corticosteroids; methenamines; NSAIDs.

Drug/Lab test interactions: Thiazides may decrease serum PBI levels without signs of thyroid disturbance. Thiazides may also cause diagnostic interference of serum electrolyte levels, blood and urine glucose levels (usually only in patients with a predisposition to glucose intolerance), serum bilirubin levels and serum uric acid levels. In uremic patients, serum magnesium levels may be increased.
Bendroflumethiazide and **trichlormethiazide** may interfere with the **phenolsulfonphthalein test** due to decreased excretion. In the **phentolamine** and **tyramine tests,** bendroflumethiazide may produce false-negative and trichlormethiazide may produce false-positive results.

Adverse Reactions:

Adverse Reactions of Thiazides and Related Diuretics												
Adverse reaction	Bendroflumethiazide	Benzthiazide	Chlorothiazide	Chlorthalidone	Hydrochlorothiazide	Hydroflumethiazide	Indapamide	Methyclothiazide	Metolazone	Polythiazide	Quinethazone	Trichlormethiazide
Cardiovascular												
Orthostatic hypotension	✓	✓	✓		✓	✓	<5%	✓	<2%[1]	✓	✓	✓
Palpitations							<5%		<2%[2]			✓
CNS												
Dizziness/Lightheadedness	✓	✓	✓	✓	✓	✓	≥5%	✓	10%[2]	✓	✓	✓
Vertigo	✓		✓	✓	✓	✓	<5%	✓	✓[3]	✓	✓	✓
Headache	✓	✓	✓	✓	✓	✓	≥5%	✓	9%[2]	✓	✓	✓
Paresthesias	✓	✓	✓	✓	✓	✓		✓	✓[3]	✓	✓	✓
Xanthopsia	✓	✓	✓	✓	✓	✓		✓		✓	✓	✓
Weakness	✓	✓	✓	✓	✓	✓	≥5%	✓	<2%[4]	✓	✓	✓
Restlessness/Insomnia	✓	✓	✓	✓	✓	✓	<5%	✓	✓[3]	✓	✓	✓
Drowsiness							<5%		✓[3]			✓
Fatigue/Lethargy/Malaise/Lassitude							≥5%		4%[2]			✓
Anxiety							≥5%		<2%[3]			
Depression							<5%		<2%[2]			✓
Nervousness							≥5%		<2%[3]			
Blurred vision (may be transient)	✓		✓		✓	✓	<5%		✓[3]			
GI												
Anorexia	✓	✓	✓	✓	✓	✓	<5%	✓	✓[3]	✓	✓	✓
Gastric irritation/epigastric distress	✓	✓	✓	✓	✓	✓	<5%	✓		✓	✓	✓
Nausea	✓	✓	✓	✓	✓	✓	<5%	✓	<2%[2]	✓	✓	✓
Vomiting	✓	✓	✓	✓	✓	✓	<5%	✓	<2%[4]	✓	✓	✓
Abdominal pain/cramping/bloating	✓	✓	✓	✓	✓	✓	<5%	✓	<2%[2]	✓	✓	✓
Diarrhea	✓	✓	✓	✓	✓	✓	<5%	✓	<2%[2]	✓	✓	✓
Constipation	✓	✓	✓	✓	✓	✓	<5%	✓	<2%[2]	✓	✓	✓
Jaundice (intrahepatic/ cholestatic)	✓	✓	✓	✓	✓	✓		✓	✓[3]	✓	✓	✓
Pancreatitis	✓	✓	✓	✓	✓	✓		✓	✓[3]	✓	✓	✓
Dry mouth							<5%		<2%[1]			✓
GU												
Nocturia							<5%		<2%[1]			
Impotence/Reduced libido	✓	✓	✓	✓	✓	✓	<5%	✓	<2%[2]	✓	✓	✓
Hematologic:												
Leukopenia	✓	✓	✓	✓	✓	✓		✓	✓[3]	✓	✓	✓
Thrombocytopenia	✓	✓	✓	✓	✓	✓		✓		✓	✓	✓
Agranulocytosis	✓	✓	✓	✓	✓	✓		✓	✓[3]	✓	✓	✓
Aplastic/Hypoplastic anemia	✓	✓	✓	✓	✓	✓		✓	✓[3]	✓	✓	✓
Dermatologic												
Purpura	✓	✓	✓	✓	✓	✓		✓	✓[3]	✓	✓	✓
Photosensitivity/Photosensitivity dermatitis	✓	✓	✓	✓	✓	✓		✓	✓[3]	✓	✓	✓
Rash	✓	✓	✓	✓	✓	✓	<5%	✓	<2%[2]	✓	✓	✓
Urticaria	✓	✓	✓	✓	✓	✓			✓[3]	✓	✓	✓
Necrotizing angiitis, vasculitis, cutaneous vasculitis	✓	✓	✓	✓	✓	✓	<5%	✓	✓[2]	✓	✓	✓
Pruritus	✓						<5%		<2%[1]			
Metabolic												
Hyperglycemia	✓	✓	✓	✓	✓	✓	<5%	✓	✓[3]	✓	✓	✓
Glycosuria	✓	✓	✓	✓	✓	✓	<5%	✓	✓[3]	✓	✓	✓
Hyperuricemia	✓	✓	✓	✓	✓	✓	<5%	✓		✓[3]		✓
Miscellaneous												
Muscle cramp/spasm	✓	✓	✓	✓	✓	✓	≥5%	✓	6%[2]	✓	✓	✓

[1] Percentage of occurrence refers to rapidly acting doseform, however this adverse reaction also occurred with the slow acting doseform.
[2] IV doseform.
[3] Possibly with life-threatening anaphylactic shock.
[4] Slow acting doseform only.
[5] Rapidly acting doseform only.

Administration and Dosage:

BENDROFLUMETHIAZIDE:

Edema – 5 mg once daily, preferably in the morning.

Initial: Up to 20 mg once daily or divided into 2 doses.

Maintenance: 2.5 to 5 mg daily.

Hypertension –

Initial: 5 to 20 mg daily.

Maintenance: 2.5 to 15 mg/day.

BENZTHIAZIDE:

Edema –

Initial: 50 to 200 mg daily for several days, or until dry weight is attained. If dosages exceed 100 mg/day, give in 2 doses, following morning and evening meal.

Maintenance: 50 to 150 mg daily.

Hypertension –

Initial: 50 to 100 mg daily. Give in 2 doses of 25 or 50 mg each, after breakfast and after lunch.

Maintenance: Maximal effective dose is 200 mg daily.

CHLOROTHIAZIDE:

Adults –

Edema: 0.5 to 1 g once or twice a day, orally or IV. Reserve IV route for patients unable to take oral medication or for emergency situations.

Hypertension (oral forms only): Starting dose is 0.5 to 1 g/day as a single or divided dose. Rarely, some patients may require up to 2 g/day in divided doses.

Infants and children –

Oral: 22 mg/kg/day (10 mg/lb/day) in 2 doses. Infants < 6 months may require up to 33 mg/kg/day (15 mg/lb/day) in 2 doses.

On this basis, infants up to 2 years of age may be given 125 to 375 mg daily in 2 doses. Children from 2 to 12 years of age may be given 375 mg to 1 g daily in 2 doses.

IV use is not generally recommended.

CHLORTHALIDONE: Give a single dose with food in the morning. Maintenance doses may be lower than initial doses.

Edema – Initiate therapy with 50 to 100 mg (*Thalitone*, 30 to 60 mg) daily, or 100 mg (*Thalitone*, 60 mg) on alternate days. Some patients may require 150 or 200 mg (*Thalitone*, 90 to 120 mg) at these intervals, or 120 mg *Thalitone* daily. Dosages above this level, however, do not usually create a greater response.

Hypertension – Initiate therapy with a single dose of 25 mg/day (*Thalitone*, 15 mg). If response is insufficient after a suitable trial, increase to 50 mg (*Thalitone*, increase from 30 to 50 mg). For additional control, increase dosage to 100 mg once daily (except *Thalitone*), or add a second antihypertensive.

Note: Doses > 25 mg/day are likely to potentiate potassium excretion but provide no further benefit in sodium excretion or blood pressure reduction.

HYDROCHLOROTHIAZIDE:

Adults –

Edema:

Initial – 25 to 200 mg daily for several days, or until dry weight is attained.

Maintenance – 25 to 100 mg daily or intermittently. Refractory patients may require up to 200 mg daily.

Hypertension –

Initial: 50 mg daily as a single or two divided doses. Doses > 50 mg are often associated with marked reductions in serum potassium. Patients usually do not require doses > 50 mg daily when combined with other antihypertensives.

Infants and children: Usual dosage is 2.2 mg/kg (1 mg/lb) daily in two doses. Pediatric patients with hypertension only rarely will benefit from doses > 50 mg daily.

Infants (< 6 months) – Up to 3.3 mg/kg (1.5 mg/lb) daily in two doses.

Infants (6 months to 2 years of age) – 12.5 to 37.5 mg daily in two doses. Base dosage on body weight.

Children (2 to 12 years of age) – 37.5 to 100 mg daily in two doses. Base dosage on body weight.

HYDROFLUMETHIAZIDE:

Edema –

Initial: 50 mg once or twice a day.

Maintenance: 25 mg to 200 mg daily. Administer in divided doses when dosage exceeds 100 mg daily.

Hypertension –

Initial: 50 mg twice daily.

Maintenance: 50 to 100 mg/day. Do not exceed 200 mg/day.

INDAPAMIDE:

Edema of congestive heart failure –

Adults: 2.5 mg as a single daily dose in the morning. If response is not satisfactory after 1 week, increase to 5 mg once daily.

Hypertension –

Adults: 1.25 mg as a single daily dose taken in the morning. If the response to 1.25 is not satisfactory after 4 weeks, increase the daily dose to 2.5 mg taken once daily. If the response to 2.5 mg is not satisfactory after 4 weeks, the daily dose may be increased to 5 mg taken once daily, but consider adding another antihypertensive.

METHYCLOTHIAZIDE:

Edema –

Adults: 2.5 to 10 mg once daily. Maximum effective single dose is 10 mg.

Hypertension –

Adults: 2.5 to 5 mg once daily. If blood pressure control is not satisfactory after 8 to 12 weeks with 5 mg once daily, add another antihypertensive.

METOLAZONE: Individualize dosage.

Zaroxolyn –

Mild to moderate essential hypertension: 2.5 to 5 mg once daily.

Edema of renal disease/cardiac failure: 5 to 20 mg once daily.

Mykrox –

Mild to moderate hypertension: 0.5 mg as a single daily dose taken in the morning. If response is inadequate, increase the dose to 1 mg daily. Do not increase dosage if blood pressure is not controlled with 1 mg. Rather, add another antihypertensive agent with a different mechanism of action.

Brand interchange – The metolazone formulations are not bioequivalent or therapeutically equivalent at the same doses. *Mykrox* is more rapidly and completely bioavailable. Do not interchange brands.

POLYTHIAZIDE:

Edema – 1 to 4 mg daily.

Hypertension – 2 to 4 mg daily.

QUINETHAZONE:

Adults – 50 to 100 mg once daily. Occasionally, 50 mg twice daily; 150 to 200 mg daily may be necessary infrequently.

TRICHLORMETHIAZIDE:

Edema – 2 to 4 mg once daily.

Hypertension – 2 to 4 mg once daily. In initiating therapy, doses may be given twice daily.

LOOP DIURETICS

BUMETANIDE	
Tablets: 0.5, 1 and 2 mg (*Rx*)	Various, *Bumex* (Roche)
Injection: 0.25 mg per ml (*Rx*)	
ETHACRYNIC ACID	
Tablets: 25, 50 mg (*Rx*)	*Edecrin* (Merck)
Powder for Injection: 50 mg (as ethacrynate sodium) per vial (*Rx*)	*Edecrin Sodium* (Merck)
FUROSEMIDE	
Tablets: 20, 40 and 80 mg (*Rx*)	Various, *Lasix* (Hoechst-Roussel)
Oral Solution: 10 mg/ml (*Rx*)	
Injection: 10 mg/ml (*Rx*)	
TORSEMIDE	
Tablets: 5, 10, 20 and 100 mg (*Rx*)	*Demadex* (Boehringer Mannheim)
Injection: 10 mg/ml (*Rx*)	*Demadex* (Boehringer Mannheim)

Warning:

These agents are potent diuretics; excess amounts can lead to a profound diuresis with water and electrolyte depletion.

Actions:

Pharmacology: Furosemide and ethacrynic acid inhibit primarily reabsorption of sodium and chloride, not only in proximal and distal tubules, but also the loop of Henle. In contrast, bumetanide is more chloruretic than natriuretic and may have an additional action in the proximal tubule; it does not appear to act on the distal tubule. Torsemide acts from within the lumen of the thick ascending portion of the loop of Henle, where it inhibits the $Na^+/K^+/2Cl^-$-carrier system.

Pharmacokinetics: These agents are metabolized and excreted primarily through the urine. Protein binding of these agents exceeds 90%. Furosemide is metabolized approximately 30% to 40%, and its urinary excretion is 60% to 70%. Oral administration of bumetanide revealed that 81% was excreted in urine, 45% of it as unchanged drug. Torsemide is cleared from the circulation by both hepatic metabolism (≈ 80% of total clearance) and excretion into the urine (≈ 20% of total clearance).

Pharmacokinetic Parameters of the Loop Diuretics

Diuretic	Bioavailability (%)	Half-life (min)	Onset of action (min)	Peak (min)	Duration (hr)	Dosage (mg)	Relative potency	Doses/day
Furosemide								
Oral	60-64[1]	≈ 120[2]	within 60	60-120[3]	6-8	20-80	1	1-2
IV or IM			within 5[4]	30	2	20-40	1	
Ethacrynic acid								
Oral	≈100	60	within 30	120	6-8	50-100	0.6-0.8	1-2
IV			within 5	15-30	2	50	0.6-0.8	1-2
Bumetanide								
Oral	72-96	60-90[5]	30-60	60-120	4-6	0.5-2	≈ 40	1
IV			within minutes	15-30	0.5-1	0.5-1	≈ 40	1-3
Torsemide								
Oral	≈ 80	210	within 60	60-120	6-8	5-20	2-4	1
IV			within 10	within 60	6-8	5-20	2-4	1

[1] Decreased in uremia and nephrosis.
[2] Prolonged in renal failure, uremia and in neonates.
[3] Decreased in CHF.
[4] Somewhat delayed after IM administration.
[5] Prolonged in renal disease.

Indications:

Edema associated with CHF, hepatic cirrhosis and renal disease, including the nephrotic syndrome. Particularly useful when greater diuretic potential is desired.

Parenteral administration is indicated when a rapid onset of diuresis is desired (eg, acute pulmonary edema), when GI absorption is impaired or when oral use is not practical for any reason. As soon as it is practical, replace with oral therapy.

Hypertension (furosemide, oral; torsemide, oral): Alone or in combination with other antihypertensive drugs.

Ethacrynic acid:

Ascites – Short-term management of ascites due to malignancy, idiopathic edema and lymphedema.

Congenital heart disease, nephrotic syndrome – Short-term management of hospitalized pediatric patients, other than infants.

Pulmonary edema, acute – Adjunctive therapy.

Unlabeled uses: Ethacrynic acid is being investigated for the treatment of glaucoma; a single injection into the eye may reduce intraocular pressure for a week or more.

Bumetanide may be beneficial in the treatment of adult nocturia; it is not effective in males with prostatic hypertrophy.

Contraindications:

Anuria; hypersensitivity to these compounds or to sulfonylureas; infants (ethacrynic acid); patients with hepatic coma or in states of severe electrolyte depletion until the condition is improved or corrected (bumetanide).

Warnings:

Dehydration: Excessive diuresis may result in dehydration and reduction in blood volume with circulatory collapse and the possibility of vascular thrombosis and embolism, particularly in elderly patients.

Hepatic cirrhosis and ascites: In these patients, sudden alterations of electrolyte balance may precipitate hepatic encephalopathy and coma. Do not institute therapy until the basic condition is improved.

Ototoxicity: Tinnitus, reversible and irreversible hearing impairment, deafness and vertigo with a sense of fullness in the ears have been reported. Deafness is usually reversible and of short duration (1 to 24 hours); however, irreversible hearing impairment has occurred. Usually, ototoxicity is associated with rapid injection, with severe renal impairment, with doses several times the usual dose and with concurrent use with other ototoxic drugs.

Systemic lupus erythematosus may be exacerbated or activated.

Thrombocytopenia: Since there have been rare spontaneous reports of thrombocytopenia with **bumetanide,** observe regularly for possible occurrence.

Hypersensitivity: Patients with known sulfonamide sensitivity may show allergic reactions to **furosemide, torsemide** or **bumetanide**. Bumetanide use following instances of allergic reactions to furosemide suggests a lack of cross-sensitivity. Refer to Management of Acute Hypersensitivity Reactions.

Renal function impairment: If increasing azotemia, oliguria or reversible increases in BUN or creatinine occur during treatment of severe progressive renal disease, discontinue therapy.

Pregnancy: Category B (ethacrynic acid, torsemide); *Category* C (furosemide, bumetanide). Since furosemide may increase the incidence of patent ductus arteriosus in preterm infants with respiratory-distress syndrome, use caution when administering before delivery.

Lactation: **Furosemide** appears in breast milk; such transfer of **ethacrynic acid, torsemide** and **bumetanide** is unknown.

Children: Safety and efficacy for use of **torsemide** in children, **bumetanide** in children < 18 years old, and **ethacrynic acid** in infants (oral) and children (IV) have not been established.

Furosemide stimulates renal synthesis of prostaglandin E_2 and may increase the incidence of patent ductus arteriosus when given in the first few weeks of life, to premature infants with respiratory-distress syndrome.

Precautions:

Monitoring: Observe for blood dyscrasias, liver or kidney damage or idiosyncratic reactions. Perform frequent serum electrolyte, calcium, glucose, uric acid, CO_2, creatinine and BUN determinations during the first few months of therapy and periodically thereafter.

Cardiovascular effects: Too vigorous a diuresis, as evidenced by rapid and excessive weight loss, may induce an acute hypotensive episode. In elderly cardiac patients, avoid rapid contraction of plasma volume and the resultant hemoconcentration to prevent thromboembolic episodes, such as cerebral vascular thromboses and pulmonary emboli.

Electrolyte imbalance may occur, especially in patients receiving high doses with restricted salt intake. Perform periodic determinations of serum electrolytes.

Hypokalemia prevention requires particular attention to the following: Patients receiving digitalis and diuretics for CHF, hepatic cirrhosis and ascites; in aldosterone excess with normal renal function; potassium-losing nephropathy; certain diarrheal states; or where hypokalemia is an added risk to the patient (eg, history of ventricular arrhythmias).

Hypomagnesemia – Loop diuretics increase the urinary excretion of magnesium.

Hypocalcemia – Serum calcium levels may be lowered (rare cases of tetany have occurred).

Hyperuricemia: Asymptomatic hyperuricemia can occur, and rarely, gout may be precipitated.

Glucose: Increases in blood glucose and alterations in glucose tolerance tests (fasting and 2 hour postprandial sugar) have been observed.

Lipids: Increases in LDL and total cholesterol and triglycerides with minor decreases in HDL cholesterol may occur.

Photosensitivity: Photosensitization (photoallergy or phototoxicity) may occur.

Drug Interactions:

Loop diuretics may affect the following drugs: Aminoglycosides; anticoagulants; chloral hydrate; digitalis glycosides; lithium; nondepolarizing neuromuscular blockers; propranolol; sulfonylureas; theophyllines. Loop diuretics may be affected by the following drugs: Charcoal; cisplatin; clofibrate; hydantoins; NSAIDs; probenecid; salicylates; thiazide diuretics.

Drug/Food interactions: The bioavailability of **furosemide** is decreased and its degree of diuresis reduced when administered with food. Simultaneous food intake with **torsemide** delays the time to C_{max} by about 30 minutes, but overall bioavailability and diuretic activity are unchanged.

Adverse Reactions:

Adverse reactions associated with loop diuretics include: Nausea; vomiting; diarrhea; gastric irritation; headache; fatigue; dizziness; thrombocytopenia; rash; orthostatic hypotension; hyperuricemia; hyperglycemia; electrolyte imbalance (decreased chloride, potassium and sodium); dehydration.

Furosemide: Adverse reactions may include anorexia, cramping, constipation, blurred vision, hearing loss, restlessness, fever, anemia, purpura, thrombocytopenia, agranulocytosis, photosensitivity, urticaria, pruritus, thrombophlebitis, muscle spasm, weakness.

Ethacrynic acid: Adverse reactions may include anorexia, pain, GI bleeding, severe neutropenia, agranulocytosis, fever, chills, confusion, fatigue, malaise, sense of fullness in the ears, blurred vision, tinnitus, hearing loss (irreversible), rash.

Bumetanide: Adverse reactions may include impaired hearing, ear discomfort, dry mouth, pain, renal failure, weakness, arthritic pain, muscle cramps, ECG changes, chest pain, hives, pruritus, itching, sweating, hyperventilation.

Torsemide: Adverse reactions may include excessive urination.

Administration and Dosage:

BUMETANIDE:

Oral – 0.5 to 2 mg/day, given as a single dose. If diuretic response is not adequate, give a second or third dose at 4 to 5 hour intervals, up to a maximum daily dose of 10 mg. An intermittent dose schedule, given on alternate days or for 3 to 4 days with rest periods of 1 to 2 days in between, is the safest and most effective method for the continued control of edema. In patients with hepatic failure, keep the dose to a minimum, and if necessary, increase the dose carefully.

Parenteral – Initially, 0.5 to 1 mg IV or IM. Administer IV over a period of 1 to 2 minutes. If the initial response is insufficient, give a second or third dose at intervals of 2 to 3 hours; do not exceed a daily dosage of 10 mg. End parenteral treatment and start oral treatment as soon as possible.

Renal function impairment – In patients with severe chronic renal insufficiency, a continuous infusion of bumetanide (12 mg over 12 hours) may be more effective and less toxic than intermittent bolus therapy.

ETHACRYNIC ACID:

Oral –

Initial therapy: Give minimally effective dose (usually, 50 to 200 mg daily) on a continuous or intermittent dosage schedule to produce gradual weight loss of 2.2 to 4.4 kg/day (1 to 2 lb/day). Adjust dose in 25 to 50 mg increments. Higher doses, up to 200 mg twice daily, achieved gradually, are most often required in patients with severe, refractory edema.

Children: Initial dose is 25 mg. Make careful increments of 25 mg to achieve maintenance. Dosage for infants has not been established.

Maintenance therapy: Administer intermittently after an effective diuresis is obtained using an alternate daily schedule or more prolonged periods of diuretic therapy interspersed with rest periods.

Parenteral – Do not give SC or IM because of local pain and irritation. The usual IV dose for the average adult is 50 mg, or 0.5 to 1 mg/kg. Give slowly through the tubing of a running infusion or by direct IV injection over several minutes. Usually, only one dose is necessary; occasionally, a second dose may be required; use a new injection site to avoid thrombophlebitis. A single IV dose, not exceeding 100 mg, has been used. Insufficient pediatric experience precludes recommendation for this age group.

FUROSEMIDE:

Oral –

Edema: 20 to 80 mg/day as a single dose. Depending on response, administer a second dose 6 to 8 hours later. If response is not satisfactory, increase by increments of 20 or 40 mg, no sooner than 6 to 8 hours after previous dose, until desired diuresis occurs. This dose should then be given once or twice daily (eg, at 8 am and 2 pm). Dosage may be titrated up to 600 mg/day in patients with severe edema.

Mobilization of edema may be most efficiently and safely accomplished with an intermittent dosage schedule; the drug is given 2 to 4 consecutive days each week. With doses > 80 mg/day, clinical and laboratory observations are advisable.

Hypertension: 40 mg twice a day; adjust according to response. If the patient does not respond, add other antihypertensive agents. Reduce dosage of other agents by at least 50% as soon as furosemide is added to prevent excessive drop in blood pressure.

Infants and children: 2 mg/kg. If diuresis is unsatisfactory, increase by 1 or 2 mg/kg, no sooner than 6 to 8 hours after previous dose. Doses > 6 mg/kg are not recommended. For maintenance therapy, adjust dose to the minimum effective level. A dose range of 0.5 to 2 mg/kg twice daily has also been recommended.

CHF and chronic renal failure: It has been suggested that doses as high as 2 to 2.5 g/day or more are well tolerated and effective in these patients.

Parenteral –

Edema: Initial dose: 20 to 40 mg IM or IV. Give the IV injection slowly (1 to 2 minutes). If needed, another dose may be given in the same manner 2 hours later.

The dose may be raised by 20 mg and given no sooner than 2 hours after previous dose, until desired diuretic effect is obtained. This dose should then be given once or twice daily. Administer high-dose parenteral therapy as a controlled infusion at a rate ≤ 4 mg/min.

Acute pulmonary edema: The usual initial dose is 40 mg IV (over 1 to 2 minutes). If response is not satisfactory within 1 hour, increase to 80 mg IV (over 1 to 2 minutes).

Infants and children: 1 mg/kg IV or IM given slowly under close supervision. If diuretic response after the initial dose is not satisfactory, increase the dosage by 1 mg/kg, no sooner than 2 hours after previous dose, until desired effect is obtained. Doses > 6 mg/kg are not recommended.

CHF and chronic renal failure: It has been suggested that doses as high as 2 to 2.5 g/day or more are well tolerated and effective in these patients. For IV bolus injections, the maximum should not exceed 1 g/day given over 30 minutes.

TORSEMIDE: Torsemide may be given at any time in relation to a meal.

Because of high bioavailability, oral and IV doses are therapeutically equivalent, so patients may be switched to and from the IV form with no change in dose. Administer the IV injection slowly over a period of 2 minutes.

Congestive heart failure/chronic renal failure – The usual initial dose is 10 or 20 mg once daily oral or IV. If the diuretic response is inadequate, titrate the dose upward by approximately doubling until the desired diuretic response is obtained. Single doses > 200 mg have not been adequately studied.

Hepatic cirrhosis – The usual initial dose is 5 or 10 mg once daily oral or IV, administered together with an aldosterone antagonist or a potassium-sparing diuretic. If the diuretic response is inadequate, titrate the dose upward by approximately doubling until the desired diuretic response is obtained. Single doses > 40 mg have not been adequately studied.

Hypertension – The usual initial dose is 5 mg once daily. If the 5 mg dose does not provide adequate reduction in blood pressure within 4 to 6 weeks, the dose may be increased to 10 mg once daily.

POTASSIUM-SPARING DIURETICS

Actions:

Pharmacology: In the kidney, potassium is filtered at the glomerulus and then absorbed parallel to sodium throughout the proximal tubule and thick ascending limb of the loop of Henle, so that only minor amounts reach the distal convoluted tubule. As a result, potassium appearing in urine is secreted at the distal tubule and collecting duct. The potassium-sparing diuretics interfere with sodium reabsorption at the distal tubule, thus decreasing potassium secretion. They exert a weak diuretic and antihypertensive effect when used alone. Their major use is to enhance the action and counteract the kaliuretic effect of thiazide and loop diuretics.

Spironolactone, a competitive inhibitor of aldosterone, binds to aldosterone receptors of the distal tubule and prevents the formation of a protein important in sodium transport. It is effective in both primary and secondary hyperaldosteronism. Spironolactone is effective in lowering systolic and diastolic blood pressure in both primary hyperaldosteronism and essential hypertension, although aldosterone secretion may be normal in benign essential hypertension.

Amiloride and *triamterene* not only inhibit sodium reabsorption induced by aldosterone, but they also inhibit basal sodium reabsorption. They are not aldosterone antagonists, but act directly on the renal distal tubule, cortical collecting tubule and collecting duct. They induce a reversal of polarity of the transtubular electrical-potential difference and inhibit active transport of sodium and potassium. Amiloride may inhibit sodium, potassium-ATPase.

Potassium-Sparing Diuretics: Pharmacological and Pharmacokinetic Properties

Parameters	Amiloride	Spironolactone	Triamterene
Pharmacology			
Tubular site of action	Proximal = distal	Distal	Distal
Mechanism of action	Na^+, K^+–ATPase inhibition; Na^+/H^+ exchange mecha nism inhibition (proximal tubule)	Aldosterone antagonism	Membrane effect
Action:			
Onset (hours)	2	24 to 48	2 to 4
Peak (hours)	6 to 10	48 to 72	6 to 8
Duration (hours)	24	48 to 72	12 to 16
Pharmacokinetics			
Bioavailability	15% to 25%	> 90%	30% to 70%
Protein binding	23%	≥ 98%[1]	50% to 67%
Half-life (hours)	6 to 9	20[2]	3
Active metabolites	none	canrenone	hydroxytriamterene sulfate
Peak plasma levels (hours)	3 to 4	canrenone: 2 to 4	3
Excreted unchanged in urine	≈ 50%[3]	†[4]	≈ 21%
Dosage			
Daily dose (mg)	5 to 20	25 to 400	200 to 300

[1] Canrenone > 98%.
[2] 10 to 35 hours for canrenone.
[3] 40% excreted in stool within 72 hours.
[4] Metabolites primarily excreted in urine, but also in bile.

AMILORIDE HCl

Tablets (Rx)	*Midamor* (Merck)

Indications:

Adjunctive treatment with thiazide or loop diuretics in CHF or hypertension to: Help restore normal serum potassium in patients who develop hypokalemia on the kaliuretic diuretic; prevent hypokalemia in patients who would be at particular risk if hypokalemia were to develop (eg, digitalized patients or patients with significant cardiac arrhythmias).

Unlabeled uses: Amiloride (10 to 20 mg/day) may be useful in reducing lithium-induced polyuria without increasing lithium levels as is seen with thiazide diuretics.

Aerosolized amiloride (drug dissolved in 0.3% saline delivered by nebulizer) appears to slow the progression of pulmonary function reduction in adults with cystic fibrosis.

Contraindications:

Hypersensitivity to amiloride; serum potassium > 5.5 mEq/L; antikaliuretic therapy or potassium supplementation; renal function impairment patients receiving spironolactone or triamterene.

Warnings:

> *Hyperkalemia:* Amiloride may cause hyperkalemia (serum potassium > 5.5 mEq/L) which, if uncorrected, is potentially fatal. Monitor serum potassium carefully. Symptoms of hyperkalemia include paresthesias, muscular weakness, fatigue, flaccid paralysis of the extremities, bradycardia, shock, and ECG abnormalities.

Diabetes mellitus: Avoid use of amiloride in diabetic patients. If it is used, monitor serum electrolytes and renal function frequently. Discontinue use at least 3 days before glucose tolerance testing.

Metabolic or respiratory acidosis: Cautiously institute amiloride in severely ill patients in whom respiratory or metabolic acidosis may occur, such as patients with cardiopulmonary disease or poorly controlled diabetes. Monitor acid-base balance frequently. Shifts in acid-base balance alter the ratio of extracellular/intracellular potassium; the development of acidosis may be associated with rapid increases in serum potassium.

Renal function impairment: Anuria, acute or chronic renal insufficiency and evidence of diabetic nephropathy are contraindications because potassium retention is accentuated and may result in the rapid development of hyperkalemia. Do not give to patients with evidence of renal impairment (BUN > 30 mg/dl or serum creatinine > 1.5 mg/dl) or diabetes mellitus without continuous monitoring of serum electrolytes, creatinine and BUN levels.

Hepatic function impairment: In patients with preexisting severe liver disease, hepatic encephalopathy, manifested by tremors, confusion and coma, and increased jaundice, may occur. Because amiloride is not metabolized by the liver, drug accumulation is not anticipated in patients with hepatic dysfunction, but accumulation can occur if hepatorenal syndrome develops.

Pregnancy: Category B.

Lactation: It is not known whether amiloride is excreted in breast milk. In rats, amiloride is excreted in milk in concentrations higher than those found in blood.

Children: Safety and efficacy for use in children have not been established.

Precautions:

Electrolyte imbalance and BUN increases: Hyponatremia and hypochloremia may occur when amiloride is used with other diuretics. Increases in BUN levels usually accompany vigorous fluid elimination, especially when diuretic therapy is used in seriously ill patients, such as those who have hepatic cirrhosis with ascites and metabolic alkalosis, or those with resistant edema.

Drug Interactions:
Drugs that may interact include digoxin, potassium preparations, ACE inhibitors and NSAIDs.

Adverse Reactions:
Possible adverse reactions include headache, nausea, anorexia, diarrhea, vomiting.

Administration and Dosage:
Administer with food.

Concomitant therapy: Add amiloride 5 mg/day to the usual antihypertensive or diuretic dosage of a kaliuretic diuretic. Increase dosage to 10 mg/day, if necessary; doses > 10 mg are usually not needed. If persistent hypokalemia is documented with 10 mg, increase the dose to 15 mg, then 20 mg, with careful titration of the dose and careful monitoring of electrolytes.

In patients with CHF, potassium loss may decrease after an initial diuresis; reevaluate the need or dosage for amiloride. Maintenance therapy may be intermittent.

Single drug therapy: The starting dose is 5 mg/day. Increase to 10 mg/day, if necessary; doses > 10 mg are usually not needed. If persistent hypokalemia is documented with 10 mg, increase the dose to 15 mg, then 20 mg, with careful monitoring of electrolytes.

SPIRONOLACTONE

Tablets: 25, 50 and 100 mg (Rx)	Various, *Aldactone* (Searle)

Indications:
Primary hyperaldosteronism: Diagnosis of primary hyperaldosteronism.

Short-term preoperative treatment of patients with primary hyperaldosteronism.

Long-term maintenance therapy for patients with discrete aldosterone-producing adrenal adenomas who are poor operative risks, or who decline surgery.

Long-term maintenance therapy for patients with bilateral micronodular or macronodular adrenal hyperplasia (idiopathic hyperaldosteronism).

Edematous conditions when other therapies are inappropriate or inadequate:

CHF – Management of edema and sodium retention; also indicated with digitalis.

Cirrhosis of the liver accompanied by edema or ascites for maintenance therapy in conjunction with bed rest and the restriction of fluid and sodium.

Nephrotic syndrome.

Essential hypertension, usually in combination with other drugs.

Hypokalemia and the prophylaxis of hypokalemia in patients taking digitalis.

Unlabeled uses: Spironolactone has been used in the treatment of hirsutism (50 to 200 mg/day) due to its antiandrogenic properties. One study suggested that a lower dosage (50 mg twice daily on days 4 through 21 of the menstrual cycle) may help minimize the risk of metrorrhagia that occurs with higher doses.

Symptoms of premenstrual syndrome (PMS) have been relieved at a dosage of 25 mg 4 times daily beginning on day 14 of the menstrual cycle.

The combination of spironolactone (2 mg/kg/day) and testolactone (20 to 40 mg/kg/day) for at least 6 months may be effective for short-term treatment of familial male precocious puberty.

Spironolactone 100 mg/day appears effective in short-term treatment of acne vulgaris.

Contraindications:
Anuria; acute renal insufficiency; significant impairment of renal function; hyperkalemia; patients receiving amiloride or triamterene.

Warnings:

Hyperkalemia: Carefully evaluate patients for possible fluid and electrolyte balance disturbances. Hyperkalemia may occur with impaired renal function or excessive potassium intake and can cause cardiac irregularities which may be fatal. No potassium supplement should ordinarily be given with spironolactone.

Renal function impairment: Use of spironolactone may cause a transient elevation of BUN, especially in patients with preexisting renal impairment. The drug may cause mild acidosis.

Carcinogenesis: Spironolactone was a tumorigen in chronic toxicity studies in rats.

Pregnancy: Spironolactone or its metabolites may cross the placental barrier.

Lactation: Canrenone, a metabolite of spironolactone, appears in breast milk. The labeling suggests that an alternative method of infant feeding be instituted when using spironolactone; however, the American Academy of Pediatrics considers the drug to be compatible with breast-feeding.

Precautions:

Hyponatremia may be caused or aggravated by spironolactone, especially in combination with other diuretics. Symptoms include dry mouth, thirst, lethargy, drowsiness.

Gynecomastia may develop and appears to be related to both dosage and duration of therapy. It is normally reversible when therapy is discontinued.

Reversible hyperchloremic metabolic acidosis, usually in association with hyperkalemia, occurs in some patients with decompensated hepatic cirrhosis, even in the presence of normal renal function.

Drug Interactions:

Drugs that may affect spironolactone include ACE inhibitors, salicylates and food. Drugs that may be affected by spironolactone include anticoagulants, digitalis glycosides, mitotane, digoxin and potassium preparations.

Adverse Reactions:

Adverse reactions are usually reversible upon discontinuation of the drug.

Possible adverse reactions include cramping; diarrhea; gastric bleeding; ulceration; gastritis; vomiting; drowsiness; lethargy; headache; mental confusion; ataxia; irregular menses; carcinoma of the breast.

Administration and Dosage:

Spironolactone may be administered in single or divided doses.

Diagnosis of primary hyperaldosteronism: As an initial diagnostic measure to provide presumptive evidence of primary hyperaldosteronism in patients on normal diets, as follows:

Long test – 400 mg/day for 3 to 4 weeks. Correction of hypokalemia and hypertension provides presumptive evidence for diagnosis of primary hyperaldosteronism.

Short test – 400 mg/day for 4 days. If serum potassium increases, but decreases when spironolactone is discontinued, consider a presumptive diagnosis of primary hyperaldosteronism.

Maintenance therapy for hyperaldosteronism: 100 to 400 mg daily in preparation for surgery. For patients unsuitable for surgery, employ the drug for long-term maintenance therapy at lowest possible dose.

Edema:

Adults (CHF, hepatic cirrhosis, nephrotic syndrome) – Initially, 100 mg/day (range, 25 to 200 mg/day). When given as the sole diuretic agent, continue for at least 5 days at the initial dosage level, then adjust to the optimal level. If after 5 days an adequate diuretic response has not occurred, add a second diuretic, which acts more proximally in the renal tubule. Because of the additive effect of spironolactone with such diuretics, an enhanced diuresis usually begins on the first day of combined treatment; combined therapy is indicated when more rapid diuresis is desired. Spironolactone dosage should remain unchanged when other diuretic therapy is added.

Children – 3.3 mg/kg/day (1.5 mg/lb/day) administered in single or divided doses.

Essential hypertension:

Adults – Initially, 50 to 100 mg/day in single or divided doses. May also be combined with diuretics, which act more proximally, and with other antihypertensive agents. Continue treatment for at least 2 weeks since the maximal response may not occur sooner. Individualize dosage.

Children – A dose of 1 to 2 mg/kg twice daily has been recommended.

Hypokalemia: 25 to 100 mg/day. Useful in treating diuretic-induced hypokalemia when oral potassium supplements or other potassium-sparing regimens are considered inappropriate.

TRIAMTERENE

Capsules: 50, 100 mg *(Rx)*	*Dyrenium* (SmithKline Beecham)

Indications:

Edema associated with CHF, hepatic cirrhosis and the nephrotic syndrome; steroid-induced edema, idiopathic edema and edema due to secondary hyperaldosteronism.

May be used alone or with other diuretics, either for additive diuretic effect or antikaliuretic (potassium-sparing) effect. It promotes increased diuresis in patients resistant or only partially responsive to other diuretics because of secondary hyperaldosteronism.

Contraindications:

Patients receiving spironolactone or amiloride; anuria; severe hepatic disease; hyperkalemia; hypersensitivity to triamterene; severe or progressive kidney disease or dysfunction, with the possible exception of nephrosis; preexisting elevated serum potassium (impaired renal function, azotemia) or patients who develop hyperkalemia while on triamterene.

Warnings:

Hyperkalemia: Abnormal elevation of serum potassium levels (≥ 5.5 mEq/L) can occur. Hyperkalemia is more likely to occur in patients with renal impairment and diabetes (even without evidence of renal impairment), and in the elderly or severely ill. Since uncorrected hyperkalemia may be fatal, serum potassium levels must be monitored at frequent intervals especially when dosages are changed or with any illness that may influence renal function.

When triamterene is added to other diuretic therapy, or when patients are switched to triamterene from other diuretics, discontinue potassium supplementation.

Hypersensitivity: Monitor patients regularly for blood dyscrasias, liver damage or other idiosyncratic reactions.

Renal function impairment: Perform periodic BUN and serum potassium determinations to check kidney function, especially in patients with suspected or confirmed renal insufficiency and in elderly or diabetic patients; diabetic patients with nephropathy are especially prone to develop hyperkalemia.

Hepatic function impairment: Triamterene is extensively metabolized in the liver. The overall diuretic response may not be affected.

Pregnancy: Category B.

Lactation: If the drug is essential, the patient should stop nursing.

Children: Safety and efficacy have not been established.

Precautions:

Electrolyte imbalance: In CHF, renal disease or cirrhosis, electrolyte imbalance may be aggravated or caused by diuretics. The use of full doses of a diuretic when salt intake is restricted can result in a low salt syndrome.

Renal stones: Triamterene has been found in renal stones with other usual calculus components. Use cautiously in patients with histories of stone formation.

Hematologic effects: Triamterene is a weak folic acid antagonist. Since cirrhotics with splenomegaly may have marked variations in hematological status, it may contribute to the appearance of megaloblastosis in cases where folic acid stores have been depleted. Perform periodic blood studies in these patients.

Metabolic acidosis: Triamterene may cause decreasing alkali reserve with a possibility of metabolic acidosis.

Diabetes mellitus: Triamterene may raise blood glucose levels for adult-onset diabetes; dosage adjustments of hypoglycemic agents may be necessary. Concurrent use with chlorpropamide may increase the risk of severe hyponatremia.

Photosensitivity: Photosensitization is likely to occur; avoid prolonged exposure to sunlight.

Drug Interactions:

Drugs that may affect triamterine include ACE inhibitors, cimetidine and indomethacin. Drugs that may be affected by triamterine include amantadine and potassium preparations. Triamterene will interfere with the fluorescent measurement of quinidine serum levels.

Adverse Reactions:

Diarrhea; nausea; vomiting; jaundice; liver enzyme abnormalities. Azotemia; elevated BUN/creatinine; increased serum uric acid levels (in patients predisposed to gouty arthritis); thrombocytopenia; megaloblastic anemia; weakness; dizziness; hypokalemia; headache; dry mouth; anaphylaxis.

Administration and Dosage:

Individualize dosage.

When used alone, the usual starting dose is 100 mg twice/daily after meals. When combined with other diuretics or antihypertensives, decrease the total daily dosage of each agent initially, and then adjust to the patient's needs. Do not exceed 300 mg/day.

CARBONIC ANHYDRASE INHIBITORS

ACETAZOLAMIDE	
Tablets: 125 and 250 mg (*Rx*)	Various, *Diamox* (Lederle)
Capsules, sustained release: 500 mg (*Rx*)	*Diamox Sequels* (Lederle)
DICHLORPHENAMIDE	
Tablets: 50 mg (*Rx*)	*Daranide* (Merck)
METHAZOLAMIDE	
Tablets: 25 and 50 mg (*Rx*)	Various, *GlaucTabs* (Akorn), *Neptazane* (Lederle)

Actions:

Pharmacology: These agents are nonbacteriostatic sulfonamides that inhibit the enzyme carbonic anhydrase. This action reduces the rate of aqueous humor formation, resulting in decreased intraocular pressure (IOP).

Pharmacokinetics:

Pharmacokinetics of Carbonic Anhydrase Inhibitors

Carbonic anhydrase inhibitor	IOP Lowering Effects			Relative inhibitor potency
	Onset (hours)	Peak effect (hours)	Duration (hours)	
Dichlorphenamide	within 1	2 to 4	6 to 12	30
Acetazolamide				
Tablets	1 to 1.5	1 to 4	8 to 12	1
Sustained release capsules	2	3 to 6	18 to 24	
Injection (IV)	2 min	15 min	4 to 5	
Methazolamide	2 to 4	6 to 8	10 to 18	†[1]

[1] † Quantitative data not available; reported to be more active than acetazolamide.

Indications:

Glaucoma: For adjunctive treatment of chronic simple (open-angle) glaucoma and secondary glaucoma; preoperatively in acute angle-closure glaucoma when delay of surgery is desired to lower IOP.

Acetazolamide:

Tablets, sustained release capsules and injection – For the prevention or amelioration of symptoms associated with acute mountain sickness in climbers attempting rapid ascent and in those who are susceptible to acute mountain sickness despite gradual ascent.

Tablets and injection only – For adjunctive treatment of edema due to CHF, drug-induced edema and centrencephalic epilepsy (petit mal, unlocalized seizures).

Contraindications:

Hypersensitivity to these agents; depressed sodium or potassium serum levels; marked kidney and liver disease or dysfunction; suprarenal gland failure; hyperchloremic acidosis; adrenocortical insufficiency; severe pulmonary obstruction with inability to increase alveolar ventilation since acidosis may be increased (dichlorphenamide); cirrhosis (acetazolamide, methazolamide); long-term use in chronic noncongestive angle-closure glaucoma.

Warnings:

Hepatic function impairment: Use of **methazolamide** in this condition could precipitate hepatic coma.

Pregnancy: Category C.

Lactation: Safety has not been established.

Children: Safety and efficacy for use in children have not been established.

Precautions:

Monitoring: Monitor for hematologic reactions common to sulfonamides. Obtain baseline CBC and platelet counts before therapy and at regular intervals during therapy.

Hypokalemia may develop when severe cirrhosis is present, during concomitant use of steroids or ACTH, and with interference with adequate oral electrolyte intake.

Dose increases: Increasing the dose of **acetazolamide** does not increase diuresis and may increase drowsiness or paresthesia; it often results in decreased diuresis. However, very large doses have been given with other diuretics to promote diuresis in complete refractory failure.

Pulmonary conditions: Use **dichlorphenamide** with caution in patients with severe degrees of respiratory acidosis. These drugs may precipitate or aggravate acidosis. Use with caution in patients with pulmonary obstruction or emphysema when alveolar ventilation may be impaired.

Cross-sensitivity between antibacterial sulfonamides and sulfonamide derivative diuretics, including acetazolamide and various thiazides, has been reported.

Drug Interactions:

Drugs that may interact with carbonic anhydrase inhibitors include cyclosporine, primidone, salicylates and diflunisal.

Adverse Reactions:

Sulfonamide-type adverse reactions may occur.

GI: Melena; anorexia; nausea; vomiting; constipation; taste alteration; diarrhea.

Renal: Hematuria; glycosuria; urinary frequency.

CNS: Convulsions; weakness; malaise; fatigue; nervousness; drowsiness; depression; dizziness; disorientation; confusion; ataxia; tremor; tinnitus; headache.

Hematologic: Bone marrow depression; thrombocytopenia; thrombocytopenic purpura; hemolytic anemia; leukopenia; pancytopenia; agranulocytosis.

Dermatologic: Urticaria; pruritus; skin eruptions; rash (including erythema multiforme, Stevens-Johnson syndrome, toxic epidermal necrolysis); photosensitivity.

Miscellaneous: Weight loss; fever; decreased/absent libido; impotence; electrolyte imbalance; hepatic insufficiency.

Administration and Dosage:

ACETAZOLAMIDE:

Chronic simple (open-angle) glaucoma –

Adults: 250 mg to 1 g/day, usually in divided doses for amounts > 250 mg. Dosage > 1 g daily does not usually increase the effect.

Secondary glaucoma and preoperative treatment of acute congestive (closed-angle) glaucoma –

Adults:

Short-term therapy – 250 mg every 4 hours or 250 mg twice daily.

Acute cases – 500 mg followed by 125 or 250 mg every 4 hours.

IV therapy may be used for rapid relief of increased intraocular pressure. A complementary effect occurs when used with miotics or mydriatics.

Children:

Parenteral – 5 to 10 mg/kg/dose, IM or IV, every 6 hours.

Oral – 10 to 15 mg/kg/day in divided doses, every 6 to 8 hours.

Diuresis in congestive heart failure –

Adults: Initially, 250 to 375 mg (5 mg/kg) once daily in the morning. If, after an initial response, the patient stops losing edema fluid, do not increase the dose; allow for kidney recovery by skipping medication for a day. Best diuretic results occur when given on alternate days, or for 2 days alternating with a day of rest. Failures in therapy may result from overdosage or from too frequent dosages.

Drug-induced edema – Most effective if given every other day or for 2 days alternating with a day of rest.

Adults: 250 to 375 mg once daily for 1 or 2 days.

Children: 5 mg/kg/dose, oral or IV, once daily in the morning.

Epilepsy –

Adults and Children: 8 to 30 mg/kg/day in divided doses. The optimum range is 375 to 1000 mg daily. When given in combination with other anticonvulsants, the starting dose is 250 mg once daily.

Acute mountain sickness – 500 to 1000 mg/day, in divided doses of tablets or sustained release capsules. For rapid ascent (ie, in rescue or military operations), use the higher dose (1000 mg). If possible, initiate dosing 24 to 48 hours before ascent and continue for 48 hours while at high altitude, or longer as needed to control symptoms.

Sustained release – May be used twice daily, but is only indicated for use in glaucoma and acute mountain sickness.

Parenteral – Direct IV administration is preferred; IM administration is painful because of the alkaline pH of the solution.

DICHLORPHENAMIDE:

Glaucoma – Most effective when given with miotics. In acute angle-closure glaucoma, dichlorphenamide may be used with miotics and osmotic agents to rapidly reduce intraocular tension.

Adults:

Initial dose – 100 to 200 mg, followed by 100 mg every 12 hours, until the desired response is obtained.

Maintenance dosage – 25 to 50 mg 1 to 3 times daily.

METHAZOLAMIDE:

Glaucoma – 50 to 100 mg 2 or 3 times daily. May be used with miotic and osmotic agents.

CARDIAC GLYCOSIDES

DIGITOXIN	
Tablets: 0.1, 0.2 mg (*Rx*)	Various, *Crystodigin* (Lilly)
DIGOXIN	
Capsules: 0.05, 0.1 or 0.2 mg (*Rx*)	*Lanoxicops* (Glaxo Wellcome)
Tablets: 0.125, 0.25 or 0.5 mg (*Rx*)	Various, *Lanoxin* (Glaxo Wellcome)
Elixir, pediatric: 0.05 mg/ml	Various, *Lanoxin* (Glaxo Wellcome)
Injection: 0.25 mg/ml (*Rx*)	Various, *Lanoxin* (Glaxo Wellcome)
Injection, pediatric: 0.1 mg/ml (*Rx*)	*Lanoxin* (Glaxo Wellcome)

Actions:

Pharmacology: The influence of the digitalis glycosides on the myocardium is dose-related, and involves both a direct action on cardiac muscle and the specialized conduction system, and indirect actions on the cardiovascular system mediated by the autonomic nervous system.

Direct effects include increasing the force and velocity of myocardial systolic contraction (positive inotropic action), increasing the refractory period of the AV node and increasing total peripheral resistance. In higher doses, digitalis increases sympathetic outflow from the CNS to both cardiac and peripheral sympathetic nerves, which may increase atrial or ventricular rate. This increase in sympathetic activity may be an important factor in digitalis cardiac toxicity.

Pharmacokinetics:

Pharmacokinetic Parameters of Digitalis Glycosides

Digitalis Glycoside	Route	Onset (Minutes)	Peak (Hours)	Plasma t ½ (Hours)	% GI Absorption	% Protein Binding	Major Route of Elimination
Digoxin	PO	30-120	2-6	30-40[1]	60 - 100	20-25	Renal
	IV	5-30	1-5		100		
Digitoxin	PO	60-240	8-12	118 - 216	90-100	90-97	Hepatic, ≈ 32%; Renal (metabolites)

[1] In anuric patients: 100+ hours.

Digitalis Glycoside Serum Levels

Digitalis Glycoside	Drug Serum Levels (ng/ml)	
	Therapeutic	Toxic
Digitoxin	9 to 25	>35
Digoxin	0.5 to 2	>2.5

Indications:

Congestive heart failure (CHF) all degrees: Increased cardiac output results in diuresis and general amelioration of disturbances characteristic of right heart failure (venous congestion, edema) and left heart failure (dyspnea, orthopnea, cardiac asthma).

Atrial flutter: Digitalis slows the heart; normal sinus rhythm may appear. Often, flutter is converted to atrial fibrillation with a slow ventricular rate.

Paroxysmal atrial tachycardia (PAT): Digitalis may be used, especially if tachycardia is resistant to lesser measures.

Cardiogenic shock: The value of these drugs has not been established; however, they are often employed when the condition is accompanied by pulmonary edema.

Contraindications:

Previous toxic response; ventricular fibrillation; ventricular tachycardia, unless congestive failure supervenes after protracted episode not due to digitalis; presence of digitalis toxicity; beriberi heart disease, hypersensitivity to digoxin; some cases of hypersensitive carotid sinus syndrome.

Warnings:

Long-term use in CHF: The drug is generally continued after heart failure is abolished unless some other known precipitating factor is corrected. Hemodynamic effects can be demonstrated in almost all patients, but corresponding improvement in signs and symptoms of heart failure is not necessarily apparent. In patients in whom digoxin may be difficult to regulate, or in whom risk of toxicity may be great, consider a cautious withdrawal of digoxin. If digoxin is discontinued, regularly monitor for clinical evidence of recurrent heart failure.

Digitalis toxicity: Many of the arrhythmias for which digitalis is indicated are identical with those reflecting digitalis intoxication. If digitalis intoxication cannot be excluded, cardiac glycosides should be withheld temporarily, if the clinical situation permits.

Cardiovascular disease: Electrical conversion of arrhythmias may require reduction of dosage to avoid induction of ventricular arrhythmias. However, consider the consequences of rapid increase in ventricular response to atrial fibrillation if digoxin is withheld 1 to 2 days prior to cardioversion.

Patients with incomplete AV block, especially if subject to Stokes-Adams attacks, may develop advanced or complete heart block if given digitalis.

In patients with acute or unstable chronic atrial fibrillation, digitalis may not normalize the ventricular rate even when the serum concentration exceeds the usual therapeutic level.

Patients with acute myocardial infarction (MI), severe pulmonary disease, severe carditis (eg, carditis associated with rheumatic fever or viral myocarditis) or advanced heart failure may be more sensitive to digitalis and more prone to disturbances of rhythm.

Cases of idiopathic hypertrophic subaortic stenosis must be managed with extreme care (outflow obstruction may worsen). Unless cardiac failure is severe, it is doubtful that digitalis should be employed.

In patients with Wolff-Parkinson-White Syndrome and atrial fibrillation, digoxin can enhance transmission of impulses through the accessory pathway. This may result in extremely rapid ventricular rates and even ventricular fibrillation.

In some patients with sinus node disease (ie, Sick Sinus syndrome), digoxin may worsen sinus bradycardia or sinoatrial block.

Patients with heart failure from amyloid heart disease or constrictive cardiomyopathies respond poorly to treatment with digoxin.

Renal function impairment: Renal insufficiency delays excretion of all glycosides except digitoxin; adjust dosage in patients with renal disease. Digoxin toxicity also develops more frequently and lasts longer in renal impairment because of decreased digoxin excretion. The presence of acute glomerulonephritis accompanied by CHF requires extreme care in digitalization.

Hepatic function impairment: Reduction in digitoxin dosage may be necessary.

Pregnancy: Category C. Both digoxin and digitoxin rapidly pass into the fetus in a concentration of 50% to 83% of maternal serum. Maternally administered digoxin has been used to treat fetal tachycardia and CHF; fetal toxicity and neonatal death have been a consequence of maternal overdosage.

Lactation: Digoxin is excreted into breast milk at a milk:plasma ratio of 0.6 to 0.9. The amount the infant receives is very small and no infant adverse effects have been reported. It is not known whether **digitoxin** is excreted in breast milk.

Children: Newborn infants display considerable variability in tolerance. Premature and immature infants are particularly sensitive; dosage must be reduced and digitalization should be even more individualized according to infant's degree of maturity. Digitalis glycosides are an important cause of accidental poisoning in children. Impaired renal function must also be taken into consideration.

Precautions:

Electrolyte imbalance: Hypokalemia sensitizes the myocardium to digitalis and may reduce the positive inotropic effect of digitalis. Toxicity may develop even with "normal" serum glycoside levels. Therefore, it is desirable to maintain normal serum potassium levels. In general, avoid rapid changes in serum potassium or other electrolytes; reserve treatment of CHF with IV potassium for special circumstances (see Treatment of Toxicity).

Calcium – Calcium affects cardiac contractility and excitability in a manner similar to digitalis. Calcium, particularly when administered rapidly IV, may produce serious arrhythmias in digitalized patients. However, hypocalcemia can nullify the effects of digoxin; thus, digoxin may be ineffective until serum calcium is restored to normal.

Magnesium – Hypomagnesemia may predispose to digitalis toxicity. If low magnesium levels are detected in a patient receiving digoxin, institute replacement therapy.

Thyroid dysfunction: The plasma levels of cardiac glycosides are inversely related to thyroid status. In myxedema, digitalis requirements are less because excretion rate is decreased. In thyrotoxic patients with heart failure, larger doses of the glycoside may be necessary. Results may not be satisfactory until the hyperthyroidism is corrected.

Laboratory monitoring tests: Perform periodic determinations of heart rate, electrolytes (especially potassium), ECG and renal function (BUN or serum creatinine). Digoxin may produce false positive ST-T changes in ECG during exercise testing. It may also be useful to measure glycoside serum concentrations periodically, especially if digitalis intoxication is suspected.

Drug Interactions:

Increased digoxin serum levels: The following agents may increase digoxin serum levels, possibly increasing its therapeutic and toxic effects: Aminoglycosides (oral), alprazolam, amiodarone, anticholinergics, benzodiazepines, bepridil, captopril, cyclosporine, diltiazem, diphenyoxylate, erythromycin, esmolol, felodipine, flecainide, hydroxychloroquine, ibuprofen, indomethacin, itraconazole, nifedipine, omeprazole, propafenone, propantheline, quinidine, quinine, tetracycline, tobutamide and verapamil.

Decreased GI absorption of digitalis glycosides may be caused by the following agents, possibly decreasing the serum levels and therapeutic effects: Aminoglutethimide, aminoglycosides (oral), aminosalicylic acid, antacids (aluminum or magnesium salts), antihistamines, antineoplastics, barbiturates, cholestyramine, colestipol, hydantoins, hypoglycemic agents (oral), kaolin/pectin, metoclopramide, neomycin, penicillamine, rifampin, sucralfate and sulfasalazine

Other drugs that may interact with cardiac glycosides include: Albuterol, amphotericin B, beta blockers, disopyramide, loop diuretics, nondepolarizing muscle relaxants, potassium-sparing diuretics, succinylcholine, sympathomimetics, thiazide diuretics, thioamines and thyroid hormones.

Adverse Reactions:

Overall incidence of adverse reactions is 5% to 20%, with 15% to 20% considered serious (1% to 4% of patients receiving digoxin). Evidence suggests that the incidence of toxicity has decreased since the introduction of serum digoxin assay and improved standardization of digoxin tablets. Cardiac toxicity accounts for about one-half, GI disturbances for about one-fourth, CNS, ophthalmic and other toxicity for about one-fourth of these adverse reactions.

Anorexia, nausea and vomiting may occur. These effects are central in origin, but following large oral doses, there is also a local emetic action. Abdominal discomfort or pain and diarrhea may also occur.

Administration and Dosage:

Loading doses: The use of initial large loading doses rapidly establishes effective plasma levels, but also increases risks of toxicity because of its narrow toxic-therapeutic ratio. Administration of small daily maintenance doses are then given to replace daily losses due to metabolism and excretion. Without a loading dose, slow digitalization may be achieved within 1 week with digoxin and in 10 to 14 days with digitoxin, with a much lower risk of toxicity than when giving a loading dose. For a rapid effect in acutely ill patients, parenteral administration of deslanoside or digoxin can be used. Use parenterally only when the drug cannot be taken orally or rapid digitalization is urgent.

Maintenance therapy: Maintenance dosage is determined tentatively by the amount necessary to sustain the desired therapeutic effect. Recommended dosages are practical average figures which may require considerable modification as dictated by individual sensitivity or associated conditions. Diminished renal function is the most important factor requiring modification of recommended doses of digoxin.

DIGITOXIN:

Loading dose –

Rapid: 0.6 mg initially, followed by 0.4 mg, then 0.2 mg at intervals of 4 to 6 hours.

Slow: 0.2 mg twice daily for a period of 4 days, followed by maintenance dosage.

Maintenance – Ranges from 0.05 to 0.3 mg daily, the most common dose being 0.15 mg daily.

Children – Individualize dosage. Monitor ECG to avoid toxic doses.

Generally, premature and immature infants are particularly sensitive and require a reduced dosage that must be determined by careful adjustment. Divide the total dose into 3, 4 or more portions, with 6 hours or more between doses.

After the neonatal period, the recomended digitalizing dose is as follows:

< 1 year of age – 0.045 mg/kg.

1 to 2 years of age – 0.04 mg/kg.

> 2 years of age – 0.03 mg/kg (0.75 mg/m^2).

Children (maintenance dose): Administer 1/10 (10%) of the digitalizing dose.

DIGOXIN:

Parenteral administration – The IV digitalizing dose is ≈ 20% less than an oral dose. Intramuscular injection offers no advantages and can cause severe pain at injection site; IV administration is preferred. Give injections over 5 minutes or longer, undiluted or diluted with a 4–fold or greater volume of Steril Water for Injection, 0.9% Sodium Chloride Injection, 5% Dextrose Injection or Lactated Ringer's Injection. Use of less diluent could lead to digoxin precipitation. Use diluted product immediately.

Adults – Rapid digitalization with a loading dose - Peak body digoxin stores of 8 to 12 mcg/kg should provide therapeutic effect. Larger stores (10 to 15 mcg/kg) are often required for control of ventricular rate in patients with atrial flutter or fibrillation. Use conservative projected peak body stores for patients with renal insufficiency (ie, 6 to 10 mcg/kg). Base the loading dose on the projected peak body stores and administer in several portions with roughly half the total given as the first dose. Give additional fractions at 4 to 8 hour intervals IV or orally, with careful assessment of clinical response before each additional dose.

In undigitalized patients, a single initial IV dose of 400 to 600 mcg (0.4 to 0.6 mg) usually produces a detectable effect in 5 to 30 minutes that becomes maximal in 1 to 4 hours. The usual parenteral amount for a 70 kg patient to achieve 8 to 15 mcg/kg peak body stores is 600 to 1000 mcg (0.6 to 1 mg). A single initial oral dose of 500 to 750 mcg (0.5 to 0.75 mg) usually produces a detectable effect in 0.5 to 2 hours that becomes maximal in 2 to 6 hours. The usual oral amount required for a 70 kg patient to achieve 8 to 15 mcg/kg peak body stores is 750 to 1250 mcg (0.75 to 1.25 mg).

Base the maintenance dose upon the percentage of the peak body stores lost each day through elimination. The following formula has wide clinical use:

$$\text{Maintenance dose} = \text{Peak Body Stores (ie, Loading Dose)} \times \frac{\text{\% Daily Loss}}{100} \text{ (ie, 14 = Ccr/5)}$$

Ccr is creatinine clearance, corrected to 70 kg body weight or 1.73 m^2 body surface area.

Gradual digitalization with a maintenance dose: The following table provides average oral (tablet) daily maintenance dose requirements for patients with heart failure based upon lean body weight and renal function:

Usual Digoxin Tablet Daily Maintenance Dose Requirements (mcg) For Estimated Peak Body Stores of 10 mcg/kg

Corrected Ccr (ml/min/70 kg)	Lean Body Weight (kg/lbs)						Number of Days Before Steady-State Achieved
	50/110	60/132	70/154	80/176	90/198	100/220	
0	63*[1]	125	125	125	188[2]	188	22
10	125	125	125	188	188	188	19
20	125	125	188	188	188	250	16
30	125	188	188	188	250	250	14
40	125	188	188	250	250	250	13
50	188	188	250	250	250	250	12
60	188	188	250	250	250	375	11
70	188	250	250	250	250	375	10
80	188	250	250	250	375	375	9
90	188	250	250	250	375	500	8
100	250	250	250	375	375	500	7

* 63 mcg = 0.063 mg.
[1] ½ of 125 mcg tablet or 125 mcg every other day.
[2] 1½ or 125 mcg tablet.

Usual Digoxin Solution Filled Capsule Daily Maintenance Dose Requirements (mcg) For Estimated Peak Body Stores of 10 mcg/kg

Corrected Ccr (ml/min/70 kg)	Lean Body Weight (kg/lbs)						Number of days before steady-state achieved
	50/110	60/132	70/154	80/176	90/198	100/220	
0	50	100	100	100	150	150	22
10	100	100	100	150	150	150	19
20	100	100	150	150	150	200	16
30	100	150	150	150	200	200	14
40	100	150	150	200	200	250	13
50	150	150	200	200	250	250	12
60	150	150	200	200	250	300	11
70	150	200	200	250	250	300	10
80	150	200	200	250	300	300	9
90	150	200	250	250	300	350	8
100	200	200	250	300	300	350	7

Infants and children – Individualize dosage. Divided daily dosing is recommended for infants and young children under 10 years of age. Children over 10 require adult dosages in proportion to their body weight.

Rapid digitalization with a loading dose: Administer loading dose in several portions, give roughly half the total as the first dose. Give additional fractions of total dose at 6 to 8 hr intervals (oral) or 4 to 8 hr intervals (parenteral).

Usual Digitalizing and Maintenance Dosages with Normal Renal Function Based on Lean Body Weight

Age	Digitalizing Dose[1] (mcg/kg)		Daily Maintenance Dose (mcg/kg)
	Oral	IV	
Premature	20-30	15-25	20%-30% of the loading dose[2]
Full term	25-35	20-30	25%-25% of the loading dose[2]
1-24 months	35-60	30-50	
2-5 years	30-40	25-35	
5-10 years	20-35	15-30	
Over 10 years	10-15	8-12	

[1] IV digitalizing doses are 80% of oral digitalizing doses.
[2] Projected or actual digitalizing dose providing desired clinical response.

Lanoxicaps (gelatin capsules) have greater bioavailability than standard tablets. Therefore, the 0.2 mg capsule is equivalent to 0.25 mg tablets; the 0.1 mg capsule is equivalent to 0.125 mg tablets; and the 0.05 mg capsule is equivalent to 0.0625 mg.

Use in the elderly – Since digoxin is eliminated by the kidneys, a decreased clearance may occur in elderly patients with decreased renal function. Therefore, a lower maintenance dose of digoxin may be necessary. Adjust the dose accordingly.

NITRATES

ISOSORBIDE MONONITRATE (ORAL)	
Tablets: 10 and 20 mg (*Rx*)	*Monoket* (Schwarz Pharma), *ISMO* (Wyeth-Ayerst)
Tablets, extended release: 60 and 120 mg (*Rx*)	*Imdur* (Key)
NITROGLYCERIN (IV)	
Injection: 0.5 and 5 mg/ml (*Rx*)	Various, *Tridil* (Faulding)
Injection solution: 25, 50, 100 and 200 mg in 5% Dextrose (*Rx*)	Various
NITROGLYCERIN (TRANSMUCOSAL)	
Tablets, buccal, controlled release: 1, 2 and 3 mg (*Rx*)	*Nitrogard* (Forest)
AMYL NITRITE	
Inhalant: 0.3 ml (*Rx*)	*Amyl Nitrite Vaporole* (Glaxo Wellcome)
NITROGLYCERIN (SUBLINGUAL)	
Tablets, sublingual: 0.3, 0.4 and 0.6 mg (*Rx*)	*Nitrostat* (Parke-Davis)
NITROGLYCERIN (TRANSLINGUAL)	
Spray: 0.4 mg/dose (*Rx*)	*Nitrolingual* (Rhone-Poulenc Rorer)
NITROGLYCERIN (SUSTAINED RELEASE)	
Tablets, sustained release: 2.6, 6.5 and 9 mg (*Rx*)	*Nitrong* (Rhone-Poulence Rorer)
Capsules, sustained release: 2.5, 6.5, 9 and 13 mg (*Rx*)	Various, *Nitroglyn* (Kenwood), *Nitro-Time* (Time-Cap Labs)
NITROGLYCERIN TRANSDERMAL SYSTEMS	
Patch: 0.1, 0.2, 0.3, 0.4, 0.6 and 0.8 mg/hr (*Rx*)	*Nitro-Dur* (Key)
NITROGLYCERIN (TOPICAL)	
Ointment: 2% in a lanolin-petroleum base (*Rx*)	Various, *Nitrol* (Adria)
ISOSORBIDE DINITRATE (SUBLINGUAL AND CHEWABLE)	
Tablets, sublingual: 2.5, 5 and 10 mg (*Rx*)	Various, *Isordil* (Wyeth-Ayerst)
Tablets, chewable: 5 and 10 mg (*Rx*)	*Sorbitrate* (ICI Pharma)
ISOSORBIDE DINITRATE (ORAL)	
Tablets: 5, 10, 20, 30 and 40 mg (*Rx*)	Various, *Isordil Titradose* (Wyeth-Ayerst)
Tablets, sustained release: 40 mg (*Rx*)	Various, *Isordil Tembids* (Wyeth-Ayerst)
Capsules, sustained release: 40 mg (*Rx*)	Various, *Isordil Tembids* (Wyeth-Ayerst), *Dilatrate-SR* (Schwarz Pharma)

Actions:

Pharmacology: Relaxation of vascular smooth muscle via stimulation of intracellular cyclic guanosine monophosphate production is the principal pharmacologic action of nitrates. Although venous effects predominate, nitroglycerin produces a dose-dependent dilation of both arterial and venous beds. Dilation of the postcapillary vessels, including large veins, promotes peripheral pooling of blood and decreases venous return to the heart, reducing left ventricular end-diatolic pressure (preload). Arteriolar relaxation reduces systemic vascular resistance and arterial pressure (afterload).

Pharmacokinetics:

Doseform, Onset and Duration of Available Nitrates			
Nitrates	Dosage form	Onset (minutes)	Duration
Amyl nitrate	Inhalant	0.5	3 to 5 min
Nitroglycerin	IV	1 to 2	3 to 5 min
	Sublingual	1 to 3	30 to 60 min
	Translingual spray	2	30 to 60 min
	Transmucosal tablet	1 to 2	3 to 5 hours[1]
	Oral, sustained release	20 to 45	3 to 8 hours
	Topical ointment	30 to 60	2 to 12 hours[2]
	Transdermal	30 to 60	up to 24 hours[3]
Isosorbide dinitrate	Sublingual	2 to 5	1 to 3 hours
	Oral	20 to 40	4 to 6 hours
	Oral, sustained release	up to 4 hours	6 to 8 hours
Isosorbide mononitrate	Oral	30 to 60	nd

Doseform, Onset and Duration of Available Nitrates			
Nitrates	Dosage form	Onset (minutes)	Duration
Erythrityl tetranitrate	Sublingual & chewable	5	3 hours
	Oral	15 to 30	6 hours
Pentaerythritol tetranitrate	Oral	20 to 60	≈ 5 hours
	Oral, sustained release	30	up to 12 hours

[1] A significant antianginal effect can persist for 5 hours if the tablet has not completely dissolved.
[2] Depends on total amount used per unit of surface area.
[3] Tolerance may develop after 12 hours.
nd = No data.

Indications:

Acute angina (nitroglycerin sublingual, transmucosal or translingual spray; isosorbide dinitrate sublingual; amyl nitrite): For relief of acute anginal episodes; prophylaxis prior to events likely to provoke an attack.

Angina prophylaxis (nitroglycerin topical, transdermal, translingual spray, transmucosal and oral sustained release; isosorbide dinitrate; isosorbide mononitrate; erythrityl tetranitrate; pentaerythritol tetranitrate): Prophylaxis and long-term management of recurrent angina.

Nitroglycerin IV: Control of blood pressure in perioperative hypertension associated with surgical procedures, especially cardiovascular procedures, such as endotracheal intubation, anesthesia, skin incision, sternotomy, cardiac bypass and in the immediate postsurgical period.

CHF associated with acute myocardial infarction (MI); treatment of angina pectoris unresponsive to organic nitrates or β-blockers; production of controlled hypotension during surgical procedures.

Unlabeled uses: Sublingual and topical nitroglycerin and oral nitrates have been used to reduce cardiac workload in patients with acute MI and in CHF.

Nitroglycerin ointment has been used as adjunctive treatment of Raynaud's disease and other peripheral vascular diseases.

IV nitroglycerin may be used in the treatment of hypertensive crisis, specifically in patients who have hypertension with angina or MI.

Contraindications:

Hypersensitivity or idiosyncrasy to nitrates; severe anemia; closed angle glaucoma; postural hypotension; early MI (sublingual nitroglycerin); head trauma or cerebral hemorrhage; allergy to adhesives (transdermal).

Amyl nitrate: Pregnancy.

Nitroglycerin IV: Hypotension or uncorrected hypovolemia; inadequate cerebral circulation; increased intracranial pressure; constrictive pericarditis; pericardial tamponade.

Warnings:

MI: In acute MI, use nitrates only under close clinical observation and with hemodynamic monitoring. In general, do not use a long-acting form because its effects are difficult to terminate rapidly if excessive hypotension or tachycardia develop.

Arcing: A cardioverter/defibrillator should not be discharged through a paddle electrode that overlies a transdermal nitroglycerin system.

Postural hypotension may occur, even with small doses.

Angina: Nitrates may aggravate angina caused by hypertrophic cardiomyopathy.

Nitroglycerin IV:

Hepatic or renal disease, severe – Use with caution.

Hypotension – Avoid excessive prolonged hypotension, because of possible deleterious effects on the brain, heart, liver and kidney from poor perfusion and the attendant risk of ischemia, thrombosis and altered organ function. Paradoxical bradycardia and increased angina pectoris may accompany nitroglycerin-induced hypotension.

Alcohol intoxication has developed in patients on high-dose IV nitroglycerin.

Sublingual nitroglycerin: Absorption is dependent on salivary secretion. Dry mough decreases absorption.

Transdermal nitroglycerin is not for immediate relief of anginal attacks.

Pregnancy: Category C; Category X (amyl nitrite).

Lactation: It is not know whether nitrates are excreted in breast milk.

Children: Safety and efficacy for use in children have not been established.

Precautions:

Tolerance to vascular and antianginal effects of nitrates may develop. The use of a low-nitrate or nitrate-free period should be part of the therapeutic strategy.

Nitrates that appear least likely to associated with tolerance are the short-acting formulations (eg, sublingual, translingual spray), with the exception of the IV form. The transmucosal formulation also appears to be associated with minimal tolerance.

Glaucoma: Intraocular pressure may be increased; therefore, caution is required in administering to patients with glaucoma.

Excessive dosage may produce severe headache.

Volume depletion/hypotension: Severe hypotension (particularly with upright posture) may occur with even small doses of isosorbide mononitrate.

Withdrawal: In terminating treatment of angina, gradually reduce the dosage to prevent withdrawal reactions.

Drug Interactions:

Drugs that may interact with nitrates include alcohol, aspirin, calcium channel blockers, dihydroergotamine and heparin.

Drug/Lab test interactions: Nitrates may interfere with the *Zlatkis-Zak* color reaction causing a false report of decreased serum cholesterol.

Adverse Reactions:

GI: Nausea; vomiting; diarrhea; dyspepsia; involuntary passing of urine and feces; abdominal pain.

CNS: Headache which may be severe and persistnet (up to 50%); apprehension; restlessness; weakness; vertigo; dizziness; agitation; anxiety; confusion; insomnia; nervousness.

Cardiovascular: Tachycardia; palpitations; hypotension (sometimes with paradoxical bradycardia and increased angina pectoris); postural hypotension.

Dermatologic: Drug rash or exfoliative dermatitis; cutaneous vasodilation with flushing; crusgy skin lesions; pruritus; rash.

Sublingual nitroglycerin tablets may cause a local burning or tingling sensation in the oral cavity at the point of dissolution. Absence of this effect does not indicate loss of potency; some older patients may not experience this effect. The stabilized tablets may be less likely to product these sensations.

GU: Dysuria; impotence; urinary frequency.

Miscellaneous: Arthralgia; bronchitis; muschle twiching; pallor; perspiration; cold sweat; asthenia; blurred vision; diplopia; edema; malaise; neck stiffness; increased appetite.

Administration and Dosage:

ISOSORBIDE MONONITRATE:

Tablets – 20 mg twice daily, with the two doses given 7 hours apart. A starting dose of 5 mg might be appropriate for persons of particularly small stature, but should be increased to at least 10 mg by the second or third day of therapy. Suggested regimen is to give first dose on awakining and second dose 7 hours later.

Tablets, extended release – Initially, 30 or 60 mg once daily. After several days, the dosage may be increased to 120 mg once daily. Rarely 240 mg may be required. Suggested regimen is to give in the morning on arising. Do not crush or chew extended release tablets, and swallow them with a half glassful of liquid.

AMYL NITRITE: Usual adult dose is 0.3 ml by inhalation, as required.

Crush the capsule and wave under the nose; 1 to 6 inhalations from one capsule are usually sufficient to produce the desired effect. May repeat in 3 to 5 minutes.

NITROGLYCERIN, INTRAVENOUS:

Dosage requirements – Initially, 5 mcg/min delivered through an infusion pump. Titrate to the clinical situation, initially in 5 mcg/min increments with increases every 3 to 5 minutes until some response is noted. If no response occurs at 20 mcg/min, use increments of 10 to 20 mcg/min. Once a partial blood pressure response is observed, reduce the dose and lengthen the interval between increments.

NITROGLYCERIN, TRANSMUCOSAL: 1 mg every 3 to 5 hours during waking hours. Place tablet between lip and gum above incisors, or between cheek and gum.

NITROGLYCERIN, SUBLINGUAL: Dissolve 1 tablet under tongue or in buccal pouch (between cheek and gum) at first sign of an acute anginal attack. Repeat approximately every 5 minutes until relief is obtained. Take no more than 3 tablets in 15 minutes. May be used prophylkactically 5 to 10 minutes prior to activities which might precipitate an acute attack.

NITROGLYCERIN, TRANSLINGUAL: At the onset of attack, spray 1 or 2 metered doses onto or under the tongue. No more than 3 metered doses are recommended within 15 minutes. May use prophylactically 5 to 10 minutes prior to activities which might precipitate an acute attack. Do not inhale spray.

NITROGLYCERIN SUSTAINED RELEASE: The usual starting dose is 2.5 or 2.6 mg, 3 or 4 times daily. The dose generally may be increased by 2.5 or 2.6 mg increments 2 to 4 times daily over a period of days or weeks. Doses as high as 26 mg given 4 times daily have been reported effective.

Give the smallest effective dose 2 to 4 times daily.

Capsules must be swallowed; not for chewing or sublingual use.

NITROGLYCERIN TRANSDERMAL SYSTEMS: Patient instructions for application are provided with products.

Apply once daily to a skin site free of hair and not subject to excessive movement. Do not apply to distal parts of extremities. Avoid areas with cuts/irritations.

Starting dose – 0.2 to 0.4 mg/hr. Doses between 0.4 and 0.8 mg/hr have shown continued effectiveness for 10 to 12 hours daily for at least 1 month of intermittent administration. Although the minimum nitrate-free interval has not been defined, data show that a nitrate-free interval of 10 to 12 hours is sufficient. Thus, an appropriate dosing schedule would include a daily "patch-on" period of 12 to 14 hours and a "patch-off" period of 10 to 12 hours. Tolerance is a major factor limiting efficacy when the system is used continuously for > 12 hours each day.

NITROGLYCERIN, TOPICAL:

Usual therapeutic dose – 1 to 2 inches (25 to 50 mm) every 8 hours, up to 4 to 5 inches (100 to 125 mm) every 4 hours. Start with ½ inch (12.5 mm) every 8 hours; increase by ½ inch with each application to achieve desired effects.

One inch (25 mm) of ointment contains ≈ 15 mg nitroglycerin.

ISOSORBIDE DINITRATE, SUBLINGUAL AND CHEWABLE:

Angina pectoris – Usual starting dose is 2.5 to 5 mg for sublingual tablets and 5 mg for chewable tablets.

Acute prophylaxis – 5 to 10 mg sublingual or chewable tablets every 2 to 3 hours. Limit use of sublingual or chewable isosorbide dinitrate for aborting an acute anginal attack in patients intolerant of or unresponsive to sublingual nitroglycerin.

Do not cursh or chew sublingual tablets; do not crush chewable tablets before administering.

ISOSORBIDE DINITRATE, ORAL:

Tablets – Initial dose is 5 to 20 mg; maintenance dose is 10 to 40 mg every 6 hours.

Sustained release – The initial dose is 40 mg; maintenance controlled release dose is 40 to 80 mg every 8 to 12 hours. Do not crush or chew these preparations.

Tolerance to these agents may develop. Consider administereing the short-acting preparations 2 or 3 times daily (last dose no later than 7 pm) and the sustained release preparations once daily or twice daily at 8 am and 2 pm.

ANTIARRHYTHMIC AGENTS

Optimal therapy of cardiac arrhythmias requires documentation, accurate diagnosis and modification of precipitating causes, and if indicated, proper selection and use of antiarrhythmic drugs. These drugs are classified according to their effects on the action potential of cardiac cells and their presumed mechanism of action.

Group I: Local anesthetics or membrane-stabilizing agents that depress phase 0.

IA *(quinidine, procainamide, disopyramide):* Depress phase 0 and prolong the action potential duration.

IB *(tocainide, lidocaine, phenytoin, mexiletine):* Depress phase 0 slightly and may shorten the action potential duration. Although arrhythmia is not a labeled indication for *phenytoin*, it is commonly used in treatment of digitalis-induced arrhythmias.

IC *(flecainide, encainide, propafenone):* Marked depression of phase 0. Slight effect on repolarization. Profound slowing of conduction. *Encainide* was voluntarily withdrawn from the market, but is still available on a limited basis.

Moricizine is a Group I agent that shares some of the characteristics of the Group IA, B and C agents.

Group II (propranolol, esmolol, acebutolol): Depress phase 4 depolarization.

Group III (bretylium, amiodarone): Produce a prolongation of phase 3 (repolarization).

Group IV (verapamil): Depress phase 4 depolarization and lengthen phases 1 and 2 of repolarization.

Sotalol has both Group II (beta blocking) and III properties; Class III effects are seen at doses > 160 mg.

Digitalis glycosides (digoxin) cause a decrease in maximal diastolic potential and action potential duration and increase the slope of phase 4 depolarization.

Adenosine slows conduction time through the AV node and can interrupt the reentry pathways through the AV node.

Serum drug levels: Some antiarrhythmic drugs (eg, quinidine) can produce toxic effects which can be easily confused with the symptoms for which the drug has been prescribed. Drug serum levels are important in evaluating toxic or subtherapeutic dosage regimens of most of the antiarrhythmic drugs. They are also aids in monitoring active metabolites (eg, procainamide/NAPA), suspected drug interactions and subtherapeutic response due to drug failure, noncompliance, altered clearance or altered absorption.

Proarrhythmic effects: Antiarrhythmic agents may cause new or worsened arrhythmias. Such proarrhythmic effects range from an increase in frequency of PVCs to the development of more severe ventricular tachycardia, ventricular fibrillation or torsade de pointes (ie, tachycardia that is more sustained or more rapid), which may lead to fatal consequences. It is often not possible to distinguish a proarrhythmic effect from the patient's underlying rhythm disorder. It is therefore essential that each patient be evaluated electrocardiographically and clinically prior to and during therapy to determine whether the response to the drug supports continued treatment.

Cardiac Arrhythmia Suppression Trial (CAST): In the National Heart, Lung and Blood Institute's Cardiac Arrhythmia Suppression Trial (CAST), a long-term study in patients with asymptomatic non-life-threatening ventricular ectopy who had an MI > 6 days but < 2 years previously, and demonstrated mild to moderate left ventricular dysfunction, an excessive mortality or non-fatal cardiac arrest rate was seen in patients treated with encainide or flecainide (56/730) compared with that seen in patients assigned to carefully matched placebo-treated groups (22/725). The moricizine and placebo arms of the trial were continued in CAST II; however, the study was discontinued because there was no possibility of demonstrating a benefit toward improved survival with moricizine and because of an evolving adverse trend after long-term treatment.

The applicability of these results to other populations (eg, those without recent MI) and to other antiarrhythmic drugs is uncertain, but at present it is prudent (1) to consider any IC agent (especially one documented to provoke new serious arrhythmias) to have a similar risk and (2) to consider the risks of Class IC agents, coupled with the lack of any evidence of improved survival, generally unacceptable in patients without life-threatening ventricular arrhythmias, even if the patients are experiencing unpleasant, but not life-threatening symptoms or signs.

Antiarrhythmic Electrophysiology/Electrocardiogram Effects

Anti-arrhythmic		Electrophysiology[1]										ECG changes[1]				
		Automaticity		Conduction velocity			Refractory period									
Group	Drug	SA node	Ectopic pacemaker	Atrium	AV node	His-Purkinje	Atrium	AV node	His-Purkinje	Ventricle	Accessory pathways[2]	Heart rate	PR interval	QRS complex	QT_c interval	JT interval
I	Moricizine[3]	0	↓	0	↓	↓	±	0	0	0-↑	↑	0-↑	↑	↑	0	↓
	Quinidine	±	↓	↓	±	↓	↑↑	0-↑[4]	↑↑	↑	↑	±	±	↑	↑	↑
	Procainamide	±	↓	↓	±	↓	↑	0-↑[4]	↑↑	↑	↑↑	±	±	↑	↑	↑
	Disopyramide	±	↓	↓	±	↓	↑↑	0-↑[4]	↑↑	↑	↑	±	±	↑	↑	↑
	Lidocaine	0	↓	—	0	0	0	±	±	±	↑-↓	0	0	0	0-↓	0
	Phenytoin	↓-0	↓	-	0	0	0	±	±	±	-	±	0-↓	0	↓	0
	Tocainide	0-↓	↓	0	0	0	↓	↓	±	↓	↑	0	0	0	0-↓	0
	Mexiletine	↓	↓	0	0	0	0	±	↑	↑	↑	-	0	0	0	0
	Flecainide	↓	↓	↓↓	↓	↓↓	0	0	↑	↑	↑↑	0	↑[5]	↑↑[5]	0 ↑[5]	0
	Encainide[6]	0-↓	↓	↓↓	↓	↓↓	0-↑	0-↑	↑	↑	↑↑	0	↑[5]	↑↑[5]	0-↑[5]	0
	Propafenone	0	↓	0	↓	↓	0	↑	↑	↑	↑	0	↑[5]	↑	0-↑[5]	0
II	Propranolol	↓	↓	±	↓	0-↓	±	↑	0	0	0-↑	↓	0-↑	0	0-↓	0
	Esmolol	↓	↓	±	↓	0-	±	↑	0	0	0-↑	↓	0-↑	0	0-↓	0
	Acebutolol	↓	↓	±	↓	0	±	↑	0	0	0-↑	↓	0-↑	0	0-↓	0
III	Bretylium	↑	↑	0	0	0-↑	0	↓-0-↑[7]	↑	0-↑	±	0	0	0	0	↑
	Amiodarone	↓	↓	↓	↓	↓	↑	↑	↑	↑	↑	↓	↑	↑	↑↑	↑↑
	Sotalol[8]	↓	↓	0	↓	0	↑↑	↑	↑↑	↑↑	↑	↓	↑	0	↑↑	↑↑
IV	Verapamil	↓	↓	0	↓	0	0	↑	0	0	0	↓	↑	0	0	0
—	Digoxin	0-↓	↑	±	↓	0-↓	±	↑	0	↓	↓-↑	↓	↑	0	↓	↓
—	Adenosine	↓	↓	0	↓	0	0	↑	0	0	0	↑	↑	0	0	—

[1] These values assume therapeutic levels.

[2] Accessory pathways occur in Wolff-Parkinson-White syndrome (preexcitation phenomena) and possibly other abnormal conditions.

[3] Does not belong to any of the 3 subclasses (A, B or C), but does have some properties of each.

[4] Retrograde AV node RP↑; antegrade RP not affected.

[5] Dose-related increases.

[6] Withdrawn from the market; however, available on a limited basis.

[7] Due to a complex balance of direct and indirect autonomic effects.

[8] Has both Group II (beta blocking) and III properties; Class III effects are seen at doses > 160 mg.

Antiarrhythmic Pharmacokinetics

Antiarrhythmics: Group		Antiarrhythmics: Drug	Onset (hrs) (oral)[1]	Duration (hrs)	Half-life (hrs)	Protein binding (%)	Excreted unchanged (%)	Therapeutic serum level (mcg/ml)	Toxic serum levels (mcg/ml)
I	A	Moricizine	2	10-24	1.5-3.5[2]	95	< 1	Not applicable	—
		Quinidine	0.5	6-8	6-7	80-90	10-50	2-6	> 8
		Procainamide	0.5	3+	2.5-4.7	14-23	40-70	4-8	> 16
		Disopyramide	0.5	6-7	4-10	20-60[3]	40-60	2-8	> 9
	B	Lidocaine	—	0.25[4]	1-2	40-80	< 3	1.5-6	> 7
		Phenytoin	0.5-1	24+	22-36[5]	87-93	< 5	10-20	> 20
		Tocainide	—	—	11-15	10-20	28-55	4-10	> 10
		Mexiletine	—	—	10-12	50-60	10	0.5-2	> 2
	C	Flecainide	—	—	12-27	40	30	0.2-1	> 1
		Encainide[6]	—	—	1-2[7]	75-85	< 5[8]	Not applicable	—
		MODE[9]			6-12	92		wide range	—
		ODE[9]			3-4	75-85		0.1-0.3	—
		Propafenone	—	—	2-10[10]	97	< 1	0.06-1	—
II		Propranolol	0.5	3-5	2-3	90-95	< 1	0.05-0.1	—
		Esmolol	< 5 min	very short	0.15	55	< 2	—	—
		Acebutolol	—	24-30	3-4	26	15-20	—	—
III		Bretylium	—	6-8	5-10	0-8	> 80	0.5-1.5	—
		Amiodarone	1-3 wks[11]	weeks to months	26-107 days	96	negligible	0.5-2.5	> 2.5
		Sotalol	—	—	12	0	100	—	—
IV		Verapamil	0.5	6	3-7	90	3-4	0.08-0.3	—
—		Digoxin	0.5-2	24+	30-40	20-25	60	0.5-2 ng/ml	> 2.5 ng/ml
—		Adenosine	(34 sec IV)	1-2 min	< 10 sec	—	0 (enters body pool)	Not applicable	—

[1] Within 1 to 5 minutes with IV use.
[2] Half-life may be prolonged in patients after multiple dosing.
[3] Protein binding is concentration-dependent.
[4] Very short after discontinuation of IV infusion.
[5] Half-life increases with increasing dosage.
[6] Withdrawn from the market; however, available on a limited basis.
[7] Half-life 6 to 11 hours in < 10% of patients (poor metabolizers).
[8] > 50% in poor metabolizers.
[9] MODE (3-methoxy-O-demethyl encainide) and ODE (O-demethyl encainide), metabolites more active than encainide on a per mg basis.
[10] Half-life 10 to 32 hours in < 10% of patients (slow metabolizers).
[11] Onset of action may occur in 2 to 3 days.

MORICIZINE HCl

Tablets: 200, 250 and 300 mg (Rx) — *Ethmozine* (Roberts)

Actions:

Pharmacology: Moricizine is a Class I antiarrhythmic agent with potent local anesthetic activity and myocardial membrane stabilizing effects. Moricizine reduces the fast inward current carried by sodium ions and shortens Phase 2 and 3 repolarization, resulting in a decreased action potential duration and effective refractory period. A dose-related decrease in the maximum rate of Phase 0 depolarization occurs.

Electrophysiology – In patients with ventricular tachycardia, moricizine prolongs AV conduction. AV nodal conduction time (AH interval), His-Purkinje conduction time (HV interval), PR interval and the QRS are prolonged. Prolongations in the corrected QT interval result from widening of the QRS interval.

Pharmacokinetics:

Absorption/Distribution – Following oral administration, moricizine undergoes significant first-pass metabolism resulting in an absolute bioavailability of ≈ 38%. Peak plasma concentrations are usually reached within 0.5 to 2 hours. The apparent volume of distribution after oral administration is very large (≥ 300 L). Moricizine is ≈ 95% bound to plasma proteins.

Metabolism/Excretion – Moricizine undergoes extensive biotransformation; < 1% is excreted unchanged in the urine. Moricizine induces its own metabolism. Approximately 56% is excreted in the feces and 39% is excreted in the urine. Some enterohepatic recycling occurs.

Indications:

Treatment of documented ventricular arrhythmias, such as sustained ventricular tachycardia, that are life-threatening. Because of the proarrhythmic effects of moricizine, reserve its use for patients in whom the benefits of treatment outweigh the risks.

Unlabeled uses: Moricizine appears effective in treatment of ventricular premature contractions, couplets and nonsustained ventricular tachycardia.

Contraindications:

Pre-existing second- or third-degree AV block; right bundle branch block when associated with left hemiblock (bifascicular block) unless a pacemaker is present; cardiogenic shock; hypersensitivity to the drug.

Warnings:

Mortality: Considering the lack of evidence of improved survival for any antiarrhythmic drug in patients without life-threatening arrhythmias, it is prudent to reserve the use of moricizine for patients with life-threatening ventricular arrhythmias.

Proarrhythmic effects: Refer to the Antiarrhythmics Introduction.

Electrolyte disturbances: Hypokalemia, hyperkalemia or hypomagnesemia may alter the effects. Correct electrolyte imbalances before administration of moricizine.

Sick sinus syndrome: Use with extreme caution in patients with sick sinus syndrome since it may cause sinus bradycardia, sinus pause or sinus arrest.

Renal function impairment: Plasma levels of intact moricizine are unchanged in hemodialysis patients, but a significant portion is metabolized and excreted in the urine.

Hepatic function impairment: Patients with significant liver dysfunction have reduced plasma clearance and an increased half-life of moricizine. Administer with particular care to patients with severe liver disease, if at all.

Pregnancy: Category B.

Lactation: Moricizine is present breast milk.

Children: Safety and efficacy in children < 18 years of age have not been established.

Precautions:

Congestive heart failure: Worsened heart failure has been attributed to moricizine.

ECG changes/Conduction abnormalities: Moricizine produces dose-related increases in PR and QRS intervals. Although the QTc interval is increased, this is due to QRS prolongation; the JT interval is shortened, indicating absence of significant slowing of ventricular repolarization. The degree of lengthening of PR and QRS intervals does not predict efficacy.

In patients with pre-existing conduction abnormalities, initiate therapy cautiously. If second- or third-degree AV block occurs, discontinue therapy unless a ventricular pacemaker is in place.

Effects on pacemaker threshold: Monitor pacing parameters if moricizine is used.

Drug Interactions:

Drugs that may interact with moricizine include cimetidine, digoxin, propranolol, theophylline and food.

Adverse Reactions:

Significant adverse reactions include proarrhythmia, nausea, sweating, musculoskeletal pain, dry mouth, blurred vision, palpitations, sustained ventricular tachycardia, cardiac chest pain, CHF, cardiac death, dizziness (dose-related), headache, fatigue, hypesthesias, asthenia, nervousness, paresthesias, sleep disorders, dyspnea, abdominal pain, dyspepsia, vomiting, diarrhea.

Administration and Dosage:

Usual adult dosage is between 600 and 900 mg/day, given every 8 hours in three equally divided doses. Within this range, the dosage can be adjusted as tolerated, in increments of 150 mg/day at 3 day intervals, until the desired effect is obtained. As the antiarrhythmic effect of moricizine persists for > 12 hours, some patients whose arrhythmias are well controlled on an every 8 hour regimen may be given the same total daily dose in an every 12 hour regimen to increase convenience and help assure compliance.

Hepatic or renal function impairment: Start at ≤ 600 mg/day and monitor closely, including measurement of ECG intervals, before dosage adjustment.

Transfer from another antiarrhythmic:

Transferring to Moricizine from Another Antiarrhythmic	
Agent transferred from	Start moricizine
Quinidine, disopyramide	6 to 12 hours after last dose
Procainamide	3 to 6 hours after last dose
Encainide, mexiletine, propafenone or tocainide	8 to 12 hours after last dose
Flecainide	12 to 24 hours after last dose

QUINIDINE

QUINIDINE SULFATE	
Tablets: 200 and 300 mg (*Rx*)	Various, *Quinora* (Key Pharm.)
Tablets, sustained release: 300 mg (*Rx*)	Various, *Quinidex Extentabs* (Robins)
QUINIDINE GLUCONATE	
Tablets, sustained release: 324 mg (*Rx*)	Various, *Quinaglute Dura-Tabs* (Berlex), *Quinalan* (Lannett)
Injection: 80 mg/ml (*Rx*)	Various
QUINIDINE POLYGALACTURONATE	
Tablets: 275 mg (*Rx*)	*Cardioquin* (Purdue Frederick)

Actions:

Pharmacology: Quinidine, a class IA antiarrhythmic, depresses myocardial excitability, conduction velocity and contractility. Therapeutically, it prolongs the effective refractory period and increases conduction time, thereby preventing the reentry phenomenon. In addition, quinidine exerts an indirect anticholinergic effect; it decreases vagal tone and may facilitate conduction in the atrioventricular junction.

Pharmacokinetics:

Absorption/Distribution –

Anhydrous Quinidine Alkaloid Content in Various Salts			
	Quinidine content		
Quinidine salts	Active drug	Absorbed	Time to peak plasma levels (hours)
Quinidine sulfate	83%	73%	1 to 3[1]
Quinidine gluconate	62%	70%	3-5
Quinidine polygalacturonate	80%	—	6

[1] 3 to 5 hours for sustained release form.

Quinidine is rapidly absorbed from the GI tract. Maximum effects of quinidine gluconate occur 30 to 90 minutes after IM administration; onset is more rapid after IV administration. Activity persists for 6 to 8 hours or more. The average therapeutic serum levels are reported to be 2 to 7 mcg/ml. Toxic reactions may occur at levels from 5 to ≥ 8 mcg/ml. Quinidine is 80% to 90% bound to plasma proteins; the unbound fraction may be significantly increased in patients with hepatic insufficiency.

Metabolism/Excretion – From 60% to 80% of a dose is metabolized via the liver into several metabolites; the primary metabolites are 3-hydroxyquinidine and 2-oxoquinidinone. Whether or not these or other metabolites have antiarrhythmic activity is unclear and controversial. Quinidine is excreted unchanged (10% to 50%) in the urine within 24 hours. The elimination half-life ranges from 4 to 10 hours in healthy patients, with a mean of 6 to 7 hours. Urinary acidification facilitates quinidine elimination, and alkalinization retards it. In patients with cirrhosis, the elimination half-life may be prolonged and the volume of distribution increased.

Indications:

Oral: Premature atrial, AV junctional and ventricular contractions; paroxysmal atrial (supraventricular) tachycardia; paroxysmal AV junctional rhythm; atrial flutter; paroxysmal and chronic atrial fibrillation; established atrial fibrillation when therapy is appropriate; paroxysmal ventricular tachycardia not associated with complete heart block; maintenance therapy after electrical conversion of atrial fibrillation or flutter.

Parenteral: When oral therapy is not feasible or when rapid therapeutic effect is required.

Quinidine gluconate – Life-threatening *Plasmodium falciparum* malaria.

Contraindications:

Hypersensitivity or idiosyncrasy to quinidine or other cinchona derivatives manifested by thrombocytopenia, skin eruption or febrile reactions; myasthenia gravis; history of thrombocytopenic purpura associated with quinidine administration; digitalis intoxication manifested by arrhythmias or AV conduction disorders; complete heart block; left bundle branch block or other severe intraventricular conduction defects exhibiting marked QRS widening or bizarre complexes; complete AV block with an AV nodal or idioventricular pacemaker; aberrant ectopic impulses and abnormal rhythms due to escape mechanisms; history of drug-induced torsade de pointes; history of long QT syndrome.

Warnings:

Hepatotoxicity (including granulomatous hepatitis) due to quinidine hypersensitivity has occurred.

Atrial flutter or fibrillation: Reversion to sinus rhythm may be preceded by a progressive reduction in degree of AV block to a 1:1 ratio, which results in an extremely rapid ventricular rate. Prior to use in atrial flutter, pretreat with a digitalis preparation.

Cardiotoxicity (eg, increased PR and QT intervals, 50% widening of QRS complex, ventricular tachyarrhythmias, frequent ventricular ectopic beats or tachycardia) dictates immediate discontinuation of quinidine; closely monitor the ECG.

In susceptible individuals (ie, marginally compensated cardiovascular disease), quinidine may produce clinically important depression of cardiac function such as hypotension, bradycardia or heartblock.

Large oral doses may reduce the arterial pressure by means of peripheral vasodilation. Serious hypotension is more likely with parenteral use.

Use quinidine with extreme caution in incomplete AV block, since complete block and asystole may result. The drug may cause unpredictable dysrhythmias in digitalized patients. Use cautiously in patients with partial bundle branch block, severe CHF and hypotensive states due to the depressant effects of quinidine on myocardial contractility and arterial pressure.

Parenteral therapy: The dangers of parenteral use of quinidine are increased in the presence of AV block or absence of atrial activity. Administration is more hazardous in patients with extensive myocardial damage. Use of quinidine in digitalis-induced cardiac arrhythmia is extremely dangerous because the cardiac glycoside may already have caused serious impairment of intracardiac conduction system. Too rapid IV administration of as little as 200 mg may precipitate a fall of 40 to 50 mm Hg in arterial pressure.

Syncope occasionally occurs in patients on long-term quinidine therapy, usually resulting from ventricular tachycardia or fibrillation.

Renal, hepatic or cardiac insufficiency: Use with caution in renal, cardiac or hepatic insufficiency because of potential toxicity.

Hypersensitivity: Asthma, muscle weakness and infection with fever prior to quinidine administration may mask hypersensitivity reactions to the drug.

Pregnancy: Category C. Quinidine crosses the placenta and achieves fetal serum levels similar to maternal levels. Neonatal thrombocytopenia has occurred after maternal use.

Lactation: Quinidine is excreted into breast milk with a milk:serum ratio of approximately 0.71. The American Academy of Pediatrics considers quinidine to be compatible with breast feeding.

Children: Safety and efficacy have not been established.

Precautions:

Monitoring: Perform periodic blood counts and liver and kidney function tests. Discontinue use if blood dyscrasias or signs of hepatic or renal disorders occur. Frequently measure arterial blood pressure during IV use.

Potassium balance: The effect of quinidine is enhanced by potassium and reduced if hypokalemia is present. The risk of drug-induced torsade de pointes is increased by concomitant hypokalemia.

Drug Interactions:

Drugs that may affect quinidine include amiodarone, antacids, barbiturates, cholinergic drugs, cimetidine, disopyramide, hydantoins, nifedipine, rifampin, sucralfate, urinary alkalinizers and verapamil. Drugs that may be affected by quinidine include anticholinergics, anticoagulants, beta blockers, cardiac glycosides, disopyramide, nondepolarizing neuromuscular blockers, procainamide, propafenone, succinylcholine and tricyclic antidepressants.

Drug/Lab test interactions: Triamterene and quinidine have similar fluorescence spectra; thus, triamterene will interfere with the fluorescent measurement of quinidine serum levels.

Adverse Reactions:

Adverse reactions may include: Nausea, vomiting, abdominal pain, diarrhea, anorexia; cinchonism (ringing in the ears, hearing loss, headache, nausea, dizziness, vertigo, lightheadedness, disturbed vision); headache; fever; vertigo; apprehension; excitement; confusion; delirium; dementia; depression; acute hemolytic anemia; hypoprothrombinemia; thrombocytopenic purpura; agranulocytosis; thrombocytopenia; leukocytosis; mydriasis; blurred vision; disturbed color perception; reduced vision field; night blindness, photophobia; rash; urticaria; cutaneous flushing with intense pruritus; photosensitivity; eczema; psoriasis; abnormalities of pigmentation; arthralgia; myalgia; disturbed hearing; lupus erythematosus; hepatitis; cardiac asystole; ventricular ectopy; idioventricular rhythms; paradoxical tachycardia; arterial embolism; hypotension; ventricular extrasystoles; complete AV block; ventricular flutter.

Administration and Dosage:

Test dose: Administer a single 200 mg tablet of quinidine sulfate or 200 mg IM quinidine gluconate to determine whether the patient has an idiosyncratic reaction.

Adjust the dosage to maintain the plasma concentration between 2 to 6 mcg/ml.

Oral:

Premature atrial and ventricular contractions – 200 to 300 mg 3 or 4 times daily.

Paroxysmal supraventricular tachycardias – 400 to 600 mg every 2 or 3 hours until the paroxysm is terminated.

Atrial flutter – Administer quinidine after digitalization. Individualize dosage.

Conversion of atrial fibrillation – 200 mg every 2 or 3 hours for 5 to 8 doses, with subsequent daily increases until sinus rhythm is restored or toxic effects occur. Do not exceed a total daily dose of 3 to 4 g in any regimen.

Maintenance therapy – 200 to 300 mg 3 or 4 times daily. Other patients may require larger doses or more frequent administration than the usually recommended schedule.

Sustained release forms – 300 to 600 mg every 8 or 12 hours.

Parenteral:

IM – In the treatment of acute tachycardia, the initial dose is 600 mg quinidine gluconate. Subsequently, 400 mg quinidine gluconate can be repeated as often as every 2 hours.

IV – In ≈ 50% of patients who respond successfully to quinidine, the arrhythmia can be terminated by ≤ 330 mg quinidine gluconate (or its equivalent in other salts); as much as 500 to 750 mg may be required. Inject slowly.

QUINIDINE GLUCONATE – *P falciparum malaria* – The following two regimens are effective emirically. As soon as practical, institute standard oral antiplasmodial therapy.

1) *Loading*, 15 mg/kg in 250 ml normal saline infused over 4 hours followed by: *Maintenance*, beginning 24 hours after the beginning of the loading dose, 7.5 mg/kg infused over 4 hours, every 8 hours for 7 days or until oral therapy can be instituted.

2) *Loading*, 10 mg/kg in 250 ml normal saline infused over 1 to 2 hours, followed immediately by: *Maintenance*, 0.02 mg/kg/min for up to 72 hours or until parasitemia decreases to < 1% or oral therapy can be instituted.

Children:

Oral (quinidine sulfate) – 30 mg/kg/day or 900 mg/m^2/day in 5 divided doses.

IV (quinidine gluconate) – 2 to 10 mg/kg/dose every 3 to 6 hours as needed; however, this route is not recommended.

PROCAINAMIDE

Tablets: 250, 375 and 500 mg (Rx)	Various, *Pronestyl* (Princeton Pharm.)
Capsules: 250, 375, 500 mg (Rx)	Various, *Pronestyl* (Princeton Pharm.)
Injection: 100, 500 mg/ml (Rx)	Various, *Pronestyl* (Princeton Pharm.)
Tablets, sustained release: 250, 500, 750 and 1000 mg (Rx)	Various, *Procan SR* (Parke-Davis), *Pronestyl-SR* (Princeton Pharm.)

Warning:

The prolonged administration often leads to the development of a positive antinuclear antibody (ANA) test. If a positive ANA titer develops, assess the benefit/risk ratio related to continued therapy.

Actions:

Pharmacology: Procainamide, a class IA antiarrhythmic, increases the effective refractory period of the atria, and to a lesser extent the bundle of His-Purkinje system and ventricles of the heart. It reduces impulse conduction velocity in the atria, His-Purkinje fibers, and ventricular muscle, but has variable effects on the AV node, a direct slowing action and a weaker vagolytic effect which may speed AV conduction slightly. Myocardial excitability is reduced in the atria, Purkinje fibers, papillary muscles, and ventricles by an increase in the threshold for excitation, combined with inhibition of ectopic pacemaker activity by retardation of the slow phase of diastolic depolarization, thus decreasing automaticity especially in ectopic sites. Slight reduction of cardiac output may occur. Therapeutic levels of procainamide may exert vagolytic effects and produce slight acceleration of heart rate, while high or toxic concentrations may prolong AV conduction time or induce AV block, or even cause abnormal automaticity and spontaneous firing.

Electrophysiology – The ECG may show slight sinus tachycardia and widened QRS complexes and, less regularly, prolonged QT and PR intervals, as well as some decrease in QRS and T wave amplitude.

Pharmacokinetics:

Absorption/Distribution – Oral procainamide is resistant to digestive hydrolysis, and the drug is well absorbed from the entire small intestinal surface, but individual patients vary in their completeness of absorption. Following oral use, plasma levels peak at ≈ 90 to 120 minutes. Following IM injection, plasma levels peak in 15 to 60 minutes. IV use can produce therapeutic plasma levels within minutes. About 15% to 20% is reversibly bound to plasma proteins. The apparent volume of distribution eventually reaches ≈ 2 L/kg with a half-life of ≈ 5 minutes.

Metabolism/Excretion – A significant fraction of the circulating procainamide may be metabolized in hepatocytes to N-acetylprocainamide (NAPA), ranging from 16% to 33% of an administered dose. NAPA also has significant antiarrhythmic activity and somewhat slower renal clearance than procainamide. The elimination half-life of procainamide is 3 to 4 hours in patients with normal renal function, but reduced creatinine clearance (Ccr) and advancing age each prolong the elimination half-life. Half-life and renal clearance are also reduced in infants. Thirty percent to 60% of the drug is excreted as unchanged procainamide, and 6% to 52% as the NAPA derivative. Both procainamide and NAPA are eliminated by active tubular secretion as well as by glomerular filtration.

While therapeutic plasma levels for procainamide have been reported to be 3 to 10 mcg/ml, certain patients such as those with sustained ventricular tachycardia may need higher levels for adequate control. This may justify the increased risk of toxicity. Plasma levels of NAPA that produce arrhythmia suppression range from 10 to 30 mcg/ml. Toxicity may occur with levels > 30 mcg/ml, although there appears to be overlap between the therapeutic and toxic ranges.

Indications:

Treatment of documented ventricular arrhythmias, such as sustained ventricular tachycardia, that are judged to be life-threatening.

Contraindications:

Complete heart block; idiosyncratic hypersensitivity; lupus erythematosus; torsade de pointes.

Warnings:

Blood dyscrasias: Agranulocytosis, bone marrow depression, neutropenia, hypoplastic anemia and thrombocytopenia in patients receiving procainamide have been reported at a rate of ≈ 0.5%. Fatalities have occurred (with ≈ 20% to 25% mortality in reported cases of agranulocytosis). Complete blood counts including white cell, differential and platelet counts should be performed at weekly intervals for the first 3 months of therapy, and periodically thereafter. Perform complete blood counts promptly if the patient develops any signs of infection (eg, fever, chills, sore throat, stomatitis), bruising or bleeding. If any of these hematologic disorders are identified, discontinue therapy. Blood counts usually return to normal within 1 month of discontinuation. Use caution in patients with preexisting marrow failure or cytopenia of any type.

Mortality: At present it is prudent to consider any antiarrhythmic agent to have a significant risk in patients with structural heart disease.

Complete heart block: Do not administer to patients with complete heart block because of its effects in suppressing nodal or ventricular pacemakers and the hazard of asystole. If significant slowing of ventricular rate occurs during treatment without evidence of AV conduction appearing, stop procainamide. In cases of second-degree AV block or various types of hemiblock, avoid or discontinue procainamide because of the possibility of increased severity of block, unless the ventricular rate is controlled by an electrical pacemaker.

Torsade de pointes: Procainamide may aggravate this special type of ventricular extrasystole or tachycardia instead of suppressing it.

Lupus erythematosus: If the lupus erythematosus-like syndrome develops in a patient with recurrent life-threatening arrhythmias not controlled by other agents, corticosteroid suppressive therapy may be used concomitantly with procainamide. Since the procainamide-induced lupoid syndrome rarely includes the dangerous pathologic renal changes, therapy may not necessarily have to be stopped unless the symptoms of serositis and the possibility of further lupoid effects are of greater risk than the benefit of procainamide in controlling arrhythmias. Patients with rapid acetylation capability are less likely to develop the lupoid syndrome after prolonged therapy.

Asymptomatic ventricular premature contractions: Avoid treatment of patients with this condition.

Digitalis intoxication: Exercise caution in the use of procainamide in arrhythmias associated with digitalis intoxication. Procainamide can suppress digitalis-induced arrhythmias; however, if there is concomitant marked disturbance of AV conduction, additional depression of conduction and ventricular asystole or fibrillation may result. Consider use of procainamide only if discontinuation of digitalis, and therapy with potassium, lidocaine or phenytoin, are ineffective.

First-degree heart block: Exercise caution if the patient exhibits or develops first-degree heart block while taking procainamide; dosage reduction is advised. If the block persists despite dosage reduction, continuation of procainamide must be evaluated on the basis of current benefit vs risk of increased heart block.

Predigitalization for atrial flutter or fibrillation: Cardiovert or digitalize patients with atrial flutter or fibrillation prior to procainamide administration to avoid enhancement of AV conduction which may result in ventricular rate acceleration beyond tolerable limits. Adequate digitalization reduces the possibility of sudden increase in ventricular rate.

CHF: Use with caution in patients with CHF and in those with acute ischemic heart disease or cardiomyopathy since even slight depression of myocardial contractility may further reduce cardiac output of the damaged heart.

Concurrent antiarrhythmic agents: may produce enhanced prolongation of conduction or depression of contractility and hypotension, especially in patients with cardiac decompensation. Reserve concurrent use of procainamide with other group IA antiarrhythmic agents (eg, quinidine, disopyramide) for patients with serious arrhythmias unresponsive to a single drug and use only if close observation is possible.

Myasthenia gravis: Procainamide administration in myasthenia gravis patients may be hazardous without optimal adjustment of anticholinesterase medications and other precautions. Immediately after initiation of therapy, closely observe patients for muscular weakness if myasthenia gravis is a possibility.

Renal insufficiency may lead to accumulation of high plasma levels from conventional oral doses of procainamide, with effects similar to those of overdosage unless dosage is adjusted for the individual patient.

Hypersensitivity: In patients sensitive to procaine or other ester-type local anesthetics, cross-sensitivity to procainamide is unlikely; however, consider the possibility. Do not use procainamide if it produces acute allergic dermatitis, asthma or anaphylactic symptoms.

Pregnancy: Category C.

Lactation: Both procainamide and NAPA are excreted in breast milk and absorbed by the nursing infant. Discontinue nursing or the drug, taking into account the importance of the drug to the mother.

Children: Safety and efficacy have not been established.

Precautions:

Monitoring: After achieving and maintaining therapeutic plasma concentrations and satisfactory ECG and clinical responses, continue frequent periodic monitoring of vital signs and ECG. If evidence of QRS widening of > 25% or marked prolongation of the QT interval occurs, concern for overdosage is appropriate; reduction in dosage is advisable if a 50% increase occurs. Elevated serum creatinine or urea nitrogen, reduced Ccr or history of renal insufficiency, as well as use in older patients (over age 50), provide grounds to anticipate that less than the usual dosage and longer time intervals between doses may suffice. If facilities are available for measurement of plasma procainamide and NAPA levels or acetylation capability, individual dose adjustment for optimal therapeutic levels may be easier, but close observation of clinical effectiveness is the most important criterion.

In the longer term, periodic complete blood counts are useful to detect possible idiosyncratic hematologic effects of procainamide on neutrophil, platelet or red cell homeostasis; agranulocytosis may occur occasionally in patients on long-term therapy. A rising titer of serum ANA may precede clinical symptoms of the lupoid syndrome. Laboratory tests such as ECG and serum creatinine or urea nitrogen may be indicated, depending on the clinical situation.

Embolization: In conversion of atrial fibrillation to normal sinus rhythm by any means, dislodgement of mural thrombi may lead to embolization.

Tartrazine sensitivity: Some of these products contain tartrazine which may cause allergic-type reactions (including bronchial asthma). Although the overall incidence of tartrazine sensitivity in the general population is low, it is frequently seen in patients who also have aspirin hypersensitivity.

Sulfite sensitivity: Some of these products contain sulfites that may cause allergic-type reactions including anaphylactic symptoms and life-threatening or less severe asthmatic episodes. Sulfite sensitivity is seen more frequently in asthmatic or atopic nonasthmatic persons.

Drug Interactions:

Drugs that may affect procainamide include beta blockers, ethanol, histamine H_2 antagonists, quinidine and trimethoprim. Drugs that may be affected by procainamide include lidocaine and succinylcholine. Tests that depend on fluorescence measurement may also be affected.

Adverse Reactions:

Significant adverse reactions include a lupus erythematosus-like syndrome of arthralgia, pleural or abdominal pain, and sometimes arthritis, pleural effusion, pericarditis, fever, chills, myalgia and possibly related hematologic or skin lesions (after prolonged administration); neutropenia; thrombocytopenia; agranulocytosis (after repeated use; deaths have occurred); anorexia; nausea; vomiting; abdominal pain; bitter taste; diarrhea.

Administration and Dosage:

Oral: Oral dosage forms are preferable for less urgent arrhythmias as well as for long-term maintenance after initial parenteral therapy. Individualize dosage based on clinical assessment of the degree of underlying myocardial disease, the patient's age and renal function.

As a general guide, for younger adult patients with normal renal function, an initial total daily oral dose of up to 50 mg/kg may be used, given in divided doses every 3 hours, to maintain therapeutic blood levels. For older patients, especially those > 50 years of age, or for patients with renal, hepatic or cardiac insufficiency, lesser amounts or longer intervals may produce adequate blood levels and decrease the probability of occurrence of dose-related adverse reactions. Administer the total daily dose in divided doses at 3, 4 or 6 hour intervals and adjust according to the patient's response.

Guidelines to Provide up to 50 mg/kg/day Procainamide

Weight		Dose every 3 hours (standard formulation)	Dose every 6 hours (sustained release)
lb	kg		
88-110	40-50	250 mg	500 mg
132-154	60-70	375 mg	750 mg
176-198	80-90	500 mg	1 g
> 220	> 100	625 mg	1.25 g

[1] Initial dosage schedule guide only, to be adjusted for each patient individually, based on age, cardiorenal function, blood level (if available) and clinical response.

Sustained release products are not recommended for initial therapy. Total dosage (50 mg/kg/day) may be given in divided doses every 6 hours.

Parenteral: Useful for arrhythmias that require immediate suppression and for maintenance of arrhythmia control. IV therapy allows most rapid control of serious arrhythmias, including those following MI; use in circumstances where close observation and monitoring of the patient are possible, such as in hospital or emergency facilities. IM administration is less apt to produce temporary high plasma levels but therapeutic plasma levels are not obtained as rapidly as with IV administration.

IM administration may be used as an alternative to the oral route for patients with less threatening arrhythmias but who are nauseated or vomiting, who are ordered to receive nothing by mouth preoperatively, or who may have malabsorptive problems. An initial daily dose of 50 mg/kg may be estimated. Divide this amount into fractional doses of ⅛ to ¼ to be injected IM every 3 to 6 hours until oral therapy is possible. If > 3 injections are given, assess patient factors such as age and renal function, clinical response and, if available, blood levels of procainamide and NAPA in adjusting further doses for that individual. For treatment of arrhythmias associated with anesthesia or surgery, the suggested dose is 100 to 500 mg by IM injection.

IV –

Dilutions and Rates for IV Infusions of Procainamide

Infusion	Final concentration	Infusion volume[1]	Procainamide to be added	Infusion rate
Initial loading infusion	20 mg/ml	50 ml	1000 mg	1 ml/min (for up to 25 to 30 min)
Maintenance infusion[2]	2 mg/ml	500 ml	1000 mg	1 to 3 ml/min
	or			
	4 mg/ml	250 ml	1000 mg	0.5 to 1.5 ml/min

[1] All infusions should be made up to final volume with 5% Dextrose Injection, USP.
[2] The maintenance infusion rates are calculated to deliver 2 to 6 mg/min depending on body weight, renal elimination rate and steady-state plasma level needed to maintain control of the arrhythmia. The 4 mg/ml maintenance concentration may be preferred if total infused volume must be limited.

Cautiously administer the IV injection to avoid a possible hypotensive response. Initial arrhythmia control, under blood pressure and ECG monitoring, may usually be accomplished safely within 30 minutes by either of the two methods that follow:

1) Slowly direct injection into a vein or into tubing of an established infusion line at a rate not to exceed 50 mg/min. It is advisable to dilute either the 100 or the 500 mg/ml concentrations prior to IV injection to facilitate control of dosage rate. Doses of 100 mg may be administered every 5 minutes at this rate until the arrhythmia is suppressed or until 500 mg has been administered, after which it is advisable to wait ≥ 10 minutes to allow for more distribution into tissues before resuming.

2) Alternatively, a loading infusion containing 20 mg/ml (1 g diluted to 50 ml with 5% Dextrose Injection, USP) may be administered at a constant rate of 1 ml/min for 25 to 30 minutes to deliver 500 to 600 mg. Some effects may be seen after infusion of the first 100 or 200 mg; it is unusual to require > 600 mg to achieve satisfactory antiarrhythmic effects.

The maximum advisable dosage to be given either by repeated bolus injections or such loading infusion is 1 g.

To maintain therapeutic levels, a more dilute IV infusion at a concentration of 2 mg/ml is convenient (1 g in 500 ml 5% Dextrose Injection, USP), and may be administered at 1 to 3 ml/min. If daily total fluid intake must be limited, a 4 mg/ml concentration (1 g in 250 ml of 5% Dextrose Injection, USP) administered at 0.5 to 1.5 ml/min will deliver an equivalent 2 to 6 mg/min. Assess the amount needed in a given patient to maintain the therapeutic level principally from the clinical response. Adjust for each patient based on close observation. A maintenance infusion rate of 50 mcg/kg/min to a person with a normal renal procainamide elimination half-life of 3 hours should produce a plasma level of ≈ 6.5 mcg/ml.

Terminate IV therapy if persistent conduction disturbances or hypotension develop. As soon as the patient's basic cardiac rhythm appears to be stabilized, oral antiarrhythmic maintenance therapy is preferable (if indicated and possible). A period of about 3 to 4 hours (one half-life for renal elimination, ordinarily) should elapse after the last IV dose before administering the first dose of oral procainamide.

Children: The following doses have been suggested.

Oral 15 to 50 mg/kg/day divided every 3 to 6 hours; maximum 4 g/day.

IM – 20 to 30 mg/kg/day divided every 4 to 6 hours; maximum 4 g/day.

IV – *Loading dose*, 3 to 6 mg/kg/dose over 5 minutes. *Maintenance*, 20 to 80 mcg/kg/min continuous infusion. Maximum 100 mg/dose or 2 g/day.

DISOPYRAMIDE

Capsules: 100 and 150 mg (*Rx*)	Various, *Norpace* (Searle)
Capsules, extended release: 100 and 150 mg (*Rx*)	Various, *Norpace CR* (Searle)

Actions:

Pharmacology:

Mechanism of action – Disopyramide is a class IA antiarrhythmic agent that decreases the rate of diastolic depolarization (phase 4), decreases the upstroke velocity (phase 0), increases the action potential duration of normal cardiac cells and prolongs the refractory period (phases 2 and 3). It also decreases the disparity in refractoriness between infarcted and adjacent normally perfused myocardium.

Electrophysiology – Disopyramide shortens sinus node recovery time and lengthens atrial and ventricular refractoriness. The principal metabolite, mono-N-dealkyldisopyramide (MND), exhibits little antiarrhythmic activity, but is 20 to 30 times more anticholinergic than the parent drug. Conduction in accessory pathways is prolonged.

Pharmacokinetics:

Absorption/Distribution – Following oral administration of immediate release disopyramide, the drug is rapidly and almost completely absorbed. Peak plasma levels usually occur within 2 hours. Therapeutic plasma levels of disopyramide are 2 to 4 mcg/ml. Protein binding is concentration-dependent and varies from 50% to 65%; it is difficult to predict the concentration of the free drug when total drug is measured.

Metabolism/Excretion – About 50% is excreted in the urine as the unchanged drug and 30% as metabolites (20% MND). The plasma concentration of MND is approximately one tenth that of disopyramide. The mean plasma half-life is 6.7 hours (range, 4 to 10 hours). In impaired renal function, half-life values ranged from 8 to 18 hours. Therefore, decrease the dose in renal failure to avoid drug accumulation.

Immediate release vs controlled release: Following multiple doses, steady-state plasma levels of between 2 and 4 mcg/ml were attained following either 150 mg every 6 hours (immediate release) or 300 mg every 12 hours (controlled release).

Indications:

Treatment of documented ventricular arrhythmias (eg, sustained ventricular tachycardia) considered to be life-threatening.

Unlabeled uses: Disopyramide may be beneficial in the treatment of paroxysmal supraventricular tachycardia.

Contraindications:

Cardiogenic shock; preexisting second- or third-degree AV block (if no pacemaker is present); congenital QT prolongation; sick sinus syndrome; hypersensitivity to disopyramide.

Warnings:

Proarrhythmic effects: Because of the proarrhythmic effects, use with lesser arrhythmias is generally not recommended.

Asymptomatic ventricular premature contractions: Avoid treatment of patients with this condition.

Survival: Antiarrhythmic drugs have not been shown to enhance survival in patients with ventricular arrhythmias.

Negative inotropic properties:

Heart failure/hypotension – May cause or aggravate CHF or produce severe hypotension, especially in patients with depressed systolic function. Do not use in patients with uncompensated or marginally compensated CHF or hypotension unless secondary to cardiac arrhythmia. Treat patients with a history of heart failure with careful attention to the maintenance of cardiac function, including optimal digitalization. If hypotension occurs or CHF worsens, discontinue use; restart at a lower dosage after adequate cardiac compensation has been established.

Do not give a loading dose to patients with myocarditis or other cardiomyopathy; closely monitor initial dosage and subsequent adjustments.

QRS widening (> 25%), although unusual, may occur; discontinue use in such cases.

QT_c prolongation and worsening of the arrhythmia, including ventricular tachycardia and fibrillation, may occur. Patients who have QT prolongation in response to quinidine may be at particular risk. Disopyramide has been associated with torsade de pointes. If QT prolongation > 25% is observed and if ectopy continues, monitor closely and consider discontinuing the drug.

Atrial tachyarrhythmias: Digitalize patients with atrial flutter or fibrillation prior to administration to ensure that enhancement of AV conduction does not increase ventricular rate beyond acceptable limits.

Conduction abnormalities: Use caution in patients with sick sinus syndrome, Wolff-Parkinson-White (WPW) syndrome or bundle branch block.

Heart block: If first degree heart block develops, reduce dosage. If the block persists, drug continuation must depend upon the benefit compared to the risk of higher degrees of heart block. Development of second- or third-degree AV block or unifascicular, bifascicular or trifascicular block requires discontinuation of therapy, unless ventricular rate is controlled by a ventricular pacemaker.

Concomitant antiarrhythmic therapy: Reserve concomitant use of disopyramide with other class IA antiarrhythmics or propranolol for life-threatening arrhythmias unresponsive to a single agent. Such use may produce serious negative inotropic effects or may excessively prolong conduction, particularly with cardiac decompensation.

Hypoglycemia has been reported in rare instances. Monitor blood glucose levels in patients with CHF, chronic malnutrition, hepatic disease and in those taking drugs which could compromise normal glucoregulatory mechanisms in the absence of food.

Anticholinergic activity: Do not use in patients with urinary retention, glaucoma or myasthenia gravis unless adequate overriding measures are taken. Males with benign prostatic hypertrophy are at particular risk of having urinary retention. In patients with a family history of glaucoma, measure intraocular pressure before initiating therapy. Use with special care in patients with myasthenia gravis, since disopyramide could precipitate a myasthenic crisis.

Renal function impairment: Reduce dosage in impaired renal function. Carefully monitor ECG for signs of overdosage. The controlled release form is not recommended for patients with severe renal insufficiency.

Hepatic function impairment: Impairment increases plasma half-life; reduce dosage in such patients. Carefully monitor the ECG. Patients with cardiac dysfunction have a higher potential for hepatic impairment.

Pregnancy: Category C.

Lactation: Disopyramide has been detected in breast milk.

Precautions:

Potassium imbalance: Disopyramide may be ineffective in *hypo*kalemia and its toxic effects may be enhanced in *hyper*kalemia. Correct any potassium deficit before instituting therapy.

Drug Interactions:

Drugs that may affect disopyramide include beta blockers, erythromycin, hydantoins, quinidine and rifampin. Drugs that may be affected by disopyramide include quinidine, anticoagulants and digoxin.

Adverse Reactions:

The most serious adverse reactions are hypotension and CHF. The most common reactions are anticholinergic and are dose-dependent. These may be transitory, but may be persistent or severe. Urinary retention is the most serious anticholinergic effect. Adverse reactions occurring in ≥ 3% of patients include: Urinary retention, frequency and urgency; dizziness; fatigue; headache; nausea; pain; bloating; gas; dry mouth; urinary hesitancy; constipation; blurred vision; dry nose; eyes and throat; muscle weakness; malaise; aches/pain.

Administration and Dosage:

Individualize dosage. Initiate treatment in the hospital.

Adults: 400 to 800 mg/day. The recommended dosage for most adults is 600 mg/day. For patients < 50 kg (110 pounds), give 400 mg/day. Divide the total daily dose and administer every 6 hours in the immediate release form or every 12 hours in the controlled release form.

Children: Divide daily dosage and administer equal doses every 6 hours or at intervals according to patient needs. Closely monitor plasma levels and therapeutic response. Hospitalize patients during initial treatment and start dose titration at the lower end of the ranges provided below:

Suggested Total Daily Disopyramide Dosage in Children[1]

Age (years)	Disopyramide (mg/kg/day)
<1	10 to 30
1 to 4	10 to 20
4 to 12	10 to 15
12 to 18	6 to 15

[1] Prepare a 1 to 10 mg/ml suspension by adding contents of the immediate release capsule to cherry syrup, NF. The resulting suspension, when refrigerated, is stable for 1 month; shake thoroughly before measuring dose. Dispense in an amber glass bottle. Do not use the controlled release form to prepare the solution.

Initial loading dose: For rapid control of ventricular arrhythmia, give an initial loading dose of 300 mg immediate release (200 mg for patients < 50 kg [110 lbs]). Therapeutic effects are attained in 30 minutes to 3 hours. If there is no response or no evidence of toxicity within 6 hours of the loading dose, 200 mg every 6 hours may be administered instead of the usual 150 mg. If there is no response within 48 hours, discontinue the drug or carefully monitor subsequent doses of 250 or 300 mg every 6 hours.

Do not use the controlled release form initially if rapid plasma levels are desired.

Severe refractory ventricular tachycardia: A limited number of patients have tolerated up to 1600 mg/day (400 mg every 6 hours), resulting in plasma levels up to 9 mcg/ml. Hospitalize patients for close evaluation and continuous monitoring.

Cardiomyopathy or possible cardiac decompensation: Do not administer a loading dose, and limit the initial dosage to 100 mg immediate release every 6 to 8 hours. Make subsequent dosage adjustments gradually.

Renal/Hepatic function impairment: For patients with moderate renal insufficiency (Ccr > 40 ml/min) or hepatic insufficiency, the recommended dosage is 400 mg/day given in divided doses (either 100 mg every 6 hours for immediate release or 200 mg every 12 hours for controlled release).

In severe renal insufficiency (Ccr ≤ 40 ml/min), the recommended dosage is 100 mg of the immediate release form given at the intervals shown in the table below, with or without an initial loading dose of 150 mg.

Disopyramide Dosage in Renal Impairment

Creatinine clearance (ml/min)	Loading dose (mg)	Dose (mg)	Dosage interval (hours)
40-30	150	100	8
30-15	150	100	12
<15	150	100	24

Transfer to disopyramide: Use the regular maintenance schedule, without a loading dose, 6 to 12 hours after the last dose of quinidine or 3 to 6 hours after the last dose of procainamide. Where withdrawal of quinidine or procainamide is likely to produce life-threatening arrhythmias, consider hospitalization.

When transferring from immediate to controlled release, start maintenance schedule of controlled release 6 hours after the last dose of immediate release.

LIDOCAINE HCl

Injection: (for IM administration) 300 mg/3 ml automatic injection device (*Rx*)	*LidoPen Auto-Injector* (Survival Technology)
Injection: (for direct IV administration) 1% (10 mg/ml), 2% (20 mg/ml) (*Rx*)	Various, *Xylocaine HCl IV for Cardiac Arrhythmias* (Astra)
Injection: (for IV admixtures) 10% (100 mg/ml) (*Rx*)	Various
Injection: (for IV admixtures) 4% (40 mg/ml), 20% (200 mg/ml) (*Rx*)	Various, *Xylocaine HCl IV for Cardiac Arrhythmias* (Astra)
Injection: (for IV infusion) 0.2% (2 mg/ml), 0.4% (4 mg/ml), 0.8% (8 mg/ml) (*Rx*)	Various

Actions:

Pharmacology: Therapeutic concentrations of lidocaine attenuate phase 4 diastolic depolarization, decrease automaticity and cause a decrease or no change in excitability and membrane responsiveness. Action potential duration and effective refractory period (ERP) of Purkinje fibers and ventricular muscle are decreased, while the ratio of ERP to action potential duration is increased. Lidocaine raises ventricular fibrillation threshold. AV nodal conduction time is unchanged or shortened. Lidocaine increases the electrical stimulation threshold of the ventricle during diastole.

Pharmacokinetics:

Absorption/Distribution – Lidocaine is ineffective orally; it is most commonly administered IV with an immediate onset (within minutes) and brief duration (10 to 20 minutes) of action following a bolus dose. Continuous IV infusion of lidocaine (1 to 4 mg/min) is necessary to maintain antiarrhythmic effects. Following IM administration, therapeutic serum levels are achieved in 5 to 15 minutes and may persist for up to 2 hours. Higher and more rapid serum levels are achieved by injection into the deltoid muscle. Therapeutic serum levels are 1.5 to 6 mcg/ml; serum levels > 6 to 10 mcg/ml are usually toxic. Lidocaine is ≈ 50% protein bound (concentration-dependent).

Metabolism/Excretion – Extensive biotransformation in the liver (≈ 90%) results in at least two active metabolites, monoethylglycinexylidide (MEGX) and glycinexylidide (GX). These metabolites exhibit both antiarrhythmic and convulsant properties. The hepatic extraction ratio is between 62% and 81%. Lidocaine exhibits a biphasic half-life. The distribution phase is ≈ 10 minutes. The elimination half-life is 1.5 to 2 hours; half-life may be ≥ 3 hours following infusions of > 24 hours. Any condition that alters liver function, including changes in liver blood flow, which could result from severe congestive heart failure (CHF) or shock, may alter lidocaine kinetics. Less than 10% of the parent drug is excreted unchanged in the urine. Renal elimination plays an important role in the elimination of the metabolites.

Indications:

IV: Acute management of ventricular arrhythmias occurring during cardiac manipulation, such as cardiac surgery or in relation to acute myocardial infarction (MI).

IM: Single doses are justified in the following exceptional circumstances: When ECG equipment is not available to verify the diagnosis but the potential benefits outweigh the possible risks; when facilities for IV administration are not readily available; by the patient in the prehospital phase of suspected acute MI, directed by qualified medical personnel viewing the transmitted ECG.

Unlabeled uses: In pediatric patients with cardiac arrest, < 10% develop ventricular fibrillation, and others develop ventricular tachycardia; the hemodynamically compromised child may develop ventricular couplets or frequent premature ventricular beats. In these cases, lidocaine 1 mg/kg should be administered by the IV, intraosseous or endotracheal route. A second 1 mg/kg dose may be given in 10 to 15 minutes. Start a lidocaine infusion if the second dose is required; a third bolus may be needed in 10 to 15 minutes to maintain therapeutic levels.

Contraindications:

Hypersensitivity to amide local anesthetics; Stokes-Adams syndrome; Wolff-Parkinson-White syndrome; severe degrees of sinoatrial, atrioventricular (AV) or intraventricular block in the absence of an artificial pacemaker.

Warnings:

Survival: Prophylactic single dose lidocaine administered in a monitored environment does not appear to affect mortality in the earliest phase of acute MI, and may harm some patients who are later shown not to have suffered an acute MI.

Constant ECG monitoring is essential for proper administration. Have emergency resuscitative equipment and drugs immediately available.

IV use: Signs of excessive depression of cardiac conductivity should be followed by dosage reduction and, if necessary, prompt cessation of IV infusion.

IM use: May increase creatine phosphokinase (CPK) levels. Use of the enzyme determination without isoenzyme separation, as a diagnostic test for acute MI, may be compromised.

Cardiac effects: Use with caution and in lower doses in patients with CHF, reduced cardiac output, digitalis toxicity accompanied by AV block and in the elderly.

In sinus bradycardia or incomplete heart block, lidocaine administration for the elimination of ventricular ectopy without prior acceleration in heart rate (eg, by atropine, isoproterenol or electric pacing) may promote more frequent and serious ventricular arrhythmias or complete heart block. Use with caution in patients with hypovolemia and shock, and all forms of heart block.

Acceleration of ventricular rate may occur when administered to patients with atrial flutter or fibrillation.

Hypersensitivity reactions may occur. Refer to Management of Acute Hypersensitivity Reactions.

Renal/Hepatic function impairment: Use caution with repeated or prolonged use in liver or renal disease; possible toxic accumulation may occur.

Pregnancy: Category B.

Lactation: Exercise caution when administering to a nursing woman.

Children: Safety and efficacy have not been established; reduce dosage. The IM auto-injector device is not recommended in children < 50 kg.

Precautions:

Malignant hyperthermia: Amide local anesthetic administration has been associated with acute onset of fulminant hypermetabolism of skeletal muscle known as malignant hyperthermic crisis. Recognition of early unexplained signs of tachycardia, tachypnea, labile blood pressure and metabolic acidosis may precede temperature elevation. Successful outcome depends on early diagnosis, prompt discontinuance of the triggering agent and institution of treatment, including oxygen, supportive measures and IV dantrolene sodium.

The safety of amide local anesthetics in patients with genetic predisposition of malignant hyperthermia has not been fully assessed; use lidocaine with caution in such patients. In hospitals where triggering agents for malignant hyperthermia are administered, a standard protocol for management should be available.

Drug Interactions:

Drugs that may affect lidocaine include beta blockers, cimetidine, procainamide, tocainide and succinylcholine.

Adverse Reactions:

Significant drug interactions include lightheadedness; nervousness; drowsiness; dizziness; apprehension; confusion; mood changes; hallucinations; tremors; convulsions;

unconsciousness; hypotension; bradycardia; cardiovascular collapse, which may lead to cardiac arrest; febrile response; soreness/infection at the injection site; venous thrombosis or phlebitis extending from the site of injection; extravasation; vomiting; respiratory depression/arrest

Hypersensitivity: Allergic reactions may occur characterized by cutaneous lesions, urticaria, edema or anaphylactoid reactions.

Administration and Dosage:

IM: 300 mg. The deltoid muscle is preferred. Avoid intravascular injection. Use only the 10% solution for IM injection.

The *LidoPen Auto-Injector* unit is for self-administration into the deltoid muscle or anterolateral aspect of thigh. Patient instructions are provided with the product.

Replacement therapy – As soon as possible, change patient to IV lidocaine or to an oral antiarrhythmic preparation for maintenance therapy. However, if necessary, an additional IM injection may be administered after 60 to 90 minutes.

IV: Use only lidocaine injection without preservatives, clearly labeled for IV use. Monitor ECG constantly to avoid potential overdosage and toxicity.

IV bolus is used to establish rapid therapeutic blood levels. Continuous IV infusion is necessary to maintain antiarrhythmic effects. The usual dose is 50 to 100 mg, given at a rate of 25 to 50 mg/minute. If the initial injection does not produce the desired clinical response, give a second bolus dose after 5 minutes. Give no more than 200 to 300 mg/hour.

Reduce loading (bolus) doses in patients with CHF or reduced cardiac output and in the elderly. However, some investigators recommend the usual loading dose be administered and only the maintenance dosage be reduced.

IV continuous infusion is used to maintain therapeutic plasma levels following loading doses in patients in whom arrhythmias tend to recur and who cannot receive oral antiarrhythmic drugs. Administer at a rate of 1 to 4 mg/min (20 to 50 mcg/kg/min). Reduce maintenance doses in patients with heart failure or liver disease, or who are also receiving other drugs known to decrease clearance of lidocaine or decrease liver blood flow and in patients > 70 years of age. Reassess the rate of infusion as soon as the cardiac rhythm stabilizes or at the earliest signs of toxicity. Change patients to oral antiarrhythmic agents for maintenance therapy as soon as possible. It is rarely necessary to continue IV infusions for prolonged periods. Use a precision volume control IV set for continuous IV infusion.

Children – The American Heart Association's Standards and Guidelines recommend a bolus dose of 1 mg/kg, followed by an infusion of 30 mcg/kg/min. The following dosage has also been suggested.

Loading dose, 1 mg/kg/dose given IV or intratracheally every 5 to 10 min to desired effect, maximum total dose 5 mg/kg; *maintenance,* 20 to 50 mcg/kg/min.

TOCAINIDE HCl

Tablets: 400, 600 mg (Rx)	*Tonocard* (Astra Merck)

Warning:

Blood dyscrasias: Agranulocytosis, bone marrow depression, leukopenia, neutropenia, aplastic/hypoplastic anemia, thrombocytopenia and sequelae such as septicemia and septic shock have occurred in patients receiving tocainide. Fatalities have occurred (with ≈ 25% mortality in reported agranulocytosis cases). Since most of these events have been noted during the first 12 weeks of therapy, perform complete blood counts, including white cell, differential and platelet counts, optimally, at weekly intervals for the first 3 months of therapy, and frequently thereafter. Perform complete blood counts promptly if the patient develops any signs of infection (eg, fever, chills, sore throat, stomatitis), bruising or bleeding. If any of these hematologic disorders are identified, discontinue tocainide and institute appropriate treatment if necessary. Blood counts usually return to normal within 1 month of discontinuation. Use with caution in patients with preexisting bone marrow failure or cytopenia of any type.

Pulmonary fibrosis, interstitial pneumonitis, fibrosing alveolitis, pulmonary edema and pneumonia have occurred in patients receiving tocainide. Many of these events occurred in patients who were seriously ill. Fatalities have occurred. The experiences are usually characterized by bilateral infiltrates on x-ray and are frequently associated with dyspnea and cough. Fever may be present. Instruct patients to promptly report any pulmonary symptoms (eg, exertional dyspnea, cough, wheezing). Chest x-rays are advisable at that time. If these pulmonary disorders develop, discontinue tocainide.

Actions:

Pharmacology: Tocainide produces dose-dependent decreases in sodium and potassium conductance, decreasing the excitability of myocardial cells. Most patients who respond to lidocaine also respond to tocainide. Failure to respond to lidocaine usually predicts failure to respond to tocainide.

Electrophysiology – Tocainide is a Class IB antiarrhythmic. In patients with cardiac disease, tocainide produces no clinically significant changes in sinus nodal function, effective refractory periods or intracardiac conduction times. Tocainide does not prolong QRS duration or QT intervals. It may be useful for ventricular arrhythmias associated with a prolonged QT interval.

Hemodynamics – Tocainide usually produces a small degree of depression of left ventricular function and left ventricular end diastolic pressure. Small significant increases in aortic and pulmonary arterial pressures observed are probably related to small increases in vascular resistance. Used concomitantly with a β-adrenergic blocking drug, tocainide further reduces cardiac index and left ventricular dP/dt and further increases pulmonary wedge pressure.

Tocainide has been used safely in patients with acute MI and various degrees of CHF. A small negative inotropic effect can increase peripheral resistance slightly.

Pharmacokinetics:

Absorption/Distribution – Following oral administration the bioavailability of tocainide approaches 100%; peak serum concentrations are attained in 0.5 to 2 hours. Bioavailability is unaffected by food. Tocainide undergoes negligible first-pass hepatic degradation. Approximately 10% to 20% is plasma protein bound. The therapeutic range is 4 to 10 mcg/ml.

Metabolism/Excretion – Inactivated via conjugation in the liver. The average plasma half-life is ≈ 15 hours. About 40% is excreted unchanged in urine; alkalinization of urine reduces the percent of drug excreted unchanged, yet acidification causes no alterations. Pharmacokinetics did not differ significantly with MI compared with healthy subjects. Half-life increased in severe renal dysfunction.

Indications:

Treatment of life-threatening ventricular arrhythmias.

Unlabeled uses: Tocainide may be beneficial in the treatment of myotonic dystrophy (800 to 1200 mg/day) and trigeminal neuralgia (20 mg/kg/day in 3 divided doses).

Contraindications:

Hypersensitivity to tocainide or to amide-type local anesthetics; patients with second- or third-degree AV block in the absence of an artificial ventricular pacemaker.

Warnings:

Proarrhythmia: Tocainide may increase arrhythmias in some patients.

Cardiac effects: Tocainide has not been shown to prevent sudden death in patients with serious ventricular ectopy. It has potentially serious adverse effects, including ability to worsen arrhythmias. Evaluate each patient by ECG and clinically prior to and during therapy to determine if response supports continued treatment.

In patients with known heart failure or minimal cardiac reserve, use with caution because of the potential for aggravating the degree of heart failure.

Use caution when instituting or continuing antiarrhythmic therapy in the presence of signs of increasing depression of cardiac conductivity.

Acceleration of ventricular rate occurs infrequently when tocainide is administered to patients with atrial flutter or fibrillation.

Renal/Hepatic function impairment: In patients with severe liver or kidney disease, the rate of drug elimination may be significantly decreased.

Pregnancy: Category C.

Lactation: Decide whether to discontinue nursing or the drug, taking into account importance of the drug to the mother.

Children: Safety and efficacy for use in children have not been established.

Precautions:

Hypokalemia: Since antiarrhythmic drugs may be ineffective in patients with hypokalemia, correct potassium deficits if present.

Drug Interactions:

Drugs that may interact include cimetidine, metoprolol and rifampin.

Adverse Reactions:

Adverse reactions occurring in ≥ 3% of patients include: Dizziness/vertigo; nausea; vomiting; anorexia; diarrhea/loose stools; arthritis/arthralgia; paresthesia; tremor; confusion/disorientation/hallucinations; headache; nervousness; altered mood/awareness/ ataxia; hypotension; tachycardia; worsening CHF (including arrhythmias); diaphoresis; rash/skin lesion and blurred vision/visual disturbances. Adverse reactions leading to discontinuation of therapy occurred in 21% of patients and were usually related to the CNS or GI system.

Administration and Dosage:

Individualize dosage. Guide dosage titration by clinical and ECG evaluation. Dose-related adverse effects tend to occur early in treatment, and they usually decrease in severity and frequency with time. These effects may be minimized by taking tocainide with food or by taking smaller, more frequent doses.

Initial dose: 400 mg every 8 hours. Range is 1200 to 1800 mg/day given in 3 divided doses. Doses > 2400 mg/day have been administered infrequently. Patients who tolerate the three times daily regimen may be tried on a twice-daily regimen with careful monitoring.

Some patients, particularly those with renal or hepatic impairment, may be adequately treated with < 1200 mg/day.

MEXILETINE HCl

Capsules: 150, 200 and 250 mg (Rx) Various, *Mexitil* (Boehringer Ingelheim)

Actions:

Pharmacology:

Mechanism – Mexiletine inhibits the inward sodium current, thus reducing the rate of rise of the action potential, Phase O. Mexiletine decreases the effective refractory period (ERP) in Purkinje fibers. This is of lesser magnitude than the decrease in action potential duration (APD), with a resulting increase in ERP/APD ratio.

Electrophysiology – Mexiletine is a local anesthetic and a Class IB antiarrhythmic compound. In patients with normal conduction systems, mexiletine has minimal effect on cardiac impulse generation and propagation. Mexiletine may be useful in treating ventricular arrhythmias associated with a prolonged QT interval. In patients with preexisting conduction defects, depression of the sinus rate, prolongation of sinus node recovery time, decreased conduction velocity and increased ERP of the intraventricular conduction system have occasionally been observed.

Among the patients entered into studies, about 30% in each treatment group had a ≥ 70% reduction in PVC count, and about 40% failed to complete the 3 month studies because of adverse effects. Follow-up of patients has demonstrated continued effectiveness in long-term use.

Hemodynamics – Small decreases in cardiac output and increases in systemic vascular resistance have occurred. Blood pressure and pulse rate remain unchanged.

Pharmacokinetics:

Absorption/Distribution – Mexiletine is well absorbed (≈ 90%) from the GI tract. The absorption rate is reduced in clinical situations in which gastric emptying time is increased. The first-pass metabolism of mexiletine is low. Peak blood levels are reached in 2 to 3 hours. The therapeutic range is approximately 0.5 to 2 mcg/ml. Mexiletine is 50% to 60% bound to plasma protein with a volume of distribution of 5 to 7 L/kg.

Metabolism/Excretion – Mexiletine is metabolized in the liver. The most active minor metabolite is N-methylmexiletine, which is < 20% as potent as mexiletine. In healthy subjects, the elimination half-life is 10 to 12 hours. Hepatic impairment prolongs it to a mean of 25 hours. Little change in half-life occurs with reduced renal function. Approximately 10% is excreted unchanged by the kidney. Urinary acidification accelerates excretion, while alkalinization retards it.

Indications:

Treatment of documented, life-threatening ventricular arrhythmias, such as sustained ventricular tachycardia. Because of the proarrhythmic effects of mexiletine, use with lesser arrhythmias is generally not recommended.

Unlabeled uses: The use of prophylactic mexiletine may significantly reduce the incidence of ventricular tachycardia and other ventricular arrhythmias in the acute phase of myocardial infarction (MI). However, mortality may not be reduced.

Mexiletine may be beneficial in reducing pain, dysesthesia and paresthesia associated with diabetic neuropathy.

Contraindications:

Cardiogenic shock; preexisting second- or third-degree AV block (if no pacemaker).

Warnings:

Proarrhythmia: Mexiletine can worsen arrhythmias; it is uncommon in patients with less serious arrhythmias but is of greater concern in patients with life-threatening arrhythmias, such as sustained ventricular tachycardia.

Initial therapy: As with other antiarrhythmics, initiate therapy in the hospital.

Mortality: It is prudent to consider any antiarrhythmic agent to have a significant risk in patients with structural heart disease.

Hepatic function impairment: Carefully monitor patients with liver disease. Observe caution in patients with hepatic dysfunction secondary to CHF.

Pregnancy: Category C.

Lactation: Mexiletine appears in breast milk. If mexiletine is essential, consider alternative infant feeding.

Children: Safety and efficacy in children have not been established.

Precautions:

Cardiovascular effects: If a ventricular pacemaker is operative, patients with second- or third-degree heart block may be treated with mexiletine if continuously monitored. Some patients with preexisting first-degree AV block were treated with mexiletine; none developed second- or third-degree AV block. Exercise caution in such patients or in patients with preexisting sinus node dysfunction or intraventricular conduction abnormalities.

Use with caution in patients with hypotension and severe CHF.

Hepatic effects: Elevations of AST > 3 times the upper limit of normal have occurred. These elevations were frequently associated with CHF, acute MI, blood transfusions and other medications and usually did not require discontinuation of therapy. Marked elevations of AST (> 1000 U/L) were seen before death in four patients with end-stage cardiac disease (severe CHF, cardiogenic shock).

Rare instances of severe liver injury have been reported. Carefully evaluate patients in whom an abnormal liver test has occurred, or who have signs or symptoms suggesting liver dysfunction. If persistent or worsening elevation of hepatic enzymes is detected, consider discontinuing therapy.

Hematologic effects: If significant hematologic changes are observed, carefully evaluate the patient and, if warranted, discontinue mexiletine. Blood counts usually return to normal within 1 month of discontinuation.

CNS effects: Convulsions have occurred in patients with and without a history of seizures. Use with caution in patients with a known seizure disorder.

Urinary pH: Avoid concurrent drugs or diets which may markedly alter urinary pH. Minor fluctuations in urinary pH associated with normal diet do not affect mexiletine excretion.

Drug Interactions:

Drugs that may affect mexilitine include aluminum-magnesium hydroxide, narcotics, cimetidine, hydantoins, metoclopramide, rifampin and urinary acidifiers/alkalinizers. Drugs that may be affected by mexilitine include caffeine and theophylline.

Adverse Reactions:

Adverse reactions occurring in ≥ 3% of patients include palpitations; chest pain; nausea/vomiting/heartburn; diarrhea; constipation; dizziness/lightheadedness; tremor; nervousness; coordination difficulties; changes in sleep habits; headache; blurred vision/visual disturbances; paresthesias/numbness; weakness; fatigue; rash; nonspecific edema; dyspnea/respiratory.

Administration and Dosage:

Individualize dosage. Administer with food or antacids.

Perform clinical and ECG evaluation as needed to determine whether the desired antiarrhythmic effect has been obtained and to guide titration and dose adjustment.

Initial dose: 200 mg every 8 hours when rapid control of arrhythmia is not essential, with a minimum of 2 to 3 days between adjustments. Adjust dose in 50 or 100 mg increments.

Control can be achieved in most patients with 200 to 300 mg given every 8 hours. If satisfactory response is not achieved at 300 mg every 8 hours, and the patient tolerates mexiletine well, try 400 mg every 8 hours. The severity of CNS side effects increases with total daily dose; do not exceed 1200 mg/day.

Renal/hepatic function impairment: In general, patients with renal failure will require the usual doses of mexiletine. Patients with severe liver disease, however, may require lower doses and must be monitored closely. Similarly, marked right-sided CHF can reduce hepatic metabolism and reduce the dose needed.

Loading dose: When rapid control of ventricular arrhythmia is essential, administer an initial loading dose of 400 mg, followed by a 200 mg dose in 8 hours. Onset of therapeutic effect is usually observed within 30 minutes to 2 hours.

Twice-daily dosage: If adequate suppression is achieved on a dose of ≤ 300 mg every 8 hours, the same total daily dose may be given in divided doses every 12 hours with monitoring. The dose may be adjusted to a maximum of 450 mg every 12 hours.

Transferring to mexiletine: Based on theoretical considerations, initiate with a 200 mg dose, and titrate to response as described above, 6 to 12 hours after the last dose of quinidine sulfate, 3 to 6 hours after the last dose of procainamide, 6 to 12 hours after the last disopyramide dose or 8 to 12 hours after the last tocainide dose.

Hospitalize patients in whom withdrawal of the previous antiarrhythmic agent is likely to produce life-threatening arrhythmias.

When transferring from lidocaine to mexiletine, stop the lidocaine infusion when the first oral dose of mexiletine is administered. Maintain the IV line until suppression of the arrhythmia appears satisfactory. Consider the similarity of adverse effects of lidocaine and mexiletine and the additive potential.

PROPAFENONE HCl

Tablets: 150, 225 and 300 mg (Rx)	*Rythmol* (Knoll)

Actions:

Pharmacology: Propafenone is a Class IC antiarrhythmic with local anesthetic effects and direct stabilizing action on myocardial membranes. Propafenone's electrophysiological effect manifests itself in reduction of upstroke velocity (Phase 0) of the monophasic action potential. In Purkinje fibers, and to a lesser extent myocardial fibers, propafenone reduces fast inward current carried by sodium ions. Diastolic excitability threshold is increased and effective refractory period prolonged. Propafenone reduces spontaneous automaticity and depresses triggered activity. Resting heart rate decreases of about 8% were noted at the higher end of the therapeutic plasma concentration range.

Propafenone causes a dose- and concentration-related decrease in rate of single and multiple PVCs and can suppress recurrence of ventricular tachycardia. Based on percent of patients attaining substantial (80% to 90%) suppression of ventricular ectopic activity, it appears trough levels of 0.2 to 1.5 mcg/ml can provide good suppression, with higher concentrations giving a greater rate of good response.

Electrophysiology – In electrophysiology studies in patients with ventricular tachycardia, propafenone prolongs atrioventricular (AV) conduction while having little or no effect on sinus node function. Both AV nodal conduction time (AH interval) and His Purkinje conduction time (HV interval) are prolonged. AV nodal functional and effective refractory periods are prolonged. In patients with Wolff-Parkinson-White syndrome, propafenone reduces conduction and increases the effective refractory period of the accessory pathway in both directions. Propafenone slows conduction and consequently produces dose-related changes in the PR interval and QRS duration. QTc interval does not change.

Hemodynamics – Sympathetic stimulation may be a vital component supporting circulatory function in patients with CHF, and its inhibition by the beta blockade produced by propafenone may in itself aggravate CHF. Propafenone exerts a negative inotropic effect on the myocardium. Cardiac catheterization studies in patients with moderately impaired ventricular function showed significant increases in pulmonary capillary wedge pressure, systemic and pulmonary vascular resistances and depression of cardiac output and index.

Pharmacokinetics:

Absorption/Distribution – Propafenone is nearly completely absorbed after oral administration with peak plasma levels occurring ≈ 3.5 hours after administration. It exhibits extensive first-pass metabolism resulting in a dose-dependent and dosage-form-dependent absolute bioavailability. Propafenone follows a nonlinear pharmacokinetic disposition presumably due to saturation of first-pass hepatic metabolism as the liver is exposed to higher concentrations of propafenone and shows a very high degree of interindividual variability.

Metabolism/Excretion – There are two genetically determined patterns of propafenone metabolism. In > 90% of patients, the drug is rapidly and extensively metabolized with an elimination half-life of 2 to 10 hours. These patients metabolize propafenone into two active metabolites: 5–hydroxypropafenone and N–depropylpropafenone. They both are usually present in concentrations < 20% of propafenone. The saturable hydroxylation pathway is responsible for the nonlinear pharmacokinetic disposition.

In < 10% of patients, propafenone metabolism is slower because the 5–hydroxy metabolite is not formed or is minimally formed. The estimated propafenone elimination half-life ranges from 10 to 32 hours. In these patients, the N–depropylpropafenone is present in quantities comparable to the levels measured in extensive metabolizers. In slow metabolizers, propafenone pharmacokinetics are linear.

There are significant differences in plasma concentrations of propafenone in slow and extensive metabolizers, the former achieving concentrations 1.5 to 2 times those of the extensive metabolizers at daily doses of 675 to 900 mg/day. At low doses the differences are greater, with slow metabolizers attaining concentrations > 5 times those of extensive metabolizers. The recommended dosing regimen is the same for all patients. Titrate dosage carefully with close attention paid to clinical and ECG evidence of toxicity. In addition, the beta-blocking action of propafenone appears to be enhanced in slow metabolizers.

Indications:

Treatment of documented life-threatening ventricular arrhythmias, such as sustained ventricular tachycardia.

Because of the proarrhythmic effects of propafenone, reserve its use for patients in whom the benefits of treatment outweigh the risks. The use of propafenone is not recommended in patients with less severe ventricular arrhythmias, even if the patients are symptomatic.

Unlabeled uses: Propafenone appears to be effective in the treatment of supraventricular tachycardias including atrial fibrillation and flutter and arrhythmias associated with WPW syndrome.

Contraindications:

Uncontrolled CHF; cardiogenic shock; sinoatrial, AV and intraventricular disorders of impulse generation or conduction (eg, sick sinus node syndrome, AV block) in the absence of an artificial pacemaker; bradycardia; marked hypotension, bronchospastic disorders; manifest electrolyte imbalance; hypersensitivity to the drug.

Warnings:

Mortality: An excessive mortality or non-fatal cardiac arrest rate was seen in patients treated with encainide or flecainide compared with that seen in patients assigned to carefully matched placebo-treated groups.

Proarrhythmic effects: Propafenone may cause new or worsened arrhythmias. Such proarrhythmic effects range from an increase in frequency of PVCs to the development of more severe ventricular tachycardia, ventricular fibrillation or torsade de pointes, which may lead to fatal consequences. It is essential that each patient be evaluated electrocardiographically and clinically prior to, and during therapy to determine whether response to propafenone supports continued use.

Non-life-threatening arrhythmias: Use of propafenone is not recommended in patients with less severe ventricular arrhythmias, even if the patients are symptomatic.

Survival: There is no evidence from controlled trials that the use of propafenone favorably affects survival or the incidence of sudden death.

Nonallergic bronchospasm (eg, chronic bronchitis, emphysema): In general, these patients should not receive propafenone or other agents with beta-adrenergic blocking activity.

CHF: New or worsened CHF has occurred in 3.7% of patients.

As propafenone exerts both beta blockade and a (dose-related) negative inotropic effect on cardiac muscle, patients with CHF should be fully compensated before receiving propafenone. If CHF worsens, discontinue propafenone unless CHF is due to the cardiac arrhythmia and, if indicated, restart at a lower dosage only after adequate cardiac compensation has been established.

Conduction disturbances: Propafenone causes first degree AV block. Average PR interval prolongation and increases in QRS duration are closely correlated with dosage increases and concomitant increases in propafenone plasma concentrations. Development of second- or third-degree AV block requires a reduction in dosage or discontinuation of propafenone. Bundle branch block and intraventricular conduction delay have occurred. Bradycardia has also occurred. Patients with sick sinus node syndrome should not be treated with propafenone.

Effects on pacemaker threshold: Pacing and sensing thresholds of artificial pacemakers may be altered. Monitor and program pacemakers accordingly during therapy.

Hematologic disturbances: Agranulocytosis with fever and sepsis has occurred. Unexplained fever or decrease in white cell count, particularly during the first 3 months of therapy, warrants consideration of possible agranulocytosis/granulocytopenia.

Renal function impairment: A considerable percentage of propafenone metabolites are excreted in the urine. Administer cautiously in impaired renal function.

Hepatic function impairment: Propafenone is highly metabolized by the liver; administer cautiously to patients with impaired hepatic function. The clearance of propafenone is reduced and the elimination half-life increased in patients with significant hepatic dysfunction. The dose of propafenone should be ≈ 20% to 30% of the dose given to patients with normal hepatic function.

Elderly: Because of the possible increased risk of impaired hepatic or renal function in this age group, use with caution. The effective dose may be lower in these patients.

Pregnancy: Category C.

Lactation: It is not known whether this drug is excreted in breast milk. Discontinue nursing or to discontinue the drug.

Children: The safety and efficacy in children have not been established.

Precautions:

Elevated ANA titers: Positive ANA titers have occurred. They have been reversible upon cessation of treatment and may disappear even with continued therapy. Carefully evaluate patients who develop an abnormal ANA test and, if persistent or worsening elevation of ANA titers is detected, consider discontinuing therapy.

Drug Interactions:

Drugs that may affect propafenone include local anesthetics, cimetidine, quinidine and rifampin. Drugs that may be affected by propafenone include anticoagulants, beta blockers, cyclosporine and digoxin.

Adverse Reactions:

Adverse reactions occurring in ≥ 3% of patients include angina; first degree AV block; CHF; intraventricular conduction delay; palpitations; proarrhythmia; ventricular tachycardia; dizziness; fatigue; headache; constipation; dyspepsia; nausea/vomiting; unusual taste; blurred vision; dyspnea. About 20% of patients discontinued treatment due to adverse reactions.

Administration and Dosage:

Individually titrate on the basis of response and tolerance. Initiate with 150 mg every 8 hours (450 mg/day). Dosage may be increased at a minimum of 3 to 4 day intervals to 225 mg every 8 hours (675 mg/day) and, if necessary, to 300 mg every 8 hours (900 mg/day). The safety and efficacy of dosages exceeding 900 mg/day have not been established. In those patients in whom significant widening of the QRS complex or second- or third-degree AV block occurs, consider dose reduction.

As with other antiarrhythmics, in the elderly or patients with marked previous myocardial damage, increase dose more gradually during initial treatment phase.

FLECAINIDE ACETATE

Tablets: 50, 100, 150 mg (*Rx*)	*Tambocor* (3M Pharm.)

Actions:

Pharmacology: Flecainide has local anesthetic activity and belongs to the membrane stabilizing (Class I) group of antiarrhythmic agents; it has electrophysiologic effects characteristic of the IC class of antiarrhythmics.

Electrophysiology – Flecainide produces a dose-related decrease in intracardiac conduction in all parts of the heart, with the greatest effect on the His-Purkinje system (H–V conduction). Effects upon atrioventricular (AV) nodal conduction time and intra-atrial conduction times are less pronounced than those on the ventricle. Significant effects on refractory periods were observed only in the ventricle. Sinus node recovery times (corrected) are somewhat increased; this may be significant in sinus node dysfunction.

Flecainide causes a dose-related and plasma level-related decrease in single and multiple PVCs and can suppress recurrence of ventricular tachycardia. Plasma levels of 0.2 to 1 mcg/ml may be needed to obtain the maximal therapeutic effect. Plasma levels > 0.7 to 1 mcg/ml are associated with a higher rate of cardiac adverse experiences. Dose reduction appears to lead to a reduced frequency and severity of proarrhythmic events.

Hemodynamics – Flecainide does not usually alter heart rate. Increases and decreases in ejection fraction have been observed.

Pharmacokinetics:

Absorption/Distribution – Oral absorption is nearly complete. Peak plasma levels are attained at ≈ 3 hours. The plasma half-life ranges from 12 to 27 hours after multiple oral doses. Steady-state levels are approached in 3 to 5 days; once at steady-state, no accumulation occurs during chronic therapy. Plasma levels are approximately proportional to dose. In patients with congestive heart failure (CHF; NYHA class III), the rate of flecainide elimination from plasma is moderately slower than for healthy subjects. Plasma protein binding is about 40% and is independent of plasma drug level over the range of 0.015 to about 3.4 mcg/ml.

Metabolism/Excretion – About 30% of a single oral dose (range, 10% to 50%) is excreted in urine unchanged. The two major urinary metabolites are meta-O-dealkylated flecainide (active, but about as potent) and the meta-O-dealkylated lactam (inactive). These two metabolites (primarily conjugated) account for most of the remaining portion of the dose. With increasing renal impairment, the extent of unchanged drug in urine is reduced and the half-life is prolonged. Hemodialysis removes only about 1% of an oral dose as unchanged flecainide.

Indications:

Atrial fibrillation: For the prevention of paroxysmal atrial fibrillation/flutter (PAF) associated with disabling symptoms and paroxysmal supraventricular tachycardias (PSVT), including atrioventricular nodal reentrant tachycardia, atrioventricular reentrant tachycardia and other supraventricular tachycardias of unspecified mechanism associated with disabling symptoms in patients without structural heart disease.

Ventricular arrhythmias: Prevention of documented life-threatening ventricular arrhythmias, such as sustained ventricular tachycardia.

Not recommended in patients with less severe ventricular arrhythmias even if the patients are symptomatic. Because of proarrhythmic effects of flecainide, reserve use for patients in whom benefits outweigh risks.

Contraindications:

Preexisting second- or third-degree AV block, right bundle branch block when associated with a left hemiblock (bifascicular block), unless a pacemaker is present to sustain the cardiac rhythm if complete heart block occurs; recent myocardial infarction (MI); presence of cardiogenic shock; hypersensitivity to the drug.

Warnings:

Mortality: An excessive mortality or non-fatal cardiac arrest rate was seen in patients treated with flecainide compared with that seen in a carefully matched placebo-treated group.

Ventricular pro-arrhythmic effects in patients with atrial fibrillation/flutter: Flecainide is not recommended for use in patients with chronic atrial fibrillation. Case reports of ventricular proarrhythmic effects in patients treated with flecainide for atrial fibrillation/flutter have included increased PVCs, VT, VF and death.

Patients treated with flecainide for atrial flutter have been reported with 1:1 atrioventricular conduction due to slowing the atrial rate. A paradoxical increase in the ventricular rate also may occur in patients with atrial fibrillation who receive flecainide. Concomitant negative chronotropic therapy such as digoxin or beta-blockers may lower the risk of this complication.

Non-life-threatening ventricular arrhythmias: It is prudent to consider the risks of Class IC agents, coupled with the lack of any evidence of improved survival, generally unacceptable in patients whose ventricular arrhythmias are not life-threatening, even if the patients are experiencing unpleasant but not life-threatening symptoms or signs.

Proarrhythmic effects: Flecainide can cause new or worsened arrhythmias. Such proarrhythmic effects range from an increase in frequency of PVCs to the development of more severe ventricular tachycardia.

Sick sinus syndrome: Use only with extreme caution; the drug may cause sinus bradycardia, sinus pause or sinus arrest. The frequency probably increases with higher trough plasma levels.

Heart failure: Flecainide has a negative inotropic effect and may cause or worsen CHF, particularly in patients with cardiomyopathy, preexisting severe heart failure (NYHA functional class III or IV) or low ejection fractions (< 30%). The initial dosage should be no more than 100 mg twice daily; monitor patients carefully. Give close attention to maintenance of cardiac function, including optimal digitalis, diuretic or other therapy. Where CHF has developed or worsened during treatment, the time of onset has ranged from a few hours to several months after starting therapy. Some patients who develop reduced myocardial function while on flecainide can continue with adjustment of digitalis or diuretics; others may require dosage reduction or discontinuation of flecainide. When feasible, monitor plasma flecainide levels. Keep trough plasma levels < 1 mcg/ml.

Cardiac conduction: Flecainide slows cardiac conduction in most patients to produce dose-related increases in PR, QRS and QT intervals. The degree of lengthening of PR and QRS intervals does not predict either efficacy or the development of cardiac adverse effects. Patients may develop new first-degree AV heart block. Use caution and consider dose reductions. The JT interval (QT minus QRS) only widens about 4% on the average. Rare cases of torsade de pointes-type arrhythmias have occurred.

If second-or third-degree AV block, or right bundle branch block associated with a left hemiblock occurs, discontinue therapy unless a ventricular pacemaker is in place to ensure an adequate ventricular rate.

Electrolyte disturbance: Hypokalemia or hyperkalemia may alter the effects of Class I antiarrhythmic drugs. Correct preexisting hypokalemia or hyperkalemia before administration.

Effects on pacemaker thresholds: Flecainide increases endocardial pacing thresholds and may suppress ventricular escape rhythms. These effects are reversible. Use with caution in patients with permanent pacemakers or temporary pacing electrodes. Do not administer to patients with existing poor thresholds or nonprogrammable pacemakers unless suitable pacing rescue is available.

Determine the pacing threshold in patients with pacemakers prior to instituting therapy, after 1 week of administration and at regular intervals thereafter. Generally, threshold changes are within the range of multiprogrammable pacemakers, and a doubling of either voltage or pulse width is usually sufficient to regain capture.

Hepatic function impairment: Since flecainide elimination from plasma can be markedly slower in patients with significant hepatic impairment, do not use in such patients unless the potential benefits outweigh the risks. If used, make dosage increases very cautiously when plasma levels have plateaued (after > 4 days).

Elderly: Patients up to age 80 and above have been safely treated with usual doses.

Pregnancy: *Category C.*

Lactation: Flecainide is excreted in breast milk; determine whether to discontinue nursing or discontinue the drug, taking into account the importance of the drug to the mother.

Children: Safety and efficacy for use in children < 18 years of age have not been established.

Based on several studies flecainide appears to be beneficial in treating supraventricular and ventricular arrhythmias in children. Elimination half-life is shorter and volume of distribution is smaller.

Drug Interactions:

Drugs that may affect flecainide include amiodarone, cimetidine, disopyramide, propranolol, urinary acidifiers/alkalinizers and verapamil. Smoking may also have an effect. Drugs that may be affected by flecainide include propranolol and digoxin.

Adverse Reactions:

Adverse interactions occurring in ≥ 3% of patients include: Dizziness; dyspnea; headache; nausea; fatigue; palpitation; chest pain; asthenia; tremor; constipation; edema; abdominal pain; visual disturbances

In post-MI patients with asymptomatic PVCs and non-sustained ventricular tachycardia, flecainide therapy was associated with a 5.1% rate of death and non-fatal cardiac arrest, compared with a 2.3% rate in a matched placebo group.

Administration and Dosage:

For patients with sustained ventricular tachycardia, initiate therapy in the hospital and monitor rhythm.

Do not increase dosage more frequently than once every 4 days, since optimal effect may not be achieved during the first 2 to 3 days of therapy.

An occasional patient not adequately controlled by (or intolerant of) a dose given at 12 hour intervals may be dosed at 8 hour intervals.

Once the arrhythmia is controlled, it may be possible to reduce the dose, as necessary, to minimize side effects or effects on conduction.

PSVT and PAF: The recommended starting dose is 50 mg every 12 hours. Doses may be increased in increments of 50 mg twice daily every 4 days until efficacy is achieved. For PAF patients, a substantial increase in efficacy without a substantial increase in discontinuation for adverse experiences may be achieved by increasing the flecainide dose from 50 to 100 mg twice daily. The maximum recommended dose for patients with paroxysmal supraventricular arrhythmias is 300 mg/day.

Sustained ventricular tachycardia:

Initial dose – 100 mg every 12 hours. Increase in 50 mg increments twice daily every 4 days until effective. Most patients do not require > 150 mg every 12 hours (300 mg/day). Maximum dose is 400 mg/day.

Use of higher initial doses and more rapid dosage adjustments have resulted in an increased incidence of proarrhythmic events and CHF, particularly during the first few days of dosing. A loading dose is not recommended.

Renal function impairment: In severe renal impairment (Ccr ≤ 35 ml/min/1.73 m^2), the initial dosage is 100 mg once daily (or 50 mg twice daily). Frequent plasma level monitoring is required to guide dosage adjustments. In patients with less severe renal disease, initial dosage is 100 mg every 12 hours. Increase dosage cautiously at intervals > 4 days, observing the patient closely for signs of adverse cardiac effects or other toxicity. It may take > 4 days before a new steady-state plasma level is reached following a dosage change. Monitor plasma levels to guide dosage adjustments.

Transfer to flecainide: Theoretically, when transferring patients from another antiarrhythmic to flecainide, allow at least 2 to 4 plasma half-lives to elapse for the drug being discontinued before starting flecainide at the usual dosage. Consider hospitalization of patients in whom withdrawal of a previous antiarrhythmic is likely to produce life-threatening arrhythmias.

Plasma level monitoring: The majority of patients treated successfully had trough plasma levels between 0.2 and 1mcg/ml. The probability of adverse experiences, especially cardiac, may increase with higher trough plasma levels, especially levels > 1 mcg/ml. Monitor trough plasma levels periodically, especially in patients with severe or moderate chronic renal failure or severe hepatic disease and CHF, as drug elimination may be slower.

BRETYLIUM TOSYLATE

Injection: 50 mg per ml (*Rx*)	Various, *Bretylol* (DuPont Critical Care)
Injection: 2 mg per ml (500 mg per vial) in 5% Dextrose, 4 mg per ml (1000 mg per vial) in 5% Dextrose (*Rx*)	Various

Actions:

Pharmacology: Bretylium tosylate inhibits norepinephrine release by depressing adrenergic nerve terminal excitability, inducing a chemical sympathectomy-like state. Catecholamine stores are not depleted, but the drug causes an early release of norepinephrine from the adrenergic postganglionic nerve terminals. Therefore, transient catecholamine effects on myocardium (tachycardia) and on peripheral vascular resistance (rise in blood pressure) are often seen shortly after use. Subsequently, bretylium blocks the release of norepinephrine in response to neuron stimulation. Peripheral adrenergic blockade causes orthostatic hypotension but has less effect on supine blood pressure. It has a positive inotropic effect on the myocardium.

Electrophysiology – Unknown, but postulated mechanisms include (1) increase in ventricular fibrillation threshold; (2) increase in action potential duration and effective refractory period without changes in heart rate; (3) little effect on the rate of rise or amplitude of the cardiac action potential (Phase 0) or in resting membrane potential (Phase 4) in normal myocardium. However, when cell injury slows rate of rise, decreases amplitude and lowers resting membrane potential, bretylium transiently restores these parameters toward normal; (4) decrease in disparity in action potential duration between normal and infarcted regions; (5) increase in impulse formation and spontaneous firing rate of pacemaker tissue, and in ventricular conduction velocity.

The restoration of injured myocardial cell electrophysiology toward normal, as well as the increase of the action potential duration and effective refractory period, without changing their ratio, may help suppress reentry of aberrant impulses and decrease induced dispersion of local excitable states.

Hemodynamics – The mild increase in arterial pressure, followed by a modest decrease, remain within normal limits.

Pharmacokinetics: Peak plasma concentration and peak hypotensive effects are seen within 1 hour of IM administration. However, suppression of premature ventricular beats is not maximal until 6 to 9 hours after dosing, when mean plasma concentration declines to less than one half of peak level. Antifibrillatory effects occur within minutes of an IV injection. Suppression of ventricular tachycardia and other ventricular arrhythmias develops more slowly, usually 20 min to 2 hours after parenteral administration.

The terminal half-life ranges from 6.9 to 8.1 hours. During dialysis, a twofold increase in clearance occurs. The drug is eliminated intact by the kidneys. Approximately 70% to 80% of an IM dose is excreted in the urine during the first 24 hours, with an additional 10% excreted over the next 3 days.

Indications:

For prophylaxis and therapy of ventricular fibrillation.

In the treatment of life-threatening ventricular arrhythmias (ie, ventricular tachycardia) which have failed to respond to first-line antiarrhythmic agents (eg, lidocaine).

Unlabeled uses: Bretylium is a second-line agent following lidocaine in the protocol for advanced cardiac life support during CPR. For resistant VF and VT (after lidocaine, defibrillation and procainamide failures), give bretylium 5 to 10 mg/kg IV; repeat as needed up to 30 mg/kg; use a bolus every 15 to 30 minutes, infusion 1 to 2 mg/min. For life-threatening arrhythmia use an undiluted infusion of 1 g/250 ml.

Warnings:

Hypotension (postural) occurs regularly in ≈ 50% of patients while they are supine, manifested by dizziness, lightheadedness, vertigo or faintness. Tolerance occurs unpredictably but may be present after several days. Hypotension with supine systolic pressure > 75 mmHg need not be treated unless symptomatic. If supine systolic pressure falls below 75 mmHg, infuse dopamine or norepinephrine to increase blood pressure; use dilute solution and monitor blood pressure closely because pressor effects are enhanced by bretylium. Perform volume expansion with blood or plasma and correct dehydration where appropriate.

Transient hypertension and increased frequency of arrhythmias may occur due to initial release of norepinephrine from adrenergic postganglionic nerve terminals.

Fixed cardiac output: Avoid use with fixed cardiac output since severe hypotension may result from a fall in peripheral resistance without a compensatory increase in cardiac output. If survival is threatened by arrhythmia, the drug may be used, but give vasoconstrictive catecholamines promptly if severe hypotension occurs.

Renal function impairment: Since the drug is excreted principally via the kidney, increase the dosage interval in patients with impaired renal function.

Pregnancy: Category C. Reduced uterine blood flow with fetal hypoxia (bradycardia) is a potential risk. Give to a pregnant woman only if clearly needed.

Children: Safety and efficacy for use in children have not been established.

Drug Interactions:

Drugs that may affect bretylium include catecholamines and digoxin.

Adverse Reactions:

Adverse reactions occurring in ≥ 3% of patients include hypotension and postural hypotension; nausea and vomiting, primarily after rapid IV administration.

Administration and Dosage:

For short-term use only.

Keep patient supine during therapy or closely observe for postural hypotension. The optimal dose has not been determined. Dosages > 40 mg/kg/day have been used without apparent adverse effect. As soon as possible, and when indicated, change patient to an oral antiarrhythmic agent for maintenance therapy.

Immediate life-threatening ventricular arrhythmias (eg, ventricular fibrillation, hemo dynamically unstable ventricular tachycardia): Administer undiluted, 5mg/kg by rapid IV injection. If ventricular fibrillation persists, increase dosage to 10 mg/kg and repeat as necessary.

Maintenance: For continuous suppression, administer the diluted solution by continuous IV infusion at 1 to 2 mg/minute. Alternatively, infuse the diluted solution at a dosage of 5 to 10 mg/kg over > 8 minutes, every 6 hours. More rapid infusion may cause nausea and vomiting.

Other ventricular arrhythmias:

IV – Dilute before administration. Administer 5 to 10 mg/kg by IV infusion over > 8 minutes. More rapid infusion may cause nausea and vomiting. Give subsequent doses at 1 to 2 hour intervals if the arrhythmia persists. For maintenance therapy, the same dosage may be administered every 6 hours, or a constant infusion of 1 to 2 mg/min may be given.

IM – 5 to 10 mg/kg undiluted. Do not dilute prior to injection. Give subsequent doses at 1 to 2 hour intervals if the arrhythmia persists. Thereafter, maintain with same dosage every 6 to 8 hours.

Do not give > 5 ml in any one site. Do not inject into or near a major nerve; vary injection sites. Repeated injection into the same site may cause atrophy and necrosis of muscle tissue, fibrosis, vascular degeneration and inflammatory changes.

Children: The following dosages have been suggested.

Acute ventricular fibrillation – 5 mg/kg/dose IV, followed by 10 mg/kg at 15 to 30 minute intervals, maximum total dose 30 mg/kg; *maintenance*, 5 to 10 mg/kg/dose every 6 hours.

Other ventricular arrhythmias – 5 to 10 mg/kg/dose every 6 hours.

AMIODARONE HCl

Tablets: 200 mg (*Rx*)	*Cordarone* (Wyeth-Ayerst)
Injection: 50 mg/ml (*Rx*)	

Actions:

Pharmacology: Amiodarone has predominantly Class III antiarrhythmic effects. The antiarrhythmic effect may be due to at least two major properties: A prolongation of the myocardial cell action potential duration and refractory period, and noncompetitive α- and β-adrenergic inhibition.

Electrophysiology – Amiodarone increases the cardiac refractory period without influencing resting membrane potential, except in automatic cells where slope of prepotential is reduced, generally reducing automaticity. These electrophysiologic effects are reflected in decreased sinus rate, increased PR and QT intervals, development of U waves, and changes in T wave contour. These changes should not require discontinuation, although amiodarone can cause marked sinus bradycardia or sinus arrest and heart block.

Electrophysiologic effects can be seen within hours after a parenteral dose. Effects on abnormal rhythms usually require 1 to 3 weeks, even when a loading dose is used. Time to effect may be shorter when a loading-dose regimen is used.

Hemodynamics – After IV use, amiodarone relaxes vascular smooth muscle, reduces peripheral vascular resistance ans slightly increases cardiac index. After oral dosing, however, it produces no significant change in left ventricular ejection fraction (LVEF), even in patients with depressed LVEF. After acute IV dosing, it may have a mild negative inotropic effect.

These differences between oral and IV administration suggest that the initial acute effects of IV amiodarone may be predominantly focused on the AV node, causing an intranodal conduction delay and increased nodal refractoriness due to slow channed blockade (Class IV activity) and noncompetitive adrenergic antagonism (Class II activity).

Pharmacokinetics:

Absorption – Following oral administration, amiodarone is slowly and variably absorbed; bioavailability is between 35% and 65%. Maximum plasma concentrations are attained 3 to 7 hours after a single dose. The onset of action commonly takes 1 to 3 weeks, even with loading doses. Plasma concentrations with chronic dosing at 100 to 600 mg/day are approximately dose-proportional, with a mean 0.5 mg/L increase for each 100 mg/day. These means, however, include considerable individual variability.

Peak serum concentrations after single 5 mg/kg 15–minute IV infusion in healthy subjects range between 5 and 41 mg/L. Peak concentrations after 10–minute infusions of 150 mg in patients with ventricular fibrillation (VF) or hemodynamically unstable ventricular tachycardia (VT) range between 7 and 26 mg/L. Due to rapid distribution, serum concentrations decline to 10% of peak values within 30 to 45 minutes after the end of the infusion.

Distribution – Amiodarone has a very large but variable volume of distribution, averaging about 60 L/kg,. One major metabolite, desethylamiodarone, accumulates to an even greater extent in almost all tissues. The plasma ratio of metabolite to parent compound is ≈ 1:1. The drug is highly protein bound (≈ 96%).

Metabolism – The main route of elimination is via hepatic excretion into bile. The drug has a very low plasma clearance with negligible renal excretion; it does not appear necessary to modify dose in patients with renal failure.

Excretion – Following discontinuation of chronic oral therapy, amiodarone has a biphasic elimination with an initial one-half reduction of plasma levels after 2.5 to 10 days. A much slower terminal plasma elimination phase shows a half-life of the parent compound ranging from 26 to 107 days. Steady-state plasma concentrations would therefore be reached between 130 and 535 days. For the metabolite, mean plasma elimination half-life was ≈ 61 days. The considerable intersubject variation requires attention to individual responses. Antiarrhythmic effects persist for weeks or months after the drug is discontinued. In general, when the drug is resumed after recurrence of arrhythmia, control is established rapidly compared to initial response.

Indications:

Ventricular arrhythmias:

Oral – Only for treatment of the following documented life-threatening recurrent ventricular arrhythmias that do not respond to documented adequate doses of other antiarrhythmics or when alternative agents are not tolerated:

1.) Recurrent ventricular fibrillation (VF).

2.) Recurrent hemodynamically unstable ventricular tachycardia (VT).

Parenteral – Initiation of treatment and prophylaxis of frequently recurring VF and hemodynamically unstable VT in patients refractory to other therapy. It can also be used to treat patients with VT/VF for whom oral amiodarone is indicated, but who are unable to take oral medication.

During or after treatment with IV amiodarone, patients may be transferred to oral amiodarone therapy. Use IV amiodarone for acute treatment until the patient's ventricular arrhythmias are stabilized. Most patients require this therapy for 48 to 96 hours, but IV amiodarone may be given safely for longer periods if necessary.

Unlabeled uses: Amiodarone (600 to 800 mg/day for 7 to 10 days, then 200 to 400 mg/day) appears to be beneficial in the treatment of refractory sustained or paroxysmal atrial fibrillation and paroxysmal supraventricular tachycardia. It also appears useful in symptomatic atrial flutter. Low dose amiodarone (200 mg/day) may produce benefits in left ventricular ejection fraction, exercise tolerance and ventricular arrhythmias in patients with CHF.

Contraindications:

Hypersensitivity to the drug or any of its components.

Oral: Severe sinus-node dysfunction, causing marked sinus bradycardia; second- and third-degree AV block; when episodes of bradycardia have caused syncope (except when used in conjunction with a pacemaker).

Parenteral: Marked sinus bradycardia; second- and third-degree AV block unless a functioning pacemaker is available; cardiogenic shock.

Warnings:

Potentially fatal toxicities with pulmonary toxicity have occurred with ventricular arrhythmias (at ≈ 400 mg/day), and symptomless abnormal diffusion capacity has occurred in much higher percentages. Pulmonary toxicity has been fatal ≈ 10% of the time. Hepatic injury is common, but usually mild, and evidenced by abnormal liver enzymes. Overt liver disease can occur and has been fatal. Amiodarone has made arrhythmia less well tolerated or more difficult to reverse. Significant heart block or sinus bradycardia has been seen. These events should be manageable in the proper clinical setting. Although such events do not appear more frequently with amiodarone than with other agents, effects are prolonged. in patients at high risk of arrhythmic death in whom amiodarone toxicity is an acceptable risk, amiodarone poses major management problems that could be life-threatening in a population at risk of sudden death so that every effort should be made to use alternative agents first.

Hospitalize patients while the loading dose is given; a response generally requires 2 weeks. Absorption and elimination are variable; therefore, maintenance dose selection is difficult. The time at which a life-threatening arrhythmia will recur after discontinuation or dose adjustment is unpredictable, ranging from weeks to months. The patient risk is greatest during this time. Substituting other antiarrhythmics when amiodarone must be stopped is made difficult by gradually, but unpredictably, changing amiodarone body stores. When amiodarone is ineffective, it still poses the risk of interacting with subsequent treatment.

Survival: There is no evidence that the use of amiodarone favorably affects survival.

Pulmonary toxicity:

Oral – Amiodarone may cause a clinical syndrome of cough and progressive dyspnea accompanied by functional, radiographic, gallium scan and pathological data consistent with pulmonary toxicity. The frequency varies from 2% to 17%; fatalities occur in about 10% of cases. However, in patients with life-threatening arrhythmias, discontinuation of amiodarone therapy due to suspected drug-induced pulmonary toxicity should be undertaken with caution, as the most common cause of death in these patients is sudden cardiac death. Therefore, make every effort to rule out other causes of respiratory impairment before discontinuing amiodarone. In addition, bronchoalveolar lavage, transbronchial lung biopsy or open lung biopsy may be necessary to confirm the diagnosis, especially in those cases where no acceptable alternative therapy is available.

Any new respiratory symptom suggests pulmonary toxicity, therefore repeat and evaluate the history, physical exam, chest x-ray, gallium scan and pulmonary function tests (with diffusion capacity). In some cases, rechallenge at a lower dose has not resulted in return of interstitial/alveolar pneumonitis.

Perform baseline chest x–rays and pulmonary function tests, including diffusion capacity before therapy initiation. A history and physicial exam and chest x-ray should be repeated every 3 to 6 months.

Patients with preexisting pulmonary disease have a poorer prognosis if pulmonary toxicity does develop. Pulmonary toxicity secondary to amiodarone seems to result from either indirect or direct toxicity as represented by hypersensitivity pneumonitis or interstitial/alveolar pneumonitis, respectively.

Hypersensitivity pneumonitis usually appears earlier in the course of therapy, and rechallenging these patients results in a more rapid recurrence of greater severity. Bronchoalveolar lavage is the procedure of choice to confirm this diagnosis. Institute steroid therapy and discontinue amiodarone therapy.

Interstitial/alveolar pneumonitis may result from the release of oxygen radicals or phospholipidosis and is characterized by findings of diffuse alveolar damage, interstitial pneumonitis or fibrosis in lung biopsy specimens. Phospholipidosis (foamy cells, foamy macrophages) will be present in most cases of amiodarone-induced pulmonary toxicity; however, these changes are also present in approximately 50% of all patients on amiodarone therapy. A diagnosis of amiodarone-induced interstitial/alveolar pneumonitis should lead to dose reduction or to withdrawal of amiodarone to establish reversibility, especially if other acceptable antiarrhythmic therapies are available. With these measures, a reduction in symptoms of amiodarone-induced pulmonary toxicity was usually noted within the first week. Chest x-ray changes usually resolve within 2 to 4 months.

According to some experts, steroids may prove beneficial. In some cases, rechallenge with amiodarone at a lower dose has not resulted in return of toxicity. Recent reports suggest that lower loading and maintenance doses of amiodarone are associated with a decreased incidence of amiodarone-induced pulmonary toxicity.

If a diagnosis of amiodarone-induced hypersensitivity pneumonitis is made, discontinue amiodarone and institute steroid treatment. If a diagnosis of amiodarone-induced interstitial/alveolar pneumonitis is made, institute steroid therapy and discontinue amiodarone or, at a minimum, reduce dosage.

Parenteral –

ARDS: 2% of patients were reported to have adult respiratory distress syndrome (ARDS) during clinical studies. It is not possible to determine what role, if any, amiodarone IV played in causing or exacerbating the pulmonary disorder in those patients.

Pulmonary fibrosis: Only 1 of > 1000 patients treated with amiodarone IV in clincal studies developed pulmonary fibrosis. In that patient, the condition was diagnosed 3 months after treatment with amiodarone IV, during which time she received oral amiodarone. Pulmonary toxicity is a well recognized complication of long-term amiodarone use.

Cardiac effects:

Proarrhythmias – Amiodarone can cause serious exacerbation of the presenting arrhythmia, a risk that may be enhanced by concomitant antiarrhythmics. In addition, amiodarone has caused symptomatic bradycardia, heart block or sinus arrest with suppression of escape foci. Drug-related bradycardia occurred while patients were receiving amiodarone IV for life-threatening VT/VF; it was not dose-related. Treat bradycardia by slowing the infusion rate or discontinuing amiodarone IV. In some patients, inserting a pacemaker is required.

Hypotension is the most common adverse effect seen with amiodarone IV. Clinically significant hypotension during infusions was seen most often in the first several hours of treatment and was not dose-related, but appeared to be related to the rate of infusion. Hypotension necessitating alterations in therapy was reported in 3% of patients, with permanent discontinuation required in < 2% of patients. Treat hypotension initially by slowing the infusion; additional standard therapy may be needed, including the following: Vasopressor drugs, positive inotropic agents and volume expansion. Monitor the initial rate of infusion closely and do not exceed prescribed dosage.

Hepatic effects:

Oral – Elevated hepatic enzyme levels are frequent, and in most cases are asymptomatic. If the increase exceeds 3 times normal, or doubles in a patient with an elevated baseline, consider discontinuation or dosage reduction. When a biopsy has been done, histology has resembled that of alcoholic hepatitis or cirrhosis. Hepatic failure has rarely caused death.

Elevations in liver enzymes (AST and ALT) can occur. Regularly monitor liver enzymes in patients on relatively high maintenence doses. If persistent significant elevations in the liver enzymes or hepatomegaly occur, consider reducing the maintenance dose or discontinuing therapy.

Parenteral – Elevations of blood hepatic enzyme values, ALT, AST and GGT, are seen commonly in patinets with immediately life-threatening VT/VF. Interpreting elevated AST activity can be difficult because the values may be elevated in patients who have had recent MI, CHF or multiple electrocal defibrillations. Baseline abnormalities in hepatic enzymes are not a contraindication to treatment.

Two cases of fatal hepatocellular necrosis after treament with amiodarone IV have been reported. Because the episodes of hepatic necrosis may have been due to the rapid rate of infusion with possible rate-related hypotension, monitor the initial rate of infusion closely and do not exceed the prescribed dosage.

In patients with life-threatening arrhythmias, weigh the potential risk of hepatic injury against the potential benefit of therapy. Monitor carefully for evidence of progressive hepatic injury. Give consideration to reducing the rate of administration or withdrawing amiodarone IV in such cases.

Elderly: Healthy subjects > 65 years of age show lower clearances of amiodarone than younger subjects and an increase in half-life.

Pregnancy: *Category D.*

Lactation: Amiodarone is excreted in breast milk. When amiodarone therapy is indicated, advise the mother to discontinue nursing.

Children: Safety and efficacy for use in children have not been established. Amiodarone is not recommended in children.

Precautions:

Ophthalmologic effects: Asymptomatic corneal microdeposits appear in the majority of adults treated with amiodarone > 6 months. Corneal microdeposits are reversible upon reduction of dose or drug discontinuation. Some patients develop photophobia and dry eyes. Vision is rarely affected and drug discontinuation is rarely needed.

Thyroid abnormalities: Amiodarone inhibits peripheral conversion of thyroxine (T_4) to triiodothyronine (T_3), prompting increased T_4 levels, increased levels of inactive reverse T_3 and decreased levels of T_3. It is also a potential source of large amounts of inorganic iodine. It can cause hypothyroidism or hyperthyroidism. Monitor thyroid function at baseline and periodically during therapy, particularly in the elderly and in any patient with a history of thyroid nodules, goiter or other thyroid dysfunction. High plasma iodide levels, altered thyroid function, and abnormal thyroid function tests may persist for several weeks or even months following amiodarone withdrawal.

Hypothyroidism can be identified by relevant clinical symptoms and particularly by elevated TSH. In some clinically hypothyroid amiodarone-treated patients, free thyroxine index values may be normal. Hypothyroidism is best managed by dose reduction or thyroid hormone supplement. However, therapy must be individualized, and it may be necessary to discontinue amiodarone in some patients.

Hyperthyroidism usually poses a greater hazard to the patient than hypothyroidism because of the possibility of arrhythmia breakthrough or aggravation. If any new signs of arrhythmia appear, consider the possibility of hyperthyroidism. Aggressive medical treatment is indicated, including, dose reduction or withdrawal of amiodarone. The institution of antithyroid drugs, beta-adrenergic blockers or temporary corticosteroid therapy may be necessary. The action of antithyroid drugs may be especially delayed in amiodarone-induced thyrotoxicosis. Radioactive iodine therapy is contraindicated because of the low radioiodine uptake associated with amiodarone-induced hyperthyroidism. Experience with thyroid surgery in this setting is extremely limited, and this form of therapy runs the theoretical risk of inducing thyroid storm. Amiodarone-induced hyperthyroidism may be followed by a transient period of hypothyroidism.

Electrolyte disturbances: Correct potassium or magnesium deficiency before therapy begins as these disorders can exaggerate the degree of QTc prolongation and increase the potential for torsade de pointes.

Photosensitivity: Amiodarone has induced photosensitization in about 10% of patients. During long-term treatment, a blue-gray discoloration of the exposed skin may occur; some protection may be afforded by sun barrier creams or protective clothing. This is slowly and occasionally incompletely reversible on discontinuation of drug.

Drug Interactions:

Although only a small number of drug interactions have been formally explored, most of these have shown such an interaction should be anticipated, particularly for drugs with potentially serious toxicity such as other antiarrhythmics. Drugs that may affect amiodarone include hydantoins, cholestyramine and cimetidine. Drugs that may be affected by amiodarone include anticoagulants, beta blockers, dextromethorphan, digoxin, flecainide, hydantoins, lidocaine, methotrexate, procainamide, quinidine and theophylline.

Drug/Lab test interactions: Amiodarone alters the results of thyroid function tests, causing an increase in serum T_4 and serum reverse T_3 levels and a decline in serum T_3 levels. Despite these biochemical changes, most patients remain clinically euthyroid.

Adverse Reactions:

Oral: Adverse reactions requiring discontinuation include: Pulmonary infiltrates or fibrosis; paroxysmal ventricular tachycardia; CHF; elevation of liver enzymes. Other symptoms causing discontinuation less often include: Visual disturbances; solar dermatitis; blue discoloration of skin; hyperthyroidism; hypothyroidism. Adverse reactions occurring in ≥ 3% of patients include: CHF; GI complaints (nausea, vomiting, constipation, anorexia); dermatologic reactions (photosensitivity, solar dermatitis); neurologic problems (malaise, fatigue, tremor/abnormal involuntary movements, lack of coordination, abnormal gait/ataxia, dizziness, paresthesias); abnormal liver function tests.

Parenteral: The most important treatment-emergent adverse effects were hypotension, asystole/cardiac arrest/electromechanical dissociation (EMD), cardiogenic shock, CHF, bradycardia, liver function test abnormalities, VT and AV block. The most common adverse effects leading to discontinuation of IV therapy were hypotension, asystole/cardiac arrest/ EMD, VT and cardiogenic shock. Adverse reactions occurring in ≥ 3% of patients include nausea.

Administration and Dosage:

In order to ensure that an antiarrhythmic effect will be observed without waiting several months, loading doses are required. Individual patient titration is suggested.

Life-threatening ventricular arrhythmias (ventricular fibrillation or hemodynamically unstable ventricular tachycardia): Administer the loading dose in a hospital. Loading doses of 800 to 1600 mg/day are required for 1 to 3 weeks (occasionally longer) until initial therapeutic response occurs. Administer in divided doses with meals for total daily doses of ≥ 1000 mg, or when GI intolerance occurs. If side effects become excessive, reduce the dose. Elimination of recurrence of ventricular fibrillation and tachycardia usually occurs within 1 to 3 weeks, along with reduction in complex and total ventricular ectopic beats.

When starting amiodarone therapy, attempt to gradually discontinue prior antiarrhythmic drugs (see concurrent antiarrhythmic agents). When adequate arrhythmia control is achieved, or if side effects become prominent, reduce dose to 600 to 800 mg/day for 1 month and then to the maintenance dose, usually 400 mg/day. Some patients may require larger maintenance doses, up to 600 mg/day, and some can be controlled on lower doses. May be administered as a single daily dose, or in patients with severe GI intolerance, as a twice daily dose. In each patient, determine the chronic maintenance dose according to antiarrhythmic effect as assessed by symptoms, Holter recordings or programmed electrical stimulation and by patient tolerance. Plasma concentrations may be helpful in evaluating nonresponsiveness or unexpectedly severe toxicity.

Use the lowest effective dose to prevent the occurrence of side effects. In all instances, be guided by the severity of the patient's arrhythmia and response to therapy. When dosage adjustments are necessary, closely monitor the patient for an extended time because of the long and variable half-life and the difficulty in predicting the time required to attain a new steady-state drug level.

Concurrent antiarrhythmic agents – In general, reserve the combination of amiodarone with other antiarrhythmic therapy for patients with life-threatening arrhythmias who are incompletely responsive to a single agent or incompletely responsive to amiodarone. During transfer to amiodarone, reduce the dose levels of previously administered agents by 30% to 50% several days after the addition of amiodarone when arrhythmia suppression should be beginning. Review the continued need for the other antiarrhythmic agent after the effects of amiodarone have been established, and attempt discontinuation. If the treatment is continued, carefully monitor these patients for adverse effects, especially conduction disturbances and exacerbation of tachyarrhythmias, as amiodarone is continued. In amiodarone-treated patients who require additional antiarrhythmic therapy, the initial dose of such agents should be ≈ ½ of the usual recommended dose.

Parenteral: Amiodarone shows considerable interindividual variation in response. Thus, although a starting dose adequate to suppress life-threatening arrhythmias is needed, close monitoring with adjustment of dose as needed is essential. The recommended starting dose of amiodarone IV is about 1000 mg over the first 24 hours of therapy, delivered by the following infusion regimen.

Amiodarone IV Dose Recommendations During the First 24 Hours	
Loading infusions	
First rapid	150 mg over the *first* 10 minutes (15 mg/min). Add 3 ml amiodarone IV (150 mg) to 100 ml D5W (concentration, 1.5 mg/ml). Infuse 100 ml/10 min.
Followed by slow	360 mg over the *next* 6 hours (1 mg/min). Add 18 ml amiodarone IV (900 mg) to 500 ml D5W (concentration, 1.8 mg/ml).
Maintenance infusion	540 mg over the *remaining* 18 hours (0.5 mg/min). Decrease the rate of the slow loading infusion to 0.5 mg/min.

After the first 24 hours, continue the maintenance infusion rate of 0.5 mg/min (720 mg/24 hrs) utilizing a concentration of 1 to 6 mg/ml (give amiodarone IV concentrations > 2 mgml via a central venous catheter). In the event of breakthrough episodes of VF or hemodynamically unstable VT, 150 mg supplemental infusions of amiodarone IV mixed in 100 ml D5W may be given. Administer such infusions over 10 minutes to minimize the potential for hypotension. The rate of the maintenance infusion may be increased to achieve effective arrhythmia suppression.

The first 24 hour dose may be individualized for each patient; however, in controlled clinical trials, mean daily doses > 2100 mg were associated with an increased risk of hypotension. The initial infusion rate should not exceed 30 mg/min.

Based on the experience from clincial studies, a maintenance infusion of up to 0.5 mg/min can be cautiously continued for 2 to 3 weeks regardless of the patient's age, renal function or left ventricular function. There has been limited experience in patients receiving amiodarone IV for > 3 weeks.

The surface properties of solutions containing injectable amiodarone are altered such that the drop size may be redued. This reduction may lead to underdosage of the patient by up to 30%. If drop counter infusion sets are used, amiodarone must be delivered by a volumetric infusion pump.

Amiodarone IV should, when possible, be administered through a central venous catheter for that purpose. Use and in-line filter during administration.

Amiodarone IV concentrations > 3 mg/ml in D5W have been associated with a high incidence of peripheral vein phlebitis; however, concentrations of ≤ 2.5 mg/ml appear to be less irritating. Therefore, for infusions > 1 hour, amiodarone IV concentrations should not exceed 2 mg/ml unless a central venous catheter is used.

Amiodarone IV infusions exceeding 2 hours must be administered in glass or polyolefin bottles containing D5W.

Amiodarone adsorbs to polyvinyl chloride (PVC) tubing and the clinical trial dose administration schedule was designed to account for this adsorption. All of the clinical trials were conducted using PVC tubing and its use is therefore recommended. The concentrations and rates of infusion provided in Administration and Dosage reflect doses identified in these studies. It is important that the recommended infusion regimen be followed closely.

IV to oral transition: Patients whose arrhythias have been suppressed by amiodarone IV may be switched to oral amiodarone. The optimal dose for changing from IV to oral administration will depend on the IV dose already administered, as well as the bioavailability of oral amiodarone. When changing to oral therapy, clinical monitoring is recommended, particularly for elderly patients.

The following table provides suggested doses of oral amiodarone to be initiated after varying durations of IV administration. These recommendations are made on the basis of a comparable total body amount of amiodarone delivered by the IV and oral routes, based on 50% bioavailability of oral amiodarone.

Recommendations for Oral Amiodarone Dosage After IV Infusion	
Duration of amiodarone IV infusions[1]	Initial daily dose of oral amiodarone
< 1 week	800 to 1600 mg
1 to 3 weeks	600 to 800 mg
> 3 weeks[2]	400 mg

[1] Assuming a 720 mg/day infusion (0.5 mg/min).
[2] Amiodarone IV is not intended for maintenance treatment.

ADENOSINE

Injection: 6 mg/2 ml (*Rx*)	*Adenocard* (Fujisawa)

Actions:

Pharmacology: Adenosine is an endogenous nucleoside occurring in all cells. It is not chemically related to other antiarrhythmic agents. Adenosine slows conduction time through the AV node, can interrupt the reentry pathways through the AV node and can restore normal sinus rhythm in patients with paroxysmal supraventricular tachycardia (PSVT), including PSVT associated with Wolff-Parkinson-White (WPW) Syndrome.

Hemodynamics – When larger doses are given by infusion, adenosine decreases blood pressure by decreasing peripheral resistance.

Pharmacokinetics: Following an IV bolus, adenosine is taken up by erythrocytes and vascular endothelial cells. Half-life is estimated to be < 10 seconds. Adenosine enters the body pool and is primarily metabolized to inosine and adenosine monophosphate (AMP).

Indications:

Conversion to sinus rhythm of paroxysmal supraventricular tachycardia, including that associated with accessory bypass tracts (WPW Syndrome). When clinically advisable, attempt appropriate vagal maneuvers (eg, Valsalva maneuver) prior to use.

Unlabeled uses: Adenosine has been used in the noninvasive assessment of patients with suspected coronary artery disease in conjunction with ^{201}thallium tomography; results are similar to assessment with exercise stress test or IV dipyridamole.

Contraindications:

Second- or third-degree AV block or sick sinus syndrome (except in patients with a functioning artificial pacemaker); atrial flutter, atrial fibrillation and ventricular tachycardia (the drug is not effective in converting these arrhythmias to normal sinus rhythm); hypersensitivity to adenosine.

Warnings:

Heart block: Adenosine may produce a short lasting first-, second- or third-degree heart block. In extreme cases, transient asystole may result. Institute appropriate therapy as needed. Patients who develop high-level block on one dose should not be given additional doses. These effects are generally self-limiting.

Arrhythmias: At the time of conversion to normal sinus rhythm, a variety of new rhythms may appear on the ECG. They generally last only a few seconds without intervention, and may take the form of premature ventricular contractions, atrial premature contractions, sinus bradycardia, sinus tachycardia, skipped beats and varying degrees of AV nodal block. Such findings were seen in 55% of patients.

Treatment of other arrhythmias: Adenosine is not effective in converting rhythms other than PSVT, such as atrial flutter, atrial fibrillation or ventricular tachycardia to normal sinus rhythm.

Ventricular response: In the presence of atrial flutter or atrial fibrillation, a transient modest slowing of ventricular response may occur immediately following use.

Hepatic and renal failure: Hepatic and renal failure should have no effect on the activity of a bolus adenosine injection.

Pregnancy: Category C.

Precautions:

Asthma: A limited number of patients with asthma have received adenosine and have not experienced exacerbation of their asthma. However, inhaled adenosine induces bronchoconstriction in asthmatic patients but not in healthy individuals. Be alert to the possibility that adenosine could produce bronchoconstriction in patients with asthma.

Drug Interactions:

Drugs that may interact with adenosine include carbamazepine, dipyridamole and methylxanthines.

Adverse Reactions:

Adverse reactions occurring in ≥ 3% of patients include facial flushing; shortness of breath/dyspnea; chest pressure; nausea;

Administration and Dosage:

For rapid bolus IV use only. To be certain the solution reaches the systemic circulation, administer either directly into a vein or, if given into an IV line, as proximal as possible and follow with a rapid saline flush.

Initial dose: 6 mg as a rapid IV bolus (administered over a 1 to 2 second period).

Repeat administration: If first dose does not result in elimination of the supraventricular tachycardia within 1 to 2 minutes, give 12 mg as a rapid IV bolus. This 12 mg dose may be repeated a second time if required.

Doses > 12 mg are not recommended.

CALCIUM CHANNEL BLOCKING AGENTS

AMLODIPINE	
Tablets: 2.5, 5, 10 mg (*Rx*)	*Norvasc* (Pfizer)
BEPRIDIL HCl	
Tablets: 200, 300, 400 mg (*Rx*)	*Vascor* (McNeil)
DILTIAZEM HCl	
Tablets: 30, 60, 90, 120 mg (*Rx*)	Various, *Cardizem* (Marion Merrell Dow)
Capsules, sustained release: 60, 90, 120, 180, 240, 300, 360 mg (*Rx*)	Various, *Cardizem SR* (Marion Merrell Dow), *Cardizem CD* (Marion Merrell Dow), *Dilacor XR* (Rhone-Poulenc Rorer), *Tiazac* (Forest)
Injection: 25 mg (5 mg/ml), 50 mg (5 mg/ml) (*Rx*)	*Cardizem* (Marion Merrell Dow)
FELODIPINE	
Tablets, extended release: 2.5, 5, 10 mg (*Rx*)	*Plendil* (Merck)
ISRADIPINE	
Capsules: 2.5, 5 mg (*Rx*)	*DynaCirc* (Sandoz)
NICARDIPINE HCl	
Capsules: 20, 30 mg (*Rx*)	*Cardene* (Syntex)
Capsules, sustained release: 30, 45, 60 mg (*Rx*)	*Cardene SR* (Syntex)
Injection: 2.5 mg/ml (*Rx*)	*Cardene I.V.* (Wyeth)
NIFEDIPIINE	
Capsules: 10, 20 mg (*Rx*)	Various, *Procardia* (Pfizer), *Adalat* (Bayer)
Tablets, sustained release: 30, 60, 90 mg (*Rx*)	*Procardia XL* (Pfizer), *Adalat* CC (Bayer)
NIMODIPINE	
Capsules, liquid: 30 mg (*Rx*)	*Nimotop* (Bayer)
NISOLDIPINE	
Tablets, extended release: 10, 20, 30, 40 mg (*Rx*)	*Sular* (Zeneca)
VERAPAMIL HCl	
Tablets: 40, 80, 120 mg (*Rx*)	Various, *Calan* (Searle), *Isoptin* (Knoll)
Tablets, sustained release: 120, 180, 240 mg (*Rx*)	Various, *Calan SR* (Searle), *Isoptin SR* (Knoll), *Covera-HS* (Searle)
Capsules, sustained release: 120, 180, 240 mg (*Rx*)	*Verelan* (Lederle)
Injection: 5 mg/2 ml (*Rx*)	Various, *Isoptin* (Knoll)

Actions:

Pharmacology: The calcium channel blockers share the ability to inhibit movement of calcium ions across the cell membrane. The effects on the cardiovascular system include depression of mechanical contraction of myocardial and smooth muscle and depression of both impulse formation (automaticity) and conduction velocity. **Bepridil** also inhibits fast sodium inward channels. Calcium channel blockers are classified by structure as follows: Diphenylalkylamines – verapamil; benzothiazepines – diltiazem; dihydropyridines – amlodipine, felodipine, isradipine, nicardipine, nifedipine, nimodipine, nisoldipine.

Although these agents are similar in that they all act on the slow (calcium) channel, they have different degrees of selectivity in their effects on vascular smooth muscle, myocardium or specialized conduction and pacemaker tissues. The resulting clinical effects depend on the direct activity of the drug, reflex physiological responses (primarily β-adrenergic response to vasodilation) and the patient's cardiovascular status. This heterogeneity of the calcium blockers, in part, determines their clinical application and the different side effects produced by each agent.

Pharmacokinetics:

Calcium Channel Blocking Agents: Pharmacology/Pharmacokinetics

	Parameters	Nifedipine/SR	Verapamil	Diltiazem/SR	Nicardipine	Nisoldipine
Pharmacokinetics	Extent of absorption (%)[1]	90	90	80-90	≈ 100	nd
	Absolute bioavailability (%)[1]	45-70/86	20-35	40-67	35	5
	Onset of action - oral (min)	20	30[2]	30-60	20	nd
	Time of peak plasma levels (hrs)	0.5/6	1-2.2	2-3/6-11	0.5-2	6-12
	Protein binding (%)	92-98	83-92	70-80	> 95	> 99
	Therapeutic serum levels (ng/ml)	25-100	80-300	50-200	28-50	nd
	Metabolite	Acid or lactone[3]	Norverapamil[4]	Desacetyl-diltiazem[5]	Glucuronide conjugates	5 major urinary metabolites
	Excreted unchanged in urine (%)	1-2	3-4	2-4	< 1	trace
	Half-life, elimination (hrs)	2-5	3-7[7]	3.5-6/5-7	2-4	7-12
Electrophysiology	Effective refractory period (ERP)					
	Atrium	0	0	0	0	0
	AV node	±	↑↑*	↑*	↑↓*	0
	His Purkinje	0	0	0	↓*	0
	Ventricle	0	0	0	0	0
	Accessory pathway	0	±	na	0	0
	SA node automaticity[8]	0	↓↓*	↓*	0	0
	AV node conduction[8]	±	↓↓↓*	↓↓*	0-↑*	0
	Sinus node recovery time	0	0[9]	0[9]	0	0
ECG Changes	Heart rate	↑*	↑↓*	↓*-0	↑*	±
	QRS complex	0	0	0	0	0
	PR interval	0	↑*	↑*	nd	0
	QT interval	nd	nd	nd	↑*	0
Hemodynamics	Myocardial contractility[8]	↓*	↓↓*	↓*	0	0
	Cardiac output	↑↑*	↑↓*	0-↑*	↑↑*	0
	Peripheral vascular resistance	↓↓↓*	↓↓*	↓*	↓↓↓*	↓↓↓

* ↑↑↑ or ↓↓↓ = pronounced effect; ↑↑ or ↓↓ = moderate effect; ↑ or ↓ = slight effect; ± = negligible effect; nd = no data; na = not applicable

[1] Although these agents are well absorbed (80% to 90%) following oral administration, they are subject to extensive first-pass effects, resulting in an absolute bioavailability that is considerably less.

[2] Peak therapeutic effects occur within 3 to 5 minutes after IV administration.

[3] Inactive.

[4] Pharmacologic activity 20% of verapamil.

[5] Pharmacologic activity 25% to 50% of diltiazem; plasma levels 10% to 20% of parent drug.

[6] Of 6 metabolites identified, account for > 75%.

[7] 4.5 to 12 hours with multiple dosing; may be prolonged in elderly.

[8] Direct effects may be counteracted by reflex activity.

[9] Prolonged in sick sinus syndrome.

[10] Dose-related.

Calcium Channel Blocking Agents: Pharmacology/Pharmacokinetics						
Nimodipine	Isradipine	Bepridil	Felodipine	Amlodipine	Parameters	
nd	90-95	≈ 100	≈100	nd	Extent of absorption (%)[1]	Pharmacokinetics
13	15-24	59	20	64-90	Absolute availability (%)[1]	
nd	120	60	120-300	nd	Onset of action - oral (min)	
≤1	1.5	2-3	2.5-5	6-12	Time of peak plasma levels (hrs)	
> 95	95	> 99	> 99	93	Protein binding (%)	
nd	nd	1-2	nd	nd	Therapeutic serum levels (ng/ml)	
Unknown[3]	Monoacids and cyclic lactone[6]	4-OH-N-phenyl-bepridil	Six inactive[2]	90% converted to inactive	Metabolite	
< 1	0	±	< 0.5	10	Excreted unchanged in urine (%)	
1-2	8	24	11-16	30-50	Half-life, elimination (hrs)	
					Effective refractory period	Electrophysiology
na	0	↑*	0	0	Atrium	
	0	↑*	0	0	AV node	
	0	↑*	0	0	His-Purkinje	
	0	↑*	0	0	Ventricle	
	nd	↑*	0	0	Accessory pathway	
	0	↓*	0	0	SA node automaticity	
	0	↓*	0	0	AV node conduction	
	±	nd	0	0	Sinus node recovery time	
	±	↓*	±	±	Heart rate	ECG Changes
	0	0	0	0	QRS complex	
	0	↑*	0	0	PR interval	
	↑*	↑↑[10]	0	0	QT interval	
	0	↓*	↑*	↑*	Myocardial contractility	Hemodynamics
	↑*	0	↑*	↑*	Cardiac output	
	↓↓↓*	↓*	↓↓↓*	↓↓↓*	Peripheral vascular resistance	

* ↑↑↑ or ↓↓↓ = pronounced effect; ↑↑ or ↓↓ = moderate effect; ↑ or ↓ = slight effect; ± = negligible effect; nd = no data; na = not applicable

[1] Although these agents are well absorbed (80% to 90%) following oral administration, they are subject to extensive first-pass effects, resulting in an absolute bioavailability that is considerably less.

[2] Peak therapeutic effects occur within 3 to 5 minutes after IV administration.

[3] Inactive.

[4] Pharmacologic activity 20% of verapamil.

[5] Pharmacologic activity 25% to 50% of diltiazem; plasma levels 10% to 20% of parent drug.

[6] Of 6 metabolites identified, account for > 75%.

[7] 4.5 to 12 hours with multiple dosing; may be prolonged in elderly.

[8] Direct effects may be counteracted by reflex activity.

[9] Prolonged in sick sinus syndrome.

[10] Dose-related.

Indications:

Calcium Channel Blocking Agents – Summary of Indications

Indications	Amlodipine	Bepridil	Diltiazem	Diltiazem SR	Diltiazem IV	Felodipine	Isradipine	Nicardipine	Nicardipine SR	Nicardipine IV	Nifedipine	Nifedipine SR	Nimodipine	Nisoldipine	Verapamil	Verapamil SR	Verapamil IV
Angina pectoris																	
Vasospastic	✓			✓							✓	✓			✓		
Chronic stable	✓	✓	✓	✓				✓							✓		
Unstable															✓		
Hypertension, essential	✓			✓		✓	✓	✓	✓	✓		✓		✓	✓	✓	
Arrhythmias					✓										✓		
Supraventricular tachyarrhythmias																	✓
Subarachnoid hemorrhage													✓				

[1] Refer to following section for further information on indications and additional unlabeled uses.

Unlabeled uses:

Nifedipine – Preliminary studies suggest nifedipine may be useful for hypertensive emergencies, prophylaxis in migraine headache and in the treatment of primary pulmonary hypertension, asthma, preterm labor, severe pregnancy-associated hypertension, esophageal disorders, biliary and renal colic, cardiomyopathy, to reduce progression of coronary artery disease, CHF and Raynaud's syndrome.

Verapamil (oral), has been used for PSVT. It has also been studied for the prophylaxis of migraine headache, cluster headache and exercise-induced asthma, for treatment of hypertrophic cardiomyopathy, as alternate therapy in manic depression and for recumbent nocturnal leg cramps.

Diltiazem has been investigated in the prevention of reinfarction of non-Q-wave myocardial infarction, tardive dyskinesia and Raynaud's syndrome.

Nimodipine appears to be beneficial in patients with common and classic migraine and chronic cluster headache.

Nicardipine may be useful in the treatment of congestive heart failure and in combination with aminocaproic acid for SAH.

Isradipine may be beneficial in the treatment of chronic stable angina.

Contraindications:

Hypersensitivity to the drug; sick sinus syndrome or second- or third-degree AV block except with a functioning pacemaker, hypotension < 90 mm Hg systolic (bepridil, diltiazem and verapamil).

Diltiazem: Acute MI and pulmonary congestion.

Verapamil: Severe left ventricular dysfunction; cardiogenic shock and severe CHF, unless secondary to a supraventricular tachycardia amenable to verapamil therapy and in patients with atrial flutter or atrial fibrillation and an accessory bypass tract.

Verapamil IV – Do not administer concomitantly with IV β-adrenergic blocking agents (within a few hours), since both may depress myocardial contractility and AV conduction; ventricular tachycardia, since use in patients with wide-complex ventricular tachycardia (QRS ≥ 0.12 sec) can result in marked hemodynamic deterioration and ventricular fibrillation.

Nicardipine: Advanced aortic stenosis.

Bepridil: History of serious ventricular arrhythmias; uncompensated cardiac insufficiency; congenital QT interval prolongation; use with other drugs that prolong QT interval.

Warnings:

Induction of new serious arrhythmias (bepridil): Bepridil has Class I anti-arrhythmic properties and, like other such drugs, can induce new arrhythmias, including VT/VF. In addition, because of its ability to prolong the QT interval, bepridil can cause torsades de pointes type ventricular tachycardia (VT). Because of these properties, reserve for patients in whom other anti-anginal agents do not offer a satisfactory effect.

While the safe upper limit of QT is not defined, it is suggested that the interval not be permitted to exceed 0.52 seconds during treatment. If dose reduction does not eliminate the excessive prolongation, stop the drug. If concomitant diuretics are needed, consider low doses and addition or primary use of a potassium-sparing diuretic and monitor serum potassium.

Hypotension, usually modest and well tolerated, may occasionally occur during initial therapy or with dosage increases, and may be more likely in patients taking concomitant β–blockers.

CHF has developed rarely, usually in patients receiving a β-blocker, after beginning **nifedipine.**

Oral verapamil, 1.8% developed CHF or pulmonary edema.

Use **diltiazem, nicardipine, isradipine, felodipine, amlodipine** and **bepridil** with caution in CHF patients.

Cardiac conduction: **IV verapamil** slows AV nodal conduction and SA nodes; it rarely produces second- or third-degree AV block, bradycardia, and in extreme cases, asystole. This is more likely to occur in patients with sick sinus syndrome.

Oral verapamil may lead to first-degree AV block and transient bradycardia, sometimes accompanied by nodal escape rhythms.

Premature ventricular contractions (PVCs): During conversion or marked reduction in ventricular rate, benign complexes of unusual appearance (sometimes resembling PVCs) may occur after **IV verapamil.** Verapamil IV may produce potentially fatal ventricular fibrillation in patients with atrial fibrillation (AF) and W-P-W syndrome.

Hypertrophic cardiomyopathy (IHSS): Serious adverse effects were seen in 120 patients with IHSS (most refractory or intolerant to propranolol) who received oral **verapamil** at doses up to 720 mg/day. Sinus bradycardia occurred in 11%, second-degree AV block in 4% and sinus arrest in 2%.

β-blocker withdrawal/nifedipine. Patients recently withdrawn from β-blockers may develop a withdrawal syndrome with increased angina, probably related to increased sensitivity to catecholamines. Initiation of nifedipine will not prevent this occurrence and might exacerbate it by provoking reflex catecholamine release. Taper β-blockers rather than stopping them abruptly before beginning nifedipine.

Hepatic function impairment: The pharmacokinetics, bioavailability and patient response to **verapamil** and **nifedipine** may be significantly affected by hepatic cirrhosis.

Since **amlodipine, diltiazem, nicardipine, bepridil, felodipine** and **nimodipine** are extensively metabolized by liver, use with caution in impaired hepatic function or reduced hepatic blood flow.

Renal function impairment: The pharmacokinetics of **diltiazem** and **verapamil** in patients with impaired renal function are similar to the pharmacokinetic profile of patients with normal renal function. However, caution is still advised. **Nifedipine's** plasma concentration is slightly increased in patients with renal impairment. **Nicardipine's** mean plasma concentrations, AUC and maximum concentration were ≈ 2–fold higher in patients with mild renal impairment. Use **bepridil** with caution in patients with serious renal disorders since the metabolites of bepridil are excreted primarily in the urine.

Increased angina: Occasional patients have increased frequency, duration or severity of angina on starting **nifedipine** or **nicardipine** or at the time of dosage increases.

Duchenne's muscular dystrophy: **Verapamil** may decrease neuromuscular transmission in patients with Duchenne's muscular dystrophy, and prolong recovery from the neuromuscular blocking agent vecuronium.

Elderly: **Verapamil, nifedipine** and **felodipine** may cause a greater hypotensive effect than that seen in younger patients, probably due to age-related changes in drug disposition.

Pregnancy: Category C.

Lactation: **Verapamil, diltiazem** and **bepridil** are excreted in breast milk. One report suggests that diltiazem concentrations in breast milk may approximate serum levels. Bepridil is estimated to reach about one third the concentration in serum. Significant concentrations of **nicardipine** and **nimodipine** appear in maternal milk of rats. An insignificant amount of **nifedipine** is transferred into breast milk (over 24 hours, < 5% of a dose). It is not known if **isradipine, amlodipine** or **felodipine** are excreted in breast milk.

Children: Safety and efficacy of **diltiazem, bepridil, felodipine, amlodipine** and **isradipine** have not been established.

Controlled studies of **IV verapamil** have not been conducted in pediatric patients, but uncontrolled experience indicates that results of treatment are similar to those in adults. Patients < 6 months of age may not respond to IV verapamil; this resistance may be related to a developmental difference of AV node responsiveness.

Precautions:

Acute hepatic injury: In rare instances, symptoms consistent with acute hepatic injury, as well as significant elevations in enzymes such as alkaline phosphatase, CPK, LDH, AST and ALT have occurred with **diltiazem** and **nifedipine**.

Elevations of transaminases with and without concomitant elevations in alkaline phosphatase and bilirubin have occurred with **verapamil**.

Isolated cases of elevated LDH, alkaline phosphatase and ALT levels have occurred rarely with **nimodipine.**

Clinically significant transaminase elevations have occurred in approximately 1% of patients receiving **bepridil;** however, no patient became clinically symptomatic or jaundiced, and values returned to normal when the drug was stopped.

Edema, mild to moderate, typically associated with arterial vasodilation and not due to left ventricular dysfunction, occurs in 10% of patients receiving **nifedipine**. It occurs primarily in the lower extremities and usually responds to diuretics. In patients with CHF, differentiate this peripheral edema from the effects of decreasing left ventricular function.

Peripheral edema, generally mild and not associated with generalized fluid retention, may occur with **felodipine** within 2 to 3 weeks of therapy initiation. The incidence is both age- and dose-dependent, with frequency ranging from 10% in patients < 50 years of age taking 5 mg/day to 30% in patients > 60 years of age taking 20 mg/day.

Drug Interactions:

Drugs that may affect calcium blockers include barbiturates, calcium salts, dantrolene, erythromycin, histamine H_2 antagonists, hydantoins, quinidine, rifampin, sulfinpyrazone, vitamin D and carbamazepine. Drugs that may be affected by calcium blockers include quinidine, anticoagulants, beta blockers, carbamazepine, cyclosporine, digitais glycosides, encainide, etomidate, fentanyl, lithium, magnesium sulfate (parenteral), nondepolarizing muscle relaxants, prazosin and theophyllines.

Drug/Food interactions: **Nifedipine, amlodipine** and **verapamil** may be administered without regard to meals.

Bioavailability of **felodipine** is not affected by food, but increased > 2–fold when taken with doubly concentrated grapefruit juice vs water or orange juice.

High-fat meals and grapefruit juice with **nisolodipine** should be avoided.

Adverse Reactions:

Generally not serious; rarely requires discontinuation or dosage adjustment.

Adverse Reactions of Calcium Channel Blockers (%)

	Adverse Reactions	Nifedipine[1]	Nisoldipine	Verapamil (IV)	Diltiazem[1]	Nicardipine	Nimodipine	Bepridil	Isradipine	Felodipine	Amlodipine
Central Nervous System	Dizziness/Light-headedness	4.1-27	5	3.5 (1.2)	1.5-7	4-6.9	< 1	11.6-27	7.3	5.8	1.1-3.4[2]
	Drowsiness							≥ 7	≤ 1		
	Nervousness	≤ 7			< 1	0.6		7.4-11.6	≤ 1	≤ 1.5	≤ 1
	Headache	10-23	22	2.2 (1.2)	2.1-12	6.4-8.2	1.4-4.1	7-13.6	13.7	18.6	7.3
	Weakness/Shakiness/Jitteriness	≤12		< 1	1.2	0.6			1.2		
	Asthenia	< 3		1.7	2.8-5	4.2-5.8		6.5-14		4.7	1-2
	Fatigue/Lethargy								3.9		4.5[2]
	Tremor/Hand tremor		≤ 1		< 1			≤ 9.3			≤ 1
Gastrointestinal	Nausea	3.3-11	2	2.7 (0.9)	1.6-1.9	1.9-2.2	0.6-1.4	7-26	1.8	1.9	2.9[2]
	Diarrhea	< 3	≤ 1	< 1	< 1		1.7-4.2	0-10.9	1.1	1.6	≤ 1
	Constipation	≤ 3.3		7.3	1.6	0.6		2.8	≤ 1	1.6	≤ 1
	Dry mouth/Thirst	< 3	≤ 1	< 1	< 1	0.4-1.4		3.4	≤ 1	≤ 1.5	≤ 1
	Flatulence	≤ 3	≤ 1					≤ 2		≤ 1.5	≤ 1
Cardiovascular	Pharyngitis		5								
	Peripheral edema	10-30	22	2.1	2.4-9	7.1-8	0.4-1.2	≤ 2	7.2	22.3	1.8-14.6[2]
	Hypotension	≤ 5		2.5 (1.5)	1	< 0.4	1.2-8.1		≤ 1	≤ 1.5	≤1
	Palpitations	≤7	3	< 1	< 1	3.3-4.1	< 1	≤ 6.5	42[2]	1.8	0.7-4.5[2]
	AV block (1°, 2° or 3°)		≤ 1	0.8-1.2	0.6-7.6	< 0.4				≤ 1.5	
	Bradycardia			1.4 (1.2)	1.5-6		0.6-1	≤ 2			≤ 1
	Congestive heart failure	2-6.7	≤ 1	1.8	< 1		< 1		≤ 1		
	Myocardialinfarction	4-6.7	≤ 1	< 1		< 0.4			≤ 1	≤ 1.5	
	Pulmonary edema	7		1.8							
	Angina	≤ 1	2		< 1	5.6			2.4	≤ 1.5	
	Tachycardia	≤ 1		(1)	< 1	0.8-3.4	1	≤ 2	1.5	≤ 1.5	≤ 1
	Abnormal ECG				4.1	0.6	0.6-1.4				
	Vasodilation		4								
Dermatologic	Dermatitis/Rash	≤ 3	2	1.2	1-1.5	0.4-1.2	0.6-2.4	≤ 2	1.5	1.5	1-2
	Pruritus/Urticaria	≤ 3	≤ 1	< 1 (†)	< 1		< 1		≤ 1	≤ 1.5	1-2

Adverse Reactions of Calcium Channel Blockers (%)											
	Adverse Reactions	Nifedipine[1]	Nisoldipine	Verapamil (IV)	Diltiazem[1]	Nicardipine	Nimodipine	Bepridil	Isradipine	Felodipine	Amlodipine
Other	Flushing	< 3-25	4	< 1	1.7-3	5.6-9.7	1-2.1		2.6	6.4	0.7-4.5[2]
	Nasal or chest congestion/sinusitis/rhinitis	≤ 6	≤ 3	†	<1	†		≤ 2		≤ 1.5	≤ 0.1
	Sexual difficulties	≤ 3		< 1	< 1	†		≤ 2	≤ 1	≤ 1.5	1-2
	Shortness of breath/ dyspnea/wheezing	≤ 8		1.4	< 1	0.6	1.2	≤ 8.7	1.8	≤ 1.5	1-2
	Muscle cramps/pain/ inflammation	≤ 8		< 1			0.2-1.4			≤ 1.9	1-2
	Joint stiffness/pain/ arthritis	≤ 3			< 1	†					≤ 1
	Cough	6						≤ 2	≤ 1	2.9	≤ 0.1
	Anorexia				< 1			≤ 7			≤ 1
	Respiratory infection	≤ 1						3.0		≤ 3.3	

[1] Includes data for sustained release form.
[2] Appears to be dose-related.
† Occurs, no incidence reported.

Administration and Dosage:

NISOLDIPINE: Administer nisoldipine orally once daily. Administration with a high fat meal can lead to excessive peak drug concentration and should be avoided. Avoid grapefruit products before and after dosing. Nisoldipine is an extended release dosage form; swallow whole, do not bite or divide.

Initiate therapy with 20 mg orally once daily, then increase by 10 mg per week, or longer intervals, to attain adequate control of blood pressure. The usual maintenance dosage is 20 to 40 mg once daily. Blood pressure response increases over the 10 to 60 mg daily dose range, but adverse event rates also increase. Doses > 60 mg once daily are not recommended.

Elderly/Hepatic function impairment – Patients over age 65 or patients with impaired liver function are expected to develop higher plasma concentrations of nisoldipine. Monitor blood pressure closely during any dosage adjustment. A starting dose not exceeding 10 mg daily is recommended in these patient groups.

NIFEDIPINE: Individualize dosage. Excessive doses can result in hypotension.

Initial dosage (capsule) – 10 mg 3 times/day. Usual range is 10 to 20 mg 3 times/day. Some patients, especially those with coronary artery spasm, respond only to higher doses, more frequent administration or both. In such patients, 20 to 30 mg 3 or 4 times/day may be effective. Doses > 120 mg/day are rarely necessary. More than 180 mg/day is not recommended.

Titrate throughout 7 to 14 days to assess response to each dose level; monitor blood pressure before proceeding to higher doses.

Sustained release –

Procardia XL: 30 or 60 mg once daily. Do not chew or divide tablet. Titrate over a 7 to 14 day period. Titration may proceed more rapidly if the patient is frequently assessed. Titration to doses > 120 mg is not recommended.

Angina patients maintained on the nifedipine capsule formulation may be switched to the sustained release tablet at the nearest equivalent total daily dose. Experience with doses > 90 mg in angina is limited; therefore, use with caution and only when clinically warranted.

Adalat CC: Adjust dosage according to the patient's needs. Administer once daily on an empty stomach. Swallow tablets whole; do not bite, chew or divide. In general, titrate over a 7 to 14 day period starting with 30 mg once daily. Base upward titration on therapeutic efficacy and safety. Usual maintenance dose is 30 to 60 mg once daily. Titration to doses > 90 mg daily is not recommended.

Concomitant drug therapy with β-blockers may be beneficial in chronic stable angina; however, the effects of concurrent treatment cannot be predicted, especially in patients with compromised left ventricular function or cardiac conduction abnormalities.

NICARDIPINE HCl:

Oral –

Angina (immediate release only): Usual initial dose is 20 mg 3 times/day (range, 20 to 40 mg 3 times/day). Allow at least 3 days before increasing dose to ensure achievement of steady-state plasma drug concentrations.

Hypertension:

Immediate release – Initial dose is 20 mg 3 times daily (range 20 to 40 mg 3 times daily). The maximum bp lowering effect occurs ≈ 1 to 2 hours after dosing. Allow at least 3 days before increasing dose to ensure achievement of steady-state plasma drug concentrations.

Sustained release – Initial dose is 30 mg twice daily. Effective doses have ranged from 30 to 60 mg twice daily. The maximum bp lowering effect at steady-state is sustained from 2 to 6 hours after dosing.

The total daily dose of immediate release nicardipine may not be a useful guide in judging the effective dose of the sustained release form. Titrate patients currently receiving the immediate release form with the sustained release form starting at their current daily dose of immediate release, then re-examine to assess adequacy of bp control.

Renal impairment: Titrate dose beginning with 20 mg 3 times a day (immediate release) or 30 mg twice daily (sustained release).

Hepatic impairment: Starting dose is 20 mg twice a day (immediate release) with individual titration.

Parenteral –

Dosage:

Substitute for oral nicardipine – The IV infusion rate required to produce an average plasma concentration equivalent to a given oral dose at steady-state is shown in the following table:

Equivalent Nicardipine Doses: Oral vs IV Infusion

Oral dose	Equivalent IV infusion rate
20 mg q 8 hr	0.5 mg/hr
30 mg q 8 hr	1.2 mg/hr
40 mg q 8 hr	2.2 mg/hr

Initiation in a drug free patient – The time course of blood pressure decrease is dependent on the initial rate of infusion and the frequency of dosage adjustment. Administer by slow continuous infusion at a concentration of 0.1 mg/ml. With constant infusion, blood pressure begins to fall within minutes. It reaches about 50% of its ultimate decrease in about 45 minutes and does not reach final steady-state for about 50 hours.

When treating acute hypertensive episodes in patients with chronic hypertension, discontinuation of infusion is followed by a 50% offset of action in 30 minutes but plasma levels of drug and gradually decreasing antihypertensive effects exist for ≈ 50 hours.

Titration – For gradual reduction in blood pressure, initiate therapy at 50 mg/hr (5 mg/hr). If desired reduction is not achieved at this dose, the infusion rate may be increased by 25 ml/hr (2.5 mg/hr) every 15 minutes up to a maximum of 150 ml/hr (15 mg/hr) until desired reduction of blood pressure is achieved. For more rapid reduction of blood pressure, initiate at 50 ml/hr. If desired reduction is not achieved at this dose, the infusion rate may be increased by 25 ml/hr every 5 minutes up to a maximum of 150 ml/hr until desired reduction of blood pressure is achieved. Following achievement of the blood pressure goal, decrease the infusion rate to 30 ml/hr.

Maintenance – Adjust the rate of infusion as needed to maintain desired response.

Conditions requiring infusion adjustment –

Hypotension or tachycardia: If there is concern of impending hypotension or tachycardia, discontinue the infusion. When blood pressure has stabilized, infusion may be restarted at low doses (eg, 30 to 50 ml/hr) and adjusted to maintain desired blood pressure.

Infusion site changes: Continue IV use as long as bp control is needed. Change the infusion site every 12 hours if administered via peripheral vein.

Cardiac/Renal/Hepatic function impairment: Use caution when titrating in patients with CHF or renal or hepatic function impairment

Transfer to oral antihypertensives – If treatment includes transfer to an oral antihypertensive other than nicardipine, generally initiate therapy upon discontinuation of the infusion. If oral nicardipine is to be used, administer the first dose of a 3 times daily regimen 1 hour prior to discontinuation of the infusion.

BEPRIDIL HCl: Usual initial dose is 200 mg/day. After 10 days, dosage may be adjusted upward depending on response. Most patients are maintained at 300 mg. Maximum daioly dose is 400 mg; minimum effective dose is 200 mg.

Elderly – Starting dose does not differ from that for younger patients; however, after therapeutic response is demonstrated, the elderly may require more frequent monitoring.

ISRADIPINE: Recommended initial dose is 2.5 mg twice daily. An antihypertensive response usually occurs within 2 to 3 hours; maximual response may require 2 to 4 weeks. If a satisfactory response does not occur after this period, the dose may be adjusted in increments of 5 mg/day at 2 to 4 week intervals up to a maximum of 20 mg/day. However, most patients show no additional response to doses > 10 mg/day, and adverse effects are increased in frequency above 10 mg/day.

NIMODIPINE: Commence therapy within 96 hours of the SAH, using 60 mg every 4 hours for 21 consecutive days.

If the capsule cannot be swallowed (eg, time of surgery, unconscious patient), make a hole in both ends of the capsule with an 18 gauge needle and extract the contents into a syringe. Empty the contents into the patient's in situ nasogastric tube and wash down the tube with 30 mg normal saline.

FELODIPINE: The recommended starting dose is 5 mg once daily. Depending on the patient's response the dosage can be decreased to 2.5 mg or increased to 10 mg once daily. These adjustments should occur generally at intervals of not less than 2 weeks. The recommended dosage range is 2.5 to 10 mg once daily. Because they may develop higher plasma felodipine levels, closely monitor blood pressure in patients > 65 years old and in impaired hepatic function during dosage adjustment; generally, do not consider doses > 10 mg.

Swallow whole; do not crush or chew.

AMLODIPINE: May be taken without regard to meals.

Hypertension – Usual dose is 5 mg once daily. Maximum dose is 10 mg once daily. Small, fragile or elderly patients or patients with hepatic insufficiency may be started on 2.5 mg once daily; this dose may also be used when adding amlodipine to other antihpertensive therapy. In general, titrate over 7 to 14 days; proceed more rapidly if clinically warranted with frequent assessment of the patient.

Angina (chronic stable or vasospastic) – 5 to 10 mg, using the lower dose for elderly and patients with hepatic insufficiency. Most patients require 10 mg.

DILTIAZEM HCl:

Oral –

Tablets: Start with 30 mg 4 times/day before meals and at bedtime; gradually increase dosage to 180 to 360 mg (given in divided doses 3 or 4 times/day) at 1 to 2 day intervals until optimum response is obtained.

Sustained release:

Cardizem SR – Start with 60 to 120 mg twice daily. Adjust dosage when maximum antihypertensive effect is achieved (usually by 14 days chronic therapy). Optimum dosage range is 240 to 360 mg/day, but some patients may respond to lower doses.

Cardizem CD –

Hypertension: 180 to 240 mg once daily; some patients may respond to lower doses. Maximum antihypertensive effect is usually achieved by 14 days chronic therapy; therefore, adjust dosage accordingly. Usual range is 240 to 360 mg once daily; experience with doses > 360 mg is limites.

Angina: Start with 120 or 180 mg once daily. Some patients may respond to higher doses of up to 480 mg once daily. When necessary, titration may be carried out over a 7 to 14 day period.

Dilacor XR –

Hypertension: 180 to 240 mg once daily; adjust dose as needed. Individual patients, particularly those ≥ 60 years of age, may respond to a lower dose of 120 mg. Usual range is 180 to 480 mg once daily. Although current clinical experience with the 540 mg dose is limited, the dose may be increased to 540 mg with little or no increased risk of adverse reactions. Do not exceed 540 mg once daily.

Angina: Adjust dosage to each patient's needs, starting with a dose of 120 mg once daily, which may be titrated to doses of up to 480 mg once daily. when necessary, titration may be carried out over a 7 to 14 day period.

Hypertensive or anginal patients treated with other formulations of diltiazem can safely be switched to *Dilacor XR* at the nearest equivalent total daily dose. Subsequent titration to higher or lower doses may, however, be necessary and should be initiated as clinically indicated.

Administration in the morning on an empty stomach is recommended. Do not open, chew or crush the capsules; swallow whole.

Parenteral –

Direct IV single injections (bolus): The initial dose is 0.25 mg/kg as a bolus administered over 2 minutes (20 mg is a reasonable dose for the average patient). If response is inadequate, a second dose may be administered after 15 minutes. The second bolus dose should be 0.35 mg/kg administered over 2 minutes (25 mg is a reasonable dose for the average patient). Individualize subsequent IV bolus doses. Dose patients with low body weights on a mg/kg basis. Some patients may respond to an initial dose of 0.15 mg/kg, although duration of action may be shorter.

Continuous IV infusion: For continued reduction of the heart rate (up to 24 hours) in patients with atrial fibrillation or atrial flutter, an IV infusion may be administered. Immediately following bolus administration of 20 mg (0.25 mg/kg) or 25 mg (0.35 mg/kg) and reduction of heart rate, begin an IV infusion. The recommended initial infusion rate is 10 mg/hr. Some patients may maintain response to an initial rate of 5 mg/hr. The infusion rate may be increased in 5 mg/hr increments up to 15 mg/hr as needed, if further reduction in heart rate is required. The infusion may be maintained for up to 24 hours. Therefore, infusion duration longer than 24 hours and infusion rates > 15 mg/hr are not recommended.

Concomitant therapy with β-blockers or digitalis is usually well tolerated, but the effects of coadministration cannot be predicted, especially in patients with left ventricular dysfunction or cardiac conduction abnormalities. Use caution in titrating dosages for impaired renal or hepatic function patients, since dosage requirements are not available.

VERAPAMIL HCl: If heart failure is not severe or rate-related, use digitalis and diuretics, as appropriate, before verapamil. In moderately severe to severe cardiac dysfunction (PCWP > 20 mmHg, ejection fraction < 30%), acute worsening of heart failure may occur.

Do not exceed 480 mg/day; safety and efficacy are not established. Half-life increases during chronic use; maximum response may be delayed.

Oral –

Angina at rest and chronic stable angina: Usual initial dose is 80 to 120 mg 3 times/day. However, 40 mg 3 times/day may be warranted if patients may have increased response to verapamil (eg, decreased hepatic function, elderly). Base upward titration of safety and efficacy evaluated ≈ 8 hours after dosing. Increase dosage daily (eg, unstable angina) or weekly until optimum clinical response is obtained.

Arrhythmias: Dosage range in digitalized patients with chronic atrial fibrillation is 240 to 320 mg/day in divided doses 3 or 4 times/day. Dosage range for prophylaxis of PSVT (non-digitalized patients) is 240 to 480 mg/day in divided doses 3 or 4 times/day. In general, maximum effects will be apparent during the first 48 hours of therapy.

Essential hypertension: The usual initial monotherapy dose is 80 mg 3 times/day (240 mg/day). Daily dosages of 360 and 480 mg have been used, but there is no evidence that dosages > 360 mg provide added effect. Consider beginning titration at 40 mg 3 times/day in patients who might respond to lower doses, (eg, elderly or people of small stature). Antihypertensive effects are evident within the first week of therapy. Base upward titration on therapeutic efficacy, assessed at the end of the dosing interval.

Sustained release (essential hypertension): Give with food. Usual daily dose is 240 mg/day in the morning. However, 120 mg/day may be warranted in patients who may have increased response (eg, elderly or people of small stature). Base upward titration on safety and efficacy evaluated ≈ 24 hours after dosing. If adequate response is not obtained, titrate upward to 240 mg/morning and 120 mg/evening, then 240 mg every 12 hours, if needed. When switching from immediate release tablets, total daily dose (in mg) may remain the same. Antihypertensive effects are evident within the first week.

Parenteral (supraventricular tachyarrhythmias): For IV use only. Give as slow IV injection over at least 2 minutes under continuous ECG and blood pressure monitoring. An IV infusion has been used (5 mg/hour); precede the infusion with an IV loading dose.

Initial dose – 5 to 10 mg (0.075 to 0.15 mg/kg) as an IV bolus over 2 minutes.

Repeat dose – 10 mg (0.15 mg/kg) 30 minutes after the first dose if the initial response is not adequate.

Older patients – Give over at least 3 min to minimize risk of untoward drug effects.

Children –

≤ 1 year: 0.1 to 0.2 mg/kg (usual single dose range, 0.75 to 2 mg) as an IV bolus over 2 minutes (under continuous ECG monitoring).

1 to 15 years: 0.1 to 0.3 mg/kg (usual single dose range, 2 to 5 mg) IV over 2 minutes. Do not exceed 5 mg.

Repeat dose: Repeat above dose 30 minutes after the first dose if the initial response is not adequate (under continuous ECG monitoring). Do not exceed a single dose of 10 mg in patients 1 to 15 years of age.

VASOPRESSORS USED IN SHOCK

Vasopressors: Sympathomimetic agents are used in shock to treat hypoperfusion in normovolemic patients and in patients unresponsive to whole blood or plasma volume expanders. These agents increase myocardial contractility, constrict capacitance vessels and dilate resistance vessels. In cardiogenic shock or advanced shock from other causes associated with a low cardiac output, they may be combined with vasodilators (eg, nitroprusside or nitroglycerin) to maintain blood pressure while the vasodilator improves myocardial performance. Nitroprusside is used to reduce preload and afterload and improve cardiac output. Nitroglycerin directly relaxes the venous vasculature and decreases preload.

Pharmacology: Sympathomimetic agents produce α-adrenergic stimulation (vasoconstriction), β_1-adrenergic stimulation (increase myocardial contractility, heart rate, automaticity and AV conduction), and β_2-adrenergic activity (peripheral vasodilation). Dopamine also causes vasodilation of the renal and mesenteric, cerebral and coronary beds by dopaminergic receptor activation. The relative activity and predominance of these actions result in a number of hemodynamic responses which may affect coronary perfusion, renal perfusion, cardiac output, total peripheral resistance and blood pressure. These actions are summarized in the Sites of Action/Hemodynamic Response table. The actual response of an individual patient will depend largely on clinical status at time of administration.

Monitoring shock patients and their response to drugs requires special vigilance. Monitor heart rate, blood pressure and ECG continuously. Record urine output and fluid intake frequently. Due to rapid and life-threatening changes that can occur in the hemodynamically unstable patient, optimal drug selection, dose titration and management is probably best achieved with the use of invasive hemodynamic monitoring.

Administration should only be via the IV route using a large-bore, free flowing IV in the antecubital vein or a central vein due to unpredictable absorption. Small IVs in the extremities are both unreliable and unsafe for vasopressor administration. Frequent monitoring of the IV sites for extravasation injury is essential when vasopressor agents are being used.

Prolonged, high-dose therapy can produce cyanosis and tissue necrosis of distal extremities. The principle of using the lowest dose which produces an adequate response for the shortest period of time is very important when using these agents.

Plasma volume depletion: Prolonged use of vasopressors may result in plasma volume depletion; this should be corrected by appropriate fluid and electrolyte replacement therapy. If plasma volumes are not corrected, hypotension may recur when these drugs are discontinued.

Acidosis lessens the response to vasopressors; therefore, correct acidosis if it exists or develops during the course of vasopressor therapy.

Avoid continuous IV therapy: Acute tolerance develops during continuous IV administration. High concentration/low volume (250 ml) vasopressor solutions administered with the aid of an infusion control device allows for maximum dosing flexibility since fluids and drugs can be regulated independently, and the development of tolerance is minimized.

Effects of Vasopressors Used in Shock

+++ *pronounced effect*
++ *moderate effect*
+ *slight effect*
0 *no effect*
↑ *increase*
↓ *decrease*

		Sites of action				Hemodynamic response			
		Heart		Blood vessels					
		Contractility (Inotropic)	SA Node Rate (Chronotropic)	Vasoconstriction	Vasodilatation	Renal Perfusion	Cardiac Output	Total Peripheral Risistance	Blood Pressure
		β_1	β_1	α	β_2				
Inotropic	Isoproterenol	+++	+++	0	+++	↑[1] or ↓[2]	↑	↓	↑[3]↓[4]
	Dobutamine	+++	0 to +[5]	0 to +[5]	+	0	↑	↓	↑
	Dopamine	+++	+ to ++[5]	+ to +++[5]	0 to +[6]	↑[5]	↑	↓[5] or ↑	0 to ↑
Mixed	Epinephrine	+++	+++	+++[5]	++[5]	↓	↑	↓	↑[3]↓[4]
	Norepinephrine	++	++[7]	+++	0	↓	0 or ↓	↑	↑
	Ephedrine	++	++	+	0 to +	↓	↑	↑ or ↓	↑
	Mephentermine	+	+	+	++	↑ or ↓	↑	0 to ↑	↑
Pressors	Metaraminol	+	+	++	0	↓	↓	↑	↑
	Methoxamine	0	0[7]	+++	0	↓	0 or ↓	↑	↑
	Phenylephrine	0	0[7]	+++	0	↓	↓	↑	↑

[1] Cardiogenic or septicemic shock.
[2] Normotensive patient.
[3] Systolic effect.
[4] Diastolic effect.
[5] Effects are dose dependent.
[6] Dilates renal and splanchnic beds via dopaminergic effect at doses < 10 mcg/kg/min.
[7] Decreased heart rate may result from reflex mechanisms.

Common Dilutions and Infusion Rates for Selected Drugs Used in Shock

Drug	Usual Dilution for IV Infusion	Infusion Rate
Isoproterenol	2 mg (10 ml) in 500 ml D5W (4 mcg/ml) or 1 mg (5 ml) in 250 ml D5W	5 mcg/min
Dobutamine	250 mg in 250 to 500 ml NS or D5W (500 to 1000 mcg/ml)	2.5 to 15 mcg/kg/min
Dopamine	200 to 800 mg in 250 to 500 ml NS or D5W (400 to 3200 mcg/ml)	Low dose – 2.5 to 10 mcg/kg/min High dose – 20 to 50 mcg/kg/min
Norepinephrine	4 mg in 250 ml of D5W (16 mcg/ml)	Initial: 8 to 12 mcg/min Maintenance: 2 to 4 mcg/min

ISOPROTERENOL HCl

Injection: 1:50,000 solution (0.2 mg per ml) (*Rx*) — Various, *Isuprel* (Winthrop Pharm.)

Actions:

Pharmacology: Isoproterenol has beta_1 and beta_2 adrenergic receptor activity. Primary actions are on the beta receptors of the heart and smooth muscle of the bronchi, skeletal muscle and vasculature and alimentary tract. Isoproterenol relaxes most smooth muscles, with the most pronounced effect on the bronchial and GI smooth muscle. It produces marked relaxation in the smaller bronchi.

Hemodynamics – The positive inotropic and chronotropic actions of the drug increase minute blood flow. There is an increase in heart rate, an approximately unchanged stroke volume, and an increase in ejection velocity. The rate of discharge of cardiac pacemakers is increased with isoproterenol hydrochloride injection.

Venous return to the heart is increased through a decreased compliance of the venous bed. Systemic resistance and pulmonary vascular resistance are decreased, and there is an increase in coronary and renal blood flow. Systolic blood pressure may increase and diastolic blood pressure may decrease.

Pharmacokinetics: Isoproterenol is not reliably absorbed following sublingual (SL) or oral administration. Onset of activity is ≈ 30 minutes after SL administration and immediate after IV administration; duration is < 1 to 2 hours. Oral forms are quickly inactivated in the GI tract, and rapidly and extensively metabolized in the liver; 50% of an IV dose is excreted unchanged in the urine.

Indications:

Parenteral: As an adjunct to fluid and electrolyte replacement therapy and the use of other drugs and procedures in the treatment of hypovolemic and septic shock, low cardiac output (hypoperfusion) states, congestive heart failure and cardiogenic shock.

Sublingual or rectal: Adams-Stokes syndrome and atrioventricular heart block.

Contraindications:

Tachyarrhythmias; tachycardia or heart block caused by digitalis intoxication; ventricular arrhythmias which require inotropic therapy; angina pectoris.

Warnings:

Pregnancy: Category C.

Lactation: It is not known whether isoproterenol is excreted in breast milk. Exercise caution when administering to a nursing woman.

Precautions:

Hypovolemia: Use is not a substitute for the replacement of blood, plasma, fluids and electrolytes, which should be restored promptly when loss has occurred. Hypovolemia should be corrected by suitable volume expanders before treatment.

Cardiovascular disorders: Use with caution in patients with coronary artery disease, coronary insufficiency, diabetes or hyperthyroidism and in patients sensitive to sympathomimetic amines.

Cardiac effects: If heart rate exceeds 110 bpm, it may be advisable to decrease the infusion rate or temporarily discontinue the infusion. Determinations of cardiac output and circulation time may also be helpful. Ensure adequate ventilation. Pay careful attention to acid-base balance and to correction of electrolyte disturbances. In cases of shock associated with bacteremia, suitable antimicrobial therapy is imperative. Doses sufficient to increase heart rate to > 130 bpm may induce ventricular arrhythmia. Such increases in heart rate will also tend to increase cardiac work and oxygen requirements which may adversely affect the failing heart or the heart with a significant degree of arteriosclerosis. If precordial distress or anginal-type pain occurs, discontinue the drug immediately.

Isoproterenol injection may have a deleterious effect on the injured or failing heart. Its use as the initial agent in treating cardiogenic shock following myocardial infarction is discouraged. When a low arterial pressure has been elevated by other means, isoporterenol hydrochloride injection may produce beneficial hemodynamic and metabolic effects.

In a few patients, isoproterenol has paradoxically worsened heart block or precipitated Adams-Stokes attacks during normal sinus rhythm or transient heart block.

Sulfite sensitivity: Some of these products contain sulfites which may cause allergic-type reactions including anaphylactic symptoms and life-threatening or less severe asthmatic episodes in certain susceptible persons.

Drug Interactions:

Drugs that may affect isoproterenol include bretylium, guanethidine, halogenated hydrocarbon anesthetics, oxytocic drugs and tricyclic antidepressants.

Adverse Reactions:

Significant adverse reactions include tachycardia; palpitations; hypertension; hypotension; ventricular arrhythmias; tachyarrhythmias; precordial distress; angina; mild tremors; nervousness; headache; dizziness; nausea; vomiting.

Administration and Dosage:

Parenteral: Isoproterenol injection 1:50,000 should generally be started at the lowest recommended dose and the rate of administration gradually increased if necessary while carefully monitoring the patient.

The usual route of administration is by IV injection or infusion. In dire emergencies, administer the drug by intracardiac injection. If time is not of utmost importance, initial therapy by IM or SC injection may be used. See Dosage for Adults with Heart Block, Adams-Stokes Attacks and Cardiac Arrest table below.

There are no well controlled studies in children to establish appropriate dosing; however, the American Heart Association recommends an initial infusion rate of 0.1 mcg/kg/min, with the usual range being 0.1 mcg/kg/min to 1 mcg/kg/min.

Dosage for Adults with Heart Block, Adams-Stokes Attacks and Cardiac Arrest

Route	Dilution	Initial Dose	Subsequent Dose Range
IV injection	Dilute 1 ml of 1:5000 solution (0.2mg) to 10 ml with NaCl or 5%Dextrose Injection	0.02 to 0.06 mg (1 to 3 ml of diluted solution)	0.01 to 0.2 mg (0.5 to 10 ml of diluted solution)
IV infusion	Dilute 10 ml of 1:5000 solution (2 mg) in 500 ml of D5W or dilute 5 ml of 1:5000 solution (1 mg) in 250 ml of D5W	5 mcg/min (1.25ml/min of diluted solution)	
IM	Undiluted 1:5000 solution	0.2 mg (1 ml)	0.02 to 1 mg (0.1 to 5 ml)
SC	Undiluted 1:5000 solution	0.2 mg (1 ml)	0.15 to 0.2 mg (0.75 to 1 ml)
Intracardiac	Undiluted 1:5000 solution	0.02 mg (0.1 ml)	

Sublingual or rectal: The usual route of administration of isoproterenol in emergency treatment of patients with severe heart block is IV injection or infusion. If time is not of utmost importance, initial therapy by IM or SC injection may be used. If further maintenance therapy is necessary, glossets may be administered sublingually. Always monitor the ECG.

The glossets form of isoproterenol is usually administered sublingually.

Heart block and certain ventricular arrhythmias – Sublingual or rectal administration is effective in the control of mild stabilized symptomatic heart block and ventricular arrhythmias. However, in acute symptomatic heart block, particularly in patients with postcardiac surgery block, electrical pacing is the preferred method of treatment for maintenance of an adequate ventricular rate. Moreover, in ventricular arrhythmias, electroshock may have to be used, and is usually the treatment of choice.

If given in acute symptomatic heart block, IV administration, with constant monitoring, is preferred. This avoids the irregular absorption which is possible with the sublingual and rectal routes of administration. Rectal administration is more satisfactory for long-term therapy because the effect is produced within 30 minutes and lasts for 2 to 4 hours. Sinus rhythm sometimes occurs and persists for a variable period, but often relapses again into complete block. In other cases, isoproterenol merely maintains an acceptable heart rate somewhere above 90 to 100 bpm. The table below summarizes the dosage regimen suggested for adults.

Suggested Isoproternol Dosage For Heart Block in Adults

Route of Administration	Initial Dose	Subsequent Dose Range
Sublingual	10 mg	5 to 50 mg
Rectal	5 mg	5 to 15 mg

DOBUTAMINE

Injection: 12.5 mg/ml (*Rx*)	Various, *Dobutrex* (Lilly)

Actions:

Pharmacology: Dobutamine's primary activity results from stimulation of the $beta_1$ receptors of the heart while producing comparatively mild chronotropic, hypertensive, arrhythmogenic and vasodilative effects. It has minor alpha and $beta_2$ effects.

Hemodynamics – In patients with depressed cardiac function, dobutamine increases the cardiac output. This increase is usually not accompanied by marked increases in heart rate and the cardiac stroke volume is usually increased. Dobutamine produces less increase in heart rate and less decrease in peripheral vascular resistance for a given inotropic effect than does isoproterenol.

Facilitation of atrioventricular conduction has been observed in human electrophysiologic studies and in patients with atrial fibrillation.

Systemic vascular resistance is usually decreased; occasionally, minimal vasoconstriction has been observed.

Pharmacokinetics:

Metabolism/Excretion – Routes of metabolism are methylation of the catechol and conjugation. The plasma half-life of dobutamine is 2 minutes. In urine, the major excretion products are the conjugates of dobutamine and the inactive 3–O–methyl dobutamine.

Children: Dobutamine's elimination half-life is 2 minutes in full-term neonates and older children, and may be as long as 4 to 5 minutes in preterm infants.

Onset: The onset of action is within 1 to 2 minutes; however, as much as 10 minutes may be required to obtain the peak effect of a particular infusion rate. The therapeutic plasma level is 40 to 190 ng/ml.

Indications:

Inotropic support in the short-term treatment of adults with cardiac decompensation due to depressed contractility, resulting either from organic heart disease or from cardiac surgical procedures.

In patients who have atrial fibrillation with rapid ventricular response, use a digitalis preparation prior to instituting therapy with dobutamine.

Unlabeled uses: Doses of dobutamine 2 and 7.75 mcg/kg/min infused for 10 minutes each have been used investigationally in 12 children with congenital heart disease undergoing diagnostic cardiac catheterization. The drug appears effective in augmenting cardiovascular function in children, and no adverse effects were noted.

Contraindications:

Idiopathic hypertrophic subaortic stenosis (IHSS). Patients hypersensitive to dobutamine.

Warnings:

Increase in heart rate or blood pressure: Dobutamine may cause a marked increase in heart rate or blood pressure, especially systolic pressure. Usually, reduction of dosage promptly reverses these effects. Patients with atrial fibrillation are at risk of developing rapid ventricular response. Patients with preexisting hypertension appear to face an increased risk of developing an exaggerated pressor response.

Hypotension: Precipitous decreases in blood pressure have occasionally been described in association with dobutamine therapy. Decreasing the dose or discontinuing the infusion typically results in rapid return of blood pressure to baseline values.

Ectopic activity: Dobutamine may precipitate or exacerbate ventricular ectopic activity, but it rarely has caused ventricular tachycardia.

Hypersensitivity reactions, may occur occasionally with dobutamine.

Pregnancy: Category B.

Children: Safety and efficacy for use in children have not been established.

Precautions:

Monitoring: Continuously monitor ECG and blood pressure. Monitor pulmonary wedge pressure and cardiac output whenever possible.

Hypovolemia: Use is not a substitute for the replacement of blood, plasma, fluids and electrolytes, which should be restored promptly when loss has occurred.

Usage following acute myocardial infarction – Clinical experience following myocardial infarction has been insufficient to establish the safety of the drug for this use.

Sulfite sensitivity: This product contains sulfites which may cause allergic-type reactions including anaphylactic symptoms and life-threatening or less severe asthmatic episodes in certain susceptible persons. Sulfite sensitivity is seen more frequently in asthmatic or atopic nonasthmatic persons.

Drug Interactions:

Drugs that may affect dobutamine include bretylium, guanethidine, halogenated hydrocarbon anesthetics, oxytocic drugs and tricyclic antidepressants.

Adverse Reactions:

Adverse reactions may include increased heart rate, blood pressure and ventricular ectopic activity; increased premature ventricular beats during infusions and reactions at injection site.

Administration and Dosage:

Rate of administration: The rate of infusion needed to increase cardiac output usually ranges from 2.5 to 10mcg/kg/min. Rarely, infusion rates up to 40 mcg/kg/min have been required. A metering device is recommended for controlling rate of administration.

Adjust the rate of administration and the duration of therapy according to patient response, as determined by heart rate, presence of ectopic activity, blood pressure, urine flow, and, whenever possible, measurement of central venous or pulmonary wedge pressure and cardiac output.

Concentrations up to 5000 mcg/ml have been administered (250 mg/50 ml). Determine the final volume administered by the fluid requirements of the patient.

Infusion Rates of Various Dilutions of Dobutamine

Desired Delivery Rate (mcg/kg/min)	Infusion Rate (ml/kg/min)		
	250 mcg/ml[1]	500 mcg/ml[2]	1000 mcg/ml[3]
2.5	0.01	0.005	0.0025
5	0.02	0.01	0.005
7.5	0.03	0.015	0.0075
10	0.04	0.02	0.01
12.5	0.05	0.025	0.0125
15	0.06	0.03	0.015

[1] 250 mg per liter of diluent.
[2] 500 mg per liter or 250 mg per 500 ml of diluent.
[3] 1000 mg per liter or 250 mg per 250 ml of diluent.

Admixture incompatibility: Incompatible with alkaline solutions; do not mix with products such as 5% Sodium Bicarbonate Injection. Do not use in conjunction with other agents or diluents containing both sodium bisulfite and ethanol. Dobutamine is also physically incompatible with hydrocortisone sodium succinate; cefazolin; cefamandole; neutral cephalothin; penicillin; sodium ethacrynate; sodium heparin.

Admixture compatibility: Dobutamine is compatible when administered through common tubing with dopamine, lidocaine, tobramycin, verapamil, nitroprusside, potassium chloride and protamine sulfate.

DOPAMINE HCl

Injection: 80 mg/100 ml (0.8 mg/ml), 160 mg/100 ml (1.6 mg/ml) (*Rx*), 320 mg/100 ml (3.2 mg/ml) (*Rx*)	Various
Injection: 40 mg/ml, 80 mg/ml, 160 mg/ml (*Rx*)	Various, *Intropin* (DuPont Critical Care)

Actions:

Pharmacology: Dopamine is an endogenous catecholamine and a precursor of norepinephrine. It acts both directly and indirectly (releases norepinephrine stores) on alpha and $beta_1$ receptors. $Beta_1$ actions produce an inotropic effect on the myocardium resulting in increased cardiac output. Systolic and pulse pressure usually increases. Blood flow to peripheral vascular beds may decrease while mesenteric flow increases. Dopamine dilates the renal and mesenteric vasculature presumptively by activation of a dopaminergic receptor. This action is accompanied by increases in GFR, renal blood flow and sodium excretion. An increase in urinary output produced by dopamine is usually not associated with a decrease in osmolality of the urine. The dopaminergic effect is overridden by alpha-adrenergic activity at higher doses.

Organ perfusion – Urine flow appears to be one of the better monitoring parameters of vital organ perfusion. Also, observe the patient for signs of reversal of confusion or comatose condition. Loss of pallor, increase in toe temperature or adequacy of nail bed capillary filling may also be used as indices of adequate dosage.

Renal function – When administered before urine flow has decreased to levels ≈ 0.3 ml/min, prognosis is more favorable. In oliguric or anuric patients, administration has resulted in an increase in urine flow to normal levels. Dopamine may also increase urine flow in patients whose output is within normal limits, thus reducing preexisting fluid accumulation. Above those optimal doses, urine flow may decrease, necessitating dosage reduction.

Cardiac output – Increased cardiac output is related to dopamine's direct inotropic effect on the myocardium, and at low or moderate doses appears to be related to a favorable prognosis.

Blood pressure – Manage hypotension due to inadequate cardiac output with low to moderate doses. At high doses, alpha-adrenergic activity is more prominent and may correct hypotension due to diminished SVR. As in other circulatory decompensation states, prognosis is better in patients whose blood pressure and urine flow have not undergone extreme deterioration. Administer dopamine as soon as a definite trend toward decreased systolic and diastolic pressure becomes apparent.

Pharmacokinetics:

Absorption/Distribution – Dopamine has an onset of action within 5 minutes, a plasma half-life of about 2 minutes and a duration of action of less than 10 minutes. The drug is widely distributed in the body but does not cross the blood-brain barrier.

Metabolism/Excretion – Dopamine is metabolized in the liver, kidney and plasma by MAO and catechol-O-methyltransferase to inactive compounds. About 25% of the dose is taken up into specialized neurosecretory vesicles (the adrenergic nerve terminals), where it is hydroxylated to form norepinephrine. About 80% of the drug is excreted in the urine within 24 hours, primarily as HVA and its sulfate and glucuronide conjugates and as 3,4-dihydroxy-phenylacetic acid.

Indications:

Correction of hemodynamic imbalances present in the shock syndrome due to myocardial infarction, trauma, endotoxic septicemia, open heart surgery, renal failure, and chronic cardiac decompensation as in refractory congestive failure.

Patients most likely to respond adequately are those in whom physiological parameters such as urine flow, myocardial function and blood pressure have not profoundly deteriorated. The shorter the time between onset of signs and symptoms of shock and initiation of therapy with volume correction and dopamine, the better the prognosis.

Unlabeled uses: Chronic obstructive pulmonary disease (COPD); CHF; respiratory distress syndrome in infants; improve kidney function in polyuria.

Contraindications:

Pheochromocytoma; uncorrected tachyarrhythmias or ventricular fibrillation.

Warnings:

Cardiac: Do not administer in the presence of uncorrected tachyarrhythmias or ventricular fibrillation.

Pregnancy: Category C.

Lactation: It is not known whether this drug is excreted in breast milk. Exercise caution when administering to a nursing woman.

Children: Safety and efficacy for use in children have not been established. It has been used in a limited number of pediatric patients, but such use has been inadequate to fully define proper dosage and use.

Precautions:

Monitoring: Close monitoring of urine flow, cardiac output, pulmonary wedge pressure and blood pressure during infusion is necessary.

Hypovolemia: Prior to treatment, correct hypovolemia with either whole blood or plasma as indicated. Monitoring of central venous pressure or left ventricular filling pressure may be helpful in detecting and treating hypovolemia.

Decreased pulse pressure: If a disproportionate rise in the diastolic pressure (a marked decrease in pulse pressure) is observed in patients receiving dopamine, decrease infusion rate and observe patient carefully for further evidence of predominant vasoconstriction.

Occlusive vascular disease: Closely monitor patients with a history of occlusive vascular disease for any changes in color or temperature of the skin of the extremities. If a change occurs and is thought to be the result of compromised circulation to the extremities, weigh the benefits of continued dopamine infusion against the risk of possible necrosis. This condition may be reversed by either decreasing the rate of infusion or discontinuing the drug.

Extravasation: Infuse into a large vein to prevent extravasation. Extravasation may cause necrosis and sloughing of surrounding tissue. Large veins of the antecubital fossa are preferred to veins in the hand or ankle. Monitor infusion site closely for free flow.

Antidote for extravasation – To prevent sloughing and necrosis in ischemic areas, infiltrate area as soon as possible with 10 to 15 ml 0.9% Sodium Chloride solution containing 5 to 10 mg phentolamine. Use a syringe with a fine hypodermic needle and infiltrate liberally throughout the ischemic area. Sympathetic blockade with phentolamine causes immediate and conspicuous local hyperemic changes if the area is infiltrated within 12 hours.

Discontinuing: When discontinuing the infusion, gradually decrease the dose, since sudden cessation may result in marked hypotension.

Sulfite sensitivity: Some of these products contain sulfites that may cause allergic-type reactions including anaphylactic symptoms and life-threatening or less severe asthmatic episodes in certain susceptible persons. Sulfite sensitivity is seen more frequently in asthmatic or atopic nonasthmatic persons.

Drug Interactions:

Drugs that may affect dopamine include halogenated hydrocarbon anesthetics, monoamine oxidase (MAO) inhibitors, furazolidone, oxytocic drugs and phenytoin. Drugs that may be affected by dopamine include guanethidine, oxytocic drugs and tricyclic antidepressants.

Adverse Reactions:

Adverse reactions may include ectopic beats; nausea and vomiting; tachycardia; anginal pain; palpitation; dyspnea; headache; hypotension and vasoconstriction.

Administration and Dosage:

This is a potent drug; dilute before use if not prediluted.

Rate of administration: After dilution, administer IV. A metering device is essential for controlling the rate of flow. Titrate each patient to the desired hemodynamic or renal response with dopamine. In titrating to the desired increase in systolic blood pressure, the optimum dosage rate for renal response may be exceeded, thus necessitating a reduction in rate after the hemodynamic condition is stabilized.

Administration at rates greater than 50 mcg/kg/min have been used safely in advanced circulatory decompensation states.

Suggested regimen: When appropriate, increase blood volume with whole blood or plasma until central venous pressure is 10 to 15 cm water, or pulmonary wedge pressure is 14 to 18 mm Hg.

Begin administration of diluted solution at doses of 2 to 5 mcg/kg/min in patients likely to respond to modest increments of cardiac contractility and renal perfusion.

In more seriously ill patients, begin administration of diluted solution at doses of 5 mcg/kg/min and increase gradually using 5 to 10 mcg/kg/min increments, up to a rate of 20 to 50 mcg/kg/min, as needed. If doses in excess of 50 mcg/kg/min are required, check urine output frequently. If urine flow decreases in the absence of hypotension, consider reduction of dosage. More than 50% of patients are satisfactorily maintained on doses less than 20 mcg/kg/min. In patients who do not respond to these doses, additional increments may be employed.

Treatment of all patients requires constant evaluation of therapy in terms of the blood volume, augmentation of cardiac contractility, and distribution of peripheral perfusion. Pay particular attention to diminution of established urine flow rate, increasing tachycardia or development of new dysrhythmias.

Take care to avoid inadvertent administration of a bolus of drug.

Admixture incompatibilities: DO NOT add to 5% Sodium Bicarbonate or other alkaline IV solutions, oxidizing agents or iron salts since the drug is inactivated in alkaline solution (solutions become pink to violet).

EPINEPHRINE

Suspension for Injection: 1:200 (5 mg/ml)	*Sus-Phrine* (Forest)
Solution: 1:1000 (1 mg/ml as the HCl) (*Rx*)	Various, *Adrenalin Chloride* (Parke-Davis)
Solution: 1:2000 (0.5 mg/ml as HCl)	*Epipen Jr.* (Center Labs)
Solution: 1:10,000 (0.1 mg/ml) (*Rx*)	Various
Solution: 1:10,000 (0.1 mg/ml as the HCl) (*Rx*)	Various
Solution: 1:100,000 (0.01 mg/ml) (*Rx*)	Various

Actions:

Pharmacology: The actions of epinephrine resemble the effects of stimulation of adrenergic nerves. It acts on alpha and beta receptor sites of sympathetic effector cells. Its most prominent actions are on the beta receptors of the heart and of vascular and other smooth muscle. At high doses, alpha adrenergic effects predominate. When given by rapid IV injection, epinephrine produces a rapid rise in blood pressure (mainly systolic); produces direct stimulation of cardiac muscle, which increases the strength of ventricular contraction; increases the heart rate; and constricts the arterioles in the skin, mucosa and splanchnic areas of circulation. When given by slow IV injection, epinephrine usually produces a moderate rise in systolic and a fall in diastolic pressure. Epinephrine relaxes the smooth muscle of the bronchi and iris and is a physiologic antagonist of histamine. The drug also increases blood sugar and liver glycogenolysis.

Total peripheral resistance at usually employed doses decreases by action of epinephrine on beta receptors of the skeletal muscle vasculature, and blood flow is thereby enhanced. Usually, this effect predominates so that the modest rise in systolic pressure which follows slow injection or absorption is the result of direct cardiac stimulation and increase in cardiac output.

Pharmacokinetics: Epinephrine crosses the placenta but not the blood-brain barrier. Intravenous injection produces an immediate and intensified response. The drug becomes fixed in the tissues and is rapidly inactivated chiefly by enzymatic transformation to metanephrine or normetanephrine, either of which is subsequently conjugated and excreted in the urine in the form of sulfates and glucuronides. Either sequence results in the formation of 3-methoxy-4-hydroxy-mandelic acid (vanillyl-mandelic acid; VMA) which is also detectable in the urine. Epinephrine is rapidly and systematically degraded in the liver and other tissues by the enzymes monoamine oxidase and catechol-O-methyltransferase. Virtually all of an injected dose can be accounted for by urinary excretion of inactive metabolites.

Indications:

IV: In acute attacks of ventricular standstill, apply physical measures first. When external cardiac compression and attempts to restore the circulation by electrical defibrillation or use of a pacemaker fail, intracardiac puncture and intramyocardial injection of epinephrine may be effective. However, this method of administration should only be employed as a last resort and by personnel skilled in intracardiac injection technique.

Treatment and prophylaxis of cardiac arrest and attacks of transitory atrioventricular (AV) heart block with syncopal seizures (Stokes-Adams syndrome).

Epinephrine is also used as a hemostatic agent, and to treat mucosal congestion of hay fever, rhinitis and acute sinusitis; to relieve bronchial asthmatic paroxysms; in syncope due to complete heart block or carotid sinus hypersensitivity; for symptomatic relief of serum sickness, urticaria and angioneurotic edema; for resuscitation in cardiac arrest following anesthetic accidents; in simple (open angle) glaucoma; for relaxation of uterine musculature and to inhibit uterine contractions; to prolong the action of intraspinal and local anesthetics; acute hypersensitivity (anaphylactoid reactions to drugs, animal serums, insect stings and other allergens); treatment of acute asthmatic attacks to relieve bronchospasm not controlled by inhalation or SC administration of other solutions of the drug.

Contraindications:

Hypersensitivity to the drug or any component. Narrow-angle (congestive) glaucoma; shock (nonanaphylactic); during general anesthesia with halogenated hydrocarbons or cyclopropane; individuals with cerebral arteriosclerosis or organic brain damage; with local anesthesia of certain areas (eg, fingers, toes) because of the danger of vasoconstriction producing sloughing of tissue; in labor because it may delay the second stage; in cardiac dilatation and coronary insufficiency; to counteract circulatory collapse or hypotension due to phenothiazines, since such agents may reverse the pressor effect of epinephrine, leading to a further lowering of blood pressure.

Warnings:

Nephrotoxicity: Initially, epinephrine administered parenterally may produce constriction of renal blood vessels and decrease urine formation.

Use with caution in the following: Elderly patients; cardiovascular disease; hypertension; diabetes; hyperthyroidism; psychoneurotic individuals; bronchial asthma and emphysema with degenerative heart disease; thyrotoxicosis.

Cardiovascular effects: Inadvertently induced high arterial blood pressure may result in angina pectoris (especially when coronary insufficiency is present), or aortic rupture. Epinephrine may induce potentially serious cardiac arrhythmias in patients not suffering from heart disease. In patients with organic heart disease or who are receiving drugs that sensitize the myocardium, arrhythmias, including fatal ventricular fibrillation may occur. Epinephrine causes changes in the ECG.

Epinephrine restores electrical activity in asystole and enhances defibrillation. Use with caution in patients with ventricular fibrillation. In patients with prefibrillatory rhythm, IV epinephrine must be used with extreme caution. Epinephrine may convert asystole to ventricular fibrillation if used in the treatment of anesthetic cardiac accidents.

Injection: Epinephrine solution, alone or in combination with other drugs, must be injected in areas of limited or compromised blood supply only after carefully weighing the potential advantages and risks, including the possibility of vasoconstriction-induced sloughing of tissue.

Cerebrovascular hemorrhage may occur from overdosage or inadvertent IV injection of epinephrine resulting from the sharp rise in blood pressure.

Pulmonary edema may result in fatalities because of the peripheral constriction and cardiac stimulation produced.

Pregnancy: Category C.

Labor and delivery – Parenteral administration, if used to support blood pressure during low or other spinal anesthesia for delivery, can cause acceleration of fetal heart rate and should not be used in obstetrics when maternal blood pressure exceeds 130/80 mm Hg. If administered during labor, epinephrine may delay the second stage. If administered in a dosage sufficiently high to reduce uterine contractions, it may cause prolonged uterine atony with hemorrhage. In obstetrics, if vasopressor drugs are used either to correct hypotension or added to the local anesthetic solution, some oxytocic drugs may cause severe persistent hypertension.

Lactation: Epinephrine is excreted in breast milk. Decide whether to discontinue nursing or to discontinue the drug.

Children: Administer with caution to infants and children. Syncope has occurred following the administration to asthmatic children.

Precautions:

Diabetic patients receiving epinephrine may require an increase in dosage of insulin or oral hypoglycemic agents.

Tolerance may occur with prolonged use.

Psychiatric effects: Epinephrine may induce or aggravate psychomotor agitation, disorientation, impairment of memory, assaultive behavior, panic, hallucinations, suicidal or homicidal tendencies, and schizophrenic-type thought disorder or paranoid delusions.

Hypovolemia: Blood, plasma, fluids and electrolytes should be restored promptly when loss has occurred.

Sulfite sensitivity: Sulfites may cause allergic-type reactions in certain susceptible persons. Sulfite sensitivity is seen more frequently in asthmatics or in atopic nonasthmatic persons.

Drug Interactions:

Drugs that may affect epinephrine include beta-adrenergic blockers, nonspecific; bretylium; guanethidine; halogenated hydrocarbon anesthetics, TCAs and oxytocic drugs.

Drug/Lab test interactions: After overdosage or prolonged use, elevated serum lactic acid levels with severe metabolic acidosis may occur.

Adverse Reactions:

Adverse reactions may include cerebral hemorrhage; hemiplegia; subarachnoid hemorrhage; anginal pain; restlessness; tremor; weakness; dizziness; pallor; respiratory difficulty; anxiety; headache; fear; palpitations; sweating; nausea; vomiting; "epinephrine-fastness" with prolonged use; syncope in children; urticaria, wheal; necrosis and hemorrhage at injection site; transient elevations of blood glucose.

Administration and Dosage:

Administer by IV injection or in cardiac arrest by an endotracheal tube or intracardiac injection into the left ventricular chamber.

SC is the preferred route of administration. If given IM, avoid injection into the buttocks.

SC or IM: 0.2 to 1 ml. Start with a small dose and increase if required.

Hypersensitivity reactions: For bronchial asthma and certain allergic manifestations (eg, angioedema, urticaria, serum sickness, anaphylactic shock) us epinephrine SC. The adult IV dose for hypersensitivity reactions or to relieve bronchospasm usually ranges from 0.1 to 0.25 mg injected slowly. Neonates may be given a dose of 0.01 mg/kg body weight; for the infant, 0.05 mg is an adequate initial dose and this may be repeated at 20 to 30 minute intervals in the management of asthma attacks.

Cardiac arrest: 0.5 to 1 mg (5 to 10 ml of 1:10,000 solution). A dose of 0.5 ml may be diluted to 10 ml with sodium chloride injection. During a resuscitation effort, administer 0.5 to 1 mg (5 to 10 ml) IV every 5 minutes.

Intracardiac injection should only be administered by personnel well trained in the technique, if there has not been sufficient time to establish an IV route. Follow intracardial administration with external cardiac massage to permit the drug to enter coronary circulation. Use epinephrine secondarily to unsuccessful attempts with physical or electromechanical methods.

The dose usually ranges from 0.3 to 0.5 mg (3 to 5 ml of 1:10,000 solution).

Cardiopulmonary resuscitation for cardiac arrest (Wyeth): IV or intracardiac administration of 1 to 10 ml of a 1:10,000 dilution is recommended. Artificial ventilation and cardiac compression must be continued. Doses of 1 to 10 ml of the 1:10,000 dilution may be repeated every 5 minutes as required. The IV route may be preferred since it need not interrupt cardiac compression.

Intravenous infusion: 1 mg in 250 ml of 5% Dextrose in Water (4 mcg/ml) to run at 1 to 4 mcg/min (15 to 60 ml/hr) has been recommended.

Intraspinal use: Usual dose is 0.2 to 0.4 ml of a 1:1000 solution added to anesthetic spinal fluid mixture (may prolong anesthetic action by limiting absorption).

Endotracheal tube: If IV access is not available, the drug may be injected via the endotracheal tube. Perform five rapid insufflations; forcefully expel 10 ml containing 1 mg epinephrine (0.1 mg/ml) directly into the endotracheal tube; follow with five quick insufflations.

Concomitant administration with local anesthetic: Epinephrine 1:100,000 to 1:20,000 is the usual concentration employed with local anesthetics.

Compatibility: If epinephrine and sodium bicarbonate are to be coadministered, inject individually at separate sites. Epinephrine is unstable in alkaline solution.

NOREPINEPHRINE (Levarterenol)

Injection: 1 mg /ml (as bitartrate) *(Rx)*	*Levophed* (Sanofi Winthrop)

Actions:

Pharmacology: A powerful peripheral vasoconstrictor acting on both arterial and venous beds (α-adrenergic action) and as a potent inotropic stimulator of the heart (β_1 action). Coronary vasodilation occurs secondary to enhanced myocardial contractility. These actions result in an increase in systemic blood pressure and coronary artery blood flow. Cardiac output is usually increased in hypotension when the blood pressure is raised to an optimal level. Venous return is increased and the heart tends to resume a more normal rate and rhythm than in the hypotensive state. In hypotension that persists after correction of blood volume deficits, norepinephrine helps raise the blood pressure to an optimal level and establish a more adequate circulation.

Pharmacokinetics: Norepinephrine is ineffective orally; SC absorption is poor. It is rapidly inactivated by catechol-O-methyltransferase and monoamine oxidase. Negligible amounts are normally found in urine. When given by IV infusion, the onset is rapid; duration is 1 to 2 minutes following discontinuation of infusion.

Indications:

Restoration of blood pressure in controlling certain acute hypotensive states (eg, pheochromocytomectomy, sympathectomy, poliomyelitis, spinal anesthesia, myocardial infarction (MI), septicemia, blood transfusion, and drug reactions), and as an adjunct in the treatment of cardiac arrest and profound hypotension.

Contraindications:

Do not give to patients who are hypotensive from blood volume deficits, except as an emergency measure to maintain coronary and cerebral artery perfusion until blood volume replacement therapy can be completed. If continuously administered to maintain blood pressure in the absence of blood volume replacement, the following may occur: Severe peripheral and visceral vasoconstriction, decreased renal perfusion and urine output, poor systemic blood flow despite "normal" blood pressure, tissue hypoxia, and lactic acidosis.

Do not give to patients with mesenteric or peripheral vascular thrombosis (because of the risk of increasing ischemia and extending the area of infarction) unless administration is necessary as a life saving procedure.

Use of norepinephrine during cyclopropane and halothane anesthesia is generally considered contraindicated because of the risk of producing ventricular tachycardia or fibrillation. The same type of cardiac arrhythmias may result from use in patients with profound hypoxia or hypercarbia.

Warnings:

Pregnancy: Category C.

Lactation: It is not known whether this drug is excreted in breast milk.

Children: Safety and effectiveness in children have not been established.

Precautions:

Hypovolemia: Use is not a substitute for the replacement of blood, plasma, fluids and electrolytes, which should be restored promptly when loss has occurred.

Avoid hypertension: Dangerously high blood pressure may be produced with overdoses. Monitor the blood pressure every 2 minutes from the time administration is started until the desired blood pressure is obtained, then every 5 minutes if administration is to be continued. Constantly watch flow rate. Never leave patient unattended during infusion.

Infusion site: Whenever possible, infuse into a large vein, particularly an antecubital vein, to minimize necrosis of the overlying skin from prolonged vasoconstriction. The femoral vein may also be an acceptable route of administration. Occlusive vascular diseases are more likely to occur in the lower extremity; avoid the veins of the leg in elderly patients or in those suffering from such disorders.

Extravasation: Infuse into a large vein to prevent extravasation, which may cause necrosis and sloughing of surrounding tissue. Monitor the infusion site closely for free flow. If blanching occurs, consider changing the infusion site at intervals to allow the effects of local vasoconstriction to subside.

Antidote for extravasation – To prevent sloughing and necrosis in ischemic areas, infiltrate area as soon as possible with 10 to 15 ml of saline solution containing 5 to 10 mg of phentolamine. Use a syringe with a fine hypodermic needle and infiltrate liberally throughout the ischemic area. Sympathetic blockade with phentolamine causes immediate and conspicuous local hyperemic changes if the area is infiltrated within 12 hours. Phentolamine (5 to 10 mg) added directly to the infusion may also be an effective antidote against sloughing should extravasation occur. The incidence of thrombosis in the infused vein and perivenous reactions and necrosis may be reduced if heparin is added to the infusion solution in an amount to supply 100 to 200 units/hour.

Sulfite sensitivity: Sulfites may cause allergic-type reactions in certain susceptible persons. This is more frequent in asthmatics or in atopic nonasthmatic persons.

Drug Interactions:

Drugs that may affect epinephrine include bretylium, guanethidine, halogenated hydrocarbon anesthetics, oxytocic drugs, tricyclic antidepressants and MAOIs.

Adverse Reactions:

Adverse reactions may include bradycardia, anxiety, transient headache, ischemic injury due to potent vasoconstrictor action and tissue hypoxia, respiratory difficulty, extravasation necrosis at injection site. Headache may indicate overdosage and extreme hypertension.

Administration and Dosage:

Restoration of blood pressure in acute hypotensive states: Always correct blood volume depletion as fully as possible before any vasopressor is administered. When, as an emergency measure, intraaortic pressures must be maintained to prevent cerebral or coronary artery ischemia, norepinephrine can be administered before and concurrently with blood volume replacement.

Average IV dosage – Add 4 ml of the solution to 1000 ml of 5% Dextrose Solution (4 mcg base/ml), or add 4 mg (base) to 250 ml (16 mcg base/ml). This concentration may be adjusted depending on fluid requirements. Avoid a catheter tie-in technique as this promotes stasis. After observing the response to an initial dose of 2 to 3 ml (from 8 to 12 mcg of base) per minute, adjust the rate of flow to establish and maintain a low normal blood pressure (usually 80 to 100 mm Hg systolic) sufficient to maintain the circulation to vital organs. In previously hypertensive patients, raise the blood pressure ≤ 40 mm Hg below the preexisting systolic pressure. The average maintenance dose ranges from 2 to 4 mcg per minute.

Dosage adjustments – Great individual variation in the dose occurs; titrate dosage according to patient response. Occasionally, enormous daily doses (as high as 68 mg base) may be necessary if the patient remains hypotensive, but occult blood volume depletion should always be suspected and corrected when present. Central venous pressure monitoring is usually helpful.

If large fluid volumes are needed at a flow rate involving an excessive dose of the pressor agent per unit of time, use a solution more dilute than 4 mcg/ml. When large fluid volumes are undesirable, a larger concentration may be administered.

Duration of therapy – Continue the infusion until adequate blood pressure and tissue perfusion are maintained without therapy. Reduce infusion gradually. In some cases of vascular collapse due to acute MI, treatment was required for up to 6 days.

Adjunctive treatment in cardiac arrest: Usually administered IV during cardiac resuscitation to restore and maintain an adequate blood pressure after an effective heartbeat and ventilation have been established. The powerful β-adrenergic stimulating action is also thought to increase the strength and effectiveness of systolic contractions once they occur.

Diluent: Administer in 5% Dextrose Solution in Distilled Water or 5% Dextrose in Saline Solution. Administration in saline solution alone is not recommended. If indicated, administer whole blood or plasma separately (for example, by use of a Y–tube and individual flasks if given simultaneously).

EPHEDRINE

Injection: 50 mg/ml (*Rx*)	Various

Actions:

Pharmacology: Ephedrine is a potent sympathomimetic that stimulates both alpha and beta receptors. Its peripheral actions include an increase in blood pressure, stimulation of heart muscle, constriction of arterioles, relaxation of the smooth muscle of the bronchi and GI tract, and dilation of the pupils. Tone of the trigone and vesicle sphincter is increased. Ephedrine also stimulates the cerebral cortex and subcortical centers. The cardiovascular responses include moderate tachycardia, unchanged or augmented stroke volume, enhanced cardiac output, variable alterations in peripheral resistance, and, usually, a rise in blood pressure. The action of ephedrine is more prominent on the heart than on the blood vessels. Ephedrine increases the flow of coronary, cerebral and muscle blood. Hepatic glycogenolysis is increased, and ephedrine also increases oxygen consumption and metabolic rate. Administration produces a modest increase in motor power.

Pharmacokinetics: Ephedrine is rapidly and completely absorbed following parenteral injection. Onset of action by IM route is more rapid (within 10 to 20 minutes) than by SC injection. Pressor and cardiac responses to ephedrine persist for up to 60 minutes following IM or SC administration of 25 to 50 mg. Small amounts are slowly metabolized in the liver. The drug and its metabolites are excreted in the urine, mostly as unchanged ephedrine. Elimination half-life of the drug is ≈ 3 to 6 hours.

Indications:

To combat acute hypotensive states, especially those associated with spinal anesthesia; Stokes-Adams syndrome with complete heart block; a CNS stimulant in narcolepsy and depressive states; occasionally, acute bronchospasm. Also used in enuresis and myasthenia gravis.

As a pressor agent in hypotensive states following sympathectomy or following overdosage with ganglionic-blocking agents, antiadrenergic agents, veratrum alkaloids, or other drugs used for lowering blood pressure in treating arterial hypertension.

Contraindications:

Hypersensitivity to the drug; angle closure glaucoma; patients anesthetized with cyclopropane or halothane (these agents may sensitize the heart to the arrhythmic action of sympathomimetic drugs); cases where vasopressor drugs are contraindicated.

Warnings:

Ephedrine may cause hypertension resulting in intracranial hemorrhage, anginal pain in patients with coronary insufficiency or ischemic heart disease or potentially fatal arrhythmias in patients with organic heart disease or who are receiving drugs that sensitize the myocardium. Initially, parenteral ephedrine may produce constriction of renal blood vessels and decreased urine formation.

Renal function impairment: Initially, parenteral ephedrine may produce constriction of renal blood vessels and decreased urine formation.

Pregnancy: Category C.

Labor and delivery – Parenteral administration of ephedrine to maintain blood pressure during low or other spinal anesthesia for delivery can cause acceleration of fetal heart rate and should not be used in obstetrics when maternal blood pressure exceeds 130/80 mm Hg. It is not known what effect ephedrine may have on the newborn or on the child's later growth and development when administered to the mother just before or during labor.

Lactation: Ephedrine is excreted in breast milk. Use by nursing mothers is not recommended.

Precautions:

Administer cautiously to patients with: Heart disease; coronary insufficiency; cardiac arrhythmias; angina pectoris; diabetes; hyperthyroidism; prostatic hypertrophy; hypertension; unstable vasomotor system. Also use with caution in patients on digitalis.

Prolonged use may produce a syndrome resembling an anxiety state.

Tolerance: Some measure of tolerance to ephedrine develops, but addiction does not occur. Temporary cessation of the drug restores its original effectiveness.

Hypovolemia: Use is not a substitute for the replacement of blood, plasma, fluids and electrolytes, which should be restored promptly when loss has occurred.

Prolonged abuse of ephedrine can lead to symptoms of paranoid schizophrenia.

Drug Interactions:

Drugs that may affect ephedrine include monoamine oxidase (MAO) inhibitors, halogenated anesthetics, oxytocic drugs and tricyclic antidepressants. Drugs that may be affected by ephedrine include guanethidine.

Adverse Reactions:

Adverse reactions may include palpitation; tachycardia; precordial pain; cardiac arrhythmias; headache; insomnia; sweating; vertigo; confusion; delirium; restlessness; anxiety; tension; tremor; weakness; dizziness; hallucinations; nausea; vomiting; anorexia; vesical sphincter spasm resulting in difficult and painful urination; respiratory difficulty.

Administration and Dosage:

May be adminstered SC, IM or slow IV.

Adults: The usual dose is 25 to 50 mg. The IV route may be used if an immediate effect is desired. Also, 5 to 25 mg may be administered slow IV push. Additional doses may be given at 5 to 10 minute intervals, not to exceed 150 mg in 24 hours.

Pediatric dose: 16.7 mg/m^2 SC or IM every 4 to 6 hours.

Labor: Administer only sufficient dosage to maintain blood pressure at or below 130/80 mmHg.

Acute attacks of asthma: Administer the smallest effective dose (0.25 to 0.5 ml).

PHENYLEPHRINE HCl

Injection: 1% (10 mg/ml) (*Rx*) *Neo-Synephrine* (Sanofi Winthrop)

Actions:

Pharmacology: Phenylephrine is a powerful postsynaptic alpha-receptor stimulant. The predominant actions of phenylephrine are on the cardiovascular system. Parenteral administration causes a rise in systolic and diastolic pressures due to peripheral vasoconstriction. Accompanying the pressor response to phenylephrine is a marked reflex bradycardia that can be blocked by atropine; after atropine, large doses of the drug increase the heart rate only slightly. Cardiac output is slightly decreased and peripheral resistance is considerably increased. Circulation time is slightly prolonged, and venous pressure is slightly increased. Most vascular beds are constricted; renal, splanchnic, cutaneous and limb blood flows are reduced, but coronary blood flow is increased. Pulmonary vessels are constricted, and pulmonary arterial pressure is raised.

The drug is a powerful vasoconstrictor, with properties very similar to those of norepinephrine, but almost completely lacking the chronotropic and inotropic actions on the heart. In contrast to epinephrine and ephedrine, phenylephrine produces longer lasting vasoconstriction, a reflex bradycardia and increases the stroke output, producing no disturbance in the rhythm of the pulse.

Indications:

Treatment of vascular failure in shock, shock-like states, drug-induced hypotension, or hypersensitivity; to overcome paroxysmal supraventricular tachycardia; to prolong spinal anesthesia; as a vasoconstrictor in regional analgesia; to maintain an adequate level of blood pressure during spinal and inhalation anesthesia.

Contraindications:

Hypersensitivity to the drug; severe hypertension; ventricular tachycardia.

Warnings:

Pregnancy: Category C.

Lactation: It is not known whether this drug is excreted in breast milk. Safety for use in the nursing mother has not been established.

Precautions:

Special populations: Use with extreme caution in elderly patients, patients with hyperthyroidism, bradycardia, partial heart block, myocardial disease or severe arteriosclerosis.

Hypovolemia: Use is not a substitute for the replacement of blood, plasma, fluids and electrolytes, which should be restored promptly when loss has occurred.

Extravasation: When infused, large veins of the antecubital fossa are preferred to veins in the hand or ankle to prevent extravasation. Extravasation may cause necrosis and sloughing of surrounding tissue. Monitor the infusion site closely for free flow.

Antidote for extravasation – To prevent sloughing and necrosis in ischemic areas, infiltrate area as soon as possible with 10 to 15 ml saline solution containing 5 to 10 mg phentolamine. Use a syringe with a fine hypodermic needle and infiltrate liberally throughout the ischemic area. Sympathetic blockade with phentolamine causes immediate and conspicuous local hyperemic changes if the area is infiltrated within 12 hours.

Sulfite sensitivity: Sulfites may cause allergic-type reactions in certain susceptible persons. Sulfite sensitivity is seen more frequently in asthmatics or in atopic nonasthmatic persons.

Drug Interactions:

Drugs that may affect phenylephrine include bretylium, guanethidine, halogenated hydrocarbon anesthetics, monoamine oxidase inhibitors, oxytocic drugs and tricyclic antidepressants.

Adverse Reactions:

Possible adverse reactions include headache; reflex bradycardia; excitability; restlessness.

Administration and Dosage:

Inject SC, IM, slow IV, or in dilute solution as a continuous IV infusion. In patients with paroxysmal supraventricular tachycardia and, in case of emergency, administer directly IV. Adjust dose according to the pressor response.

Phenylephrine Dosage Calculations						
Dose Required (mg)	0.1	0.2	0.5	1	5	10
Phenylephrine 1% (ml)	—	—	—	0.1	0.5	1
Diluted Phenylephrine[1] 0.1% (ml)	0.1	0.2	0.5	—	—	—

[1] For convenience in intermittent IV administration, dilute 1 ml phenylephrine 1% with 9 ml Sterile Water for Injection, USP.

Mild or moderate hypotension: SC or IM – 2 to 5 mg (range, 1 to 10 mg). Do not exceed an initial dose of 5 mg. A 5 mg IM dose should raise blood pressure for 1 to 2 hours.

IV – 0.2 mg (range, 0.1 to 0.5 mg). Do not exceed an initial dose of 0.5 mg. Do not repeat injections more often than every 10 to 15 minutes. A 0.5 mg IV dose should elevate the pressure for about 15 minutes.

To prepare a 0.1% solution of phenylephrine (0.1mg/0.1 ml), dilute 1 ml of 1% solution with 9 ml Sterile Water for Injection.

Severe hypotension and shock including drug-related hypotension: Correct blood volume depletion as completely as possible before any vasopressor is administered. When intraaortic pressures must be maintained as an emergency measure to prevent cerebral or coronary artery ischemia, phenylephrine can be administered before and concurrently with blood volume replacement.

Hypotension and occasionally severe shock may result from overdosage or idiosyncratic reactions following administration of certain drugs. Patients who receive a phenothiazine as preoperative medication are especially susceptible. As an adjunct in the management of such episodes, phenylephrine is a suitable agent for restoring blood pressure.

Higher initial and maintenance doses are required in patients with persistent or untreated severe hypotension or shock. Hypotension produced by powerful peripheral adrenergic blocking agents or pheochromocytomectomy may also require more intensive therapy.

Continuous infusion: Add 10 mg to 250 or 500 ml of Dextrose Injection or NaCl Injection (providing a 1:25,000 or 1:50,000 dilution). To raise blood pressure rapidly, start the infusion at about 100 to 180 mcg/min (based on 20 drops/ml, this would be 50 to 90 or 100 to 180 drops/min). When blood pressure is stabilized (at a low normal level for the individual), a maintenance rate of 40 to 60 mcg/min usually suffices (based on 20 drops/ml, this would be 20 to 30 or 40 to 60 drops/min). If the drop size of the infusion system varies from 20 drops/ml, adjust dose accordingly.

If a prompt initial vasopressor response is not obtained, add additional increments of the drug (10 mg or more) to the infusion bottle. Adjust the flow rate until the desired blood pressure level is obtained. (A more potent vasopressor, eg, norepinephrine, may be required.) Avoid hypertension. Check blood pressure frequently. Headache or bradycardia may indicate hypertension. Arrhythmias are rare.

Spinal anesthesia:

Hypotension – Administer SC or IM 3 or 4 minutes before injection of the spinal anesthetic. The total requirement for high anesthetic levels is usually 3 mg, and for lower levels, 2 mg. For hypotensive emergencies during spinal anesthesia, phenylephrine may be injected IV beginning with a dose of 0.2 mg. Any subsequent dose should not exceed the previous dose by more than 0.1 to 0.2 mg; do not administer more than 0.5 mg in a single dose.

Pediatric dose – To combat hypotension during spinal anesthesia in children, administer 0.5 to 1 mg/25 lbs, SC or IM.

Prolongation of spinal anesthesia – The addition of 2 to 5 mg phenylephrine to the anesthetic solution increases the duration of motor block by as much as 50% without an increase in the incidence of complications.

Vasoconstrictor for regional analgesia: Concentrations about 10 times those of epinephrine are recommended. The optimum strength is 1:20,000 (made by adding 1 mg phenylephrine to every 20 ml of local anesthetic solution). Some pressor responses may be expected when 2 mg or more are injected.

Paroxysmal supraventricular tachycardia: Rapid IV injection (within 20 to 30 seconds) is recommended; do not exceed an initial dose of 0.5 mg. Subsequent doses, which are determined by the initial blood pressure response, should not exceed the preceding dose by more than 0.1 to 0.2 mg, and should never exceed 1 mg.

IV compatibility: Phenylephrine at a concentration of 1 mg/L was found to be physically compatible with the following IV solutions: Dextrose-Ringer's combinations; Dextrose-Lactated Ringer's combinations; Dextrose-saline combinations; Dextrose 2½%, 5% and 10% in Water; Ringer's Injection; Lactated Ringer's Injection; 0.45% and 0.9% Sodium Chloride Injection; ⅙M Sodium Lactate Injection.

BETA-ADRENERGIC BLOCKING AGENTS

ATENOLOL	
Tablets: 25, 50 and 100 mg (*Rx*)	Various, *Tenormin* (ICI Pharma)
Injection: 5 mg/10 ml (*Rx*)	*Tenormin* (ICI Pharma)
ESMOLOL HCl	
Injection: 10 or 250 mg/ml (*Rx*)	*Brevibloc* (Ohmeda)
BETAXOLOL HCl	
Tablets: 10 and 20 mg (*Rx*)	*Kerlone* (Searle)
PENBUTOLOL SULFATE	
Tablets: 20 mg (*Rx*)	*Levatol* (Schwarz Pharma)
CARTEOLOL HCl	
Tablets: 2.5 and 5 mg (*Rx*)	*Cartrol* (Abbott)
BISOPROLOL FUMARATE	
Tablets: 5 and 10 mg (*Rx*)	*Zebeta* (Lederle)
PINDOLOL	
Tablets: 5 and 10 mg (*Rx*)	Various, *Visken* (Sandoz)
METOPROLOL	
Tablets: 50 and 100 mg (*Rx*)	Various, *Lopressor* (Geigy)
Tablets, extended release: 50, 100 and 200 mg (*Rx*)	*Toprol XL* (Astra)
Injection: 1 mg/ml (*Rx*)	Various, *Lopressor* (Geigy)
TIMOLOL MALEATE	
Tablets: 5, 10 and 20 mg (*Rx*)	Various, *Blocadren* (Merck)
SOTALOL HCl	
Tablets: 80, 120, 160 and 240 mg (*Rx*)	*Betapace* (Berlex)
ACEBUTOLOL HCl	
Capsules: 200 and 400 mg (*Rx*)	Various, *Sectral* (Wyeth-Ayerst)
NADOLOL	
Tablets: 20, 40, 80, 120 and 160 mg (*Rx*)	Various, *Corgard* (Bristol-Myers Squibb)
PROPRANOLOL	
Tablets: 10, 20, 40, 60, 80 and 90 mg (*Rx*)	Various, *Inderal* (Wyeth-Ayerst)
Capsules, sustained release: 60, 80, 120 and 160 mg (*Rx*)	Various, *Inderal LA* (Wyeth-Ayerst), *Betachron E-R* (Inwood)
Solution, oral: 4 or 8 mg/ml (*Rx*)	Various
Solution, concentrated oral: 80 mg/ml (*Rx*)	*Propranolol Intensol* (Roxane)
Injection: 1 mg/ml (*Rx*)	Various, *Inderal* (Wyeth-Ayerst)

Actions:

Pharmacology:

Pharmacologic/Pharmacokinetic Properties of Beta-Adrenergic Blocking Agents

0–none +-low ++-moderate +++-high Drug	Adrenergic receptor blocking activity	Membrane stabilizing activity	Intrinsic sympathomimetic activity	Lipid solubility	Extent of absorption (%)	Absolute oral bioavailability (%)	Half-life (hrs)	Protein binding (%)	Metabolism/Excretion
Acebutolol	β_1[1]	+	+	Low	90	20-60	3-4	26	Hepatic; renal excretion 30% to 40%; non-renal excretion 50% to 60% (bile; intestinal wall)
Atenolol	β_1[1]	0	0	Low	50	50-60	6-9	16-16	≈ 50% excreted unchanged in feces
Betaxolol	β_1[1]	+	0	Low	≈ 100	89	14-22	≈ 50	Hepatic; > 80% recovered in urine, 15% unchanged

Pharmacologic/Pharmacokinetic Properties of Beta-Adrenergic Blocking Agents

0–none +-low ++-moderate +++-high Drug	Adrenergic receptor blocking activity	Membrane stabilizing activity	Intrinsic sympathomimetic activity	Lipid solubility	Extent of absorption (%)	Absolute oral bioavailability (%)	Half-life (hrs)	Protein binding (%)	Metabolism/Excretion
Bisoprolol	β_1[1]	0	0	Low	≥ 90	80	9-12	≈ 30	≈ 50% excreted unchanged in urine, remainder as inactive metabolites; < 2% excreted in feces.
Esmolol	β_1[1]	0	0	Low	na[2]	na[2]	0.15	55	Rapid metabolism by esterases in cytosol of red blood cells
Metoprolol	β_1[1]	0[3]	0	Moderate	95	40-50	3-7	12	Hepatic; renal excretion, < 5% unchanged
Metoprolol, long-acting						77			
Carteolol	β_1 β_2	0	++	Low	80	85	6	23-30	50% to 70% excreted unchanged in urine
Nadolol	β_1 β_2	0	0	Low	30	30-50	20-24	30	Urine, unchanged
Penbutolol	β_1 β_2	0	+	High	≈100	≈100	5	80-98	Hepatic (conjugation, oxidation); renal excretion of metabolites (17% as conjugate)
Pindolol	β_1 β_2	+	+++	Moderate	95	≈100	3-4[4]	40	Urinary excretion of metabolites (60% to 65%) and unchanged drug (35% to 40%)
Propranolol	β_1 β_2	++	0	High	90	30	3-5	90	Hepatic; < 1% excreted unchanged in urine
Propranolol, long-acting						9-18	8-11		
Sotalol	β_1 β_2	0	0	Low	nd[5]	90-100	12	0	Not metabolized; excreted unchanged in urine
Timolol	β_1 β_2	0	0	Low to moderate	90	75	4	10	Hepatic; urinary excretion of metabolites and unchanged drug
Labetalol	β_1 β_2 α_1	0	0	Moderate	100	30-40	5.5-8	50	55% to 60% excreted in urine as conjugates or unchanged drug

[1] Inhibits β_2 receptors (bronchial and vascular) at higher doses.
[2] na = Not applicable (available IV only).
[3] Detectable only at doses much greater than required for beta blockade.
[4] In elderly hypertensive patients with normal renal function, t½ variable: 7 to 15 hours.
[5] nd = No data.

Indications:

Beta-Adrenergic Blocking Agents – Summary of Indications														
Indications ✓ = labeled x = unlabeled	Acebutolol	Atenolol	Betaxolol	Bisoprolol	Carteolol	Esmolol	Labetalol	Metoprolol	Nadolol	Penbutolol	Pindolol	Propranolol	Sotalol	Timolol
Hypertension	✓	✓	✓	✓	✓		✓	✓	✓	✓	✓	✓		✓
Angina pectoris		✓		x	x	x		✓	✓			✓		
Cardiac arrhythmias														
Supraventricular arrhythmias/ tachycardias		x		x		✓						✓		
Sinus tachycardia						✓								
Ventricular arrhythmias/ tachycardias		x						x	x		x	✓	x	✓
PVCs	✓			x								✓		
Digitalis-induced tachyarrhythmias												✓		
Resistant tachyarrhythmias (during anesthesia)												✓		
Atrial ectopy								x						
Myocardial infarction		✓						✓				✓		✓
Pheochromocytoma							x					✓		
Migraine prophylaxis		x						x	x			✓		x
Hypertrophic subaortic stenosis												✓		
Tremors														
Essential								x	x			✓		x
Lithium-induced									x					
Parkinsonism									x			x		
Alcohol withdrawal syndrome		x										x		
Aggressive behavior								x	x			x		
Antipsychotic-induced akathisia								x	x		x	x		
Esophageal varices rebleeding		x							x			x		
Anxiety (including situational)		x							x		x	x		x
Enhanced cognitive performance								x						
Schizophrenia/Acute panic												x		
Gastric bleeding in portal hypertension												x		
Vaginal contraceptive												x		
Intraocular pressure reduction									x					
Thyrotoxicosis symptoms												x		
Congestive heart failure								x						

Contraindications:

Sinus bradycardia; greater than first degree heart block; cardiogenic shock; congestive heart failure (CHF) unless secondary to a tachyarrhythmia treatable with β-blockers; overt cardiac failure; hypersensitivity to β-blocking agents.

Acebutolol, carteolol: Persistently severe bradycardia.

Propranolol, nadolol, timolol, penbutolol, carteolol, sotalol and pindolol: Bronchial asthma or bronchospasm, including severe chronic obstructive pulmonary disease.

Metoprolol: Treatment of MI in patients with a heart rate < 45 beats/min; significant heart block greater than first degree (PR interval ≥ 0.24 sec); systolic blood pressure < 100 mm Hg; moderate to severe cardiac failure.

Sotalol: Congenital or acquired long QT syndromes.

Warnings:

Proarrhythmia: Like other antiarrhythmic agents, **sotalol** can provoke new or worsened ventricular arrhythmias in some patients, including sustained ventricular tachycardia or ventricular fibrillation, with potentially fatal consequences. Because of its effect on cardiac repolarization, is the most common form of proarrhythmia associated with **sotalol**, occurring in about 4% of high risk patients.

Cardiac failure: Sympathetic stimulation is a vital component supporting circulatory function in CHF, and β-blockade carries the potential hazard of further depressing myocardial contractility and precipitating more severe failure.

Wolff-Parkinson-White syndrome: In several cases, the tachycardia was replaced by a severe bradycardia requiring a demand pacemaker after **propranolol** administration with as little as 5 mg.

Abrupt withdrawal: The occurrence of a β-blocker withdrawal syndrome is controversial. However, hypersensitivity to catecholamines has been observed in patients withdrawn from β-blocker therapy. Exacerbation of angina, MI, ventricular arrhythmias and death have occurred after abrupt discontinuation of therapy. Reduce dosage gradually over 1 to 2 weeks and carefully monitor the patient.

Because coronary artery disease may be unrecognized, do not discontinue therapy abruptly, even in patients treated only for hypertension, as abrupt withdrawal may result in transient symptoms.

Peripheral vascular disease: Treatment with β-antagonists reduces cardiac output and can precipitate or aggravate the symptoms of arterial insufficiency in patients with peripheral or mesenteric vascular disease.

Nonallergic bronchospasm (eg, chronic bronchitis, emphysema): In general, do not administer β-blockers to patients with bronchospastic diseases. Administer **nadolol, timolol, penbutolol, propranolol, sotalol** and **pindolol** with caution, since they may block bronchodilation produced by endogenous or exogenous catecholamine stimulation of β_2 receptors.

Because of their relative β_1 selectivity, low doses of **metoprolol, acebutolol, bisoprolol** and **atenolol** may be used with caution in patients with bronchospastic disease who do not respond to, or cannot tolerate, other antihypertensive treatment.

Bradycardia: **Metoprolol** produces a decrease in sinus heart rate in most patients; this decrease is greatest among patients with high initial heart rates and least among patients with low initial heart rates.

Pheochromocytoma: It is hazardous to use **propranolol** unless α-adrenergic blocking drugs are already in use, since this would predispose to serious blood pressure elevation.

Sinus bradycardia (heart rate < 50 bpm) occurred in 13% of patients receiving **sotalol** in clinical trials, and led to discontinuation in about 3%. Bradycardia itself increases risk of torsade de pointes.

Electrolyte disturbances: Do not use **sotalol** in patients with hypokalemia or hypomagnesemia prior to correction of imbalance.

Hypotension: If hypotension (systolic blood pressure ≤ 90 mmHg) occurs, discontinue drug and carefully assess patient's hemodynamic status and extent of myocardial damage.

Anaphylaxis has occurred and may include symptoms such as profound hypotension, bradycardia with or without AV nodal block, severe sustained bronchospasm, hives and angioedema. Deaths have occurred. Refer to Management of Acute Hypersensitivity Reactions.

Anesthesia and major surgery: Necessity, or desirability, of withdrawing β-blockers prior to major surgery is controversial. β-blockade impairs the heart's ability to respond to β-adrenergically mediated reflex stimuli. While this might help prevent arrhythmic response, risk of excessive myocardial depression during general anesthesia may be enhanced, and difficulty restarting and maintaining heart beat has occurred. If β-blockers are withdrawn, allow 48 hours between the last dose and anesthesia. Others may recommend withdrawal of β-blockers well before surgery takes place.

AV block: **Metoprolol** slows AV conduction and may produce significant first (PR interval ≥ 0.26 sec), second, or third-degree heart block. Acute MI also produces heart block.

Sick sinus syndrome: Use **sotalol** only with extreme caution in patients with sick sinus syndrome associated with symptomatic arrhythmias, because it may cause sinus bradycardia, sinus pauses or sinus arrest.

Renal/Hepatic function impairment: Use with caution.

Pregnancy: Category C (atenolol, labetalol, esmolol, metoprolol, nadolol, timolol, propranolol, penbutolol, carteolol, bisoprolol).

Category B (acebutolol, pindolol, sotalol).

Lactation: In general, nursing should not be undertaken by mothers receiving these drugs.

Children: Safety and efficacy for use in children have not been established.

IV administration of **propranolol** is not recommended in children; however, oral propranolol has been used.

Precautions:

Diabetes/Hypoglycemia: β-adrenergic blockade may blunt premonitory signs and symptoms (eg, tachycardia, blood pressure changes) of acute hypoglycemia. Nonselective β-blockers may potentiate insulin-induced hypoglycemia.

Thyrotoxicosis: β-adrenergic blockers may mask clinical signs (eg, tachycardia) of developing or continuing hyperthyroidism. Abrupt withdrawal may exacerbate symptoms of hyperthyroidism, including thyroid storm.

In contrast, propranolol may be beneficial in reducing the symptoms of thyrotoxicosis.

Serum lipid concentrations: β-blockers may alter serum lipids including an increase in the concentration of total triglycerides, total cholesterol and LDL and VLDL cholesterol, and a decrease in the concentration of HDL cholesterol.

Muscle weakness: β-blockade has potentiated muscle weakness consistent with certain myasthenic symptoms (eg, diplopia, ptosis, generalized weakness).

Drug Interactions:

Drugs that may affect beta-blockers include aluminum salts, barbiturates, calcium salts, cholestyramine, colestipol, NSAIDs, penicillins (ampicillin), rifampin, salicylates, sulfinpyrazole, calcium blockers, oral contraceptives, ethanol, flecainide, haloperidol, H_2 antagonists, hydralazine, loop diuretics, MAO inhibitors, phenothiazines propafenone, quinidine, quinolones (ciprofloxacin), thioamines and thyroid hormones.

Drugs that may be affected by beta-blocers include flecainide, haloperidol, hydralazine, acetaminophen, phenothiazines, anticoagulants, benzodiazepines, clonidine, disopyramide, epinephrine, ergot alkaloids, lidocaine, nondepolarizing muscle relaxants, prazosin, sulfonylureas and theophylline.

Drug/Lab test interactions: These agents may produce hypoglycemia and interfere with **glucose** or **insulin** tolerance tests. Propranolol may interfere with the glaucoma screening test due to a reduction in intraocular pressure.

Drug/Food interactions: Food enhances the bioavailability of **metoprolol** and **propranolol**; this effect is not noted with **nadolol, bisoprolol** or **pindolol**. The rate of **carteolol** and **penbutolol** absorption is slowed by the presence of food; however, extent of absorption is not appreciably affected. **Sotalol** absorption is reduced approximately 20% by a standard meal.

Adverse Reactions:

Most adverse effects are mild and transient and rarely require withdrawal of therapy.

Hypersensitivity: Pharyngitis; photosensitivity reaction; erythematous rash; fever combined with aching and sore throat; laryngospasm; respiratory distress; angioedema; anaphylaxis.

Cardiovascular: Bradycardia; torsade de pointes and other serious new ventricular arrhythmias; chest pain; hypertension; hypotension; peripheral ischemia; pallor; flushing; worsening of angina and arterial insufficiency; shortness of breath; peripheral vascular insufficiency; CHF; edema; pulmonary edema; vasodilation; presyncope and syncope; tachycardia; palpitations; first, second and third degree heart block; abnormal ECG; supraventricular tachycardia.

CNS: Dizziness; vertigo; tiredness/fatigue; headache; mental depression; peripheral neuropathy; paresthesias; lethargy; anxiety; nervousness; diminished concentration/memory; somnolence; restlessness; insomnia; sleep disturbances; sedation; change in behavior; mood change; incoordination; hallucinations; acute mental changes in the elderly; increase in signs and symptoms of myasthenia gravis.

It has been suggested that the more lipophilic the β-blocker, the higher the CNS penetration and subsequent incidence of adverse CNS effects.

Endocrine: Hyperglycemia; hypoglycemia; unstable diabetes.

GI: Gastric/epigastric pain; flatulence; gastritis; constipation; nausea; diarrhea; dry mouth; vomiting; heartburn; appetite disorder; anorexia; bloating; abdominal discomfort/pain; dyspepsia; taste distortion.

GU: Sexual dysfunction; impotence or decreased libido; dysuria; nocturia; urinary retention or frequency.

Hematologic: Agranulocytosis; nonthrombocytopenic or thrombocytopenic purpura; bleeding; thrombocytopenia; eosinophilia; leukopenia; hyperlipdemia.

Dermatologic: Rash; pruritus; skin irritation; increased pigmentation; sweating/hyperhidrosis; alopecia; dry skin; psoriasis; acne; eczema; flushing; purpura; erythematous rash.

Ophthalmic: Eye irritation/discomfort; dry/burning eyes; blurred vision; conjunctivitis; ocular pain/pressure; abnormal lacrimation.

Respiratory: Bronchospasm; dyspnea; cough; bronchial obstruction; wheeziness; nasal stuffiness; pharyngitis; laryngospasm with respiratory distress; asthma; rhinitis; sinusitis.

Musculoskeletal: Joint pain; arthralgia; muscle cramps/pain; back/neck pain; arthritis; twitching/tremor; localized pain; extremity pain; myalgia.

Miscellaneous: Facial swelling; weight gain; weight loss; Raynaud's phenomenon; speech disorder; earache; asthenia; malaise; fever; death.

Lab test abnormalities: **Propranolol** may elevate blood urea levels in patients with severe heart disease. **Propranolol** and **metoprolol** may cause elevated serum transaminase, alkaline phosphatase and LDH.

Minor persistent elevations in AST and ALT have occurred in 7% of patients treated with **pindolol**. Elevations of AST and ALT of 1 to 2 times normal have occurred with **bisoprolol** (3.9% to 6.2%).

Administration and Dosage:

ATENOLOL:

Hypertension (oral) –

Initial dosage: 50 mg once daily, used alone or added to a diuretic. If an optimal response is not achieved, increase to 100 mg/day. Dosage > 100 mg/day is unlikely to produce any further benefit.

Angina pectoris (oral) –

Initial dosage: 50 mg/day. If an optimal response is not achieved within 1 week, increase to 100 mg/day. Some patients may require 200 mg/day for optimal effect.

Acute myocardial infarction –

IV: Initiate treatment as soon as possible after the patient's arrival in the hospital and after eligibility is established. Begin treatment with 5 mg over 5 minutes followed by another 5 mg IV injection 10 minutes later.

Oral: In patients who tolerate the full 10 mg IV dose, initiate 50 mg tablets 10 minutes after the last IV dose followed by another 50 mg dose 12 hours later. Thereafter, administer 100 mg once daily or 50 mg twice daily for a further 6 to 9 days or until discharge from the hospital.

Renal function impairment –

Atenolol Dosage Adjustments in Severe Renal Impairment

Creatinine clearance (ml/min/1.73 m^2)	Elimination half-life (hrs)	Maximum dosage
15 to 35	16 to 27	50 mg/day
< 15	> 27	50 mg every other day

Hemodialysis – Give 50 mg after each dialysis.

ESMOLOL HCl:

Supraventricular tachycardia – 50 to 200 mcg/kg/min; average dose is 100 mcg/kg/min although dosages as low as 25 mcg/kg/min have been adequate. Dosages as high as 300 mcg/kg/min provide little added effect and an increased rate of adverse effects, and are not recommended.

Esmolol Dosage in Supraventricular Tachycardia

		1 minute loading infusion (mcg/kg/min)	4 minute maintenance infusion (mcg/kg/min)					
		500	50	100	150	200	250	300
Suggested Administration for Supraventricular Tachycardia								
Patient wt		Infusion rates (ml/min)	Infusion rates (ml/hr)					
lbs	kg							
110	50	2.5	15	30	45	60	175	190
121	55	2.75	16.5	33	49.5	66	182.5	199
132	60	3	18	36	54	72	190	108
143	65	3.25	19.5	39	58.5	78	197.5	117
154	70	3.5	21	42	63	84	105	126
165	75	3.75	22.5	45	67.5	90	112.5	135
176	80	4	24	48	72	96	120	144
187	85	4.25	25.5	51	76.5	102	127.5	153
198	90	4.5	27	54	81	108	135	162
209	95	4.75	28.5	57	85.5	114	142.5	171
220	100	5	30	60	90	120	150	180
231	105	5.25	31.5	63	94.5	126	157.5	189
242	110	5.5	33	66	99	132	165	198

Maintenance dosages > 200 mcg/kg/min do not significantly increase benefits. The safety of dosages > 300 mcg/kg/min has not been studied.

Transfer to alternative agents – After achieving adequate heart rate control and stable clinical status, transition to alternative antiarrhythmatic agents may be accomplished.

Withdrawal effects – The use of esmolol infusions up to 24 hours has been well documented. Limited data indicate that esmolol is well tolerated up to 48 hours.

BETAXOLOL HCl:

Initial dose – 10 mg once daily, alone or added to diuretic therapy. If the desired response is not achieved the dose can be doubled. Increasing the dose > 20 mg has not produced a statistically significant additional hypertensive effect; however, the 40 mg dose is well tolerated.

Elderly – Cosider reducing the starting dose to 5 mg.

PENBUTOLOL SULFATE: Usual starting and maintenance dose is 20 mg once daily. Doses of 40 to 80 mg have been well tolerated but have not shown greater antihypertensive effect. A dose of 10 mg also lowers blood pressure, but the full effect is not seen for 4 to 6 weeks.

CARTEOLOL HCl:

Initial dose – 2.5 mg as a single daily dose, either alone or with a diuretic. If adequate response is not achieved, gradually increase to 5 and 10 mg as single daily doses. Doses > 10 mg/day are unlikely to produce further benefit, and may decrease response.

Maintenance – 2.5 to 5 mg once daily.

Renal function impairment –

Carteolol Dosage in Renal Impairment	
Creatinine clearance (ml/min/1.73 m^2)	Dosage interval (hrs)
> 60	24
20 to 60	48
< 20	72

BISOPROLOL FUMARATE: May be given without regard to meals.

Initial dose – 5 mg once daily. In some patients, 2.5 mg may be appropriate. If the antihypertensive effect of 5 mg is inadequate, the dose may be increased to 10 mg and then, if necessary, to 20 mg once daily.

Renal/Hepatic function impairment – In patients with renal dysfunction (creatinine clearance < 40 ml/min) or hepatic impairment (hepatitis or cirrhosis), use an initial daily dose of 2.5 mg and use caution in dose titration.

Elderly – Dose adjustment is not necessary.

PINDOLOL:

Initial dose – 5 mg twice daily, alone or with other antihypertensive agents. If a satisfactory reduction in blood pressure does not occur within 3 to 4 weeks, adjust dose in increments of 10 mg/day at 3 to 4 week intervals, to a maximum of 60 mg/day.

METOPROLOL:

Tablets (immediate release) and injection –

Hypertension: Initial dosage - 100 mg/day in single or divided doses, used alone or added to a diuretic. The dosage may be increased at weekly (or longer) intervals until optimum blood pressure reduction is achieved.

Maintenance dosage - 100 to 450 mg/day. Dosages > 450 mg/day have not been studied. While once daily dosing is effective and can maintain a reduction in blood pressure throughout the day, lower doses (especially 100 mg) may not maintain a full effect at the end of the 24 hour period; larger or more frequent daily doses may be required.

Angina pectoris: Initial dosage - 100 mg/day in two divided doses. Dosage may be gradually increased at weekly intervals until optimum clinical response is obtained or a pronounced slowing of heart rate occurs. Effective dosage range is 100 to 400 mg/day. Dosages above 400 mg/day have not been studied.

Myocardial infarction (MI): Early treatment -During the early phase of definite or suspected acute MI, initiate treatment as soon as possible. Administer 3 IV bolus injections of 5 mg each at ≈ 2 minute intervals.

In patients who tolerate the full IV dose (15 mg), give 50 mg orally every 6 hours 15 minutes after the last IV dose and continue for 48 hours. Thereafter, administer a maintenance dosage of 100 mg twice daily.

In patients who do not tolerate the full IV dose, start with 25 or 50 mg orally every 6 hours (depending on the degree of intolerance) 15 minutes after the last IV dose or as soon as the clinical condition allows.

Late treatment - Patients with contraindications to early treatment, patients who do not tolerate the full early treatment and patients in whom therapy is delayed for any other reason should be started at 100 mg orally, twice daily, as soon as their clinical condition allows. Continue for at least 3 months.

Tablets, extended release – The extended release tablets are for once daily administration. When switching from immediate release metoprolol tablets to extended release, use the same daily dose.

Hypertension: The usual initial dosage is 50 to 100 mg/day in a single dose whether used alone or added to a diuretic. The dosage may be increased at weekly (or longer) intervals until optimum blood pressure reduction is achieved. Dosages > 400 mg/day have not been studied.

Angina pectoris: The usualy initial dosage is 100 mg/day in a single dose. The dosage may be gradually increased at weekly intervals until optimum clinical response has been obtained or there is a pronounced slowing of the heart rate. Dosages > 400 mg/day have not been studied.

TIMOLOL MALEATE:

Hypertension –

Initial dosage: 10 mg twice daily used alone or added to a diuretic.

Maintenance dosage: 20 to 40 mg/day. Titrate, depending on blood pressure and heart rate. Increases to a maximum of 60 mg/day divided into 2 doses may be necessary. There should be an interval of at least 7 days between dosage increases.

Myocardial infarction (long-term prophylactic use in patients who have survived the acute phase of MI) – 10 mg twice daily.

Migraine – Initial dosage is 10 mg twice daily. During maintenance therapy the 20 mg daily dosage may be given as a single dose. Total daily dosage may be increased to a maximum of 30 mg in divided doses or decreased to 10 mg once daily depending on clinical response and tolerability. Discontinue if a satisfactory response is not obtained after 6 to 8 weeks of the maximum daily dosage.

SOTALOL HCl: The recommended initial dose is 80 mg twice daily. This dose may be increased if necessary, after appropriate evaluation, to 240 or 320 mg/day. In most patients, a therapeutic response is obtained at a total daily dose of 160 to 320 mg/day, given in two or three divided doses. Some patients with life-threatening refractory ventricular arrhythmias may require doses as high as 480 to 640 mg/day.

Renal function impairment –

Sotalol Dosing Interval in Renal Impairment

Creatinine clearance (ml/min)	Dosing interval (hours)
> 60	12
30 to 60	24
10 to 30	36 to 48
< 10	Individualize dosage

Transfer to sotalol – Before starting sotalol, generally withdraw previous antiarrhythmatic therapy.

ACEBUTOLOL HCl:

Hypertension –

Initial dose: 400 mg in uncomplicated mild to moderate hypertension. May be given as a single daily dose, but 200 mg twice daily may be required for adequate control. Optimal response usually occurs with 400 to 800 mg/day (range, 200 to 1200 mg/day given twice daily).

Vetricular arrhythmia –

Initial dose: 400 mg (200 mg twice daily). Increase dosage gradually until optimal response is obtained, usually 600 to 1200 mg/day.

Elderly – Since bioavailability increases about 2–fold, older patients may require lower maintenance doses. Avoid doses > 800 mg/day.

Renal/Hepatic function impairment – Reduce the daily dose by 50% when creatinine clearance is < 50 ml/min/1.73^2. Reduce by 75% when it is < 25 ml/min/1.73^2. Use cautiously in impaired hepatic function.

NADOLOL:

Angina pectoris –

Initial dose: 40 mg/day. Gradually increase dosage in 40 to 80 mg increments at 3 to 7 day intervals until optimum clinical response is obtained or there is pronounced slowing of the heart rate.

Maintenance dosage: Usual dose is 40 to 80 mg once daily. Up to 240 to 320 mg once daily may be needed.

Hypertension –

Initial dose: 40 mg once daily, alone or in addition to diuretic therapy. Gradually increase dosage in 40 to 80 mg increments until optimum blood pressure reduction is achieved.

Maintenance dose: Usual dose is 40 to 80 mg once daily. Up to 240 to 320 mg once daily may be needed.

Renal function impairment –

Nadolol Dosage Adjustments in Renal Failure	
Creatinine clearance ($ml/min/1.73^2$)	Dosage interval (hours)
> 50	24
31 to 50	24 to 36
10 to 30	24 to 48
< 10	40 to 60

PROPRANOLOL HCl:

Propranolol Dosage Based on Indication

Indication	Initial dosage	Usual range	Maximum daily dosage
Arrhythmias		10 - 30 mg tid-qid (given ac-hs)	
Hypertension	40 mg bid or 80 mg once daily (SR)	120 - 240 mg/day (given bid-tid) or 120 - 160 mg once daily (SR)	640 mg
Angina	80 - 320 mg bid, tid, qid or 80 mg once daily (SR)	160 mg once daily (SR)	320 mg
MI		180 - 240 mg/day (given tid - qid)	240 mg
IHSS		20 - 40 mg tid - qid (given ac-hs) or 8 - 160 mg once daily (SR)	
Pheochromocytoma		60 mg/day x 3 days preoperatively (in divided doses)	
Inoperable tumor		30 mg/day (in divided doses)	
Migraine	80 mg/day once daily (SR) or in divided doses	160 - 240 mg/day (in divided doses)	
Essential tremor	40 mg bid	120 mg/day	320 mg

Parenteral –

Usual dose: 1 to 3 mg. Do not exceed 1 mg/min. If necessary, give a second dose after 2 minutes. Thereafter, do not give additional drug in < 4 hour. Transfer to oral therapy as soon as possible.

Pediatrics – IV use is not recommended.

Oral dosage for treating hypertension requires titration, beginning with a 1 mg/kg/day dosage regimen (eg, 0.5 mg/kg twice daily). May be increased at 3 to 5 day intervals to a maximum of 2 mg/kg/day.

The usual pediatric dosage range is 2 to 4 mg/kg/day in two equally divided doses (eg, 1 to 2 mg/kg twice daily). Dosage calculated by weight generally produces plasma levels in a therapeutic range similar to that in adults. Do not use doses > 16 mg/kg/day.

LABETALOL HCl

Tablets: 100, 200 and 300 mg (*Rx*)	*Normodyne* (Schering), *Trandate* (Glaxo Wellcome)
Injection: 5 mg/ml (*Rx*)	*Normodyne* (Schering), *Trandate* (Glaxo Wellcome)

Actions:

Pharmacology: Labetalol combines both selective, competitive postsynaptic α_1-adrenergic blocking and nonselective, competitive β-adrenergic blocking activity. The α- and β-blocking actions decrease blood pressure (BP). Standing BP is lowered more than supine.

Pharmacokinetics:

Absorption/Distribution – Oral labetalol is completely absorbed; peak plasma levels occur in 1 to 2 hours. Steady-state plasma levels during repetitive dosing are reached by about the third day. Due to an extensive first-pass effect, absolute bioavailability is 25%. Protein binding is ≈ 50%.

Metabolism/Excretion – Metabolism is mainly through conjugation to glucuronide metabolites, which are excreted in urine and in feces (via bile). Elimination half-life is 5.5 to 8 hours. About 55% to 60% of a dose appears in urine as conjugates or unchanged drug in the first 24 hours.

Onset/Peak/Duration –

Oral: The peak effects of single oral doses occur within 2 to 4 hours and lasts 8 to 12 hours. The maximum, steady-state BP response upon oral, twice-a-day dosing occurs within 24 to 72 hours.

IV: The maximum effect of each IV injection of labetalol at each dose level occurs within 5 minutes. Following discontinuation of IV therapy, PB approaches pretreatment baseline values in 16 to 18 hours.

Indications:

Oral: Hypertension, alone or with other agents, especially thiazide and loop diuretics.

Parenteral: For control of blood pressure in severe hypertension.

Unlabeled uses: Labetalol has effectively lowered BP and relieved symptoms in patients with pheochromocytoma; higher IV doses may be required.

Labetalol has also been used in clonidine withdrawal hypertension.

Contraindications:

Bronchial asthma; overt cardiac failure; greater than first degree heart block; cardiogenic shock; severe bradycardia.

Warnings:

Cardiac failure: Avoid use in overt CHF; may be used with caution in patients with a history of heart failure who are well compensated. CHF has been observed in patients receiving labetalol.

Patients without history of cardiac failure (latent cardiac insufficiency): Continued depression of myocardium with β-blockers can lead to cardiac failure.

Withdrawal: Hypersensitivity to catecholamines has been seen in patients withdrawn from β-blockers. Exacerbation of angina and, in some cases, myocardial infarction and ventricular dysrhythmias have occurred after abrupt discontinuation of such therapy. When discontinuing chronic labetalol, particularly in ischemic heart disease, gradually reduce dosage over 1 to 2 weeks and carefully monitor.

Nonallergic bronchospasm (eg, chronic bronchitis and emphysema): Patients with bronchospastic disease should, in general, not receive β-blockers.

Diabetes mellitus and hypoglycemia: β-blockade may prevent the appearance of premonitory signs and symptoms of acute hypoglycemia. β-blockade also reduces insulin release; it may be necessary to adjust antidiabetic drug dose.

Major surgery: Withdrawing β-blockers prior to major surgery is controversial. Protracted severe hypotension and difficulty restarting or maintaining heartbeat have been reported with beta-blockers.

Rapid decreases of BP: Observe caution when reducing severely elevated BP. Achieve desired BP lowering over as long a time as possible.

Hepatic function impairment: Drug metabolism may be diminished.

Jaundice or hepatic dysfunction has rarely been associated with labetalol.

Elderly: Bioavailability is increased in elderly patients.

Pregnancy: Category C.

Lactation: Small amounts are excreted in breast milk.

Children: Safety and efficacy for use in children have not been established.

Precautions:

Hypotension: Symptomatic postural hypotension is most likely to occur 2 to 4 hours after a dose, especially following a large initial dose or upon large changes in dose. It is likely to occur if patients are tilted or allowed to assume the upright position within 3 hours of receiving labetalol injection.

Drug Interactions:

Drugs that may interact with labetalol include beta-adrenergic agonists, cimetidine, glutethimide, halothane and nitroglycerin.

Drug/Lab test interactions: A labetalol metabolite may falsely increase urinary catecholamine levels when measured by a nonspecific trihydroxyindole reaction.

Drug/Food interactions: Food may increase bioavailability of the drug.

Adverse Reactions:

Significant adverse reactions include: Fatigue; headache; drowsiness; paresthesias; difficulty in micturition; diarrhea; reversible increases in serum transaminases; dyspnea; bronchospasm; asthenia; muscle cramps; nausea; vomiting; fever with aching and sore throat; toxic myopathy; rashes; systemic lupus erythematosus; vision abnormality; hypoesthesia; ventricular arrhythmias; intensification of AV block; mental depression; scalp tingling.

Administration and Dosage:

Oral: Initial dose - 100 mg twice daily, alone or added to a diuretic. After 2 or 3 days, using standing BP as an indicator, titrate dosage in increments of 100 mg twice daily, every 2 or 3 days.

Maintenance dose – 200 to 400 mg twice daily. Patients with severe hypertension may require 1.2 to 2.4 g/day. Should side effects (principally nausea or dizziness) occur with twice daily dosing, the same total daily dose given 3 times/day may improve tolerability. Titration increments should not exceed 200 mg twice/day.

Parenteral:

Repeated IV injection – Initially, 20 mg (0.25 mg/kg for an 80 kg patient) slowly over 2 minutes. Additional injections of 40 or 80 mg can be given at 10 minute intervals until a desired supine BP is achieved or a total of 300 mg has been injected. The maximum effect usually occurs within 5 minutes of each injection.

Slow continuous infusion – Give at a rate of 3 ml/min (2 mg/min). Continue infusion until satisfactory response is obtained; then discontinue infusion and start oral labetalol. Effective IV dose range is 50 to 200 mg, up to 300 mg.

Transfer to oral dosing (hospitalized patients): Begin oral dosing when supine diastolic BP begins to rise. Recommended initial dose is 200 mg, then 200 or 400 mg, 6 to 12 hours later, depending on BP response. Thereafter, proceed as follows:

Inpatient Titration Instructions

IV Regimen	Oral Daily Dose*
200 mg bid	400 mg
400 mg bid	800 mg
800 mg bid	1600 mg
1200 mg bid	2400 mg

* Total daily dose may be given in 3 divided doses.

CARVEDILOL

Tablets: 6.25, 12.5 and 25 mg (*Rx*)	*Coreg* (SmithKline Beecham)

Actions:

Pharmacology: Carvedilol, an antihypertensive agent, is a racemic mixture in which nonselective β-adrenoreceptor blocking activity is present in the S(-) enantiomer and α-adrenergic blocking activity is present in both R(+) and S(-) enantiomers at equal potency. Carvedilol has no intrinsic sympathomimetic activity.

Carvedilol (1) reduces cardiac output, (2) reduces exercise- or isoproterenol-induced tachycardia and (3) reduces reflex orthostatic tachycardia. Significant β-blocking effect is usually seen within 1 hour of drug administration. The mechanism by which β-blockade produces an antihypertensive effect has not been established.

Carvedilol also (1) attenuates the pressor effects of phenylephrine, (2) causes vasodilation and (3) reduces peripheral vascular resistance. These effects contribute to the reduction of blood pressure and usually are seen within 30 minutes of drug administration.

Pharmacokinetics:

Absorption/Distribution – Carvedilol is rapidly and extensively absorbed following oral administration, with absolute bioavailability of ≈ 25% to 35% due to a significant degree of first pass metabolism. Following oral administration, the apparent mean terminal elimination half-life generally ranges from 7 to 10 hours. Plasma concentrations achieved are proportional to the oral dose administered.

Carvedilol is > 98% bound to plasma proteins (primarily albumin). It has a steady-state volume of distribution of ≈ 115 L, indicating substantial distribution into extravascular tissues. Plasma clearance ranges from 500 to 700 ml/min.

Metabolism/Excretion – Carvedilol is extensively metabolized. Following oral administration in healthy volunteers, carvedilol accounted for only about 7% of the total in plasma as measured by area under the curve. Less than 2% of the dose was excreted unchanged in the urine. The metabolites of carvedilol are excreted primarily via the bile into the feces.

Indications:

Essential hypertension: Management of essential hypertension. It can be used alone or in combination with other antihypertensive agents, especially thiazide-type diuretics.

Unlabeled uses: Carvedilol appears to be beneficial in the treatment of the following conditions: Congestive heart failure (12.5 to 50 mg twice daily); angina pectoris (25 to 50 mg twice daily); idiopathic cardiomyopathy (6.25 to 25 mg twice daily).

Contraindications:

Patients with NYHA Class IV decompensated cardiac failure; bronchial asthma (two cases of death from status asthmaticus have been reported in patients receiving single doses of carvedilol) or related bronchospastic conditions; second- or third-degree AV block; cardiogenic shock; severe bradycardia; hypersensitivity to the drug.

Warnings:

Cardiac failure: Hypertensive patients who have CHF controlled with digitalis, diuretics or an angiotensin converting enzyme inhibitor should use carvedilol with caution. Both digitalis and carvedilol slow AV conduction.

Hepatic injury: Mild hepatocellular injury, confirmed by rechallenge, has occurred rarely with carvedilol therapy. At the first symptom/sign of liver dysfunction (eg, pruritus, dark urine, persistent anorexia, jaundice, right upper quadrant tenderness, unexplained flu-like symptoms) perform laboratory testing. If the patient has laboratory evidence of liver injury or jaundice, stop therapy and do not restart.

Peripheral vascular disease: β-blockers can precipitate or aggravate symptoms of arterial insufficiency in patients with peripheral vascular disease. Exercise caution in such individuals.

Anesthesia and major surgery: If carvedilol treatment is to be continued perioperatively, take particular care when anesthetic agents which depress myocardial function (eg, ether, cyclopropane, trichloroethylene) are used.

Diabetes and hypoglycemia: β-blockers may mask some of the manifestations of hypoglycemia, particularly tachycardia. Nonselective β-blockers may potentiate insulin-induced hypoglycemia and delay recovery of serum glucose levels. Caution patients subject to spontaneous hypoglycemia, or diabetic patients receiving insulin or oral hypoglycemic agents about these possibilities and use carvedilol with caution.

Thyrotoxicosis: β-adrenergic blockade may mask clinical signs of hyperthyroidism, such as tachycardia. Abrupt withdrawal of β-blockade may be followed by an exacerbation of the symptoms of hyperthyroidism or may precipitate thyroid storm.

Renal/Hepatic function impairment: Although carvedilol is metabolized primarily by the liver, plasma concentrations of carvedilol have been reported to be increased in patients with renal impairment. Based on mean AUC data, ≈ 40% to 50% higher plasma concentrations of carvedilol were observed in hypertensive patients with moderate to severe renal impairment compared to a control group of hypertensive patients with normal renal function. Changes in mean peak plasma levels were less pronounced, ≈ 12% to 26% higher in patients with impaired renal function. Consistent with its high degree of plasma protein-binding, carvedilol does not appear to be cleared significantly by hemodialysis.

Compared to healthy subjects, patients with cirrhotic liver disease exhibit significantly higher concentrations of carvedilol (≈ 4- to 7-fold) following single dose therapy. Use of carvedilol in patients with clinically manifest hepatic impairment is not recommended.

Elderly: Plasma levels of carvedilol average about 50% higher in the elderly compared to young subjects. With the exception of dizziness (8.8% in the elderly vs 6% in younger patients), there were no events for which the incidence in the elderly exceeded that in the younger population by > 2%.

Pregnancy: Category C.

Lactation: It is not known whether this drug is excreted in breast milk. Because of the potential for serious adverse reactions in nursing infants from β-blockers, especially bradycardia, decide whether to discontinue nursing or to discontinue the drug, taking into account the importance of the drug to the mother.

Children: Safety and efficacy in patients < 18 years of age have not been established.

Precautions:

Cardiovascular effects: Since carvedilol has β-blocking activity, it should not be discontinued abruptly, particularly in patients with ischemic heart disease. Instead, discontinue over 1 to 2 weeks.

In clinical trials, carvedilol caused bradycardia in about 2% of patients. If pulse rate drops below 55 beats/min, reduce the dosage.

Anaphylactic reaction: While taking β-blockers, patients with a history of severe anaphylactic reaction to a variety of allergens may be more reactive to repeated challenge, either accidental, diagnostic or therapeutic. Such patients may be unresponsive to the usual doses of epinephrine used to treat allergic reaction.

Bronchospasm, nonallergic (eg, chronic bronchitis, emphysema): In general, patients with bronchospastic disease should not receive β-blockers. Carvedilol may be used with caution, however, in patients who do not respond to, or cannot tolerate, other antihypertensive agents. It is prudent, if carvedilol is used, to use the smallest effective dose so that inhibition of endogenous or exogenous β-agonists is minimized.

Drug Interactions:

Drugs that may affect carvedilol include cimetidine and rifampin.

Drugs that may be affected by carvedilol include antidiabetic agents, calcium blockers, clonidine and digoxin.

Drug/Food interactions: When taken with food, rate of absorption is slowed but extent of bioavailability is not affected. Taking with food minimizes the risk of orthostatic hypotension.

Adverse Reactions:

Adverse reactions may include: Dizziness; fatigue; chest pain; dyspepsia; headache; nausea; pain; sinusitis; upper respiratory tract infection.

Administration and Dosage:

The recommended starting dose is 6.25 mg twice daily. If this dose is tolerated, using standing systolic pressure measured about 1 hour after dosing as a guide, maintain the dose for 7 to 14 days, and then increase to 12.5 mg twice daily, if needed, based on trough blood pressure, again using standing systolic pressure 1 hour after dosing as a guide for tolerance. This dose should also be maintained for 7 to 14 days and can then be adjusted upward to 25 mg twice daily if tolerated and needed. The full antihypertensive effect of carvedilol is seen within 7 to 14 days. Total daily dose should not exceed 50 mg. Carvedilol should be taken with food to slow the rate of absorption and reduce the incidence of orthostatic effects.

Addition of a diuretic to carvedilol or carvedilol to a diuretic can be expected to produce additive effects and exaggerate the orthostatic component of carvedilol action.

ANTIHYPERTENSIVES

Agents used in hypertension therapy are listed in the following tables:

Pharmacological Effects of Antihypertensive Agents

↑ = increase ⇧ = slight increases 0 = no change ⇩ = slight decrease ↓ = decrease	Onset (min)	Peak effect[1] (hrs)	Duration of action[2] (hrs)	Plasma volume	Plasma renin activity	RBF GFR[3]	Peripheral resistance	Cardiac output	Heart rate	LVH	Total cholesterol	HDL	LDL	Triglycerides
Antiadrenergic Agents – Centrally Acting														
Methyldopa	120	2-6	12-24	↑	⇩/0	⇩/0	↓	⇩/0	⇩/0	↓	0	0	0	0
Clonidine	30-60	2-5	12-24	↑	⇩	⇩/0	↓	⇩/0	↓	↓	0	0	0	0
Guanabenz	60	2-4	6-12	0	↓	0	↓	0	↓	↓	0	0	0	0
Guanfacine		1-4	24	⇩/0	↓		↓	0	⇩	↓	0	0	0	0
Antiadrenergic Agents – Peripherally Acting														
Reserpine	days	6-12	6-24	↑	⇩/0	⇩/0	↑	0/↓	↑					
Guanethidine		6-8	24-48	↑	⇩/0	⇩/0	↓	0/↓	↑					
Guanadrel	30-120	4-6	9-14	↑		0	↑	0	↓					
Doxazosin		2-3								↓	↓	↑	0/↓	↓
Prazosin	120-130	1-3	6-12	0/⇧	⇩/0	0	↓	0/⇧	0/⇧	↓	↓	↑	0/↑	↓
Terazosin	15	1-2	12-24	0	0	0	↑	⇧	⇧	↓	↓	↑	0/↓	↓
Antiadrenergic Agents – Beta-Adrenergic Blockers														
Acebutolol		3-8	24 30				⇩	↓	↓	0/↓	0/↑	↓	↑	0/↑
Atenolol		2-4	24 +	⇩/0	↓	↓/0	0	↓	↓	↓	0/↑	↓	↑	0/↑
Betaxolol								↓	↓		0/↑	↓	↑	0/↑
Bisoprolol								↓	↓		0			0
Carteolol		1-3	24 +					↓	↓		0			0
Metoprolol		1.5	13-19	⇩/0	↓	⇩/0	0/↓	↓	↓	↓	0/↑	↓	↑	0/↑
Nadolol		3-4	17-24	⇩/0	↓	0	0	↓	↓	↓	0/↑	↓	↑	0/↑
Penbutolol		1.5-3	20 +		↓	⇩	0	↓	↓		0	0/↑	0	↑/↓
Pindolol		1	24 +		0	0	↓	⇩	↓	0/↓	0	0/↑	0	↑/↓
Propranolol		2-4	8-12	⇩/0	↓	↓	⇩/0	↓	↓	↓	0	0/↑	0	↑/↓
Timolol		1-3	12	⇩/0	↓		0	↓	↓	↓	0	0/↑	0	↑/↓
Antiadrenergic Agents – Alpha/Beta-Adrenergic Blocker														
Labetalol		2-4	8-12	↑	↓	0/↑	↓	0	↓	↓				
Carvedilol	30						↓	↓	↓					
Angiotensin Converting Enzyme (ACE) Inhibitors														
Benazepril	60	0.5-1	24		↑	RBF ↑ GFR 0	↓	0/↑	0	↓	0	0	0	0
Captopril	15-30	0.5-1.5	6-12	⇧	↑	RBF ↑ GFR 0	↓	0/↑	0	↓	0	0	0	0
Enalapril	60	4-6	24	0/⇧	↑	RBF ↑ GFR 0	↓	↑	0	↓	0	0	0	0
Enalaprilat	15	3-4	≈ 6		↑	RBF ↑ GFR 0	↓	↑	0	↓	0	0	0	0
Fosinopril	60	≈ 3	24		↑	RBF ↑ GFR 0	↓	0/↑	0	↓	0	0	0	0
Lisinopril	60	≈ 7	24		↑	RBF ↑ GFR 0	↓	0	0	↓	0	0	0	0
Quinapril	60	1	24		↑	RBF ↑ GFR 0	↓	0/↑	0	↓	0	0	0	0
Ramipril	60-120	1	24		↑	RBF ↑ GFR 0	↓	0/↑	0	↓	0	0	0	0
Calcium Channel Blocking Agents														
Amlodipine	gradual	6-12	> 24	0	0	↑	↓↓↓	0	0	↓	0	0	0	0
Diltiazem SR	30-60	6-11					↓	0-↑	↓-0	↓	0	0	0	0
Felodipine	120-300	2.5-5					↓↓↓	↑	↑	↓	0	0	0	0

Pharmacological Effects of Antihypertensive Agents

↑ = increase ⇧ = slight increases 0 = no change ⇩ = slight decrease ↓ = decrease	Onset (min)	Peak effect[1] (hrs)	Duration of action[2] (hrs)	Plasma volume	Plasma renin activity	RBF GFR[3]	Peripheral resistance	Cardiac output	Heart rate	LVH	Total cholesterol	HDL	LDL	Triglycerides
Isradipine	120	1.5					↓↓↓	↑	↑/↓	↓	0	0	0	0
Nicardipine	20	0.5-2			⇧/↑	⇧	↓	↑	↑	↓	0	0/⇧	0	0
Nifedipine SR	20	6					↓↓↓	↑↑	↑	↓	0	0	0	0
Verapamil	30	1-2.2			0/⇧	0	↓	↑/↓	↑/↓	↓	0	0/⇧	0	0
Diuretics														
Thiazides & deriv.	60-120	4-12	6-72	↓	↑	↓	↓	↓	0	0/??	↑	0	↑	↑
Loop diuretics	within 60	1-2	4-8	↓	↑	↓	↓	↓	0	0/??	↑	0	↑	↑
Amiloride	120	6-10	24	↓	↑	0	↓	↓	0					
Spironolactone	24-48 hr	48-72	48-72	↓	↑	0	↓	0	0					
Triamterene	2-4 hr	6-8	12-16											
Vasodilators														
Hydralazine	45	0.5-2	6-8	↑	↑	↑	↓	↑	↑	↑				
Minoxidil	30	2-3	24-72	↑	↑	0	↓	↑	↑	↑				
Agents For Hypertensive Emergencies/Urgencies														
Phentolamine	immed.		5-10 min	⇧	↑	↑	↓	0/↑	↑					
Phenoxybenzamine	gradual	2-3	24 +	⇧	↑	↑	↓	↑	↓					
Metyrosine		6 +	2-3 days				↓		↓					
Agents For Pheochromocytoma														
Nitroprusside	0.5-1		3-5 min	↑	↑	0	↓	⇩	⇧		NA			
Diazoxide	1-2	5 min	< 12	↑	↑	↑	↓	↑	↑					
Trimethaphan camsylate	1-2		10-15 min	↑	↓	0	↓	↓	↓					
Nitroglycerin (IV)	immed.		transient	0	0		↓	↑	↑					
Captopril[4]				⇧	↑	RBF ↑ GFR 0	↓	0/↑	0					
Enalaprilat[4]					↑	RBF ↑ GFR 0	↓	↑	0					
Hydralazine[4]	10-20		3-6											
Labetalol[4]	5-10		3-6	↑	↓	0/↑	↓	0	↓					
Nicardipine[4]	1-5		3-6		⇧/↑	⇧	↓	↑	↑					
Nifedipine[4]							↓↓↓	↑↑	↑					
Phentolamine[4]	1-2		3-10 min											
Miscellaneous Agents														
Mecamylamine	30-120		6-12+	↑	↓	↓	↓	↓	↑					
Pargyline		4-21 days	3 weeks			↓	↓	0	0					
Tolazoline							↓							

[1] Peak clinical effect following a single oral dose, except where indicated.
[2] Duration of action is frequently dose-dependent.
[3] Renal blood flow and glomerular filtration rate.
[4] Unlabeled use.
[5] NA = Not applicable.

Stepped-Care Antihypertensive Regimen†: Experience in treating essential hypertension (systolic blood pressure [BP] ≥ 140 mmHg and/or diastolic BP ≥ 90 mmHg) demonstrates the benefits of pharmacotherapy. Reducing BP decreases cardiovascular mortality and morbidity in patients with hypertension. Antihypertensive therapy protects against stroke, left ventricular hypertrophy, congestive heart failure and progression to more severe hypertension. In addition to drug therapy, lifestyle modifications of adjunctive value include weight reduction, sodium and alcohol restriction, smoking cessation, regular exercise and a diet low in saturated fat.

Hypertension Categories

Range (mmHg)		
Systolic	Diastolic	Category[1]
< 130	< 85	Normal BP
130-139	85-89	High normal BP
140-159	90-99	Stage 1 (mild) hypertension
160-179	100-109	Stage 2 (moderate) hypertension
180-209	110-119	Stage 3 (severe) hypertension
≥ 210	≥ 120	Stage 4 (very severe) hypertension

[1] When systolic and diastolic BP fall into different categories, select the higher category to classify the patient's BP (eg, classify 165/95 mmHg as Stage 2, 170/115 mmHg as Stage 3). Isolated systolic hypertension is systolic BP ≥ 140 mmHg and diastolic BP < 90 mmHg (stage appropriately).

For purposes of risk classification and management, specify presence or absence of target-organ disease and additional risk factors in addition to classifying hypertension stages. For example, classify a diabetic patient with Stage 3 hypertension and left ventricular hypertrophy as "Stage 3 hypertension with target-organ disease (left ventricular hypertrophy) and with one additional risk factor (diabetes)."

The *stepped-care approach* begins with lifestyle modifications. If BP remains ≥ 140/90 mmHg for 3 to 6 months, start antihypertensive therapy, especially in patients with target-organ disease or other risk factors for cardiovascular disease. Initiate therapy with one agent, increase the dosage gradually, then add or substitute agents with gradual increases in doses until the therapeutic goal is achieved, side effects become intolerable or maximum dosages are reached. Try lifestyle modifications first.

† The Fifth-Report of the Joint National Committee on Detection, Evaluation, and Treatment of High Blood Pressure. *Arch Intern Med* 1993;153:154-83.

Stepped-Care Approach		
I. Lifestyle modifications	Weight reduction Moderation of alcohol intake Regular physicial activity	Reduction of sodium intake Smoking cessation
II. Inadequate response	Continue lifestyle modifications Initial pharmacological selection[1] 1) Diuretics or beta blockers[2] 2) ACE inhibitors, calcium blockers, alpha$_1$-blockers, alpha-beta blocker[3]	
III. Inadequate response	1) Increase drug dose, or; 2) Substitute another drug, or; 3) Add a second agent from a different class.[4]	
IV. Inadequate response	Add a second or third agent or diuretic if not already prescribed.[4]	

[1] Initial drug therapy is monotherapy for Stage 1 and Stage 2 hypertension.
[2] Preferred because a reduction in morbidity and mortality has been demonstrated.
[3] Equally effective in reducing BP; however, these have not been tested in long-term controlled trials to demonstrate reduction of morbidity and mortality. Reserve for special indications or when preferred agents are unacceptable or ineffective.
[4] Supplemental antihypertensive agents, which include centrally acting alpha$_2$-agonists (clonidine, guanabenz, guanfacine, methyldopa), peripheral-acting adrenergic antagonists (guanadrel, guanethidine, rauwolfia alkaloids) and direct vasodilators (hydralazine, minoxidil), are not routinely well suited for initial monotherapy.

Diuretics: Generally initiate therapy with a thiazide or other oral diuretic. Thiazide-type diuretics are drugs of choice; hydrochlorothiazide or chlorthalidone are generally preferred. Reserve loop diuretics for selected patients. This therapy alone may control many cases of mild hypertension. Diuretics exert an indirect antihypertensive effect by decreasing vascular tone as well as increasing sodium and water excretion. Black people are generally more responsive to diuretics, and these agents are effective in older patients as well. Diuretics are also added or substituted as therapy when blood pressure response to another agent is inadequate. Consider treating diuretic-induced hypokalemia (< 3.5 mEq/L) with potassium supplementation or by adding a potassium-sparing diuretic to therapy.

Beta-adrenergic blocking agents may also be used as initial drug monotherapy. Beta blockers are effective in older patients, but less effective in black people. Beta-adrenergic blocking agents decrease cardiac output without effects on vascular resistance. In addition, they inhibit renin release.

Calcium channel blockers, ACE inhibitors, labetalol and alpha$_1$-blockers may be used as initial monotherapy, although they are not routinely preferred over diuretics and beta blockers. Black people tend to respond better to calcium blockers than ACE inhibitors; labetalol may be more effective in black people than other beta blockers.

Antiadrenergic agents (central and peripheral adrenergic inhibitors) are considered supplemental agents and are used when the initial drug therapy fails to achieve the desired effect. Diuretics are usually continued to provide synergistic effects and to prevent secondary fluid accumulation that may occur with use of antiadrenergic agents alone. Combination therapy may also minimize untoward reactions which are more common at the higher doses necessary when a single drug is used alone.

Decreased adrenergic tone results in reduced cardiac output or decreased peripheral vascular resistance. Methyldopa, guanabenz, guanfacine and clonidine act mainly in the CNS. Although reserpine has been used for years, other agents are preferred. Guanadrel is a peripheral antiadrenergic similar to guanethidine.

Vasodilators are also considered supplemental agents and are not suited for initial monotherapy. A three drug regimen should include agents acting by different mechanisms. Hydralazine and minoxidil have direct vasodilating actions. In order to prevent reflex tachycardia caused by decreased peripheral resistance, these agents are most effective when used with a diuretic and a β-blocker. Minoxidil's undesirable side effects limit its use to severely hypertensive patients who do not respond to minimum doses of a diuretic and two other agents.

Antihypertensive drug withdrawal syndrome may occur after discontinuation of antihypertensives. Patients may experience symptoms associated with catecholamine excess, with or without a rapid rise in blood pressure, including nervousness, agitation, tremors, palpitations, insomnia, headache, sweating, flushing, nausea and vomiting; rarely, malignant hypertension, angina, myocardial infarction and cardiac arrhythmias occur. Most often reported with clonidine, the syndrome also occurs with other agents including centrally acting, peripherally acting and β-blocking drugs. The typical patient is young, has severe hypertension and is taking multiple drugs in high doses for prolonged periods.

To circumvent problems, encourage patient compliance, avoid excessive doses, avoid combining sympatholytics and β-blockers and maintain antihypertensive medication in surgical patients. When discontinuing medication, taper the dose slowly, one drug at a time; use special caution in patients with coronary artery or cerebrovascular disease.

Treatment generally includes reinstitution of therapy, bed rest/sedation and, perhaps, therapy similar to treatment of malignant hypertension.

Step-down therapy: Attempt to decrease the dosage or the number of antihypertensive agents in patients; have them maintain lifestyle modifications. It may be possible to accomplish this in a deliberate, slow, progressive manner if the patient has been effectively controlled for one year and at least four visits.

Patient Information: Consider compliance to weight reduction, sodium and alcohol restriction, discontinuation of smoking, regular exercise and behavior modification.

Do not discontinue medication unless directed by physician; do not stop abruptly.

Avoid cough, cold or allergy medications containing sympathomimetics.

If dizziness (orthostatic hypotension) occurs, avoid sudden changes in posture. Taking a hot bath or shower may aggravate the dizziness.

Many of these medications may cause drowsiness, especially during the first days of therapy or when dose is increased. Observe caution while driving or performing other tasks requiring alertness, coordination or physical dexterity.

If dehydration occurs due to nausea, vomiting, diarrhea, etc., the hypotensive effect may be increased. If this occurs, contact the physician; a lower dose may be necessary.

METHYLDOPA AND METHYLDOPATE HCl

Tablets: 125 mg, 250 mg, 500 mg methyldopa (*Rx*)	Various, *Aldomet* (Merck)
Oral Suspension: 250 mg methyldopa/5 ml (*Rx*)	Various, *Aldomet* (Merck)
Injection: 250 mg methyldopate HCl/5 ml (*Rx*)	Various, *Aldomet* (Merck)

Actions:

Pharmacology: The mechanism of action of methyldopa has not been conclusively demonstrated, but is probably due to the drug's metabolism to alpha-methyl norepinephrine, which lowers arterial pressure by the stimulation of central inhibitory α-adrenergic receptors, false neurotransmission or reduction of plasma renin activity. Methyldopa reduces blood pressure. It usually produces highly effective lowering of supine pressure with infrequent symptomatic postural hypotension. Methyldopate HCl, the ethyl ester of methyldopa HCl, is pharmacologically equal.

Pharmacokinetics:

Absorption/Distribution – Oral absorption of methyldopa is variable (range 8% to 62%); peak plasma levels are achieved in 2 to 4 hours. There is no correlation between plasma concentration and antihypertensive effect. Approximately 2 days are required to establish maximal antihypertensive effects and for hypertension to return after discontinuation of therapy. Effective IV doses cause a decline in blood pressure which may begin in 4 to 6 hours and last 10 to 16 hours.

Metabolism – The elimination half-life is ≈ 2 hours; however, antihypertensive activity persists for up to 24 hours. The main metabolite, an inactive O-sulfate conjugate, is formed in intestinal cells. Approximately 70% of the drug which is absorbed is excreted in the urine as methyldopa and its mono-O-sulfate conjugate. The renal clearance is diminished in renal insufficiency. The plasma half-life of methyldopa is 105 minutes. After oral doses, excretion is essentially complete in 36 hours. Blood pressure reduction is pronounced and prolonged in renal failure. The drug is removed by dialysis.

Indications:

Hypertension.

Methyldopate HCl may be used to initiate treatment of acute hypertensive crises; however, due to its slow onset of action, other agents may be preferred for rapid reduction of blood pressure.

Contraindications:

Active hepatic disease, such as acute hepatitis or active cirrhosis; if previous methyldopa therapy has been associated with liver disorders; hypersensitivity to any component of these formulations.

Warnings:

Positive Coombs' test/hemolytic anemia: With prolonged therapy, 10% to 20% of patients develop a positive direct Coombs' test, usually between 6 and 12 months of therapy. This is associated rarely with hemolytic anemia, which could lead to potentially fatal complications and is difficult to predict. If a positive direct Coombs' test develops during therapy, determine whether hemolytic anemia exists and whether the positive Coombs' test may be a problem. Perform baseline and periodic blood counts to detect hemolytic anemia. A direct Coombs' test may be useful before therapy and at 6 and 12 months later. If Coombs'-positive hemolytic anemia occurs, discontinue methyldopa; anemia usually remits promptly. If not, give corticosteroids and consider other causes. If hemolytic anemia is related to methyldopa, do not reinstitute. The positive Coombs' test may not revert to normal until weeks to months after methyldopa is stopped.

Liver disorders: Fever has occasionally occurred within the first 3 weeks of therapy, sometimes associated with eosinophilia or abnormalities in one or more liver function tests. Jaundice with or without fever may occur, usually within the first 2 to 3 months of therapy. In some patients, the findings are consistent with cholestasis. Fatal hepatic necrosis has been reported rarely. Incidence of elevated serum transaminase levels and impaired hepatic function ranges from 1% to 27%.

Perform periodic determinations of hepatic function, particularly during the first 6 to 12 weeks of therapy or when an unexplained fever occurs. If fever, abnormalities in liver function tests or jaundice appear, discontinue therapy; temperature and abnormalities in liver function revert to normal when the drug is discontinued. Do not reinstitute methyldopa therapy in such patients.

Hematologic disorders: Rarely, a reversible reduction of the white blood cell (WBC) count with a primary effect on granulocytes has been seen.

Renal function impairment: The active metabolites of methyldopa accumulate in uremia. Use with caution in renal failure. Prolonged hypotension has been reported.

Hypertension has recurred occasionally after dialysis in patients given methyldopa because the drug is removed by this procedure.

Hepatic function impairment: Use with caution in patients with previous liver disease or dysfunction.

Pregnancy: Category B.

Lactation: Methyldopa is excreted in breast milk, with a reported milk:plasma ratio of 1. The possibility of effects on the nursing infant cannot be excluded.

Precautions:

Paradoxical pressor response has been reported with IV methyldopa.

Involuntary choreoathetotic movements have been observed rarely in patients with severe bilateral cerebrovascular disease. Should these occur, discontinue methyldopa therapy.

Sedation, usually transient, may occur during initial therapy or whenever the dose is increased; patients should observe caution while performing tasks requiring alertness during these periods.

Urine discoloration: Rarely, when urine is exposed to air, it may darken because of breakdown of methyldopa or its metabolites.

Sulfite sensitivity: These products contain sulfites that may cause allergic-type reactions in certain susceptible persons. Sulfite sensitivity is seen more frequently in asthmatic or atopic nonasthmatic persons.

Drug Interactions:

Drugs that may affect methyldopa include haloperidol, levodopa, lithium, propranolol.

Drugs that may be affected by methyldopa include haloperidol, levodopa, lithium, sympathomimetics and tolbutamide.

Drug/Lab test interactions: Methyldopa may interfere with tests for: **Urinary uric acid**by phosphotungstate method; **serum creatinine**by alkaline picrate method; **AST** by colorimetric methods. Since methyldopa causes fluorescence in urine samples at the same wavelengths as catecholamines, falsely high levels of **urinary catecholamines**-may occur and will interfere with the diagnosis of pheochromocytoma.

Adverse Reactions:

Possible adverse reactions include fever; lupus-like syndrome; rise in BUN; myalgia; septic shock-like syndrome; headache; asthenia; weakness; dizziness; symptoms of cerebrovascular insufficiency; paresthesias; parkinsonism; Bell's palsy; decreased mental acuity; involuntary choreoathetotic movements; psychic disturbances; verbal memory impairment; bradycardia; prolonged carotid sinus hypersensitivity; aggravation of angina pectoris; pericarditis; myocarditis (fatal); orthostatic hypotension; edema/weight gain (usually relieved by a diuretic; discontinue methyldopa if edema progresses or signs of heart failure appear); nausea; vomiting; constipation; diarrhea; colitis; sore or "black" tongue; pancreatitis; liver disorders; Positive Coombs' test, bone marrow depression; leukopenia; granulocytopenia; thrombocytopenia; positive tests for antinuclear antibody, LE cells and rheumatoid factor; rash; toxic epidermal necrolysis; gynecomastia; lactation; amenorrhea.

Administration and Dosage:

Impaired renal function: Methyldopa is largely excreted by the kidneys; patients with impaired renal function may respond to smaller doses.

Elderly: Syncope in older patients may be related to an increased sensitivity and advanced arteriosclerotic vascular disease. May be avoided by lower doses.

Adults: Initial therapy: 250 mg, 2 or 3 times a day in the first 48 hours. Adjust dosage at intervals of not less than 2 days until adequate response is achieved. To minimize sedation, increase dosage in the evening. By adjustment of dosage, morning hypotension may be prevented without sacrificing control of afternoon blood pressure.

Maintenance therapy – 500 mg to 3 g daily in 2 to 4 doses. Methyldopa is usually administered in 2 divided doses; some patients may be controlled with a single daily dose given at bedtime.

Concomitant drug therapy – When methyldopa is given with antihypertensives other than thiazides, limit the initial dosage to 500 mg/day in divided doses; when added to a thiazide, the dosage of thiazide need not be changed.

Children: Individualize dosage. Initial oral dosage is based on 10 mg/kg/day in 2 to 4 doses. The maximum daily dosage is 65 mg/kg or 3 g, whichever is less.

Tolerance may occur, usually between the second and third month of therapy. Adding a diuretic or increasing the dosage of methyldopa frequently restores blood pressure control. A thiazide is recommended if therapy was not started with a thiazide or if effective control of blood pressure cannot be maintained on 2 g methyldopa daily.

Discontinuation: Methyldopa has a relatively short duration of action; therefore, withdrawal is followed by return of hypertension, usually within 48 hours. This is not complicated by an overshoot of blood pressure above pretreatment levels.

IV: Add dose to 100 ml of 5% Dextrose or give in 5% Dextrose in Water in a concentration of 10 mg/ml. Administer over 30 to 60 minutes. When control has been obtained, substitute oral therapy starting with the same parenteral dosage schedule.

Adults – 250 to 500 mg every 6 hours as required (maximum 1 g every 6 hours).

Children – 20 to 40 mg/kg/day in divided doses every 6 hours. The maximum daily dosage is 65 mg/kg or 3 g, whichever is less.

CLONIDINE HCl

Tablets: 0.1 mg, 0.2 mg, 0.3 mg (*Rx*)	Various, *Catapres* (Boehringer-Ingelheim)
Transdermal system: 2.5 mg (release rate 0.1 mg/24 hrs) (*Rx*)	*Catapres-TTS-1* (Boehringer-Ingelheim)
Transdermal system: 5 mg (release rate 0.2 mg/24 hrs) (*Rx*)	*Catapres-TTS-2* (Boehringer-Ingelheim)
Transdermal system: 7.5 mg (release rate 0.2 mg/24 hrs) (*Rx*)	*Catapres-TTS-3* (Boehringer-Ingelheim)

Actions:

Pharmacology: Initially, clonidine stimulates peripheral α-adrenergic receptors producing transient vasoconstriction. Stimulation of alpha-adrenergic in the brain stem results in reduced sympathetic outflow from the CNS and a decrease in peripheral resistance, renal vascular resistance, heart rate and blood pressure.

Orthostatic effects are mild and infrequent since supine pressure is reduced to essentially the same extent as standing pressure. The coadministration of a diuretic enhances antihypertensive efficacy of clonidine.

Plasma renin activity and excretion of aldosterone and catecholamines is reduced.

Pharmacokinetics: Blood pressure declines within 30 to 60 minutes after an oral dose. The peak plasma level occurs in ≈ 3 to 5 hours with a plasma half-life of 12 to 16 hours. About 50% of the absorbed dose is metabolized in the liver. In patients with impaired renal function, half-life increases to 30 to 40 hours. Clonidine and its metabolites are excreted mainly in the urine. About 40% to 60% of the absorbed dose is recovered in the urine as unchanged drug in 24 hours.

Transdermal System – The system, a 0.2 mm thick film with four layers, contains a drug reservoir of clonidine, released at an approximately constant rate for 7 days.

Therapeutic plasma levels, achieved 2 to 3 days after initial application, are lower than during oral therapy with equipotent doses. When system is removed, therapeutic plasma clonidine levels persist for ≈ 8 hours and then decline slowly over several days; blood pressure returns gradually to pretreatment levels. Elimination half-life is ≈ 19 hours.

Indications:

Hypertension.

Unlabeled uses: Clonidine has been evaluated for use in the following conditions:

Clonidine Unlabeled Uses

Use	Dosage[1]
Alcohol withdrawal	0.3 to 0.6 mg every 6 hours
Constitutional growth delay in children	0.0375 to 0.15 mg/m²/day
Diabetic diarrhea	0.15 to 1.2 mg/day or 0.3 mg/ 24 hr patch (1 to 2 patches/week)
Gilles de la Tourette syndrome	0.15 to 0.2 mg/day
Hypertensive "urgencies" (diastolic > 120 mmHg)	initially 0.1 to 0.2 mg, followed by 0.05 to 0.1 mg every hour to a maximum of 0.8 mg
Menopausal flushing	0.1 to 0.4 mg/day or 0.1 mg/24 hr patch
Methadone/opiate detoxification	15 to 16 mcg/kg/day

Clonidine Unlabeled Uses	
Use	Dosage[1]
Pheochromocytoma diagnosis (overnight clonidine suppression test)	0.3 mg
Postherpetic neuralgia	0.2 mg/day
Reduction of allergen-induced inflammatory reactions in patients with extrinsic asthma	0.15 mg for 3 days
Smoking cessation facilitation	0.15 to 0.4 mg/day or 0.2 mg/24 hour patch
Ulcerative colitis	0.3 mg 3 times a day

[1] Dosage given as oral unless otherwise specified.

Contraindications:

Hypersensitivity to clonidine or any component of adhesive layer of transdermal system.

Warnings:

Use with caution in patients with severe coronary insufficiency, recent myocardial infarction (MI), cerebrovascular disease or chronic renal failure.

Tolerance may develop, necessitating a reevaluation of therapy.

Pregnancy: Category C.

Lactation: Clonidine is excreted in breast milk; following a 0.15 mg oral dose, milk concentrations of 1.5 ng/ml may be achieved (milk-plasma ratio 1.5).

Children: Safety and efficacy for use in children have not been established.

Precautions:

Rebound hypertension: Do not discontinue therapy without consulting a physician. Discontinue therapy by reducing the dose gradually over 2 to 4 days to avoid a rapid rise in blood pressure. Abrupt withdrawal of clonidine may result in subjective symptoms such as nervousness, agitation, headache and elevated catecholamine concentrations in the plasma, but such occurrences have usually been associated with previous administration of high oral doses (> 1.2 mg/day) or with continuation of concomitant β-blocker therapy. Tachycardia, rebound hypertension, flushing, nausea, vomiting and cardiac arrhythmias have also occurred. The risk may be dose-related, and the risk may be increased with multiple drug therapy.

If an excessive rise in blood pressure occurs, it can be reversed by resumption of therapy or by IV phentolamine, phenoxybenzamine or prazosin. Direct vasodilators and captopril have also been used. If therapy is to be discontinued in patients receiving β-blockers and clonidine concurrently, β-blockers should be discontinued several days before the gradual withdrawal of clonidine.

Rebound hypertension has also occurred following discontinuation of the transdermal patch.

Ophthalmologic effects: Perform periodic eye examinations, since retinal degeneration has been noted in animal studies.

Perioperative use: Continue administration of clonidine to within 4 hours of surgery and resume as soon as possible thereafter. Carefully monitor blood pressure and institute appropriate measures to control it. If transdermal therapy is started during the perioperative period, note that therapeutic plasma levels are not achieved until 2 to 3 days after initial application.

Sensitization to transdermal clonidine: In patients who develop an allergic reaction to transdermal clonidine, oral clonidine HCl substitution may elicit a similar reaction.

Drug Interactions:

Drugs that may interact with clonidine include beta-adrenergic blocking agents and tricyclic antidepressants.

Adverse Reactions:

Oral: Adverse reactions may include: Dry mouth; drowsiness; dizziness; sedation; constipation; anorexia; malaise; nausea and vomiting; parotid pain; mild transient abnormalities in liver function tests; gynecomastia; congestive heart failure; orthostatic symptoms; palpitations, tachycardia and bradycardia; Raynaud's phenomenon; ECG abnormalities; conduction disturbances, arrhythmias, sinus bradycardia; dreams or nightmares; insomnia; hallucinations; delirium; nervousness; anxiety; depression; headache; rash, angioneurotic edema, hives, urticaria; hair thinning and alopecia; pruritus; impotence; decreased sexual activity; difficulty in micturition; weakness; muscle or joint pain; increased sensitivity to alcohol; dryness, itching or burning of the eyes; dryness of the nasal mucosa; pallor; fever; weakly positive Coombs' test.

Transdermal system: Adverse reactions may include: Dry mouth, drowsiness (the most frequent systemic reactions); constipation; nausea; change in taste; fatigue; headache; sedation; insomnia; nervousness; dizziness; impotence/sexual dysfunction; transient localized skin reactions; hyperpigmentation; edema; excoriation; burning; papules; throbbing; generalized macular rash.

Administration and Dosage:

Oral: Individualize dosage.

Initial dose – 0.1 mg twice daily. The elderly may benefit from a lower initial dose.

Maintenance dose – Increments of 0.1 or 0.2 mg/day may be made until desired response is achieved; most common range is 0.2 to 0.8 mg/day given in divided doses. The maximum dose is 2.4 mg/day. Minimize sedative effects by slowly increasing the daily dosage and giving the majority of the daily dose at bedtime.

Children – 5 to 25 mcg/kg/day in divided doses every 6 hours; increase at 5 to 7 day intervals.

Unlabeled route of administration – Sublingual clonidine, using a dosage of 0.2 to 0.4 mg/day, may be effective in hypertensive patients unable to take oral medication. The onset occurs within 30 to 60 minutes and blood pressure appears to be maintained on a twice daily regimen.

Renal Impairment – Adjust dosage according to degree of renal impairment and carefully monitor patients. Since only a minimal amount of clonidine is removed during hemodialysis, there is no need to give supplemental clonidine following dialysis.

Transdermal: Apply to a hairless area of intact skin on upper arm or torso, once every 7 days. Use a different skin site from the previous application. If the system loosens during the 7 day wearing, apply the adhesive overlay directly over the system to ensure good adhesion.

For initial therapy, start with the 0.1 mg system. If, after 1 or 2 weeks, desired blood pressure reduction is not achieved, add another 0.1 mg system or use a larger system. Dosage > two 0.3 mg systems usually does not improve efficacy. Note that the antihypertensive effect of the system may not commence until 2 to 3 days after application. Therefore, when substituting the transdermal system in patients on prior antihypertensive therapy, a gradual reduction of prior drug dosage is advised. Previous antihypertensive treatment may have to be continued, particularly in patients with severe hypertension.

GUANFACINE HCl

Tablets: 1 mg, 2 mg (*Rx*)	*Tenex* (Robins)

Actions:

Pharmacology: Guanfacine is a centrally acting oral antihypertensive with α_2-adrenoreceptor agonist properties. Guanfacine reduces sympathetic nerve impulses from the vasomotor center to the heart and blood vessels, resulting in a decrease in peripheral vascular resistance and a reduction in heart rate.

Hemodynamics – The decrease in blood pressure observed after single dose or long-term oral treatment with guanfacine was accompanied by a significant decrease in peripheral resistance and a slight reduction in heart rate (5 bpm).

Pharmacokinetics:

Absorption/Distribution – Relative to a 3 mg IV dose, the absolute oral bioavailability of guanfacine is about 80%. Peak plasma concentrations occur from 1 to 4 hours with an average of 2.6 hours after single oral doses or at steady state. The area under the concentration time-curve increases linearly with the dose. The drug is ≈ 70% bound to plasma proteins, independent of drug concentration. The whole body volume of distribution is high (mean, 6.3 L/kg).

Metabolism/Excretion – In individuals with normal renal function, the average elimination half-life is ≈ 17 hours (range, 10 to 30 hours). Younger patients tend to have shorter elimination half-lives (13 to 14 hours) while older patients tend to have half-lives at the upper end of the range. Steady-state blood levels were attained within 4 days in most subjects. Approximately 50% (40% to 75%) of the dose is eliminated in the urine as unchanged drug; the remainder is eliminated mostly as conjugates of metabolites produced by oxidative metabolism of the aromatic ring. The guanfacine to creatinine clearance ratio is > 1, suggesting that tubular secretion of drug occurs.

Indications:

Hypertension: Management of hypertension, alone or in combination with other antihypertensives, especially thiazide-type diuretics.

Unlabeled uses: Guanfacine (0.03 to 1.5 mg/day) may be beneficial in ameliorating withdrawal symptoms in patients discontinuing heroin usage.

In a small study, guanfacine (1 mg/day for 12 weeks) significantly reduced the frequency of migraine headache and reduced nausea and vomiting.

Contraindications:

Hypersensitivity to guanfacine.

Warnings:

Renal function impairment: Guanfacine clearance in patients with renal insufficiency is reduced, but drug plasma levels are only slightly increased compared to patients with normal renal function. Use the low end of the dosing range in patients with renal impairment. Patients on dialysis can be given usual doses of guanfacine.

Pregnancy: *Category B.*

Labor and delivery – Not recommended in the treatment of acute hypertension associated with toxemia of pregnancy.

Lactation: It is not known whether guanfacine is excreted in human breast milk. Use caution when administering to a nursing mother.

Children: Safety and efficacy in children < 12 years of age have not been demonstrated. Use in this age group is not recommended.

Precautions:

Special risk patients: Use guanfacine with caution in patients with severe coronary insufficiency, recent myocardial infarction, cerebrovascular disease or chronic renal or hepatic failure.

Sedation: Like other centrally active oral α_2-adrenergic agonists, guanfacine causes dose-related sedation or drowsiness, especially when beginning therapy. When used with other centrally active depressants, consider potential for additive sedative effects.

Rebound: Abrupt cessation of therapy with centrally active oral α_2-adrenergic agonists may be associated with increases in plasma and urinary catecholamines, symptoms of nervousness and anxiety and, less commonly, increases in blood pressure to levels significantly greater than those prior to therapy.

The frequency of rebound hypertension is low, but when rebound occurs, it does so after 2 to 4 days, which is delayed compared with clonidine. This is consistent with guanfacine's longer half-life. In most cases, after abrupt withdrawal of guanfacine, blood pressure returns to pretreatment levels slowly (in 2 to 4 days) without ill effects.

Adverse Reactions:

Adverse reactions include dry mouth; somnolence; asthenia; constipation; impotence; fatigue; headache. While the reactions are common, most are mild and tend to disappear on continued dosing.

Administration and Dosage:

The recommended dose, alone or with other antihypertensives, is 1 mg/day given at bedtime to minimize daytime somnolence.

If 1 mg does not produce a satisfactory result after 3 to 4 weeks of therapy, doses of 2 mg may be given, although most of the drug's effect is seen at 1 mg.

Higher daily doses have been used, but adverse reactions increase significantly with doses > 3 mg/day.

GUANABENZ ACETATE

Tablets: 4 mg, 8 mg (*Rx*)	Various, *Wytensin* (Wyeth-Ayerst)

Actions:

Pharmacology: Guanabenz is an orally active central α_2-adrenergic agonist, resulting in decreased sympathetic outflow from the brain. The chronic effect appears to be a decrease in peripheral resistance. Blood pressure decreases in both the supine and standing positions without alterations of normal postural mechanisms. Guanabenz decreases pulse rate by about 5 bpm.

Pharmacokinetics:

Absorption/Distribution – About 75% of an oral dose is absorbed. Peak plasma concentrations of unchanged drug occur between 2 and 5 hours after a single dose. The onset of action begins within 60 minutes after a single oral dose and reaches a peak effect within 2 to 4 hours.

Metabolism/Excretion – The average half-life is about 6 hours. Less than 1% of unchanged drug is recovered in the urine.

Renal/Hepatic Impairment: Mean plasma concentrations of guanabenz were higher in hepatic impaired patients than in healthy subjects. In renal impaired patients, half-life is prolonged and clearance decreased, especially in patients on hemodialysis.

Indications:

Treatment of hypertension, alone or in combination with a thiazide diuretic.

Contraindications:

Known sensitivity to guanabenz.

Warnings:

Pregnancy: Category C.

Lactation: No information is available on excretion in breast milk; therefore, do not administer to nursing mothers.

Children: Safety and efficacy for use in children less than 12 years of age have not been demonstrated; therefore, use in this age group is not recommended.

Precautions:

Sedation: Guanabenz causes sedation or drowsiness in a large fraction of patients.

Use with caution in patients with severe coronary insufficiency, recent myocardial infarction, cerebrovascular disease or severe hepatic or renal failure.

Monitor blood pressure carefully when administering guanabenz to patients with coexisting hypertension and chronic hepatic dysfunction or renal impairment.

Rebound: Sudden cessation of therapy with central α-agonists like guanabenz may rarely result in "overshoot" hypertension and more commonly produces an increase in serum catecholamines and subjective symptomatology.

Laboratory tests: During long-term administration, there is a small decrease in serum cholesterol and total triglycerides without any change in the high density lipoprotein fraction. Rarely, a nonprogressive increase in liver enzymes has been observed.

Adverse Reactions:

Adverse reactions occurring in ≥ 3% of patients include drowsiness/sedation; dry mouth; dizziness; weakness; headache. These effects led to treatment discontinuation ≈ 15% of the time. Side effects appear to be dose-related.

Administration and Dosage:

Initial dose: 4 mg twice a day, whether used alone or with a thiazide diuretic; increase in increments of 4 to 8 mg per day every 1 to 2 weeks.

The maximum dose studied has been 32 mg twice daily, but doses this high are rarely needed.

ALPHA-1-ADRENERGIC BLOCKERS

PRAZOSIN
Capsules: 1, 2 and 5 mg (*Rx*) — Various, *Minipress* (Pfizer)

TERAZOSIN
Tablets: 1, 2, 5 and 10 mg (*Rx*) — *Hytrin* (Abbott/Glaxo Wellcome)

DOXAZOSIN MESYLATE
Tablets: 1, 2, 4 and 8 mg (*Rx*) — *Cardura* (Roerig)

Actions:

Pharmacology: Prazosin, terazosin and doxazosin selectively block postsynaptic α-1-adrenergic receptors. These peripherally acting drugs dilate both resistance (arterioles) and capacitance (veins) vessels. Both supine and standing blood pressure are lowered. The effect is most pronounced on diastolic blood pressure.

In the treatment of benign prostatic hyperplasia (BPH), the reduction in symptoms and improvement in urine flow rates following use of terazosin, is related to relaxation of smooth muscle produced by blockade of $alpha_1$ adrenoceptors in the bladder neck and prostate.

Pharmacokinetics: Prazosin is extensively metabolized. The metabolites of prazosin are active. Duration of antihypertensive effect is 10 hours.

Terazosin undergoes minimal hepatic first-pass metabolism; nearly all of the circulating dose is in the form of parent drug.

Doxazosin is extensively metabolized in the liver.

Pharmacokinetics of Alpha-1-Adrenergic Blockers

Parameters	Prazosin	Terazosin	Doxazosin
Oral bioavailability	48% to 68%	90%	65%
Affected by food	No	No	nd[1]
Peak plasma level, time	1 to 3 hrs	1 to 2 hrs	2 to 3 hrs
Protein binding	92% to 97%	90% to 94%	98%
Half-life	2 to 3 hrs	9 to 12 hrs	22 hrs
Excretion: Bile/feces	< 90%	60%	63%
Excretion: Urine	< 10%	40%	9%

[1] nd = no data

Indications:

Hypertension: For the treatment of hypertension, alone or in combination with other antihypertensive agents (eg, diuretics or β-adrenergic blocking agents).

Terazosin: Treatment of symptomatic benign prostatic hyperplasia.

Unlabeled uses:

Prazosin – Refractory CHF.
Management of Raynaud's vasospasm.
Treatment of prostatic outflow obstruction.

Doxazosin – Treatment of CHF with concurrent digoxin and diuretics.

Contraindications:

Hypersensitivity to quinazolines (eg, doxazosin, prazosin, terazosin).

Warnings:

"First-dose" effect: Prazosin, terazosin and doxazosin, like other α-adrenergic blocking agents, can cause marked hypotension (especially postural hypotension) and syncope with sudden loss of consciousness with the first few doses. Anticipate a similar effect if therapy is interrupted for more than a few doses, if dosage is increased rapidly, or if another antihypertensive drug is introduced.

The "first-dose" phenomenon may be minimized by limiting the initial dose to 1 mg of terazosin or prazosin (given at bedtime) or doxazosin.

Hepatic function impairment: Administer doxazosin with caution to patients with evidence of impaired hepatic function or to patients receiving drugs known to influence hepatic metabolism.

Pregnancy: *Category* C (prazosin, terazosin); *Category* B (doxazosin).

Lactation: Safety has not been established.

Children: Safety and efficacy for use in children have not been established.

Precautions:

Weight gain: There was a tendency for patients to gain weight during terazosin therapy.

Cholesterol: During controlled clinical studies prazocin, terazosin and doxazosin were associated with small decreases in LDL and cholesterol.

Drug Interactions:

Drugs that interact may include beta blockers, indomethacin, verapamil and clonidine.

Drug/Lab test interactions: False-positive results may occur in screening tests for pheochromocytoma in patients who are being treated with prazosin.

Adverse Reactions:

Alpha-1-Adrenergic Blocker Adverse Reactions

	Hypertension			BPH
Adverse Reaction	Prazosin	Terazosin	Doxazosin	Terazosin
Cardiovascular				
Palpitations	5.3%	4.3%	2%	0.9%
Postural hypotension/ hypotension	✔[1]	1.3%	0.3% to 1%	0.6% to 3.9%
GI				
Nausea	4.9%	4.4%	3%	1.7%
Respiratory				
Dyspnea	✔[1]	3.1%	1%	1.7%
Nasal congestion	✔[1]	5.9%	no report	1.9%
Pharyngitis/rhinitis	no report	1%	3%	1.9%
Musculoskeletal				
Shoulder/neck/back/ extremity pain	no report	1% to 3.5%	<0.5% to 2%	
CNS				
Dizziness	10.3%	19.3%	19%	9.1%
Somnolence	no report	5.4%	5%	3.6%
Asthenia	≈ 7%	11.3%	1% to 12%	7.4%
Drowsiness	7.6%	✔[1]	✔[1]	
Miscellaneous				
Headache	7.8%	16.2%	14%	4.9%
Edema	✔[1]	< 1%	4%	
Peripheral edema	no report	5.5%	no report	0.9%

[1] Reactions associated with the drug, incidence unknown.

Administration and Dosage:

PRAZOSIN:

Initial dose – 1 mg 2 or 3 times daily. When increasing dosages, give the first dose of each increment at bedtime to reduce syncopal episodes.

Maintenance dose – 6 to 15 mg/day in divided doses. Doses > 20 mg usually do not increase efficacy; however, a few patients may benefit from up to 40 mg/day. After initial adjustment, some patients can be maintained on a twice-daily regimen.

Children – A dose of 0.5 to 7 mg 3 times a day has been suggested.

Concomitant therapy – When adding a diuretic or other antihypertensive agent, reduce dosage to 1 or 2 mg 3 times a day and then retitrate.

TERAZOSIN:

Hypertension – Adjust dose and the dose interval (12 or 24 hours) individually. The following is a guide.

Initial dose: 1 mg at bedtime for all patients. Do not exceed this dose. Strictly observe this initial dosing regimen to avoid severe hypotensive effects.

Subsequent doses: Slowly increase the dose to achieve the desired blood pressure response. The recommended dose range is 1 to 5 mg daily; however, some patients may benefit from doses as high as 20 mg/day. If response is substantially diminished at 24 hours, consider an increased dose or a twice-daily regimen.

Benign prostatic hyperplasia –

Initial dose: 1 mg at bedtime is the starting dose for all patients; do not exceed as an initial dose. Closely monitor patients to minimize the risk of severe hypotensive response.

Subsequent doses: Increase the dose in a stepwise fashion to 2, 5 or 10 mg daily to achieve desired improvement of symptoms or flow rates. Doses of 10 mg once daily are generally required for clinical response; therefore, treatment with 10 mg for a minimum of 4 to 6 weeks may be required to assess whether a beneficial response has been achieved. There is insufficient data to support the use of doses > 20 mg in patients who do not respond.

Concomitant therapy – Observe caution when terazosin is administered concomitantly with other antihypertensive agents (eg, calcium antagonists) to avoid the possibility of significant hypotension. When adding a diuretic or other antihypertensive agent, dosage reduction and retitration may be necessary.

DOXAZOSIN MESYLATE:

Initial dosage – 1 mg once daily. Postural effects are most likely to occur between 2 and 6 hours after a dose.

Maintenance dose – Depending on the standing blood pressure response, dosage may be increased to 2 mg and thereafter, if necessary, to 4, 8 and 16 mg to achieve the desired reduction in blood pressure. Increases in dose beyond 4 mg increase the likelihood of excessive postural effects.

HYDRALAZINE HCl

Tablets: 10, 25, 50 and 100 mg (*Rx*)	Various, *Apresoline* (Ciba)
Injection: 20 mg/ml (*Rx*)	Various, *Apresoline* (Ciba)

Actions:

Pharmacology: Hydralazine exerts a peripheral vasodilating effect through a direct relaxation of vascular smooth muscle.

The peripheral vasodilating effect of hydralazine results in decreased arterial blood pressure (diastolic more than systolic); decreased peripheral vascular resistance; and an increased heart rate, stroke volume and cardiac output. Hydralazine is commonly used in combination with a drug which inhibits sympathetic activity.

Pharmacokinetics: Hydralazine is rapidly absorbed after oral use. Half-life is 3 to 7 hours. Protein binding is 87%, and bioavailability is 30% to 50%. Plasma levels vary widely among individuals. Peak plasma concentrations occur 1 to 2 hours after ingestion; duration of action is 6 to 12 hours. Hypotensive effects are seen 10 to 20 minutes after parenteral use and last 2 to 4 hours. Slow acetylators generally have higher plasma levels of hydralazine and require lower doses to maintain control of blood pressure. Hydralazine undergoes extensive hepatic metabolism; it is excreted in the urine as active drug (12% to 14%) and metabolites.

Indications:

Oral: Essential hypertension, alone or in combination with other agents.

Parenteral: Severe essential hypertension when the drug cannot be given orally or when the need to lower blood pressure is urgent.

Unlabeled uses: Hydralazine in doses up to 800 mg 3 times daily has been effective in reducing afterload in the treatment of congestive heart failure (CHF), severe aortic insufficiency and after valve replacement.

Contraindications:

Hypersensitivity to hydralazine; coronary artery disease; mitral valvular rheumatic heart disease.

Warnings:

Lupus erythematosus: Hydralazine may produce a clinical picture simulating systemic lupus erythematosus including glomerulonephritis. Symptoms usually regress when the drug is discontinued, but residual effects have been detected years later. Long-term treatment with steroids may be necessary. Lupus occurs more frequently in "slow acetylators". The syndrome usually occurs after at least 6 months of continuous therapy. The likelihood increases with larger doses and with long duration of therapy.

Perform complete blood counts and antinuclear antibody (ANA) titer determinations before and during prolonged therapy, even in the asymptomatic patient. These studies are also indicated if the patient develops arthralgia, fever, chest pain, continued malaise or other unexplained signs or symptoms. If the ANA titer reaction is positive, carefully weigh benefits to be derived from hydralazine.

Renal function impairment: In hypertensive patients with normal kidneys who are treated with hydralazine, there is evidence of increased renal blood flow and a maintenance of glomerular filtration rate. Renal function may improve where control values were below normal prior to administration. Use with caution in patients with advanced renal damage.

Pregnancy: Category C.

Lactation: Hydralazine is excreted in breast milk. Exercise caution when administering to a nursing woman. Hydralazine is compatible with breastfeeding according to the American Academy of Pediatrics.

Children: Safety and efficacy for use in children have not been established.

Precautions:

Cardiovascular: The "hyperdynamic" circulation caused by hydralazine may accentuate specific cardiovascular inadequacies. It may reduce the pressor responses to epinephrine. Postural hypotension may result from hydralazine. Use with caution in patients with cerebral vascular accidents.

Coronary artery disease – Myocardial stimulation produced by hydralazine can cause anginal attacks and ECG changes of myocardial ischemia. The drug has been implicated in the production of myocardial infarction. Use with caution in patients with suspected coronary artery disease.

Pulmonary hypertension – Use hydralazine with caution in patients with pulmonary hypertension. Severe hypotension may result. Monitor carefully.

Lipids – Hydralazine may cause some decrease in total cholesterol.

Peripheral neuritis evidenced by paresthesias, numbness and tingling, has been observed. Add pyridoxine to the regimen if symptoms develop.

Hematologic effects: Blood dyscrasias consisting of reduction in hemoglobin and red cell count, leukopenia, agranulocytosis and purpura have been reported. If such abnormalities develop, discontinue therapy. Periodic blood counts are advised.

Tartrazine sensitivity: Some of these products contain tartrazine, which may cause allergic-type reactions in susceptible individuals. Tartrazine sensitivity is frequently seen in patients who also have aspirin hypersensitivity.

Drug Interactions:

Drugs that may interact with hydralazine include beta blockers (eg, metoprolol, propranolol) and indomethacin.

Drug/Food interactions: Taking with food results in higher plasma hydralazine levels.

Adverse Reactions:

Possible adverse reactions include headache; anorexia; nausea; vomiting; diarrhea; palpitations; tachycardia; angina pectoris; toxic reactions (particularly the LE cell syndrome); lacrimation; conjunctivitis; dizziness; tremors; psychotic reactions; rash; urticaria; pruritus; fever; chills; arthralgia; eosinophilia; constipation; paralytic ileus; lymphadenopathy; splenomegaly; nasal congestion; flushing; edema; muscle cramps; hypotension; paradoxical pressor response; dyspnea; urination difficulty; Adverse reactions with hydralazine are usually reversible when dosage is reduced. However, it may be necessary to discontinue the drug.

Administration and Dosage:

Bioavailability of hydralazine tablets is enhanced by the concurrent ingestion of food.

Initiate therapy in gradually increasing dosages; individualize dosage. Start with 10 mg 4 times daily for the first 2 to 4 days, increase to 25 mg 4 times daily for the balance of the first week.

Second and subsequent weeks: Increase dosage to 50 mg 4 times daily.

Maintenance: Adjust dosage to lowest effective level. Twice daily dosage may be adequate. In a few resistant patients, up to 300 mg/day may be required for a significant antihypertensive effect. In such cases, consider a lower dosage of hydralazine combined with a thiazide and/or reserpine or a beta blocker. However, when combining therapy, individual titration is essential to ensure the lowest possible therapeutic dose of each drug.

Children – Initial: 0.75 mg/kg/day in 4 divided doses. Dosage may be increased gradually over the next 3 to 4 weeks to a maximum of 7.5 mg/kg or 200 mg daily.

Parenteral: Therapy in the hospitalized patient may be initiated IV or IM. Use parenterally only when the drug cannot be given orally. Usual dose is 20 to 40 mg, repeated as necessary. Certain patients (especially those with marked renal damage) may require a lower dose. Check blood pressure frequently; it may begin to fall within a few minutes after injection; average maximal decrease occurs in 10 to 80 minutes. Where there is a previously existing increased intracranial pressure, lowering the blood pressure may increase cerebral ischemia. Most patients can transfer to the oral form in 24 to 48 hrs.

Children – 0.1 to 0.2 mg/kg/dose every 4 to 6 hours as needed.

Eclampsia – A dose of 5 to 10 mg every 20 minutes as an IV bolus has been recommended. If there is no effect after 20 mg, try another agent.

Stability: Use hydralazine injection as quickly as possible after drawing through a needle into a syringe. Hydralazine changes color after contact with a metal filter.

MINOXIDIL

Tablets: 2.5 mg, 10 mg (*Rx*) — Various, *Loniten* (Upjohn)

Warning:

Minoxidil may produce serious adverse effects. It can cause pericardial effusion, occasionally progressing to tamponade, and it can exacerbate angina pectoris. Reserve for hypertensive patients who do not respond adequately to maximum therapeutic doses of a diuretic and two other antihypertensive agents.

Administer under close supervision, usually concomitantly with a beta-adrenergic blocking agent, to prevent tachycardia and increased myocardial workload. Usually, it must be given with a diuretic, frequently one acting in the ascending limb of the loop of Henle, to prevent serious fluid accumulation. When first administering minoxidil, hospitalize and monitor patients with malignant hypertension and those already receiving guanethidine to avoid too rapid or large orthostatic decreases in blood pressure.

Actions:

Pharmacology: Minoxidil is a direct-acting peripheral vasodilator. The exact mechanism of action on the vascular smooth muscle is unknown.

Antihypertensive effects – Minoxidil reduces elevated blood pressure (BP) by decreasing peripheral vascular resistance. The BP response to minoxidil is dose-related and proportional to the extent of hypertension. Forearm and renal vascular resistance decline; forearm blood flow increases while renal blood flow and glomerular filtration rate (GFR) are preserved.

Hemodynamics – Minoxidil triggers sympathetic, vagal inhibitory and renal homeostatic mechanisms, including an increase in renin secretion, which leads to increased cardiac rate and output, and salt and water retention. These adverse effects can usually be minimized by coadministration of a diuretic and a β-adrenergic blocking agent or other sympathetic nervous system suppressant.

Pharmacokinetics:

Absorption/Distribution – Minoxidil is at least 90% absorbed from the GI tract. Plasma levels of the parent drug reach a maximum within the first hour and decline rapidly thereafter. Minoxidil is not protein bound; it concentrates in arteriolar smooth muscle.

Onset/Duration: The extent and time course of BP reduction by minoxidil do not correspond closely to its plasma concentration. When minoxidil is administered chronically, once or twice a day, the time required to achieve maximum effect on blood pressure is inversely related to the size of the dose. Thus, maximum effect is achieved on 10 mg/day within 7 days, on 20 mg/day within 5 days and on 40 mg/day within 3 days.

Metabolism/Excretion – 90% is metabolized, predominantly by conjugation with glucuronic acid. Average plasma half-life is 4.2 hours.

Indications:

Severe hypertension that is symptomatic or associated with target organ damage, and is not manageable with maximum therapeutic doses of a diuretic plus two other antihypertensives.

Topical minoxidil is used for the treatment of male pattern baldness (alopecia androgenetica) of the vertex of the scalp. Use of the tablets, in any formulation, to promote hair growth is not an approved use.

Contraindications:

Hypersensitivity to any component of the product; pheochromocytoma (because the drug may stimulate secretion of catecholamines from the tumor through its antihypertensive action); acute myocardial infarction; dissecting aortic aneurysm.

Warnings:

Mild hypertension: Due to potential for serious adverse effects, use in milder degrees of hypertension is not recommended.

Cardiac lesions: Autopsies did not reveal right atrial or other hemorrhage pathology of the kind seen in animals.

ECG changes: Rarely, a large negative amplitude of the T wave may encroach upon the ST segment, but the ST segment is not independently altered. These changes usually disappear with continuance of treatment and revert to the pretreatment state if therapy is discontinued.

Fluid and electrolyte balance: Monitor fluid and electrolyte balance and body weight. Give with a diuretic to prevent fluid retention and possible CHF; a loop diuretic is usually required. If used without a diuretic, retention of several hundred mEq salt and corresponding volumes of water can occur in a few days, leading to increased plasma and interstitial fluid volume and local or generalized edema. Diuretics alone, or with restricted salt intake, usually minimize fluid retention, but reversible edema developed in ≈ 10% of nondialysis patients so treated. Ascites has also occurred. Diuretic effectiveness is limited by impaired renal function. Condition of patients with preexisting CHF occasionally deteriorates due to fluid retention, but because of the fall in BP (afterload reduction), more than twice as many improve rather than worsen.

Refractory fluid retention rarely may require discontinuation of minoxidil. Under close medical supervision, it may be possible to resolve refractory salt retention by discontinuing the drug for 1 or 2 days, and then resuming treatment in conjunction with vigorous diuretic therapy.

Tachycardia: Minoxidil increases heart rate; this can be prevented by concomitant administration of a β-adrenergic blocking drug or other sympathetic nervous system suppressants. In addition, angina may worsen or appear for the first time during treatment, probably because of the increased oxygen demands associated with increased heart rate and cardiac output. This can usually be prevented by sympathetic blockade.

Pericardial effusion, occasionally with tamponade, has occurred in about 3% of treated patients not on dialysis, especially those with inadequate or compromised renal function. Many cases were associated with connective tissue disease, the uremic syndrome, CHF or fluid retention, but were instances in which these potential causes of effusion were not present. Observe patients closely for signs of pericardial disorder. Perform echocardiographic studies if suspicion arises. More vigorous diuretic therapy, dialysis, pericardiocentesis or surgery may be required. If the effusion persists, consider drug withdrawal.

Hazard of rapid control of blood pressure: In patients with very severe BP elevation, too rapid control of blood pressure can precipitate syncope, cerebrovascular accidents, MI and ischemia of special sense organs with resulting decrease or loss of vision or hearing. Patients with compromised circulation or cryoglobulinemia may also suffer ischemic episodes of affected organs. Although such events have not been unequivocally associated with minoxidil use, experience is limited.

Hospitalize any patient with malignant hypertension during initial treatment to assure that blood pressure is not falling more rapidly than intended.

Renal function impairment: Renal failure or dialysis patients may require smaller doses; closely supervise to prevent cardiac failure or exacerbation of renal failure.

Pregnancy: Category C.

Lactation: Safety for use in the nursing mother has not been established. Minoxidil is excreted in breast milk; do not nurse while taking minoxidil.

Children: Use in children is limited, particularly in infants. The recommendations under Administration and Dosage are only a rough guide; careful titration is essential.

Precautions:

Myocardial infarction: Minoxidil has not been used in patients who have had an MI within the preceding month. A reduction in arterial pressure with the drug might further limit blood flow to the myocardium, although this might be compensated by decreased oxygen demand because of lower BP.

Hypertrichosis: Elongation, thickening and enhanced pigmentation of fine body hair develops within 3 to 6 weeks after starting therapy in ≈ 80% of patients. It is usually first noticed on the temples, between the eyebrows, between the hairline and the eyebrows or in the sideburn area of the upper lateral cheek, later extending to the back, arms, legs and scalp. After discontinuation, 1 to 6 months may be required for restoration to pretreatment appearance. No endocrine abnormalities have been found to explain the abnormal hair growth; thus, it is hypertrichosis without virilism.

Laboratory tests: Repeat tests that are abnormal at initiation of minoxidil therapy to ascertain whether improvement or deterioration is occurring under therapy. Initially, perform such tests frequently, at 1 to 3 month intervals, and as stabilization occurs, at 6 to 12 month intervals.

Drug Interactions:

Drugs that may interact with minoxidil include guanethidine.

Adverse Reactions:

Adverse reactions may include: Stevens-Johnson syndrome; pericardial effusion; rebound hypertension (following gradual withdrawal in children); decreased initial hematocrit, hemoglobin and erythrocyte counts; nausea; vomiting; temporary edema; alkaline phosphatase/serum creatinine/BUN increase.

Administration and Dosage:

Adults and children (≥ 12 years of age): Initial dosage is 5 mg/day as a single dose. Daily dosage can be increased to 10, 20, then 40 mg in single or divided doses if required. Effective range is usually 10 to 40 mg/day. Maximum dosage is 100 mg/day.

Children: Initial dosage is 0.2 mg/kg/day as a single dose. Dose may be increased in 50% to 100% increments until optimum BP control is achieved. Effective range is usually 0.25 to 1 mg/kg/day. Maximum dosage is 50 mg daily.

Dose frequency: If supine diastolic pressure has been reduced < 30 mmHg, administer the drug only once a day; if reduced > 30 mmHg, divide the daily dosage into 2 equal parts.

Dosage adjustment intervals, which must be carefully titrated, should be at least 3 days because the full response to a given dose is not obtained until then.

ACE INHIBITORS

BENAZEPRIL HCl	
Tablets: 5, 10, 20, 40 mg (*Rx*)	*Lotensin* (Ciba)
CAPTOPRIL	
Tablets: 12.5, 25, 50, 100 mg (*Rx*)	Various, *Capoten* (Bristol-Myers Squibb)
ENALAPRIL MALEATE	
Tablets: 2.5, 5, 10, 20 mg (*Rx*)	*Vasotec* (Merck)
Injection: 1.25 mg enalaprilat/ml (*Rx*)	*Vasotec I.V.* (Merck)
FOSINOPRIL SODIUM	
Tablets: 10, 20 mg (*Rx*)	*Monopril* (Mead Johnson)
LISINOPRIL	
Tablets: 2.5, 5, 10, 20, 40 mg (*Rx*)	*Prinivil* (Merck, *Zestril* (Zeneca)
MOEXIPRIL HCl	
Tablets: 7.5, 15 mg (*Rx*)	*Univasc* (Schwarz Pharma)
QUINAPRIL HCl	
Tablets: 5, 10, 20, 40 mg (*Rx*)	*Accupril* (Parke-Davis)
RAMIPRIL	
Capsules: 1.25, 2.5, 5, 10 mg (*Rx*)	*Altace* (Hoechst-Roussel/Upjohn)

Warning:

Pregnancy: When used in pregnancy during the second and third trimesters, ACE inhibitors can cause injury and even death to the developing fetus. When pregnancy is detected, discontinue the ACE inhibitor as soon as possible.

Actions:

Pharmacology: The angiotensin converting enzyme inhibitors (ACEIs) appear to act primarily through suppression of the renin-angiotensin-aldosterone system; however, no consistent correlation has been described between renin levels and drug response.

Synthesized by the kidneys, renin is released into the circulation where it acts on a plasma globulin substrate to produce angiotensin I, a relatively inactive decapeptide. Angiotensin I is then converted by angiotensin converting enzyme (ACE) to angiotensin II, a potent endogenous vasoconstrictor that also stimulates aldosterone secretion from the adrenal cortex, contributing to sodium and fluid retention. These agents prevent the conversion of angiotensin I to angiotensin II by inhibiting ACE. ACEIs may also inhibit local angiotensin II at vascular and renal sites and attenuate the release of catecholamines from adrenergic nerve endings.

Inhibiting ACE results in decreased plasma angiotensin II and increased plasma renin activity (PRA), the latter resulting from loss of negative feedback on renin release caused by reduction in angiotensin II. This leads to decreased aldosterone secretion, resulting in small increases in serum potassium and sodium and fluid loss.

Increased prostaglandin synthesis may also play a role in the antihypertensive action of captopril.

Pharmacokinetics:

Pharmacokinetics of ACEIs								
ACEI	Onset/ Duration (hrs)	Time to peak serum levels (hrs)	Percent absorbed	Active metabolite	t½ Normal renal function	t½ Impaired renal function	Elimination 24 hr: Total	Elimination 24 hr: Unchanged
Benazepril	1/24	0.5 to 1	37%[1]	Benazeprilat	10 to 11[2] hr	Prolonged	nd[3]	trace
Captopril	0.25/ dose-related	0.5 to 1.5	75%[4]		< 2 hr	3.5 to 32 hr	> 95%	40% to 50% in urine
Enalapril	1/24	0.5 to 1.5 (enalaprilat 3 to 4)	60%[1]	Enalaprilat	1.3 hr	nd[3]	94% urine and feces	54% in urine (40% enalaprilat)
Enalaprilat	0.25/ ≈ 6	na[5]	na[5]		11 hr	Prolonged	nd[3]	> 90% (urine)
Fosinopril	1/24	≈ 3	36%[1]	Fosinoprilat	12 hr (fosinoprilat IV)	Prolonged	50% urine, 50% feces	negligible
Lisinopril	1/24	≈ 7	25%[1]		12 hr	Prolonged	nd[3]	urine, 100%
Quinapril	1/24	1	60%[4]	Quinaprilat	2 hr (quinaprilat)	Prolonged	≈ 60% urine, ≈37% feces	trace
Ramipril	1 to 2/24	1 (ramiprilat 2 to 4)	50% to 60%[1]	Ramiprilat	13 to 17 hr (ramiprilat)	Prolonged	60% urine, 40% feces	< 2%

[1] Absorption not influenced by food.
[2] Effective t½ of accumulation of metabolite following multiple dosing.
[3] nd – No data.
[4] Absorption reduced by food (see Drug Interactions).
[5] na – Not applicable (available IV only).

Indications:

Hypertension: The ACEIs are effective alone and in combination with other antihypertensive agents, especially thiazide-type diuretics.

Heart failure: Captopril, enalapril, lisinopril and quinapril.

Left ventricular dysfunction (LVD):

Captopril – To improve survival following myocardial infarction (MI) in clinically stable patients with LVD manifested as an ejection fraction ≤ 40% and to reduce the incidence of overt heart failure and subsequent hospitalizations for CHF in these patients.

Enalapril – For clinically stable asymptomatic patients with LVD (ejection fraction ≤ 35%); enalapril decreases the rate of development of overt heart failure and decreases the incidence of hospitalization for CHF.

Diabetic nephropathy:

Captopril – Treatment of diabetic nephropathy (proteinuria > 500 mg/day) in patients with type I insulin-dependent diabetes mellitus and retinopathy.

Unlabeled uses:

Captopril – Management of hypertensive crises. Sublingual captopril 25 mg has also been used effectively.

Neonatal and childhood hypertension; rheumatoid arthritis; diagnosis of anatomic renal artery stenosis ("captopril test"); hypertension related to scleroderma renal crisis; diagnosis of primary aldosteronism; idiopathic edema; Bartter's syndrome; Raynaud's syndrome (symptomatic relief); hypertension of Takayasu's disease.

Enalapril – Diabetic nephropathy (reduction of proteinuria, albuminuria and glomerular hypertension).

Childhood hypertension and hypertension related to scleroderma renal crisis.

Enalaprilat – May be used for hypertensive emergencies, but the effects are often variable.

Ramipril – Congestive heart failure.

Contraindications:

Hypersensitivity to these products.

Warnings:

Neutropenia/Agranulocytosis: Neutropenia (< 1000/mm^3) with myeloid hypoplasia resulted from use of captopril. About half of the neutropenic patients developed systemic or oral cavity infections or other features of agranulocytosis. Neutropenia/agranulocytosis has occurred rarely with enalapril or lisinopril and in one patient on quinapril.

Angioedema has occurred. It may occur at any time during treatment, especially following the first dose of enalapril (0.2%), captopril, lisinopril or quinapril (0.1%). Angioedema associated with laryngeal edema may be fatal.

Proteinuria: Total urinary proteins > 1 g/day were seen in 0.7% of captopril patients. Nephrotic syndrome occurred in about 20% of these cases.

Hypotension:

First-dose effect – ACE inhibitors may cause a profound fall in blood pressure following the first dose.

In heart failure, where the blood pressure was either normal or low, transient decreases in mean blood pressure > 20% occurred in about half of the patients.

Renal function impairment: Some hypertensive patients with renal disease, particularly those with severe renal artery stenosis, have developed increases in BUN and serum creatinine after reduction of blood pressure.

In patients with severe CHF whose renal function may depend on the activity of the renin-angiotensin-aldosterone system, treatment with ACEIs may be associated with oliguria or progressive azotemia and, rarely, with acute renal failure or death.

Impaired renal function decreases lisinopril elimination. The elimination half-life of quinaprilat increases as Ccr decreases. Dosage adjustment may be necessary for quinapril, benazepril, ramipril and lisinopril. Impaired renal function decreases total clearance of fosinoprilat and approximately doubles the AUC.

Hepatic function impairment: Patients with impaired liver function could develop markedly elevated plasma levels of unchanged fosinopril or ramipril. In patients with alcoholic or biliary cirrhosis, the rate, but not extent of fosinopril hydrolysis was reduced. Quinaprilat concentrations are reduced in patients with alcoholic cirrhosis.

Elderly: Elderly patients may have higher lisinopril blood levels and AUC, and higher peak ramiprilat and quinaprilat levels and AUC than younger patients. This may relate to decreased renal function rather than to age itself.

Pregnancy: Category C (first trimester); Category D (second and third trimesters). See Warning Box.

Lactation: Ingestion of 20 mg/day fosinopril resulted in detectable fosinoprilat levels in breast milk; do not administer to nursing mothers. Concentrations of captopril in breast milk are approximately 1% of those in maternal blood. Benazepril, enalapril and enalaprilat are detected in breast milk in trace amounts; a newborn would receive < 0.1% of the mg/kg maternal dose of benazepril and benazeprilat. It is not known whether lisinopril, quinapril or ramipril is excreted in breast milk.

Children: Safety and efficacy have not been established. Use captopril in children only when other measures for controlling blood pressure have not been effective.

Precautions:

Hyperkalemia: Elevated serum potassium (> 5.7 mEq/L) was observed in approximately 1% of hypertensive patients given benazepril, enalapril or ramipril, 2.2% of hypertensive patients given lisinopril, 2.6% of hypertensive patients given fosinopril, and 4% of CHF patients given lisinopril. Hyperkalemia also occurred with captopril.

Valvular stenosis: Theoretically, patients with aortic stenosis might be at risk of decreased coronary perfusion when treated with vasodilators, because they do not develop as much afterload reduction as others.

Surgery/Anesthesia: In patients undergoing major surgery or during anesthesia with agents that produce hypotension, ACEIs will block angiotensin II formation secondary to compensatory renin release.

Cough: Chronic cough has occurred with the use of all ACE inhibitors. Characteristically, the cough is nonproductive, persistent and resolves within 1 to 4 days after therapy discontinuation.

The incidence of cough, although still reported as 0.5% to 3% by some manufacturers, appears to range from 5% to 25% and has been reported to be as high as 39%, resulting in discontinuation rates as high as 15%.

Drug Interactions:

Drugs that may affect ACE inhibitors may include antacids, capsaicin, indomethacin, phenothiazines, probenecid and rifampin. Drugs that may be affected by ACE inhibitors include allopurinol, digoxin, lithium, potassium preparations/potassium-sparing diuretics and tetracycline.

Drug/Lab test interactions: Captopril may cause a false-positive test for *urine acetone*.

Fosinopril may cause a false low measurement of serum digoxin levels with the *Digi-Tab RIA Kit for Digoxin* other kits such as the *Coat-A-Count RIA Kit*, may be used.

Drug/Food interactions: Food significantly reduces the bioavailability of captopril by 30% to 40%. Administer captopril 1 hour before meals. The rate and extent of quinapril absorption are diminished moderately (25% to 30%) when administered during a high-fat meal. The rate, but not extent, of ramipril and fosinopril absorption is reduced by food. Food does not reduce the GI absorption of benazepril, enalapril and lisinopril.

Adverse Reactions:

Adverse reactions may include: Chest pain; hypotension; headache; dizziness; fatigue; diarrhea; dysgeusia; cough; rash.

Administration and Dosage:

BENAZEPRIL HCl:

Initial dose – 10 mg once daily.

Maintenance dosage – 20 to 40 mg/day as a single dose or two divided doses. A dose of 80 mg gives an increased response, but experience is limited.

Renal function impairment – 5 mg once daily in patients with Ccr of < 30 ml/min/1.73 m^2 (serum creatinine > 3 mg/dl). Dosage may be titrated upward until blood pressure is controlled or to a maximum of 40 mg/day.

CAPTOPRIL: Administer 1 hour before meals.

Hypertension –

Initial: 25 mg 2 or 3 times/day. If satisfactory blood pressure reduction is not achieved after 1 or 2 weeks, increase to 50 mg 2 or 3 times/day. If blood pressure is not controlled after 1 or 2 weeks at this dose (and patient is not already on a diuretic), add a modest dose of a thiazide diuretic.

If further blood pressure reduction is required, increase to 100 mg captopril 2 or 3 times/day and then, if necessary, to 150 mg 2 or 3 times/day (while continuing diuretic). Usual dose is 25 to 150 mg 2 or 3 times/day. Do not exceed daily dose of 450 mg.

Accelerated or malignant hypertension: Promptly initiate captopril at 25 mg 2 or 3 times daily under close supervision. Increase dose every 24 hours until a satisfactory response is obtained or the maximum dose is reached.

Heart failure – Usual initial dosage is 25 mg 3 times daily. After 50 mg 3 times daily is reached, delay further dosage increases, where possible, for at least 2 weeks to determine if a satisfactory response occurs. Most patients have had a satisfactory clinical improvement at 50 or 100 mg 3 times daily. Do not exceed a daily dose of 450 mg.

LVD after MI – 50 mg 3 times daily is the target maintenance dose. Thereapy may be initiated as early as 3 days following an MI. After a single 6.25 mg dose, initiate at 12.5 mg 3 times daily, then increase to 25 mg 3 times daily during the next several days and to a target of 50 mg 3 times daily over the next several weeks as tolerated.

Diabetic nephropathy – Recommended dose for long-term use is 25 mg 3 times daily.

Renal impairment – Reduce initial dosage and use smaller increments for titration, which should be quite slow (1 to 2 week intervals). After the desired therapeutic effect is achieved, slowly back-titrate to the minimal effective dose.

ENALAPRIL MALEATE:

Oral –

Hypertension:

Patients not taking diuretics – Discontinue the diuretic, if possible, for 2 to 3 days before beginning therapy with lisinopril to reduce the likelihood of hypertension. If the diuretic cannot be discontinued, use an initial dose of 2.5 mg under medical supervision for at least 2 hours and until blood pressure has stabilized for at least an additional hour.

Patients taking diuretics – Initial dose is 5 mg once a day. The usual dosage range is 10 to 40 mg/day as a single dose or in 2 divided doses.

Impaired renal function – Titrate the dosage upward until blood pressure is controlled or until a maximum dose of 40 mg/day is reached. Use initial dose of 5 mg/day in normal renal function and mild impairment (creatinine clearance [Ccr] 30 to 80 ml/min, serum creatinine < 3 mg/dl); 2.5 mg/day in moderate to severe renal impairment (Ccr ≤ 30 ml/min, serum creatinine ≥ 3 mg/dl) and in dialysis patients on dialysis days.

Heart failure: As adjunctive therapy with diuretics and digitalis, the recommended starting dose is 2.5 mg once or twice daily. The usual therapeutic dosing range for the treatment of heart failure is 5 to 20 mg/day given in two divided doses. The maximum daily dose is 40 mg.

Renal impairment or hyponatremia –

Serum sodium < 130 mEq/L or with serum creatinine > 1.6 mg/dl: Initiate at 2.5 mg/day under close medical supervision. the dose may be increased to 2.5 mg twice daily, then 5 mg twice daily and hither as needed, usually at intervals of ≥ 4 days. The maximum daily dose is 40 mg.

Asymptomatic left ventricular dysfunction: 2.5 mg twice daily, titrated as tolerated to the targeted daily dose of 20 mg in divided doses.

Parenteral (enalaprilat) – For IV administration only.

Hypertension: 1.25 mg every 6 hours IV over 5 minutes.

The dose for patients being converted to IV from oral therapy is 1.25 mg every 6 hours. For conversion from IV to oral therapy, the recommended initial dose of tablets is 5 mg once a day with subsequent dosage adjustments as necessary.

Patients taking diuretics: Starting dose for hypertension is 0.625 mg IV over 5 minutes. If there is inadequate clinical response after 1 hour, repeat the 0.625 dose. Give additional doses of 1.25 mg at 6 hour intervals.

For conversion from IV to oral therapy, the recommended initial dose of enalapril maleate tablets for patients who have responded to 0.625 mg enalaprilat every 6 hours is 2.5 mg once a day with subsequent dosage adjustment as necessary.

Renal function impairment: Administer 1.25 mg every 6 hours for patients with Ccr > 30 ml/min. For Ccr ≤ 30 ml/min, initial dose is 0.625 mg. If there is inadequate clinical response after 1 hour, the 0.625 mg dose may be repeated. May give additional 1.25 mg doses at 6 hour intervals. For dialysis patients, initial dose is 0.625 mg every 6 hour.

For conversion from IV to oral therapy, the recommended initial dose is 5 mg once a day for patients with Ccr > 30 ml/min and 2.5 mg once daily for patients with Ccr ≤ 30 ml/min.

FOSINOPRIL SODIUM:

Initial dose – 10 mg once daily.

Maintenance dosage – Usual range needed to maintain a response is 20 to 40 mg/day but some patients appear to have a further response to 80 mg. If trough response is inadequate, consider dividing the daily dose.

LISINOPRIL:

Hypertension –

Initial therapy: 10 mg once/day in patients with uncomplicated essential hypertension not on diuretic therapy. The usual dosage range is 20 to 40 mg/day as a single daily dose.

Diuretic-treated patients: Discontinue the diuretic, if possible, for 2 to 3 days before beginning therapy with lisinopril to reduce the likelihood of hypertension. If the diuretic cannot be discontinued, use an initial dose of 5 mg under medical supervision for at least 2 hours and until blood pressure has stabilized for at least an additional hour.

CHF –

Initial dose: 5 mg once daily with diuretics and digitalis. Usual effective dosage range is 5 to 20 mg/day as a single dose. In patients with hyponatremia (serum sodium < 130 mEq/L), initiate dose at 2.5 mg once daily. If used with diuretics, initial dose is 5 mg/day.

Elderly – Make dosage adjustments with particular caution.

Renal function impairment – For hypertension, titrate dosage upward until blood pressure is controlled or to a maximum of 40 mg daily.

In acute MI, initiate lisinopril with caution in patients with evidence of renal dysfunction (serum creatinine concentration exceeding 2 mg/dl).

Lisinopril Dosage in Renal Impairment

Renal status	Creatinine clearance (ml/min)	Serum creatinine (mg/dl)	Initial dose (mg/day)
Normal function to mild impairment	> 30	≤ 3	10 mg
Moderate to severe impairment	≥ 10 ≤ 30	≥ 3	5 mg
Dialysis patients	< 10	—	2.5 mg

Acute myocardial infarction – In hemodynamically stable patients within 24 hours of the onset of symptoms of acute MI, the first dose is 5 mg, followed by 5 mg after 24 hours, 10 mg after 48 hours and then 10 mg once daily. Continue dosing for 6 weeks. Patients with a low systolic blood pressure (≤ 120 mmHg) when treatment is started or during the first 3 days after the infarct should be given a lower 2.5 mg dose. If hopytension occurs (systolic blood pressure ≤ 100 mmHg), a daily maintenance dose of 5 mg may be given with temporary reductions to 2.5 mg if needed. If prolonged hypotension occurs (systolic blood pressure < 90 mmHg for > 1 hour), withdraw lisinopril.

MOEXIPRIL HCl:

Initial dose – In patients not receiving diuretics, 7.5 mg 1 hour prior to meals once daily. If control is not adequate, increase the dose of divide the dosing.

Maintenance dose – 7.5 to 30 mg daily in 1 or 2 divided doses 1 hour before meals.

Renal function impairment – Cautiously use 3.75 mg once daily in patients with Ccr of ≤ 40 ml/min/1.73 m^2. Dosage may be titrated upward to a maximum of 15 mg/day.

QUINAPRIL HCl:

Hypertension –

Initial dose: 10 mg once daily.

Elderly (≥ 65 years old): 10 mg once daily followed by titration to the optimal response.

Renal function impairment: Initial dose is 10 mg with Ccr > 60 ml/min, 5 mg with Ccr 30 to 60 ml/min and 2.5 mg with Ccr 10 to 30 ml/min.

CHF – The recommended starting dose is 5 mg twice daily. If the initial dose is well tolerated, titrate patients at weekly intervals until and effective dose, usually 20 to 40 mg daily given in 2 equally divided doses, is reached or undesirable hypotension, orthostasis or azotemia prohibit reaching this dose.

Renal impairment or hyponatremia: In patients with heart failure and renal impairment, the recomended initial dose is 5 mg with Ccr > 30 ml/min and 2.5 mg with Ccr 10 to 30 ml/min. There is insufficient data for dosage recommendation in patients with Ccr < 10 ml/min.

RAMIPRIL:

Initial dose – 2.5 mg once daily in patients not receiving a diuretic.

Maintenance dosage – 2.5 to 20 mg/day as a single dose or in two equally divided doses.

Alternative route of administration – Ramipril capsules are usually swallowed whole. However, the capsules may be opened and the contents sprinkled on a small amount of ≈ 4 oz applesauce or mixed in apple juice or water.

Renal function impairment – 1.25 mg once daily in patients with Ccr of < 40 ml/min/1.73 m^2 (serum creatinine > 2.5 mg/dl). Dosage may be titrated upward until blood pressure is controlled or to a maximum of 5 mg/day.

LOSARTAN POTASSIUM

Tablets: 25 and 50 mg (*Rx*)	*Cozaar* (Merck)

Warning:

Pregnancy: When used in pregnancy during the second and third trimesters, drugs that act directly on the renin-angiotensin system can cause injury and even death to the developing fetus. When pregnancy is detected, discontinue losartan as soon as possible.

Actions:

Pharmacology: Losartan is an angiotensin II receptor (type AT_1) antagonist. Losartan and its principal active metabolite block the vasoconstrictor and aldosterone-secreting effects of angiotensin II by selectively blocking the binding of angiotensin II to the AT_1 receptor found in many tissues.

Pharmacokinetics:

Absorption/Distribution – Losartan is well absorbed and undergoes substantial first-pass metabolism by cytochrome P450 enzymes; the systemic bioavailability is ≈ 33%. About 14% of an orally administered dose is converted to the active metabolite. While maximum plasma concentrations of losartan and its active metabolite are approximately equal, the AUC of the metabolite is about 4 times as great as that of losartan. The terminal half-life is about 2 hours and about 6 to 9 hours for the metabolite. Both losartan and its active metabolite are highly bound to plasma proteins, primarily albumin, with plasma free fractions of 1.3% and 0.2%, respectively.

Metabolism/Excretion – In addition to the active carboxylic acid metabolite, several inactive metabolites are formed. The volume of distribution is about 34 L and that of the active metabolite is about 12 L. About 4% of the dose is excreted unchanged in the urine and about 6% is excreted in urine as active metabolite. Biliary excretion contributes to the elimination of losartan and its metabolites. Following an oral dose, about 35% is recovered in the urine and about 60% in the feces.

Indications:

Hypertension: Treatment of hypertension, alone or in combination with other antihypertensive agents.

Contraindications:

Hypersensitivity to any component of this product.

Warnings:

Hypotension/Volume-depleted patients: In patients who are intravascularly volume-depleted, symptomatic hypotension may occur after initiation of therapy with losartan.

Monotherapy: Losartan had an effect on blood pressure that was notably less in African-American patients than in non-African-Americans, a finding similar to the small effect of ACE inhibitors in African-Americans.

Gender: Plasma concentrations were about twice as high in female hypertensives as male hypertensives, but concentrations of the active metabolite were similar in males and females. No dosage adjustment is necessary.

Renal function impairment: In patients whose renal function may depend on the activity of the renin-angiotensin-aldosterone system, treatment with ACE inhibitors has been associated with oliguria or progressive azotemia and (rarely) with acute renal failure or death. Losartan would be expected to behave similarly. In studies of ACE inhibitors in patients with unilateral or bilateral renal artery stenosis, increases in serum creatinine or BUN may occur.

Plasma concentrations of losartan are not altered in patients with creatinine clearance (Ccr) > 30 ml/min. In patients with lower Ccr, AUCs are about 50% greater and they are doubled in hemodialysis patients. Neither losartan nor its active metabolite can be removed by hemodialysis. No dosage adjustment is necessary for patients with renal impairment unless they are volume-depleted.

Hepatic function impairment: Compared to healthy subjects, the total plasma clearance in patients with hepatic insufficiency was about 50% lower and the oral bioavailability was about 2 times higher.

Fertility impairment: The administration of toxic dosage levels in females was associated with a significant decrease in the number of corpora lutea/female, implants/female and live fetuses/female at C-section.

Elderly: Plasma concentrations of losartan and its active metabolite are similar in elderly and young hypertensives. No initial dosage adjustment is necessary for elderly patients.

Pregnancy: Category C (*first trimester*); Category D (*second and third trimesters*).

Lactation: It is not known whether losartan is excreted in breast milk.

Children: Safety and efficacy in children have not been established.

Precautions:

Laboratory tests: Minor increases in BUN or serum creatinine were observed in < 0.1% of patients with essential hypertension treated with losartan alone.

Small decreases in hemoglobin and hematocrit occurred frequently in patients treated with losartan alone, but were rarely of clinical importance.

Occasional elevations of liver enzymes or serum bilirubin have occurred.

Drug Interactions:

Drugs that may interact with losartan include cimetidine and phenobarbital.

Drug/Food interactions: A meal slows absorption of losartan and decreases its C_{max} but has only minor effects on losartan AUC or on the AUC of the metabolite (about 10% decreased).

Adverse Reactions:

Adverse reactions occurring in ≥ 3% of patients include dizziness; cough; upper respiratory infection.

Administration and Dosage:

The usual starting dose is 50 mg once daily, with 25 mg used in patients with possible depletion of intravascular volume and patients with a history of hepatic impairment. Losartan can be administered once or twice daily with total daily doses ranging from 25 to 100 mg, and it may be administered with or without food.

If the antihypertensive effect measured at trough using once-a-day dosing is inadequate, a twice daily regimen at the same total daily dose or an increase in dose may give a more satisfactory response.

ANTIHYPERLIPIDEMIC AGENTS

Lowering cholesterol levels can arrest or reverse atherosclerosis in all vascular beds and can significantly decrease the morbidity and mortality associated with atherosclerosis. Each 10% reduction in cholesterol levels is associated with an ≈ 20% to 30% reduction in the incidence of coronary heart disease. Hyperlipidemia, particularly elevated serum cholesterol and low density lipoprotein (LDL) levels, is a risk factor in the development of atherosclerotic cardiovascular disease.

Treatment of hyperlipidemia is based on the assumption that lowering serum lipids decreases morbidity and mortality of atherosclerotic cardiovascular disease.

The cornerstone of treatment in primary hyperlipidemia is diet restriction and weight reduction. Limit or eliminate alcohol intake. Use drug therapy in conjunction with diet, and after maximal efforts to control serum lipids by diet alone prove unsatisfactory, when tolerance to or compliance with diet is poor or when hyperlipidemia is severe and risk of complications is high. Treat contributory diseases such as hypothyroidism or diabetes mellitus.

Classification of Total and HDL Cholesterol Levels

Level (mg/dl)	Classification
< 200 (5.2 mmol/L)	desirable
200-239 (5.2 - 6.2 mmol/L)	borderline-high
≥ 240 (6.2 mmol/L)	high
HDL < 35 (0.9 mmol/L)	low

Classification of LDL- Cholesterol Levels

Level (mg/dl)	Classification
< 130 (3.4 mmol/L)	desirable
130 -159 (3.4 - 4.1 mmol/L)	borderline-high
≥ 160 (4.1 mmol/L)	high

Elevations and treatment associated with each type of hyperlipidemia follow:

Hyperlipidemias and Their Treatment[1]

	Hyperlipidemia type					
	I	IIa	IIb	III	IV	V
Lipids						
Cholesterol	N-⇧	↑	↑	N-↑	N-⇧	N-↑
Triglycerides	↑	N	↑	N-↑	↑	↑
Lipoproteins						
Chylomicrons	↑	N	N	N	N	↑
VLDL (pre-β)	N-⇧	N-↓	↑	N-⇧	↑	↑
ILDL (broad-β)[2]				↑		
LDL (β)	↓	↑	↑	↑	N-⇩	↓
HDL (α)	↓	N	N	N	N-⇩	↓
Treatment	Diet	Diet Bile acid sequestrants Dextrothyroxine Nicotinic acid Probucol HMG-CoA reductase inhibitors	Diet Bile acid sequestrants[3] Probucol[3] Clofibrate[4] Gemfibrozil[5] Nicotinic acid HMG-CoA reductase inhibitors	Diet Clofibrate Gemfibrozil Nicotinic acid	Diet Clofibrate Gemfibrozil Nicotinic acid	Diet Clofibrate Gemfibrozil Nicotinic acid

[1] N = normal ↑ = increase ↓ = decrease ⇧ = slight increase ⇩ = slight decrease
[2] An abnormal lipoprotein.
[3] Particularly useful if hypercholesterolemia predominates.
[4] With high serum triglyceride levels and moderately elevated cholesterol.
[5] In patients with inadequate response to weight loss, bile acid sequestrants and nicotinic acid.

Antihyperlipidemic Drug Effects[1]

Drug	Lipids		Lipoproteins		
	Cholesterol	Triglycerides	VLDL (pre-β)	LDL (β)	HDL
Atorvastatin	↓	↓	↓	↓	↑
Cholestyramine	↓	→↑	→↑	↓	→↑
Clofibrate[2]	↓	↓	↓	→↓	→↑
Colestipol	↓	→↑	↑	↓	→↑
Dextrothyroxine[2]	↓	→	→	↓	→
Fluvastatin	↓	↓	↓	↓	↑
Gemfibrozil	↓	↓	↓	→↓	↑
Lovastatin	↓	↓	↓	↓	↑
Nicotinic Acid	↓	↓	↓	↓	↑
Pravastatin	↓	↓	↓	↓	↑
Simvastatin	↓	↓	↓	↓	↑

[1] ↓ = decrease ↑ = increase → = unchanged
[2] These agents are no longer commonly used as antihyperlipidemics.

BILE ACID SEQUESTRANTS

CHOLESTYRAMINE
Powder: 4 g/9 g, 4 g/5 g and 4 g/5.5 g (*Rx*) — *Questran*, *Questran Light* (Bristol Labs)

COLESTIPOL HCl
Tablets: 1g (*Rx*) — *Colestid* (Pharmacia & Upjohn)
Granules: 5 g/7.5 g (*Rx*)

Actions:

Pharmacology: Bile acid sequestering resins bind bile acids in the intestine to form an insoluble complex which is excreted in the feces. This results in a partial removal of bile acids from the enterohepatic circulation, preventing their absorption. The lipid-lowering effect of 4 g cholestyramine equals 5 g colestipol.

Treatment with anion-exchange resins may result in a 20% reduction in LDL. The decline in serum cholesterol is usually evident by 1 month.

Indications:

Hyperlipoproteinemia: Adjunctive therapy for the reduction of elevated serum cholesterol in patients with primary hypercholesterolemia (elevated LDL) who do not respond adequately to diet.

Biliary obstruction (cholestyramine only): Relief of pruritus associated with partial biliary obstruction.

Unlabeled uses: Cholestyramine in vitro binds the toxin produced by *Clostridium difficile*, the causative organism of antibiotic-induced pseudomembranous colitis, with variable success. It is also effective in bile salt-mediated and postvagotomy diarrhea.

Cholestyramine has been used in the treatment of chlordecone (*Kepone*) pesticide poisoning.

Cholestyramine and colestipol have been used in the treatment of digitalis toxicity.

Cholestyramine may be useful to treat an overdose with thyroid hormones.

Contraindications:

Hypersensitivity to bile acid sequestering resins or any components of the products; complete biliary obstruction.

Warnings:

Powder: To avoid accidental inhalation or esophageal distress, do not take dry. Mix with fluids.

Pregnancy: These agents are not absorbed systemically and are not expected to cause fetal harm when given during pregnancy in recommended doses.

Lactation: Exercise caution when administering to a nursing woman. The possible lack of proper vitamin absorption may have an effect on nursing infants.

Children: Dosage schedules have not been established.

Precautions:

Diet: Before instituting therapy, vigorously attempt to control serum cholesterol by an appropriate dietary regimen and weight reduction.

Malabsorption: Because they sequester bile acids, these resins may interfere with normal fat absorption and digestion and may prevent absorption of fat-soluble vitamins such as A, D, E and K.

Chronic use of resins may be associated with increased bleeding tendency due to hypoprothrombinemia associated with vitamin K deficiency.

Reduced folate: Reduction of serum or red cell folate has been reported over long-term administration of cholestyramine. Consider supplementation with folic acid.

Hyperchloremic acidosis: Prolonged use may cause hyperchloremic acidosis, especially in younger and smaller patients where relative dosage may be higher.

Constipation: These agents may produce or severely worsen preexisting constipation. Fecal impaction may occur and hemorrhoids may be aggravated.

Drug Interactions:

These resins may delay or reduce the absorption of concomitant oral medication by binding the drugs in the gut. Take other drugs at least 1 hour before or 4 to 6 hours after these agents.

Drugs that may be affected by bile acid sequestrants include anticoagulants, aspirin, clindamycin, clofibrate, diclofenac, digitalis glycosides, furosemide, gemfibrozil, glipizide, hydrocortisone, imipramine, iopanoic acid, methyldopa, mycophenolate, nicotinic acid (niacin), penicillin G, phenytoin, phosphate supplements, piroxicam, propranolol, tetracyclines, thiazide diuretics, thyroid hormones, tolbutamide, ursodiol and vitamins A, D, E and K.

Adverse Reactions:

GI:

Most common – Constipation.

Less frequent – Abdominal pain/distention/cramping; GI bleeding; belching; bloating; flatulence; nausea; vomiting; diarrhea; loose stools; indigestion; heartburn; anorexia, steatorrhea.

Miscellaneous: Transient and modest elevations of AST, ALT and alkaline phosphatase, (colestipol); liver function abnormalities (cholestyramine); headache (including migraine and sinus); anxiety; vertigo; dizziness; lightheadedness; insomnia; fatigue; tinnitus; syncope; drowsiness; urticaria; dermatitis; asthma; wheezing; rash; backache; muscle/joint pains; hematuria; dysuria; burnt odor to urine; diuresis; uveitis; anorexia; weight loss/gain; increased libido; swollen glands; edema; weakness; shortness of breath; swelling of hands/feet.

Administration and Dosage:

Although generally given 3 to 4 times daily, there appears to be no advantage to dosing more frequently than twice daily.

CHOLESTYRAMINE:

Powder –

Adults: 4 g 1 to 2 times daily.

Maintenance dose: 8 to 16 g/day divided into 2 doses. Use gradual increases in dose with periodic assessment of lipid/lipoprotein levels at intervals of ≥ 4 weeks. Maximum recommended daily dose is 24 g.

Suggested time of administration is at mealtime but may be modified to avoid interference with absorption of other medications. Although the recommended dosing scedule is twice daily, it may be given in 1 to 6 per day.

COLESTIPOL HCl:
Granules –
Adults: 5 to 30 g colestipol per day given once or in divided doses. The starting dose should be 5 g once or twice daily with a daily increment of 5 g at 1 or 2 month intervals.
Tablets – 2 to 16 g/day given once or in divided doses. The starting dose should be 2 g once or twice daily. Dosage increases of 2 g, once or twice daily, should occur at 1 or 2 month intervals.
Swallow tablets whole; do not cut, chew or crush.

HMG-CoA REDUCTASE INHIBITORS

LOVASTATIN (Mevinolin)
Tablets: 10, 20 and 40 mg (*Rx*) — *Mevacor* (Merck)

SIMVASTATIN
Tablets: 5, 10, 20 and 40 mg (*Rx*) — *Zocor* (Merck)

PRAVASTATIN SODIUM
Tablets: 10, 20 and 40 mg (*Rx*) — *Pravachol* (Bristol-Myers Squibb)

FLUVASTATIN
Capsules: 20 and 40 mg (*Rx*) — *Lescol* (Sandoz)

ATORVASTATIN CALCIUM
Tablets: 10, 20 and 40 mg — *Lipitor* (Parke-Davis)

Actions:
Pharmacology: These agents specifically competitively inhibit 3-hydroxy-3-methylglutaryl-coenzyme A (HMG-CoA) reductase, the enzyme which catalyzes the early rate-limiting step in cholesterol biosynthesis, conversion of HMG-CoA to mevalonate.

Pharmacokinetics:

Pharmacokinetics of HMG-CoA Reductase Inhibitors

	Bioavailability	Excretion	t½ (hrs)	Protein binding	Effects of renal/hepatic impairment
Fluvastatin	> 90% absorbed; absolute bioavailability 24%; extensive first-pass hepatic extraction	5% (urine) 90% (feces)	< 1	> 98%	nd[1]
Lovastatin	≈ 35% absorbed; extensive first-pass hepatic extraction (liver is primary site of action); < 5% of oral dose reaches general circulation as active inhibitors	10% (urine) 83% (feces)	3-4	> 95%	nd[1]
Pravastatin	≈ 34% absorbed; absolute bioavailability 17%; extensive first-pass hepatic extraction; plasma levels may not correlate with lipid-lowering efficacy	≈20% (urine) 70% (feces)	1.8	≈ 50%	Mean AUC varied 18-fold in cirrhotic patients and peak values varied 47-fold
Simvastatin	60% to 80% absorbed; extensive first-pass metabolism; < 5% of oral dose reaches general circulation as active inhibitors	13% (urine) 60% (feces)	3	≈ 95%	Higher systemic exposure may occur in severe renal insufficiency
Atorvastatin	≈ 12% absolute bioavailability; first pass metabolism (CYP3A4)	< 2% (urine)	14	≥ 98%	Plasma levels not affected by renal disease; markedly increased with chronic alcoholic liver disease.

[1] nd = no data.

Indications:

Adjunct to diet for the reduction of elevated total and LDL cholesterol levels in patients with primary hypercholesterolemia (Types IIa and IIb), when the response to diet and other nonpharmacological measures alone has been inadequate.

Atherosclerosis (lovastatin/pravastatin): To slow the progression of coronary atherosclerosis in patients with CHD as part of a treatment strategy to lower total-C and LDL-C to target levels; to reduce the risk of acute coronary events.

Coronary heart disease (simvastatin/pravastatin): To reduce the risk of total mortality by reducing coronary death; to reduce the risk of non-fatal myocardial infarction; reduce the risk of undergoing myocardial revascularization procedures.

Unlabeled uses:

Lovastatin – Diabetic dyslipidemia, nephrotic hyperlipidemia, familial dysbetalipoproteinemia and familial combined hyperlipidemia.

Pravastatin or simvastatin can significantly lower elevated cholesterol levels in patients with: Heterozygous familial hypercholesterolemia; familial combined hyperlipidemia; diabetic dyslipidemia in non-insulin dependent diabetics; hypercholesterolemia secondary to the nephrotic syndrome; homozygous familial hypercholesterolemia in patients who are not completely devoid of LDL receptors but have a reduced level of LDL receptor activity (pravastatin only); homozygous familial hypercholesterolemia in patients with defective, rather than absent, LDL receptors (simvastatin only).

Fluvastatin – To slow progression of coronary atherosclerosis in patients with CHD.

Contraindications:

Hypersensitivity to any component of these products; active liver disease or unexplained persistent elevated liver function tests; pregnancy, lactation.

Warnings:

Liver dysfunction: Use with caution in patients who consume substantial quantities of alcohol or who have a history of liver disease.

Pravastatin and **fluvastatin** plasma clearance is decreased but no dose adjustment is needed.

Skeletal muscle effects: Rhabdomyolysis with renal dysfunction secondary to myoglobinuria has occurred with some drugs in this class. Myalgia has occurred with **lovastatin**. Uncomplicated myalgia has been reported in **atorvastatin**-treated patients.

Consider myopathy in any patient with diffuse myalgias, muscle tenderness or weakness, or marked elevation of CPK. Advise patients to report promptly muscle pain, tenderness or weakness, particularly with malaise or fever. Discontinue the drug if markedly elevated CPK levels occur or if myopathy is diagnosed.

Hypersensitivity: An apparent hypersensitivity syndrome has occurred. Refer to Management of Acute Hypersensitivity Reactions.

Elderly: In patients > 70 years of age, the AUC of **lovastatin** and **simvastatin** is increased. **Pravastatin** does not need dosage adjustment. The safety and efficacy of **atorvastatin** in patients ≥ 70 years of age were similar to those of patients < 70 years of age. Elderly patients (≥ 65 years old) demonstrated a greater treatment response in respect to LDL-C, total-C and LDL/HDL ratio than patients < 65 years old.

Pregnancy: Category X.

Lactation: It is not known whether **lovastatin** and **simvastatin** are excreted in breast milk; a small amount of **pravastatin** is excreted in breast milk; **fluvastatin** is present in breast milk in a 2:1 ratio (milk: plasma).

Children: Safety and efficacy in individuals < 18 years old have not been established; treatment in this age group is not recommended at this time.

Precautions:

Monitoring: Perform liver function tests before initiating therapy, at 6 and 12 weeks after initiation of therapy or after dose elevation and periodically thereafter (≈ 6 month intervals). Pay special attention to patients who develop elevated serum transaminase levels. If transaminase levels progress, particularly if they rise to 3 times the upper limit of normal and are persistent, discontinue the drug. Consider liver biopsy if elevations persist beyond drug discontinuation.

Diet: Before instituting therapy, attempt to control hypercholesterolemia with diet, exercise, and weight reduction in obese patients. Treat underlying medical problems.

Homozygous familial hypercholesterolemia: **Lovastatin** and **simvastatin** are less effective in patients with the rare homozygous familial hypercholesterolemia, possibly because these patients have no functional LDL receptors. **Pravastatin** may be useful in these patients who are not completely devoid of LDL receptors but have a reduced level of LDL receptor activity.

Sleep disturbance: **Lovastatin** and **simvastatin** may interfere with sleep, causing insomnia, whereas **pravastatin** does not appear to disturb sleep.

Photosensitivity: Photosensitization (photoallergy or phototoxicity) may occur.

Drug Interactions:

Lovastatin is metabolized by CYP3A; it may interact with CYP3A inhibitors.

Fluvastatin is metabolized by CYP2C; it may interact with CYP2C inhibitors.

Drugs that may affect HMG-CoA reductase inhibitors include alcohol, antacids, bile acid sequestrants, colestipol, cyclosporine, erythromycin gemfibrozil, isradipine, itraconazole, niacin, nicotinic acid, propranolol, digoxin and rifampin.

Drugs that may be affected by HMG-CoA reductase inhibitors include oral contraceptives, digoxin and warfarin.

Adverse Reactions:

HMG-CoA Reductase Inhibitor Adverse Reactions (%)[1]

Adverse reaction	Atorvastatin (n = 36)	Fluvastatin (n = 620)	Lovastatin (n = 613)	Pravastatin (n = 900)	Simvastatin (n = 1583)
GI					
Nausea/Vomiting	—	3.2	1.9 - 4.7	7.3	1.3
Diarrhea	0	4.9	2.6 - 5.5	6.2	1.9
Abdominal pain/cramps	0	5.5	2 - 5.7	5.4	3.2
Constipation	0	2.6	2 - 4.9	4	2.3
Flatulence	2.8	2.6	3.7 - 6.4	3.3	1.9
Dyspepsia	2.8	8.1	1 - 3.9	—	1.1
Musculoskeletal					
Localized pain	—	—	0.5 - 1	10	—
Myalgia	5.6	5	2.4-2.6	2.7	—
Back pain	0	5.7	—	—	—
Arthralgia	0	4	0.5-1	—	—
CNS					
Headache	16.7	8.9	2.6 - 9.3	6.2	3.5
Dizziness	—	2.2	0.7 - 2	3.3	—
Respiratory					
Upper respiratory infection	—	16.2	—	—	2.1
Common cold	—	—	—	7	—
Rhinitis	—	4.7	—	4	—
Pharyngitis	0	3.8	—	—	—
Other					
Chest pain	—	—	0.5 - 1	3.7	—
Rash/Pruritus	2.8	2.3	0.8 - 5.2	4	—
Cardiac chest pain	—	—	—	4	—
Fatigue	—	2.7	—	3.8	—
Influenza	0	5.1	—	2.4	—

[1] All events. Data are pooled from separate studies and are not necessarily comparable.

Administration and Dosage:

LOVASTATIN (MEVINOLIN): Give lovastatin with meals.

Initial dose – 20 mg/day with the evening meal.

For those patients with severly elevated serum cholesterol levels (eg, > 300 mg/dl [7.8 mmol/L] on diet), initiate dosage at 40 mg/day.

Dose range – 10 to 80 mg/day in single or 2 divided doses. Adjust at intervals of at least 4 weeks.

Immunosuppressive therapy – In patients taking immunosuppressive drugs concomitantly with lovastatin, therapy should begin with 10 mg/day and should not exceed 20 mg/day.

Concomitant therapy – Cholesterol-lowering effects of lovastatin and the bile acid sequestrant, cholestyramine, are additive.

Renal function impairment – In patients with severe renal insufficiency (creatinine clearance < 30 ml/min), use dosage > 20 mg/day with caution.

SIMVASTATIN: May give without regard to meals.

Initial dose – 5 to 10 mg once daily in the evening. Consider starting dose of 5 mg/day for patients with LDL ≤ 190 mg/dl; 10 mg/day for patients with LDL > 190 mg/dl.

Elderly – Consider starting dose of 5 mg/day; maximum LDL reductions may be achieved with ≤ 20 mg/day.

Dose range – 5 to 40 mg/day as single dose in the evening. Adjust the dose at intervals of at least 4 weeks.

PRAVASTATIN SODIUM: May be taken without regard to meals.

Initial dose – 10 to 20 mg once daily at bedtime.

Elderly – In the elderly, maximum reductions in LDL-cholesterol may be achieved with daily doses of ≤ 20 mg.

Dose range – 10 to 40 mg once daily at bedtime.

Concomitant therapy – In patients taking concomitant immunosuppressive drugs (eg, cyclosporine), start pravastatin at 10 mg once daily at bedtime; titrate to higher doses with caution. Most patients treated with this combination received a maximum pravastatin dose of 20 mg/day.

Renal/Hepatic function impairment – A starting dose of 10 mg/day at bedtime is recommended.

FLUVASTATIN: May be taken without regard to meals.

Initial dose – 20 to 40 mg once daily at bedtime.

Dose range – 20 to 80 mg/day as a single dose in the evening. Administer the daily regimen of 80 mg in divided doses (eg, 40 mg twice a day) to those whose LDL-cholesterol response is inadequate at 40 mg/day.

ATORVASTATIN CALCIUM:

Initial dose – 10 mg/day.

Dose range – 10 to 80 mg/day. Can be administered as a single dose at any time of the day, with or without food.

Concomitant therapy – Atorvastatin may be used in combination with a bile acid binding resin for additive effect. Avoid the combination of HMG-CoA reductase inhibitors and fibrates.

GEMFIBROZIL

Tablets: 600 mg (*Rx*)	*Gemcor* (Upsher-Smith), *Lopid* (Parke-Davis)
Capsules: 300 mg (*Rx*)	Various

Actions:

Pharmacology: Gemfibrozil is a lipid regulating agent which decreases serum triglycerides and very low density lipoprotein (VLDL) cholesterol, and increases high density lipoprotein (HDL) cholesterol. While modest decreases in total and low density lipoprotein (LDL) cholesterol may be observed with gemfibrozil therapy, treatment of patients with elevated triglycerides due to Type IV hyperlipoproteinemia often results in a rise in LDL-cholesterol. Gemfibrozil usually raises HDL-cholesterol significantly in Type IIb patients with elevations of both serum LDL-cholesterol and triglycerides.

Pharmacokinetics:

Absorption/Distribution – Gemfibrozil is well absorbed from the GI tract. Peak plasma levels occur in 1 to 2 hours.

Metabolism/Excretion – Gemfibrozil mainly undergoes oxidation to form a hydroxymethyl and a carboxyl metabolite. It has a plasma half-life of 1.5 hours following multiple doses. Biological half-life is considerably longer, as some of the drug undergoes enterohepatic circulation and is reabsorbed in the GI tract. Approximately 70% is excreted in the urine, mostly as the glucuronide conjugate.

Indications:

Hypertriglyceridemia in adult patients (Types IV and V hyperlipidemia) who present a risk of pancreatitis and who do not respond to diet. Consider therapy for those with triglyceride elevations between 1000 and 2000 mg/dl,and who have a history of pancreatitis or of recurrent abdominal pain typical of pancreatitis.

Reducing coronary heart disease risk: Consider gemfibrozil therapy in those Type IIb patients who have low HDL-cholesterol levels in addition to elevated LDL-cholesterol and triglycerides and who have not responded to weight loss, dietary therapy, exercise and other pharmacologic agents.

Gemfibrozil is not useful for the hypertriglyceridemia of Type I hyperlipidemia.

Contraindications:

Hepatic or severe renal dysfunction, including primary biliary cirrhosis; preexisting gallbladder disease; hypersensitivity to gemfibrozil.

Warnings:

Cholelithiasis: If cholelithiasis is suspected, perform gallbladder studies. Discontinue therapy if gallstones are found.

Concomitant therapy with gemfibrozil and lovastatin has been associated with rhabdomyolysis, markedly elevated creatine kinase (CK) levels and myoglobinuria, leading in a high proportion of cases to acute renal failure. In most subjects who have had an unsatisfactory lipid response to either drug alone, the possible benefit of combined therapy does not outweigh the risks. The use of gemfibrozil may occasionally be associated with myositis. If myositis is suspected or diagnosed, withdraw therapy.

Renal function impairment: There have been reports of worsening renal insufficiency upon the addition of gemfibrozil therapy in individuals with baseline plasma creatinine > 2 mg/dl. In such patients, consider the use of alternative therapy against the risks and benefits of a lower dose of gemfibrozil.

Pregnancy: Category C.

Lactation: Decide whether to discontinue nursing or discontinue the drug, taking into account the importance of the drug to the mother.

Children: Safety and efficacy in children have not been established.

Precautions:

Estrogen therapy is sometimes associated with massive rises in plasma triglycerides, especially in subjects with familial hypertriglyceridemia.

Contributory diseases such as hypothyroidism or diabetes mellitus should be adequately treated.

Monitoring therapy: Perform adequate pretreatment laboratory studies. Obtain periodic determinations of serum lipids during administration. Withdraw the drug after 3 months if response is inadequate.

Hematologic – Mild hemoglobin, hematocrit and white blood cell decreases have been observed. Perform periodic blood counts during the first 12 months of administration.

Liver function – Abnormal elevations of AST, ALT, LDH, bilirubin and alkaline phosphatase have occurred, and are usually reversible on drug discontinuation. Perform periodic liver function studies and terminate therapy if abnormalities persist.

Blood glucose – Gemfibrozil has a moderate hyperglycemic effect; carefully monitor blood glucose levels during therapy.

Hazardous tasks: May produce drowsiness (dizziness or blurred vision); patients should observe caution while driving or performing other tasks requiring alertness, coordination and physical dexterity.

Drug Interactions:

Drugs that may interact with gemfibrozil include oral anticoagulants and lovastatin.

Adverse Reactions:

Adverse reactions occurring in ≥ 3% of patients include dyspepsia, abdominal pain; diarrhea; fatigue.

Administration and Dosage:

Adults: 1200 mg/daily in 2 divided doses, 30 minutes before the morning and evening meals.

Chapter 5
RESPIRATORIES

SYMPATHOMIMETICS

SALMETEROL	
Aerosol: 25 mcg salmeterol base (as salmeterol xinafoate) from actuator per actuation; 25 mcg salmeterol base (as salmeterol xinafoate) per actuation (*Rx*)	*Serevent* (Glaxo Wellcome)
ALBUTEROL	
Tablets: 2 and 4 mg (*Rx*)	Various, *Proventil* (Schering), *Ventolin* (Glaxo Wellcome)
Tablets, extended release: 4 mg (*Rx*)	*Proventil Repetabs* (Schering), *Volmax* (Muro)
Syrup: 2 mg per 5 ml (*Rx*)	Various, *Proventil* (Schering), *Ventolin* (Glaxo Wellcome)
Aerosol: Each actuation delivers 90 mcg (*Rx*)	Various, *Proventil* (Schering), *Ventolin* (Glaxo Wellcome)
Solution for Inhalation: 0.083%, 0.5% (*Rx*)	Various, *Airet* (Adams), *Proventil* (Schering), *Ventolin Nebules* (Allen & Hanburys)
Capsules for Inhalation: 200 mcg (*Rx*)	*Ventolin Rotacaps* (GlaxoWellcome)
METAPROTERENOL	
Tablets: 10 and 20 mg (*Rx*)	Various, *Alupent* (Boehringer-Ingelheim)
Syrup: 10 mg per 5 ml (*Rx*)	Various, *Alupent* (Boehringer-Ingelheim), *Prometa* (Muro)
Aerosol: 75 mg (100 inhalations). Each dose delivers 0.65 mg; 150 mg (200 inhalations). Each dose delivers 0.65 mg (*Rx*)	*Alupent* (Boehringer Ingelheim)
Solution for Inhalation: 0.4% 0.6%, 5% (*Rx*)	Various, *Alupent* (B-I), *Arm-a-Med Metaproterenol Sulfate* (Astra)
ISOETHARINE	
Solution for inhalation: 0.062%, 0.08%, 0.1%, 0.125%, 0.167%, 0.17%, 0.2%, 0.25%, 1% (*Rx*)	Various, *Arm-a-Med Isoetharine HCl* (Astra), *Beta-2* (Nephron), *Bronkosol* (Winthrop),
Aerosol: 0.61% (as mesylate). Delivers 340 mcg isoetharine per metered dose (*Rx*)	*Bronkometer* (Winthrop)
TERBUTALINE	
Tablets: 2.5 and 5 mg (*Rx*)	*Brethine* (Geigy), *Bricanyl* (Marion Merrell Dow)
Aerosol: 0.2 mg per actuation (*Rx*)	*Brethaire* (Geigy)
Injection: 1 mg/ml (*Rx*)	*Brethine* (Geigy), *Bricanyl* (Marion Merrell Dow)
ISOPROTERENOL	
Solution for inhalation: 0.25% (1:400), 0.5% (1:200), 1% (1:100) (*Rx*)	Various, *Dispos-a-Med Isoproterenol HCl* (Parke-Davis), *Isuprel* (Winthrop Pharm.)
Aerosol: 0.25% (1:400) (*Rx*)	Various
131 mcg /dose in fine mist (*Rx*)	*Isuprel Mistometer* (Winthrop Pharm.)
0.2%; delivers 80 mcg/measured dose (*Rx*)	*Medihaler-Iso* (3M)
Injection: (1:5000 solution) 0.2 mg/ml (*Rx*)	Various, *Isuprel* (Winthrop Pharm.)
ISOEPHEDRINE AND PHENYLEPHRINE	
Aerosol: 0.16 mg isoproterenol HCl and 0.24 mg phenylephrine bitartrate (*Rx*)	*Duo-Medihaler* (3M)
BITOLTEROL	
Aerosol: 0.8%; 0.37 mg/actuation (*Rx*)	*Tornalate* (Dura)
Solution for Inhalation: 0.2% (*Rx*)	*Tornalate* (Dura)
EPINEPHRINE	
Solution for inhalation: 1:100 (*Rx*)	*Adrenalin Chloride* (Parke-Davis)
Solution for inhalation: 2.25% racepinephrine HCl (equivalent to 1.125% epinephrine base); 2% racepinephrine base (equivalent to 1% epinephrine base) (*Rx*)	*AsthmaNefrin* (Menley & James), *microNefrin* (Bird), *Nephron* (Nephron), *S-2* (Nephron), *Vaponefrin* (Fisons)
Aerosol: 0.3 mg epinephrine bitartrate (equivalent to 0.16 mg epinephrine base per spray) (*Rx*)	*AsthmaHaler Mist* (Menley & James), *Bronitin Mist* (Whitehall), *Medihaler-Epi* (3M), *Primatene Mist Suspension* (Whitehall)
0.5% (equivalent to 0.25 mg epinephrine per spray) (*Rx*)	*Bronkaid Mist* (Sterling Health)
0.2 mg per spray (*Rx*)	*Primatene Mist* (Whitehall)
Injection: 1:1000 (1 mg/ml) (*Rx*)	Various, *Adrenalin Chloride Solution* (Parke-Davis)
1:200 (5 mg/ml) (*Rx*)	*Sus-Phrine* (Forest)
EPHEDRINE	

Capsules: 25 (*otc*) and 50 mg (*Rx*)	Various
Injection: 25 and 50 mg/ml (*Rx*)	Various
PIRBUTEROL	
Aerosol: Delivers 0.2 mg/actuation	*Maxair* (3M Pharm.)

Actions:

Pharmacology: These agents are used to produce bronchodilation. They relieve reversible bronchospasm by relaxing the smooth muscles of the bronchioles in conditions associated with asthma, bronchitis, emphysema or bronchiectasis. Bronchodilation may additionally facilitate expectoration.

The pharmacologic actions of these agents include: Alpha-adrenergic stimulation (vasoconstriction, nasal decongestion, pressor effects); β_1-adrenergic stimulation (increased myocardial contractility and conduction); and β_2-adrenergic stimulation (bronchial dilation and vasodilation).

The relative selectivity of action of sympathomimetic agents is the primary determinant of clinical usefulness; it can predict the most likely side effects. The β_2 selective agents provide the greatest benefit with minimal side effects. Direct administration via inhalation provides prompt effects and minimizes systemic activity. These drugs also inhibit histamine release from mast cells, produce vasodilation and increase ciliary motility. Bitolterol functions as a prodrug which must first be hydrolyzed by esterases in tissue and blood to its active moiety, colterol. Isoproterenol is one of the most potent bronchodilators available.

Sympathomimetic Bronchodilators: Pharmacologic Effects and Pharmacokinetic Properties

Sympathomimetic	Adrenergic receptor activity	Route	Onset (minutes)	Duration (hrs)
Albuterol[1]	β_1 < β_2	PO Inh[2]	within 30 within 5	4-8 3-8
Bitolterol[1]	β_1 < β_2	Inh	3-4	5 ≥ 8
Isoetharine[1]	β_1 < β_2	Inh[2]	within 5	1-3
Metaproterenol[1]	β_1 < β_2	PO Inh[2]	≈ 30 5-30	4 2-6
Pirbuterol[1]	β_1 < β_2	Inh	within 5	5
Salmeterol[1]	β_1 < β_2	Inh	within 20	12
Terbutaline[1]	β_1 < β_2	PO SC Inh	30 5-15 5-30	4-8 1.5-4 3-6
Isoproterenol	β_1 β_2	SL IV Inh[2]	≈ 30 immediate 2-5	1-2 < 1 0.5-2
Ephedrine	α β_1 β_2	PO SC IM IV	within 60 > 20 10-20 —	3-5 ≤ 1 ≤ 1 —
Epinephrine	α β_1 β_2	SC IM Inh[2]	5-15 — 1-5	1-4 1-4 1-3

[1] These agents all have minor β_1 activity.
[2] May be administered via aerosol nebulizer, bulb nebulizer or IPPB administration.

Indications:

Salmeterol:

Asthma/Bronchospasm – Long-term, twice-daily (morning and evening) administration in the maintenance treatment of asthma and in the prevention of bronchospasm in patients ≥ 12 years of age with reversible obstructive airway disease, including patients with symptoms of nocturnal asthma, who require regular treatment with inhaled, short-acting beta$_2$-agonists. It should not be used in patients whose asthma can be managed by occasional use of short-acting, inhaled $beta_2$-agonists. Salmeterol may be used with or without concurrent inhaled or systemic corticosteroid therapy.

Exercise-induced bronchospasm – Prevention of exercise-induced bronchospasm in patients ≥ 12 years of age.

Albuterol: Relief and prevention of bronchospasm in patients with reversible obstructive airway disease; prevention of exercise-induced bronchospasm.

Metaproterenol: For bronchial asthma and reversible bronchospasm; treatment of acute asthmatic attacks in children ≥ 6 years of age (Alupent solution for inhalation *only*).

Isoetharine: For bronchial asthma and reversible bronchospasm that occurs with bronchitis and emphysema.

Terbutaline: A bronchodilator for bronchial asthma and for reversible bronchospasm which may occur with bronchitis and emphysema.

Isoproterenol:

Inhalation – Treatment of bronchospasm associated with acute and chronic bronchial asthma, pulmonary emphysema, bronchitis and bronchiectasis.

Injection – Management of bronchospasm during anesthesia.

Sublingual – Management of patients with bronchopulmonary disease.

Isoproterenol and Phenylephrine Bitartrate: Treatment of bronchospasm associated with acute and chronic asthma; reversible bronchospasm which may be associated with emphysema or chronic bronchitis.

Bitolterol: Prophylaxis and treatment of bronchial asthma and reversible bronchospasm. May be used with or without concurrent theophylline or steroid therapy.

Epinephrine:

Inhalation – Temporary relief from acute paroxysms (eg, shortness of breath, tightness of chest, wheezing) of bronchial asthma; postintubation and infectious croup.

MicroNefrin: Chronic obstructive lung disease, chronic bronchitis, broncheolitis, bronchial asthma and other peripheral airway diseases.

Injection – To relieve respiratory distress in bronchial asthma or during acute asthma attacks and for reversible bronchospasm in patients with chronic bronchitis, emphysema and other obstructive pulmonary diseases.

Treatment of hypersensitivity reactions to drugs, sera, insect stings or other allergens, including such symptoms as bronchospasm, urticaria, pruritus, angioneurotic edema, or swelling of the lips, eyelids, tongue and nasal mucosa.

Ephedrine: Treatment of allergic disorders, such as bronchial asthma, and for local treatment of nasal congestion in acute coryza, vasomotor rhinitis, acute sinusitis and hay fever.

Parenteral ephedrine is sometimes used to relieve acute bronchospasm, but it is less effective than epinephrine for this purpose and has been given as a CNS stimulant in narcolepsy and depressive states.

Pirbuterol: Prevention and reversal of bronchospasm in patients with reversible bronchospasm including asthma. Use with or without concurrent theophylline or steroid therapy.

Unlabeled uses: Oral and IV terbutaline have successfully inhibited premature labor. Initiate IV use at 10 mcg/minute; titrate upward to a maximum of 80 mcg/minute. Maintain IV dosage at the minimum effective dose for 4 hours. Oral doses of 2.5 mg every 4 to 6 hours have been used as maintenance therapy until term.

Contraindications:

Hypersensitivity to any component (allergic reactions are rare); cardiac arrhythmias associated with tachycardia; tachycardia or heart block caused by digitalis intoxication, angina (isoproterenol); narrow angle glaucoma, shock, during general anesthesia with halogenated agents or cyclopropane, organic brain damage (epinephrine).

Warnings:

Special risk patients: Administer with caution to patients with diabetes mellitus, hyperthyroidism, prostatic hypertrophy (ephedrine) or history of seizures; elderly; psychoneurotic individuals, patients with long-standing bronchial asthma and emphysema who have developed degenerative heart disease (epinephrine).

In patients with status asthmaticus and abnormal blood gas tensions, improvement in vital capacity and blood gas tensions may not accompany apparent relief of bronchospasm following isoproterenol.

Cardiovascular effects: Use with caution in patients with cardiovascular disorders including coronary insufficiency, ischemic heart disease, history of stroke, coronary artery disease, cardiac arrhythmias, CHF and hypertension. These agents may cause toxic symptoms through idiosyncratic response or overdosage. If cardiac rate increases sharply, angina patients may experience anginal pain until the cardiac rate decreases.

Closely monitor patients receiving **epinephrine**. Inadvertently induced high arterial blood pressure may result in angina pectoris, aortic rupture or cerebral hemorrhage. Cardiac arrhythmias develop in some individuals even after therapeutic doses. Epinephrine causes changes in the ECG even in healthy persons, including a decrease in amplitude of the T wave.

Large doses of inhaled or oral **salmeterol** (12 to 20 times the recommended dose) have been associated with clinically significant prolongation of the QTc interval, which has the potential for producing ventricular arrhythmias.

Significant changes in systolic and diastolic blood pressure can occur in some patients after use of any beta-adrenergic aerosol bronchodilator.

Paradoxical bronchospasm: Occasional patients have developed severe paradoxical airway resistance with repeated, excessive use of inhalation preparations; the cause is unknown. Discontinue the drug immediately and institute alternative therapy, since patients may not respond to other therapy until the drug is withdrawn.

Excessive use of inhalants: Deaths have been reported; the exact cause is unknown, but cardiac arrest following an unexpected severe acute asthmatic crisis and subsequent hypoxia is suspected.

Usual dose response: Advise patients to contact a physician if they do not respond to their usual dose of a sympathomimetic amine.

Reduce **epinephrine** dose if bronchial irritation, nervousness, restlessness or sleeplessness occurs. Do not continue to use epinephrine, but seek medical assistance immediately if symptoms are not relieved within 20 min or become worse.

CNS effects: Sympathomimetics may produce CNS stimulation.

Long-term use: Prolonged use of **ephedrine** may produce a syndrome resembling an anxiety state; many patients develop nervousness; a sedative may be needed. After prolonged use or overdosage, elevated serum lactic acid levels with severe metabolic acidosis have occurred, as have transient blood glucose elevations.

Acute symptoms: Do not use **salmeterol** to relieve acute asthma symptoms. If the patient's short-acting, inhaled β_2-agonist becomes less effective (eg, the patient needs more inhalations than usual), medical evaluation must be obtained immediately and increasing use of salmeterol in this situation is inappropriate. Do not use salmeterol more frequently than twice daily (morning and evening) at the recommended dose. When prescribing salmeterol, patients must be provided with a short-acting, inhaled β_2-agonist (eg, albuterol) for treatment of symptoms that occur despite regular twice-daily (morning and evening) use of salmeterol.

Use with short-acting β_2-agonists – When patients begin treatment with salmeterol, advise those who have been taking short-acting, inhaled β_2-agonists on a regular daily basis to discontinue their regular daily-dosing regimen and clearly instruct them to use short-acting, inhaled β_2-agonists only for symptomatic relief if they develop asthma symptoms while taking salmeterol.

Overdosage or inadvertent IV injection of conventional SC **epinephrine** doses may cause severe or fatal hypertension or cerebrovascular hemorrhage resulting from the sharp rise in blood pressure. Fatalities may also occur from pulmonary edema resulting from peripheral constriction and cardiac stimulation.

Hypersensitivity (allergic) reactions can occur after administration of **bitolterol, albuterol, metaproterenol, terbutaline, ephedrine, salmeterol** and possibly other bronchodilators. See Management of Acute Hypersensitivity Reactions.

Elderly: Lower doses may be required due to increased sympathomimetic sensitivity. Observe special caution when using in elderly patients who have concomitant cardiovascular disease that could be adversely affected by this class of drug.

Pregnancy: Category B (terbutaline). *Category* C (albuterol, bitolterol, ephedrine, epinephrine, isoetharine, isoproterenol, metaproterenol, salmeterol).

Labor and delivery – Use of β_2 active sympathomimetics inhibits uterine contractions. Other reactions include increased heart rate, transient hyperglycemia, hypokalemia, cardiac arrhythmias, pulmonary edema, cerebral and myocardial ischemia and increased fetal heart rate and hypoglycemia in the neonate. Although these effects are unlikely with aerosol use, consider the potential for untoward effects.

Lactation: **Terbutaline** and **epinephrine** are excreted in breast milk. It is not known whether other agents are excreted in breast milk.

Children:

Inhalation – Safety and efficacy for use of **bitolterol, pirbuterol, isoetharine, isoproterenol, salmeterol, terbutaline** and **albuterol** in children ≤ 12 years of age (*Ventolin* – < 4 years) have not been established. **Metaproterenol** may be used in children ≥ 6 years of age.

Injection – Parenteral **terbutaline** is not recommended for use in children < 12 years old. Administer **epinephrine** with caution to infants and children. Syncope has occurred following administration to asthmatic children.

Oral – **Metaproterenol** is not recommended for use in children < 6 years old. **Terbutaline** is not recommended for use in children < 12 years old. **Albuterol:** Safety and efficacy have not been established for children < 2 years (syrup), < 6 years (tablets) and < 12 years (tablets, timed release) old.

In children, **ephedrine** is effective in the oral therapy of asthma. Because of its CNS-stimulating effect, it is rarely used alone. This effect is usually countered by an appropriate sedative; however, its rationale has been questioned.

Precautions:

Tolerance may occur with prolonged use of sympathomimetic agents, but temporary cessation of the drug restores its original effectiveness.

Hypokalemia: Decreases in serum potassium levels have occurred, possibly through intracellular shunting which can produce adverse cardiovascular effects. The decrease is usually transient, not requiring supplementation.

Parkinson's disease: Epinephrine may temporarily increase rigidity and tremor.

Parenteral use: Administer **epinephrine** with great caution and in carefully circumscribed quantities in areas of the body served by end arteries or with otherwise limited blood supply (eg, fingers, toes, nose, ears, genitals) or if peripheral vascular disease is present to avoid vasoconstriction-induced tissue sloughing.

Combined therapy: Concomitant use with other sympathomimetic agents is not recommended, as it may lead to deleterious cardiovascular effects. This does not preclude the judicious use of an adrenergic stimulant aerosol bronchodilator in patients receiving tablets. Do not give on a routine basis. If regular coadministration is required, consider alternative therapy.

Patients must be warned not to stop or reduce corticosteroid therapy without medical advice, even if they feel better when they are being treated with β_2 agonists.

Drug Interactions:

Most interactions listed apply to sympathomimetics when used as vasopressors; however, consider the interaction when using the bronchodilator sympathomimetics. Drugs that may interact include beta blockers furazolidine, guanethidine, lithium, methyldopa, MAO inhibitors, oxytocic drugs, rauwolfia alkaloids, tricyclic antidepressants, digoxin, theophylline, insulin or oral hypoglycemic agents.

Drug/Lab test interactions: Isoproterenol causes false elevations of bilirubin as measured in vitro by a sequential multiple analyzer. Isoproterenol inhalation may result in enough absorption of the drug to produce elevated urinary epinephrine values. Although small with standard doses, the effect is likely to increase with larger doses.

Adverse Reactions:

Sympathomimetic Bronchodilator Adverse Reactions (%)[1]

	Adverse reaction	Albuterol	Bitolterol	Ephedrine	Epinephrine	Isoetharine	Isoproterenol	Metapro-terenol	Pirbuterol	Salmeterol	Terbutaline
Cardiovascular	Palpitations	1-10	1.5- 3	✓[2]	7.8-30	✓	5-22	0.3-4	1.3-1.7	1-3	7.8-23
	Tachycardia	1-10	< 1	–	≤ 2.6	–	2-10	< 17	1.3	1-3	1.3-3
	Blood pressure changes/ hypertension	3.1-5			✓	✓	2-5	0.3			< 1
	PVCs, arrhythmias, skipped beats		0.5	–	✓		1-3		< 1		≈ 4
CNS	Tremor	1-20	9-14		16-18	–	< 15	3.3-33	1.3-6	4	5-38
	Dizziness/vertigo	1-7	1-3	–	3.3-7.8	–	1.5-5	1-4	0.6-1.2	≥ 3	1.3-10
	Shakiness/nervousness/tension	1-20	1.5-5	–	8.5-31	–	< 15	2.6-14	4.5-7	1-3	5-31
	Drowsiness	< 1			8.2-14		< 5	0.7			5-11.7
	Hyperactivity/Hyperkinesia, excitement	1-20	< 1			–	✓		< 1		
	Headache	2-27	≈ 4	–	3.3-10	–	1.5-10	≤ 4	1.3-2	28	7.8-10
	Insomnia	1-3.1	< 1	–	✓	–	1.5		< 1		✓
	Nausea/Vomiting	2-15	≤ 3	–	1-11.5	–	< 15	< 14	≤ 1.7	1-3	1.3-10
	Heartburn/GI distress/disorder	≤ 5					5-10	≤ 4		1-4	< 10
	Diarrhea	≤ 1						0.7	< 1.3	1-3	
Respiratory	Cough	1-5	4.1				1-5	≤ 4	1.2	7	
	Bronchospasm	1-15.4	≤ 1				≤ 18				✓
	Throat dryness/irritation, pharyngitis	≤ 6	3-5				3.1	≤ 4	< 1	≥ 3	✓

[1] Data pooled for all routes of administration and all age groups. Data are pooled from separate studies and are not necessarily comparable.

[2] ✓ Reported; no incidence given.

Adverse reactions are generally transient, and no cumulative effects have been reported. It is usually not necessary to discontinue treatment; however, in selected cases temporarily reduce dosage.

Albuterol:

Respiratory – Bronchitis (1.5% to 4%); epistaxis (1% to 3%).

Miscellaneous – Increased appetite (3%); muscle cramps (1% to 3%).

Bitolterol: Lightheadedness (3%). The overall incidence of cardiovascular effects was ≈ 5%.

Isoproterenol: Bronchitis (5%).

Metaproterenol: Asthma exacerbation (1% to 4%).

Salmeterol:

Respiratory – Upper respiratory tract infection, nasopharyngitis (14%); nasal cavity/sinus disease (6%); sinus headache, lower respiratory tract infection (4%); allergic rhinitis (> 3%); rhinitis, laryngitis, tracheitis/bronchitis (1% to 3%).

Musculoskeletal – Joint/back pain, muscle cramp/contraction, myalgia/myositis, muscular soreness (1% to 3%).

Miscellaneous – Giddiness, influenza (> 3%); viral gastroenteritis, urticaria, dental pain, malaise/fatigue, rash/skin eruption, dysmenorrhea (1% to 3%).

Administration and Dosage:

SALMETEROL: Administer by the orally inhaled route only (see Patient's Instructions for Use).

Asthma/Bronchospasm – For maintenance of bronchodilatation and prevention of symptoms of asthma, including the symptoms of nocturnal asthma, the usual dosage for adults and children ≥ 12 years of age is 2 inhalations (42 mcg) twice daily (morning and evening, approximately 12 hours apart). Adverse effects are more likely to occur with higher doses of salmeterol, and more frequent administration or administration of a larger number of inhalations is not recommended.

To gain full therapeutic benefit, administer twice daily (morning and evening) in the treatment of reversible airway obstruction.

Prevention of exercise-induced bronchospasm – Two inhalations at least 30 to 60 minutes before exercise protects against exercise-induced bronchospasm in many patients for up to 12 hours. Additional doses of salmeterol should not be used for 12 hours after the administration of this drug. Patients who are receiving salmeterol twice daily (morning and evening) should not use additional salmeterol for prevention of exercise-induced bronchospasm.

ALBUTEROL:

Inhalation aerosol – Adults and children ≥ 12 years (Ventolin – ≥ 4 years) - 2 inhalations every 4 to 6 hours. In some patients, 1 inhalation every 4 hours may be sufficient. More frequent administration or a larger number of inhalations is not recommended. If previously effective dosage fails to provide relief, seek medical advice immediately. This is often a sign of seriously worsening asthma; reassess therapy.

Prevention of exercise-induced bronchospasm:

Adults and children ≥ 12 years – 2 inhalations 15 minutes prior to exercise.

Inhalation solution – Adults, children ≥ 12 years - 2.5 mg 3 to 4 times/day nebulization. Dilute 0.5 ml 0.5% solution with 2.5 ml sterile normal saline. Deliver over ~ 5 to 15 min (if needed)

Inhalation capsules – Adults and children ≥ 4 years - Usual dose is 200 mcg inhaled every 4 to 6 hours using a Rotahaler device. Some patients may need 400 mcg every 4 to 6 hours.

Prevention of exercise-induced bronchospasm:

Adults and children ≥ 12 years – 200 mcg inhaled using a Rotahaler inhalation device 15 minutes before exercise.

Tablets – Adults and children ≥ 12 years - Usual starting dosage is 2 or 4 mg 3 or 4 times daily. Do not exceed a total daily dose of 32 mg. Use doses > 4 mg 4 times daily only when the patient fails to respond. If a favorable response does not occur, cautiously increase stepwise, up to a max of 8 mg 4 times daily, as tolerated.

Children 6 to 12 years: Usual starting dosage is 2 mg 3 to 4 times/day. For those who fail to respond to the initial starting dosage, cautiously increase stepwise, but do not exceed 24 mg/day in divided doses.

Elderly patients and those sensitive to β-adrenergic stimulants: Start with 2 mg 3 or 4 times daily. If adequate bronchodilation is not obtained, increase dosage gradually to as much as 8 mg 3 or 4 times daily.

Tablets, extended release – Adults and children ≥ 12 years - Usual starting dosage is 4 or 8 mg every 12 hours. Use doses > 8 mg twice/day only when the patient fails to respond. If a favorable response does not occur with the 4 mg initial dosage, cautiously increase stepwise up to a maximum of 16 mg twice a day. Do not exceed 32 mg/day.

Switching to extended release tablets: Patients maintained on regular release albuterol can be switched to *Proventil Repetabs*. A 4 mg extended release tablet every 12 hours is equivalent to a regular 2 mg tablet every 6 hours. Multiples of this regimen up to the maximum recommended dose also apply.

Syrup – Adults and children > 14 years - Usual dose is 2 or 4 mg 3 or 4 times/day. Give doses > 4 mg 4 times/day only when patient fails to respond. If a favorable response does not occur, cautiously increase, but do not exceed 8 mg 4 times/day.

Children (6 to 14): Usual starting dose is 2 mg 3 or 4 times/day. If patient does not respond to 2 mg 4 times/day, cautiously increase step-wise. Do not exceed 24 mg/day in divided doses.

Children (2 to 6): Initiate at 0.1 mg/kg 3 times daily. Do not exceed 2 mg 3 times daily. If the patient does not respond to the initial dose, increase step-wise to 0.2 mg/kg 3 times a day. Do not exceed 4 mg 3 times a day.

Elderly patients and those sensitive to β-adrenergic stimulation – Restrict initial dose to 2 mg 3 or 4 times daily. Individualize dosage thereafter.

METAPROTERENOL:

Metered dose inhaler – 2 to 3 inhalations every 3 to 4 hours. Do not exceed 12 inhalations/day. Not recommended for children < 12 years of age.

Inhalant solutions – Usually, treatment need not be repeated more often than every 4 hours to relieve acute bronchospasm attacks. In chronic bronchospastic pulmonary diseases, give 3 to 4 times a day. A single dose of nebulized metaproterenol in the treatment of an acute attack of asthma may not completely abort an attack. Not recommended for children < 12 years of age.

Dosage and Dilution for Metaproterenol Inhalant Solutions			
Administration	Usual dose	Range	Dilution
Hand bulb nebulizer	10 inhalations	5-15 inhalations	No dilution
IPPB	0.3 ml	0.2-0.3 ml	In ≈ 2.5 ml saline or other diluent

Oral –

Adults and children (> 9 years or > 60 lbs): 20 mg 3 or 4 times a day.

Children (> 6 to 9 years or < 60 lbs): 10 mg 3 or 4 times a day.

Children (< 6 years): Doses of ≈ 1.3 to 2.6 mg/kg/day in divided doses of syrup were well tolerated in 78 children. Tablets are not recommended for this age group.

Isoetharine Doses (Volume) Based on Strength of Solution		
Solution strength	Usual dose (IPPB[1] or oxygen aerosolization[2])	Equivalent isoetharine 1% dose
1%	0.25 to 1 ml (IPPB) or 0.25 to 0.5 ml (0_2 aerosolization) diluted 1:3 with salineor other diluent	same
0.25%	2 ml	0.5 ml
0.2%	1.25 to 2.5 ml	0.25 to 0.5 ml
0.17%	3 ml	0.5 ml
0.167%	3 ml	0.25 to 0.5 ml
0.125%	2 to 4 ml	0.25 to 0.5 ml
0.1%	2.5 to 5 ml	0.25 to 0.5 ml
0.08%	3 ml	0.25 ml
0.062%	4 ml	0.25 ml

[1] Usually an inspiratory flow rate of 15 L/min at a cycling pressure of 15 cm H_2O; may adjust flow rate to 6 to 30 L/min, cycling pressure to 10 to 15 cm H_2O.

[2] When given with oxygen, adjust flow to 4 to 6 L/min over 15 to 20 minutes.

Hand nebulizer – 3 to 7 inhalations undiluted.

Aerosol nebulizer – 1 or 2 inhalations. Occasionally, more may be required; however, wait 1 full minute after the initial dose to be certain another dose is necessary.

Usually, treatment need not be repeated more often than every 4 hours, although in severe cases more frequent administration may be necessary.

TERBUTALINE:

Inhalation –

Adults and children ≥ 12 years: 2 inhalations separated by 60 seconds every 4 to 6 hours. Do not repeat more often than every 4 to 6 hours.

Oral –

Adults and children > 15 years: 5 mg, given at 6 hour intervals, 3 times daily during waking hours. If side effects are pronounced, dose may be reduced to 2.5 mg 3 times daily. Do not exceed 15 mg in 24 hours.

Children (12 to 15 years): 2.5 mg 3 times daily. Do not exceed 7.5 mg in 24 hours. Not recommended for children < 12 years of age.

Parenteral – Usual dose is 0.25 mg SC into the lateral deltoid area. If significant improvement does not occur in 15 to 30 minutes, administer a second 0.25 mg dose. Do not exceed a total dose of 0.5 mg in 4 hours. If a patient fails to respond to a second 0.25 mg dose within 15 to 30 minutes, consider other therapeutic measures.

ISOPROTERENOL:

Inhalation –

Acute bronchial asthma:

Hand bulb nebulizer – In adults and children, administer the 1:200 solution in a dosage of 5 to 15 deep inhalations. In adults, the 1:100 solution may be used if a stronger solution seems indicated. The dose is 3 to 7 deep inhalations. If no relief is evident after 5 to 10 minutes, repeat doses one more time. If acute attack recurs, repeat treatment up to 5 times daily if necessary.

Metered dose inhaler – The usual dose is 1 to 2 inhalations. Start with 1 inhalation. If no relief is evident after 2 to 5 minutes, a second inhalation may be taken. For daily maintenance, use 1 to 2 inhalations 4 to 6 times daily. Do not take more than 2 inhalations at any one time, nor more than 6 inhalations per hour.

Bronchospasm in chronic obstructive lung disease:

Hand bulb nebulizer – Usually 5 to 15 deep inhalations using the 1:200 solution. Some patients with severe attacks may require 3 to 7 inhalations using the 1:100 solution. Do not use at less than 3 to 4 hour intervals.

Nebulization by compressed air or oxygen – 0.5 ml of a 1:200 solution is diluted to 2 to 2.5 ml with appropriate diluent for a concentration of 1:800 to 1:1000. Deliver the solution over 10 to 20 minutes. May repeat up to 5 times daily.

IPPB – 0.5 ml of a 1:200 solution diluted to 2 to 2.5 ml with water or isotonic saline. Deliver over 15 to 20 minutes. May repeat up to 5 times daily.

Metered dose inhaler – 1 or 2 inhalations; repeat at no less than 3 to 4 hour intervals (4 to 6 times daily).

Children: Administration is similar to that of adults, since children's smaller ventilatory exchange capacity automatically provides proportionally smaller aerosol intake. The 1:200 solution is recommended for an acute attack of bronchospasm. Do not use more than 0.25 ml of the 1:200 solution for each 10 to 15 minute programmed treatment.

Injection – For the management of bronchospasm during anesthesia, dilute 1 ml of a 1:5000 solution to 10 ml with Sodium Chloride Injection or 5% Dextrose Injection. Administer an initial dose of 0.01 to 0.02 mg IV and repeat when necessary.

ISOPROTERENOL and PHENYLEPHRINE BITARTRATE:

Relief of dyspnea – Acute episode, 1 to 2 inhalations. Start with one inhalation; if not relieved in 2 to 5 minutes, administer a second.

Daily maintenance: 1 to 2 inhalations, 4 to 6 times daily. Do not take > 2 inhalations at any one time or > 6 in any 1 hour within 24 hours.

BITOLTEROL:

Bronchospasm –

Adults and children > 12 years of age: 2 inhalations at an interval of at least 1 to 3 minutes, followed by a third inhalation if needed.

Prevention of bronchospasm – 2 inhalations every 8 hours.

Do not exceed 3 inhalations every 6 hours or 2 inhalations every 4 hours.

EPINEPHRINE:

Inhalation aerosol – Start treatment at the first symptoms of bronchospasm. Individualize dosage. Wait 1 to 5 minutes between inhalations.

Nebulization – Place 8 to 15 drops into the nebulizer reservoir. Place the nebulizer nozzle into the partially opened mouth. Squeeze the bulb 1 to 3 times. Inhale deeply.

If relief does not occur within 5 minutes, administer 2 to 3 additional inhalations. Nebulizer use, 4 to 6 times daily, is usually sufficient to maintain comfort.

IPPB: Add 0.5 ml epinephrine to 20 ml water just prior to treatment. Administer for 15 minutes every 3 to 4 hours.

Injection –

Solution (1:1000): The initial adult: SC or IM dose is 0.3 to 0.5 ml (0.3 to 0.5 mg); repeat every 20 min to 4 hours.

For infants and children – (except premature infants and full-term newborns), give 0.01 ml/kg or 0.3 ml/m^2 (0.01 mg/kg or 0.3 mg/m^2) SC. Do not exceed 0.5 ml (0.5 mg) in a single pediatric dose. Repeat every 20 minutes to 4 hours or more often if necessary.

Suspension (1:200) – For SC use only. Administer subsequent doses only when necessary and not more often than every 6 hours.

Adults – 0.1 to 0.3 ml (0.5 to 1.5 mg) SC.

Infants and children (1 month to 12 years) – 0.005 ml/kg (0.025 mg/kg) SC.

Children ≤ 30 kg – The maximum single dose is 0.15 ml (0.75 mg).

EPHEDRINE:

Adults – The usual oral dose is 25 to 50 mg, 2 or 3 times a day. The usual parenteral dose is 25 to 50 mg, administered SC, IM or slowly IV.

Children – 3 mg/kg/day or 100 mg/m^2/day divided into 4 to 6 doses by the oral, SC or IV route.

PIRBUTEROL:

Adults and children ≥ 12 years of age – 2 inhalations (0.4 mg) repeated every 4 to 6 hours. One inhalation (0.2 mg) may be sufficient for some patients.

Do not exceed a total daily dose of 12 inhalations.

XANTHINE DERIVATIVES

THEOPHYLLINE

Tablets: 100, 125, 200, 250 and 300 mg (*Rx*)	Various, *Slo-Phyllin* (Rhone-Poulenc Rorer), *Theolair* (3M Pharm), *Quibron-T Dividose* (Bristol Labs)
Capsules: 100 and 200 mg (*Rx*)	*Bronkodyl* (Winthrop),
Syrup: 80 mg or 150 mg/15 ml (26.7 or 50 mg/5 ml) (*Rx*)	*Aquaphyllin* (Ferndale), *Accurbron* (Marion Merrell Dow)
Elixir: 80 mg/15 ml (26.7 mg/5 ml) (*Rx*)	Various, *Asmalix* (Century), *Elixomin* (Cenci), *Elixophyllin* (Forest), *Theolair* (3M Pharmaceuticals), *Lanophyllin*(Lannett)
Solution: 80 mg/15 ml (26.7 mg/5 ml) (*Rx*)	Various, *Theolair* (3M Pharm)
Capsules, timed release (8 to 12 hours): 50, 60, 65, 75, 100, 125, 130, 200, 250, 260 and 300 mg (sustained reoease) (*Rx*)	*Aerolate* (Fleming), *Slo-bid Gyrocaps* (Rhone-Poulenc Rorer), *Slo-Phyllin Gyrocaps* (Rhone-Poulenc Rorer)
Capsules, timed release (24 hours): 100, 200 and 300 mg (*Rx*)	*Theo-24* (Whitby)
Capsules, timed release (12 hours): 125, 130, 250 and 260 mg (*Rx*)	*Theovent*(Schering), *Theoclear* L.A.(Central), *Teospan SR*(Laser)
Capsules, extended release: 100, 125, 200 and 300 mg (*Rx*)	Various
Tablets, timed release (12 to 24 hours): 100, 200, 300 and 450 mg (*Rx*)	Various
Tablets, extended release: 450 mg (*Rx*)	Various
Tablets, extended release (12 to 24 hours): 100, 200 and 300 mg (*Rx*)	*Theochron* (Various)
Tablets, extended release (24 hours): 400 and 600 mg (*Rx*)	*Uni-Dur*(Key)
Tablets, timed release (8 to 12 hours): 200, 250, 300 and 500 mg (*Rx*)	*Theolair-SR* (3M Pharm), *T-Phyl* (Purdue Frederick), *Quibron-T/SR* (Roberts), *Respbid* (Boehringer-Ingelheim)
Tablets, sustained release (8 to 12 hours): 100 and 300 mg (*Rx*)	*Sustaire* (Pfizer Labs)

Tablets, timed release (8 to 24 hours): 100, 200, 300 and 450 mg (*Rx*)	*Theo-Dur* (Key)
Tablets, controlled release (12 to 24 hours): 100, 200 and 300 mg (*Rx*)	*Theo-X* (Carnrick)
Tablets, timed release (24 hours): 400 mg (*Rx*)	*Uniphyl* (Purdue Frederick)
OXTRIPHYLLINE	
Tablets: 100 mg (equiv. to 64 mg theophylline), 200 mg (equiv. to 127 mg theophylline) (*Rx*)	Various, *Choledyl* (Parke-Davis)
Tablets, sustained action: 400 mg (equiv. to 254 mg theophylline), 600 mg (equiv. to 382 mg theophylline) (*Rx*)	*Choledyl SA* (Parke-Davis)
Syrup, pediatric: 50 mg (equiv. to 32 mg theophylline) per 5 ml (*Rx*)	Various, *Choledyl* (Parke-Davis)
Elixir: 100 mg (equiv. to 64 mg theophylline) per 5 ml (*Rx*)	Various, *Choledyl* (Parke-Davis)
THEOPHYLLINE AND DEXTROSE	
Injection: 200, 400 and 800 mg/container (*Rx*)	Various
AMINOPHYLLINE	
Tablets: 100 mg (equiv. to 79 mg theophylline), 200 mg (equiv. to 158 mg theophylline) (*Rx*)	Various
Tablets, controlled release (12 hours): 225 mg (equiv. to 178 mg theophylline) (*Rx*)	*Phyllocontin* (Purdue Frederick)
Oral Liquid: 105 mg (equiv. to 90 mg theophylline) per 5 ml (*Rx*)	Various
Injection: 250 mg (equiv. to 197 mg theophylline) per 10 ml (*Rx*) For IV use.	Various
Suppositories: 250 mg (equiv. to 197.5 mg theophylline), 500 mg (equiv. to 395 mg theophylline) (*Rx*)	Various, *Truphylline* (G & W)
DYPHYLLINE	
Tablets: 200 or 400 mg (*Rx*)	Various, *Dilor* (Savage)
Elixir: 100 or 160 mg/15 ml (33.3 or mg/5 ml) (*Rx*)	*Lufyllin* (Wallace), *Dilor* (Savage)
Injection: 250 mg per ml (*Rx*)	*Lufyllin* (Wallace)

Actions:

Pharmacology: The methylxanthines (theophylline, its soluble salts and derivatives) directly relax the smooth muscle of the bronchi and pulmonary blood vessels, stimulate the CNS, induce diuresis, increase gastric acid secretion, reduce lower esophageal sphincter pressure and inhibit uterine contractions. Theophylline is also a central respiratory stimulant. Aminophylline has a potent effect on diaphragmatic contractility in healthy persons and may then be capable of reducing fatigability and thereby improve contractility in patients with chronic obstructive airways disease.

Other effects that appear to occur at therapeutic concentrations and may collectively play a role in the mechanism of the xanthines include: Inhibition of extracellular adenosine (which causes bronchoconstriction), although it is unlikely that this is a main mechanism; stimulation of endogenous catecholamines, although this also does not appear to be a major mechanism; antagonism of prostaglandins PGE_2 and $PGF_2\alpha$; direct effect on mobilization of intracellular calcium resulting in smooth muscle relaxation; beta-adrenergic agonist activity on the airways. None of these mechanisms has been proven.

Pharmacokinetics:

Absorption – Theophylline is well absorbed from oral liquids and uncoated plain tablets; maximal plasma concentrations are reached in 2 hours. Rectal absorption from suppositories is slow and erratic, the oral route is generally preferred. Enteric coated tablets and some sustained release dosage forms may be unreliably absorbed.

Distribution – Average volume of distribution is 0.45 L/kg (range, 0.3 to 0.7 L/kg). Theophylline does not distribute into fatty tissue. Approximately 40% is bound to plasma protein. Therapeutic serum levels generally range from 10 to 20 mcg/ml. Although some bronchodilatory effect occurs at lower concentrations, stabilization of hyperreactive airways is most evident at levels > 10 mcg/ml, and adverse effects are uncommon at levels < 20 mcg/ml.

Metabolism/Excretion – Xanthines are biotransformed in the liver (85% to 90%) to 1, 3–dimethyluric acid, 3–methylxanthine and 1–methyluric acid; 3–methylxanthine accumulates in concentrations approximately 25% of those of theophylline.

Excretion is by the kidneys; < 15% of the drug is excreted unchanged. Elimination kinetics vary greatly. Plasma elimination half-life averages about 3 to 15 hours in adult nonsmokers, 4 to 5 hours in adult smokers (1 to 2 packs per day), 1 to 9 hours in children and 20 to 30 hours for premature neonates. In the neonate, theophylline is metabolized partially to caffeine. The premature neonate excretes about 50% unchanged theophylline and may accumulate the caffeine metabolite.

Equivalent dose: Because of differing theophylline content, the various salts and derivatives are not equivalent on a weight basis.

Theophylline Content and Equivalent Dose of Various Theophylline Salts		
Theophylline salts	Theophylline %	Equivalent dose
Theophylline anhydrous	100	100 mg
Theophylline monohydrate	91	110 mg
Aminophylline anhydrous	86	116 mg
Aminophylline dihydrate	79	127 mg
Oxtriphylline	64	156 mg

Dyphylline, a chemical derivative of theophylline, is not a theophylline salt as are the other agents. It is about one-tenth as potent as theophylline. Following oral administration, dyphylline is 68% to 82% bioavailable. Peak plasma concentrations are reached within 1 hour, and its half-life is 2 hours. The minimal effective therapeutic concentration is 12 mcg/ml. It is not metabolized to theophylline and 83% ± 5% is excreted unchanged in the urine.

Indications:

Symptomatic relief or prevention of bronchial asthma and reversible bronchospasm associated with chronic bronchitis and emphysema.

Unlabeled uses: Treatment of apnea and bradycardia of prematurity.

Theophylline 10 mg/kg/day may significantly improve pulmonary function and dyspnea in patients with chronic obstructive pulmonary disease.

Contraindications:

Hypersensitivity to any xanthine; peptic ulcer; underlying seizure disorders (unless receiving appropriate anticonvulsant medication).

Aminophylline: Hypersensitivity to ethylenediamine.

Aminophylline rectal suppositories: Irritation or infection of rectum or lower colon.

Warnings:

Status asthmaticus is a medical emergency and is not rapidly responsive to usual doses of conventional bronchodilators. Optimal therapy frequently requires both parenteral medication and close monitoring, preferably in an intensive care setting. Oral theophylline products alone are not appropriate for status asthmaticus.

Toxicity: Excessive doses may cause severe toxicity; monitor serum levels to assure maximum benefit with minimum risk. Incidence of toxicity increases significantly at serum levels > 20 mcg/ml. Serum levels > 20 mcg/ml are rare after appropriate use of recommended doses. However, if theophylline plasma clearance is reduced for any reason (eg, hepatic impairment; patients > 55 years old, particularly males and those with chronic lung disease; cardiac failure; sustained high fever; infants < 1 year old), even conventional doses may result in increased serum levels and potential toxicity. Frequently, such patients have markedly prolonged levels following drug discontinuation.

Serious side effects such as ventricular arrhythmias, convulsions or even death may appear as the first sign of toxicity without any previous warning. Less serious signs of toxicity (eg, nausea, restlessness) may occur frequently when initiating therapy, but are usually transient; when such signs are persistent during maintenance therapy, they are often associated with serum concentrations > 20 mcg/ml. Serious toxicity is not reliably preceded by less severe side effects.

Cardiac effects: Theophylline may cause dysrhythmias or worsen pre-existing arrhythmias. Any significant change in cardiac rate or rhythm warrants monitoring and further investigation. Many patients who require theophylline may exhibit tachycardia due to underlying disease; the relationship to elevated serum theophylline concentrations may not be appreciated.

Pregnancy: *Category* C. Theophylline has been found in cord serum and crosses the placenta; newborns may have therapeutic serum levels.

Lactation: Theophylline distributes readily into breast milk with a milk:plasma ratio of 0.7 and may cause irritability or other signs of toxicity in nursing infants.

Children: Sufficient numbers of infants < 1 year of age have not been studied in clinical trials to support use in this age group; however, there is evidence that the use of dosage recommendations for older infants and young children may result in the development of toxic serum levels.

Precautions:

Use with caution in: Cardiac disease; hypoxemia; hepatic disease; hypertension; congestive heart failure (CHF); alcoholism; elderly (particularly males); and neonates.

GI effects: Use cautiously in peptic ulcer. Local irritation may occur; centrally mediated GI effects may occur with serum levels > 20 mcg/ml. Reduced lower esophageal pressure may cause reflux, aspiration and worsening of airway obstruction.

Drug Interactions:

Agents that may decrease theophylline levels include aminoglutethimide, barbiturates, charcoal, hydantoins, ketoconazole, rifampin, smoking (cigarettes and marijuana), sulfinpyrazone, sympathomimetics (β-agonists), thioamines, carbamazepine, isoniazid and loop diuretics.

Agents that may increase theophylline levels include allopurinol, beta blockers (nonselective), calcium channel blockers, cimetidine, oral contraceptives, corticosteroids, disulfiram, ephedrine, influenza virus vaccine, interferon, macrolides, mexiletine, quinolones, thiabendazile, thyroid hormones, carbamazepine, isoniazid and loop diuretics.

The following agents may be affected by theophylline: Benzodiazepines, halothane, ketamine, lithium, nondepolarizing muscle relaxants and propofol. Probenecid may increase the effects of dyphylline.

Drug/Food interactions: Theophylline elimination is increased (half-life shortened) by a low carbohydrate, high protein diet and charcoal broiled beef (due to a high polycyclic carbon content). Conversely, elimination is decreased (prolonged half-life) by a high carbohydrate low protein diet. Food may alter the bioavailability and absorption pattern of certain sustained release preparations. Some sustained release preparations may be subject to rapid release of their contents when taken with food, resulting in toxicity. It appears that consistent administration in the fasting state allows predictability of effects.

Adverse Reactions:

Adverse reactions/toxicity are uncommon at serum theophylline levels < 20 mcg/ml.

Levels > 20 mcg/ml: 75% of patients experience adverse reactions (eg, nausea, vomiting, diarrhea, headache, insomnia, irritability).

Levels > 35 mcg/ml: Hyperglycemia; hypotension; cardiac arrhythmias; tachycardia (> 10 mcg/ml in premature newborns); seizures; brain damage; death.

Other: Fever; flushing; hyperglycemia; inappropriate antidiuretic hormone syndrome; rash; alopecia. Ethylenediamine in aminophylline can cause sensitivity reactions, including exfoliative dermatitis and urticaria.

CNS: Irritability; restlessness; headache; insomnia; reflex hyperexcitability; muscle twitching; convulsions.

GI: Nausea; vomiting; epigastric pain; hematemesis; diarrhea; rectal irritation or bleeding (aminophylline suppositories). Therapeutic doses of theophylline may induce gastroesophageal reflux during sleep or while recumbent, increasing the potential for aspiration which can aggravate bronchospasm.

Cardiovascular: Palpitations; tachycardia; extrasystoles; hypotension; circulatory failure; life-threatening ventricular arrhythmias.

Respiratory: Tachypnea; respiratory arrest.

Renal: Proteinuria; potentiation of diuresis.

Administration and Dosage:

THEOPHYLLINE: Individualize dosage. Base dosage adjustments on clinical response and improvement in pulmonary function with careful monitoring of serum levels. If possible, monitor serum levels to maintain levels in the therapeutic range of 10 to 20 mcg/ml. Levels > 20 mcg/ml may produce toxicity, and it may even occur with levels between 15 to 20 mcg/ml, particularly when factors known to reduce theophylline clearance are present (see Warnings). Once stabilized on a dosage, serum levels tend to remain constant.

Calculate dosages on the basis of lean body weight, since theophylline does not distribute into fatty tissue. Regardless of salt used, dosages should be equivalent based on anhydrous theophylline content.

Individualize frequency of dosing. With immediate release products, dosing every 6 hours is generally required, especially in children; intervals up to 8 hours may be satisfactory in adults. Some children and adults requiring higher than average doses (those having rapid rates of clearance; eg, half-lives < 6 hours) may be more effectively controlled during chronic therapy with sustained release products. Determine dosage intervals to produce minimal fluctuations between peak and trough serum theophylline concentrations. Consider the absorption profile and the elimination rate. When converting from an immediate release to a sustained release product, the total daily dose should remain the same, and only the dosing interval adjusted.

Acute symptoms requiring rapid theophyllinization in patients not receiving theophylline – To achieve a rapid effect, an initial loading dose is required. Dosage recommendations are for theophylline anhydrous.

Dosage Guidelines for Rapid Theophyllinization		
Patient Group	Oral loading	Maintenance
Children 1 to 9 years	5 mg/kg	4 mg/kg q 6 h
Children 9 to 16 and young adult smokers	5 mg/kg	3 mg/kg q 6 h
Otherwise healthy non-smoking adults	5 mg/kg	3 mg/kg q 8 h
Older patients, patients with cor pulmonale	5 mg/kg	2 mg/kg q 8 h
Patients with congestive heart failure	5 mg/kg	1-2 mg/kg q 12 h

Infants (preterm to < 1 year) –

Theophylline Dosage Guidelines for Infants	
Age	Initial maintenance dose
Premature infants	
≤ 24 days postnatal	1 mg/kg q 12 h
> 24 days postnatal	1.5 mg/kg q 12 h
Infants (6 to 52 weeks)	[(0.2 x age in weeks) = 5] x kg = 24 hr dose in mg
Up to 26 weeks	Divide into q 8 h dosing
26 to 52 weeks	Divide into q 6 h dosing

Acute symptoms requiring rapid theophyllinization in patients receiving theophylline – Each 0.5 mg/kg theophylline administered as a loading dose will increase the serum theophylline concentration by approximately 1 mcg/ml. Ideally, defer the loading dose if a serum theophylline concentration can be obtained rapidly.

If this is not possible, exercise clinical judgment. When there is sufficient respiratory distress to warrant a small risk, then 2.5 mg/kg of theophylline administered in rapidly absorbed form is likely to increase serum concentration by approximately 5 mcg/ml. If the patient is not experiencing theophylline toxicity, this is unlikely to result in dangerous adverse effects.

Chronic therapy – Slow clinical titration is generally preferred.

Initial dose: 16 mg/kg/24 hours or 400 mg/24 hours, whichever is less, of anhydrous theophylline in divided doses at 6 or 8 hour intervals.

Increasing dose: The above dosage may be increased in approximately 25% increments at 3 day intervals so long as the drug is tolerated or until the maximum dose (indicated below) is reached.

Maximum dose (where the serum concentration is not measured) – Do not attempt to maintain any dose that is not tolerated.

Maximum Daily Theophylline Dose Based on Age	
Age	Maximum daily dose[1]
1 to 9 years	24 mg/kg/day
9 to 12 years	20 mg/kg/day
12 to 16 years	18 mg/kg/day
> 16 years	13 mg/kg/day

[1] Not to exceed listed dose or 900 mg, whichever is less.

Exercise caution in younger children who cannot complain of minor side effects. Older adults and those with cor pulmonale, CHF or liver disease may have unusually low dosage requirements; they may experience toxicity at the maximal dosages recommended.

Measurement of serum theophylline concentrations during chronic therapy is recommended. The table below provides guidance to dosage adjustments based on serum theophylline level determinations:

Dosage Adjustment After Serum Theophylline Measurement		
If serum theophylline is:		Directions
Too low	5 to 10 mcg/ml	Increase dose by about 25% at 3 day intervals until either the desired clinical response or serum concentration is achieved.[1]
Within desired range	10 to 20 mcg/ml	Maintain dosage if tolerated. Recheck serum theophylline concentration at 6 to 12 month intervals.[2]
Too high	20 to 25 mcg/ml	Decrease doses by about 10%. Recheck serum theophylline concentration after 3 days.[2]
	25 to 30 mcg/ml	Skip next dose and decrease subsequent doses by about 25%. Recheck serum theophylline after 3 days.
	> 30 mcg/ml	Skip next 2 doses and decrease subsequent doses by 50%. Recheck serum theophylline after 3 days.

[1] The total daily dose may need to be administered at more frequent intervals if asthma symptoms occur repeatedly at the end of a dosing interval.
[2] Finer adjustments in dosage may be needed for some patients.

Timed Release Capsules – These dosage forms gradually release the active medication so that the total daily dosage may be administered in 1 to 3 doses divided by 8 to 24 hours, depending on the patient's pharmacokinetic profile, thus reducing the number of daily doses required. These products are not necessarily interchangeable. If patients are switched from one brand to another, closely monitor their theophylline serum levels; serum concentrations may vary greatly following brand interchange.

OXTRIPHYLLINE:

Adults – 4.7 mg/kg every 8 hours.

Children (9 to 16 years) and adult smokers – 4.7 mg/kg every 6 hours.

Children (1 to 9 years) – 6.2 mg/kg every 6 hours.

Sustained action – If total daily maintenance dosage is established at approximately 800 or 1200 mg, 1 sustained action tablet every 12 hours may be substituted.

THEOPHYLLINE and DEXTROSE: Substitute oral therapy for IV theophylline as soon as adequate improvement is achieved.

Children – Due to marked variation in theophylline metabolism, use this drug only if clearly needed in infants < 6 months of age.

AMINOPHYLLINE:

IV – The loading dose may be infused into 100 to 200 ml of 5% Dextrose Injection or 0.9% Sodium Chloride Injection. Do not exceed 25 mg/min infusion rate.

Parenteral administration – Inject aminophylline slowly, not more than 25 mg/min, when given IV. Substitute oral therapy for IV aminophylline as soon as adequate improvement is achieved.

Loading dose:

In patients currently not receiving theophylline products – 6 mg/kg.

In patients currently receiving theophylline products – Each 0.5 mg/kg theophylline (0.6 mg/kg aminophylline) will increase the serum theophylline concentration by approximately 1 mcg/ml. When respiratory distress warrants a small risk, 2.5 mg/kg theophylline (3.1 mg aminophylline IV) increases serum concentration by approximately 5 mcg/ml. If the patient is not experiencing theophylline toxicity, this is unlikely to result in dangerous side effects.

Maintenance infusions Administer by a large volume infusion to deliver the desired amount of drug each hour.

Aminophylline Maintenance Infusion Rates (mg/kg/hr)		
Patient Group	First 12 hours	Beyond 12 hours
Neonates to infants < 6 months	Not recommended	
Children 6 months to 9 years	1.2	1
Children ages 9 to 16 and young adult smokers	1	0.0
Otherwise healthy nonsmoking adults	0.7	0.5
Older patients and those with cor pulmonale	0.6	0.3
Patients with CHF, liver disease	0.5	0.1-0.2

DYPHYLLINE: Dyphylline is a derivative of theophylline; it is not a theophylline salt, and is not metabolized to theophylline in vivo. Although dyphylline is 70% theophylline by molecular weight ratio, the amount of dyphylline equivalent to a given amount of theophylline is not known. Specific dyphylline serum levels may be used to monitor therapy; serum theophylline levels will NOT measure dyphylline. The minimal effective therapeutic concentration is 12 mcg/ml.

Oral –

Adults: Up to 15 mg/kg every 6 hours.

IM – (Not for IV administration.)

Adults: 250 to 500 mg injected slowly every 6 hours. Do not exceed 15 mg/kg every 6 hours.

Children: Safety and efficacy have not been established.

CORTICOSTEROIDS

BECLOMETHASONE	
Aerosol: Each actuation delivers approx. 42 mcg (Rx)	*Beclovent* (Glaxo Wellcome), *Vanceril* (Schering)
DEXAMETHASONE	
Aerosol: Each activation releases dexamethasone sodium phosphate equivalent to approximately 84 mcg dexamethasone (Rx)	*Dexacort Phosphate in Respihaler* (Adams)
TRIAMCINOLONE	
Aerosol: Each actuation delivers approx. 100 mcg. Contains 60 mg triamcinolone acetonide (Rx)	*Azmacort* (Rhone-Poulenc Rorer)
FLUNISOLIDE	
Aerosol: Each actuation delivers approx. 250 mcg (Rx)	*AeroBid* (Forest), *AeroBid-M* (Forest)

Warning:

Adrenal insufficiency: Deaths due to adrenal insufficiency have occurred in asthmatic patients during and after transfer from systemic corticosteroids to aerosol steroids. After withdrawal from systemic corticosteroids, several months are required for recovery of hypothalamic-pituitary-adrenal (HPA) function. During this period of HPA suppression, patients may exhibit symptoms of adrenal insufficiency when exposed to trauma, surgery or infections, particularly gastroenteritis. Although aerosolized glucocorticoids may control asthmatic symptoms during these episodes, they do NOT provide the systemic steroid necessary for the treatment of these emergencies.

Stress/Severe asthma attack: During periods of stress or a severe asthmatic attack, patients withdrawn from systemic corticosteroids should resume them (in large doses) immediately and contact physician. Patients should carry a warning card indicating they may need supplementary systemic steroids during such periods.

Actions:

Pharmacology: These agents are synthetic adrenocortical steroids with basic glucocorticoid actions and effects. The mechanism responsible for the potent anti-inflammatory activity and the precise mechanism of action of aerosolized drug in the lung is unknown. Glucocorticoids may decrease number and activity of inflammatory cells, enhance effect of beta-adrenergic drugs on cyclic AMP production, inhibit bronchoconstrictor mechanisms or produce direct smooth muscle relaxation. Inhaler use provides effective local steroid activity with minimal systemic effect.

Pharmacokinetics:

Beclomethasone dipropionate – Systemic absorption occurs rapidly with all routes of administration. There is no evidence of tissue storage of beclomethasone or its metabolites. Lung slices can metabolize beclomethasone dipropionate rapidly to beclomethasone 17-monopropionate, and more slowly to free beclomethasone. The principal route of excretion of drug and metabolites is via feces; < 10% in urine.

Dexamethasone sodium phosphate – Because of the high water solubility of dexamethasone sodium phosphate, the aerosolized particles dissolve readily in bronchial and bronchiolar mucous membrane secretions. On 12 inhalations daily, the patient absorbs ≈ 0.4 to 0.6 mg dexamethasone (≈ 40% to 60% absorption) or 3 to 4 mg or 11 to 16 mg prednisone or hydrocortisone equivalent, respectively.

Triamcinolone acetonide – Studies demonstrate rapid disappearance from the lungs. Peak blood levels occur in 1 to 2 hours. Three metabolites have been identified; the major portion of the dose is eliminated in the feces.

Flunisolide – After inhalation of 1mg flunisolide, systemic availability was 40%. The absorbed flunisolide is rapidly and extensively metabolized during the first pass through the liver. Plasma half-life is approximately 1.8 hours.

Indications:

For control of bronchial asthma in patients requiring chronic treatment with corticosteroids. Such patients include those already receiving systemic corticosteroids, and those inadequately controlled on a nonsteroid regimen in whom steroid therapy has been withheld because of concern over potential adverse effects.

For related corticosteroid-responsive bronchospastic states intractable to adequate trial of conventional therapy.

NOT indicated for relief of asthma which can be controlled by bronchodilators and other nonsteroid medications, in patients who require systemic corticosteroid treatment infrequently, or in the treatment of nonasthmatic bronchitis.

Contraindications:

Primary treatment of status asthmaticus or other acute episodes of asthma when intensive measures are required; hypersensitivity to any ingredient; systemic fungal infections; persistently positive sputum cultures for *Candida albicans*.

Warnings:

Infections: Localized fungal infections with *Candida albicans* or *Aspergillus niger* have occurred in the mouth, pharynx and occasionally in the larynx. Positive cultures for oral *Candida* may be present in up to 75% of patients. The incidence of clinically apparent infection is low, and may require treatment with appropriate antifungal therapy or discontinuance of aerosol steroid treatment.

Acute asthma: These products are not bronchodilators and are not for rapid relief of bronchospasm. Contact a physician immediately when episodes of asthma do not respond to bronchodilators. Patients may require systemic corticosteroids.

There is no evidence that control of asthma can be achieved by administration of inhaled corticosteroids in amounts greater than recommended doses.

Replacement therapy: Transfer from systemic steroid therapy may unmask allergic conditions previously suppressed. During withdrawal from oral steroids, some patients may experience withdrawal symptoms despite maintenance or improvement of respiratory function.

Pregnancy: (Triamcinolone – Category D. Flunisolide – Category C).

Lactation: Glucocorticoids are excreted in breast milk. It is not known whether inhaled corticosteroids are excreted in breast milk, but it is likely.

Children: Insufficient information is available to warrant use in children < 6 years old.

Precautions:

Adrenal effects: In responsive patients, inhaled corticosteroids may permit control of asthmatic symptoms without HPA suppression. Since these agents are absorbed and can be systemically active, the beneficial effects in minimizing or preventing HPA dysfunction may be expected only when recommended dosages are not exceeded.

Long-term effects of inhaled glucocorticoids are unknown; although there is no clinical evidence of adverse effects, the local effects on developmental or immunologic processes in the mouth, pharynx, trachea and lung are unknown.

There is also no information about effects on pulmonary infection (including active or quiescent tuberculosis), or effects of long-term use administration on lung or other tissues.

Pulmonary infiltrates with eosinophilia may occur with beclomethasone or flunisolide. This may become manifest due to systemic steroid withdrawal when inhalational agents are used, but a causative role for either agent or vehicle cannot be ruled out.

Dysphonia: A relatively common occurrence, intermittent dysphonia has occurred in $\leq 50\%$ of patients and may be due to laryngeal candidiasis or a bilateral adductor vocal cord deformity induced by the corticosteroid. This symptom may be dose-related.

Coughing and wheezing may be more common with the use of beclomethasone and appears to be due to the dispersant rather than the drug. An alternative agent may diminish these effects. Also, pretreatment with an aerosol bronchodilator is effective in reducing coughing and wheezing in some patients.

Adverse Reactions:

Local: Throat irritation; hoarseness/dysphonia, coughing (see Precautions); dry mouth; rash; wheezing; facial edema.

Systemic: Suppression of HPA function has occurred in adults who used beclomethasone 1600 mcg/day for 1 month and 4000 mcg/day triamcinolone or recommended doses for 6 to 12 weeks. Deaths due to adrenal insufficiency have occurred during and after transfer from systemic to aerosol corticosteroids.

Beclomethasone: Rare cases of immediate and delayed hypersensitivity reactions, including urticaria, angioedema, rash and bronchospasm.

Administration and Dosage:

Patients receiving concomitant systemic steroids: Transfer to steroid inhalant and subsequent management may be more difficult because of slow HPA function recovery which may last up to 12 months. These agents may be effective and may permit replacement or significant reduction in corticosteroid dosage.

Stabilize the patient's asthma before treatment is started. Initially, use aerosol concurrently with usual maintenance dose of systemic steroid. After ≈ 1 week, start gradual withdrawal of the systemic steroid by reducing the daily or alternate daily dose. Make the next reduction after 1 to 2 weeks, depending on response. These decrements should not exceed 2.5 mg prednisone or equivalent. A slow rate of withdrawal cannot be overemphasized.

During withdrawal, some patients may experience symptoms of steroid withdrawal despite maintenance or even improvement of respiratory function. Encourage continuance with the inhaler, but observe for objective signs of adrenal insufficiency. If adrenal insufficiency occurs, increase the systemic steroid dose temporarily and continue further withdrawal more slowly.

During periods of stress or severe asthma attack, transfer patients will require supplementary systemic steroids.

BECLOMETHASONE: 50 mcg released at the valve delivers ≈ 42 mcg to the patient.

Adults – 2 inhalations (84 mcg) 3 or 4 times daily. Alternatively, 4 inhalations (168 mcg) given twice daily has been effective in some patients. In patients with severe asthma, start with 12 to 16 inhalations a day and adjust dosage downward according to response. Do not exceed 20 inhalations (840 mcg) daily.

Children – 1 or 2 inhalations (42 to 84 mcg) 3 or 4 times daily according to response. Alternatively, 2 to 4 inhalations (84 to 168 mcg) given twice daily has been effective in some patients. Do not exceed 10 inhalations (420 mcg) daily. Clinical data are insufficient with respect to administration in children < 6 years if age.

Patients not receiving systemic steroids – Follow above directions. In responsive patients, pulmonary function usually improves within 1 to 4 weeks.

DEXAMETHASONE:

Recommended initial dosage –

Adults: 3 inhalations 3 or 4 times per day; maximum 12 inhalations/day.

Children: 2 inhalations 3 or 4 times per day; maximum 8 inhalations/day.

TRIAMCINOLONE: 200 mcg released with each actuation delivers ≈ 100 mcg to the patient.

Adults – The usual dosage is 2 inhalations (≈ 200 mcg) 3 to 4 times a day. Do not exceed a maximum daily intake of 16 inhalations (1600 mcg). Higher initial doses (12 to 16 inhalations per day) may be advisable in patients with more severe asthma, the dosage then being adjusted downward according to patient response. In some patients, maintenance can be accomplished when the total daily dose is administered twice a day.

Children – The usual dosage is 1 or 2 inhalations (100 to 200 mcg) 3 to 4 times a day. Do not exceed a maximum daily intake of 12 inhalations (1200 mcg). Clinical data are insufficient with respect to use in children < 6 years of age.

Patients not receiving systemic steroids – Follow above directions. In responsive patients, an improvement in pulmonary function is usually apparent within 1 to 2 weeks.

FLUNISOLIDE: Each actuation delivers ≈ 250 mcg flunisolide to the patient.

Adults – 2 inhalations (500 mcg) twice daily, morning and evening (total daily dose 1000 mcg). Do not exceed 4 inhalations twice daily (2000 mcg).

Children (6 to 15 years) – 2 inhalations twice daily, morning and evening (total daily dose 1000 mcg). Higher doses have not been studied. Safety and efficacy for use in children < 6 years have not been established. With chronic use, monitor children for growth as well as for effects on the HPA axis.

Patients not receiving systemic steroids – In responsive patients, pulmonary function usually improves within 1 to 4 weeks.

ACETYLCYSTEINE (N-Acetylcysteine)

Solution: 10% and 20% (*Rx*)	Various, *Mucomyst* (Apothecon), *Mucosil-10* (Dey Labs)

Actions:

Pharmacology: The mucolytic action of acetylcysteine is related to the sulfhydryl group in the molecule, which acts directly to split disulfide linkages between mucoprotein molecular complexes, resulting in depolymerization and a decrease in mucus viscosity. The mucolytic activity of acetylcysteine increases with increasing pH.

Acetylcysteine also reduces the extent of liver injury following acetaminophen overdose. It is thought that acetylcysteine protects the liver by maintaining or restoring glutathione levels, or by acting as an alternate substrate for conjugation with, and thus, detoxification of, the reactive metabolite of acetaminophen.

Pharmacokinetics: Following a 200 to 400 mg oral dose, peak plasma concentrations of 0.35 to 4 mg/L are achieved within 1 to 2 hours. Protein binding is ≈ 50% 4 hours post-dose. Volume of distribution is 0.33 to 0.47 L/kg. The terminal half-life of reduced acetylcysteine is 6.25 hours. Approximately 70% of total body clearance is nonrenal.

Indications:

Mucolytic: Adjuvant therapy for abnormal, viscid or inspissated mucus secretions in chronic bronchopulmonary disease (chronic emphysema, emphysema with bronchitis, chronic asthmatic bronchitis, tuberculosis, bronchiectasis, primary amyloidosis of lung).

Acute bronchopulmonary disease (pneumonia, bronchitis, tracheobronchitis).

Pulmonary complications of cystic fibrosis.

Tracheostomy care.

Pulmonary complications associated with surgery.

Use during anesthesia.

Posttraumatic chest conditions.

Atelectasis due to mucus obstruction.

Diagnostic bronchial studies (bronchograms, bronchospirometry, bronchial wedge catheterization).

Antidote: To prevent or lessen hepatic injury which may occur following ingestion of a potentially hepatotoxic quantity of acetaminophen.

Unlabeled uses: As an ophthalmic solution to treat keratoconjunctivitis sicca. It has been used as an enema to treat bowel obstruction due to meconium ileus or its equivalent.

Contraindications:

Hypersensitivity to acetylcysteine. As an antidote, there are no contraindications.

Warnings:

Bronchial secretions: An increased volume of liquefied bronchial secretions may occur; when cough is inadequate, maintain an open airway by mechanical suction if necessary. When there is a large mechanical block due to a foreign body or local accumulation, clear the airway by endotracheal aspiration, with or without bronchoscopy.

Asthmatics: Carefully observe asthmatics under treatment with acetylcysteine. If bronchospasm progresses, discontinue medication immediately.

Antidotal use:

Allergic effects – Generalized urticaria has been observed rarely. If this or other allergic symptoms appear, discontinue treatment unless it is deemed essential and the allergic symptoms can be otherwise controlled.

Hepatic effects – If encephalopathy due to hepatic failure occurs, discontinue treatment to avoid further administration of nitrogenous substances. No data indicate that acetylcysteine adversely influences hepatic failure, but this is theoretically possible.

Vomiting, occasionally severe and persistent, occurs as a symptom of acute acetaminophen overdose. Treatment with oral acetylcysteine may aggravate vomiting. Evaluate patients at risk of gastric hemorrhage concerning the risk of upper GI hemorrhage vs the risk of developing hepatic toxicity. Diluting acetylcysteine minimizes its propensity to aggravate vomiting.

Pregnancy: Category B.

Lactation: It is not known whether this drug is excreted in breast milk.

Precautions:

Disagreeable odor: Administration may initially produce a slight disagreeable odor which soon disappears.

Face mask use: A face mask may cause stickiness on the face after nebulization; remove with water.

Solution color may change in the opened bottle, but does not significantly impair the drug's safety or efficacy.

Continued nebulization of acetylcysteine with a dry gas results in concentration of drug in the nebulizer due to evaporation. Extreme concentration may impede nebulization and drug delivery. Dilute with Sterile Water for Injection as concentration occurs.

Adverse Reactions:

Stomatitis; nausea; vomiting; fever; rhinorrhea; drowsiness; clamminess; chest tightness; bronchoconstriction; bronchospasm; irritation to the tracheal and bronchial tracts.

Antidotal use: Large doses of oral acetylcysteine may result in nausea, vomiting and other GI symptoms. Rash (with or without mild fever), pruritus, angioedema, bronchospasm, tachycardia, hypotension and hypertension have occurred.

Administration and Dosage:

Nebulization (face mask, mouth piece, tracheostomy): 1 to 10 ml of the 20% solution or 2 to 20 ml of the 10% solution every 2 to 6 hours; the dose for most patients is 3 to 5 ml of the 20% solution or 6 to 10 ml of the 10% solution 3 to 4 times a day.

Nebulization (tent, croupette): Very large volumes are required, occasionally up to 300 ml during a treatment period. The dose is the volume of solution that will maintain a very heavy mist in the tent or croupette for the desired period. Administration for intermittent or continuous prolonged periods, including overnight, may be desirable.

Instillation:

Direct – 1 to 2 ml of a 10% to 20% solution as often as every hour.

Tracheostomy – 1 to 2 ml of a 10% to 20% solution every 1 to 4 hours by instillation into the tracheostomy.

May be introduced directly into a particular segment of the bronchopulmonary tree by inserting (under local anesthesia and direct vision) a plastic catheter into the trachea. Instill 2 to 5 ml of the 20% solution by a syringe connected to the catheter.

Percutaneous intratracheal catheter – 1 to 2 ml of the 20% solution or 2 to 4 ml of the 10% solution every 1 to 4 hours by a syringe attached to the catheter.

Diagnostic bronchograms: 2 or 3 administrations of 1 to 2 ml of the 20% solution or 2 to 4 ml of the 10% solution by nebulization or by instillation intratracheally, prior to the procedure.

Equipment compatibility: Certain materials in nebulization equipment react with acetylcysteine, especially certain metals (notably iron and copper) and rubber. Where materials may come into contact with acetylcysteine solution, use parts made of the following materials: Glass, plastic, aluminum, anodized aluminum, chromed metal, tantalum, sterling silver or stainless steel. Silver may become tarnished after exposure, but this is not harmful to the drug action or to the patient.

Acetaminophen overdosage: Administer acetylcysteine immediately if ≤ 24 hours have elapsed from the reported time of acetaminophen ingestion. Do not await results of assays for acetaminophen level before initiating treatment. The following procedures are recommended:

1.) Empty the stomach promptly by lavage or by inducing emesis with syrup of ipecac. Repeat the ipecac dose if emesis does not occur in 20 minutes.
2.) If activated charcoal has been administered, lavage before administering acetylcysteine. Activated charcoal may adsorb acetylcysteine, thereby reducing its effectiveness.
3.) Draw blood for acetaminophen plasma assay and for baseline AST, ALT, bilirubin, prothrombin time, creatinine, BUN, blood sugar and electrolytes. If an assay cannot be obtained or if the acetaminophen level is clearly in the toxic range, continue acetylcysteine for the full course of therapy. Monitor hepatic and renal function and electrolyte and fluid balance.
4.) Administer a 140 mg/kg loading dose of acetylcysteine.
5.) Administer the first maintenance dose (70 mg/kg) 4 hours after the loading dose. Repeat the maintenance dose at 4 hour intervals for a total of 17 doses unless the acetaminophen assay reveals a nontoxic level.
6.) If the patient vomits the loading dose or any maintenance dose within 1 hour of administration, repeat that dose.
7.) If the patient is persistently unable to retain the orally administered acetylcysteine, administer by duodenal intubation. Acetylcysteine may also be administered IV. Although there is no FDA-approved commercially available acetylcysteine IV formulation, the 20% solution can be diluted in D5W and administered at the previously mentioned dosage for acetaminophen overdosage. Adverse reactions to IV administration appear to be rate-dependent; infuse the dose slowly over 1 hour.
8.) Repeat AST, ALT, bilirubin, prothrombin time, creatinine, BUN, blood sugar and electrolytes daily if the acetaminophen plasma level is in the potentially toxic range.

Acetaminophen assays – The acute ingestion of acetaminophen in quantities of ≥ 150 mg/kg may result in hepatic toxicity. However, the reported history of the quantity of a drug ingested as an overdose is often inaccurate and is not a reliable guide to antidotal therapy. Therefore, determine plasma or serum acetaminophen concentrations as early as possible, but no sooner than 4 hours following an acute overdose to assess the potential risk of hepatotoxicity. If an acetaminophen assay cannot be obtained, assume that the overdose is potentially toxic.

Interpretation of acetaminophen assays (refer to the following nomogram) – When results of the plasma acetaminophen assay are available, refer to the nomogram. Values above the solid line connecting 200 mcg/ml at 4 hours with 50 mcg/ml at 12 hours are associated with a possibility of hepatic toxicity if an antidote is not administered. Do not wait for assay results to begin treatment.

If the plasma level is above the broken line, continue with maintenance doses of acetylcysteine. It is better to err on the safe side; thus, the broken line is plotted 25% below the solid line which defines possible toxicity.

If the plasma level is below the broken line described above, there is minimal risk of hepatic toxicity and acetylcysteine treatment can be discontinued.

Estimating potential for hepatotoxicity – The following nomogram estimates the probability that plasma levels in relation to intervals postingestion will result in hepatotoxicity.

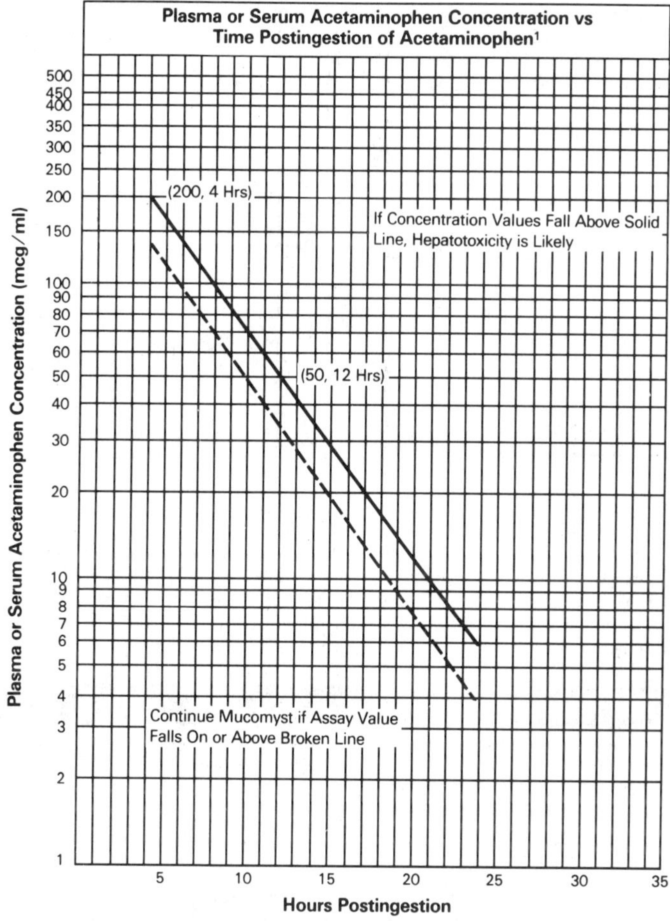

[1] Adapted from Rumack and Matthews, *Pediatrics* 1975;55:871-76.

Supportive treatment: Maintain fluid and electrolyte balance. Treat as necessary for hypoglycemia. Administer vitamin K_1 if prothrombin time ratio exceeds 1.5; administer fresh frozen plasma if the prothrombin time ratio exceeds 3. Avoid diuretics and forced diuresis.

Acetylcysteine Dosage Guide and Preparation					
Loading dose (140 mg/kg)*					
Body weight (kg)	Body weight (lb)	Acetylcysteine (g)	20% solution (ml)	Diluent (ml)	5% solution (ml)
100-109	220-240	15	75	225	300
90-99	198-218	14	70	210	280
80-89	176-196	13	65	195	260
70-79	154-174	11	55	165	220
60-69	132-152	10	50	150	200
50-59	110-130	8	40	120	160
40-49	88-108	7	35	105	140
30-39	66-86	6	30	90	120
20-29	44-64	4	20	60	80
Maintenance dose (70 mg/kg)*					
(kg)	(lb)				
100-109	220-240	7.5	37	113	150
90-99	198-218	7	35	105	140
80-89	176-196	6.5	33	97	130
70-79	154-174	5.5	28	82	110
60-69	132-152	5	25	75	100
50-59	110-130	4	20	60	80
40-49	88-108	3.5	18	52	70
30-39	66-86	3	15	45	60
20-29	44-64	2	10	30	40

* If patient weighs < 20 kg (usually patients < 6 years of age), calculate the dose. Each ml of 20% solution contains 200 mg acetylcysteine. Add 3 ml of diluent to each ml of 20% solution. Do not decrease the proportion of diluent.

Admixture incompatibility: Tetracycline, chlortetracycline, oxytetracycline, erythromycin lactobionate, amphotericin B and sodium ampicillin are incompatible when mixed in the same solution with acetylcysteine. Administer from separate solutions. Iodized oil, chymotrypsin, trypsin and hydrogen peroxide are also incompatible.

IPRATROPIUM BROMIDE

Aerosol: Each actuation delivers 18 mcg (*Rx*) — *Atrovent* (Boehringer Ingelheim)
Solution for Inhalation: 0.02% (500 mcg per vial) (*Rx*)
Nasal spray: 0.03% (21 mcg/spray), 0.06% (42 mcg/spray) (Rx)

Actions:

Pharmacology: Ipratropium for oral inhalation is a synthetic quaternary anticholinergic (parasympatholytic) ammonium compound chemically related to atropine. It appears to inhibit vagally mediated reflexes by antagonizing the action of acetylcholine.

The bronchodilation following inhalation is primarily a local, site-specific effect, not a systemic one. Much of an inhaled dose is swallowed as shown by fecal excretion studies. Ipratropium is not readily absorbed into the systemic circulation either from the surface of the lung or from the GI tract as confirmed by blood levels and renal excretion studies.

Pharmacokinetics: The elimination half-life is about 1.6 hours.

Indications:

Bronchospasm: As a bronchodilator for maintenance treatment of bronchospasm associated with chronic obstructive pulmonary disease (COPD), including chronic bronchitis and emphysema.

Rhinorrhea:

Perennial rhinitis (0.03% nasal spray) – Symptomatic relief of rhinorrhea associated with allergic and nonallergic perennial rhinitis in adults and children ≥ 12 years of age.

Common cold (0.06% nasal spray) – Symptomatic relief of rhinorrhea associated with the common cold in adults and children ≥ 12 years of age.

Contraindications:

Hypersensitivity to ipratropium, atropine or its derivatives; a history of hypersensitivity to soya lecithin or related food products such as soy bean or peanut (inhalation aerosol).

Warnings:

Acute bronchospasm: Use of itratropium as a single agent for relief of bronchospasm in acute COPD exacerbation has not been adequately studied. Drugs with faster onset may be preferable as initial therapy in this situation. Combination with beta agonists is no more effective than either drug alone in reversing the bronchospasm associated with acute COPD exacerbation.

Special risk patients: Use with caution in patients with narrow-angle glaucoma, prostatic hypertrophy or bladder neck obstruction.

Pregnancy: Category B.

Lactation: It is not known whether this drug is excreted in breast milk. Although lipid-insoluble quaternary bases pass into breast milk, it is unlikely that ipratropium would reach the infant to an important extent, especially when taken by inhalation.

Children: Safety and efficacy in children < 12 years old have not been established.

Drug Interactions:

Ipratropium has been used concomitantly with other drugs, including sympathomimetic bronchodilators, methylxanthines, steroids and cromolyn sodium, commonly used in the treatment of chronic obstructive pulmonary disease, without adverse drug reactions.

Adverse Reactions:

Adverse reactions from **inhalational aerosol** may include nervousness, cough, dryness of the oropharynx, irritation from aerosol, exacerbation of symptoms, dizziness, headache, GI distress and dry mouth.

Adverse reactions from **inhalational solution** may include headache, influenza-like symptoms, back or chest pain, dry mouth, nausea, cough, dyspnea, bronchitis, upper respiratory tract infection and pharyngitis.

Adverse reactions from **inhalational spray** may include headache, upper respiratory infection, epistaxis, pharyngitis, nasal dryness and miscellaneous nasal symptoms.

Administration and Dosage:

Aerosol: The usual dose is 2 inhalations (36 mcg) 4 times a day. Patients may take additional inhalations as required; however, do not exceed 12 inhalations in 24 hours.

Solution: The usual dose is 500 mcg (1 unit dose vial) administered 3 to 4 times a day by oral nebulization, with doses 6 to 8 hours apart. The solution can be mixed in the nebulizer with albuterol if used within 1 hour.

Nasal spray:

0.03% – The usual dose is 2 sprays (42 mcg) per nostril 3 or 4 times daily (total dose, 504 to 672 mcg/day). Optimum dosage varies with the response of the individual patient.

0.06% – The recommended dose is 2 sprays (84 mcg) per nostril 3 or 4 times daily (total dose 504 to 672 mcg/day). Optimum dosage varies with the response of the individual patient.

The safety and efficacy of use beyond 4 days in patients with the common cold have not been established.

CROMOLYN SODIUM (Disodium Cromoglycate)

Inhalation: 20 mg /2 ml (*Rx*)	Various
Solution for nebulization: 20 mg/vial (*Rx*)	Various
Solution (for nebulizer only): 20 mg per amp (*Rx*)	*Intal* (Fisons)
Aerosol spray: Each actuation delivers 800 mcg (*Rx*)	
Nasal Solution: 40 mg/ml. Each actuation delivers 5.2 mg (*Rx*)	*Nasalcrom* (Fisons)
Capsules (Oral): 100 mg (*Rx*)	*Gastrocrom* (Fisons)

Actions:

Pharmacology: Cromolyn is an antiasthmatic, antiallergic and mast cell stabilizer. It has no intrinsic bronchodilator, antihistaminic, anticholinergic, vasoconstrictor or anti-inflammatory activity. In animal studies, cromolyn inhibits the degranulation of sensitized and nonsensitized mast cells which occurs after exposure to specific antigens. The drug inhibits the release of histamine and SRS-A (the slow-reacting substance of anaphylaxis, a leukotriene) from the mast cell.

Pharmacokinetics: After inhalation, about 7% to 8% is absorbed from the lung and is rapidly excreted unchanged in bile and urine. The remainder is either exhaled, or deposited in the oropharynx, swallowed and excreted via the alimentary tract.

Cromolyn is poorly absorbed from the GI tract. No more than 1% of an administered dose is absorbed after oral administration, the remainder being excreted in the feces.

Indications:

Severe bronchial asthma (nebulization solution, inhalation capsules, aerosol): Prophylactic management of severe bronchial asthma where the frequency, intensity and predictability of episodes indicate the continued use of symptomatic medication. Such patients must have a significant bronchodilator-reversible component to their airway obstruction as demonstrated by pulmonary function tests.

Improvement ordinarily occurs within the first 4 weeks of administration, manifested by a decrease in the severity of clinical symptoms, or the need for concomitant therapy or both. Long-term use is justified if the drug produces a significant reduction in the severity of symptoms of asthma, permits a significant reduction in, or elimination of, steroid dosage or improves management of those who have intolerable side effects to sympathomimetic agents or methylxanthines.

Prevention of exercise-induced bronchospasm (nebulization solution, capsules, aerosol): Prevention of acute bronchospasm induced by toluene diisocyanate, environmental pollutants and known antigens (aerosol).

Allergic rhinitis (nasal solution): Prevention and treatment of allergic rhinitis.

Mastocytosis (oral): Improves diarrhea, flushing, headaches, vomiting, urticaria, abdominal pain, nausea and itching in some patients.

Unlabeled uses: Oral use is being evaluated in patients with food allergies to prevent GI and systemic reactions and for use in eczema, dermatitis, ulcerations, urticaria pigmentosa, chronic urticaria, hay fever and postexercise bronchospasm.

Contraindications:

Hypersensitivity to cromolyn or to any ingredient contained in these products.

Warnings:

Acute asthma: Cromolyn has no role in the treatment of acute asthma, especially status asthmaticus; it is a prophylactic drug with no benefit for acute situations.

Hypersensitivity: Severe anaphylactic reactions may occur rarely with oral cromolyn.

Renal/Hepatic function impairment: In view of the biliary and renal routes of excretion, decrease the dose or discontinue the drug in these patients.

Pregnancy: Category B.

Lactation: Safety for use in the nursing mother has not been established.

Children: Inhalation capsules – Clinical experience in children < 5 years of age is limited due to administration by inhalation. Capsule use is not recommended.

Aerosol – Safety and efficacy in children < 5 years old are not established.

Nebulizer sol – Safety and efficacy in children < 2 years old not established.

Nasal solution – Safety and efficacy in children < 6 years old are not established.

Oral capsule – Reserve use in children < 2 years for patients with severe disease in which potential benefits clearly outweigh risks.

Precautions:

Bronchospasm: Occasionally, patients experience cough or bronchospasm following inhalation and, at times, may not be able to continue treatment despite prior bronchodilator administration. Very severe bronchospasm has occurred rarely.

Asthma may recur if drug is reduced below recommended dosage or discontinued.

Eosinophilic pneumonia (pulmonary infiltrates with eosinophilia): If this occurs during the course of therapy, discontinue the drug.

Nasal stinging or sneezing may be experienced by some patients immediately following instillation of the nasal solution. This has rarely caused discontinuation of therapy.

Aerosol: Because of the propellants in this preparation, use with caution in patients with coronary artery disease or cardiac arrhythmias.

Drug Interactions:

Drugs that may interact with cromolyn sodium incude isoproterenol.

Adverse Reactions:

Adverse reactions associated with **inhalation capsules and aerosol** may include lacrimation, swollen parotid gland, dysuria, urinary frequency, dizziness, headache, rash, urticaria, angioedema, joint swelling and pain, and nausea.

Reactions from the **nebulizer solution** may include cough, nasal congestion, wheezing, sneezing, nasal itching, epistaxis, nose burning and abdominal pain.

Adverse events associated with the **nasal solution** may include sneezing, nasal stinging, nasal burning, nasal irritation, headache and bad taste in mouth.

Adverse reactions from oral capsules may include headache and diarrhea.

Administration and Dosage:

Nebulizer solution and inhalation capsules: Adults and children (≤ 5 years for capsules; ≥ 2 years for nebulizer solution) – Initially, 20 mg inhaled 4 times daily at regular intervals. Carefully instruct patients in the use of the inhaler. The effectiveness of therapy depends upon administration at regular intervals.

Administer solution from a power operated nebulizer having an adequate flow rate and equipped with a suitable face mask. *Hand operated nebulizers are not suitable.*

Introduce cromolyn into the patient's therapeutic regimen when the acute episode has been controlled and the patient is able to inhale adequately.

The Spinhaler (inhalation capsule) route delivers more drug to the lungs compared to nebulization of the solution, but there is no difference in effectiveness.

Prevention of exercise-induced bronchospasm: Inhale one 20 mg capsule or 20 mg of the nebulizer solution no more than 1 hour before anticipated exercise. The drug's protective effect will be stronger the shorter the interval between inhalation and exercise. Repeat inhalation as required for protection during prolonged exercise.

Concomitant corticosteroid treatment and bronchodilators should be continued following the introduction of cromolyn. If the patient improves, attempt to decrease corticosteroid dosage. Even if the steroid-dependent patient fails to improve following cromolyn use, attempt gradual tapering of steroid dosage while maintaining close patient supervision. Consider reinstituting steroid therapy for a patient subjected to significant stress while being treated or within 1 year (occasionally up to 2 years) after steroid treatment has been terminated, in case of adrenocortical insufficiency. When the inhalation of cromolyn is impaired, a temporary increase in the amount of steroids or other agents may be required.

Cautiously withdraw cromolyn in cases where its use has permitted a reduction in the maintenance dose of steroids as there may be a sudden reappearance of asthma which will require immediate therapy and possible reintroduction of corticosteroids.

Aerosol: For management of bronchial asthma in adults and children ≥ 5 years of age, the usual starting dose is two metered sprays inhaled 4 times daily at regular intervals. Do not exceed this dose. Not all patients will respond to the recommended dose, and a lower dose may provide efficacy in younger patients.

Advise patients with chronic asthma that the effect of therapy is dependent upon its administration at regular intervals, as directed. Introduce therapy into the patient's therapeutic regimen when the acute episode has been controlled, the airway has been cleared and the patient is able to inhale adequately.

For the prevention of acute bronchospasm which follows exercise, exposure to cold dry air or environmental agents, the usual dose is inhalation of two metered dose sprays shortly, (ie, 10 to 15 minutes but not more than 60 minutes), before exposure to the precipitating factor.

Nasal solution:

Adults and children ≥ 6 years – One spray in each nostril 3 to 6 times daily at regular intervals. Clear the nasal passages before administering the spray and inhale through the nose during administration.

Seasonal (pollenotic) rhinitis, and for prevention of rhinitis caused by exposure to other types of specific inhalant allergens – Treatment will be more effective if started prior to contact with the allergen. Continue treatment throughout exposure period.

Perennial allergic rhinitis – Effects of treatment may require 2 to 4 weeks of treatment. Concomitant use of antihistamines or nasal decongestants may be necessary during the initial phase of treatment, but the need for this medication should diminish and may be eliminated when the full benefit of therapy is achieved.

Use with Nasalmatic metered spray device. Replace pump device every 6 months.

Oral:

Adults – Two capsules 4 times daily, one-half hour before meals and at bedtime.

Children –

Premature to term infants: Not recommended.

Term to 2 years: 20 mg/kg/day in four divided doses. Use of this product in children < 2 years old is not recommended and should be attempted only in those patients with severe incapacitating diseases where benefits clearly outweigh risks.

2 to 12 years: One capsule 4 times daily one-half hour before meals and bedtime.

If satisfactory control of symptoms is not achieved within 2 to 3 weeks, the dosage may be increased but should not exceed 40 mg/kg/day (30 mg/kg/day for children 6 months to 2 years).

The effect of therapy is dependent upon its administration at regular intervals as directed.

Maintenance – Once a therapeutic response has been achieved the dose may be reduced to the minimum required to maintain the patient with a lower degree of symptomatology. To prevent relapses, maintain the dosage.

Administer as a solution in water at least one-half hour before meals after preparation according to the following directions.

1.) Open capsule(s) and pour powder contents into one-half glass of hot water.
2.) Stir until completely dissolved (clear solution).
3.) Add equal quantity of cold water while stirring.
4.) Do not mix with fruit juice, milk or foods.
5.) Drink all of the liquid.

Each capsule contains a precisely measured dose. The capsules are intentionally oversized to prevent the powder from spilling when the capsule is opened.

Oral capsules are not for inhalation.

Compatibility: Cromolyn **nebulizer solution** is compatible with metaproterenol sulfate, isoproterenol HCl, 0.25% isoetharine HCl, epinephrine HCl, terbutaline sulfate and 20% acetylcysteine solution for at least 1 hour after their admixture.

NEDOCROMIL SODIUM

Aerosol: 1.75 mg per actuation (*Rx*)	*Tilade* (Fisons)

Actions:

Pharmacology: Nedocromil is an inhaled anti-inflammatory agent for the preventive management of asthma. It inhibits the in vitro activation of, and mediator release from, a variety of inflammatory cell types associated with asthma, including eosinophils, neutrophils, macrophages, mast cells, monocytes and platelets. In vitro, nedocromil inhibits the release of mediators including histamine, leukotriene C_4 and prostaglandin D_2. Similar studies with human bronchoalveolar cells showed inhibition of histamine release from mast cells and beta-glucuronidase release from macrophages.

Nedocromil inhibits the development of early and late bronchoconstriction responses to inhaled antigen. The development of airway hyper-responsiveness to nonspecific bronchoconstrictors was also inhibited. Nedocromil reduced antigen-induced increases in airway, microvasculature leakage when administered IV.

Pharmacokinetics: Systemic bioavailability is low. In a single-dose study involving 20 healthy subjects who were administered a 3.5 mg dose, the mean AUC was 5 ng•hr/ml and the mean Cmax was 1.6 ng/ml attained about 28 minutes after dosing. The mean half-life was 3.3 hours. Urinary excretion over 12 hours averaged 3.4% of the administered dose, of which ≈ 75% was excreted in the first 6 hours of dosing.

Similarly, in a multiple dose study of 12 asthmatic patients, each given a 3.5 mg single dose followed by 3.5 mg 4 times a day for 1 month, both single dose and multiple dose inhalations gave a mean high plasma concentration of 2.8 ng/ml between 5 and 90 minutes, mean AUC of 5.6 ng•hr/ml and a mean terminal half-life of 1.5 hours. The mean 24 hour urinary excretion after either single- or multiple-dose administration represented ≈ 5% of the administered dose.

Nedocromil is ≈ 89% bound to plasma protein over a concentration range of 0.5 to 50 mcg/ml. This binding is reversible. It is not metabolized after IV administration and is excreted unchanged.

Indications:

Bronchial asthma: Maintenance therapy in the management of patients with mild to moderate bronchial asthma.

Contraindications:

Hypersensitivity to nedocromil or other ingredients in the preparation.

Warnings:

Acute bronchospasm: Nedocromil is not a bronchodilator and, therefore, should not be used for the reversal of acute bronchospasm, particularly status asthmaticus. Ordinarily continue nedocromil during acute exacerbations, unless the patient becomes intolerant to the use of inhaled dosage forms.

Pregnancy: Category B.

Lactation: It is not known whether this drug is excreted in breast milk.

Children: Safety and efficacy in children < 12 years of age have not been established.

Precautions:

Coughing/Bronchospasm: Inhaled medications can cause coughing and bronchospasm in some patients. If this should occur with nedocromil, discontinue use and institute alternative therapy as appropriate.

Corticosteroids: If systemic or inhaled steroid therapy is at all reduced, monitor patients carefully. Nedocromil has not been shown to be able to substitute for the total dose of steroids.

Adverse Reactions:

Adverse reactions associated with nedocromil may include coughing, pharyngitis, rhinitis, upper respiratory tract infection, bronchospasm, nausea, headache, chest pain and unpleasant taste.

Administration and Dosage:

The recommended dosage for symptomatic adults and children (≥ 12 years of age) is 2 inhalations 4 times a day at regular intervals to provide 14 mg/day. Initiate maintenance therapy at the same dose. In patients under good control on 4 times daily dosing (ie, patients whose only medication need is occasional [not more than twice a week] inhaled or oral beta-agonists, and who have no serious exacerbations with respiratory infections), a lower dose can be tried. If use of lower doses is attempted, first reduce to a 3 times daily regimen (10.5 mg/day) then, after several weeks on continued good control, to twice a day (7 mg/day).

Add nedocromil to the patient's existing treatment regimen (eg, bronchodilators). When a clinical response to nedocromil is evident and if the asthma is under good control, an attempt may be made to decrease concomitant medication usage gradually.

Proper inhalational technique is essential.

Advise patients that the optimal effect of nedocromil therapy depends on its administration at regular intervals, even during symptom-free periods.

NASAL DECONGESTANTS

PHENYLPROPANOLAMINE	
Tablets: 25 mg (*otc*)	Various, *Propagest* (Reed & Carnrick)
50 mg (*otc*)	Various
Capsules, timed release: 75 mg (*otc*)	Various
PSEUDOEPHEDRINE SULFATE	
Tablets, extended release: 120 mg (60 mg immediate release/60 mg delayed release) (*otc*)	*Afrin* (Schering-Plough), *Drixoral Non-Drowsy Formula* (Schering-Plough)
PSEUDOEPHEDRINE HCl	
Tablets: 30 mg (*otc*)	Various, *Halofed* (Halsey), *Sudafed* (Burroughs Wellcome), *Sudex* (Roberts)
60 mg (*otc*)	Various, *Cenafed* (Century Pharm.), *Halofed* (Halsey), *Sudafed* (Burroughs Wellcome)
240 mg (*otc*)	*Efidac/24* (Ciba)
Tablets, extended release: 120 mg (*otc*)	*Sudafed 12 Hour Caplets* (Burroughs Wellcome)
Capsules: 60 mg (*otc*)	*Allermed* (Murdock), *Sinustop Pro* (Murdock)
Capsules, timed release: 120 mg (*Rx*)	*Novafed* (Marion Merrell Dow)
Liquid: 15 mg per 5 ml (*otc*)	*Dorcol Children's Decongestant* (Sandoz), *Triaminic AM Decongestant Formula* (Sandoz)
30 mg per 5 ml (*otc*)	Various, *Cenafed Syrup* (Century Pharm.), *Children's Sudafed* (Burroughs Wellcome)
Drops: 7.5 mg per 0.8 ml (*otc*)	*PediaCare Infants' Decongestant* (McNeil)
PHENYLEPHRINE	
Solution: 0.125% (*otc*)	*Neo-Synephrine* (Sterling Health)
0.16% (*otc*)	*Alconefrin 12* (PolyMedica)
0.25% (*otc*)	Various, *Alconefrin 25* (PolyMedica), *Neo-Synephrine* (Sterling Health). *Children's Nostril* (Ciba), *Rhinall* (Scherer)
0.5% (*otc*)	*Alconefrin* (PolyMedica), *Neo-Synephrine* (Sterling Health), *Nostril* (Ciba), *Sinex* (Richardson-Vicks)
1% (*otc*)	Various, *Neo-Synephrine* (Sterling Health)
EPINEPHRINE	
Solution: 0.1% (*otc*)	*Adrenalin Chloride* (Parke-Davis)
EPHEDRINE	
Spray: 0.25% ephedrine sulfate (*otc*)	*Pretz-D* (Parnell)
Drops: 0.5% ephedrine sulfate (*otc*)	*Vicks Vatronol* (Richardson-Vicks)
Jelly: 1% ephedrine alkaloid (*otc*)	*Kondon's Nasal* (Kondon)
NAPHAZOLINE	
Drops: 0.05% solution (*otc*)	*Privine* (Ciba Consumer)
Spray: 0.05% solution (*otc*)	
OXYMETAZOLINE	
Solution: 0.025% (*otc*)	*Afrin Children's Nose Drops* (Schering-Plough)
0.05% (*otc*)	Various, *Afrin* (Schering-Plough), *Afrin Sinus* (Schering-Plough), *Allerest 12 Hour Nasal* (Ciba Cons.), *Cheracol Nasal* (Roberts), *Chlorphed-LA* (Roberts-Hauck), *Dristan 12 Hr Nasal* (Whitehall), *Duramist Plus* (Pfeiffer), *Duration* (Schering-Plough), *4-Way Long Lasting Nasal* (Bristol-Myers), *Nostrilla* (Ciba Consumer), *NTZ Long Acting Nasal* (Sterling Health), *Sinarest 12 Hour* (Ciba Cons.), *Vicks Sinex 12-Hour* (Richardson-Vicks)
TETRAHYDROZOLINE	
Solution: 0.05% (*Rx*)	*Tyzine Pediatric Drops* (Kenwood/Bradley)
0.1% (*Rx*)	*Tyzine* (Kenwood/Bradley)
XYLOMETAZOLINE	
Solution: 0.05% (*otc*)	*Otrivin Pediatric Nasal Drops* (Ciba Consumer)
0.1% (*otc*)	*Otrivin* (Ciba Consumer)

MISCELLANEOUS NASAL DECONGESTANTS	
Capsules: 5 mg phenylephrine HCl, 40 mg phenylpropanolamine HCl, 40 mg pseudoephedrine HCl (*Rx*)	*No-Hist* (Dunhall)
MISCELLANEOUS NASAL DECONGESTANT INHALERS	
Inhaler: 250 mg propylhexedrine (*otc*)	*Benzedrex* (Menley & James)
50 mg l-desoxyephedrine (*otc*)	*Vicks Inhaler* (Richardson-Vicks)
MISCELLANEOUS NASAL DECONGESTANT COMBINATIONS	
Solution: 0.25% phenylephrine HCl, 0.15% pyrilamine maleate (*otc*)	*Myci-Spray* (Misemer)
Solution: 0.5% phenylephrine HCl and 0.2% pheniramine maleate (*otc*)	*Dristan Nasal* (Whitehall)
Solution: 0.5% phenylephrine HCl, 0.05% naphazoline HCl and 0.2% pyrilamine maleate (*otc*)	*4-Way Fast Acting Original* (Bristol-Myers)

Actions:

Pharmacology: Decongestants stimulate α-adrenergic receptors of vascular smooth muscle (vasoconstriction, pressor effects, nasal decongestion), although some retain β-adrenergic properties (eg, ephedrine, pseudoephedrine). Other alpha effects include contraction of the GI and urinary sphincters, mydriasis and decreased pancreatic beta cell secretion. The α-adrenergic effects cause intense vasoconstriction when applied directly to mucous membranes; systemically, the products have similar muted effects and decongestion occurs without drastic changes in blood pressure, vascular redistribution or cardiac stimulation. Constriction in the mucous membranes results in their shrinkage; this promotes drainage, thus improving ventilation and the stuffy feeling.

Decongestants are sympathomimetic amines administered directly to swollen membranes (eg, via spray, drops) or systemically via the oral route. They are used in acute conditions such as hay fever, allergic rhinitis, vasomotor rhinitis, sinusitis and the common cold to relieve membrane congestion.

Oral agents are not as effective as topical products, especially on an immediate basis, but generally have a longer duration of action, cause less local irritation and are not associated with rebound congestion (rhinitis medicamentosa).

Routes, Doses and Strengths of the Nasal Decongestants

	Drug and route	Usual adult dose	Strengths
Arylalkylamines	Phenylpropanolamine Oral	25 mg q 4 hrs; 50 mg q 8 hrs	25 mg, 50 mg
	Oral-SR	75 mg q 12 hrs	75 mg
	Pseudoephedrine Oral	60 mg q 4 to 6 hrs	30 mg, 60 mg, 7.5 mg/0.8 ml, 15 mg/5 ml, 30 mg/5 ml, 30 mg/ml
	Oral-SR	120 mg q 12 hrs	120 mg
	Phenylephrine – Topical	1 to 2 sprays or a few drops q 3 to 4 hrs	0.125%, 0.16%, 0.2%, 0.25%, 0.5%, 1%, 0.5% jelly
	Epinephrine – Topical	Maximum 1 ml/15 min[1]	0.1%
	Ephedrine – Topical	2 to 3 drops q 4 hrs	0.5%, 0.6% jelly
	Desoxyephedrine – Topical	2 inhalations per nostril q 2 h	50 mg inhaler
Imidazolines	Naphazoline – Topical	2 drops q 3 hrs	0.05%
	Oxymetazoline – Topical	2 to 3 sprays twice daily	0.025%, 0.05%
	Tetrahydrozoline – Topical	2 to 4 drops or 3 or 4 sprays q 3 hrs	0.05%, 0.1%
	Xylometazoline – Topical	2 to 3 drops q 8 to 10 hrs	0.05%, 0.1%

Routes, Doses and Strengths of the Nasal Decongestants			
	Drug and route	Usual adult dose	Strengths
Cycloalkyl-amine	Propylhexedrine – Topical	2 inhalations through each nostril. Use as needed, but avoid excessive use	250 mg inhaler

[1] Refer to manufacturer's directions.

Indications:

Oral: For temporary relief of nasal congestion due to the common cold, hay fever or other upper respiratory allergies, and nasal congestion associated with sinusitis; to promote nasal or sinus drainage; relief of eustachian tube congestion.

Phenylpropanolamine is also used as an anorexiant.

Topical: Symptomatic relief of nasal and nasopharyngeal mucosal congestion due to the common cold, sinusitis, hay fever or other upper respiratory allergies.

Adjunctive therapy of middle ear infections by decreasing congestion around the eustachian ostia. Nasal inhalers may relieve ear block and pressure pain in air travel.

Contraindications:

Monoamine oxidase inhibitor (MAOI) therapy; hypersensitivity or idiosyncrasy to sympathomimetic amines manifested by insomnia, dizziness, weakness, tremor or arrhythmias.

Oral: Severe hypertension and coronary artery disease.

Phenylpropanolamine, sustained release – Nursing mothers.

Sustained release phenylpropanolamine and pseudoephedrine, naphazoline – Children < 12 years of age.

Topical:

Tetrahydrozoline – 0.1% solution in children < 6 years of age; 0.05% solution in infants < 2 years of age.

Naphazoline – Glaucoma.

Systemic effects are less likely from topical use, but use caution in the conditions listed for oral agents. Adverse reactions are more likely with excessive use, in the elderly and in children.

Warnings:

Special risk patients: Administer with caution to patients with hyperthyroidism, diabetes mellitus, cardiovascular disease, coronary artery disease, ischemic heart disease, increased intraocular pressure or prostatic hypertrophy. Sympathomimetics may cause CNS stimulation and convulsions or cardiovascular collapse with hypotension.

Hypertension: Hypertensive patients should use these products only with medical advice, as they may experience a change in blood pressure because of the added vasoconstriction. Studies suggest pseudoephedrine is the drug of choice and that phenylpropanolamine should be avoided; however, some studies report that lower doses of phenylpropanolamine do not significantly increase blood pressure in normotensive and hypertensive patients. Sustained action preparations may affect the cardiovascular system less.

Excessive use of decongestants may cause systemic effects (eg, nervousness, dizziness, sleeplessness) which are more likely in infants and in the elderly. Habituation and toxic psychosis have followed long-term high-dose therapy.

Rebound congestion (rhinitis medicamentosa) following topical application may occur after the vasoconstriction subsides. Patients may increase the amount of drug and frequency of use, producing toxicity and perpetuating the rebound congestion.

Treatment – A simple but uncomfortable solution is to completely withdraw the topical medication. A more acceptable method is to gradually withdraw therapy by initially discontinuing the medication in one nostril, followed by total withdrawal. Substituting an oral decongestant for a topical one may also be useful.

Elderly: Patients ≥ 60 years of age are more likely to experience adverse reactions to sympathomimetics. Overdosage may cause hallucinations, convulsions, CNS depression and death. Demonstrate safe use of a short-acting sympathomimetic before use of a sustained action formulation in elderly patients.

Pregnancy: Category C.

Lactation: Oral pseudoephedrine and phenylpropanolamine are contraindicated in the nursing mother because of the higher than usual risks to infants from sympathomimetic agents.

Other oral preparations – Consult a physician before using.

Topical – It is not known if these agents are excreted in breast milk.

Children: Use in children is product specific.

Precautions:

Acute use: Use topical decongestants only in acute states and not longer than 3 to 5 days. Use sparingly (especially the imidazolines) in all patients, particularly infants, children and patients with cardiovascular disease.

Stinging sensation: Some individuals may experience a mild, transient stinging sensation after topical application. This often disappears after a few applications.

Drug Interactions:

Most interactions listed apply to sympathomimetics when used as vasopressors; however, consider the interaction when using the nasal decongestants.

Drugs that may affect nasal decongestants include beta blockers, furazolidone, guanethidine, indomethacin, methyldopa, MAO inhibitors, rauwolfia alkaloids, tricyclic antidepressants, urinary acidifiers and urinary alkalinizers.

Drugs that may be affected by nasal decongestants include bromocriptine, caffeine, guanethidine, insulin or oral hypoglycemic agents, and theophylline.

Adverse Reactions:

Adverse reactions may include fear, anxiety, tenseness, restlessness, headache, lightheadedness, dizziness, drowsiness, tremor, insomnia, hallucinations, psychological disturbances, prolonged psychosis, convulsions, CNS depression, weakness, arrhythmias and cardiovascular collapse with hypotension, palpitatins, nausea, vomiting, pallow, respiratory difficulty, orofacial dystonia, sweating, dysuria and blepharospasm.

Reactions associated with topical use include burning, stinging, sneezing, dryness, local irritation and rebound congestion.

Administration and Dosage:

PHENYLPROPANOLAMINE:

Adults – 25 mg every 4 hours, not to exceed 150 mg/day (or 75 mg sustained release every 12 hours).

Children (6 to 12 years) – 12.5 mg every 4 hours. Do not exceed 75 mg/day.

Children (2 to 6 years) – 6.25 mg every 4 hours.

PSEUDOEPHEDRINE SULFATE:

Adults and children 12 years and over – 120 mg every 12 hours.

Do not crush or chew sustained release preparations.

PSEUDOEPHEDRINE HCl:

Adults – 60 mg every 4 to 6 hours (120 mg sustained release every 12 hours). Do not exceed 240 mg in 24 hours.

Children – 30 mg every 4 to 6 hours. Do not exceed 120 mg in 24 hours.

(2 to 5 years): 15 mg every 4 to 6 hours. Do not exceed 60 mg in 24 hours.

(1 to 2 years): 7 drops (0.2 ml)/kg every 4 to 6 hours up to 4 doses/day.

(3 to 12 months): 3 drops/kg every 4 to 6 hours up to 4 doses/day.

PHENYLEPHRINE HCl:

Adults – (≥ 12 years old) - 2 to 3 sprays or drops in each nostril. Repeat every 3 to 4 hours (0.25% and 0.5%). The 1% solution should be repeated no more often than every 4 hours. The 0.25% solution is adequate in most cases. However, in resistant cases or if more powerful decongestion is desired, use the 0.5% or 1% solution.

Children (6 to 12 yrs) – 0.25% – 2 to 3 sprays or drops in each nostril every 3 to 4 hours.

Infants (> 6 months old) – 0.16% – 1 or 2 drops in each nostril every 3 hours.

EPINEPHRINE:

Adults and children (≥ 6 years) – Apply locally as drops or spray, or with a sterile swab, as required. Do not use in children < 6 years of age, except on physician's advice.

EPHEDRINE: Dosage is product-specific; see labeling.

NAPHAZOLINE:

Adults and children (≥ 12 years) – 1 or 2 drops or sprays in each nostril as needed, no more than every 6 hours (spray). Do not use in children < 12, unless directed by physician.

OXYMETAZOLINE:

Adults and children (≥ 6 years) – 2 or 3 sprays or 2 or 3 drops of 0.05% solution in each nostril twice daily, morning and evening or every 10 to 12 hours *(Allerest)*.

Children (2 to 5 years) – 2 or 3 drops of 0.025% solution in each nostril twice daily, morning and evening.

TETRAHYDROZOLINE:

Adults and children (≥ 6 years) – 2 to 4 drops of 0.1% solution in each nostril every 3 to 4 hours as needed, or 3 to 4 sprays in each nostril every 4 hours as needed.

Children (2 to 6 years) – 2 to 3 drops of 0.05% solution in each nostril every 4 to 6 hours, as necessary. Do not use the 0.1% solution in children < 6 years.

XYLOMETAZOLINE:

Adults (≥ 12 years) – 2 to 3 drops or 2 to 3 sprays (0.1%) in each nostril every 8 to 10 hours.

Children (2 to 12 years) – 2 to 3 drops (0.05%) in each nostril every 8 to 10 hours.

MISCELLANEOUS NASAL DECONGESTANT INHALER:

Adults and children (≥ 6 years) – 1 to 2 inhalations in each nostril (while blocking the other nostril) not more than every 2 hours. Do not exceed recommended dosage. Do not use propylhexedrine for > 3 days or l-desoxyephedrine for > 7 days. If symptoms persist beyond this time, consult physician.

Abuse – Propylhexedrine has been extracted from inhalers and injected IV as an amphetamine substitute. It has also been ingested by soaking the fibrous interior in hot water. Chronic abuse has caused cardiomyopathy (severe left and right ventricular failure), pulmonary hypertension, foreign body granuloma (emboli), dyspnea and sudden death.

INTRANASAL STEROIDS

DEXAMETHASONE SODIUM PHOSPHATE	
Aerosol: ≈ 84 mcg dexamethasone (170 sprays per cartridge) (*Rx*)	*Dexacort Phosphate Turbinaire* (Adams)
FLUNISOLIDE	
Spray: ≈ 25 mcg flunisolide (*Rx*)	*Nasalide* (Syntex)
BECLOMETHASONE DIPROPIONATE	
Aerosol: 42 mcg (*Rx*)	*Beconase Inhalation* (Allen & Hanburys), *Vancenase Nasal Inhaler* (Schering)
Spray: 0.042% (*Rx*)	*Beconase AQ Nasal* (Allen & Hanburys), *Vancenase AQ Nasal* (Schering)
TRIAMCINOLONE	
Spray:≈ 55 mcg triamcinolone acetonide per actuation (*Rx*)	*Nasacort* (RPR)
BUDESONIDE	
Aerosol: 32 mcg budesonide per actuation (*Rx*)	*Rhinocort* (Astra)
FLUTICASONE	
Spray: 50 mcg actuation (100 mg) (*Rx*)	*Flonase* (Allen & Hanbury's)

Actions:

Pharmacology: These drugs have potent glucocorticoid and weak mineralocorticoid activity. The mechanisms responsible for the anti-inflammatory action of corticosteroids on the nasal mucosa are unknown. However, glucocorticoids have a wide range of inhibitory activities against multiple cell types and mediators involved in allergic and nonallergic/irritant-mediated inflammation. These agents, when administered topically in recommended doses, exert direct local anti-inflammatory effects with minimal systemic effects. Exceeding the recommended dose may result in systemic effects, including hypothalamic-pituitary-adrenal (HPA) function suppression.

Pharmacokinetics: The amount of an intranasal dose that reaches systemic circulation is generally low, and metabolism is rapid.

Indications:

Dexamethasone Sodium Phosphate: Allergic or inflammatory nasal conditions; nasal polyps (excluding polyps originating within the sinuses).

Flunisolide: Relief of the symptoms of seasonal or perennial rhinitis when effectiveness of or tolerance to conventional treatment is unsatisfactory.

Beclomethasone Dipropionate: Relief of the symptoms of seasonal or perennial rhinitis in those cases poorly responsive to conventional treatment.

Prevention of recurrence of nasal polyps following surgical removal.

Spray formulations – For nonallergic (vasomotor) rhinitis.

Triamcinolone: Treatment of seasonal and perennial allergic rhinitis symptoms.

Budesonide: Management of symptoms of seasonal or perennial allergic rhinitis in adults and children and nonallergic perennial rhinitis in adults.

Fluticasone: Management of seasonal and perennial allergic rhinitis in patients ≥ 12 years.

Contraindications:

Untreated localized infections involving the nasal mucosa; hypersensitivity to the drug or any component of the product.

Warnings:

Systemic corticosteroids: The combined administration of alternate day systemic prednisone with these products may increase the likelihood of HPA suppression.

During withdrawal from oral corticosteroids, some patients may experience symptoms (eg, joint or muscular pain, lassitude, depression). Carefully monitor patients previously treated for prolonged periods with systemic corticosteroids and transferred to intranasal steroids to avoid acute adrenal insufficiency in response to stress. This is particularly important in patients who have asthma or other conditions where too rapid a decrease in systemic corticosteroids may cause a severe exacerbation of their symptoms.

Excessive doses/sensitivity: If recommended doses of intranasal beclomethasone are exceeded or if individuals are particularly sensitive or predisposed by virtue of recent systemic steroid therapy, symptoms of hypercorticism may occur, including, very rarely, menstrual irregularities, acneiform lesions and cushingoid features.

Hypersensitivity: Rare cases of immediate and delayed hypersensitivity reactions, including angioedema and bronchospasm, have occurred. Have epinephrine 1:1000 immediately available. Refer to Management of Acute Hypersensitivity Reactions.

Pregnancy: Category C.

Carefully observe infants born of mothers who have received substantial doses of corticosteroids during pregnancy for signs of adrenal insufficiency.

Lactation: Advise mothers taking pharmacologic doses not to nurse. **Dexamethasone** appears in breast milk and could suppress growth, interfere with endogenous corticosteroid production or cause other unwanted effects.

Beclomethasone, budesonide, flunisolide, triamcinolone – It is not known whether these drugs are excreted in breast milk.

Children: Safety and efficacy for use in children < 6 years or < 12 years (**triamcinolone**) have not been established. Use in children < 6 years is not recommended; carefully follow growth and development if prolonged therapy is used.

Precautions:

Infections: Localized infections of the nose and pharynx with *Candida albicans* have developed only rarely. When such an infection occurs, it may require treatment with appropriate local therapy or discontinuation of steroid treatment.

Use with caution in patients with active or quiescent tuberculosis infections of the respiratory tract, or in untreated fungal, bacterial or systemic viral infections or ocular herpes simplex. Avoid exposure to chicken pox or measles.

Wound healing: Because of the inhibitory effect of corticosteroids on wound healing in patients who have experienced recent nasal septal ulcers, recurrent epistaxis, nasal surgery or trauma, use nasal steroids with caution until healing has occurred.

Vasoconstrictors: In the presence of excessive nasal mucosa secretion or edema of the nasal mucosa, the drug may fail to reach the site of intended action. In such cases, use a nasal vasoconstrictor during the first 2 to 3 days of therapy.

Systemic effects: Although systemic absorption is low when used in recommended dosage, HPA suppression and other systemic effects may occur, especially with excessive doses.

Long-term treatment: Examine patients periodically over several months or longer for possible changes in the nasal mucosa.

Adverse Reactions:

Adverse reactions associated with intranasal steroids include mild nasopharyngeal irritation, nasal irritation, burning, stinging, dryness and headache.

Those associated with budesonide in particular include epistaxis, pharyngitis and increased cough.

Administration and Dosage:

DEXAMETHASONE SODIUM PHOSPHATE:

Adults – 2 sprays (168 mcg) into each nostril 2 or 3 times a day. Maximum daily dose is 12 sprays (1008 mcg).

Children – 1 or 2 sprays (84 to 168 mcg) into each nostril 2 times a day. Maximum daily dose is 8 sprays (672 mcg).

When improvement occurs, reduce dosage. Some patients will be symptom free on 1 spray into each nostril 2 times a day. Do not exceed the recommended dosage. Discontinue therapy as soon as feasible. Reinstitute if symptoms recur.

FLUNISOLIDE:

Adults – Starting dose is 2 sprays (50 mcg) in each nostril 2 times a day (total dose 200 mcg/day). May increase to 2 sprays in each nostril 3 times a day (total dose 300 mcg/day). Maximum daily dose is 8 sprays in each nostril (400 mcg/day).

Children – Starting dose is 1 spray (25 mcg) in each nostril 3 times a day or 2 sprays (50 mcg) in each nostril 2 times a day (total dose 150 to 200 mcg/day). Maximum daily dose is 4 sprays in each nostril (200 mcg/day).

Improvement in symptoms usually becomes apparent within a few days. However, relief may not occur in some patients for as long as 3 weeks. Do not continue beyond 3 weeks in absence of significant symptomatic improvement.

Maintenance dose – After desired clinical effect is obtained, reduce maintenance dose to smallest amount necessary to control symptoms. Approximately 15% of patients with perennial rhinitis may be maintained on 1 spray in each nostril per day.

BECLOMETHASONE DIPROPIONATE:

Adults and children ≥ 12 years – 1 inhalation (42 mcg) in each nostril 2 to 4 times a day (total dose 168 to 336 mcg/day). Patients can often be maintained on a maximum dose of 1 inhalation in each nostril 3 times a day (252 mcg/day).

Children 6 to 12 years of age – 1 inhalation in each nostril 3 times a day (252 mcg/day). Not recommended for children < 6 years of age since safety and efficacy studies have not been conducted in this age group.

Improvement in symptoms usually becomes apparent within a few days. Results from two clinical trials showed significant symptomatic relief within 3 days. Relief may not occur in some patients for as long as 2 weeks. Do not continue therapy beyond 3 weeks in the absence of symptomatic improvement.

Nasal polyps – Treatment may have to be continued for several weeks or more before a therapeutic result can be fully assessed. Recurrence of symptoms due to polyps can occur after stopping treatment, depending on the severity of the disease.

TRIAMCINOLONE:

Adults and children > 12 years – Individual patients will experience a variable time to onset and degree of symptom relief. Starting dose is 2 sprays (110 mcg) in each nostril once a day (total dose 220 mcg/day). Assess the effect in 4 to 7 days; some relief can be expected in approximately two-thirds of patients within that time. May increase to 440 mcg/day either as once-a-day dosage or divided up to 4 times a day (ie, twice a day [2 sprays/nostril] or 4 times a day [1 spray/nostril]). The degree of relief does not seem to be significantly different when comparing 2 or 4 times a day dosing with once-a-day dosing. After desired effect is obtained, some patients (≈ 50%) may be maintained on as little as 1 spray in each nostril once a day.

A dose response between 110 and 440 mcg/day is not clearly discernible. In general, the highest dose tends to provide relief sooner. This suggests an alternative approach to starting therapy: Start treatment with 440 mcg (4 sprays/nostril/day), and then, depending on response, decrease the dose by 1 spray per day every 4 to 7 days.

A decrease in symptoms may occur as soon as 12 hours after starting steroid therapy and generally can be expected to occur within a few days of initiating therapy in allergic rhinitis. If improvement is not evident after 2 to 3 weeks, re-evaluate the patient.

BUDESONIDE:

Adults and children ≥ 6 years of age – Recommended starting dose is 256 mcg daily, given as either 2 sprays in each nostril in the morning and evening or as 4 sprays in each nostril in the morning. Doses exceeding 256 mcg daily (4 sprays/nostril) are not recommended. After the desired clinical effect has been obtained, reduce the maintenance dose to the smallest amount necessary for control of symptoms; gradually decrease the dose every 2 to 4 weeks as long as desired effect is maintained. If symptoms return, the dose may briefly be increased to the starting dose.

A decrease in symptoms may occur as soon as 24 hours after onset of treatment, but it generally takes 3 to 7 days to reach maximum benefit. If no improvement occurs by the third week of treatment, discontinue therapy.

Children < 6 years of age or with nonallergic perennial rhinitis – Not recommended because adequate numbers of these children have not been studied.

FLUTICASONE:

Adults – Recommended starting dose is 2 sprays (50 mcg each) per nostril once daily (total daily dose, 200 mcg). The same dosage divided into 100 mcg given twice daily (eg, 8:00 am and 8:00 pm) is also effective. After the first few days, dosage may be reduced to 100 mcg (1 spray per nostril) once daily for maintenance therapy. Maximum total daily dosage should not exceed 200 mcg/day.

Adolescents ≥ 12 years of age – Start most adolescents with 100 mcg (1 spray/nostril). Patients not adequately responding to 100 mcg or patients with more severe symptoms may use 200 mcg (2 sprays/nostril). Depending on response, dosage may be decreased to 100 mcg daily. Total daily dosage should not exceed 200 mcg/day.

Children < 12 years of age or patients with nonallergic rhinitis – Use not recommended.

ANTIHISTAMINES

DIPHENHYDRAMINE HCl	
Capsules: 25 and 50 mg (otc/Rx[1])	Various, *Benadryl* (Warner Wellcome), *Benadryl Allergy* (Warner Wellcome)
Tablets: 25 and 50 mg (otc/Rx[1])	Various, *Benadryl 25* (Warner Wellcome), *Benadryl Allergy* (Warner Wellcome)
Tablets, chewable: 12.5 mg (otc)	*Benadryl Allergy* (Warner Wellcome)
Liquid: 6.25 mg/5 ml and 12.5 mg/5 ml (otc)	*Scot-Tussin Allergy Relief Formula* (Scot-Tussin), *Benadryl Allergy* (Warner Wellcome), *Benadryl Allergy Dye-Free* (Warner Wellcome)
Elixir: 12.5 mg/5 ml (otc/Rx[1])	Various, *Benadryl* (Warner Wellcome), *Siladryl* (Silarx)
Syrup: 12.5 mg/5 ml (otc/Rx[1])	Various, *Benylin Cough* (Warner Wellcome)
Injection: 10 mg/ml and 50 mg/ml	Various, *Benadryl* (Warner Wellcome)
CLEMASTINE FUMARATE	
Tablets: 1.34 mg (otc/Rx[1])	Various, *Tavist-1* (Sandoz)
Tablets: 2.68 mg (Rx)	Various, *Tavist* (Sandoz)
Syrup: 0.67 mg/5 ml (Rx)	Various, *Tavist* (Sandoz)
TRIPELENNAMINE HCl	
Tablets: 25 and 50 mg (Rx)	Various, *PBZ* (Geigy)
Tablets, sustained release: 100 mg (Rx)	*PBZ-SR* (Geigy)
Elixir: 37.5 mg tripelennamine citrate (equiv. to 25 mg HCl)/5 ml (Rx)	*PBZ* (Geigy)
PYRILAMINE MALEATE	
Tablets: 25 mg (otc)	Various
CHLORPHENIRAMINE MALEATE	
Tablets, chewable: 2 mg (otc)	*Chlo-Amine* (Hollister-Stier)
Tablets: 4, 8 and 12 mg (otc/Rx[1])	Various, *Chlor-Trimeton Allergy* (Schering-Plough)
Tablets, timed release: 8 and 12 mg (otc/Rx[1])	Various, *Chlor-Trimeton 8 Hour allergy*, *Chlor-Trimeton 12 Hour Allergy*(Schering-Plough)
Tablets, extended release: 16 mg (otc)	*Efidac 24 Chlorpheniramine* (Ciba)
Capsules: 12 mg (otc)	Various
Capsules, timed release: 8 and 12 mg (otc/Rx[1])	Various, *Teldrin* (SmithKline Consumer)
Liquid: 1 mg/5 ml (otc)	*Pedia Care Allergy Formula* (McNeil-CPC)
Syrup: 2 mg/5 ml (otc/Rx[1])	Various, *Chlor-Trimeton* (Schering)
Injection: 10 mg/ml and 100 mg/ml (Rx)	Various, *Chlor-Trimeton* (Schering)
DEXCHLORPHENIRAMINE	
Tablets: 2 mg (Rx)	*Polarmine* (Schering)
Tablets, timed release: 4 and 6 mg (Rx)	Various, *Polarmine* (Schering)
Syrup: 2 mg/5 ml (Rx)	*Polarmine* (Schering)
BROMPHENIRAMINE MALEATE	
Tablets: 4, 8 and 12 mg (otc/Rx[1])	Various, *Dimetane* (Robins)
Tablets, timed release: 8 and 12 mg (otc/Rx[1])	*Dimetane Extentabs* (Robins)
Elixir: 2 mg/5 ml (otc)	Various, *Dimetane* (Robins)
Injection: 10 mg/ml (Rx)	Various, *ND Stat* (Hyrex)
TRIPROLIDINE HCL	
Syrup: 1.25 mg/5 ml (Rx)	Various
PROMETHAZINE HCl	
Tablets: 12.5, 25 and 50 mg (Rx)	Various, *Phenergan* (Wyeth-Ayerst)
Syrup: 6.25 mg/5 ml, 25 mg/5 ml (Rx)	Various, *Phenergan Plain* (Wyeth-Ayerst), *Phenergan Fortis* (Wyeth-Ayerst)
Suppositories: 12.5, 25 and 50 mg (Rx)	Various, *Phenergan* (Wyeth-Ayerst)
Injection: 25 mg/ml, 50 mg/ml (Rx)	Various, *Phenergan* (Wyeth-Ayerst), *Anergan 50* (Forest)
METHDILAZINE HCl	
Tablets, chewable: 4 mg (Rx)	*Tacaryl* (Westwood-Squibb)
Tablets: 8 mg (Rx)	*Tacaryl* (Westwood-Squibb)
Syrup: 4 mg/5 ml (Rx)	*Tacaryl* (Westwood-Squibb)

CYPROHEPTADINE HCl	
Tablets: 4 mg (Rx)	Various, *Periactin* (Merck)
Syrup: 2 mg/5 ml (Rx)	Various, *Periactin* (Merck)
AZATADINE MALEATE	
Tablets: 1 mg (Rx)	*Optimine* (Schering)
PHENINDAMINE TARTRATE	
Tablets: 25 mg (Rx)	*Nolahist* (Carnrick)
ASTEMIZOLE	
Tablets: 10 mg (Rx)	*Hismanal* (Janssen)
LORATADINE	
Tablets: 10 mg (Rx)	*Claritin* (Schering)
CETIRIZINE HCl	
Tablets: 5 and 10 mg (Rx)	*Zyrtec* (Pfizer)
Syrup: 5 mg/ml	*Zyrtec* (Pfizer)
TERFENADINE	
Tablets: 60 mg (Rx)	*Seldane* (Hoechst Marion Roussel)
FEXOFENADINE HCl	
Capsules: 60 mg (Rx)	*Allegra* (Hoechst Marion Roussel)

Warning:

Astemizole and terfenadine:

QT interval prolongation/ventricular arrhythmias – Rare cases of serious cardiovascular adverse events, including death, cardiac arrest, torsade de pointes and other ventricular arrhythmias, have been observed in the following clinical settings, frequently in association with increased terfenadine and astemizole (including metabolite) levels which lead to electrocardiographic QT prolongation:

1.) Overdose including single terfenadine doses as low as 360 mg and astemizole doses as low as 20 to 30 mg/day.

2.) Significant hepatic dysfunction

3.) Concomitant administration of erythromycin, ketoconazole or itraconazole.

Terfenadine and astemizole are contraindicated in patients taking ketoconazole, itraconazole or erythromycin and in patients with significant hepatic dysfunction.

Do not exceed recommended dose.

In some cases, severe arrhythmias have been preceded by episodes of syncope. Syncope in patients receiving astemizole or terfenadine should lead to discontinuation of treatment and full evaluation of potential arrhythmias, including ECG testing (looking for QT prolongation and ventricular arrhythmias).

Actions:

Pharmacology:

Antihistamines: Dosage and Effects

Antihistamine	Dose[1] (mg)	Dosing interval[2] (hrs)	Sedative effects[3]	Antihistaminic activity[3]	Anticholinergic activity[3]	Antiemetic effects[3]
Ethanolamines						
Clemastine	1	12	++	+ to ++	+++	++ to +++
Diphenhydramine	25 to 50	6 to 8	+++	+ to ++	+++	++ to +++
Ethylenediamines						
Pyrilamine	25 to 50	6 to 8	+	+ to ++	±	—
Tripelennamine	25 to 50	4 to 6	++	+ to ++	±	—
Alkylamines						
Brompheniramine	4	4 to 6	+	+++	++	—
Chlorpheniramine	4	4 to 6	+	++	++	—
Dexchlorpheniramine	2	4 to 6	+	+++	++	—

Antihistamines: Dosage and Effects

Antihistamine	Dose[1] (mg)	Dosing interval[2] (hrs)	Sedative effects[3]	Antihistaminic activity[3]	Anticholinergic activity[3]	Antiemetic effects[3]
Triprolidine	2.5	4 to 6	+	++ to +++	++	—
Phenothiazines						
Methdilazine	8	6 to 12	+	++ to +++	+++	++++
Promethazine	12.5 to 25	6 to 24	+++	+++	+++	++++
Piperidines						
Azatadine	1 to 2	12	++	++	++	—
Cyproheptadine	4	8	+	++	++	—
Phenindamine	25	4 to 6	—[4]	++	++	—
Miscellaneous						
Astemizole	10	24	±	++ to +++	±	—
Cetirizine	5 to 10	24	±	++ to +++	±	—
Loratadine	10	24	±	++ to +++	±	—
Terfenadine	60	12	±	++ to +++	±	—

[1] Usual single oral adult dose.
[2] For conventional dosage forms.
[3] ++++ = very high, +++ = high, ++ = moderate, + = low, ± = low to none.
[4] Stimulation possible.

Antihistamines competitively antagonize histamine at the H_1 receptor site, but do not bind with histamine to inactivate it. Antihistamines do not block histamine release, antibody production or antigen-antibody interactions. They antagonize in varying degrees most pharmacological effects of histamine. Most also have anticholinergic (drying), antipruritic and sedative effects. Antihistamines with predominant sedative effects are used as nonprescription sleep aids. Cyproheptadine and azatadine also have antiserotonin activity. Antihistamines with antiemetic effects are useful in management of nausea, vomiting and motion sickness. Conversely, GI upset is a frequent side effect of the ethylenediamines.

Although common cold symptoms might be modified by antihistamines, they do not prevent or cure colds, nor do they shorten the course of the disease.

Switching from one class of antihistamine to another may restore responsiveness when a patient becomes refractory to the effects of a particular agent.

Pharmacokinetics:

Pharmacokinetics have not been extensively studied. With a few exceptions, these agents are well absorbed following oral administration use, have an onset of action within 15 to 30 minutes, are maximal within 1 to 2 hours and have a duration of about 4 to 6 hours, although some are much longer acting (see table). Most are metabolized by liver. Antihistamine metabolites and small amounts of unchanged drug are excreted in urine. Small amounts may be excreted in breast milk.

Indications:

Oral: Symptomatic relief of symptoms associated with: Perennial and seasonal allergic rhinitis; vasomotor rhinitis; allergic conjunctivitis; temporary relief of runny nose and sneezing due to the common cold; allergic and non-allergic pruritic symptoms; mild, uncomplicated urticaria and angioedema; amelioration of allergic reactions to blood or plasma; dermatographism; adjunctive therapy in anaphylactic reactions; idiopathic chronic urticaria; lacrimation.

Parenteral: Amelioration of allergic reactions to blood or plasma; in anaphylaxis as an adjunct to epinephrine and other measures; for other uncomplicated allergic conditions of the immediate type when oral therapy is not possible.

Diphenhydramine: In addition to the general uses, diphenhydramine is indicated for active and prophylactic treatment of motion sickness; as a nighttime sleep aid; for parkinsonism (including drug-induced) in the elderly intolerant of more potent agents, for mild cases in other age groups and incombination with centrally-acting anticholinergics. As a nonnarcotic cough suppressant; however, only the "syrup" formulations are labeled for this indication.

Promethazine: In addition to uses discussed in the general monograph, promethazine is indicated for: Active and prophylactic treatment of motion sickness; preoperative, postoperative or obstetric sedation; prevention and control of nausea and vomiting associated with anesthesia and surgery; an adjunct to analgesics for control of postoperative pain; sedation and relief of apprehension, and to produce light sleep; antiemetic effect in postoperative patients.

IV – Special surgical situations such as repeated bronchoscopy, ophthalmic surgery, poor risk patients and with reduced amounts of meperidine or other narcotic analgesics as an adjunct to anesthesia and analgesia.

Cyproheptadine: In addition to the general uses discussed in the antihistamine monograph, cyproheptadine is also indicated for cold urticaria.

Unlabeled uses: One study suggested the combination of an H_1 and H_2 antagonist may be useful in patients with chronic idiopathic urticaria who do not adequately respond to an H_1 antagonist alone.

Terfenadine may be useful in some lower respiratory conditions such as histamine-induced bronchoconstriction in asthmatics and exercise and hyperventilation-induced bronchospasm.

Cyproheptadine has been used with variable success to stimulate appetite in underweight patients and in those with anorexia nervosa. It has also been used to treat vascular cluster headaches.

Contraindications:

Hypersensitivity to antihistamines; newborn or premature infants; nursing mothers; narrow-angle glaucoma; stenosing peptic ulcer; symptomatic prostatic hypertrophy; asthma attack; bladder neck obstruction; pyloro-duodenal obstruction; monoamine oxidase inhibitor (MAOI) use.

Phenothiazine antihistamines (promethazine and methdilazine): Comatose patients; CNS depression from barbiturates, general anesthetics, tranquilizers, alcohol, narcotics or narcotic analgesics; previous phenothiazine idiosyncrasy, jaundice or bone marrow depression; acutely ill or dehydrated children because there is greater susceptibility to dystonias.

Astemizole/Terfenadine: Significant hepatic dysfunction; concomitant erythromycin, ketoconazole or itraconazole therapy.

Warnings:

Cardiovascular effects: Cases of torsades de pointes have been reported following **terfenadine** use. It is possible that terfenadine, but not its metabolite, has quinidine-like actions that may induce arrhythmias.

Respiratory disease: In general, antihistamines are not recommended to treat *lower* respiratory tract symptoms including asthma, as their anticholinergic (drying) effects may cause thickening of secretions and impair expectoration.

Promethazine may lower the seizure threshold.

Sedatives/CNS depressants: Avoid sedatives and CNS depressants in patients with a history of sleep apnea.

Hypersensitivity reactions may occur, and any of the usual manifestations of drug allergy may develop. Refer to Management of Acute Hypersensitivity Reactions.

Hepatic function impairment: Use caution in patients with cirrhosis or other liver diseases. **Astemizole** and **terfenadine** are contraindicated in patients with significant hepatic dysfunction (see Warning Box). Use a lower initial dose of loratadine (10 mg every other day).

Elderly: Antihistamines are more likely to cause dizziness, excessive sedation, syncope, toxic confusional states and hypotension in elderly patients. Dosage reduction may be required.

The phenothiazine side effects are more prone to develop in the elderly.

Pregnancy: (*Category B – chlorpheniramine, dexchlorpheniramine, diphenhydramine, cyproheptadine, clemastine, azatadine, methdilazine, loratadine. Category C – astemizole, brompheniramine, promethazine, carbinoxamine, terfenadine, triprolidine*). Do not use during the third trimester; newborn and premature infants may have severe reactions (eg, convulsions).

Lactation: Qualitative tests have documented the excretion of **diphenhydramine, pyrilamine** and **tripelennamine** in breast milk. **Loratadine** and its metabolite pass easily into breast milk and achieve concentrations that are equivalent to plasma levels with an AUC milk/AUC plasma ratio of 1.17 and 0.85, respectively. Due to the higher risk of adverse effects for infants generally, and for newborns and prematures in particular, antihistamine therapy is contraindicated in nursing mothers.

Children: Antihistamine overdosage may cause hallucinations, convulsions and death. Antihistamines may diminish mental alertness. In the young child, they may produce paradoxical excitation.

Avoid using **phenothiazines** in children with a history of sleep apnea, a family history of sudden infant death syndrome (SIDS) or hepatic diseases. Avoid use in a child with Reye's syndrome.

Safety and efficacy for use of **promethazine** and **cyproheptadine** in children < 2 years, **methdilazine** in children < 3 years, 4 mg **dexchlorpheniramine** in children < 6 years, and **terfenadine, azatadine, dexchlorpheniramine, loratadine** and **astemizole** in children < 12 years of age have not been established.

Precautions:

Hematologic: Use **promethazine** with caution in bone marrow depression. Leukopenia and agranulocytosis have been reported, usually when used with other toxic agents.

Anticholinergic effects: Antihistamines have varying degrees of atropine-like actions; use with caution in patients with a predisposition to urinary retention, history of bronchial asthma, increased intraocular pressure, hyperthyroidism, cardiovascular disease or hypertension. Antihistamines may thicken bronchial secretions due to anticholinergic (drying) properties and may inhibit expectoration and sinus drainage.

Phenothiazines: Use phenothiazines with caution in patients with cardiovascular disease, liver dysfunction or ulcer disease. Promethazine has been associated with cholestatic jaundice.

Use cautiously in persons with acute or chronic respiratory impairment, particularly children, since phenothiazines may suppress the cough reflex. If hypotension occurs, epinephrine is not recommended since phenothiazines may reverse its usual pressor effect and cause a paradoxical further lowering of blood pressure. Since these drugs have an antiemetic action, they may obscure signs of intestinal obstruction, brain tumor or overdosage of toxic drugs.

Parenteral use: Do not give **promethazine** intra-arterially because of possible severe arteriospasm and resultant gangrene. Do not give SC; chemical irritation and necrotic lesions have resulted.

Hazardous tasks: May cause drowsiness and reduce mental alertness; patients should not drive or perform other tasks requiring alertness, coordination or physical dexterity. Astemizole, loratadine and terfenadine appear to cause less sedation.

Photosensitivity: Photosensitization may occur.

Drug Interactions:

Drugs that may affect antihistamines include MAO inhibitors. Drugs that may affect antihistamines, specifically astemizole and terfenadine, include azole antifungals, fluconazole, itraconazole, ketoconazole, miconazole and macrolide antibiotics. Drugs that may be affected by antihistamines include MAO inhibitors, alcohol and CNS depressants.

See the Antipsychotic Agents monograph for drug interactions that relate to the three phenothiazine antihistamines: Promethazine, trimeprazine and methdilazine.

Drug/Lab test interactions: **Diagnostic pregnancy tests** based on immunological reactions between HCG and anti-HCG may result in false-negative or false-positive interpretations in patients on promethazine. Increased **blood glucose** has occurred in promethazine patients.

In patients on phenothiazines, the following have occurred: Increased **serum cholesterol, blood glucose, spinal fluid protein** and **urinary urobilinogen levels;** decreased **protein bound iodine (PBI);** false-positive **urine bilirubin tests;** interference with **urinary ketone determinations, pregnancy tests** and **steroid determinations.**

Discontinue antihistamines about 4 days prior to **skin testing procedures;** these drugs may prevent or diminish otherwise positive reactions to dermal reactivity indicators.

Drug/Food interactions: **Astemizole** absorption is reduced by 60% when taken with food. Take at least 2 hours after a meal, with no food for 1 hour after taking the drug. In a single-dose study, food increased the AUC of **loratadine** by ≈ 40% and the metabolite by ≈ 15%. The time to peak plasma concentration of parent and metabolite was delayed by 1 hour with a meal. Although not expected to be clinically important, take on an empty stomach.

Adverse Reactions:

Adverse reactions may include: Peripheral, angioneurotic and laryngeal edema; dermatitis; asthma; lupus erythematosus-like syndrome; urticaria drug rash; postural hypotension; palpitations; bradycardia; tachycardia; faintness; increases and decreases in blood pressure; drowsiness (often transient); sedation; dizziness; faintness; disturbed coordination; epigastric distress, especially ethylenediamines; urinary frequency; dysuria; urinary retention; decreased libido; impotence; anemias; thrombocytopenia; leukopenia; agranulocytosis; pancytopenia; thickening of bronchial secretions; tingling, heaviness and weakness of the hands; excessive perspiration; chills.

Terfenadine: Alopecia; arrhythmia; visual disturbances; angioedema; skin eruption and itching; bronchospasm; cough; depression; musculoskeletal pain; nightmares.

Astemizole: Headache (6.7%); appetite increase (3.9%); weight gain (3.6%, average gain 3.2 kg).

Loratadine: Altered salivation; increased sweating; altered lacrimation; thirst; flushing; conjunctivitis; blurred vision; earache; eye pain; leg cramps; malaise; fever; aggravated allergy; migraine; flatulence; gastritis; dyspepsia; stomatitis; altered taste; arthralgia; myalgia; anxiety; depression; agitation; amnesia; impaired concentration; pharyngitis; dyspnea; coughing; rhinitis; sinusitis; sneezing; bronchospasm; bronchitis; laryngitis; dry hair; dry skin; pruritus; purpura; urinary discoloration.

Administration and Dosage:

DIPHENHYDRAMINE HCl:

Oral –

Adults: 25 to 50 mg, every 6 to 8 hours.

Children (over 10 kg): 12.5 to 25 mg, 3 or 4 times daily or 5 mg/kg/day or 150 mg/m^2/day. Maximum daily dosage is 300 mg.

In motion sickness, give full dosage for prophylactic use; give the first dose 30 minutes before exposure to motion and similar doses before meals and at bedtime for the duration of exposure.

Nighttime sleep aid:

Adults – 50 mg at bedtime.

Parenteral: Administer IV or deeply IM.

Adults – 10 to 50 mg; 100 mg if required; maximum daily dosage is 400 mg.

Children – 5 mg/kg/day or 150 mg/m^2/day. Maximum daily dosage is 300 mg divided into 4 doses.

CLEMASTINE FUMARATE:

Adults and children (over 12) – 1.34 mg twice daily to 2.68 mg 3 times daily. Do not exceed 8.04 mg/day. For dermatologic conditions, use 2.68 mg dosage only.

TRIPELENNAMINE HCl:

Tablets and elixir –

Adults: 25 to 50 mg every 4 to 6 hours. As little as 25 mg may control symptoms; as much as 600 mg daily may be given in divided doses.

Children and infants: 5 mg/kg/day or 150 mg/m^2/day divided into 4 to 6 doses. Maximum total dose is 300 mg/day.

Sustained release tablets –

Adults: 100 mg in the morning and evening. In difficult cases, 100 mg every 8 hours may be required.

Children: Do not use in children.

PYRILAMINE MALEATE:

Adults – 25 to 50 mg, 3 or 4 times daily.

CHLORPHENIRAMINE MALEATE:

Tablets or syrup –

Adults and children over 12: 4 mg every 4 to 6 hours. Do not exceed 24 mg in 24 hours.

Children:

6 to 12 – 2 mg every 4 to 6 hours. Do not exceed 12 mg in 24 hours.

2 to 6 – 1 mg every 4 to 6 hours. Do not exceed 4 mg in 24 hours.

Sustained release forms:

Adults (12 years and older) – 8 to 12 mg at bedtime or every 8 to 12 hours during the day. Do not exceed 24 mg in 24 hours.

Children –

6 to 12 years: 8 mg at bedtime or during the day, as indicated.

< 6 years: Not recommended for this age group.

Parenteral: The 10 mg/ml injection is intended for IV, IM or SC administration. The 100 mg/ml injection is intended for IM or SC use only.

Allergic reactions to blood or plasma – 10 to 20 mg as a single dose. The maximum recommended dose is 40 mg per 24 hours.

Anaphylaxis – 10 to 20 mg IV as a single dose.

Uncomplicated allergic conditions – 5 to 20 mg as a single dose.

DEXCHLORPHENIRAMINE MALEATE:

Adults – 2 mg every 4 to 6 hours, or 4 to 6 mg timed release tablets at bedtime, or ever 8 to 10 hours during the day.

Children –

6 to 11 years: 1 mg every 4 to 6 hours or a 4 mg timed release tablet once daily at bedtime.

2 to 5 years: 0.5 mg every 4 to 6 hours. Do not use timed release form.

BROMPHENIRAMINE MALEATE:

Oral –

Adults (12 and older): 4 mg every 4 to 6 hours, or 8 or 12 mg sustained release every 8 to 12 hours. Do not exceed 24 mg in 24 hours.

Children (6 to 12): 2 mg every 4 to 6 hours. Do not exceed 12 mg in 24 hours.

Children (< 6 years): Use only as directed by a physician.

Parenteral – Give IM or SC without dilution. Give IV, either undiluted or diluted 1 to 10 with Sterile Saline for Injection. Administer slowly, preferably to recumbent patient.

Adults: Usual dose, 10 mg (range 5 to 20 mg). Duration of action, 3 to 12 hours; twice daily administration is usually sufficient. Maximum dose is 40 mg/24 hours.

Children (< 12 years): 0.5 mg/kg/day or 15 mg/m^2/day, in 3 or 4 divided doses.

TRIPROLIDINE HCl:

Adults (12 and older) – 2.5 mg every 4 to 6 hours.

Children (6 to 12 years) – 1.25 mg every 4 to 6 hours.

Children (< 6 years) – Consult physician.

Do not exceed 4 doses in 24 hours.

PROMETHAZINE HCl:

Oral and Rectal – Tablets and suppositories are not recommended for children < 2 years of age.

Allergy – Average dose is 25 mg at bedtime. Give 12.5 mg before meals and at bedtime, if necessary. Children may be given 25 mg at bedtime or 6.25 to 12.5 mg 3 times daily. When the oral route is not feasible, use 25 mg suppositories. Repeat dose in 2 hours if necessary, but resume oral therapy when circumstances permit.

Motion sickness – 25 mg twice daily. Take initial dose ½ to 1 hour before travel; repeat in 8 to 12 hours, if necessary. Thereafter, give 25 mg doses on arising and before the evening meal. For children, 12.5 to 25 mg twice daily, oral or rectal.

Nausea and vomiting – 25 mg orally. Repeat doses of 12.5 to 25 mg, as necessary, at 4 to 6 hour intervals. When oral medication cannot be tolerated, administer parenterally or rectally. For prophylaxis of nausea and vomiting (as during surgery and the postoperative period) the average dose is 25 mg every 4 to 6 hours. For children, adjust the dose to the age and weight of the patient (0.5 mg/lb or 1 mg/kg).

Sedation –

Adults: 25 to 50 mg.

Children: 12.5 to 25 mg orally or rectally.

Preoperative use – 12.5 to 25 mg for children and 50 mg for adults, given the night before surgery.

Children: 0.5 mg/lb (1 mg/kg) in combination with an equal dose of meperidine and the appropriate dose of an atropine-like drug.

Adults: 50 mg with an equal amount of meperidine and the required amount of belladonna alkaloid.

Postoperative sedation and adjunctive use with analgesics – 25 to 50 mg in adults and 12.5 to 25 mg in children.

Parenteral – The preferred route is deep IM injection. Proper IV administration is well tolerated, but not without hazard. Administer IV in a concentration no greater than 25 mg/ml and at a rate not to exceed 25 mg/minute.

Adults:

Allergy (including allergic reactions to blood or plasma – 25 mg, repeated within 2 hours if necessary.

Nausea and vomiting – 12.5 to 25 mg, not to be repeated more frequently than every 4 hours.

Nighttime sedation – 25 to 50 mg.

Preoperative and postoperative use – 25 to 50 mg in adults may be combined with appropriately reduced doses of analgesics and anticholinergics.

Labor – 50 mg in early stages of labor. When labor is established, give 25 to 75 mg IM or IV with a reduced dose of narcotic. A maximum total dose in 24 hours is 100 mg.

Children (< 12 years): Dosage should not exceed one-half the adult dose. As an adjunct to premedication, the dose is 0.5 mg/lb (1 mg/kg) in combination with a narcotic or barbiturate and the appropriate dose of an anticholinergic drug.

METHDILAZINE HCl:

Adults – 8 mg 2 to 4 times daily.

Children – 4 mg 2 to 4 times daily.

CYPROHEPTADINE HCl:

Adults – 4 to 20 mg daily. Initiate therapy with 4 mg 3 times daily. A majority of patients require 12 to 16 mg per day and occasionally as much as 32 mg per day. Do not exceed 0.5 mg/kg/day (0.23 mg/lb/day).

Children – Calculate total daily dosage as approximately 0.25 mg/kg (0.11 mg/lb) or 8 mg/m^2.

Children (7 to 14 years): 4 mg 2 or 3 times daily. Do not exceed 16 mg/day.

Children (2 to 7 years): 2 mg 2 or 3 times daily. Do not exceed 12 mg/day.

AZATADINE MALEATE:

Adults – 1 or 2 mg twice a day.

Children – Not intended for use in children < 12 years old.

PHENINDAMINE TARTRATE:

Adults – 25 mg every 4 to 6 hours. Do not exceed 150 mg in 24 hours.

Children (6 to < 12 years) – 12.5 mg every 4 to 6 hours. Do not exceed 150 mg in 24 hours.

Children (under 6 years) – As directed by physician.

ASTEMIZOLE:

Adults and children ≥ 12 years of age – 10 mg daily. Do not exceed the recommended dose.

Take on an empty stomach at least 2 hours after a meal. There should be no additional food intake for at least 1 hour post-dosing.

Children 6 to 12 years of age – 5 mg daily.

Children < 6 years of age – Safety and efficacy have not been established.

Hepatic function impairment – Since astemizole is extensively metabolized by the liver, generally avoid use in these patients.

LORATADINE:

Adults and children ≥ 12 years of age – 10 mg once daily on an empty stomach.

Children 2 to 12 years of age (< 30 kg) – 5 mg daily.

Hepatic function impairment (GFR< 30 *kg)* – 10 mg every other day.

CETIRIZINE HCl: The recommended initial dose is 5 or 10 mg per day in adults and children ≥ 6 years of age, depending on symptom severity. Cetirzine is given as a single daily dose, with or without food.

Renal/Hepatic function impairment – In patients with decreased renal function, hemodialysis patients and in hepatically impaired patients, 5 mg once daily is recommended.

TERFENADINE:

Adults and children ≥ 12 years of age – 60 mg twice daily.

Children – The following doses have been suggested:

(6 to 12 years of age): 30 to 60 mg twice daily.

(3 to 6 years of age): 15 mg twice daily.

FEXOFENADINE:

Adults and children ≥ 12 years of age – 60 mg twice daily.

Renal function impairment – 60 mg once daily.

CODEINE

Tablets: 15, 30 and 60 mg (*c-II*)	Various

Actions:

Pharmacology: Codeine has good antitussive activity; side effects are infrequent at the usual antitussive dose. The dose required to suppress coughing is lower than the dose required for analgesia.

Pharmacokinetics: Codeine and its salts are well absorbed. Codeine is metabolized primarily in the liver and is excreted primarily in the urine within 24 hours, 5% to 15% as unchanged codeine and the remainder as the products of glucuronide conjugation and metabolites. The plasma half-life of codeine is about 2.9 hours.

Indications:

Cough: For suppression of cough induced by chemical or mechanical respiratory tract irritation.

Pain: Relief of mild to moderate pain.

Contraindications:

Hypersensitivity to the drug; premature infants or during labor when delivery of a premature infant is anticipated.

Warnings:

Head injury and increased intracranial pressure: The respiratory depressant effects of the opiates and their capacity to elevate cerebrospinal fluid pressure may be markedly exaggerated in the presence of head injury, intracranial lesions or a preexisting increase in intracranial pressure. Usual oral doses of codeine produce little respiratory depression; however, exercise caution, particularly with larger doses. Furthermore, opiates may produce adverse reactions which may obscure the clinical course of patients with head injuries.

Asthma and other respiratory conditions: Use with extreme caution in patients having an acute asthmatic attack, patients with chronic obstructive pulmonary disease or cor pulmonale, patients having a substantially decreased respiratory reserve and patients with preexisting respiratory depression, hypoxia or hypercapnia.

Acute abdominal conditions: Administration of codeine or other opiates may obscure the diagnosis or clinical course in patients with acute abdominal conditions.

Pregnancy: Category C. Dependence has been reported in newborns whose mothers took opiates regularly during pregnancy. Withdrawal signs include irritability, excessive crying, tremors, hyperreflexia, fever, vomiting and diarrhea. Signs usually appear during the first few days of life.

Labor and delivery – Opiates cross the placental barrier. The closer to delivery and the larger the dose used, the greater the possibility of respiratory depression in the newborn. Avoid use during labor if a premature infant is anticipated. If the mother has received opiates during labor, closely observe newborn for signs of respiratory depression. Resuscitation and, in severe depression, naloxone may be required. Codeine may also prolong labor.

Lactation: Some studies have reported detectable amounts of codeine in breast milk. The levels are probably not clinically significant after usual therapeutic dosage. Clinically important amounts may be excreted in breast milk in individuals abusing codeine.

Children: Do not use opiates, including codeine, in premature infants. Give opiates to infants and small children only with great caution and carefully monitor dosage. Safety and efficacy of codeine in newborn infants have not been established.

Precautions:

Administer with caution, and reduce the initial dose in patients with acute abdominal conditions, convulsive disorders, significant hepatic or renal impairment, fever, hypothyroidism, Addison's disease, ulcerative colitis, prostatic hypertrophy, urethral stricture, patients with recent GI or urinary tract surgery and in very young, elderly or debilitated patients.

Drug abuse and dependence:

Abuse – The abuse potential of codeine is less than that of heroin or morphine.

Most patients who receive opiates for medical indications do not develop drug-seeking behavior or compulsive drug use. However, give under close supervision to patients with a history of drug abuse or dependence.

Dependence – Psychological dependence, physical dependence and tolerance may occur.

The severity of the abstinence syndrome is related to degree of dependence, abruptness of withdrawal and the drug used. If the syndrome is precipitated by a narcotic antagonist, symptoms appear in a few minutes and are maximal within 30 minutes.

While codeine can partially suppress the symptoms of morphine withdrawal, the codeine withdrawal syndrome (after 1.2 to 1.8 g codeine/day), though similar to that seen with morphine, is less intense. Withdrawal symptoms in patients dependent on codeine include yawning, sweating, lacrimation, rhinorrhea, a restless sleep, dilated pupils, gooseflesh, irritability, tremor, nausea, vomiting and diarrhea. Treatment is primarily symptomatic and supportive, including maintenance of proper fluid and electrolyte balance.

Drug Interactions:

CNS depressants and **alcohol**. Use codeine cautiously and in reduced dosage to avoid additive effects when given concomitantly.

Drug/Lab test interactions: Because opiates may increase biliary tract pressure, with resultant increases in plasma amylase or lipase levels, determination of these enzyme levels may be unreliable for 24 hours after an opiate has been given.

Adverse Reactions:

Adverse reactions associated with codeine may include nausea, vomiting, sedation, dizziness, constipation, lightheadedness, euphoria, dysphoria, weakness, headache, hallucinations, disorientation, visual disturbances, convulsions, pruritus, giant urticaria and laryngeal edema.

Administration and Dosage:

Adults: 10 to 20 mg every 4 to 6 hours. Maximum 120 mg/day.

Children:

6 to 12 years – 5 to 10 mg every 4 to 6 hours. Maximum 60 mg/day.

2 to 6 years – 2.5 to 5 mg every 4 to 6 hours. Maximum 30 mg/day.

Codeine is also available in many multi-ingredient respiratory preparations as an antitussive.

DEXTROMETHORPHAN HBr

Capsules: 30 mg (*otc*)	*Drixoral Cough Liquid Caps* (Schering-Plough)
Lozenges: 2.5, 5, 7.5 and 15 mg (*otc*)	*Scot-Tussin DM Cough Chasers* (Scot-Tussin), *Children's Hold* (Menley & James), *Hold DM* (Menley & James), *Robitussin Cough Calmers* (Robins), *Sucrets Cough Control* (SK-Beecham), *Suppress* (Ferndale), *Trocal* (Hauck), *Sucrets 4-Hour Cough* (SK-Beecham)
Liquid: 10 mg per 15 ml (3.33 mg/5 ml) (*otc*)	*Creo-Terpin* (Lee)
3.5, 7.5 and 15 mg per 5 ml (*otc*)	*Pertussin CS* (Pertussin), *Robitussin Pediatric* (Robins), *Benylin Pediatric* (Warner Wellcome), *St. Joseph Cough Suppressant* (Schering–Plough), *Benylin Adult* (Warner Wellcome), *Pertussin ES* (Pertussin), *Vicks Dry Hacking Cough* (Richardson-Vicks)
10 mg per 5 ml (*otc*)	Various, *Benylin DM* (Parke-Davis), *Silphen DM* (Silarx)
Liquid, sustained action: Dextromethorphan polistirex equivalent to 30 mg dextromethorphan HBr/5 ml (*otc*)	*Delsym* (Fisons)

Actions:

Pharmacology: Dextromethorphan is the d–isomer of the codeine analog of levorphanol; it lacks analgesic and addictive properties. Its cough suppressant action is due to a central action on the cough center in the medulla. Dextromethorphan 15 to 30 mg equals 8 to 15 mg codeine as an antitussive.

Indications:

To control nonproductive cough.

Contraindications:

Hypersensitivity to any component.

Warnings:

Do not use for persistent or chronic cough or cough accompanied by excessive secretions. Persons with high fever, rash, persistent headache, nausea or vomiting should use only under medical supervision.

Drug Abuse and Dependence: Anecdotal reports of abuse of dextromethorphan-containing cough/cold products has increased, especially among teenagers.

Drug Interactions:

Drugs that may interact with dextromethorphan include MAO inhibitors.

Administration and Dosage:

Liquid, lozenges and syrup: Adults and children (> 12 years of age) - 10 to 30 mg every 4 to 8 hours. Do not exceed 120 mg in 24 hours.

Children (6 to 12 years) – 5 to 10 mg every 4 hours or 15 mg every 6 to 8 hours. Do not exceed 60 mg in 24 hours.

Children (2 to 6 years) – 2.5 to 7.5 mg every 4 to 8 h. Do not exceed 30 mg/day.

Children (< 2 years) – Use only as directed by a physician.

Sustained action liquid: Adults - 60 mg every 12 hours.

Children (6 to 12 years) – 30 mg every 12 hours.

Children (2 to 5 years) – 15 mg every 12 hours.

DIPHENHYDRAMINE HCl

Syrup: 12.5 mg per 5 ml (*otc*)[1]	Various, *Silphen Cough* (Silarx), *Tusstat* (Century)

[1] Products available *otc* or *Rx* depending on product labeling.

Indications:

For the control of cough due to colds or allergy.

Administration and Dosage:

Adults: 25 mg every 4 hours, not to exceed 150 mg in 24 hours.

Children (6 to 12 years): 12.5 mg every 4 hours, not to exceed 75 mg in 24 hours.

Children (2 to 6 years): 6.25 mg every 4 hours, not to exceed 25 mg in 24 hours.

BENZONATATE

Capsules: 100 mg (*Rx*)	Various, *Tessalon Perles* (Forest)

Actions:

Pharmacology: Benzonatate is related to tetracaine. It anesthetizes stretch receptors in respiratory passages, lungs and pleura, dampening their activity, and reducing the cough reflex at its source. It has no inhibitory effect on the respiratory center in recommended dosage. Onset of action is 15 to 20 minutes; effects last 3 to 8 hours.

Indications:

Symptomatic relief of cough.

Contraindications:

Hypersensitivity to benzonatate or related compounds (eg, tetracaine).

Warnings:

Pregnancy: Category C.

Lactation: It is not known whether this drug is excreted in breast milk.

Precautions:

Local anesthesia: Release of benzonatate in the mouth can produce a temporary local anesthesia of the oral mucosa. Swallow the capsules without chewing.

Adverse Reactions:

Sedation; headache; mild dizziness; constipation; nausea; GI upset; pruritus; skin eruptions; nasal congestion; sensation of burning in the eyes; a vague "chilly" sensation; chest numbness; hypersensitivity.

Administration and Dosage:

Adults and children (> 10 years): 100 mg 3 times daily, up to 600 mg/day.

DEXTROMETHORPHAN HBr and BENZOCAINE

Lozenges: 10 mg dextromethorphan HBr and 10 mg benzocaine	*Spec-T* (Apothecon)
5 mg dextromethorphan and 2 mg benzocaine	*Cough-X* (Ascher)
5 mg dextromethorphan HBr and 1.25 mg benzocaine	*Vicks Formula 44 Cough Control Discs* (Richardson-Vicks)
2.5 mg dextromethorphan HBr, 1 mg benzocaine	*Vicks Cough Silencers* (Richardson-Vicks)

Administration and Dosage:

Vicks Formula 44:

Adults and children ≥ 12 years – 2 lozenges dissolved in mouth, one at a time, every 4 hours. Do not exceed 12 lozenges in 24 hours.

Children 3 to 12 years – 1 lozenge every 4 hours. Do not exceed 6 in 24 hours.

Children < 3 years – Use only as directed by physician.

Vicks Cough Silencers:

Adults and children ≥ 12 years – 4 lozenges dissolved in mouth, one at a time, every 4 hours. Do not exceed 48 lozenges in 24 hours.

Children 6 to < 12 yrs – 2 to 4 lozenges every 4 hrs. Do not exceed 24 in 24 hrs.

Children 2 to < 6 yrs – 1 to 2 lozenges every 4 hours. Do not exceed 12 in 24 hrs.

Children < 2 – Use only as directed by physician.

Spec-T: *Adults and children ≥ 6 years* - 1 every 3 hrs. Do not exceed 6 in 24 hrs.

Children < 6 years – Use only as directed.

Cough-X:

Adults and children ≥ 6 years – 1 every 2 hours, up to 12/day.

Children 2 to 6 years – 1 every 4 hours, up to 6/day.

Children < 2 – Use only as directed by physician.

ZAFIRLUKAST

ZAFIRLUKAST
Tablets: 20 mg — *Accolate* (Zeneca)

Actions:

Pharmacology: Zafirlukast is a selective and competitive leukotreine receptor antagonist (LTRA) of leukotreine D_4 and E_4 (LTD_4 and LTE_4), components of slow-reacting substance of anaphylaxis (SRSA). Cysteinyl leukotreine production and receptor occupation have been correlated with the pathophysiology of asthma, including airway edema, smooth muscle constriction and altered cellular activity associated with the inflammatory process, which contribute to the signs and symptoms of asthma.

Pharmacokinetics: Zafirlukast is rapidly absorbed following oral administration. Peak plasma concentrations are achieved 3 hours after dosing. The mean terminal elimination half-life of zafirlukast is ≈ 10 hours in both normal subjects and patients with asthma. Zafirlukast is > 99% bound to plasma proteins, predominantly albumin.

Zafirlukast is extensively metabolized. Urinary excretion accounts for ≈ 10% of the dose and the remainder is excreted in the feces. Liver microsomes that hydroxylate metabolites of zafirlukast are formed through the cytochrome P450 2C9 (CYP2C9) enzyme pathway. Zafirlukast inhibits the cytochrome P450 CYP3A4 and CYP2C9 isoenzymes.

Indications:

Asthma: Prophylaxis and chronic treatment of asthma in adults and children ≥ 12 years of age.

Contraindications:

Hypersensitivity to zafirlukast or any of its inactive ingredients.

Warnings:

Acute asthma attacks: Zafirlukast is not indicated for use in the reversal of bronchospasm in acute asthma attacks, including status asthmaticus. Therapy with zafirlukast can be continued during acute exacerbations of asthma.

Infection: An increased proportion of zafirlukast patients > 55 years old reported infections as compared to placebo-treated patients. These infections were mostly mild or moderate in intensity and predominantly affected the respiratory tract.

Hepatic function impairment: The clearance of zafirlukast is reduced in patients with stable alcoholic cirrhosis such that the C_{max} and AUC are ≈ 50% to 60% > those of normal adults.

Elderly: The clearance of zafirlukast is reduced in elderly patients (≥ 65 years old), such that C_{max} and AUC are ≈ twice those of younger adults.

Pregnancy: Category B.

Lactation: Zafirlukast is excreted in breast milk.

Children: The safety and effectiveness of zafirlukast in patients < 12 years of age have not been established.

Drug Interactions:

Due to zafirlukast's inhibition of cytochrome P450 2C9 and 3A4 isoenzymes, use caution with coadministration of drugs known to be metabolized by these isoenzymes.

Drugs that may affect zafirlukast include: Aspirin, erythromycin, terfenadine and theophylline.

Drugs that may be affected by zafirlukast include warfarin.

Drug/Food interactions: The bioavailability of zafirlukast may be decreased when taken with food. Take zafirlukast at least 1 hour before or 2 hours after meals.

Adverse Reactions:

Adverse reactions occurring in ≥ 3% of patients include: Headache, nausea, infection.

Administration and Dosage:

The recommended dose of zafirlukast is 20 mg twice daily in adults and children ≥ 12 years old. Because food reduces bioavailability of zafirlukast, take at least 1 hour before or 2 hours after meals.

ZILEUTON

Tablets: 600 mg	*Zyflo* (Abbott)

Actions:

Pharmacology: Zileuton is a specific inhibitor of 5-lipoxygenase and thus inhibits leukotriene (LTB_1, LTC_1, LTD_1, LTe_1) formation. Both the R(+) and S(-) enantiomers are pharmacologically active as 5-lipoxygenase inhibitors. Leukotrienes are substances that induce numerous biological effects including augmentation of neutrophil and eosinophil migration, neutrophil and monocyte aggregation, leukocyte adhesion, increased capillary permeability and smooth muscle contraction. These effects contribute to inflammation, edema, mucus secretion and bronchoconstriction in the airways of asthmatic patients.

Zileuton inhibits leukotriene-dependent smooth muscle contractions. Pretreatment with zileuton attenuated bronchoconstriction caused by cold air challenge in patients with asthma.

Pharmacokinetics:

Absorption – Zileuton is rapidly absorbed upon oral administration with a mean time to peak plasma concentration (T_{max}) of 1.7 hours and a mean peak level (C_{max}) of 4.98 mcg/ml. Systemic exposure (mean AUC) following 600 mg zileuton administration is 19.2 mcg•hr/ml. Plasma concentrations of zileuton are proportional to dose.

Distribution – The apparent volume of distribution of zileuton is ≈ 1.2 L/kg. Zileuton is 93% bound to plasma proteins, primarily to albumin, with minor binding to alpha-acid glycoprotein.

Metabolism – Several zileuton metabolites have been identified in plasma and urine. These include two diastereomeric O-glucuronide conjugates (major metabolites) and an N-dehydroxylated metabolite and unchanged zileuton each accounted for < 0.5% of the dose. Liver microsomes have shown that zileuton and its N-dehydroxylated metabolite can be oxidatively metabolized by the cytochrome P450 isoenzymes 1A2, 2C9 and 3A4 (CYP1A2, CYP2C9 and CYP3A4).

Excretion – Elimination of zileuton is predominantly via metabolism with a mean terminal half-life of 2.5 hours. Apparent oral clearance of zileuton is 7 ml/min/kg. Zileuton activity is primarily because of the parent drug. Orally administered zileuton is well absorbed into the systemic circulation with 94.5% and 2.2% of the dose recovered in urine and feces, respectively.

Indications:

Asthma: The prophylaxis and chronic treatment of asthma in adults and children ≥ 12 years of age.

Contraindications:

Active liver disease or transaminase elevations ≥ 3 times the upper limit of normal, hypersensitivity to zileuton or any of its inactive ingredients.

Warnings:

Hepatotoxicity: Elevations of one or more liver function tests may occur during zileuton therapy. These laboratory abnormalities may progress, remain unchanged or resolve with continued therapy. The frequency of ALT elevations (≥ 3×ULN) was ≥ 1.9%.

Acute asthma attacks: Zileuton is not indicated for use in the reversal of bronchospasm in acute asthma attacks, including status asthmaticus. Therapy with zileuton can be continued during acute exacerbations of asthma.

Hematologic: Occurrences of low white blood cell count ($\leq 2.8 \times 10^9$/L) were observed in 1% of 1678 patients taking zileuton and 0.6% of 1056 patients taking placebo. These findings were transient, and the majority of cases returned toward normal or baseline with continued zileuton therapy.

Elderly: Zileuton pharmacokinetics were similar in healthy elderly subjects (> 65 years) compared with healthy younger adults (18 to 40 years).

Hepatic function impairment: Because treatment with zileuton may result in increased hepatic transaminases, use with caution in patients who consume substantial quantities of alcohol or have a past history of liver disease.

Pregnancy: Category C.

Lactation: Zileuton and its metabolites are excreted in rat milk. It is not known if zileuton is excreted in breast milk. Decide whether to discontinue nursing or to discontinue the drug.

Children: The safety and effectiveness of zileuton in pediatric patients < 12 years of age have not been established.

Precautions:

Monitoring: Evaluate hepatic transaminases at initiation of and during therapy with zileuton. Monitor serum ALT before treatment begins, once-a-month for the first 3 months, every 2 to 3 months for the remainder of the first year and periodically thereafter for patients receiving long-term zileuton therapy. If symptoms of liver dysfunction develop or transaminase elevations > 5 time the ULN occur, discontinue therapy and follow transaminase levels until normal.

Drug Interactions:

Liver microsomes have shown that zileuton and its N-dehydroxylated metabolite can be oxidatively metabolized by the cytochrome P450 isoenzymes 1A2, 2C9 and 3A4. Use caution when prescribing a medication that inhibits any of these enzymes.

Drugs that may be affected by zileuton include: Propranolol, terfenadine, theophylline and warfarin.

Drugs that may affect zileuton include: Digoxin, oral contraceptives, phenytoin and prednisone.

Adverse Reactions:

Adverse reactions occurring ≥ 3% of patients include: Headache; pain; abdominal pain; asthenia; accidental injury; dyspepsia; nausea; ALT elevation; myalgia.

Administration and Dosage:

The recommended dosage of zileuton for the symptomatic treatment of patients with asthma is 600 mg 4 times a day for a total daily dose of 2400 mg. For ease of administration, zileuton may be taken with meals and at bedtime.

Chapter 6

CNS DRUGS

AMPHETAMINES

AMPHETAMINE SULFATE (Racemic Amphetamine Sulfate)	
Tablets: 5 and 10 mg (*c-ii*)	Various
DEXTROAMPHETAMINE SULFATE	
Tablets: 5 mg (*c-ii*)	Various, *Dexedrine* (SmithKline Beecham)
Tablets: 10 mg (*c-ii*)	Various
Capsules, sustained release: 5 and 10 mg (*c-ii*)	*Dexedrine Spansules* (SmithKline Beecham)
Capsules, sustained release: 15 mg (*c-ii*)	Various, *Dexedrine Spansules* (SmithKline Beecham)
METHAMPHETAMINE HCl (Desoxyephedrine HCl)	
Tablets: 5 mg (*c-ii*)	*Desoxyn* (Abbott)
Tablets, long-acting: 5, 10 and 15 mg (*c-ii*)	*Desoxyn Gradumet* (Abbott)
AMPHETAMINE MIXTURES	
Tablets: 10 and 20 mg mixed salts of a single entity amphetamine product (*c-ii*)	*Adderall* (Richwood)

Warning:

Drug dependence: Amphetamines have a high potential for abuse. Abrupt cessation following prolonged high dosage results in extreme fatigue, mental depression and changes on the sleep EEG. Use in weight reduction programs only when alternative therapy has been ineffective. Administration for prolonged periods may lead to drug dependence. Prescribe or dispense sparingly.

Actions:

Pharmacology: Amphetamines are sympathomimetic amines with CNS stimulant activity. CNS effects are mediated by release of norepinephrine from central noradrenergic neurons. At higher doses, dopamine may be released in the mesolimbic system. Peripheral alpha and beta activity includes elevation of systolic and diastolic blood pressures and weak bronchodilator and respiratory stimulant action. The site of action for appetite suppression is thought to be the lateral hypothalamic feeding center.

Pharmacokinetics:

Absorption/Distribution – Following oral use, amphetamines are completely absorbed within 3 hours. They are widely distributed in the body, with high concentrations in the brain. Therapeutic blood levels of amphetamine range from 5 to 10 mcg/dl.

Metabolism/Excretion – Amphetamine is metabolized in the liver. Accumulated hydroxylated metabolites have been implicated in the development of amphetamine psychosis. Urinary excretion of the unchanged drug is pH dependent. Urinary acidification to a pH < 5.6 yields a plasma half-life of 7 to 8 hours; alkalinization increases half-life (range, 18.6 to 33.6 hours).

Indications:

Narcolepsy.

Attention deficit disorder with hyperactivity: Indicated as an integral part of a total treatment program which includes other remedial measures (psychological, educational, social) for a stabilizing effect in children with a behavioral syndrome characterized by moderate to severe distractibility, short attention span, hyperactivity, emotional lability and impulsivity.

Exogenous obesity: As a short-term adjunct in a regimen of weight reduction based on caloric restriction, for patients refractory to alternative therapy.

Contraindications:

Advanced arteriosclerosis; symptomatic cardiovascular disease; moderate to severe hypertension; hyperthyroidism; hypersensitivity or idiosyncrasy to the sympathomimetic amines; glaucoma; agitated states; history of drug abuse; during or within 14 days following administration of MAO inhibitors (hypertensive crises may result).

Warnings:

Tolerance: When tolerance to the anorectic effect develops, do not exceed recommended dose in an attempt to increase the effect; rather, discontinue the drug.

Pregnancy: *Category* C. Infants born to mothers dependent on amphetamines have an increased risk of premature delivery and low birth weight. Also, these infants may experience symptoms of withdrawal as demonstrated by dysphoria, including agitation and significant lassitude.

Lactation: Amphetamines are excreted in breast milk.

Children: Do not use as anorectic agents in children < 12 years of age. Amphetamine and dextroamphetamine are not recommended in children < 3 years of age for attention deficit disorder.

Precautions:

Hypertension: Use cautiously.

Potentially hazardous tasks: May cause dizziness. Observe caution while driving or performing other tasks requiring alertness.

Attention deficit disorders (ADD): Drug treatment is not indicated in all cases. Amphetamine use should depend on the chronicity and severity of the child's symptoms and appropriateness for his/her age. Use should not depend solely on the presence of one or more of the behavioral characteristics.

Drug Interactions:

Drugs that may interact with amphetamines include guanethidine, monoamine oxidase (MAO) inhibitors, tricyclic antidepressants, urinary acidifiers and urinary alkalinizers

Drug/Lab test interactions: Plasma **corticosteroid** levels may be increased. This increase is greatest in the evening. **Urinary steroid** determinations may be altered by amphetamines.

Adverse Reactions:

Adverse reactions that may occur include: Palpitations; tachycardia; elevation of blood pressure; reflex decrease in heart rate; arrhythmias (at larger doses); overstimulation; restlessness; dizziness; insomnia; euphoria; dysphoria; tremor; headache; changes in libido; dry mouth; unpleasant taste; diarrhea; constipation; urticaria; impotence.

Administration and Dosage:

Administer at the lowest effective dosage and adjust individually. Avoid late evening doses, particularly with the long-acting form, because of the resulting insomnia.

ADD: When treating the attention deficit disorder in children, occasionally interrupt drug administration to determine if there is a recurrence of behavioral symptoms sufficient to require continued therapy.

Obesity: When used for obesity, intermittent or interrupted courses of therapy may be useful. A 3 to 6 week course of therapy followed by a discontinuation period of half the original treatment length has been suggested.

AMPHETAMINE SULFATE:

Narcolepsy – 5 to 60 mg/day in divided doses.

Children (6 to 12 years): Narcolepsy seldom occurs in children < 12. When it does, initial dose is 5 mg daily; increase in increments of 5 mg at weekly intervals until optimal response is obtained (maximum 60 mg/day).

Adults (≥ 12 years and older): Start with 10 mg daily; raise in increments of 10 mg/day at weekly intervals. If adverse reactions appear (eg, insomnia, anorexia), reduce dose. Long-acting forms may be used for once-a-day dosage. With tablets or elixir, give first dose on awakening; additional doses (1 or 2) at intervals of 4 to 6 hours.

ADD – Not recommended for children < 3 years of age.

Children (3 to 5 years): 2.5 mg daily; increase in increments of 2.5 mg/day at weekly intervals until optimal response is obtained. Usual range is 0.1 to 0.5 mg/kg/dose every morning.

Children (≥ 6 years): 5 mg once or twice daily; increase in increments of 5 mg/day at weekly intervals until optimal response is obtained. Dosage will rarely exceed 40 mg/day. Usual range is 0.1 to 0.5 mg/kg/dose every morning.

Long-acting forms may be used for once-a-day dosage. With tablets or elixir, give first dose on awakening; additional doses (1 or 2) may be given at intervals of 4 to 6 hours.

Exogenous obesity – 5 to 30 mg daily in divided doses of 5 to 10 mg, 30 to 60 minutes before meals. Long-acting form: 10 or 15 mg in the morning. Not recommended for children < 12 years of age.

DEXTROAMPHETAMINE SULFATE: Refer to Administration and Dosage for Amphetamine Sulfate.

METHAMPHETAMINE HCl:

ADD – Initially, 5 mg once or twice a day; increase in increments of 5 mg/day at weekly intervals until an optimum response is achieved. Usual effective dose is 20 to 25 mg daily.

Total daily dose may be given as conventional tablets in 2 divided doses, or once daily using the long-acting form. Do not use the long-acting form for initiation of dosage or until the titrated daily dose is equal to or greater than the dosage provided in a long-acting tablet.

Obesity – 5 mg, 30 minutes before each meal.

Long-acting form: 10 to 15 mg in the morning.

Treatment duration should not exceed a few weeks. Do not use in children < 12 years old.

AMPHETAMINE MIXTURES: These mixtures contain various salts of amphetamine and dextroamphetamine. Refer to Administration and Dosage for Amphetamine Sulfate.

ANOREXIANTS

BENZPHETAMINE HCL	
Tablets: 25 mg, 50 mg (c-III)	*Didrex* (Upjohn)
DIETHYLPROPION HCl	
Tablets: 25 mg (c-IV)	Various, *Tenuate* (Hoescht-Marion Roussel)
Tablets, sustained release: 75 mg (c-IV)	Various, *Tenuate Dospan* (Hoescht-Marion Roussel)
FENFLURAMINE HCL	
Tablets: 20 mg (c-IV)	*Pondimin* (Robins)
MAZINDOL	
Tablets: 1 and 2 mg (c-IV)	*Mazanor* (Wyeth), *Sanorex* (Sandoz)
PHENDIMETRAZINE TARTRATE	
Tablets: 35 mg (c-III)	Various, *Bontril PDM* (Carnrick)
Capsules: 35 mg (c-III)	Various
Capsules, sustained release: 105 mg (c-III)	Various, *Prelu-2* (Boehringer-Ingelheim), *Rexigen Forte* (ION Labs)
PHENTERMINE HCl	
Tablets: 8 mg, 30 mg, 37.5 mg (c-IV)	Various, *Phentrol* (Vortech), *Zantryl* (Ion), *Adipex-P* (Lemmon), *OBY-CAP* (Richwood)
Capsules: 15 mg, 18.75 mg, 37.5 mg (c-IV)	Various, *Adipex-P* (Lemmon), *Obe-Nix 30* (Holloway)
Capsules: 30 mg (c-IV)	Various, *Ionamin* (Pennwalt)

Actions:

Pharmacology: The nonamphetamine anorexiants, commonly known as "anorectics" or "anorexigenics", are indirect-acting sympathomimetic amines. Except for mazindol (an imidazoline), phenmetrazine and phendimetrazine (morpholines), all are phenethylamine (amphetamine-like) analogs, and are pharmacologically similar to the amphetamines.

Although the exact mechanism of action has not been established, it is thought that appetite suppression is produced by a direct stimulant effect on the satiety center in the hypothalamic and limbic regions. Diethylpropion and phentermine act primarily on adrenergic pathways; mazindol acts on both adrenergic and dopaminergic pathways; fenfluramine influences serotonin pathways. Secondary actions include CNS stimulation and blood pressure elevation. Fenfluramine differs from other drugs of this class since it produces CNS depression. Fenfluramine's mechanism of action may be related to brain levels (or turnover rates) of serotonin or to increased glucose utilization.

Pharmacokinetics:

Absorption – After oral administration, the immediate release dosage forms generally exert their effects for 4 to 6 hours, except for mazindol (8 to 15 hours).

Distribution – Fenfluramine is widely distributed in body tissues. It is lipid soluble and crosses the blood-brain barrier. Diethylpropion and its active metabolites cross the blood brain barrier and the placenta.

Excretion – Most of the drug and metabolites are excreted via the kidneys.

The half-life of fenfluramine is about 20 hours compared with 5 hours for amphetamines and from 1.9 to 9.8 hours for phendimetrazine tartrate. Fenfluramine's half-life can be reduced to 11 hours if urinary excretion is rapid and the pH is acidic (< pH 5). Fenfluramine reaches steady-state concentrations in plasma within 3 to 4 days following chronic dosage.

Indications:

Exogenous obesity: As a short-term (8 to 12 weeks) adjunct in a regimen of weight reduction based on caloric restriction. Measure the limited usefulness of these agents against their inherent risks.

Unlabeled uses: Preliminary studies suggest fenfluramine may be useful in treating autistic children with elevated serotonin levels.

Contraindications:

Advanced arteriosclerosis; symptomatic cardiovascular disease; moderate to severe hypertension; hyperthyroidism; known hypersensitivity or idiosyncrasy to sympathomimetic amines; glaucoma; agitated states; history of drug abuse; during or within 14 days following the administration of MAO inhibitors (hypertensive crises may result); coadministration with other CNS stimulants; pregnancy (benzphetamine HCl).

Do not administer fenfluramine to alcoholics, since psychiatric symptoms (paranoia, depression, psychosis) have been reported in a few such patients.

Warnings:

Concomitant surgical anesthesia: Fenfluramine may have a catecholamine-depleting effect when administered for prolonged periods; administer potent anesthetics cautiously to patients taking fenfluramine.

Tolerance to the anorectic effects may develop within a few weeks; cross tolerance is almost universal. Discontinue the drug rather than increase the dosage. It has been suggested that therapy may be continued past 12 weeks if the patient continues to lose weight, does not develop dependence or side effects, and does not require an increased dosage. However, patients should be closely monitored and therapy should not exceed 6 months duration.

Drug dependence: These drugs are chemically and pharmacologically related to the amphetamines, and have abuse potential. Intense psychological or physical dependence and severe social dysfunction may be associated with long-term therapy or abuse. If this occurs, gradually reduce the dosage to avoid withdrawal symptoms.

Pregnancy: (Category X - benzphetamine HCl; category C – fenfluramine; category B - diethylpropion).

Lactation: Safety for use in the nursing mother has not been established.

Diethylpropion and its metabolites are excreted in breast milk. Exercise caution when administering to a nursing woman.

Children: Not recommended for use in children under 12 years of age.

Precautions:

Potentially hazardous tasks: May produce dizziness, extreme fatigue and depression after abrupt cessation of prolonged high dosage therapy; patients should observe caution while driving or performing other tasks requiring alertness.

Psychological disturbances occurred in patients who received an anorectic agent together with a restrictive diet.

Cardiovascular disease: Use with caution and monitor blood pressure in patients with mild hypertension. Not recommended for patients with symptomatic cardiovascular disease, including arrhythmias.

Convulsions may increase in some epileptics receiving **diethylpropion**.

Depression: **Fenfluramine's** central effects are mediated by 5-hydroxytryptamine (5-HT) in the brain stem. A rapid reduction in 5-HT in the brain can lead to depression. This commonly occurs immediately following abrupt withdrawal of fenfluramine; therefore, do not discontinue abruptly.

Blood glucose levels: **Mazindol** and **fenfluramine** moderately lower blood glucose levels independent of appetite suppressant effects by increasing glucose uptake in human skeletal muscle.

Drug Interactions:

Drugs that may affect anorexiants include MAO inhibitors, furazolidone and tricyclic antidepressants. Drugs that may be affected by anorexiants include guanethidine, insulin and sulfonylureas.

Adverse Reactions:

Cardiovascular: Palpitations; tachycardia; arrhythmias; hypertension or hypotension; fainting.

CNS: Overstimulation; nervousness; restlessness; dizziness; insomnia; weakness or fatigue; malaise; anxiety; tension; euphoria; elevated mood; drowsiness; depression;

agitation; dysphoria; tremor; dyskinesia; dysarthria; confusion; incoordination; tremor; headache; change in libido.

GI: Dry mouth; unpleasant taste; nausea; vomiting; abdominal discomfort; diarrhea; constipation; stomach pain.

Hypersensitivity: Urticaria; rash; erythema; burning sensation.

Ophthalmic: Mydriasis; eye irritation; blurred vision.

GU: Dysuria; polyuria; urinary frequency; impotence; menstrual upset.

Hematologic: Bone marrow depression; agranulocytosis; leukopenia.

Miscellaneous: Hair loss; ecchymosis; muscle pain; chest pain; excessive sweating; clamminess; chills; flushing; fever; myalgia; gynecomastia.

Administration and Dosage:

Intermittent or interrupted courses of therapy may be useful in the treatment of obesity. A 3 to 6 week course of therapy followed by a discontinuation period of half the original treatment length has been suggested.

BENZPHETAMINE HCl: Initiate dosage with 25 to 50 mg once daily; increase according to response. Dosage ranges from 25 to 50 mg, 1 to 3 times daily.

DIETHYLPROPION HCl:

Tablets – 25 mg 3 times daily, 1 hour before meals, and in midevening if needed to overcome night hunger.

Sustained release tablets – 75 mg once daily, in midmorning

FENFLURAMINE HCl:

Usual dose – 20 mg 3 times daily, before meals. May increase at weekly intervals by 20 mg daily to a maximum of 40 mg 3 times daily, depending on the degree of effectiveness and side effects. Total dosage should not exceed 120 mg/day.

Sustained release tablets – 75 mg once daily in midmorning.

MAZINDOL: Usual dose is 1 mg 3 times daily, 1 hour before meals, or 2 mg once daily, 1 hour before lunch. Initiate therapy at 1 mg once a day and adjust to patient response. Take with meals to avoid GI discomfort.

PHENDIMETRAZINE TARTRATE:

Tablets and capsules – 35 mg 2 or 3 times daily, 1 hour before meals.

Sustained release capsules – 105 mg once daily in the morning before breakfast.

PHENTERMINE HCl: Take 8 mg 3 times daily, one-half hour before meals, or 15 to 37.5 mg as a single daily dose before breakfast or 10 to 14 hours before retiring.

DEXFENFLURAMINE

Capsules: 15 mg (c-iv)	*Redux* (Wyeth-Ayerst)

Actions:

Pharmacology: Dexfenfluramine, an anti-obesity drug, is a serotonin reuptake inhibitor and releasing agent. The action of dexfenfluramine in treating obesity is primarily via decreased caloric intake associated with increased serotonin levels in brain synapses. In vitro, the drug inhibits serotonin reuptake by axon terminals and causes the release of serotonin from synaptosomes. Unlike amphetamines and other serotonin-active agonists and antagonists, dexfenfluramine neither enhances nor suppresses dopamine-mediated neuro-transmission.

Pharmacokinetics:

Absorption/Distribution – Dexfenfluramine is completely absorbed after oral dosing with a systemic bioavailability of ≈ 68% because of first-pass metabolism by the liver. Following doses of 15 mg twice a day for 15 days, mean maximal plasma concentrations ranging from 15 to 92 ng/ml were observed, and steady-state plasma levels were achieved 8 days after the initial dose. The major active metabolite, d-norfenfluramine accumulated to maximal plasma concentrations of about 26 ng/ml, with steady state plasma levels occurring at ≈ 9 days. The d-norfenfluramine plasma half-life is estimated to be 32 hours. Plasma concentrations of dexfenfluramine increase in proportion to the administered dose.

At a dexfenfluramine plasma concentration of 100 ng/ml, 36% is bound to plasma proteins. Dexfenfluramine is distributed into body tissue in non-obese subjects with a volume of distribution of 839 L.

Metabolism/Excretion – Dexfenfluramine is metabolized in the liver. The first steps in the metabolism are dealkylation, resulting in formation of the active metabolite, d-norfen-fluramine and deamination to an inactive hydroxy derivative.

Mean steady-state plasma concentrations of dexfenfluramine and d-norfenfluramine after 6 months of treatment (15 mg twice daily) to 18 obese patients > 60 years old were 27.3 and 14 ng/ml, respectively, compared to values of 24.1 and 15.6, respectively, in 268 patients < 60 years old.

Indications:

Obesity: Management of obesity including weight loss and a reduced-calorie diet. Dexfenfluramine is recommended for obese patients with an initial body mass index ≥ 30 kg/m^2 or ≥ 27 kg/m^2 in the presence of other risk factors (eg, hypertension, diabetes, hyperlipidemia).

Contraindications:

Diagnosed pulmonary hypertension; patients receiving monoamine oxidase inhibitors; hypersensitivity to dexfenfluramine, fenfluramine or related compounds.

Warnings:

Primary pulmonary hypertension: In one study, the use of anorexigens for more than 3 months was associated with an increased risk of developing PPH. The increase risk of PPH was concentrated in persons who had used the drugs within the preceding year; there was no significant increase in risk for persons who had taken the drugs for > 1 year previously or for persons who had used these agents for ≤ 3 months.

The initial symptom of pulmonary hypertension is generally dyspnea. Other initial symptoms include: Angina pectoris, syncope or lower extremity edema. Advise patients to report immediately any deterioration in exercise tolerance or any of the above symptoms. Treatment should be discontinued and patients should be evaluated for the etiology of these symptoms and the possible presence of pulmonary hypertension.

Long-term use: The safety and efficacy of dexfenfluramine use for > 1 year have not been determined.

Diagnosis: Exclude organic causes of obesity (eg, hypothyroidism) before prescribing dexfenfluramine.

Glaucoma: Use with caution in patients with glaucoma.

Elderly: As with all CNS-active medications, exercise caution in treating elderly patients with dexfenfluramine.

Pregnancy: Category C.

Lactation: It is not known whether dexfenfluramine is excreted in breast milk. Therefore, do not administer to a nursing woman.

Children: Safety and efficacy in children have not been established.

Precautions:

Drowsiness: Dexfenfluramine may potentiate the sedative effects of alcohol or other drugs with CNS action.

Intolerance: If the patient develops any symptoms of intolerance, reduce the dosage or discontinue the drug.

Misuse potential: As with any weight-loss agent, the potential exists for misuse of dexfenfluramine in inappropriate patient populations (eg, patients with anorexia nervosa or bulimia).

Combination therapy is not recommended.

Special risk patients: Weight loss has been associated with a reduction in hyperglycemia in obese diabetic patients, a reduction of blood pressure in obese hypertensive patients, and an improvement in the lipid profile in obese hyperlipidemic patients.

Therefore, when dexfenfluramine is used for the management of obesity associated with hypertension, diabetes or dyslipidemia there may be changes in these conditions and the medications used to treat them should be monitored, and adjusted, if necessary.

Drug Interactions:

Drugs that may interact with dexfenfluramine include MAOIs, sumatriptan and dihydroergotamine.

Drug/Lab test interactions: False-positive urine drug tests for amphetamines by ELISA have been observed for up to 24 hours following a 30 mg dose.

Adverse Reactions:

Adverse reactions occurring in ≥ 3% of patients include: Abdominal pain; diarrhea; vomiting; dry mouth; somnolence; dizziness; depression; vertigo; emotional lability; pharyngitis; increased cough; bronchitis; asthenia; insomnia; headache.

Administration and Dosage:

The usual dosage is 15 mg twice daily with meals. Doses > 30 mg/day are not recommended. If a patient has not lost at least 4 pounds in the first 4 weeks of treatment, consider re-evaluation of therapy which may include discontinuation of dexfenfluramine.

Body mass index (BMI): Below is a chart based on various heights and weights which may be useful when determining candidates for dexfenfluramine therapy.

Body Mass Index (BMI; kg/m^2)

Weight		Height (feet, inches)					
lbs	kg	5'0"	5'3"	5'6"	5'9"	6'	6'3"
140	64	**27**	25	23	21	19	18
150	69	**29**	**27**	24	22	20	19
160	73	31	**28**	26	24	22	20
170	77	33	30	**28**	25	23	21
180	82	35	32	**29**	**27**	25	23
190	86	37	34	31	**28**	26	24
200	91	39	36	32	30	**27**	25
210	95	41	37	34	31	**29**	26
220	100	43	39	36	33	30	**28**
230	105	45	41	37	34	31	**29**
240	109	47	43	39	36	33	30
250	113	49	44	40	37	34	31

NARCOTIC AGONIST ANALGESICS

ALFENTANIL HCL	
Injection: 500 mcg (as HCl)/ml (*c-ii*)	*Alfenta* (Janssen)
CODEINE	
Tablets: 15, 30, 60 mg (*c-ii*)	Various
Injection: 30 mg, 60 mg (*c-ii*)	Various
FENTANYL	
Injection: 0.05 mg base (as citrat)/ml (*c-ii*)	Various, *Sublimaze* (Janssen)
FENTANYL TRANSDERMAL SYSTEM	
Patch: 25 mcg/hr, 50 mcg/hr, 75 mcg/hr, 100 mcg/hr (*c-ii*)	*Duragesic-25*, *Duragesic-50*[1], *Duragesic-75*[1], *Duragesic-100*[1] (Janssen)
FENTANYL TRANSMUCOSAL SYSTEM	
Lozenges: 100 mcg, 200 mcg, 300 mcg, 400 mcg (*c-ii*)	*Fentanyl Oralet* (Abbott)
HYDROMORPHONE HCl	
Injection: 1 mg/ml, 2 mg/ml, 3 mg/ml, 4 mg/ml, 10 mg/ml (*c-ii*)	Various, *Dilaudid* (Knoll), *HydroStat IR* (Richwood)
Tablets: 1, 2, 3, 4, 8 mg (*c-ii*)	Various, *Dilaudid* (Knoll), *HydroStat IR* (Richwood)
Liquid:5 mg/5 ml (*c-ii*)	*Dilaudid-5* (Knoll)
Suppositories: 3 mg	*Dilaudid* (Knoll)
LEVOMETHADYL ACETATE HCl	
Solution: 10 mg/ml (*c-ii*)	ORLAAM (BioDevelopment)
LEVORPHANOL TARTRATE	
Injection: 2 mg/ml (*c-ii*)	*Levo-Dromoran* (Roche)
Tablets: 2 mg (*c-ii*)	*Levo-Dromoran* (Roche)
MEPERIDINE HCl	
Tablets: 50 mg, 100 mg (*c-ii*)	Various, *Demerol HCl* (Winthrop)
Syrup: 50 mg/5 ml (*c-ii*)	
Injection: 10 mg/ml, 50 mg/ml, 100 mg/ml (*c-ii*)	
Injection: 25 mg/dose, 50 mg/dose, 75 mg/dose, 100 mg/dose (*c-ii*)	
METHADONE HCl	
Injection: 10 mg/ml (*c-ii*)	*Dolophine HCl* (Lilly)
Tablets: 5 mg, 10 mg (*c-ii*)	*Methadone HCl* (Roxane), *Dolophine HCl* (Lilly)
Dispersible Tablets: 40 mg (*c-ii*)	*Methadone HCl Diskets*[1] (Lilly)
Oral Solution: 5 mg/5 ml, 10 mg/5 ml and 10 mg/10 ml (*c-ii*)	*Methadone HCl* (Roxane)
Oral Concentrate: 10 mg/ml (*c-ii*)	*Methadone HCl Intensol* (Roxane)
MORPHINE SULFATE	
Injection: 0.5, 1, 2, 3, 4, 5, 8, 10, 15, 25, 50 mg/ml (*c-ii*)	Various, *Astramorph PF* (Astra), *Duramorph* (Elkins-Sinn), *Infumorph* (Elkins-Sinn)
Soluble Tablets: 10, 15, 30 mg (*c-ii*)	Various
Tablets: 15, 30 mg (*c-ii*)	Various, *MSIR* (Purdue Frederick)
Tablets, controlled release: 15, 30, 60, 100, 200 mg (*c-ii*)	*MS Contin* (Purdue Frederick), *Oramorph SR* (Roxane)
Solution: 10 mg/5 mg, 10 mg/2.5 mg, 20 mg/5 ml, 20 mg/ml, 100 mg/5 ml (*c-ii*)	Various, *MSIR* (Purdue Frederick), *Roxanol* (Roxane), *OMS Concentrate* (Upsher-Smith), *MS/L* (Richwood)
Rectal Suppositories:5, 10, 20, 30 mg (*c-ii*)	Various, *RMS* (Upsher-Smith), *Roxanol* (Roxane), *MS/S* (Richwood)
OPIUM	
Injection: 20 mg/ml (equiv. to 15 mg morphine) (*c-ii*)	*Pantopon* (Roche)
Liquid: 10% (*c-ii*)	*Opium Tincture, Deodorized* (Lilly)
Liquid (samphorated tincture of opium):2 mg morphine equiv. per 5 ml (*c-iii*)	*Paregoric* (Various)
OXYCODONE HCl	
Tablets: 5 mg (*c-ii*)	*Roxicodone* (Roxane)
Tablets, controlled release: 10, 20, 40 mg (*c-ii*)	OxyContin (Purdue Pharma)
Oral Solution: 5 mg/5 ml (*c-ii*)	*Roxicodone* (Roxane)

Solution, concentrate: 20 mg/ml *(c-ii)*	*Roxicodone Intensol* (Roxane)
OXYMORPHONE HCl	
Injection: 1 mg/ml, 1.5 mg/ml *(c-ii)*	*Numorphan* (DuPont)
Suppositories: 5 mg *(c-ii)*	*Numorphan* (DuPont)
PROPOXYPHENE HCl	
Capsules: 32, 65 mg *(c-iv)*	Various, *Darvon Pulvules* (Lilly), *Dolene* (Lederle)
PROPOXYPHENE NAPSYLATE	
Tablets: 100 mg *(c-iv)*	*Darvon-N* (Lilly)
SUFENTANIL CITRATE	
Injection: 50 mcg (as citrate)/ml *(c-ii)*	Various, *Sufenta* (Janssen)

[1] For use in opioid tolerant patients only.

Warning:

Fentanyl transmucosal: Fentanyl transmucosal contains the potent narcotic fentanyl citrate in a formulation which:

- Should only be used as an anesthetic premedication or for inducing conscious sedation prior to a diagnostic or therapeutic procedure in a monitored anesthesia care setting.
- Should only be given in hospital settings such as the operating room, emergency department, ICU or other monitored anesthesia care settings where there is immediate access to life support equipment, oxygen, facilities for endotracheal intubation, IV fluids and opioid antagonists.
- Can only be used safely in patients being monitored by both 1) direct visual observation by a health professional whose sole responsibility is observation of the patients and 2) by some means of measuring respiratory function such as pulse oximetry until patients has completely recovered. Fentanyl transmucosal use is contraindicated in:
- Use at any other setting outside a hospital.
- Children who weigh < 10 kg (22 lbs).
- Doses > 15 mcg/kg in children, and > 5 mcg/kg in adults., Due to the excessive frequency of significant hypoventilation at higher doses, the maximum dose any child or adult should receive is 400 mcg, regardless of weight.

Levomethadyl Acetate HCl: Levomethadyl acetate HCl, used for the treatment of narcotic addiction, shall be dispensed only by treatment programs approved by the FDA, the DEA and the designated state authority. Approved treatment programs shall dispense and use levomethadyl in oral form only and according to the treatment requirements stipulated in federal regulations. Failure to abide by these requirements may result in injection precluding operation of the program, seizure of the drug supply, revocation of the program approval and possible criminal prosecution.

Levomethadyl is only recommended for treatment of opiate addiction.

Actions:

Pharmacology: Narcotic analgesics are classified as agonists, mixed agonist-antagonists, or partial agonists by their activity at opioid receptors. Five major categories of opioid receptors are known: mu (μ), *kappa* (κ), *sigma* (σ), *delta* (δ) and *epsilon* (ε). Actions of the narcotic analgesics now available can be defined by their activity at three specific receptor types: μ, κ and σ.

The μ receptors mediate morphine-like supraspinal analgesia, euphoria and respiratory and physical depression. The κ receptors mediate pentazocine-like spinal analgesia, sedation and miosis. The σ receptors mediate dysphoria, psychotomimetic effects (ie, hallucinations), and respiratory and vasomotor stimulation caused by drugs with antagonist activity.

Morphine-like **narcotic agonists** have activity at the μ and κ receptors, and possibly at the δ. Narcotic agonists include natural opium alkaloids (eg, morphine, codeine), semisynthetic analogs (eg, hydromorphone, oxymorphone, oxycodone) and synthetic compounds (eg, meperidine, levorphanol, methadone).

Mixed *agonist-antagonist* drugs (eg, nalbuphine, pentazocine) have agonist activity at some receptors and antagonist activity at other receptors; also included are the *partial agonists* (eg, butorphanol, buprenorphine).

Narcotic Agonist Comparative Pharmacology[1]

Drug	Analgesic	Antitussive	Constipation	Respiratory Depression	Sedation	Emesis	Physical Dependence
Phenanthrenes							
Codeine	+	+++	+	+	+	+	+
Hydrocodone	+	+++	nd[2]	+	nd[2]	nd[2]	+
Hydromorphone	++	+++	+	++	+	+	++
Levorphanol	++	++	++	++	++	+	++
Morphine	++	+++	++	++	++	++	++
Oxycodone	++	+++	++	++	++	++	++
Oxymorphone	++	+	++	+++	nd[2]	+++	+++
Phenylpiperidines							
Alfentanil	++	nd[2]	nd[2]	nd[2]	nd[2]	nd[2]	nd[2]
Fentanyl	++	nd[2]	nd[2]	+	nd[2]	+	nd[2]
Meperidine	++	+	+	++	+	nd[2]	++
Sufentanil	+++	nd[2]	nd[2]	nd[2]	nd[2]	nd[2]	nd[2]
Diphenylheptanes							
Methadone	++	++	++	++	+	+	+
Propoxyphene	+	nd[2]	nd[2]	+	+	+	+

[1] Table adapted from Catalano RB. The medical approach to management of pain caused by cancer. *Semin Oncol* 1975;2:379-92 and Reuler JB, et al. The chronic pain syndrome: Misconceptions and management. *Ann Intern Med* 1980;93:588-96.

[2] nd – No data available.

Pharmacokinetics: Pharmacokinetic profiles are summarized in the table below using morphine as the standard. Data based on IM administration unless otherwise noted.

Pharmacokinetics of Narcotic Agonist Analgesics

Drug	Onset (minutes)	Peak (hours)	Duration[1] (hours)	t 1/2 (hours)	Equianalgesic Doses: Parenteral	Equianalgesic Doses: Other
Alfentanil	immediate	nd[2]	nd[2]	1-2[3]	IM 0.4 to 0.8	nd[2]
Codeine	10 to 30	0.5 to 1	4 to 6	3	IM 120 to 130 SC 120	Oral 200[4]
Fentanyl	7 to 8	nd[2]	1 to 2	1.5 to 6	IM 0.1 to 0.2	Transdermal 100 mcg/hr
Hydrocodone	nd[2]	nd[2]	4 to 8	3.3 to 4.5	nd[2]	Oral 5 to 10
Hydromorphone	15 to 30	0.5 to 1	4 to 5	2 to 3	IM 1.3 to 1.5 SC 1 to 1.5	Oral 7.5
Levorphanol	30 to 90	0.5 to 1	6 to 8	12 to 16	IM 2 SC 2	Oral 4
Meperidine	10 to 45	0.5 to 1	2 to 4	3 to 4	IM 75 SC 75 to 100	Oral 300[4]
Methadone	30 to 60	0.5 to 1	4 to 6[5]	15 to 30	IM 10 SC 8 to 10	Oral 10 to 20
Morphine	15 to 60[6]	0.5 to 1	3 to 7	1.5 to 2	IM 10 SC 10	Oral 30 to 60
Oxycodone	15 to 30	1	4 to 6	nd[2]	IM 10 to 15 SC 10 to 15	Oral 30[4]
Oxymorphone	5 to 10	0.5 to 1	3 to 6	nd[2]	IM 1 SC 1 to 1.5	Rectal 5, 10
Propoxyphene (PO)	30 to 60	2 to 2.5	4 to 6	6 to 12	nd[2]	Oral 130[7]
Sufentanil	1.3 to 3[3]	nd[2]	nd[2]	2.5	IM 0.1 to 0.4	nd[2]

[1] After IV administration, peak effects may be more pronounced but duration is shorter. Duration of action may be longer with the oral route.

[2] nd – No data available.

[3] Data based on IV administration.

[4] Starting doses lower (codeine, 30 mg; oxycodone, 5 mg; meperidine, 50 mg).

[5] Duration and half-life increase with repeated use due to cumulative effects.

[6] Data based on intrathecal or epidural administration.

[7] Starting doses lower (propoxyphene, 65 to 130 mg).

Administration IV is most reliable and rapid; IM or SC use may delay absorption and peak effect, especially with impaired tissue perfusion. Many agents undergo a significant first-pass effect. All are metabolized by the liver and excreted primarily in urine. Meperidine is metabolized to normeperidine, a metabolite with significant pharmacologic activity. The half-life of normeperidine is 15 to 30 hours and accumulates with chronic dosing, especially in renal dysfunction. Accumulation of this metabolite may lead to CNS excitation (eg, tremors, twitches, seizures).

Indications:

ALFENTANIL HCl: As an analgesic adjunct given in incremental doses in the maintenance of anesthesia with barbiturate/nitrous oxide/oxygen.

As an analgesic administered by continuous infusion with nitrous oxide/oxygen in the maintenance of general anesthesia.

As a primary anesthetic for induction of anesthesia in general surgery when endotracheal intubation and mechanical ventilation are required.

Analgesic component for monitored anesthesia care (MAC).

CODEINE: Relief of mild to moderate pain and for coughing induced by chemical or mechanical irritation of the respiratory system.

FENTANYL:

Pain – For analgesic action of short duration during anesthesia (premediaction, induction, maintenance), and in the immediate postoperative period (recovery room) as needed.

For use as a narcotic analgesic supplement in general or regional anesthesia.

For administration with a neuroleptic such as droperidol as an anesthetic premedication, for induction of anesthesia and as an adjunct in maintenance of general and regional anesthesia.

For use as an anesthetic agent with oxygen in selected high-risk patients (open heart surgery or certain complicated neurological or orthopedic procedures.

FENTANYL TRANSDERMAL SYSTEM:

Pain – Management of chronic pain in patients requiring opioid analgesia.

FENTANYL TRANSMUCOSAL SYSTEM:

Anesthesia – Only indicated for use in a hospital setting 1) as an anesthetic premedication in the operating room setting or 2) to induce conscious sedation prior to a diagnostic or therapeutic procedure in other monitored anesthesia care settings in the hospital.

HYDROMORPHONE HCl: Relief of moderate to severe pain.

LEVOMETHADYL ACETATE HCl: Management of opiate dependence.

LEVORPHANOL TARTRATE: Relief of moderate to severe pain. Preoperatively to allay apprehension, provide prolonged analgesia, reduce thiopental requirements and shorten recovery time.

MEPERIDINE HCl:

Oral and parenteral – Relief of moderate to severe pain.

Parenteral – For preoperative medication, support of anesthesia and obstetrical analgesia.

METHADONE HCl: For relief of severe pain; detoxification and temporary maintenance treatment of narcotic addiction. Methadone is ineffective for the relief of general anxiety.

MORPHINE SULFATE: Relief of moderate to severe acute and chronic pain. Preoperatively to sedate patient, allay apprehension, facilitate induction of anesthesia, reduce anesthetic dosage.

Unlabeled uses – Dyspnea associated w/acute left ventricular failure, pulmonary edema.

OPIUM: For all disorders in which the analgesic, sedative-hypnotic narcotic or antidiarrheal effect of an opiate is needed; for relief of severe pain in place of morphine.

OXYCODONE HCl: Relief of moderate to moderately severe pain.

OXYMORPHONE HCl: Relief of moderate to severe pain.

Parenterally for preoperative medication, support of anesthesia, obstetrical analgesia and for relief of anxiety in patients with dyspnea associated with acute left ventricular failure and pulmonary edema.

PROPOXYPHENE (Dextropropoxyphene): Relief of mild to moderate pain.

SUFENTANIL CITRATE: Analgesic adjunct at dosages ≤ 8 mcg/kg to maintain balanced general anesthesia.

A primary anesthetic agent at dosages ≥ 8 mcg/kg to induce and maintain anesthesia with 100% oxygen in patients undergoing major surgical procedures, such as cardiovascular surgery or neurosurgical procedures in the sitting position, to provide favorable myocardial and cerebral wxygen balance or when extended postoperative ventilation is anticipated.

Pain – For analgesic action of short duration during anesthesia (premedication, induction, maintenance), and in the immediate postoperative period (recovery room) as needed.

For use as a narcotic analgesic supplement in general or regional anesthesia.

For administration with a neuroleptic such as droperidol as an anesthetic premedication, for induction of anesthesia and as an adjunct in maintenance of general and regional anesthesia.

For use as an anesthetic agent with oxygen in selected high-risk patients (open heart surgery or certain complicated neurological or orthopedic procedures).

Contraindications:

Hypersensitivity to narcotics; diarrhea caused by poisoning until the toxic material has been eliminated; acute bronchial asthma; upper airway obstruction.

Morphine, epidural or intrathecal: Presence of infection at injection site; anticoagulant therapy; bleeding diathesis; parenterally administered corticosteroids within a 2 week period or other concomitant drug therapy or medical condition that would contraindicate the technique of epidural or intrathecal analgesia.

Levorphanol: Acute alcoholism; bronchial asthma; increased intracranial pressure; respiratory depression; anoxia.

Meperidine: In patients taking monoamine oxidase inhibitors (MAOIs) or in those who have received such agents within 14 days.

Hydromorphone injection: In patients not already receiving large amounts of parenteral narcotics; patients with respiratory depression in the absence of resuscitative equipment; status asthmaticus; use as obstetrical analgesia.

Warnings:

Propoxyphene: These products given in excessive doses, either alone or in combination with other CNS depressante (including alcohol), are a major cause of drug-related deaths. Consider nonnarcotic analgesics for depressed or suicidal patients. Advise patients of the additive depressant effects of these combinations with alcohol.

Suicide: Do not prescribe **propoxyphene** for patients who are suicidal or addiction-prone.

Head injury and increased intracranial pressure: Narcotics may obscure the clinical course of patients with head injuries. The respiratory depressant effects and the capacity to elevate cerebrospinal fluid pressure may be markedly exaggerated in the presence of head injury, brain tumor, other intracranial lesions or a preexisting elevated intracranial pressure.

Parenteral therapy: Give by very slow IV injection, preferably as a diluted solution. The patient should be lying down. Rapid IV injection increases the incidence of adverse reactions. Use caution when injecting SC or IM in chilled areas or in patients with hypotension or shock, since impaired perfusion may prevent complete absorption.

Limit epidural or intrathecal administration of **morphine** to the lumbar area.

Hydrochlorides of opium alkaloids – Do not administer IV.

Asthma and other respiratory conditions: Use with extreme caution in patients with acute asthma, bronchial asthma, chronic obstructive pulmonary disease or cor pulmonale, a substantially decreased respiratory reserve, and with preexisting respiratory depression, hypoxia or hypercapnia. Even therapeutic doses of narcotics may decrease respiratory drive while simultaneously increasing airway resistance to the point of apnea.

Hypotensive effect: Narcotic analgesics may cause severe hypotension in individuals whose ability to maintain blood pressure has been compromised by a depleted blood volume, or coadministration of drugs such as phenothiazines or general anesthetics.

Renal/Hepatic function impairment: Renal and hepatic dysfunction may cause a prolonged duration and cumulative effect; smaller doses may be necessary.

Meperidine – In patients with renal dysfunction, normeperidine (an active metabolite of meperidine) may accumulate, resulting in increased CNS adverse reactions.

Pregnancy: Category C. The placental transfer of narcotics is rapid. Maternal addiction and neonatal withdrawal occurs following illicit use.

Labor – Narcotics cross the placental barrier and can produce depression of respiration and psycho-physiologic effects in the neonate.

Lactation: Most of these agents appear in breast milk, but effects on the infant may not be significant. Some recommend waiting 4 to 6 hours after use before nursing.

Children: Safety and efficacy of **sufentanil** in children < 2 years undergoing cardiovascular surgery have been documented in a limited number of cases. Safety and efficacy of **fentanyl** in children < 2 years is not established. Hypotension has occurred in neonates with respiratory distress syndrome receiving **alfentanil** 20 mcg/kg.

Do not use **oxycodone** in children; **propoxyphene** use is not recommended in children. **Methadone** is not recommended as an analgesic in children; documented clinical experience is insufficient to establish suitable dosage regimens. Safety of **oxymorphone** and **hydromorphone** are not established in children.

Precautions:

Acute abdominal conditions: Narcotics may obscure diagnosis or clinical course.

Special risk patients: Exercise caution in elderly and debilitated patients and in those suffering from conditions accompanied by hypoxia or hypercapnia when even moderate therapeutic doses may dangerously decrease pulmonary ventilation. Also exercise caution in patients sensitive to CNS depressants, including those with cardiovascular disease; myxedema; convulsive disorders; increased ocular pressure; acute alcoholism; delirium tremens; cerebral arteriosclerosis; ulcerative colitis; fever; decreased respiratory reserve (eg, emphysema, severe obesity); hypothyroidism; kyphoscoliosis; Addison's disease; prostatic hypertrophy; urethral stricture; CNS depression; coma; gallbladder disease; recent GI or GU tract surgery; toxic psychosis.

Supraventricular tachycardias: Use with caution in atrial flutter and other supraventricular tachycardias; vagolytic action may increase the ventricular response rate.

Seizures may be aggravated or may occur in individuals without a history of convulsive disorders if dosage is substantially increased because of tolerance.

Cough reflex is suppressed. Exercise caution when using narcotic analgesics postoperatively and in patients with pulmonary disease.

Tolerance: Some patients develop tolerance to the narcotic analgesic. This may occur after days or months of continuous therapy. The dose generally needs to be increased to obtain adequate analgesia.

Cross-tolerance is not complete. Switching to another narcotic agonist, starting with half the predicted equianalgesic dose, may circumvent the cross-tolerance.

Drug abuse and dependence: Narcotic analgesics have abuse potential. Psychological dependence and physical tolerance and dependence may develop upon repeated use. However, most patients who receive opiates for medical reasons do not develop dependence syndromes.

Infants born to mothers physically dependent on narcotics will also be physically dependent and may exhibit respiratory difficulties and withdrawal symptoms.

Acute abstinence syndrome (withdrawal) – Severity is related to the degree of dependence, the abruptness of withdrawal and the drug used. Generally, withdrawal symptoms develop at the time the next dose would ordinarily be given.

Hazardous tasks: May produce drowsiness or dizziness; observe caution while driving or performing other tasks requiring alertness or physical dexterity.

Drug Interactions:

Drug/Lab test interactions: Drugs that may affect narcotic analgesics include barbiturate anesthetics, cimetidine, chlropromazine, hycantoins, diazepam, droperidol and rifampin. Charcoal and cigarette smoking may also affect narcotic analgesics. Drugs that may be affected by narcotic analgesics include carbamazepine, warfarin, MAOIs, furazolidone and nitrous oxide.

Determinations of plasma amylase or lipase levels may be unreliable for 24 hours after narcotic administration.

Adverse Reactions:

Most frequent: Lightheadedness; dizziness; sedation; nausea; vomiting; sweating.

CNS: Euphoria; dysphoria; delirium; insomnia; agitation; anxiety; fear; hallucinations; disorientation; drowsiness; sedation; lethargy; impairment of mental and physical performance; skeletal or uncoordinated movements; coma; mood changes; weakness; headache; mental cloudiness; blurred vision; visual disturbances; diplopia; miosis; tremor; convulsions; psychic dependence; toxic psychoses; depression; increased intracranial pressure; miosis.

GI: Nausea; vomiting; diarrhea; cramps; abdominal pain; taste alterations; dry mouth; anorexia; constipation.

Cardiovascular: Facial flushing; chills; faintness; peripheral circulatory collapse; tachycardia; bradycardia; arrhythmia; palpitations; hypertension; hypotension; orthostatic hypotension; syncope.

GU: Ureteral spasm and spasm of vesical sphincters; urinary retention or hesitancy; oliguria; antidiuretic effect; reduced libido or potency.

Hypersensitivity: Pruritus; urticaria; other skin rashes; diaphoresis; laryngospasm; edema; hemorrhagic urticaria (rare).

Miscellaneous: Bronchospasm; depression of cough reflex; interference with thermal regulation; laryngospasm; muscular rigidity; paresthesia.

Administration and Dosage:

ALFENTANIL HCl: In obese patients (> 20% above ideal total body weight), determine dosage on the basis of lean body weight. Reduce dose in elderly or debilitated patients.

Children < 12 years of age – Use is not recommended.

Alfentanil Dosage Range

Indication	≈ Duration of Anesthesia	Induction (Initial Dose)	Maintenance (Increments/ Infusion)	Total Dose	Effects
Incremental injection	≤ 30 min	8-20 mcg/kg	3-5 mcg/kg or 0.5-1 mcg/kg/ min	8-40 mcg/kg	Spontaneous breathing or assisted ventilation when required.
Incremental injection	30-60 min	20-50 mcg/kg	5-15 mcg/kg	up to 75 mcg/kg	Assisted or controlled ventilation required. Attenuation of response to laryngoscopy and intubation.

Alfentanil Dosage Range					
Indication	≈ Duration of Anesthesia	Induction (Initial Dose)	Maintenance (Increments/ Infusion)	Total Dose	Effects
Anesthetic induction	> 45 min	130-245 mcg/kg	0.5-1.5 mcg/kg/ min or general anesthetic	dependent on duration of procedure	Assisted or controlled ventilation required. Give slowly (over 3 min). Reduce concentration of inhalation agents by 30%-50% for initial hour.
Continuous infusion[1]	> 45 min	50-75 mcg/kg	0.5-3 mcg/kg/ min. Average infusion rate 1-1.5 mcg/kg/ min	dependent on duration of procedure	Assisted or controlled ventilation required. Some attenuation of response to intubation and incision, with intraoperative stability.
MAC	≤ 30 min	3-8 mcg/kg	3-5 mcg/kg every 5-20 min to 1 mcg/kg/ min	3-40 mcg/kg	Assisted or controlled ventilation required

[1] 0.5–3 mcg/kg/min with nitrous oxide/oxygen in general surgery. Following anesthetic induction dose, reduce infusion rate requirements by 30% to 50% for first hour of maintenance. Vital sign changes that indicate response to surgical stress or lightening of anesthesia may be controlled by increasing rate to a max of 4 mcg/kg/min or administering bolus doses of 7 mcg/kg. If changes are not controlled after three bolus doses given over 5 minutes, use a barbiturate, vasodilator or inhalation agent. Always adjust infusion rates downward in the absence of these signs until there is some response to surgical stimulation. Rather than an increase in infusion rate, administer 7 mcg/kg bolus doses of alfentanil or a potent inhalation agent in response to signs of lightening of anesthesia within the last 15 minutes of surgery. Discontinue infusion at least 10 to 15 minutes prior to the end of surgery.

CODEINE:

Analgesic –

Adults: 15 to 60 mg every 4 to 6 hours, orally, IM, IV or SC. Usual dose is 30 mg. Do not exceed 360 mg in 24 hours.

Children (≥ 1 year of age): 0.5 mg/kg or 15 m^2 of body surface every 4 to 6 hours SC, IM or orally. Do not use IV in children

Antitussive – (See also Respiratories chapter).

Adults: 10 to 20 mg every 4 to 6 hours. Do not exceed 120 mg in 24 hours.

Children (6 to 12 years): 5 to 10 mg orally every 4 to 6 hours. Do not exceed 60 mg in 24 hours.

(2 to 6 years) – 2.5 to 5 mg orally every 4 to 6 hours. Do not exceed 30 mg in 24 hours.

FENTANYL:

Premedication – 0.05 to 0.1 mg IM, 30 to 60 minutes prior to surgery.

Adjunct to general anesthesia –

Total low dosage: 0.002 mg/kg in small doses for minor, painful surgical procedures and postoperative pain relief; *maintenance low dosage:* Infrequently needed.

Total low dosage: 0.002 to 0.02 mg/kg.

Maintenance moderate dosage: 0.025 to 0.1 mg IV or IM when movement or changes in vital signs indicate surgical stress or lightening of analgesia.

Total high dosage: 0.02 to 0.05 mg/kg. For "stress free" anesthesia. Use during open heart surgery and complicated neurosurgical and orthopedic procedures where surgery is prolonged and the stress response is detrimental.

Maintenance high dosage: Ranging from 0.025 mg to half the initial loading dose.

Adjunct to regional anesthesia – 0.05 to 0.1 mg IM or slowly IV over 1 to 2 minutes as required.

Postoperatively (recovery room) – 0.05 to 0.1 mg IM for the control of pain, tachypnea and emergence delirium; repeat dose in 1 to 2 hours as needed.

Children (2 to 12 years) – For induction and maintenance, a reduced dose as low as 2 to 3 mcg/kg is recommended. Safety and efficacy in children < 2 years of age have not been established.

General anesthetic: 0.05 to 0.1 mg/kg with oxygen and a muscle relaxant when attenuation of the responses to surgical stress is especially important. Up to 0.15 mg/kg may be necessary.

FENTANYL TRANSDERMAL SYSTEM: The most important factor to be considered in determining the appropriate dose is the extent of pre-existing opioid tolerance. Reduce initial doses in elderly or debilitated patients.

Application – Each system may be worn continuously for 72 hours. If analgesia for > 72 hours is required, apply a new system to a different skin site after removal of the previous transdermal system.

Dose selection – Maintain each patient at the lowest dose providing acceptable pain control. Unless the patient has pre-existing opioid tolerance, use the lowest dose, 25 mcg/hr, as the initial dose.

Upwards titration may be done 3 days after the initial dose; thereafter, it may be donse no more frequently than every 6 days. For delivery rates in excess of 100 mcg/hr, multiple systems may be used.

Fentanyl Transdermal Dose Based on Daily Morphine Equivalence Dose[1]

Oral 24 hour morphine (mg/day)	IM 24 hour morphine (mg/day)	Fentanyl transdermal (mcg/hr)
45-134	8-22	25
135-224	23-37	50
225-314	38-52	75
315-404	53-67	100
405-494	68-82	125
495-584	83-97	150
585-674	98-112	175
675-764	113-127	200
765-854	128-142	225
855-944	143-157	250
945-1034	158-172	275
1035-1124	173-187	300

[1] A 10 mg IM or 60 mg oral dose of morphine every 4 hours for 24 hours for 24 hours (total of 60 mg/day IM or 360 mg/day IM or 360 mg/day oral) was considered approximately equivalent to fentanyl transdermal 100 mcg/hr.

The majority of patients are adequately maintained with transdermal fentanyl administered every 72 hours. A small number of patients may require systems to be applied every 48 hours.

During the initial application, patients should use short-acting analgesics for the first 24 hours as needed until analgesic efficacy with the transdermal system is attained. Thereafter, some patients still may require periodic supplemental doses of other short-acting analgesics for breakthrough pain.

Dose titration – Base appropriate dosage increments on the daily dose of supplementary opioids, using the ratio of 90 mg/24 hours of oral morphine to a 25 mcg/hr increase in transdermal fentanyl dose.

Discontinuation – Some patients will require a change to other methods of opioid administration when the dose exceeds 300 mcg/hr. To convert patients to another opioid, remove the system and initiate treatment with half the equinanalgesic dose of the new opioid 12 to 18 hours later (it takes ≥ 17 hours for the fentanyl serum concentration to fall by 50% after system removal).

FENTANYL TRANSMUCOSAL SYSTEM: Fentanyl transmucosal doses of 5 mcg/kg provide effects similar to usual doses of fentanyl given IM (0.75 to 1.25 mcg/kg). Larger doses have not been shown to increase efficacy. Adults should not receive doses > 5 mcg/kg (400 mcg), and most children not apprehensive at onset may be managed with the same 5 mcg/kg dose. Children apprehensive at onset and some younger children may need doses of 5 to 15 mcg/kg with an attendant increased risk of hypoventilation.

Children – Due to the excessive frequency of significant hypoventilation at higher doses, doses > 5 mcg/kg (maximum, 400 mcg) are contraindicated in adults.

Adults – Because of the excessive frequency of significant hypoventilation at higher doses, doses > 5 mcg/kg (maximum, 400 mcg) are contraindicated in aduts.

Vulnerable patients – Cosider selection of a lower dose for vulnerable patients (eg, patients with head injury, cardiovascular or pulmonary disease, hepatic disease, liver dysfunction). If signs of excessive opioid effects appear before the unit is consumed, remove the dosage unit from the patient's mouth immediately.

Elderly – If fentanyl transmucosal is to be sued in patients over age 65, reduce the dose to 2.5 to 5 mcg/kg.

Administration – Administration of the unit should begin 20 to 40 minutes prior to the anticipated need of desired effect. Patients typically take 10 to 20 minutes for complete consumption. Peak effect occurs ≈ 20 to 30 minutes after the start of administration.

HYDROMORPHONE HCl:

Oral – 2 mg every 4 to 6 hours; ≥ 4 mg every 4 to 6 hours for more severe pain.

Parenteral – 1 to 2 mg SC or IM every 4 to 6 hours as needed. For severe pain, administer 3 to 4 mg every 4 to 6 hours as needed. May be given by slow IV injection over 2 to 5 minutes.

Rectal – 3 mg every 6 to 8 hours.

Children – Safety and efficacy have not been established.

LEVORPHANOL TARTRATE: The average adult dose is 2 mg orally or SC; increase to 3 mg, if necessary. It has been given by slow IV injection.

LEVOMETHADYL ACETATE HCl:

Dosing schedules – Usually administer 3 times a week, either on Monday, Wednesday and Friday, or on Tuesday, Thursday and Saturday. If withdrawal is a problem during the 72 hour inter-dose interval, the receding dose may be increased. In some cases, an every-other-day schedule may be appropriate. The usual doses must not be given on consecutive days because of the risk of fatal overdose. No dose mentioned in this section is ever meant to be given as a daily dose.

Induction – The initial dose for street addicts should be 20 to 40 mg. Each subsequent dose, administered at 48 or 72 hour intervals, may be adjusted in increments of 5 to 10 mg until steady-state is reached, usually within 1 or 2 weeks.

Patients dependent on methadone may require higher initial doses of levomethadyl. The suggested initial 3 times a week dose for such patients is 1.2 to 1.3 times the daily methadone maintenance dose being replaced. This initial dose should not exceed 120 mg; adjust subsequent doses, administered at 48 or 72 hour intervals, according to clinical response.

Maintenance – Most patients will be stabilized on doses in the range of 60 to 90 mg 3 times a week. Doses as low as 10 mg and as high as 140 mg 3 times a week have been given in clinical studies. Supplemental dosing over the 72 hour inteer-dose interval (weekend) is rarely needed.

The maximum *total* amount of levomethadyl recommended for any patient is 140–140–140 mg or 130–130–180 mg on a thrice-weekly schedule or 140 mg every other day.

Transfer from levomethadyl to methadone – Patients maintained on levomethadyl may be transferred directly to methadone. Because of the difference between the two compounds' metabolites and their pharmacological half-lives, it is recommended that methadone be started on a dily dose at 80% of the levomethadyl dose being replaced; the initial methadone dose must be given no sooner than 48 hours after the last levomethadyl dose. Subsequent increses or decresses of 5 to 10 mg in the daily methadone dose may be given to control symptoms of withdrawal or, less likely, symptoms of excessive sedation, in accordance with clinical observations.

MEPERIDINE HCl:

Relief of pain – While SC administration is suitable for occasional use, IM administration is preferred for repeated doses. If IV administration is required, decrease dosage and inject very slowly, preferably using a diluted solution. Meperidine is less effective when administered orally than when given parenterally.

Adults: 50 to 150 mg IM, SC or orally every 3 to 4 hours, as necessary.

Children: 1 to 1.8 mg/kg (0.5 to 0.8 mg/lb) IM, SC or orally up to adult dose, every 3 or 4 hours, as necessary.

Preoperative medication –

Adults: 50 to 100 mg IM or SC, 30 to 90 minutes before beginning anesthesia.

Children: 1 to 2 mg/kg (0.5 to 1 mg/lb) IM or SC, up to adult dose, 30 to 90 minutes before beginning anesthesia.

Support of anesthesia – Meperidine may be administered in repeated doses diluted to 10 mg/ml by slow IV injection, or by continuous IV infusion of solution diluted to 1 mg/ml.

Obstetrical analgesia – When pains become regular, administer 50 to 100 mg IM or SC; repeat at 1 to 3 hour intervals.

METHADONE HCl: Oral methadone is ≈ ½ as potent as parenteral.

Pain –

Adults: 2.5 to 10 mg IM, SC or orally every 3 or 4 hours as necessary.

Children: Not for analgesic use, due to insufficient documentation.

Detoxification treatment should not exceed 21 days and may not be repeated earlier than 4 weeks after completion of the preceding course.

Initially, 15 to 20 mg will often suppress withdrawal symptoms. When patients are physically dependent on high doses, 40 mg/day in single or divided doses is usually an adequate stabilizing dose. Continue stabilization for 2 to 3 days, then gradually decrease the dose on a daily basis or at 2 day intervals.

Maintenance treatment – Initial dosage should control abstinence symptoms following narcotic withdrawal, but should not cause sedation, respiratory depression or other effects of acute intoxication. Adjust dosage as tolerated and required, up to 120 mg/day.

For a complete description of detoxification and maintenance regulations and dosage protocols, consult a local approved methadone program.

MORPHINE SULFATE:

Oral – 10 to 30 mg every 4 hours or as directed by physician.

Controlled release: 30 mg every 8 to 12 hours or as directed by physician. Do not crush or chew.

SC/IM –

Adults: 10 mg (5 to 20 mg)/70 kg every 4 hours.

Children: 0.1 to 0.2 mg/kg (up to 15 mg) every 4 hours.

IV –

Adults: 2.5 to 15 mg/70 kg in 4 to 5 ml of Water for Injection, administered over 4 to 5 minutes.

Continuous IV infusion: 0.1 to 1 mg/ml in 5% Dextrose in Water by controlled-infusion device; higher concentrations have been used.

Rectal – 10 to 20 mg every 4 hours or as directed by physician.

Epidural –

Adults: Initial injection of 5 mg in the lumbar region may provide satisfactory pain relief for up to 24 hours. If adequate pain relief is not achieved within 1 hour, carefully administer incremental doses of 1 to 2 mg at intervals sufficient to assess effectiveness. Give no more than 10 mg/24 hr.

For continuous infusion, an initial dose of 2 to 4 mg/24 hours is recommended. Further doses of 1 to 2 mg may be given if pain relief is not achieved initially.

Aged or debilitated patients: Administer with extreme caution. Doses < 5 mg may provide satisfactory pain relief for up to 24 hours.

Intrathecal: Adult – Intrathecal dosage is usually 1/10 that of epidural dosage. A single injection of 0.2 to 1 mg may provide satisfactory pain relief for up to 24 hours.

Aged or debilitated: Use extreme caution. A lower dosage is usually satisfactory.

Intraventricular – Currently available data indicate that this route of administration is effective in select patients with intractable pain and short life expectancy. One to two doses per day are generally administered.

OPIUM: The activity of opium is primarily due to its morphine content. The major medical use of opium has been for its antiperistaltic activity, particularly in diarrhea. Opium alkaloids (eg, morphine, codeine) have replaced opium in medical use.

OXYCODONE HCl:

Adults – 5 mg or 5 ml every 6 hours as needed.

Children – Not recommended for use in children.

OXYMORPHONE HCl:

IV – Initially, 0.5 mg.

SC or IM – Initially, 1 to 1.5 mg every 4 to 6 hours, as needed. For analgesia during labor, give 0.5 to 1 mg IM.

Rectal – 5 mg every 4 to 6 hours.

Safety for use in children < 12 years of age has not been established.

PROPOXYPHENE HCl:

Usual dose – 65 mg every 4 hours as needed. Do not exceed 390 mg/day.

In hepatic or renal impairment, consider reducing total daily dosage.

PROPOXYPHENE NAPSYLATE: Because of differences in molecular weight, 100 mg of propoxyphene napsylate is required to supply propoxyphene equivalent to 65 mg of the HCl. In hepatic or renal impairment, consider reducing total daily dosage.

Usual dose – 100 mg every 4 hours as needed. Do not exceed 600 mg per day.

SUFENTANIL CITRATE: In obese patients (> 20% above ideal total body weight), determine dosage on the basis of lean body weight. Reduce dosage in the elderly or debilitated. Monitor vital signs routinely.

For IV injection.

Adult dosage range: Total dosage –

1 to 2 mcg/kg: Administer with nitrous oxide/oxygen in patients undergoing general surgery ≤ 8 hours in which endotracheal intubation and mechanical ventilation are required. Expected duration of anesthesia is 1 to 2 hours.

Maintenance – 10 to 25 mcg (0.2 to 0.5 ml) as needed for surgical stress or lightening of analgesia.

2 to 8 mcg/kg: Administer with nitrous oxide/oxygen in more complicated major surgical procedures. Expected duration of anesthesia is 2 to 8 hours.

Maintenance – 10 to 50 mcg (0.2 to 1 ml) for stress or lightening of analgesia.

8 to 30 mcg/kg (Anesthetic doses): Administer with 100% oxygen and a muscle relaxant. Sufentanil produces sleep at dosages ≥ 8 mcg/kg and maintains a deep level of anesthesia without additional agents.

Maintenance – 25 to 50 mcg (0.5 to 1 ml) for stress and lightening of anesthesia.

Children (< 12 years of age) – For induction and maintenance of anesthesia in children undergoing cardiovascular surgery, a dose of 10 to 25 mcg/kg administered with 100% oxygen is recommended. Supplemental dosages of up to 25 to 50 mcg are recommended for maintenance.

NARCOTIC AGONIST-ANTAGONIST ANALGESICS

Narcotic agonist-antagonist analgesics compete with other substances at the mu (μ) receptor. The μ receptors mediate morphine-like supraspinal analgesia, euphoria and respiratory and physical depression. There are two types of narcotic agonist-antagonists: 1) Drugs which are antagonists at the μ receptor and are agonists at other receptors (ie, pentazocine), 2) Partial agonists (ie, buprenorphine) which have limited agonist activity at the μ receptor. The narcotic agonist-antagonist analgesics are potent analgesic agents with a lower abuse potential than pure narcotic agonists. Because of their narcotic antagonist activity, these agents may precipitate withdrawal symptoms in those with opiate dependence.

Narcotic Agonist-Antagonist Pharmacokinetics

Agonist/Antagonist		Onset (min)	Peak (min)	Duration (hrs)	$t_{1/2}$ (hrs)	Equivalent Dose[1] (mg)	Relative Antagonist Activity
Buprenorphine	IM	15	60	6	2.2-3.5	0.3	Equipotent with Naloxone
	IV[2]						
Butorphanol	IM	<10	30-60	3-4	2.5-4	2-3	30x Pentazocine or 1/40 Naloxone
Dezocine	IM	≤ 30	30-150	2-4[3]	nd	10	Greater than Pentazocine
	IV	≤ 15			2.4[4]		
Nalbuphine	IM	< 15[5]	60	3-6	5	10	10x Pentazocine
	IV	12-30[2]	30				
Pentazocine	IM	15-20[2]	15-601	3	2.2-3.5	30	Weak
	IV	12-30[2]	nd				
	Oral	15-30[2]	60-180				

[1] Parenteral dose equivalent to 10 mg morphine.
[2] Time to onset and peak effect shorter.
[3] Dose related.
[4] For 10 or 20 mg dose; 1.7 hr for 5 mg dose.
[5] Also for subcutaneous administration.
* nd – no data

DEZOCINE

Injection: 5, 10 and 15 mg/ml (*Rx*) — *Dalgan* (Astra)

Actions:

Pharmacology: Dezocine is a strong synthetic opioid agonist-antagonist parenteral analgesic of the aminotetralin series. Its analgesic potency, onset and duration of action in the relief of postoperative pain are comparable to morphine.

Pharmacokinetics:

Absorption/Distribution – Dezocine is completely and rapidly absorbed following IM injection, with an average peak serum concentration of 19 ng/ml (range, 10 to 38 ng/ml) occurring between 10 and 90 minutes after a 10 mg IM injection. Following a 10 mg IV infusion over 5 minutes, the average terminal half-life of dezocine is 2.4 hours (range, 1.2 to 7.4 hours). The average volume of distribution is 10.1 L/kg (range, 4.7 to 20.1 L/kg), and the average total body clearance is 3.3 L/hr/kg (range, 1.7 to 7.2 L/hr/kg).

Metabolism/Excretion – Approximately two-thirds of a dose is recovered in the urine with about 1% being excreted as unchanged dezocine and the remainder as the glucuronide conjugate.

Cardiovascular effects: Dezocine is not associated with significant changes.

Indications:
Management of pain when the use of an opioid analgesic is appropriate.

Contraindications:
Hypersensitivity to the drug.

Warnings:
Drug dependence/abuse: Because of its opioid antagonist properties, dezocine is not recommended for patients physically dependent on narcotics.

Renal/Hepatic function impairment: Dezocine undergoes extensive hepatic metabolism and renal excretion of the glucuronide metabolite. Give cautiously with reduced doses to patients with hepatic or renal dysfunction.

Elderly: Like all strong, mixed opioid agonist-antagonist analgesics, dezocine can depress respiration and reduce ventilatory drive to a clinically significant extent. It also can alter mental status or induce delirium in elderly patients. Reduce the initial dose of dezocine in the geriatric population to assess its relative risk and individualize subsequent doses.

Pregnancy: Category C.

Lactation: The use of dezocine in nursing mothers is not recommended.

Children: Safety and efficacy in patients < 18 years old have not been established.

Precautions:
Head injury and increased intracranial pressure: Use only when essential and with extreme caution.

Chronic obstructive pulmonary disease: Because strong opioids cause some respiratory depression, administer only with caution and in low doses to patients with preexisting respiratory depression, severely limited respiratory reserve, bronchial asthma, obstructive respiratory conditions or cyanosis. Respiratory depression induced by dezocine can be reversed by naloxone.

Biliary surgery: Use with caution in such settings.

Ambulatory patients: Strong opioid analgesics impair the mental or physical abilities required for the performance of potentially dangerous tasks such as driving a car or operating machinery. Patients who have been given dezocine should not drive or operate dangerous machinery until the effects of the drug are no longer present.

Drug Interactions:
Drugs that may interact with dezocine include: Opioid analgesics; general anesthetics; sedatives; tranquilizers; hypnotics or other CNS depressants (including alcohol).

Adverse Reactions:
Adverse reactions occuring in ≥ 3% of patients include: Nausea; vomiting; sedation; injection site reactions.

Administration and Dosage:
Adults:

IM – Single dose of 5 to 20 mg (usual, 10 mg). Adjust dosage according to the patient's weight, age, severity of pain, physical status and other medications that the patient may be receiving. Repeat every 3 to 6 hours as necessary.

Maximum dose – 20 mg; probable upper limit of 120 mg/day. There is insufficient information regarding the risk of chronic use of dezocine to establish limits for the maximum recommended duration of treatment with the drug.

IV – 2.5 to 10 mg repeated every 2 to 4 hours. The usual initial IV dose is 5 mg.

SC – Not recommended.

PENTAZOCINE

Injection: 30 mg (as lactate) per ml (*c-iv*)	*Talwin* (Sanofi Winthrop)
Tablets: 50 mg (as HCl) and 0.5 mg naloxone HCl (*c-iv*)	*Talwin NX* (Sanofi Winthrop)

Warning:

Talwin Nx is intended for oral use only. Severe, potentially lethal reactions (eg, pulmonary emboli, vascular occlusion, ulceration and abscesses, withdrawal symptoms in narcotic-dependent individuals) may result from misuse of this drug by injection or in combination with other substances.

Actions:

Pharmacology: Pentazocine, a potent analgesic, weakly antagonizes the effects of morphine, meperidine and other opiates at the μ-opioid receptor. Pentazocine, presumed to exert its agonistic actions at the kappa (κ) and sigma (σ) opioid receptors, may precipitate withdrawal symptoms in patients taking narcotic analgesics regularly. In addition, it produces incomplete reversal of cardiovascular, respiratory and behavioral depression induced by morphine and meperidine. Pentazocine also has sedative activity.

Talwin NX tablets, which contain naloxone, produce analgesic effects when administered orally because naloxone has poor bioavailability.

Pharmacokinetics: Pentazocine is well absorbed from the GI tract and from SC and IM sites. However, it undergoes extensive first-pass hepatic metabolism. Oral bioavailability is < 20%, and was increased threefold in cirrhotic patients. Concentrations in plasma coincide closely with onset, intensity and duration of analgesia. Pentazocine passes into fetal circulation. It is excreted via the kidney, < 5% unchanged.

Indications:

Oral and parenteral: Relief of moderate to severe pain.

Parenteral: For preoperative or preanesthetic medication; supplement to surgical anesthesia.

Contraindications:

Hypersensitivity to pentazocine, naloxone (in *Talwin NX*) or any product component.

Warnings:

Drug dependence: Exercise special care in prescribing to emotionally unstable patients and to those with history of drug abuse; closely supervise when therapy exceeds 4 or 5 days.

"Ts and Blues" – Injection IV of oral preparations of**pentazocine** (*Talwin*, "Ts") and **tripelennamine** (PBZ, "Blues"), an H_1-blocking antihistamine has become a common form of drug abuse as a "substitute" for heroin.

Tissue damage: Severe sclerosis of skin, subcutaneous tissues and underlying muscle has occurred at injection sites following multiple doses of pentazocine lactate. Rotate injection sites; IM may be tolerated better than SC.

Head injury and increased intracranial pressure: Pentazocine can produce effects which may obscure the clinical course of head injury patients. The potential for elevating cerebrospinal fluid pressure may be attributed to CO_2 retention due to the respiratory depressant effects of the drug. These effects may be exaggerated in the presence of head injury, other intracranial lesions or a preexisting increase in intracranial pressure. Use with extreme caution and only if essential.

Myocardial infarction (MI): Exercise caution in the IV use of pentazocine for patients with acute MI accompanied by hypertension or left ventricular failure. Pentazocine IV elevates systemic and pulmonary arterial pressure, systemic vascular resistance and left ventricular end-diastolic pressure, causing increased cardiac workload. Use the oral form with caution in MI patients who have nausea or vomiting.

Acute CNS manifestations: Patients receiving therapeutic doses have experienced hallucinations (usually visual), disorientation and confusion which have cleared spontaneously. If the drug is reinstituted, acute CNS manifestations may recur.

Seizures have occurred with the use of pentazocine.

Renal/Hepatic function impairment: The drug is metabolized in liver and excreted by the kidney; administer with caution to patients with such impairment. Extensive liver disease predisposes to greater side effects and may be the result of decreased drug metabolism.

Pregnancy: Category C. Pentazocine rapidly crosses the placenta with cord blood levels 40% to 70% of maternal serum levels. Chronic maternal ingestion of pentazocine may result in neonatal withdrawal symptoms.

Labor – Use with caution in women delivering premature infants.

Lactation: Safety for use in the nursing mother has not been established.

Children: Safety and efficacy in children < 12 years old have not been established.

Precautions:

Respiratory conditions: Use caution and low dosage in patients with respiratory depression, severely limited respiratory reserve, severe bronchial asthma, obstructive respiratory conditions, cyanosis.

Biliary tract pressure elevation generally occurs for varying periods following narcotic use. However, some evidence suggests pentazocine causes little or no elevation in biliary tract pressures.

Patients receiving narcotics: Pentazocine is a mild narcotic antagonist. Some patients previously given narcotics, including methadone for the daily treatment of narcotic dependence, have experienced withdrawal symptoms after receiving pentazocine.

Hazardous tasks: May produce sedation, dizziness and occasional euphoria; observe caution while driving or performing other tasks requiring alertness, coordination or physical dexterity.

Drug Interactions:

Drugs that may interact with pentazocine include: Alcohol and barbiturate anesthetics.

Adverse Reactions:

Significant adverse reactions include: Nausea; dizziness or lightheadedness; drowsiness; vomiting; euphoria; constipation; cramps; abdominal distress; anorexia; diarrhea; dry mouth; taste alteration; sedation; headache; weakness or faintness; depression; disturbed dreams; insomnia; syncope; hallucinations; tremor; irritability; excitement; tinnitus; disorientation; confusion; blurred vision; focusing difficulty; nystagmus; diplopia; miosis; edema of the face; sweating; anaphylactic reaction; rash; urticaria; soft tissue induration; nodules; cutaneous depression; ulceration (sloughing); severe sclerosis of the skin, subcutaneous tissues and, rarely, underlying muscle at the injection site; diaphoresis; stinging on injection; flushed skin; dermatitis; pruritus; toxic epidermal necrolysis; hypotension; decrease in blood pressure; tachycardia; circulatory depression; shock; hypertension; respiratory depression; dyspnea; transient apnea in newborns whose mothers received parenteral pentazocine during labor; Depression of white blood cells (especially granulocytes), usually reversible; moderate transient eosinophilia; urinary retention; paresthesia; chills; neuromuscular and psychiatric muscle tremors; alterations in rate or strength of uterine contractions during labor (parenteral form).

Administration and Dosage:

Oral:

Adults – Initially, 50 mg every 3 or 4 hours; increase to 100 mg if necessary. Do not exceed a total daily dosage of 600 mg. When anti-inflammatory or antipyretic effects are desired in addition to analgesia, aspirin can be administered concomitantly.

Children (< 12 years old) – Clinical experience is limited; use is not recommended.

Pentazocine tablets are intended for oral use only. Severe, potentially lethal reactions may result from misuse by injection or when combined with other substances.

Oral pentazocine tablets contain 0.5 mg naloxone, a narcotic antagonist, to aid in elimination of the abuse potential.

Parenteral:

Adults – 30 mg IM, SC or IV; may repeat every 3 to 4 hours. Doses in excess of 30 mg IV or 60 mg IM or SC are not recommended. Do not exceed a total daily dosage of 360 mg.

Use SC only when necessary; severe tissue damage is possible at injection sites. When frequent injections are needed, administer IM, constantly rotating injection sites.

Patients in labor – A single 30 mg IM dose is most common. A 20 mg IV dose, given 2 or 3 times at 2 to 3 hour intervals, has resulted in adequate pain relief when contractions become regular.

Children (< 12 years old) – Clinical experience is limited; use is not recommended.

Admixture incompatibility – Do not mix pentazocine in the same syringe with soluble barbiturates because precipitation will occur.

PENTAZOCINE COMBINATIONS

Tablets: 12.5 mg (as HCl) and 325 mg aspirin (*c-iv*)	*Talwin Compound Caplets* (Sanofi Winthrop)
Tablets: 25 mg (as HCl) and 650 mg acetaminophen (*c-iv*)	*Talacen Capets* (Sanofi Winthrop)

Administration and Dosage:

Adults:

Pentazocine and aspirin – 2 tablets 3 or 4 times daily.

Pentazocine and acetaminophen – 1 tablet every 4 hours, up to 6 tablets per day.

Children: Not recommended for children < 12 years old.

BUTORPHANOL TARTRATE

Injection: 1 mg per ml and 2 mg per ml (1 mg of tartrate salt is equal to 0.68 mg base) (*Rx*)	*Stadol* (Mead Johnson)
Nasal spray: 10 mg/ml (*Rx*)	*Stadol NS* (Mead Johnson)

Actions:

Pharmacology: Butorphanol is a potent analgesic with both narcotic agonist and antagonist effects. The exact mechanism of action is unknown.

Narcotic antagonist activity – Butorphanol's narcotic antagonist activity is ≈ 30 times that of pentazocine and 1⁄40 that of naloxone.

Effect on respiration – A parenteral dose of 2 to 3 mg butorphanol produces analgesia and respiratory depression approximately equal to that of 10 mg morphine or 80 mg meperidine. However, butorphanol appears to have a ceiling effect at 30 to 60 mcg/kg in the degree of respiratory depression produced; it is reversible by naloxone.

Cardiovascular effects – Hemodynamic changes after IV administration, similar to those seen with pentazocine, include increased pulmonary artery pressure, pulmonary wedge pressure, left ventricular end-diastolic pressure, systemic arterial pressure, pulmonary vascular resistance and increased cardiac workload.

Pharmacokinetics:

Butorphanol Pharmacokinetics Based on Route of Administration			
Parameter	IV	IM	Nasal
Onset (min)	rapid	10-15	within 15
Peak (hrs)	0.5-1	0.5-1	1-2
Duration (hrs)	3-4	3-4	4-5
Half-life (hrs)	2.1-8.8	—	2.9-9.2
AUC (hr • ng/ml)	4.4-13	—	0.3-10.3

Butorphanol is extensively metabolized in the liver. The elimination half-life of hydroxybutorphanol may be greater than the parent compound. Elimination occurs in the urine (70% to 80%) and feces (≈ 15%). In the urine, ≈ 5% is excreted unchanged, 49% as hydroxybutorphanol and < 5% as norbutorphanol. and in patients with decreased creatinine clearance. Protein binding is ≈ 80%.

Indications:

Parenteral/Nasal: Management of pain (including postoperative analgesia).

Parenteral: For preoperative or preanesthetic medication; to supplement balanced anesthesia; for relief of pain during labor.

Contraindications:

Hypersensitivity to butorphanol or any components of the products.

Warnings:

Physically dependent narcotic patients should not receive butorphanol prior to detoxification; it may precipitate withdrawal.

Drug dependence: Although butorphanol has low physical dependence liability, exercise care in administering to emotionally unstable patients and to those prone to drug misuse and abuse.

Head injury and increased intracranial pressure: Butorphanol may elevate cerebrospinal fluid pressure; use in cases of head injury can produce effects (eg, miosis) which may obscure the clinical course of these patients. Use with extreme caution and only if essential.

Cardiovascular disease: Butorphanol increases the cardiac workload; limit its use in acute myocardial infarction or in ventricular dysfunction or coronary insufficiency to those situations where the benefits outweigh the risk.

Severe hypertension has occurred rarely. Discontinue butorphanol and treat the hypertension.

Renal/Hepatic function impairment: The drug is metabolized in the liver and excreted by the kidneys; increase the dosage interval.

Elderly: The mean half-life of butorphanol is increased by 25% (to > 6 hours) and elimination half-life is also increased in patients > 65 years of age. Elderly patients may be more sensitive to its side effects, especially dizziness.

Pregnancy: Category C.

Labor and delivery – Butorphanol injection may be used during labor. Reports of infant respiratory distress/apnea following butorphanol use during labor have been associated with administration of a dose ≤ 2 hours prior to delivery, use of multiple doses, use with additional analgesic or sedative drugs or use in preterm pregnancies. Use with caution in the presence of an abnormal fetal heart rate pattern.

Nasal spray is not recommended during labor/delivery.

Lactation: Butorphanol appears in breast milk following the injectable route; assume the drug will appear in breast milk following the nasal route as well. The amount an infant would receive is probably clinically insignificant (estimated at 4 mcg/L of milk using 2 mg IM 4 times daily).

Children: Safety and efficacy for use in children < 18 years of age have not been established. Not recommended for use in this age group.

Precautions:

Respiratory conditions: Butorphanol causes some respiratory depression. Administer with caution and in low dosage to patients with respiratory depression, severely limited respiratory reserve, bronchial asthma, obstructive respiratory conditions or cyanosis.

Hazardous tasks: May cause dizziness or drowsiness; observe caution while driving or performing other tasks requiring alertness, coordination or physical dexterity.

Drug Interactions:

Barbiturate anesthetics may increase the respiratory and CNS depression of butorphanol because of additive pharmacologic activity.

Adverse Reactions:

Adverse reactions occuring in ≥ 3% of patients include: Nausea; vomiting; dry mouth; somnolence; dizziness; confusion; sweating; clammy skin; asthenia; lethargy; headache; vasodilation; anorexia; constipation; insomnia; nasal congestion; dyspnea; epistaxis; nasal irritation; pharyngitis; rhinitis; sinus congestion; upper respiratory infection; tinnitus; unpleasant taste.

Administration and Dosage:

Pain:

IV – 1 mg (dosage range, 0.5 to 2 mg) repeated every 3 to 4 hours as necessary.

IM – 2 mg (dosage range, 1 to 4 mg) every 3 to 4 hours as necessary in patients who will be able to remain recumbent. Do not exceed single doses of 4 mg.

Nasal – 1 mg (1 spray in one nostril). If adequate pain relief is not achieved within 60 to 90 minutes, an additional 1 mg dose may be given. The initial 2 dose sequence may be repeated in 3 to 4 hours as needed. Depending on the pain severity, an initial 2 mg dose (1 spray in each nostril) may be used in patients who will be able to remain recumbent. Do not give additional 2 mg doses for 3 to 4 hours.

Preoperative/Preanesthetic use: Individualize dosage. Usual dose is 2 mg IM 60 to 90 minutes before surgery.

Labor: 1 to 2 mg IV or IM in patients at full term in early labor; repeat after 4 hours.

Children: Not recommended in children < 18 years of age.

Elderly:

Parenteral – Use one-half the usual dose at twice the usual interval. Base subsequent doses and intervals on patient response.

Nasal – 1 mg initially. Allow 90 to 120 minutes to elapse before deciding whether a second 1 mg dose is needed.

Renal/Hepatic function impairment: Increase the initial dosage interval to 6 to 8 hours. Determine subsequent doses by patient response.

NALBUPHINE HCl

Injection: 10 and 20 mg per ml (*Rx*)	Various, *Nubain* (DuPont)

Actions:

Pharmacology: Nalbuphine, a potent analgesic with narcotic agonist and antagonist actions, has a chemical structure similar to phenanthrene derivatives, oxymorphone and naloxone. Its analgesic potency is essentially equivalent to that of morphine and about 3 times that of pentazocine on a milligram basis. Nalbuphine does not significantly increase pulmonary artery pressure or systemic vascular resistance or cardiac work.

Pharmacokinetics: Onset of action occurs within 2 to 3 minutes after IV administration, and in < 15 minutes following SC or IM injection. Nalbuphine is metabolized in the liver; plasma half-life is 5 hours. The duration of analgesic activity ranges from 3 to 6 hours. Approximately 7% is excreted unchanged in the urine.

The narcotic antagonist activity of nalbuphine is 10 times that of pentazocine.

Indications:

Relief of moderate to severe pain.

For preoperative analgesia, as a supplement to balanced analgesia, to surgical and postsurgical anesthesia and for obstetrical analgesia during labor and delivery.

Contraindications:

Hypersensitivity to nalbuphine.

Warnings:

Drug dependence: Nalbuphine's low abuse potential is less than codeine and propoxyphene. Psychological and physical dependence and tolerance may follow nalbuphine abuse. Cautiously prescribe to emotionally unstable patients or to individuals with a history of narcotic abuse.

Abrupt discontinuation after prolonged use has been followed by symptoms of narcotic withdrawal.

Head injury and increased intracranial pressure: The possible respiratory depressant effects and the potential of potent analgesics to elevate cerebrospinal fluid pressure may be markedly exaggerated in the presence of head injury, intracranial lesions or a preexisting increase in intracranial pressure. Therefore, use with extreme caution and only if deemed essential.

Renal function impairment: The drug is metabolized in the liver and excreted by the kidneys; patients with renal or liver dysfunction may overreact to customary doses. Therefore, use with caution and administer in reduced amounts.

Pregnancy: Safe use in pregnancy has not been established. Prolonged use during pregnancy could result in neonatal withdrawal. Administer to pregnant women only when the potential benefits outweigh the possible hazards.

Labor and delivery – May produce respiratory depression in the neonate. Use with caution in women delivering premature infants.

Children: Not recommended in patients < 18 years old.

Precautions:

Respiratory depression: At the usual adult dose of 10 mg/70 kg, nalbuphine causes respiratory depression approximately equal to that produced by equal doses of morphine. However, nalbuphine exhibits a ceiling effect; increases in dosage beyond 30 mg produce no further respiratory depression. Respiratory depression induced by nalbuphine can be reversed by naloxone. Administer with caution at low doses to patients with impaired respiration.

Myocardial infarction: Use with caution in patients with myocardial infarction who have nausea or vomiting.

Biliary tract surgery: Use with caution in patients about to undergo biliary tract surgery since it may cause spasm of the sphincter of Oddi.

Hazardous tasks: May produce drowsiness. Observe caution while driving or performing other tasks requiring alertness, coordination or physical dexterity.

Drug Interactions:

Drugs that may interact with nalbuphine HCl include: Barbiturate anesthetics.

Adverse Reactions:

Adverse reactions occuring in ≥ 3% of patients include: Sedation; sweaty/clammy feeling; nausea; vomiting; dizziness; vertigo; dry mouth; headache.

Administration and Dosage:

Adults: Usual dose is 10 mg/70 kg administered SC, IM or IV every 3 to 6 hours as necessary. Individualize dosage. In nontolerant individuals, the recommended single maximum dose is 20 mg, with a maximum total daily dose of 160 mg.

Patients dependent on narcotics may experience withdrawal symptoms upon the administration of nalbuphine. If unduly troublesome, control by slow IV administration of small increments of morphine until relief occurs. If the previous analgesic was morphine, meperidine, codeine or another narcotic with similar duration of activity, administer ¼ the anticipated nalbuphine dose initially. Observe for signs of withdrawal. If untoward symptoms do not occur, progressively increase doses at appropriate intervals until analgesia is obtained.

BUPRENORPHINE HCl

Injection: 0.324 mg (equiv. to 0.3 mg buprenorphine) per ml (c-v) — *Buprenex* (Reckitt & Colman)

Actions:

Pharmacology: Buprenorphine is a semisynthetic centrally-acting opioid analgesic derived from thebaine; a 0.3 mg dose is approximately equivalent to 10 mg morphine in analgesic effects. Buprenorphine exerts its analgesic effect via high affinity binding of CNS opiate receptors. It has a high affinity for the μ receptors and dissociates from them slowly, which may contribute to its long duration of action and low physical dependence.

Its narcotic antagonist activity is approximately equipotent to naloxone.

Cardiovascular – Buprenorphine may cause a decrease or, rarely, an increase in pulse rate and blood pressure in some patients.

Respiratory effects – A therapeutic dose of 0.3 mg buprenorphine can decrease respiratory rate similarly to an equianalgesic dose of morphine (10 mg).

Pharmacokinetics: Onset of analgesic effect occurs 15 minutes after IM injection, peaks in about 1 hour, and persists up to 6 hours. When given IV, the time to onset and peak is shortened.

Plasma protein binding is about 96%. Buprenorphine is metabolized by the liver and its clearance is related to hepatic blood flow. Terminal half-life is 2 to 3 hours. The drug is excreted predominantly in the feces as free buprenorphine with traces of the N–dealkyl metabolite.

Indications:

Relief of moderate to severe pain.

Contraindications:

Hypersensitivity to buprenorphine.

Warnings:

Narcotic-dependent patients: Because of the narcotic antagonist activity of buprenorphine, use in physically dependent individuals may result in withdrawal effects. Buprenorphine, a partial agonist, has opioid properties which may lead to psychic dependence due to a euphoric component of the drug. The drug may not be substituted in acutely dependent narcotic addicts due to its antagonist component.

Respiratory effects: There have been occasional reports of clinically significant respiratory depression associated with buprenorphine. Use with caution in patients with compromised respiratory function and those given other respiratory depressants. In such cases, reduce the dose by one half. The use of assisted or controlled ventilation may be necessary.

Head injury/increased intracranial pressure: Buprenorphine may elevate cerebrospinal fluid (CSF) pressure; use with caution in head injury, intracranial lesions and other states where CSF pressure may be increased. Buprenorphine can produce miosis and changes in consciousness levels which may interfere with patient evaluation.

Hepatic function impairment: Buprenorphine is metabolized by the liver; the activity may be altered in those individuals with impaired hepatic function.

Pregnancy: Category C.

Labor and Delivery – Safety and efficacy have not been established.

Lactation: It is not known whether buprenorphine is excreted in breast milk.

Children: Safety and efficacy for use in children have not been established.

Precautions:

Use with caution in the following: Elderly or debilitated; severe impairment of hepatic, pulmonary or renal function; myxedema or hypothyroidism; adrenal cortical insufficiency; CNS depression or coma; toxic psychoses; prostatic hypertrophy or urethral stricture; acute alcoholism; delirium tremens or kyphoscoliosis. Naloxone may not be effective in reversing respiratory depression.

Biliary tract dysfunction: Buprenorphine increases intracholedochal pressure to a similar degree as other opiates; administer with caution.

Potentially hazardous tasks: May cause dizziness or drowsiness; observe caution while driving or performing other tasks requiring alertness.

Drug Interactions:

Drugs that may interact with buprenorphine HCl include: Barbiturate anesthetics; diazepam.

Adverse Reactions:

Adverse reactions occurring in ≥ 3% of patients include: Sedation; dizziness/vertigo; headache; hypotension; nausea/vomiting; hypoventilation; miosis; sweating.

Administration and Dosage:

Patients ≥ 13 years of age: 0.3 mg IM or slow IV, every 6 hours, as needed. Repeat once (up to 0.3 mg) if required, 30 to 60 minutes after initial dosage, giving consideration to previous dose pharmacokinetics; use thereafter only as needed. In high-risk patients (eg, elderly, debilitated, presence of respiratory disease) or in patients where other CNS depressants are present, such as in the immediate postoperative period, reduce dose by approximately one-half. Exercise extra caution with the IV route of administration, particularly with the initial dose.

Occasionally, it may be necessary to give up to 0.6 mg. Data are insufficient to recommend single IM doses > 0.6 mg for long-term use.

IV compatibility: Buprenorphine is compatible with: Isotonic saline, Lactated Ringer's Solution, 5% Dextrose and 0.9% Saline, 5% Dextrose, scopolamine HBr, haloperidol, glycopyrrolate, droperidol and hydroxyzine HCl.

IV incompatibility: Buprenorphine is incompatible with diazepam and lorazepam.

METHOTRIMEPRAZINE

Injection: 20 mg (as HCl) per ml (*Rx*)	*Levoprome* (Lederle)

This agent acts by central mechanisms and is therefore distinct from the salicylates and other nonsteroidal anti-inflammatory agents which act peripherally.

Actions:

Pharmacology: A phenothiazine derivative and potent CNS depressant which produces suppression of sensory impulses, reduction of motor activity, sedation and tranquilization. Methotrimeprazine raises the pain threshold and produces amnesia. It also has antihistaminic, anticholinergic and antiadrenergic effects.

It produces an analgesic effect comparable to morphine and meperidine with a marked sedative effect. Respiratory depression in the patient or in the newborn during or following preanesthetic or obstetrical use occurs infrequently. The drug does not appear to affect the cough reflex. Its use has not been reported to result in addiction, dependence or withdrawal symptoms even with large doses or with prolonged administration.

Pharmacokinetics: Peak plasma concentrations occur 30 to 90 minutes after injection. Maximum analgesic effect usually occurs within 20 to 40 minutes after IM injection and is maintained for about 4 hours. Methotrimeprazine is metabolized into sulfoxides and glucuronic conjugates and largely excreted in the urine as such. Elimination half-life is 15 to 30 hours. Small amounts of unchanged drug are excreted in the feces and in the urine (1%). Elimination into the urine usually continues for several days after IM administration is discontinued.

Indications:

Relief of moderate to marked pain in nonambulatory patients.

For obstetrical analgesia and sedation where respiratory depression is to be avoided.

Preanesthetic for producing sedation, somnolence and relief of apprehension and anxiety.

Contraindications:

Concurrent administration with antihypertensive agents including MAO inhibitors; history of phenothiazine hypersensitivity; presence of overdosage of CNS depressants or comatose states; severe myocardial, renal or hepatic disease; clinically significant hypotension; patients <12 years of age.

Warnings:

Following administration, orthostatic hypotension, sedation, fainting or dizziness may occur. Avoid or carefully supervise ambulation for at least 6 hours following the initial dose. Once this effect is tolerated, it will usually be maintained unless more than several days elapse between subsequent doses. Therapy with vasopressors has been required very rarely. Phenylephrine and methoxamine are suitable vasopressors; however, do not use epinephrine since a paradoxical decrease in blood pressure may result. Reserve norepinephrine for hypotension not reversed by other vasopressors.

Elderly: Elderly and debilitated patients with heart disease are more sensitive to phenothiazine effects. Therefore, give a low initial dose and individualize dosage thereafter. Monitor pulse, blood pressure and general circulatory status until dosage requirements and response are stabilized.

Pregnancy: Use with caution in women of childbearing potential and during early pregnancy. There is no evidence of adverse developmental effects when administered during late pregnancy and labor.

Children: Do not use in children < 12 years of age.

Precautions:

Prolonged administration for > 30 days is usually unnecessary, and is only advised when narcotic drugs are contraindicated or in terminal illnesses. When long-term use is anticipated, perform periodic blood counts and liver function studies.

Drug Interactions:

Drugs that may interact with methotrimeprazine include: CNS depressants; atropine; scopolamine; succinylcholine.

Adverse Reactions:

Adverse reactions may include: Orthostatic hypotension; fainting; syncope; weakness; fall in blood pressure; disorientation; dizziness; excessive sedation; weakness; slurring of speech; abdominal discomfort; nausea; vomiting; difficult urination; uterine inertia; local inflammation; swelling; agranulocytosis; jaundice; chills; dry mouth; nasal congestion; pain at injection site.

Administration and Dosage:

Administer by deep IM injection into a large muscle mass. Rotate injection sites. Do not administer SC, as local irritation may occur. Do not administer IV.

Analgesia (adult): 10 to 20 mg (0.5 to 1 ml) IM every 4 to 6 hours as required (range, 5 to 40 mg [0.5 to 2 ml] at intervals of 1 to 24 hours). A flexible dosage schedule and initial dose of 10 mg are advisable until individual patient response and tolerance have been determined.

Elderly: Initial dose of 5 to 10 mg (0.25 to 0.5 ml). Gradually increase subsequent doses if needed.

Analgesia for acute or intractable pain: Initially, 10 to 20 mg, with adjustment of subsequent doses every 4 to 6 hours for pain relief.

Obstetrical analgesia: During labor, an initial dose of 15 to 20 mg may be repeated or adjusted as needed.

Preanesthetic medication: Administer 2 to 20 mg 45 minutes to 3 hours before surgery. Adose of 10 mg is often satisfactory, and 15 to 20 mg may be used for more sedation. Atropine sulfate or scopolamine HBr may be used concurrently in lower than usual doses.

Postoperative analgesia: In the immediate postoperative period, give an initial dosage of 2.5 to 7.5 mg, since residual effects of anesthetic agents and other medications may be additive. Administer at intervals of 4 to 6 hours as needed. Supervise ambulation.

TRAMADOL HCl

Tablets: 50 mg (*Rx*)	*Ultram* (Ortho-McNeil)

Actions:

Pharmacology: Tramadol is a centrally acting synthetic analgesic compound. Although its mode of action is not completely understood, from animal tests two complementary mechanisms appear applicable: Binding to μ-opioid receptors and inhibition of reuptake of norepinephrine and serotonin.

Onset of analgesia is evident within 1 hour after administration and reaches a peak in ≈ 2 to 3 hours.

Pharmacokinetics:

Absorption – Tramadol is rapidly and almost completely absorbed after oral administration. The mean absolute bioavailability of a 100 mg oral dose is ≈ 75%.

Steady state is achieved after 2 days of a 100 mg four times daily dosing regimen (maximum plasma concentration was 592 ± 177 ng/ml). The plasma half-life of tramadol, following single and multiple dosing, was 6 and 7 hours, respectively.

Distribution – The volume of distribution was 2.6 and 2.9 L/kg in male and female subjects, respectively, following a 100 mg IV dose. Binding to human plasma proteins is ≈ 20% and appears to be independent of concentration up to 10 mcg/ml.

Metabolism – Tramadol is extensively metabolized after oral administration. Approximately 30% of the dose is excreted in the urine as unchanged drug, whereas 60% of the dose is excreted as metabolites.

Excretion – The plasma elimination half-life of tramadol increased from ≈ 6 to 7 hours upon multiple dosing.

Indications:

Pain: Management of moderate to moderately severe pain.

Contraindications:

Hypersensitivity to tramadol; acute intoxication with alcohol, hypnotics, centrally acting analgesics, opioids or psychotropic drugs.

Warnings:

Seizure: Administration of tramadol may enhance the seizure risk in patients taking MAO inhibitors, neuroleptics, other drugs that reduce the seizure threshold, patients with epilepsy or patients otherwise at increased risk for seizure.

Anaphylactoid reactions: Serious and rarely fatal anaphylactoid reactions have been reported in patients receiving tramadol therapy. Other reported reactions include pruritus, hives, bronchospasm and angioedema. Patients with a history of anaphylactoid reactions to codeine and other opioids may be at increased risk and therefore should not receive tramadol.

Concomitant CNS depressants: Use with caution and in reduced dosages when administering to patients receiving CNS depressants such as alcohol, opioids, anesthetic agents, phenothiazines, tranquilizers or sedative hypnotics.

Concomitant MAO inhibitors: Use with great caution in patients taking MAO inhibitors, since tramadol inhibits the uptake of norepinephrine and serotonin.

Pregnancy: Category C.

Lactation: Tramadol is not recommended for obstetrical preoperative medication or for post-delivery analgesia in nursing mothers because its safety in infants and newborns has not been studied.

Children: Not recommended in children because safety and efficacy in patients < 16 years of age have not been established.

Precautions:

Respiratory depression: When large doses of tramadol are administered with anesthetic medications or alcohol, respiratory depression may result. Such cases should be treated as overdoses. Administer cautiously in patients at risk for respiratory depression.

Increased intracranial pressure or head trauma: Use with caution in patients with increased intracranial pressure or head injury. Pupillary changes (miosis) from tramadol may obscure the existence, extent or course of intracranial pathology. Clinicians should also maintain a high index of suspicion for adverse drug reactions when evaluating altered mental status in these patients if they are receiving tramadol.

Acute abdominal conditions: Tramadol may complicate the clinical assessment of patients with acute abdominal conditions.

Opioid dependence: Tramadol is not recommended for patients who are dependent on opioids.

Drug abuse and dependence: Do not use tramadol in opioid-dependent patients. Tramadol has been shown to reinitiate physical dependence in some patients that have been previously dependent on other opoids.

Drug Interactions:

Drugs that may interact with tramadol include carbamazepine, MAO inhibitors and quinidine.

Drug/Food interactions: Food does not affect rate or extent of absorption; tramadol can be administered without regard to meals.

Adverse Reactions:

Adverse reactions occurring in ≥ 3% of patients include dizziness/vertigo; nausea; constipation; headache; somnolence; vomiting; pruritus; CNS stimulation; asthenia; sweating; dyspepsia; dry mouth; diarrhea; malaise; vasodilation; abdominal pain; anorexia; flatulence; rash; visual disturbance; urinary retention/frequency; menopausal symptoms; hypertonia.

Administration and Dosage:

For the treatment of painful conditions, 50 to 100 mg can be administered as needed for relief every 4 to 6 hours, not to exceed 400 mg/day. For moderate pain, 50 mg may be adequate as the initial dose, and for more severe pain, 100 mg is usually more effective as the initial dose.

Elderly: Available data do not suggest that a dosage adjustment is necessary in elderly patients 65 to 75 years of age unless they also have renal or hepatic impairment. For elderly patients > 75 years old, < 300 mg/day in divided doses as above is recommended.

Renal function impairment: In all patients with creatinine clearance < 30 ml/min, it is recommended that the dosing interval be increased to 12 hours, with a maximum daily dose of 200 mg. Since only 7% of an administered dose is removed by hemodialysis, dialysis patients can receive their regular dose on the day of dialysis.

Hepatic function impairment: The recommended dose for patients with cirrhosis is 50 mg every 12 hours.

ACETAMINOPHEN (N-Acetyl-P-Aminophenol, APAP)

ACETAMINOPHEN	
Suppositories: 80, 120, 125, 300, 325 and 650 mg (*otc*)	Various, *Acetaminophen Uniserts* (Upsher-Smith), *Acephen* (G & W Labs) *Neopap* (PolyMedica)
Tablets, chewable: 80 mg (*otc*)	Various, *St. Joseph Aspirin-Free for Children* (Plough), *Tylenol, Children's*, *Tylenol, Junior Strength* (McNeil-CPC)
Capsules: 80, 160 and 500 mg (*otc*)	Various, *Feverall Sprinkle Caps* (Upsher-Smith), *Dapa Extra Strength* (Ferndale)
Granules: 80 mg (*otc*)	*Snaplets-FR Granules* (Baker Cummins)
Caplets: 160 mg (*otc*)	*Junior Strength Panadol* (Sterling Health)
Caplets, extended release: 650 mg (*otc*)	*Tylenol Extended Relief* (McNeil-CPC)
Tablets: 160, 325, 500 and 650 mg (*otc*)	Various, *Tylenol Regular Strength Tablets* (McNeil-CPC), *Aspirin Free Anacin Maximum Strength* (Whitehall)
Elixir: 80, 120, 130, 160 and 325 mg/5 ml (*otc*)	Various, *Ridenol* (RID), *Dolanex* (Lannett), *Oraphen-PD* (Great Southern), *Tylenol, Children's* (McNeil-CPC)
Liquid: 160 mg/5 ml and 500 mg/15 ml (*otc*)	Various, *St. Joseph Aspirin-Free Fever Reducer for Children* (Plough), *Tylenol Extra Strength* (McNeil-CPC)
Solution: 100 mg/ml and 120 mg/2.5 ml (*otc*)	Various, *Tempra Drops* (Mead Johnson Nutritional), *Liquiprin Infants' Drops* (Menley & James)
Suspension: 80 mg/0.8 ml and 160 mg/5 ml (*otc*)	*Tylenol Infants' Drops* (McNeil-CPC), *Tylenol, Children's* (McNeil-CPC)
ACETAMINOPHEN, BUFFERED	
Effervescent Granules: 325 mg w/2.781 g sodium bicarbonate & 2.224 g citric acid/dose measure (*otc*)	*Bromo Seltzer* (Warner-Lambert)

Actions:

Pharmacology: Acetaminophen (APAP) is the principal active metabolite of phenacetin and acetanilid, but has less toxicity in usual recommended dosages.

The site and mechanism of the analgesic effect is unclear. APAP reduces fever by a direct action on the hypothalamic heat-regulating centers, which increases dissipation of body heat (via vasodilatation and sweating). APAP is almost as potent as aspirin in inhibiting prostaglandin synthetase in the CNS, but its peripheral inhibition of prostaglandin synthesis is minimal, which may account for its lack of clinically significant antirheumatic or anti-inflammatory effects.

Generally, antipyretic and analgesic effects of APAP and aspirin are comparable. Aspirin is clearly superior to APAP for pain of inflammatory origin. APAP does not inhibit platelet aggregation, affect prothrombin response or produce GI ulceration.

Pharmacokinetics:

Absorption of acetaminophen is rapid and almost complete from the GI tract. Peak plasma concentrations occur within 0.5 to 2 hours, with slightly faster absorption of liquid preparations. The rate and extent of acetaminophen absorption from suppositories varies.

Distribution Usual analgesic doses produce total serum concentrations of 5 to 20 mcg/ml. Serum protein binding varies from 20% to 50% at toxic concentrations.

Metabolism/Excretion Acetaminophen is extensively metabolized and excreted in urine primarily as inactive glucuronate and sulfate conjugates (94%). Average elimination half-life is 1 to 3 hrs; half-life is slightly prolonged in neonates (2.2 to 5 hrs) and in cirrhotics.

Indications:

An analgesic-antipyretic in the presence of aspirin allergy, hemostatic disturbances (including anticoagulant therapy), bleeding diatheses (eg, hemophilia), upper GI disease (eg, ulcer, gastritis, hiatus hernia) and gouty arthritis; variety of arthritic and rheumatic conditions involving musculoskeletal pain, as well as in other painful disorders; diseases accompanied by discomfort and fever such as the common cold, "flu" and other bacterial or viral infections.

Unlabeled uses: Prophylactic APAP use in children receiving DTP vaccination appears to decrease incidence of fever and injection site pain. A dose immediately following vaccination and every 4 to 6 hrs thereafter for 48 to 72 hrs is suggested.

Contraindications:

Hypersensitivity to acetaminophen.

Warnings:

Do not exceed recommended dosage. Consult physician for use in children < 3 years old, or for oral use longer than 5 days (children), 10 days (adults) or 3 days for fever. Chronic excessive use (> 4 g/day) eventually may lead to transient hepatotoxicity. The kidneys may undergo tubular necrosis; the myocardium may be damaged.

Hepatic function impairment: Hepatotoxicity and severe hepatic failure occurred in chronic alcoholics following therapeutic doses. The hepatotoxicity is believed to be caused by induction of hepatic microsomal enzymes resulting in an increase in toxic metabolites, or by the reduced amount of glutathione responsible for conjugating toxic metabolites. Caution chronic alcoholics to limit acetaminophen intake to ≤ 2 g/day.

Pregnancy: Acetaminophen crosses the placenta. It is routinely used during all stages of pregnancy; when used in therapeutic doses, it appears safe for short-term use.

Lactation: Acetaminophen is excreted in breast milk in low concentrations with reported milk:plasma ratios of 0.91 to 1.42 at 1 and 12 hours, respectively. No adverse effects in nursing infants were reported.

Precautions:

If a sensitivity reaction occurs, discontinue use.

Severe or recurrent pain or high or continued fever may indicate serious illness. If pain persists for more than 5 days, if redness is present or in arthritic and rheumatic conditions affecting children < 12 years old, consult physician immediately.

Drug Interactions:

Drugs that may affect APAP include barbiturates, carbamazepine, hydantoins, isoniazid, rifampin, sulfinpyrazone, ethyl alcohol and activated charcoal.

Drug/Lab test interactions: Acetaminophen may interfere with *Chemstrip bG*, *Dextrostix* and *Visidex II* home blood glucose measurement systems; decreases of > 20% in mean glucose values may be noted. This effect appears to be drug, concentration and system dependent.

Adverse Reactions:

Used as directed, acetaminophen rarely causes severe toxicity or side effects.

Administration and Dosage:

Oral:

Adults – 325-650 mg every 4 to 6 hrs, or 1 g 3-4 times/day. Do not exceed 4 g/day.
Children – May repeat doses 4 or 5 times daily; do not exceed 5 doses in 24 hours.

Acetaminophen Dosage for Children

Age	Dosage (mg)	Age (years)	Dosage (mg)
0-3 months	40	4-5	240
4-11 months	80	6-8	320
1-2 years	120	9-10	400
2-3 years	160	11	480

A 10 mg/kg/dose schedule has also been recommended.

Suppositories:

Adults – 650 mg every 4 to 6 hrs. Give no more than 6 in 24 hours.
Children –
(3 to 11 months): 80 mg every 6 hours.
(1 to 3 years): 80 mg every 4 hours.
(3 to 6 years): 120 to 125 mg every 4 to 6 hours. Give no more than 720 mg in 24 hrs.
(6 to 12 years): 325 mg every 4 to 6 hours. Give no more than 2.6 g in 24 hours.

SALICYLATES

ASPIRIN	
Tablets, chewable: 81 mg (*otc*)	*Bayer Children's Aspirin* (Glenbrook), *St. Joseph Adult Chewable Asprin* (Schering-Plough)
Gum Tablets: 227.5 mg (*otc*)	*Aspergum* (Schering-Plough)
Tablets: 325 and 500 mg (*otc*)	Various, *Genuine Bayer Aspirin Tablets and Caplets* (Glenbrook), *Empirin* (Burroughs Wellcome), *Genprin* (Goldline), *Arthritis Foundation Pain Reliever* (McNeil-CPC), *Maximum Bayer Aspirin Tablets and Caplets* (Glenbrook), *Norwich Extra-Strength* (Procter & Gamble Pharm.)
Tablets, enteric coated: 325 mg (*otc*)	Various, *Ecotrin Tablets and Caplets* (SmithKline Beecham), *Regular Strength Bayer Enteric Coated Caplets* (Sterling Health)
Tablets, enteric coated: 81, 165, 500, 650, 975 mg (*otc*)	Various, *Bayer Low Adult Strength* (SK-Beecham), *½ Halfprin* (Kramer), *Ecotrin Maximum Strength Tablets and Caplets* (SK Beecham), *Extra Strength Bayer Enteric 500 Aspirin* (Sterling Health), *Easprin* (Parke-Davis)
Tablets, timed release: 650 mg (*otc*)	*8-hour Bayer Timed-Release Caplets* (Glenbrook)
Tablets, controlled release: 800 mg (*Rx*)	*ZORprin* (Boots)
Suppositories: 120 mg, 200 mg, 300 mg, 600 mg (*otc*)	Various
ASPIRIN (Acetylsalicylic Acid; ASA), BUFFERED	
Tablets: 325 mg with buffers (*otc*)	Various, *Bayer Buffered Aspirin* (Sterling Health), *Magnaprin* (Rugby), *Regular Strength Ascriptin* (Rhone-Poulenc Rorer), *Bufferin* (Bristol-Myers), *Asprimox* (Invamed), *Adprin-B* (Pfeiffer), *Asprimox Extra Protection for Arthritis Pain* (Bristol-Myers), *Buffex* (Roberts Med.)
Tablets, coated: 500 mg with buffers (*otc*)	*Extra Strength Adprin-B* (Pfeiffer), *Extra Strength Bayer Plus Caplets* (Sterling Health), *Ascriptin Extra Strength* (Rhone-Poulenc Rorer), *Cama Arthritis Pain Reliever* (Sandoz), *Arthritis Pain Formula* (Whitehall)
Tablets, effervescent: 325 and 500 mg with buffers (*otc*)	*Alka-Seltzer with Asprin, Alka-Seltzer Extra Strength with Aspirin* (Miles)
SALSALATE (Salicylsalicyclic Acid)	
Capsules: 500 mg (*Rx*)	*Amigesic* (Amide), *Disalcid* (3M)
Tablets: 500 mg (*Rx*)	Various, *Disalcid* (3M), *Salflex* (Carnrick), *Salsitab* (Upsher-Smith)
Tablets: 750 mg (*Rx*)	Various, *Disalcid* (3M), *Salsitab* (Upsher-Smith), *Salflex* (Carnrick), *Marthritic* (Marnel)
SODIUM SALICYLATE	
Tablets, enteric coated: 325 mg and 650 mg (*otc*)	Various
SODIUM THIOSALICYLATE	
Injection: 50 mg per ml (*Rx*)	Various, *Rexolate* (Hyrex)
CHOLINE SALICYLATE	
Liquid: 870 mg per 5 ml (*otc*)	*Arthropan* (Purdue Frederick)
MAGNESIUM SALICYLATE	
Tablets: 325, 467, 500, 545, 580 and 600 mg (*otc*)	*Original Doan's* (Ciba Consumer), *Backache Maximum Strength Relief* (B-M Squibb), *Extra Strength Doan's* (Ciba Consumer), *Magan* (Adria), *Bayer Select Maximum Strength Backache* (Sterling Health), *Mobidin*, (Ascher)
SALICYLATE COMBINATIONS	
Tablets: 500 mg salicylate (as 293 mg choline salicylate and 362 mg Mg salicylate), 750 mg salicylate (as 440 mg choline salicylate and 544 mg Mg salicylate), 1000 mg salicylate (as 587 mg choline salicylate, 725 mg Mg salicylate) (*Rx*)	*Choline Magnesium Trisalicylate* (Sidmak), *Tricosal* (Invamed), *Trilisate* (Purdue Frederick)
Liquid: 500 mg salicylate (as 293 mg choline salicylate and 362 mg Mg salicylate) per 5 ml (*Rx*)	*Trilisate* (Purdue Frederick)

Warning:

Children and teenagers should not use salicylates for chickenpox or flu symptoms before a doctor is consulted about Reye's syndrome, a rare but serious illness.

Actions:

Pharmacology: Salicylates have analgesic, antipyretic, anti-inflammatory and antirheumatic effects. The pharmacological effects of these agents are qualitatively similar. Salicylates lower elevated body temperature through vasodilation of peripheral vessels, thus enhancing dissipation of excess heat. The anti-inflammatory and analgesic activity may be mediated through inhibition of the prostaglandin synthetase enzyme complex.

Aspirin differs from the other agents in this group in that it more potently inhibits prostaglandin synthesis, has greater anti-inflammatory effects and irreversibly inhibits platelet aggregation.

Irreversible inhibition of platelet aggregation (aspirin) – Single analgesic aspirin doses prolong bleeding time. Acetylation of platelet cyclo-oxygenase prevents synthesis of thromboxane A_2, a prostaglandin derivative, which is a potent vasoconstrictor and inducer of platelet aggregation and platelet release reaction. Aspirin (no other salicylates) inhibits platelet aggregation for the life of the platelet (7–10 days).

Aspirin has shown some success as an antiplatelet agent in patients with thromboembolic disease. Low doses of aspirin inhibit platelet aggregation and may be more effective than higher doses. Larger doses inhibit cyclo oxygenase in arterial walls, interfering with prostacyclin production, a potent vasodilator and inhibitor of platelet aggregation.

Pharmacokinetics:

Absorption/Distribution – Salicylates are rapidly and completely absorbed after oral use. Bioavailability is dependent on the dosage form, presence of food, gastric emptying time, gastric pH, presence of antacids or buffering agents and particle size. Bioavailability of some enteric coated products may be erratic. Food slows the absorption of salicylates. Absorption from rectal suppositories is slower, resulting in lower salicylate levels. Aspirin is partially hydrolyzed to salicylic acid during absorption and is distributed to all body tissues and fluids, including fetal tissues, breast milk and CNS. Highest concentrations are found in plasma, liver, renal cortex, heart and lungs. Protein binding of salicylates is concentration-dependent. At low therapeutic concentrations (100 mcg/ml), about 90% is bound; at higher plasma concentrations (400 mcg/ml), 76% is bound. Signs of salicylism (eg, tinnitus) occur at serum levels > 200 mcg/ml; severe toxic effects may occur at levels > 400 mcg/ml (see Adverse Reactions).

Metabolism/Excretion – Salicylic acid is eliminated by renal excretion and by oxidation and conjugation of metabolites. Aspirin has a half-life of ≈ 15 to 20 min. Salicylic acid has a half-life of 2 to 3 hrs at low doses; at higher doses, it may exceed 20 hrs. In therapeutic anti-inflammatory doses, half-life ranges from 6 to 12 hrs. Plasma salicylate levels increase disproportionately as dosage is increased. Elimination is determined by zero order kinetics. Renal excretion of unchanged drug depends upon urine pH. As urinary pH changes from 5 to 8, renal clearance of free ionized salicylate increases from 2% to 3% of amount excreted to > 80%.

Indications:

Mild to moderate pain; fever; various inflammatory conditions such as rheumatic fever, rheumatoid arthritis and osteoarthritis.

Aspirin, for reducing the risk of recurrent transient ischemic attacks (TIAs) or stroke in men who have had transient ischemia of the brain due to fibrin platelet emboli. It has not been effective in women and is of no benefit for completed strokes.

To reduce the risk of death or nonfatal myocardial infarction (MI) in patients with previous infarction or unstable angina pectoris.

Unlabeled uses: Possible effect of long-term aspirin-like analgesics to prevent cataract formation is being studied. Low-dose aspirin may help prevent toxemia of pregnancy and may be beneficial in pregnant women with inadequate uteroplacental blood flow (eg, systemic lupus erythematosus).

Contraindications:

Hypersensitivity to salicylates or nonsteroidal anti-inflammatory drugs (NSAIDs). Use extreme caution in patients with history of adverse reactions to salicylates. Cross-sensitivity may exist between aspirin and other NSAIDs which inhibit prostaglandin synthesis, and aspirin and tartrazine. Aspirin cross-sensitivity does not appear to occur with sodium salicylate, salicylamide or choline salicylate. Aspirin hypersensitivity is more prevalent in those with asthma, nasal polyposis, chronic urticaria.

In hemophilia, bleeding ulcers and hemorrhagic states.

Magnesium salicylate in advanced chronic renal insufficiency due to Mg^{++} retention.

Warnings:

Otic effects: Discontinue use if dizziness, ringing in ears (tinnitus) or impaired hearing occurs. Tinnitus probably represents blood salicylic acid levels reaching or exceeding the upper limit of the therapeutic range.

Use in surgical patients: Avoid aspirin, if possible, for 1 week prior to surgery because of the possibility of postoperative bleeding.

Hypersensitivity: Aspirin intolerance, manifested by acute bronchospasm, generalized urticaria/angioedema, severe rhinitis or shock occurs in 4% to 19% of asthmatics. Symptoms occur within 3 hours after ingestion. Have epinephrine 1:1000 immediately available.

Foods may contribute to a reaction. Some foods with 6 mg/100 g salicylate include curry powder, paprika, licorice, Benedictine liqueur, prunes, raisins, tea, gherkins. A typical American diet contains 10 to 200 mg/day salicylate.

Hepatic function impairment: Use caution in liver damage, preexisting hypoprothrombinemia and vitamin K deficiency.

Pregnancy: Category D (aspirin); Category C (salsalate, magnesium salicylate). Aspirin may produce adverse maternal effects: Anemia, ante- or postpartum hemorrhage, prolonged gestation and labor. Salicylates readily cross placenta. By inhibiting prostaglandin synthesis, salicylates may cause constriction of ductus arteriosus, and, possibly, other untoward fetal effects. Maternal aspirin use during later stages of pregnancy may cause adverse fetal effects: Low birth weight, increased incidence of intracranial hemorrhage in premature infants, stillbirths, neonatal death. Salicylates may be teratogens. Avoid use during pregnancy, especially in third trimester.

Lactation: Salicylates are excreted in breast milk in low concentrations, producing peak milk levels ranging from 1.1 to 10 mcg/ml.

Children: Safety and efficacy of **magnesium salicylate** or **salsalate** have not been established. Administration of **aspirin** to children (including teenagers) with acute febrile illness has been associated with the development of Reye's syndrome. Dehydrated febrile children appear more prone to salicylate intoxication.

Precautions:

Renal effects: Use with caution in chronic renal insufficiency; aspirin may cause a transient decrease in renal function, and may aggravate chronic kidney diseases (rare).

In patients with renal impairment, take precautions when administering **magnesium salicylate**.

GI effects: Use caution in those intolerant to salicylate because of GI irritation, and in gastric ulcers, peptic ulcer, mild diabetes, gout, erosive gastritis or bleeding tendencies. **Salsalate** and **choline salicylate** may cause less GI irritation than aspirin.

Although fecal blood loss is less with enteric coated aspirin than with uncoated, give enteric coated aspirin with caution to patients with GI distress, ulcer or bleeding problems.

Hematologic effects: Aspirin interferes with hemostasis. Avoid use if patients have severe anemia, history of blood coagulation defects, or take anticoagulants.

Long-term therapy: To avoid potentially toxic concentrations, warn patients on long-term therapy not to take other salicylates (nonprescription analgesics, etc). Periodically monitor plasma salicylic acid concentrations during long-term treatment to aid maintenance of therapeutic levels (100 to 300 mcg/ml).

Salicylism may require dosage adjustment.

Controlled release aspirin, because of its relatively long onset of action, is not recommended for antipyresis or short-term analgesia. Not recommended in children > 12; contraindicated in all children with fever accompanied by dehydration.

Drug Interactions:

Drugs that may affect aspirin include activated charcoal, ammonium chloride, ascorbic acid or methionine, antacids and urinary alkalinizers, carbonic anhydrase inhibitors, corticosteroids and nizatidine. Drugs that may be affected by aspirin include alcohol, ACE inhibitors, anticoagulants (oral), beta-adrenergic blockers, heparin, loop diuretics, methotrexate, nitroglycerin, NSAIDs, probenecid and sulfinpyrazone, spironolactone, sulfonylureas and exogenous insulin and valproic acid.

Drug/Lab test interactions: Salicylates compete with thyroid hormone for binding sites on thyroid binding pre-albumin and possibly thyroid binding globulin resulting in increases in **protein bound iodine (PBI).** Salicylates probably do not interfere with T_3 resin uptake.

Serum uric acid levels are elevated by salicylate levels < 10 mg/dl and decreased by levels > 10 mg/dl.

Salicylates in moderate to large (anti-inflammatory) doses cause false-negative readings for **urine glucose** by the glucose oxidase method and false-positive readings by the copper reduction method.

Salicylates in the urine interfere with **5–HIAA** determinations by fluorescent methods, but not by the nitrosonaphthol colorimetric method.

Salicylates in the urine interact with **urinary ketone** determinations by the ferric chloride (Gerhardt) method producing a reddish color.

Large doses may decrease urinary excretion of **PSP (phenolsulfonphthalein).**

Salicylates in the urine result in falsely elevated **VMA (vanillylmandelic acid)** with most tests, but falsely decrease VMA determinations by the Pisano method.

Adverse Reactions:

GI: Nausea, dyspepsia (5% to 25%), heartburn, epigastric discomfort, anorexia, massive GI bleeding, occult blood loss. Aspirin may potentiate peptic ulcer.

Chronic aspirin use may cause a persistent iron deficiency anemia.

Dermatologic: Hives, rashes, angioedema.

Hematologic: Prolongation of bleeding time, leukopenia, thrombocytopenia, purpura, decreased plasma iron concentration, shortened erythrocyte survival time.

Miscellaneous: Fever, thirst, dimness of vision.

Mild "salicylism" may occur after repeated use of large doses and consists of dizziness, tinnitus, difficulty hearing, nausea, vomiting, diarrhea, mental confusion, CNS depression, headache, sweating, hyperventilation and lassitude. Salicylate serum concentrations correlate with pharmacological actions and adverse effects observed.

Serum Salicylate: Clinical Correlations		
Serum Salicylate Concentration (mcg/ml)	Desired Effects	Adverse Effects/ Intoxication
≈ 100	Antiplatelet Antipyresis Analgesia	GI intolerance and bleeding, hypersensitivity, hemostatic defects
150-300	Anti-inflammatory	Mild salicylism
250-400	Treatment of rheumatic fever	Nausea/vomiting, hyperventilation, salicylism, flushing, sweating, thirst, headache, diarrhea and tachycardia
> 400-500		Respiratory alkalosis, hemorrhage, excitement, confusion, asterixis, pulmonary edema, convulsions, tetany, metabolic acidosis, fever, coma, cardiovascular collapse, renal and respiratory failure

Administration and Dosage:

ASPIRIN (Acetylsalicylic Acid; ASA):

Minor aches and pains – 325 to 650 mg every 4 hours as needed. Some extra strength (500 mg) products suggest 500 mg every 3 hours or 1000 mg every 6 hours.

Arthritis, other rheumatic conditions (eg, osteoarthritis) – 3.2 to 6 g/day in divided doses.

Juvenile rhematoid arthritis: 60 to 110 mg/kg/day in divided doses (every 6 to 8 hours). When starting at lower doses (eg, 60 mg/kg/day), may increase by 20 mg/kg/day after 5 to 7 days, followed by 10 mg/kg/day after another 5 to 7 days.

Maintain a serum salicylate level of 150 to 300 mcg/ml.

Acute rheumatic fever –

Adults: 5 to 8 g/day, initially.

Children: 100 mg/kg/day for 2 weeks, then decreased to 75 mg/kg/day for 4 to 6 weeks.

Therapeutic salicylate level is 150 to 300 mcg/ml.

Transient ischemic attacks in men – 1300 mg/day in divided doses (650 mg 2 times daily, or 325 mg 4 times daily). One study indicated that a dose of 300 mg/day is as effective as the larger dose and may be associated with fewer side effects.

Mycardial infarction prophylaxis – 300 or 325 mg/day. This use applies to solid oral doseforms (buffered and plain) and to buffered aspirin in solution.

Children –

Analgesic/antipyretic dosage: 10 to 15 mg/kg/dose every 4 hours (see table), up to 60 to 80 mg/kg/day.

Recommended Aspirin Dosage in Children					
Age (years)	Weight		Dosage (mg every 4 hours)	No. of 81 mg tablets (every 4 hours)	No. of 325 mg tablets (every 4 hours)
	lbs	kg			
2-3	24-35	10.6-15.9	162	2	½
4-5	36-47	16-21.4	243	3	
6-8	48-59	21.5-26.8	324	4	1
9-10	60-71	26.9-32.3	405	5	
11	72-95	32.4-43.2	486	6	1½
12-14	≥ 96	≥ 43.3	648	8	2

Kawasaki disease (mucocutaneous lymph node syndrome): For acute febrile period, 80 to 180 mg/kg/day; very high doses may be needed to achieve therapeutic levels. After the fever resolves, dosage may be adjusted to 10 mg/kg/day.

ASPIRIN, BUFFERED: The addition of small amounts of antacids may decrease GI irritation and increase the dissolution and absorption rates of these products. Dosing is the same as with unbuffered aspirin.

CHOLINE SALICYLATE: Has fever GI side effects than aspirin.

Adults and children (over 12 years) – 870 mg every 3 to 4 hours; maximum 6 times/day. Rhematoid arthritis patients may start with 5 to 10 ml, up to 4 times/day.

MAGNESIUM SALICYLATE: A sodium free salicylate derivative that may have a low incidence of GI upset. The product labeling and dosage are expressed as magnesium salicylate anhydrous. The possibility of magnesium toxicity exists in persons with renal insufficiency.

Usual dose is 650 mg every 4 hours or 1090 mg, 3 times a day. May increase to 3.6 to 4.8 g/day in 3 or 4 divided doses.

Safety and efficacy for use in children have not been established.

SALSALATE (Salicylsalicylic Acid): After absorption, the drug is partially hydrolyzed into two molecules of salicylic acid. Insoluble in gastric secretions, it is not absorbed until it reaches the small intestine.

Usual adult dose is 300 mg/day given in divided doses.

SODIUM SALICYLATE: Less effective than an equal dose of aspirin in reducing pain or fever. Patients hypersensitive to aspirin may be able to tolerate sodium salicylate. Each gram contains 6.25 mEq sodium.

Usual dose – 325 to 650 mg every 4 hours.

SODIUM THIOSALICYLATE: Intramuscular administration is preferred.

Acute gout – 100 mg every 3 to 4 hours for 2 days, then 100 mg/day until asymptomatic.

Muscular pain, musculoskeletal disturbances – 50 to 100 mg/day or on alternate days.

Rheumatic fever – 100 to 150 mg every 4 to 8 hours for 3 days, then reduce to 100 mg twice daily. Continue until patient is aymptomatic.

DIFLUNISAL

Tablets: 250 mg, 500 mg (*Rx*)	Various, *Dolobid* (Merck)

Actions:

Pharmacology: Diflunisal, a salicylic acid derivative, is a nonsteroidal, peripherally-acting, nonnarcotic analgesic with anti-inflammatory and antipyretic properties. Chemically, it differs from aspirin and is not metabolized to salicylic acid. Its mechanisms are unknown. Diflunisal is a prostaglandin synthetase inhibitor.

Pharmacokinetics:

Absorption/Distribution – Diflunisal is rapidly and completely absorbed following oral administration; peak plasma concentrations occur between 2 to 3 hours, producing significant analgesia within 1 hour and maximum analgesia within 2 to 3 hours. The first dose tends to have a slower onset of pain relief than other drugs achieving comparable peak effects. Time required to achieve steady-state increases with dosage, from 3 to 4 days with 125 mg twice daily to 7 to 9 days with 500 mg twice daily, because of its long half-life and nonlinear pharmacokinetics. An initial loading dose shortens the time to reach steady-state levels; 2 to 3 days of observation are necessary for evaluating changes in treatment regimens if a loading dose is not used. More than 99% is bound to plasma proteins.

Metabolism – Concentration-dependent pharmacokinetics prevail; doubling the dosage more than doubles drug accumulation. The plasma half-life of diflunisal is 8 to 12 hours; it increases in renal impairment. The drug is excreted in the urine as glucuronide conjugates which account for about 90% of the dose. Less than 5% is recovered in the feces.

Indications:

Acute or long-term symptomatic treatment of mild to moderate pain, rheumatoid arthritis and osteoarthritis.

Contraindications:

Hypersensitivity to diflunisal.

Patients in whom acute asthmatic attacks, urticaria or rhinitis are precipitated by aspirin or other nonsteroidal anti-inflammatory drugs.

Warnings:

Peptic ulceration and GI bleeding have been reported. Fatalities occurred rarely. In patients with active GI bleeding or an active peptic ulcer, weigh the benefits of therapy against possible hazards; institute an appropriate ulcer treatment regimen and monitor progress. When administered to patients with a history of GI disease, monitor closely.

Renal function impairment: Since diflunisal is eliminated primarily by the kidneys, monitor patients with significant renal impairment; use a lower daily dosage.

Pregnancy: Category C.

Lactation: Diflunisal is excreted in breast milk in concentrations 2% to 7% of that in plasma. Because of the potential for adverse reactions in nursing infants, discontinue either nursing or the drug.

Children: Use in children below 12 years of age is not recommended. Safety and efficacy in infants and children have not been established.

Precautions:

Platelet function and bleeding time are inhibited by diflunisal at higher doses.

Ophthalmologic effects have been reported with these agents; perform ophthalmologic studies in patients who develop eye complaints during treatment.

Peripheral edema has been observed. Use with caution in patients with compromised cardiac function, hypertension or other conditions predisposing to fluid retention.

Acetylsalicylic acid has been associated with Reye's syndrome. Since diflunisal is a salicylic acid derivative, the possibility of its association with Reye's syndrome cannot be excluded.

Drug Interactions:

Drug interactions with diflusinol include: acetaminophen; anticoagulants, oral; hydrochlorothiazide; indomethacin; sulindac.

Adverse Reactions:

Adverse reactions that occur in ≥ 3% include: Nausea; dyspepsia; GI pain; diarrhea; vomiting; headache; rash; fatigue/tiredness; tinnitus.

Patient Information:

May cause GI upset; may be taken with water, milk or meals.

Do not take aspirin or **acetaminophen** with diflunisal, except on professional advice.

Swallow tablets whole; do not crush or chew.

Administration and Dosage:

Mild to moderate pain: Initially, 1 g, followed by 500 mg every 8 to 12 hours. A lower dosage may be appropriate; for example, 500 mg initially, followed by 250 mg every 8 to 12 hours.

Osteoarthritis/rheumatoid arthritis: 500 mg to 1 g daily in 2 divided doses. Individualize dosage. Do not exceed maintenance doses higher than 1.5 g daily.

NONSTEROIDAL ANTI-INFLAMMATORY AGENTS

Product	Brand (Manufacturer)
FLURBIPROFEN	
Tablets: 50 or 100 mg (*Rx*)	Various, *Ansaid* (Upjohn)
FENOPROFEN	
Capsules: 200 or 300 mg (*Rx*)	Various, *Nalfon Pulvules* (Dista)
Tablets: 600 mg (*Rx*)	Various
NABUMETONE	
Tablets: 500 or 750 mg (*Rx*)	*Relafen* (SK-Beecham)
IBUPROFEN	
Tablets: 100 mg (*Rx*)	*Motrin* (McNeil)
Tablets: 200 mg (*otc*)	Various, *Advil* (Whitehall), *Motrin IB* (Upjohn), *Nuprin* (Bristol-Myers Squibb)
Tablets: 300, 400, 600 or 800 mg (*Rx*)	Various, *Motrin* (McNeil)
Tablets, chewable: 50 or 100 mg (*Rx*)	*Motrin* (McNeil)
Suspension: 100 mg/5 ml (*Rx*)	Various, *Children's Advil* (Wyeth-Ayerst)
Suspension: 100 mg/5 ml (*otc*)	*Children's Motrin* (McNeil-CPC)
Oral drops: 40 mg/ml (*Rx*)	*Children's Motrin* (McNeil)
KETOPROFEN	
Tablets: 12.5 mg (*otc*)	*Orudis KT* (Whitehall-Robins), *Actron* (Bayer)
Capsules: 25, 50 or 75 mg (*Rx*)	Various, *Orudis* (Wyeth-Ayerst)
Capsules, extended release: 100, 150 or 200 mg (*Rx*)	*Oruvail* (Wyeth-Ayerst)
PIROXICAM	
Capsules: 10 or 20 mg (*Rx*)	Various, *Feldene* (Pfizer)
NAPROXEN	
Tablets: 200, 250 or 500 mg (as naproxen sodium) (*otc, Rx*)	Various, *Aleve* (Procter & Gamble), *Anaprox* (Syntex)
Tablets: 250, 375 or 500 mg (*Rx*)	Various, *Naprosyn* (Syntex)
Tablets, delayed release: 375 or 500 mg (*Rx*)	*EC-Naprosyn* (Syntex)
Tablets, controlled release: 375 or 500 mg (as naproxen sodium) (*Rx*)	*Naprelan* (Wyeth-Ayerst)
Suspension: 125 mg/5 ml (*Rx*)	Various, *Naprosyn* (Syntex)
DICLOFENAC	
Tablets: 50 mg (as potassium) (*Rx*)	*Cataflam* (Geigy)
Tablets, delayed release (enteric coated): 25, 50 or 75 mg (as sodium) (*Rx*)	Various, *Voltaren* (Geigy)
Tablets, extended release: 100 mg (*Rx*)	*Voltaren-XR* (Geigy)
INDOMETHACIN	
Capsules: 25 or 50 mg (*Rx*)	Various, *Indocin* (Merck)
Capsules, sustained release: 75 mg (*Rx*)	Various, *Indocin SR* (Merck)
Oral suspension: 25 mg per 5 ml (*Rx*)	Various, *Indocin* (Merck)
Suppositories: 125 mg/5 ml (*Rx*)	*Indocin* (Merck)
SULINDAC	
Tablets: 150 or 200 mg (*Rx*)	Various, *Clinoril* (Merck)
TOLMETIN SODIUM	
Tablets: 200 or 600 mg (*Rx*)	Various, *Tolectin 200 or 600* (McNeil Pharm.)
Capsules: 400 mg (*Rx*)	Various, *Tolectin DS* (McNeil Pharm.)
MECLOFENAMATE SODIUM	
Capsules: 50 or 100 mg (*Rx*)	Various, *Meclomen* (Parke-Davis)
MEFENAMIC ACID	
Capsules: 250 mg (*Rx*)	*Ponstel* (Parke-Davis)
ETODOLAC	
Capsules: 200 or 300 mg (*Rx*)	*Lodine* (Wyeth-Ayerst)
Tablets: 400 mg (*Rx*)	*Lodine* (Wyeth-Ayerst)
KETOROLAC	
Tablets: 10 mg (*Rx*)	*Toradol* (Syntex)
Injection: 15 or 30 mg/ml (*Rx*)	*Toradol* (Syntex)
OXAPROZIN	
Tablets: 600 mg (*Rx*)	*Daypro* (Searle)

Actions:

Pharmacology: Nonsteroidal anti-inflammatory drugs have analgesic and antipyretic activities. Major mechanism is believed to be inhibition of cyclooxygenase activity and prostaglandin synthesis.

Pharmacokinetics:

Pharmacokinetic Parameters/Maximum Dosage Recommendations of NSAIDS

NSAID	Time to peak levels (hrs)[1]	Half-life (hrs)	Analgesic action		Antirheumatic action		Maximum recommended daily dose (mg)
			Onset (hrs)	Duration (hrs)	Onset (days)	Peak (weeks)	
Propionic acids							
Fenoprofen	1 to 2	2 to 3	—	—	2	2 to 3	3200
Flurbiprofen	1.5	5.7	—	—	—	—	300
Ibuprofen	1 to 2	1.8 to 2.5	0.5	4 to 6	within 7	1 to 2	3200
Ketoprofen	0.5 to 2	2 to 4	—	—	—	—	300
Naproxen	2 to 4	12 to 15	1	up to 7	within 14	2 to 4	1500
Naproxen sodium	1 to 2	12 to 13	1	up to 7	within 14	2 to 4	1375
Oxaprozin	3 to 5	42 to 50	—	—	within 7	—	1800 mg
Acetic acids							
Diclofenac sodium	2 to 3	1 to 2	—	—	—	—	200
Etodolac	1 to 2	7.3	0.5	4 to 12	—	—	1200
Indomethacin	1 to 2 SR: 2 to 4	4.5 SR: 4.5 to 6	0.5	4 to 6	within 7	1 to 2	200 SR: 150
Ketorolac	0.5 to 1	2.4 to 8.6	IM: 10 min	IM: up to 6	—	—	IM: 120[2] Oral: 40
Nabumetone[3]	2.5 to 4	22.5 to 30[4]	—	—	—	—	2000
Sulindac	2 to 4	7.8 (16.4)[4]	—	—	within 7	2 to 3	400
Tolmetin	0.5 to 1	1 to 1.5	—	—	within 7	1 to 2	2000
Fenamates (anthranilic acids)							
Meclofenamate	0.5 to 1	2 (3.3)[5]	—	—	few days	2 to 3	400
Mefenamic acid	2 to 4	2 to 4	—	—	—	—	1000
Oxicams							
Piroxicam	3 to 5	30 to 86	1	48 to 72	7 to 12	2 to 3	20

[1] Food decreases the rate of absorption and may delay the time to peak levels.
[2] 150 mg on the first day.
[3] The active metabolite of nabumetone is an acetic acid.
[4] Half-life of active metabolite.
[5] Half-life with multiple doses.

Indications:

NSAIDs: Summary of Indications

Indications (✓ -Labeled X- Unlabeled)	Diclofenac	Etodolac	Fenoprofen	Flurbiprofen	Ibuprofen	Indomehtacin /SR	Ketoprofen	Ketorolac	Meclofenamate	Mefenamic acid	Nabumetone	Naproxin/ Naproxen Sod.	Oxaprozin	Piroxicam	Sulindac	Tolmetin
Rheumatoid arthritis	✓	X	✓	✓	✓	✓	✓		✓		✓	✓	✓	✓	✓	✓
Osteoarthritis	✓	✓	✓	✓	✓	✓	✓		✓		✓	✓	✓	✓	✓	✓
Ankylosing spondylitis	✓	X		X		✓						✓			✓	
Mild to moderate pain	X	✓	✓	X	✓		✓	✓	✓	✓[1]		✓				
Primary dysmenorrhea				X	✓	X	✓			✓		✓		X		
Juvenile rheumatoid arthritis	X		X		X		X					✓/		X	X	✓
Tendinitis		X		X		✓						✓			✓	
Bursitis		X		X		✓						✓			✓	
Acute painful shoulder	X	X		X		✓										
Acute gout		X		X		✓/						✓			✓	
Fever					✓							X				
Sunburn	X		X	X	X	X[2]	X		X	X		X		X	X	X
Migraine																
Abortive (acute attack)				X					X	X		/X				
Prophylactic			X			X/	X					X				
Menstrual			X				X		X	X		X				
Cluster headache						X/										
Polyhydramnios						X/										
Acne vulgaris, resistant					X[3]											
Menorrhagia									X							
Premenstrual syndrome										X		X				
Cystoid macular edema						X[4]										
Closure of persistent patent ductus arteriosus						X[5]										

[1] If therapy will be ≤ 1 week.
[2] Topical indomethacin may prevent and treat sunburn.
[3] With tetracycline.
[4] Topical eye drops 0.5% to 1%.
[5] Indomethacin IV approved for this indication (see Agents for Patent Ductus Arteriosus).

Contraindications:

NSAID hypersensitivity: Because of potential cross-sensitivity to other NSAIDs, do not give these agents to patients in whom aspirin, iodides or other NSAIDs have induced symptoms of asthma, rhinitis, urticaria, nasal polyps, angioedema, bronchospasm and other symptoms of allergic or anaphylactoid reactions.

Fenoprofen or mefenamic acid: Preexisting renal disease.

Mefenamic acid: Active ulceration or chronic inflammation of either the upper or lower GI tract.

Indomethacin suppositories: History of proctitis or recent rectal bleeding.

Ketoprofen: See Warnings.

Warnings:

Ketorolac tromethamine: Ketorolac is indicated for the short-term (up to 5 days) management of moderately severe acute pain that requires analgesia at the opioid level. It is not indicated for minor or chronic painful conditions. Increasing the dose beyond the label recommendations will not provide better efficacy but will result in increasing risk of developing serioud adverse events.

GI effects – Ketorolac can cause peptic ulcers, GI bleeding or perforation.

Renal effects – Ketorolac is contraindicated in patients with advanced renal impairment and in patients at risk for renal failure due to volume depletion.

Risk of bleeding – Ketorolac inhibits platelet function and is therefore contraindicated in patients with suspected or confirmed cerebrovascular bleeding, hemorrhagic diathesis, incomplete hemostasis and those at high risk of bleeding.

Ketorolac is contraindicated as prophylactic analgesia before any major surgery and is contraindicated intra-operatively when hemostasis is critical because of the increased risk of bleeding.

Hypersensitivity – Hypersensitivity reactions, ranging from bronchospasm to anaphylactic shock, have occurred, and appropriate counteractive measures must be available when administering the first dose of ketorolac.

Intrathecal or epidural administration – Ketorolac is contraindicated for intrathecal or epidural administration due to its alcohol content.

Labor, delivery and lactation – Use in labor and delivery and lactation is contraindicated.

Concomitant use with NSAIDs – Ketorolac is contraindicated in patients currently receiving aspirin or other NSAIDs because of the cumulative risk of inducing serious NSAID-related side effects.

Administration and dosage – Ketorolac (oral) is indicated only as continuation therapy to ketorolac IV/IM; the combined duration of use of IV/IM and oral is not to exceed 5 days because of the increased risk of serious adverse events.

Special populations – Adjust dosage for patients ≥ 65 years old, for patients < 50 kg (110 lbs) and for patients with moderately elevated serum creatinine. IV/IM doses are not to exceed 60 mg/day in these patients.

GI effects: Serious GI toxicity such as bleeding, ulceration and perforation can occur at any time, with or without warning symptoms, in patients treated chronically with NSAID therapy.

CNS effects: **Indomethacin** may aggravate depression or other psychiatric disturbances, epilepsy and parkinsonism. Some of these agents may also cause headaches (highest incidence with fenoprofen, indomethacin and ketorolac).

Renal effects: Acute renal insufficiency, interstitial nephritis, hyperkalemia, hyponatremia and renal papillary necrosis may occur.

Hypersensitivity: A potentially fatal apparent hypersensitivity syndrome has occurred with **sulindac**. Severe hypersensitivity reactions with fever, rashes, abdominal pain, headache, nausea, vomiting, signs of liver damage and meningitis have occurred in **ibuprofen** patients, especially those with systemic lupus erythematosus (SLE) or other collagen diseases.

Renal function impairment: NSAID metabolites are eliminated primarily by kidneys; use with caution.

Hepatic function impairment: Naproxen may exhibit an increase in unbound fraction and a reduced clearance of free drug in cirrhotic liver patients, suggesting an increased potential for toxicity in this group; may need to reduce dose.

Elderly: Age appears to increase the possibility of adverse reactions to NSAIDs. The risk of serious ulcer disease is increased; this risk appears to increase with dose.

Pregnancy: *Category B (ketoprofen, naproxen, flurbiprofen, diclofenac). Category C (etodolac, ketorolac, mefenamic acid, nabumetone, oxaprozin, tolmetin).* Some NSAIDs may prolong pregnancy if given before onset of labor. Avoid during pregnancy, especially in the third trimester.

Lactation: Most NSAIDs are excreted in breast milk. In general, do not use in nursing mothers because of effects on infant's cardiovascular system.

Children: **Mefenamic acid** and **meclofenamate** are not recommended in children < 14 years old. **Indomethacin's** is not recommended in children ≤ 14 years old, except in circumstances that warrant the risk. When using in children ≥ 2 years old, closely monitor liver function. Suggested starting dose is 2 mg/kg/day in divided doses. Do not exceed 4 mg/kg/day or 150 to 200 mg/day, whichever is less. **Tolmetin** and **naproxen** are the only agents labeled for juvenile rheumatoid arthritis, although studies are being conducted with other agents. Safety and efficacy of tolmetin in infants < 2 years old are not established. Safety and efficacy of other NSAIDs in children are not established.

Precautions:

Steroid dosage: If reduced or eliminated during therapy, reduce slowly and observe patient closely for evidence of adverse effects, including adrenal insufficiency and exacerbation of symptoms.

Platelet aggregation: NSAIDs can inhibit platelet aggregation; the effect is quantitatively less and of shorter duration than that seen with aspirin. These agents prolong bleeding time (within normal range) in healthy subjects.

Hematologic effects: Decreased hemoglobin or hematocrit levels have rarely required discontinuation.

Cardiovascular effects: May cause fluid retention and peripheral edema.

Ophthalmologic effects: Effects include blurred or diminished vision, scotomata, changes in color vision, corneal deposits and retinal disturbances, including maculas.

Infection: NSAIDs may mask the usual signs of infection.

Hepatic effects: Borderline liver function test elevations may occur in ≈ 15% of patients and may progress, remain essentially unchanged or become transient with continued therapy.

Pancreatitis: has occurred in patients receiving **sulindac**.

Auditory effects: Perform periodic auditory function tests during chronic **fenoprofen** therapy in patients with impaired hearing.

Dermatologic effects: Promptly discontinue **mefenamic acid** if rash occurs.

Concomitant therapy: Do not use **naproxen sodium** and **naproxen** concomitantly; both drugs circulate as naproxen anion.

Photosensitivity may occur.

Drug Interactions:

Drugs that affect NSAIDs include cimetidine, probenecid, salicylates and DMSO.

Drugs that may be affected by NSAIDs include anticoagulants, ACE inhibitors, beta blockers, cyclosporine, digoxin, dipyridamole, hydantoins, lithium, loop diuretics, methotrexate, penicillamine, sympathomimetics and thiazide diuretics.

Drug/Lab test interactions: Naproxen use may result in increased urinary values for 17-ketogenic steroids. Although 17-hydroxycorticosteroid measurements (Porter-Silber test) do not appear to be artificially altered, temporarily discontinue naproxen therapy 72 hours before **adrenal function tests** are performed.

Naproxen may interfere with some urinary assays of 5-hydroxy indoleacetic acid.

Tolmetin metabolites in urine give positive tests for **proteinuria** using acid precipitation tests (eg, sulfosalicylic acid).

Mefenamic acid – A false-positive reaction for urinary bile, using the **diazo tablet test,** may result.

Fenoprofen – Amerlex-M kit assay values of total and free triiodothyronine in patients on fenoprofen have been reported as falsely elevated.

Drug/Food interactions: Administration of **tolmetin** with milk decreased total tolmetin bioavailability by 16%. When tolmetin was taken immediately after a meal, peak plasma concentrations were reduced by 50%, while total bioavailability was again decreased by 16%. Peak concentration of **etodolac** is reduced by ≈ ½ and the time to peak is increased by 1.4 to 3.8 hours following administration with food; however, the extent of absorption is not affected. Food may reduce the rate of absorption of **oxaprozin,** but the extent is unchanged.

Adverse Reactions:

GI:

Common NSAID GI Adverse Reactions (%)																
GI adverse reactions	Diclofenac	Etodolac	Fenoprofen	Flurbiprofen	Ibuprofen	Indomethacin	Ketoprofen	Ketorolac	Meclofenamate	Mefenamic acid	Nabumetone	Naproxen	Oxaproxen	Piroxicam	Sulindac	Tolmetin
Nausea (with or without vomiting)	3-9	3-9	3-9	3-9	3-9	3-9	> 3	12	11	†	3-9	3-9	3-9	3-9	3-9	11
Vomiting	< 1	1-3	3-9	1-3			> 1	< 3			1-3	< 1	< 3	< 1		3-9
Diarrhea	3-9	3-9		3-9	< 3	< 3	> 3	3-9	10-33	5	14	< 3	3-9	1-3	3-9	3-9
Constipation	3-9	1-3	3-9	1-3	< 3	< 3	> 3	< 3	1-3	†	3-9	3-9	3-9	1-3	3-9	< 3
Abdominal distress/ cramps/pain	3-9	3-9	< 3	3-9	< 3	< 3	> 3	13	3-9	†	12	3-9	< 3	1-3	10	3-9
Dyspepsia	3-9	10	3-9	3-9	3-9	3-9	11.5	12			13	3-9	3-9	3-9	3-9	3-9
Flatulence	1-3	3-9	< 3	1-3	< 3	< 1	> 3	< 3	3-9	†	3-9		< 3	1-3	1-3	3-9
Anorexia		< 1	< 3			< 1	> 1		1-3	†	< 1		< 3	< 3	1-3	1-3
Stomatitis	< 1	< 1		< 1		< 1	> 1	< 3	1-3		1-3	< 3	< 1	1-3	< 1	< 1

† Occurs, no incidence reported.

CNS: Dizziness (3% to 9%; **flurbiprofen** and **diclofenac** 1% to 3%); headache; **ketorolac** 17%; **fenoprofen** 15%; **indomethacin** 11%; **diclofenac, flurbiprofen, meclofenamate, nabumetone, naproxen** and **tolmetin** 3% to 9%; **ketoprofen** > 3%); somnolence/drowsiness (**fenoprofen** 15%; **naproxen** 3% to 9%; **oxaprozin** < 3%).

Cardiovascular: Congestive heart failure; hypotension; hypertension; palpitations; arrhythmias; tachycardia; vasodilation; peripheral edema and fluid retention.

Renal: Hematuria; cystitis; azotemia; nocturia; proteinuria; polyuria; dysuria; urinary frequency; pyuria; oliguria; anuria.

Hematologic: Neutropenia; eosinophilia; leukopenia; pancytopenia; thrombocytopenia; agranulocytosis; granulocytopenia; aplastic anemia; hemolytic anemia; epistaxis; menorrhagia; hemorrhage; bruising.

Special senses: Blurred vision; photophobia; amblyopia; swollen, dry or irritated eyes; conjunctivitis; iritis; reversible loss of color vision; hearing disturbances or loss; ear pain; change in taste (metallic or bitter); diplopia; tinnitus.

Respiratory: Dyspnea; pharyngitis; bronchospasm; rhinitis; shortness of breath.

Dermatologic: Rash/dermatitis, including maculopapular type (3% to 9%; **ibuprofen, sulindac** and **meclofenamate**); erythema; urticaria; desquamation; angioneurotic edema; ecchymosis; petechiae; purpura; alopecia; pruritus; eczema; skin discoloration; hyperpigmentation; skin irritation; peeling.

Metabolic: Decreased or increased appetite; weight decrease or increase (3% to 9% with **tolmetin**); glycosuria; hyperglycemia; hypoglycemia; hyperkalemia; hyponatremia; flushing or sweating.

Miscellaneous: Thirst; pyrexia (fever and chills); sweating; breast changes; gynecomastia; muscle cramps; facial edema; menstrual disorders; impotence; vaginal bleeding.

Administration and Dosage:

FLURBIPROFEN:

Rheumatoid arthritis and osteoarthritis – Initial recommended total daily dose is 200 to 300 mg; administer in divided doses 2, 3 or 4 times daily. The largest recommended single dose in a multiple-dose daily regimen is 100 mg. Doses > 300 mg per day are not recommended.

FENOPROFEN: Do not exceed 3.2 g/day. If GI upset occurs, take with meals or milk.

Rheumatoid arthritis and osteoarthritis – 300 to 600 mg 3 or 4 times daily.

Mild to moderate pain – 200 mg every 4 to 6 hours, as needed.

NABUMETONE: Recommended starting dose is 1000 mg as a single dose with or without food. Some patients may obtain more symptomatic relief from 1500 to 2000 mg/day. Nabumetone can be given either once or twice daily. Dosages > 2000 mg/day have not been studied.

IBUPROFEN:

Adults – Do not exceed 3.2 g/day. If GI upset occurs, take with meals or milk.

Rheumatoid arthritis and osteoarthritis: 1.2 to 3.2 g/day (300 mg 4 times daily or 400, 600 or 800 mg 3 or 4 times daily).

Mild to moderate pain: 400 mg every 4 to 6 hours, as necessary.

Primary dysmenorrhea: 400 mg every 4 hours, as necessary.

OTC use (minor aches and pains, dysmenorrhea, fever reduction): 200 mg every 4 to 6 hours while symptoms persist. If pain or fever do not respond to 200 mg, 400 mg may be used. Do not exceed 1.2 g in 24 hours. Do not take for pain for > 10 days or for fever for > 3 days, unless directed.

Children –

Juvenile arthritis: Usual dose is 30 to 70 mg/kg/day in 3 or 4 divided doses; 20 mg/kg/day may be adequate for milder disease.

Fever reduction in children 6 months to 12 years old: Adjust dosage on the basis of the initial temperature level. If baseline temperature is ≤ 39.2°C (102.5°F), recommended dose is 5 mg/kg; if baseline temperature is > 39.2°C (102.5°F), recommended dose is 10 mg/kg. Duration of fever reduction is longer with the higher dose. Maximum daily dosage is 40 mg/kg.

KETOPROFEN: Take with antacids, food or milk to minimize adverse GI effects.

Rheumatoid arthritis and osteoarthritis – Do not exceed 300 mg/day.

Daily dose: 150 to 300 mg divided into 3 or 4 doses.

Starting dose: 75 mg 3 times daily or 50 mg 4 times daily. Reduce initial dose to ½ to ⅓ in elderly or debilitated patients or those with impaired renal function.

Mild to moderate pain, primary dysmenorrhea – 25 to 50 mg every 6 to 8 hours as needed. Give smaller dosages initially to smaller patients, the elderly and those with renal or liver disease. Doses > 50 mg may be given, but doses > 75 mg do not display added therapeutic effects. Do not exceed 300 mg/day.

OTC –

Adults: 12.5 mg with a full glass of liquid every 4 to 6 hours. If pain or fever persists after 1 hour, follow with 12.5 mg. With experience, some patients may find an initial dose of 25 mg will give better relief. Do not exceed 25 mg in a 4 to 6 hour period or 75 mg in a 24 hour period.

Children: Do not give to those < 16 years of age unless directed by a physician.

PIROXICAM: Initiate and maintain at a single daily dose of 20 mg. May divide daily dose.

Children – Use in children has not been established.

NAPROXEN:

Rx – Do not exceed 1.25 g naproxen (1.375 g naproxen sodium) per day.

Rheumatoid srthritis, osteoarthritis, ankylosing spondylitis, pain, dysmenorrhea, acute tendinitis and bursitis:

Naproxen – 250 to 500 mg twice/day. May increase to 1.5 g/day for limited periods.

Delayed release naproxen (EC-Naprosyn) – 375 to 500 mg twice/day. Do not break, crush or chew tablets.

Controlled release (Naprelan) – 750 mg or 1000 mg once daily. Do not exceed 1000 mg/day.

Naproxen Sodium – 275 to 550 mg twice daily. May increase to 1.65 g for limited periods.

Juvenile arthritis:

Naproxen – Total daily dose is ≈ 10 mg/kg in 2 divided doses.

Suspension: Use the following as a guide:

Naproxen Suspension: Children's Dose	
Child's weight	Dose
13 kg (29 lb)	2.5 ml (0.5 tsp) bid
25 kg (55 lb)	5 ml (1 tsp) bid
38 kg (84 lb)	7.5 ml (1.5 tsp) bid

Acute gout:

Naproxen – 750 mg, followed by 250 mg every 8 hours until the attack subsides.

Naproxen sodium – 825 mg, then 275 mg every 8 hours until attack subsides.

Controlled release (Naprelan) – 1000 mg to 1500 mg once daily on the first day followed by 1000 mg once daily until the attack has subsided.

Mild to moderate pain; primary dysmenorrhea; acute tendinitis and bursitis:

Naproxen – 500 mg, followed by 250 mg every 6 to 8 hours. Do not exceed a 1.25 g total daily dose.

Naproxen sodium – 550 mg, followed by 275 mg every 6 to 8 hours. Do not exceed a 1.375 g total daily dose.

Controlled release (Naprelan) – 1000 mg once daily. For patients requiring greater analgesic benefit, 1500 mg/day may be used for a limited period.

Children: Safety and efficacy in children < 2 years of age have not been established.

OTC –

Adults: 200 mg with a full glass of liquid every 8 to 12 hours while symptoms persist. With experience, some patients may find that an initial dose of 400 mg followed by 200 mg 12 hours later, if necessary, will give better relief. Do not exceed 600 mg in 24 hours unless otherwise directed.

Elderly (> 65 years of age): Do not take > 200 mg every 12 hours.

Children: Do not give to children < 12 years of age except under the advice and supervision of a physician.

DICLOFENAC:

Osteoarthritis – 100 to 150 mg/day in divided doses (50 mg twice daily or 3 times daily [diclofenac sodium or potassium] or 75 mg twice daily [diclofenac sodium]). Dosages > 150 mg/day have not been studied.

Rheumatoid arthritis – 150 to 200 mg/day in divided doses (50 mg 3 or 4 times daily [diclofenac sodium or potassium] or 75 mg twice daily [diclofenac sodium]). Dosages > 225 mg/day are not recommended.

Ankylosing spondylitis – 100 to 125 mg/day as 25 mg 4 times/day, with an extra 25 mg dose at bedtime, if necessary. Dosages > 125 mg/day have not been studied.

Analgesia and primary dysmenorrhea (diclofenac potassium only) – Recommended starting dose is 50 mg 3 times daily. In some patients, an initial dose of 100 mg followed by 50 mg doses will provide better relief. After the first day, when the maximum recommended dose may be 200 mg, the total daily dose should generally not exceed 150 mg.

INDOMETHACIN:

Moderate to severe rheumatoid arthritis (including acute flares of chronic disease), ankylosing spondylitis and osteoarthritis – 25 mg 2 or 3 times daily. If this is well tolerated, increase the daily dose by 25 or 50 mg (if required by continuing symptoms) at weekly intervals until a satisfactory response is obtained or until a daily dose of 150 to 200 mg is reached. Doses above this amount generally do not increase the effectiveness of the drug.

In patients who have persistent night pain or morning stiffness, giving a large portion, up to a maximum of 100 mg of the total daily dose at bedtime, may help to relieve pain. The total daily dose should not exceed 200 mg.

In acute flares of chronic rheumatoid arthritis, it may be necessary to increase the dosage by 25 or 50 mg daily.

Acute painful shoulder (bursitis or tendinitis) – 75 to 150 mg daily in 3 or 4 divided doses. Discontinue the drug after inflammation has been controlled for several days. Usual course of therapy is 7 to 14 days.

Acute gouty arthritis – 50 mg 3 times daily until pain is tolerable, then rapidly reduce the dose to complete cessation of the drug. Definite relief of pain usually occurs within 2 to 4 hours. Tenderness and heat usually subside in 24 to 36 hours, and swelling gradually disappears in 3 to 5 days. Do not use sustained release form.

Sustained release form – Do not crush. The 75 mg sustained release capsule can be taken once a day as an alternative to the 25 mg capsule 3 times daily. In addition, one 75 mg sustained release capsule twice daily can be substituted for the 50 mg capsule 3 times daily. Do not use sustained release form in acute gouty arthritis.

Children – Efficacy in children ≤ 14 years of age has not been established.

SULINDAC: Administer twice a day with food. The usual maximum dosage is 400 mg/day. Dosages above 400 mg/day are not recommended.

Osteoarthritis, rheumatoid arthritis and ankylosing spondylitis – Initial dosage is 150 mg twice a day.

Acute painful shoulder (acute subacromial bursitis/supraspinatus tendinitis); acute gouty arthritis – 200 mg twice/day. After satisfactory response, reduce dosage accordingly.

Children – Safety and efficacy have not been established.

TOLMETIN SODIUM:

Adults –

Rheumatoid arthritis and osteoarthritis: Initially, 400 mg 3 times/day; preferably include dose on arising and at bedtime. Control is usually achieved at doses of 600 to 1800 mg/day generally in 3 divided doses. Doses > 1800 mg/day are not recommended.

Children –

(≥ 2 years): Initially, 20 mg/kg/day in 3 or 4 divided doses. When control is achieved, usual dosage ranges from 15 to 30 mg/kg/day. Doses > 30 mg/kg/day are not recommended.

MECLOFENAMATE SODIUM:

Mild to moderate pain – 50 mg every 4 to 6 hours. Doses of 100 mg may be required for optimal pain relief. Do not exceed daily dosage of 400 mg.

Excessive menstrual blood loss and primary dysmenorrhea – 100 mg 3 times daily for up to 6 days, starting at the onset of menstrual flow.

Rheumatoid arthritis and osteoarthritis –

Usual dosage: 200 to 400 mg per day in 3 or 4 equal doses.

Initial dosage: Initiate at lower dosage; increase as needed to improve response. Do not exceed 400 mg/day.

Children – Safety and efficacy in children < 14 years of age are not established.

MEFENAMIC ACID:

Acute pain –

Adults (≥ 14 yrs): 500 mg, then 250 mg every 6 hours, as needed, usually not to exceed 1 week. Give with food.

Primary dysmenorrhea – 500 mg, then 250 mg every 6 hours. Start with the onset of bleeding and associated symptoms. Should not be necessary for > 2 to 3 days.

Children – Safety and efficacy in children < 14 years have not been established.

ETODOLAC:

Osteoarthritis – Initially 800 to 1200 mg/day in divided doses, followed by adjustment in the range of 600 to 1200 mg/day in divided doses (400 mg 2 or 3 times/day; 300 mg 2, 3 or 4 times/day; 200 mg 3 or 4 times/day). Do not exceed 1200 mg/day.

Patients ≤ 60 kg: Do not exceed 20 mg/kg.

Analgesia –

Acute pain: 200 to 400 mg every 6 to 8 hrs. Do not exceed 1200 mg/day.

Patients ≤60 kg: Do not exceed 20 mg/kg.

KETOROLAC TROMETHAMINE: The combined duration of ketorolac IV/IM and oral is not to exceed 5 days. Oral use is only indicated as combination therapy to IV/IM.

IV/IM – When administering IV/IM, the IV bolus must be given over no less than 15 seconds. Give IM administration slowly and deeply into the muscle.

Single-dose treatment: Limit the following regimen to single administration use only

IM dosing –

< 65 years old: One 60 mg dose.

≥ 65 years old, renal impairment or < 50 kg (110 lbs): One 30 mg dose.

IV dosing –

< 65 years old: One 30 mg dose.

≥ 65 years old, renal impairment or < 50 kg (110 lbs): One 15 mg dose.

Multiple-dose treatment:

< 65 years old – The recommended dose is 30 mg every 6 hours. The maximum daily dose should not exceed 120 mg.

≥ 65 years old, renal impairment or < 50 kg (110 lbs) – The recommended dose is 15 mg every 6 hours. The maximum daily dose for these populations should not exceed 60 mg.

Oral – Indicated only as continuation therapy to ketorolac IV/IM.

Transition from IV/IM to oral:

< 65 years old – 20 mg as a first oral dose for patients who received 60 mg IM single dose, 30 mg single IV dose or 30 mg multiple dose IV/IM followed by 10 mg every 4 to 6 hours, not to exceed 40 mg/24 hours.

≥ 65 years old, renal impairment or < 50 kg (110 lbs) – 10 mg as a first oral dose for patients who received a 30 mg IM single dose, 15 mg IV single dose or 15 mg multiple dose IV/IM followed by 10 mg every 4 to 6 hours, not to exceed 40 mg/24 hours.

OXAPROZIN:

Rheumatoid arthritis – 1200 mg once a day.

Osteoarthritis – 1200 mg once a day. For patients of low body weight or with milder disease, an initial dosage of 600 mg once a day may be appropriate.

Maximum dose – 1800 mg/day (or 26 mg/kg, whichever is lower) in divided doses.

AGENTS FOR GOUT

In addition to the agents in this section, sulindac and indomethacin (see Nonsteroidal Anti-inflammatory Agents monograph) and phenylbutazone and oxyphenbutazone (see individual monographs) are indicated for the treatment of gout.

PROBENECID

Tablets: 0.5 g (*Rx*)	Various, *Benemid* (Merck), *Probalan* (Lannett)

Actions:

Pharmacology: A uricosuric and renal tubular blocking agent, probenecid inhibits the tubular reabsorption of urate, thus increasing the urinary excretion of uric acid and decreasing serum uric acid levels. Effective uricosuria reduces the miscible urate pool, retards urate deposition and promotes resorption of urate deposits.

Probenecid also inhibits the tubular secretion of most penicillins and cephalosporins and usually increases plasma levels by any route the antibiotic is given. A 2– to 4–fold plasma elevation has been demonstrated.

Pharmacokinetics: Probenecid is well absorbed after oral administration and produces peak plasma concentrations in 2 to 4 hours. It is highly protein bound (85% to 95%) to plasma albumin. The half-life is dose-dependent and varies from < 5 to > 8 hours. Probenecid is hydroxylated to active metabolites and is excreted in the urine primarily as metabolites.

Indications:

Hyperuricemia: Treatment of hyperuricemia associated with gout and gouty arthritis.

Plasma levels: Adjuvant to therapy with penicillins or cephalosporins, for elevation and prolongation of plasma levels of the antibiotic.

Contraindications:

Hypersensitivity to probenecid; children < 2 years of age; blood dyscrasias or uric acid kidney stones. Do not start therapy until an acute gouty attack has subsided.

Warnings:

Exacerbation of gout following therapy with probenecid may occur; in such cases, colchicine or other appropriate therapy is advisable.

Salicylates: Use of salicylates is contraindicated in patients on probenecid therapy. Salicylates antagonize probenecid's uricosuric action.

Sulfa drug allergy: Probenecid is a sulfonamide; patients with a history of allergy to sulfa drugs may react to probenecid. Use with caution.

Hypersensitivity: Rarely, severe allergic reactions and anaphylaxis have occurred. Most of these occur within several hours after readministration following prior use of the drug. The appearance of hypersensitivity reactions requires cessation of therapy. Refer to Management of Acute Hypersensitivity Reactions.

Renal function impairment: Dosage requirements may be increased in renal impairment. Probenecid may not be effective in chronic renal insufficiency, particularly when the glomerular filtration rate is ≤ 30 ml/minute. Probenecid is not recommended in conjunction with a penicillin in the presence of known renal impairment.

Pregnancy: Category B.

Children: Do not use in children < 2 years of age.

Precautions:

Alkalinization of urine: Hematuria, renal colic, costovertebral pain and formation of urate stones associated with use in gouty patients may be prevented by alkalization of urine and liberal fluid intake; monitor acid-base balance.

Peptic ulcer history: Use with caution.

Drug Interactions:

Drugs that may affect probenecid include: Salicylates.

Drugs that may be affected by probenecid include: Acyclovir; allopurinol; barbiturates; benzodiazepines; clofibrate; dapsone; dyphylline; methotrexate; NSAIDs; pantothenic acid; penicillamine; rifampin; sulfonamides; sulfonylureas; zidovudine; salicylates.

Drug/Lab test interactions: A reducing substance may appear in the urine during therapy. Although this disappears with discontinuation, a false diagnosis of glycosuria may be made. Confirm suspected glycosuria by using a test specific for glucose.

Falsely high determination of **theophylline** has occurred in vitro using the Schack and Waxler technique, when therapeutic concentrations of theophylline and probenecid were added to human plasma.

Probenecid may inhibit the renal excretion of: **Phenolsulfonphthalein (PSP), 17–ketosteroids** and **sulfobromophthalein (BSP).**

Adverse Reactions:

Adverse reactions may include: Headache; anorexia; nausea; vomiting; urinary frequency; hypersensitivity reactions; sore gums; flushing; dizziness; anemia; hemolytic anemia (possibly related to G-6-PD deficiency); nephrotic syndrome; hepatic necrosis; aplastic anemia; exacerbation of gout; uric acid stones with or without hematuria; renal colic or costovertebral pain.

Administration and Dosage:

Gout: Do not start therapy until an acute gouty attack has subsided. However, if an acute attack is precipitated during therapy, probenecid may be continued. Give full therapeutic doses of colchicine or other appropriate therapy to control the acute attack.

Adults – 0.25 g twice daily for 1 week, followed by 0.5 g twice daily thereafter. Gastric intolerance may indicate overdosage, and may be reduced by decreasing dosage.

Renal impairment – Some degree of renal impairment may be present in patients with gout. A daily dosage of 1 g may be adequate. However, if necessary, the daily dosage may be increased by 0.5 g increments every 4 weeks within tolerance (usually not > 2 g/day) if symptoms of gouty arthritis are not controlled or the 24 hour urate excretion is not > 700 mg. Probenecid may not be effective in chronic renal insufficiency, particularly when the glomerular filtration rate is ≤ 30 ml/minute.

Urinary alkalinization – Urates tend to crystallize out of an acid urine; therefore, a liberal fluid intake is recommended, as well as sufficient sodium bicarbonate (3 to 7.5 g/day) or potassium citrate (7.5 g/day) to maintain an alkaline urine; continue alkalization until the serum uric acid level returns to normal limits and tophaceous deposits disappear. Thereafter, urinary alkalization and the restriction of purine-producing foods may be relaxed.

Maintenance therapy – Continue the dosage that maintains normal serum uric acid levels. When there have been no acute attacks for ≥ 6 months and serum uric acid levels have remained within normal limits, decrease the daily dosage by 0.5 g every 6 months. Do not reduce the maintenance dosage to the point where serum uric acid levels increase.

Penicillin or cephalosporin therapy: The PSP excretion test may be used to determine the effectiveness of probenecid in retarding penicillin excretion and maintaining therapeutic levels. The renal clearance of PSP is reduced to about the normal rate when dosage of probenecid is adequate.

Adults – 2 g/day in divided doses. Reduce dosage in older patients in whom renal impairment may be present. Not recommended in conjunction with penicillin or a cephalosporin in the presence of known renal impairment.

Children (2 to 14 yrs) – Initial dose 25 mg/kg or 0.7 g/m^2. Maintenance dose 40 mg/kg/day or 1.2 g/m^2, divided into 4 doses. For children weighing > 50 kg (110 lb), use the adult dosage. Do not use in children < 2 years of age.

Gonorrhea (uncomplicated) – Give probenecid as a single 1g dose immediately before or with 4.8 million units penicillin G procaine, aqueous, divided into at least two doses.

Neurosyphilis – Aqueous procaine penicillin G, 2 to 4 million units/day IM plus probenecid 500 mg 4 times daily, both for 10 to 14 days†.

Pelvic inflammatory disease (PID) – Cefoxitin 2 g IM plus probenecid, 1 g orally in a single dose concurrently.

ALLOPURINOL

Tablets: 100 and 300 mg *Rx*	Various, *Zyloprim* (Burroughs Wellcome)

Actions:

Pharmacology: Allopurinol inhibits xanthine oxidase, the enzyme responsible for the conversion of hypoxanthine to xanthine to uric acid. Allopurinol is metabolized to oxipurinol (alloxanthine), which is also an inhibitor of xanthine oxidase. Allopurinol acts on purine catabolism, reducing the production of uric acid, without disrupting the biosynthesis of vital purines.

Administration generally results in a fall in both serum and urinary uric acid within 2 to 3 days. The magnitude of this decrease is dose-dependent. One week or more of treatment may be required before the full effects of the drug are manifested; likewise, uric acid may return to pretreatment levels slowly following cessation of therapy.

Pharmacokinetics: Allopurinol is approximately 90% absorbed from the GI tract. Peak plasma levels occur at 1.5 hours and 4.5 hours for allopurinol and oxipurinol, respectively. Allopurinol has a plasma half-life of about 1 to 2 hours.

Oxipurinol, however, has a plasma half-life of approximately 15 hours. Therefore, effective xanthine oxidase inhibition is maintained over 24 hours with single daily doses. Allopurinol is cleared essentially by glomerular filtration; oxipurinol is reabsorbed in the kidney tubules in a manner similar to the reabsorption of uric acid. Approximately 20% is excreted in the feces.

Indications:

Gout: Management of signs and symptoms of primary or secondary gout.

Malignancies: Management of patients with leukemia, lymphoma and malignancies receiving therapy which causes elevations of serum and urinary uric acid. Discontinue allopurinol when the potential for overproduction of uric acid is no longer present.

Calcium oxalate calculi: Management of patients with recurrent calcium oxalate calculi whose daily uric acid excretion exceeds 800 mg/day (males) or 750 mg/day (females). Carefully assess therapy initially and periodically to determine that treatment is beneficial and that the benefits outweigh the risks.

Unlabeled uses: In a limited number of patients, the use of an allopurinol mouthwash (20 mg in 3% methylcellulose; 1 mg/ml) after fluorouracil administration prevented stomatitis, a major dose-limiting toxicity of fluorouracil. However, another report indicated that allopurinol mouthwash is not effective. Further study is needed.

Recent studies suggest a role for allopurinol in the prevention of ischemic reperfusion tissue damage; to reduce the incidence of perioperative mortality and postoperative arrhythmias in coronary artery bypass surgery patients; to reduce relapse rates of *H. pylori-* induced duodenal ulcers and treatment of hematemesis from NSAID-induced erosive gastritis; ex vivo preservation and function of organs for liver and kidney transplantation; and to reduce rejection episodes in adult cadaver renal transplant recipients.

Contraindications:

Patients who have developed a severe reaction should not be restarted on the drug.

Warnings:

Asymptomatic hyperuricemia: Generally, do not use to treat asymptomatic hyperuricemia. Treatment should be considered with persitent hyperuricemia characterized by a serum urate concentration of > 13 mg/dl. High serum urate may be nephrotoxic.

Hepatotoxicity: A few cases of reversible clinical hepatotoxicity have occurred; in some patients, asymptomatic rises in serum alkaline phosphatase or serum transaminase levels have been observed. If anorexia, weight loss or pruritis develop in patients on allopurinol, evaluation of liver function should be part of their diagnostic workup. Perform periodic liver function tests during early stages of therapy, particularly in patients with preexisting liver disease.

Hypersensitivity: Discontinue at first appearance of skin rash or other signs of allergic reactions. In some instances, rash may be followed by more severe hypersensitivity reactions such as exfoliative, urticarial or purpuric lesions, or Stevens-Johnson syndrome, generalized vasculitis, irreversible hepatotoxicity and rarely, death.

Renal function impairment: Some patients with preexisting renal disease or poor urate clearance have increased BUN during allopurinol administration. Although the mechanism has not been established, patients with impaired renal function require less drug and careful observation during the early stages of treatment; reduce dosage or discontinue therapy if increased abnormalities in renal function appear and persist.

Renal failure in association with allopurinol has been observed among patients with hyperuricemia secondary to neoplastic diseases. Concurrent conditions such as multiple myeloma and congestive myocardial disease were present. Renal failure is also frequently associated with gouty nephropathy and rarely with allopurinol-associated hypersensitivity reactions. Albuminuria has occurred among patients who developed clinical gout following chronic glomerulonephritis and chronic pyelonephritis.

In patients with severely impaired renal function or decreased urate clearance, the plasma half-life of oxipurinol is greatly prolonged. A dose of 100 mg/day or 300 mg twice a week, or less, may be sufficient to maintain adequate xanthine oxidase inhibition to reduce serum urate levels.

Pregnancy: Category C.

Lactation: Allopurinol and oxipurinol have been found in the breast milk of a mother who received allopurinol. Exercise caution when administering to a nursing woman.

Children: Allopurinol is rarely indicated for use in children, with the exception of those with hyperuricemia secondary to malignancy or to certain rare inborn errors of purine metabolism.

Precautions:

Monitoring: Periodically determine liver and kidney function especially during the first few months of therapy. Perform BUN, serum creatinine or creatinine clearance and reassess the patient's dosage.

Acute attacks of gout have increased during the early stages of allopurinol administration when normal or subnormal serum uric acid levels have been attained; in general, give maintenance doses of colchicine prophylactically when allopurinol is begun. In addition, start patient at a low dose of allopurinol (100 mg daily) and increase at weekly intervals by 100 mg until a serum uric acid level of ≤ 6 mg/dl is attained without exceeding the maximum recommended dose. The attacks usually become shorter and less severe after several months of therapy.

Fluid intake sufficient to yield a daily urinary output of at least 2 L and the maintenance of a neutral or slightly alkaline urine are desirable to avoid the theoretical possibility of formation of xanthine calculi under the influence of allopurinol therapy and to help prevent renal precipitation of urates in patients receiving concomitant uricosurics.

Drowsiness has occurred occasionally. Patients should observe caution while driving or performing other tasks requiring alertness, coordination or physical dexterity.

Bone marrow depression has occurred in patients receiving allopurinol, most of whom received concomitant drugs with the potential for causing this reaction. This has occurred as early as 6 weeks to as long as 6 years after the initiation of therapy. Rarely, a patient may develop varying degrees of bone marrow depression, affecting one or more cell lines, while receiving allopurinol alone.

Drug Interactions:

Drugs that may affect allopurinol include: ACE inhibitors; aluminum salts; thiazide diuretics; uricosuric agents.

Drugs that may be affected by allopurinol include: Ampicillin; anticoaggulants; cyclophosphamide; theophyllines; thiopurines.

Adverse Reactions:

Adverse reactions may include: Skin rash; fever; chills; arthralgias; cholestatic jaundice; eosinophilia; mild leukocytosis; leukopenia; vesicular bullous dermatitis; eczematoid dermatitis; pruritus; urticaria; onycholysis; lichen planus; Stevens-Johnson syndrome; purpura; toxic epidermal necrolysis; nausea; vomiting; diarrhea; intermittent abdominal pain; gastritis; dyspepsia; increased alkaline phosphatase; AST and ALT; hepatomegaly; cholestatic jaundice; granulomatous hepatitis; hepatic necrosis; leukopenia; leukocytosis; eosinophilia; thrombocytopenia; headache; peripheral neuropathy; neuritis; paresthesia; somnolence; arthralgia; acute attacks of gout; ecchymosis; fever; myopathy; epistaxis; taste loss or perversion; renal failure; uremia; alopecia; hypersensitivity vasculitis; necrotizing angiitis.

Administration and Dosage:

Control of gout and hyperuricemia: The average dose is 200 to 300 mg/day for mild gout and 400 to 600 mg/day for moderately severe tophaceous gout. Divide doses in excess of 300 mg. The minimum effective dose is 100 to 200 mg daily; the maximum recommended dose is 800 mg/day.

Children (6 to 10 years of age) – In secondary hyperuricemia associated with malignancy, give 300 mg daily; those < 6 years old are generally given 150 mg/day. Evaluate response after approximately 48 hours of therapy and adjust dosage if necessary.

Another suggested dose is 1 mg/kg/day divided every 6 hours, to a maximum of 600 mg/day. After 48 hours of treatment, titrate dose according to serum uric acid levels.

Prevention of uric acid nephropathy during vigorous therapy of neoplastic disease: 600 to 800 mg daily for 2 to 3 days together with a high fluid intake. Similar considerations govern dosage regulation for maintenance purposes in secondary hyperuricemia.

To reduce the possibility of flare-up of acute gouty attacks: Start with 100 mg daily and increase at weekly intervals by 100 mg (without exceeding the maximum recommended dosage) until a serum uric acid level of ≤ 6 mg/dl is attained.

Serum uric acid levels: Normal serum urate levels are usually achieved in 1 to 3 weeks. The upper limit of normal is about 7 mg/dl for men and postmenopausal women and 6 mg/dl for premenopausal women. Do not rely on a single reading since estimation of uric acid may be difficult. By selecting the appropriate dose, and using uricosuric agents in certain patients, it is possible to reduce the serum uric acid level to normal and, if desired, to hold it as low as 2 to 3 mg/dl indefinitely.

Renal impairment: Accumulation of allopurinol and its metabolites can occur in renal failure; consequently, reduce the dose. With a creatinine clearance (Ccr) of 10 to 20 ml/min, 200 mg/day is suitable. When the Ccr is < 10 ml/min, do not exceed 100 mg/day. With extreme renal impairment (Ccr < 3 ml/min) the interval between doses may also need to be increased. The correct dosage is best determined by using the serum uric acid level as an index.

Other suggested doses include: Ccr 60 ml/min, 200 mg/day; Ccr 40 ml/min, 15 mg/day; Ccr 20 ml/min, 100 mg/day; Ccr 10 ml/min, 100 mg on alternate days. Ccr < 10 ml/min, 100 mg 3 times a week.

Concomitant therapy: In patients treated with colchicine or anti-inflammatory agents, continue therapy while adjusting the allopurinol dosage until a normal serum uric acid level and freedom from acute attacks have been maintained for several months.

Replacement therapy: In transferring a patient from a uricosuric agent to allopurinol, gradually reduce the dose of the uricosuric agent over several weeks and gradually increase the dose of allopurinol until a normal serum uric acid level is maintained.

Recurrent calcium oxalate stones: For hyperuricosuric patients, 200 to 300 mg/day in single or divided doses. Adjust dose up or down depending upon the resultant control of the hyperuricosuria based upon subsequent 24 hour urinary urate determinations. Patients may also benefit from dietary changes such as reduction of animal protein, sodium, refined sugars, oxalate-rich foods and excessive calcium intake as well as increase in oral fluids and dietary fiber.

COLCHICINE

Tablets: 0.5 mg (1/120 gr), 0.6 mg (1/100 gr)	Various, *Colchicine* (Abbott)
Injection: 1 mg (1/60 gr)	*Colchicine* (Lilly)

Actions:

Pharmacology: The exact mechanism of action of colchicine in gout is not known. It is involved in leukocyte migration inhibition; reduction of lactic acid production by leukocytes which results in a decreased deposition of uric acid; interference with kinin formation; and reduction of phagocytosis with inflammatory response abatement.

Colchicine apparently exerts its effect by reducing the inflammatory response to the deposited crystals and also by diminishing phagocytosis. Colchicine diminishes lactic acid production by leukocytes directly and by diminishing phagocytosis and thereby interrupts the cycle of urate crystal deposition and inflammatory response that sustains the acute attack.

Colchicine can produce a temporary leukopenia, followed by leukocytosis.

Pharmacokinetics: Colchicine is rapidly absorbed after oral administration; peak plasma concentrations occur in 0.5 to 2 hours. Large amounts of drug and metabolites enter the intestinal tract in bile and intestinal secretions. High colchicine concentrations are found in kidney, liver and spleen. It is metabolized in the liver. Excretion occurs primarily by biliary and renal routes; 10% to 20% is eliminated unchanged in urine.

Indications:

Gout: Relieves pain of acute attacks, especially if adequate doses are given early in the attack. Many therapists use colchicine as interval therapy to prevent acute attacks. Recommended for regular prophylactic use between attacks and is often effective in aborting an attack when taken at the first sign of articular discomfort.

Colchicine IV is used when rapid response is desired or GI side effects interfere with oral use. Occasionally, it is effective when the oral preparation is not. After the acute attack has subsided, the patient can usually be given oral colchicine.

Unlabeled uses: Orphan drug designation for arresting the progression of neurologic disability due to chronic progressive multiple sclerosis.

Familial Mediterranean fever; to lessen frequency and severity of acute febrile episodes and to prevent amyloidosis.

Hepatic cirrhosis.

Primary biliary cirrhosis. Further study is needed.

Adjunctive treatment of primary amyloidosis.

Treatment of Behcet's disease.

Pseudogout due to chondrocalcinosis.

Refractory idiopathic thrombocytopenic purpura.

Skin manifestations of scleroderma.

Various dermatologic disorders including: Psoriasis; palmo-plantar pustulosis; dermatitis herpetiformis; pyoderma gangrenosum associated with Crohn's disease.

Contraindications:

Hypersensitivity to colchicine; serious GI, renal, hepatic or cardiac disorders; blood dyscrasias.

Warnings:

Hepatic function impairment: Increased colchicine toxicity may occur. IV colchicine is not recommended in patients with severe renal/hepatic dysfunction.

Fertility impairment: Colchicine arrests cell division in animals and plants. It has adversely affected spermatogenesis in humans and in some animal species.

Elderly: Administer colchicine with great caution to elderly and debilitated patients.

Pregnancy: Category C (Parenteral – Category D).

Lactation: It is not known whether this drug is excreted in breast milk. Exercise caution when administering colchicine to a nursing woman.

Children: Safety and efficacy for use in children have not been established.

Precautions:

Monitoring: Perform periodic blood counts in patients receiving long-term therapy.

GI effects: Vomiting, diarrhea, abdominal pain and nausea may occur, especially with maximum doses. These may be particularly troublesome in the presence of peptic ulcer or spastic colon. At toxic doses, colchicine may cause severe diarrhea, generalized vascular damage and renal damage with hematuria and oliguria. GI symptoms may occur with IV therapy, usually large doses. To avoid more serious toxicity, discontinue use when these symptoms appear, regardless of whether joint pain has been relieved.

Thrombophlebitis rarely occurs at the site of IV injection.

Myopathy and neuropathy: Colchicine myoneuropathy appears to be a common cause of weakness in patients on standard therapy who have elevated plasma levels due to altered renal function. It is often unrecognized and misdiagnosed as polymyositis or uremic neuropathy. Proximal weakness and elevated serum creatine kinase are generally present, and resolve in 3 to 4 weeks following drug withdrawal.

Malabsorption of vitamin B_{12}: Colchicine induces reversible malabsorption of vitamin B_{12}, apparently by altering the function of ileal mucosa.

Drug Interactions:

Drug/Lab test interactions: Decreased **thrombocyte** values may be obtained. Colchicine may cause false-positive results when testing **urine** for **RBC** or **hemoglobin.**

Adverse Reactions:

Adverse reactions may include: Bone marrow depression with aplastic anemia; agranulocytosis or thrombocytopenia (long-term therapy); peripheral neuritis; purpura; myopathy; loss of hair; reversible azoospermia; dermatoses; hypersensitivity; vomiting; diarrhea; abdominal pain; nausea; elevated alkaline phosphatase; AST.

Administration and Dosage:

Oral:

Acute gouty arthritis – Begin at the first warning of an acute attack. Usual initial dose is 1 to 1.2 mg; follow with 0.5 to 1.2mg every 1 to 2 hours, until pain is relieved, or nausea, vomiting or diarrhea occurs. (Opiates may be needed to control diarrhea.) After one or more attacks, a patient can often judge his requirement accurately enough to stop before the"diarrheal dose."

The total amount of colchicine needed to control pain and inflammation during an acute attack is 4 to 8 mg. Articular pain and swelling typically abate within 12 hours and are usually gone in 24 to 48 hours. Wait 3 days before initiating a second course to minimize the possibility of cumulative toxicity.

If ACTH is used to treat a gouty arthritis attack, give colchicine at least 1 mg/day, and continue for a few days after ACTH is withdrawn.

Prophylaxis during intercritical periods – To reduce the frequency and severity of paroxysms, administer continuously. If patients have < 1 attack/year, usual dose is 0.5 or 0.6 mg/day for 3 or 4 days a week; if > 1 attack/year, usual dose is 0.5 or 0.6 mg/day. Severe cases may require 1 to 1.8 mg/day.

Prophylaxis in patients undergoing surgery – In patients with gout, an attack may be precipitated by even a minor surgical procedure. Administer 0.5 or 0.6 mg 3 times daily for 3 days before and 3 days after surgery.

Parenteral: For IV use only. Severe local irritation occurs if given SC or IM. If leakage into surrounding tissue or outside the vein should occur, considerable irritation and possible tissue damage may follow. There is no specific antidote. Local application of heat or cold, as well as use of analgesics, may afford relief.

Administer over 2 to 5 minutes. Do not dilute with 5% Dextrose in Water. If a decrease in concentration of colchicine is required, use 0.9% Sodium Chloride Injection which does not contain a bacteriostatic agent. Do not use turbid solutions.

Treatment of acute gouty arthritis – Average initial dose is 2 mg. This may be followed by 0.5 mg every 6 hours until a satisfactory response is achieved. In general, do not exceed a total dosage of 4 mg for a 24 hour period. Do not exceed total dosage of 4 mg for one course of treatment. Some clinicians recommend a single IV dose of 3 mg, while others recommend ≤ 1 mg IV for the initial dose, followed by 0.5 mg once or twice daily if needed.

If pain recurs, it may be necessary to give 1 to 2 mg/day for several days; however, do not give more colchicine by any route for at least 7 days after a full course of IV therapy (4 mg). Transfer to oral colchicine in a dose similar to that given IV.

Prophylaxis or maintenance of recurrent or chronic gouty arthritis – 0.5 to 1 mg once or twice daily. Oral colchicine is preferable, usually in conjunction with a uricosuric agent.

AGENTS FOR MIGRAINE

In addition to the agents on the following pages, propanolol and timolol are indicated for migraine prophylaxis.

SUMATRIPTAN SUCCINATE

Injection: 12 mg/ml (*Rx*)	*Imitrex* (Glaxo Wellcome)
Tablets: 25 and 50 mg (*Rx*)	

Actions:

Pharmacology: Sumatriptan is a selective agonist for a vascular 5-hydroxytryptamine$_1$ (serotonin) receptor subtype. The vascular 5-HT$_1$ receptor subtype to which sumatriptan binds selectively and through which it presumably exerts its antimigrainous effect is present on the human basilar artery and in vasculature of the isolated human dura mater. In these tissues, sumatriptan activates this receptor to cause vasoconstriction, an action in humans correlating with the relief of migraine.

Pharmacokinetics:

Injection – Following a 6 mg SC injection, distribution half-life was 15 minutes, terminal half-life was 115 minutes, and volume of distribution central compartment was 50 L. Of this dose, 22% was excreted in the urine as unchanged sumatriptan and 38% as the indole acetic acid metabolite. The T_{max} or amount absorbed were not significantly altered by either the site or technique of injection (deltoid vs thigh).

Oral – Sumatriptan is rapidly absorbed after oral administration, with low absolute bioavailability (≈ 15%). The apparent volume of distribution is 2.4 L/kg. Elimination half-life is ≈ 2.5 hours. Sumatriptan is largely renally excreted (≈ 60%) with ≈ 40% found in the feces.

Indications:

Migraine: Acute treatment of migraine attacks with or without aura.

Unlabeled uses: In one study, sumatriptan SC was effective in treating cluster headache in 74% of patients (vs 26% with placebo).

Contraindications:

IV use (because of its potential to cause coronary vasospasm); SC use in patients with ischemic heart disease (angina pectoris, history of myocardial infarction [MI] or documented silent ischemia) or in patients with Prinzmetal's angina; patients with symptoms or signs consistent with ischemic heart disease; patients with uncontrolled hypertension; with concurrent ergotamine-containing preparations; hypersensitivity to sumatriptan; management of hemiplegic or basilar migraine.

Warnings:

Migraine diagnosis: Use oral sumatriptan only where a clear diagnosis of migraine has been established. Do not administer to patients with basilar or hemiplegic migraine.

Cardiac events/Coronary constriction: Serious coronary events following sumatriptan can occur but are extremely rare. If symptoms consistent with angina occur, carry out ECG evaluation to look for ischemic changes.

Sumatriptan may cause coronary vasospasm in patients with a history of CAD, who are known to be more susceptible to coronary artery vasospasm, and, rarely, in patients without history suggestive of CAD.

There have been rare reports of serious or life-threatening arrhythmias. In addition, there have been rare, but more frequent, reports of chest and arm discomfort thought to represent angina pectoris.

Fatalities: Deaths have been reported following the use of sumatriptan. In most cases, these have occurred well after sumatriptan use (ie, ≥ 3 hours postinjection) and probably reflect underlying disease and spontaneous events. Advise patients not to administer sumatriptan if a headache being experienced is atypical.

Hypersensitivity reactions have occurred on rare occasions, and severe anaphylaxis/anaphylactoid reactions have occurred. Such reactions can be life-threatening or fatal.

Renal/Hepatic function impairment: Administer with caution to patients with diseases that may alter the absorption, metabolism or excretion of drugs. The liver plays an important role in the presystemic clearance of orally administered sumatriptan. Accordingly, the bioavailability may be markedly increased in patients with liver disease.

Elderly: Pharmacokinetics in the elderly are similar to those seen in younger adults.

Pregnancy: Category C.

Lactation: Sumatriptan is excreted in breast milk.

Children: Safety and efficacy in children have not been established.

Precautions:

Chest, jaw or neck tightness is relatively common after sumatriptan, and atypical sensations over the precordium (tightness, pressure, heaviness) have occurred, but has only rarely been associated with ischemic ECG changes.

Blood pressure changes: Sumatriptan injection may cause mild, transient elevation of blood pressure and peripheral vascular resistance.

Seizures: There have been rare reports of seizures following sumatriptan use.

Binding to melanin-containing tissues: Because sumatriptan binds to melanin, it could accumulate in melanin-rich tissues (such as the eye) over time, raising the possibility that toxicity in these tissues could occur after extended use.

Corneal opacities: Sumatriptan causes corneal opacities and defects in the dog, raising the possibility that these changes may occur in humans.

Drug Interactions:

Sumatriptan may be affected by MAOIs and ergot-containing drugs.

Adverse Reactions:

Adverse reactions occuring in IV sumatriptan patients includet tingling; warm/hot sensation; burning sensation; feeling of heaviness; pressure sensation; feeling of tightness; numbness; dizziness/vertigo; musculoskeletal weakness; nech pain/stiffness; chest discomfort; throat discomfort; injection site reaction; flushing.

Adverse reactions associated with oral sumatriptan may include tingling; warm/hot sensation; flushing; nasal discomfort; visual disturbance.

Administration and Dosage:

Injection: The maximum single adult dose is 6 mg injected SC.

The maximum recommended dose that may be given in 24 hours is two 6 mg injections separated by at least 1 hour. Although the recommended dose is 6 mg, if side effects are dose limiting, then lower doses may be used.

Oral: Rcommended adult dose is 25 mg taken with fluids; maximum recommended single dose is 100 mg. There is no evidence that an initial dose of 100 mg provides substantially greater relief than 25 mg.

If satisfactory response has not been obtained at 2 hours, as second dose of up to 100 mg may be given. If headache returns, additional doses may be taken at intervals of at least 2 hours up to a daily maximum of 300 mg. If headache returns following an initial treatment with the injection, additional doses of single tablets (up to 200 mg/day) may be given with an interval of at least 2 hours between tablet doses.

Sumatriptan is equally effective at whatever stage of the attack they are administered, although it is advisable to take as early as possible after the onset of a migraine attack.

METHYSERGIDE MALEATE

Tablets: 2 mg (*Rx*)	*Sansert* (Sandoz)

> **Warning:**
> Retroperitoneal fibrosis, pleuropulmonary fibrosis and fibrotic thickening of cardiac valves may occur in patients receiving long-term methysergide therapy. Reserve this drug for prophylaxis in patients whose vascular headaches are frequent or severe and uncontrollable and who are under close medical supervision.

Actions:

Pharmacology: Methysergide is a semisynthetic ergot derivative. It has no intrinsic vasoconstrictor properties and its mechanism of action has not been established. It inhibits or blocks the effects of serotonin.

Allow 1 to 2 days for the protective effects to develop; following termination, 1 to 2 days are required before the effects subside.

Indications:

Vascular headache:

Prevention or reduction of intensity and frequency in patients suffering from one or more severe vascular headaches per week or from vascular headaches that are so severe that preventive therapy is indicated, regardless of the frequency of the attack.

Prophylaxis of vascular headache. Not for management of acute attacks.

Contraindications:

Pregnancy; peripheral vascular disease; severe arteriosclerosis; severe hypertension; coronary artery disease; phlebitis or cellulitis of the lower limbs; pulmonary disease; collagen diseases or fibrotic processes; impaired liver or renal function; valvular heart disease; debilitated states; serious infections.

Warnings:

Prolonged therapy: With long-term, uninterrupted administration, retroperitoneal fibrosis or related conditions have occurred. Continuous administration should not exceed 6 months.

Pleuropulmonary fibrosis, a similar nonspecific fibrotic process limited to pleural and immediately subjacent pulmonary tissues, usually presents with dyspnea, chest tightness/pain, pleural friction rubs and pleural effusion.

Cardiac fibrosis – Nonrheumatic fibrotic thickenings of the aortic root and of the aortic and mitral valves usually present clinically with cardiac murmurs and dyspnea.

Other fibrotic complications – Fibrotic plaques simulating Peyronie's disease.

Pregnancy: Category X. Contraindicated in pregnancy due to oxytocic properties.

Lactation: Ergot derivatives in breast milk have caused symptoms of ergotism.

Children: Not recommended for use in children.

Drug Interactions:

Beta blockers may interact with methysergine maleate.

Adverse Reactions:

Adverse reactions may include encroachment of retroperitoneal fibrosis on the aorta; inferior vena cava and their common iliac branches; intrinsic vasoconstriction of large and small arteries which may present with chest pain, abdominal pain or cold, numb, painful extremities with or without paresthesias and diminished or absent pulses; postural hypotension; tachycardia; nausea; vomiting; diarrhea; heartburn; abdominal pain; constipation; insomnia; drowsiness; mild euphoria; dizziness; ataxia; weakness; lightheadedness; hyperesthesia; facial flush; telangiectasia; increased hair loss; peripheral edema; neutropenia; eosinophilia; arthralgia; myalgia; weight gain.

Administration and Dosage:

Adults: 4 to 8 mg daily; take with meals. There must be a drug free interval of 3 to 4 weeks after every 6 month course of treatment.

ERGOTAMINE DERIVATIVES

ERGOTAMINE TARTRATE	
Tablets, sublingual: 2 mg (*Rx*)	*Ergomar* (Lotus), *Ergostat* (Parke-Davis)
DIHYDROERGOTAMINE	
Injection: 1 mg per ml (*Rx*)	*D.H.E. 45* (Sandoz)

Actions:

Pharmacology: Ergotamine has partial agonist or antagonist activity against tryptaminergic, dopaminergic and alpha-adrenergic receptors, depending upon their site; it is a highly active uterine stimulant. It constricts peripheral and cranial blood vessels and depresses central vasomotor centers.

Ergotamine reduces extracranial blood flow, causes a decline in the amplitude of pulsation in the cranial arteries and decreases hyperperfusion of the basilar artery territory. It does not reduce cerebral hemispheric blood flow. It may inhibit receptor reuptake of norepinephrine at sympathetic nerve endings, increasing the vasoconstrictive action. Ergotamine is a potent emetic that stimulates the chemoreceptor trigger zone. Small doses increase force and frequency of uterine contractions; larger doses increase resting uterine tone. The gravid uterus is more sensitive to these effects.

Dihydroergotamine, a hydrogenated derivative of ergotamine, differs mainly in its degree of activity. It has less vasoconstrictive action than ergotamine, is 12 times less active as an emetic and has less oxytocic effect.

Pharmacokinetics:

Absorption/Distribution – GI absorption of ergotamine is incomplete and erratic; following oral administration, peak blood levels are reached in ≈ 2 hours. Caffeine administered concurrently increases absorption rate and peak plasma levels of ergotamine.

Onset of action occurs in 15 to 30 minutes following IM administration of dihydroergotamine and persists for 3 to 4 hours. Repeat dosage at 1 hour intervals; up to 3 hours may be required to obtain maximal effect.

Metabolism/Excretion – Ergotamine is metabolized by the liver; 90% of the metabolites are excreted in the bile. Unmetabolized drug is erratically secreted in saliva, and only trace amounts of unmetabolized drug are excreted in the feces and urine. Although plasma half-life is about 2 hours, ergotamine has long-lasting effects which may be due to tissue storage.

Indications:

Headache: To abort or prevent vascular headaches such as migraine, migraine variant and cluster headache (histaminic cephalalgia).

Dihydroergotamine is used when rapid control is desired or when other routes of administration are not feasible.

Contraindications:

Pregnancy (ergotamine's powerful uterine stimulant actions may cause fetal harm); hypersensitivity to ergot alkaloids; peripheral vascular disease (eg, thromboangiitis obliterans, leutic arteritis, severe arteriosclerosis, thrombophlebitis, Raynaud's disease); hepatic or renal impairment; severe pruritus; coronary artery disease; hypertension; sepsis; malnutrition.

Warnings:

Pregnancy: Category X. Although no specific teratogenic effects have been found, the fetus suffers if ergotamine is given to the mother.

Lactation: Ergotamine is secreted into breast milk and has caused symptoms of ergotism (eg, vomiting, diarrhea) in the infant. Excessive dosing or prolonged administration may inhibit lactation.

Children: Safety and efficacy for use in children have not been established.

Precautions:

Avoid prolonged administration or excessive dosage because of the danger of ergotism and gangrene.

Drug abuse and dependence: Patients who take ergotamine for extended periods of time may become dependent upon it and require progressively increasing doses for relief of vascular headaches and for prevention of dysphoric effects which follow withdrawal.

Drug Interactions:

Drugs that may interact with ergot alkaloids include beta blockers, macrolides, nitrates and vasodilators.

Adverse Reactions:

Nausea and vomiting (10%) may be relieved by atropine or phenothiazine antiemetics.

Miscellaneous: Numbness and tingling of fingers and toes; muscle pain in the extremities; pulselessness; weakness in the legs; precordial distress and pain; transient tachycardia or bradycardia; localized edema; itching.

Large doses raise arterial pressure, produce coronary vasoconstriction and slow the heart by both a direct action and a vagal effect.

Administration and Dosage:

ERGOTAMINE: Initiate therapy as soon as possible after the first symptoms of an attack. Place 1 tablet under the tongue; take subsequent doses at 30 minute intervals if necessary. Do not exceed 3 tablets/24 hours. Do not exceed 10 mg/week.

DIHYDROERGOTAMINE:

IM – Inject 1 mg at first sign of headache; repeat at 1 hour intervals to a total of 3 mg. For optimal results, adjust the dose for several headaches to determine the minimal effective dose; use this dose at the onset of subsequent attacks.

IV – Where more rapid effect is desired, administer IV to a maximum of 2 mg. Do not exceed 6 mg/week.

ISOMETHEPTENE MUCATE/DICHLORALPHENAZONE/ ACETAMINOPHEN

Capsules: 65 mg isometheptene mucate, 100 mg dichloralphenazone, 325 mg APAP (*Rx*)	Various, *Isocom* (Nutripharm), *Isopap* (Geneva), *Midchlor* (Schein), *Midrin* (Carnrick), *Migratine* (Major)

Actions:

Pharmacology: Isometheptene mucate is an unsaturated aliphatic amine with sympathomimetic properties. It acts by constricting dilated cranial and cerebral arterioles, thus reducing the stimuli that lead to vascular headaches.

Pharmacokinetics: Dichloralphenazone, a mild sedative, reduces the patient's emotional reaction to the pain of both vascular and tension headaches.

Acetaminophen raises the threshold to painful stimuli, thus exerting an analgesic effect against all types of headaches.

Indications:

For relief of tension and vascular headaches.

Based on a review of this drug (isometheptene mucate) by the National Academy of Sciences-National Research Council or other information, FDA has classified the other indication as "possibly" effective in the treatment of migraine headache. Final classification of the less-than-effective indication requires further investigation.

Contraindications:

Glaucoma; severe cases of renal disease; hypertension; organic heart disease; hepatic disease; MAO inhibitor therapy.

Precautions:

Observe caution in hypertension, peripheral vascular disease and after recent cardiovascular attacks.

Drug Interactions:

Drugs that may interact include MAO inhibitors.

Adverse Reactions:

Adverse reactions may include transient dizziness and skin rash.

Administration and Dosage:

Migraine headache: Usual dosage is 2 capsules at once followed by 1 capsule every hour until relieved, up to 5 capsules within a 12 hour period.

Tension headache: Usual dosage is 1 or 2 capsules every 4 hours, up to 8 capsules per day.

ANTIEMETIC/ANTIVERTIGO AGENTS

Product	Manufacturer
CHLORPROMAZINE	
Tablets: 10, 25, 50, 100 and 200 mg (*Rx*)	Various, *Thorazine* (SmithKline Beecham)
Capsules, sustained release: 30, 75, 150, 200 and 300 mg (*Rx*)	*Thorazine Spansules* (SmithKline Beecham)
Syrup: 10 mg/5 ml (*Rx*)	*Chlorpromazine HCl* (Geneva), *Thorazine* (SmithKline Beecham)
Concentrate: 30 and 100 mg/ml (*Rx*)	Various, *Thorazine* (SmithKline Beecham)
Suppositories (as base): 25 and 100 mg (*Rx*)	*Thorazine* (SmithKline Beecham)
Injection: 25 mg/ml (*Rx*)	Various, *Ormazine* (Hauck), *Thorazine* (SmithKline Beecham)
PERPHENAZINE	
Tablets: 2, 4, 8 and 16 mg (*Rx*)	Various, *Trilafon* (Schering)
Concentrate: 16 mg/5 ml (*Rx*)	*Trilafon* (Schering)
Injection: 5 mg/ml (*Rx*)	*Trilafon* (Schering)
TRIFLUPROMAZINE	
Injection: 10 and 20 mg/ml (*Rx*)	*Vesprin* (Princeton)
PROCHLORPERAZINE	
Tablets (as maleate): 5, 10 and 25 mg (*Rx*)	Various, *Compazine* (SmithKline Beecham)
Capsules, sustained release: 10, 15 and 30 mg (*Rx*)	*Compazine Spansules* (SmithKline Beecham)
Suppositories: 2.5, 5 and 25 mg (*Rx*)	Various, *Compazine* (SmithKline Beecham)
Syrup: 5 mg/5 ml (*Rx*)	*Compazine* (SmithKline Beecham)
Injection (as edisylate): 5 mg/ml (*Rx*)	Various, *Prochlorperazine* (Wyeth-Ayerst), *Compazine* (SmithKline Beecham)
THIETHYLPERAZINE	
Tablets: 10 mg (*Rx*)	*Norzine* (Purdue Frederick), *Torecan* (Roxane)
Suppositories: 10 mg (*Rx*)	
Injection: 5 mg/ml (*Rx*)	
METOCLOPRAMIDE	
Tablets: 5 mg (*Rx*)	Various, *Reglan* (Robins)
Tablets: 10 mg (*Rx*)	Various, *Clopra* (Quantum), *Maxolon* (Beecham), *Octamide* (Adria), *Reclomide* (Major), *Reglan* (Robins)
Syrup: 5 mg/5 ml (*Rx*)	Various, *Reglan* (Robins), *Maxolon* (Beecham)
Concentrated solution: 10 mg/ml (*Rx*)	*Metoclopramide Intensol* (Roxane)
Injection: 5 mg/ml (*Rx*)	Various, *Octamide PFS* (Adria), *Reglan* (Robins)

For complete listing of promethazine products refer to Antihistamine Product Pages.

Actions:

Pharmacology: Drug-induced vomiting (eg, drugs, radiation, metabolic disorders) is generally stimulated through the chemoreceptor trigger zone (CTZ), which in turn stimulates the vomiting center (VC) in the brain. Nausea of motion sickness is initiated by stimulation of labyrinthine mechanism of the ear, which sends impulses to CTZ. VC may also be stimulated directly by GI irritation, motion sickness, vestibular neuritis.

The following table indicates manufacturers' recommended uses for agents in this group. Several of these are indicated for uses other than as antiemetic/antivertigo agents.

Recommended Uses for Antiemetic/Antivertigo Agents

	Drug	Indications		
		Nausea and Vomiting	Motion Sickness	Vertigo
ANTIDOPAMINERGICS				
Phenothiazines	Chlorpromazine [1]	✓		
	Triflupromazine	✓		
	Perphenazine [1]	✓		
	Prochlorperazine	✓		
	Promethazine	✓	✓	
	Thiethylperazine	✓		
Other	Metoclopramide	✓		
ANTICHOLINERGICS				
Antihistamines	Cyclizine	✓	✓	
	Meclizine	✓	✓	✓[2]
	Buclizine	✓	✓	
	Diphenhydramine		✓	
	Dimenhydrinate	✓	✓	✓
Other	Trimethobenzamide	✓		
	Scopolamine		✓	
MISCELLANEOUS				
Miscellaneous	Diphenidol	✓		✓
	Benzquinamide	✓		
	PhosphoratedCarbohydrate Solution	✓		
	Hydroxyzine HCl	✓[3]		
	Corticosteroids	✓[3]		
	Cannabinoids	✓		

[1] Also indicated for relief of intractable hicoughs.
[2] Classified "possibly effective" by the FDA.
[3] This is an *unlabeled* use.

Warnings:

Children: Not recommended for uncomplicated vomiting in children; limit use to prolonged vomiting of known etiology for three principal reasons:

1.) Although there is no confirmatory evidence, centrally-acting antiemetics may contribute, in combination with viral illnesses (a possible cause of vomiting in children), to the development of Reye's syndrome, a potentially fatal acute childhood encephalopathy.
2.) The extrapyramidal symptoms that can occur secondary to some drugs may be confused with the CNS signs of an undiagnosed primary disease responsible for the vomiting, eg, Reye's syndrome or other encephalopathy.
3.) Drugs with hepatotoxic potential may unfavorably alter the course of Reye's syndrome. Avoid such drugs in children whose signs and symptoms (vomiting) could represent Reye's syndrome.

Children with acute illnesses (eg, chickenpox, CNS infections, measles, gastroenteritis) or dehydration seem to be much more susceptible to neuromuscular reactions, particularly dystonias, than are adults. In such patients, use antiemetics only under close supervision. Do not use dimenhydrinate in children under 2 years of age unless directed by a doctor.

Severe emesis should not be treated with an antiemetic drug alone; where possible, establish cause of vomiting. Direct primary emphasis toward restoration of body fluids and electrolyte balance, and relief of fever and causative disease process. Avoid overhydration which may result in cerebral edema.

Administration and Dosage:

CHLORPROMAZINE HCl:

Adults –

Nausea and vomiting:

Oral – 10 to 25 mg every 4 to 6 hours, as needed; increase if necessary.

Rectal – 50 to 100 mg every 6 to 8 hours, as needed.

IM – 25 mg. If no hypotension occurs, give 25 to 50 mg every 3 to 4 hours, as needed, until vomiting stops. Then switch to oral dosage.

Intractable hiccoughs: Orally, 25 to 50 mg 3 or 4 times/day. If symptoms persist 2 to 3 days, give 25 to 50 mg IM. If still persistent, use slow IV infusion with patient flat in bed. Give 25 to 50 mg in 500 to 1000 ml saline. Monitor blood pressure.

Children –

Nausea and vomiting: Do not use in children < 6 months of age except where potentially lifesaving. Do not use in conditions for which specific children's dosages have not been established. The activity following IM use may last 12 hours.

Oral – 0.25 mg/lb (0.55 mg/kg) every 4 to 6 hours.

Rectal – 0.5 mg/lb (1.1 mg/kg) every 6 to 8 hours, as needed.

IM – 0.25 mg/lb (0.55 mg/kg) every 6 to 8 hours, as needed.

Maximum IM dosage –

Children up to 5 years of age: 40 mg/day.

Children 5 to 12 years of age: 75 mg/day, except in severe cases.

PERPHENAZINE:

Oral – 8 to 16 mg daily in divided doses; occasionally, 24 mg may be necessary. Early dosage reduction is desirable.

IM – Give to seated or recumbent patient; observe patient for a short period afterward.

Adults: 5 mg repeated every 6 hours as necessary. Do not exceed 15 mg in ambulatory or 30 mg in hospitalized patients. For severe conditions, an initial dose of 10 mg may be given. Place patients on oral therapy as soon as possible, usually within 24 hours. In general, reserve higher dosages for hospitalized patients.

Children (> 12): The lowest adult dose (5 mg). Pediatric dose not established.

IV – Use only when necessary to control severe vomiting, intractable hiccoughs or acute conditions such as violent retching during surgery. Limit use to recumbent hospitalized adults in doses not exceeding 5 mg. Give as a diluted solution by either fractional injection or slow drip infusion. In the surgical patient, slow infusion is preferred. When administered in divided doses, dilute to 0.5 mg/ml (1 ml mixed with 9 ml saline solution) and give not more than 1 mg per injection at not less than 1 to 2 minute intervals. Discontinue as soon as symptoms are controlled. Do not exceed 5 mg.

TRIFLUPROMAZINE HCl:

Adults –

IM (range): 5 to 15 mg repeated every 4 hours, up to 60 mg maximum daily dose.

Elderly or debilitated – 2.5 mg; maximum daily dose, 15 mg.

IV (range): 1 mg, up to 3 mg total daily dose.

Children (over 2½ years of age) –

IM: 0.2 to 0.25 mg/kg; maximum 10 mg/day. The duration of activity following IM administration may last up to 12 hours. Do not administer IV.

PROCHLORPERAZINE: Do not crush or chew sustained release preparations.

Adults: Control of severe nausea and vomiting –

Oral: Usually, 5 or 10 mg, 3 or 4 times daily; *sustained release* —15 mg on arising or 10 mg every 12 hours.

Rectal: 25 mg twice daily.

IM: Initially, 5 to 10 mg. If necessary, repeat every 3 or 4 hours. Do not exceed 40 mg/day.

SC: Do not administer SC because of local irritation.

Adult surgery: Control of severe nausea and vomiting – Total parenteral dosage should not exceed 40 mg/day. Hypotension may occur if the drug is given IV or by infusion.

IM: 5 to 10 mg, 1 to 2 hours before induction of anesthesia (may repeat once in 30 minutes), or to control acute symptoms during and after surgery (may repeat once).

IV injection: 5 to 10 mg, 15 to 30 minutes before induction of anesthesia, or to control acute symptoms during or after surgery. Repeat once if necessary. Prochlorperazine may be administered either undiluted or diluted in isotonic solution, but do not exceed 10 mg in a single dose of the drug. Do not exceed 5 mg/ml/min. Do not use bolus injection.

IV infusion: 20 mg/L of isotonic solution. Do not dilute in less than 1 L of isotonic solution. Add to IV infusion 15 to 30 minutes before induction.

Children (over 20 pounds or 2 years of age): Control of severe nausea and vomiting –

Oral or rectal: More than one day of therapy is seldom necessary.

9.1 to 13.2 kg – 2.5 mg 1 or 2 times/day (not to exceed 7.5 mg/day).

13.6 to 17.7 kg – 2.5 mg 2 or 3 times/day (not to exceed 10 mg/day).

18.2 to 38.6 kg – 2.5 mg 3 times/day or 5 mg twice daily (not to exceed 15 mg/day).

IM: 0.06 mg/lb (0.132 mg/kg). Give by deep IM injection. Control is usually obtained with one dose. Duration of action may be 12 hours. Subsequent doses may be given if necessary.

PROMETHAZINE:

Oral and rectal –

Motion sickness: The average adult dose is 25 mg twice daily. Take the initial dose 1 hour before travel, and repeat 8 to 12 hours later, if necessary. On succeeding days, administer 25 mg on arising and again before the evening meal. For children, administer 12.5 to 25 mg twice daily.

Nausea and vomiting: The average dose for active therapy in children or adults is 25 mg. Repeat as necessary in doses of 12.5 to 25 mg at 4 to 6 hour intervals.

Children – 0.25 to 0.5 mg/kg every 4 to 6 hours rectally, as needed. Do not use in children < 2 yrs. Adjust dose based on age, weight and severity of condition.

Parenteral – Administer preferably by deep IM injection. Proper IV administration is well tolerated, but hazardous. When used IV, give in a concentration no greater than 25 mg/ml, and at a rate not to exceed 25 mg/min; it is preferable to inject through an appropriate site in tubing of an IV infusion set.

Motion sickness: 12.5 to 25 mg; may repeat as necessary 3 or 4 times a day.

Nausea and vomiting: 12.5 to 25 mg; do not repeat more frequently than every 4 hours. For postoperative nausea and vomiting, administer IM or IV.

In children < 12 years, do not exceed half the adult dose. As an adjunct to premedication, use 0.5 mg/lb (1.1 mg/kg) with an equal dose of narcotic or barbiturate and the appropriate dose of an atropine-like drug. Do not use in premature infants or neonates or in vomiting of unknown etiology in children.

THIETHYLPERAZINE MALEATE: Do not use IV (may cause severe hypotension).

When used for nausea or vomiting associated with anesthesia and surgery, administer by deep IM injection at, or shortly before, termination of anesthesia.

Adults –

Oral and rectal: 10 to 30 mg daily in divided doses.

IM: 2 ml, 1 to 3 times daily.

Children – Dosage not determined. Not recommended in children < 12 years old.

THIETHYLPERAZINE: Do not use IV (may cause severe hypotension). Use of this drug has not been studied following intracardiac or intracranial surgery.

When used for nausea or vomiting associated with anesthesia and surgery, administer by deep IM injection at, or shortly before, termination of anesthesia.

Adults –

Oral and Rectal: 10 to 30 mg daily in divided doses.

IM: 2 ml, 1 to 3 times daily.

Children – Dosage not determined. Not recommended in children < 12 years old.

METOCLOPRAMIDE:

Prevention of chemotherapy-induced emesis – For doses in excess of 10 mg, dilute injection in 50 ml of a parenteral solution (Dextrose 5% in Water, Sodium Chloride Injection, Dextrose 5% in 0.45% Sodium Chloride, Ringer's or Lactated Ringer's Injection). Infuse slowly IV over not less than 15 minutes, 30 minutes before beginning cancer chemotherapy; repeat every 2 hours for 2 doses, then every 3 hours for 3 doses.

The initial 2 doses should be 2 mg/kg if highly emetogenic drugs such as cisplatin or dacarbazine are used alone or in combination. For less emetogenic regimens, 1 mg/kg/dose may be adequate.

Metoclopramide may have some potential value (10 mg orally or IV 30 minutes before each meal and at bedtime) in nausea and vomiting of a variety of etiologies (uncontrolled studies report 80% to 90% efficacy), including emesis during pregnancy and labor (5 to 10 mg orally or 5 to 20 mg IV or IM, 3 times a day).

CYCLIZINE AND MECLIZINE

CYCLIZINE	
Tablets: 50 mg (as HCl) (*otc*)	*Marezine* (Himmel)
MECLIZINE	
Tablets: 12.5, 25 and 50 mg (*Rx*)	Various, *Antivert* (Roerig), *Ru-Vert-M* (Solvay), *Dramamine II* (Upjohn)
Tablets, chewable: 25 mg (*Rx*)	Various
Tablets, chewable: 25 mg (*otc*)	Various, *Bonine* (Leeming)
Capsules: 25 mg (*Rx*)	Various, *Meni-D* (Seatrace)
Capsules: 30 mg (*otc*)	*Vergon* (Marnel)

Actions:

Pharmacology: Cyclizine and meclizine have antiemetic, anticholinergic and antihistaminic properties.

Cyclizine and meclizine have an onset of action of 30 to 60 minutes, depending on dosage; their duration of action is 4 to 6 hours and 12 to 24 hours, respectively.

Indications:

Motion sickness, vestibular system disease: Prevention and treatment of nausea, vomiting and dizziness of motion sickness.

Meclizine is "possibly effective" for the management of vertigo associated with diseases affecting the vestibular system.

Contraindications:

Hypersensitivity to cyclizine or meclizine.

Warnings:

Pregnancy: Category B. Meclizine presents the lowest risk of teratogenicity and is the drug of first choice in treating nausea and vomiting during pregnancy.

Lactation: Safety for use in the nursing mother has not been established.

Children: Safety and efficacy for use in children have not been established. Not recommended for use in children < 12 years of age.

Precautions:

Hazardous tasks: May produce drowsiness; patients should observe caution while driving or performing other tasks requiring alertness.

Because of the anticholinergic action of these agents, use with caution and with appropriate monitoring in patients with glaucoma, obstructive disease of the GI or GU tract and in elderly males with possible prostatic hypertrophy. These drugs may have a hypotensive action, which may be confusing or dangerous in postoperative patients.

May have additive effects with alcohol and other CNS depressants (eg, hypnotics, sedatives, tranquilizers, antianxiety agents); use with caution.

Adverse Reactions:

CNS: Drowsiness; restlessness; excitation; nervousness; insomnia; euphoria; blurred vision; diplopia; vertigo; tinnitus; auditory and visual hallucinations (particularly when dosage recommendations are exceeded).

Dermatologic: Urticaria; rash.

GI: Dry mouth; anorexia; nausea; vomiting; diarrhea; constipation; cholestatic jaundice (cyclizine).

GU: Urinary frequency; difficult urination; urinary retention.

Cardiovascular: Hypotension; palpitations; tachycardia.

Miscellaneous: Dry nose and throat.

Administration and Dosage:

CYCLIZINE:

Oral –

Adults: 50 mg taken ½ hour before departure; repeat every 4 to 6 hours. Do not exceed 200 mg daily.

Children (6 to 12 years of age): 25 mg, up to 3 times daily.

Parenteral – For IM use only. Not recommended for use in children.

Adults: 50 mg every 4 to 6 hours, as necessary.

MECLIZINE:

Motion sickness – Take an initial dose of 25 to 50 mg, 1 hour prior to travel. May repeat dose every 24 hours for the duration of the journey.

Vertigo – 25 to 100 mg daily in divided doses.

BUCLIZINE HCl

Tablets: 50 mg (*Rx*)	*Bucladin-S Softabs* (Stuart)

Actions:

Pharmacology: Acts centrally to suppress nausea and vomiting.

Indications:

For the control of nausea, vomiting and dizziness of motion sickness.

Contraindications:

Hypersensitivity to buclizine HCl; pregnancy (see Warnings).

Warnings:

Pregnancy: When administered to the pregnant rat at doses above the human therapeutic range, buclizine induced fetal abnormalities. Clinical data are not adequate to establish safety in early pregnancy.

Children: Safety and efficacy for use in children have not been established.

Adverse Reactions:

Drowsiness, dry mouth, headache and jitteriness.

Administration and Dosage:

Tablets can be taken without swallowing water. Place tablet in mouth and allow to dissolve, or chew or swallow whole.

Adults: A 50 mg dose usually alleviates nausea. In severe cases, 150 mg/day may be taken. Usual maintenance dose is 50 mg, 2 times daily. In prevention of motion sickness, take 50 mg at least hour before beginning travel. For extended travel, a second 50 mg dose may be taken after 4 to 6 hours.

DIPHENHYDRAMINE

For complete prescribing information and product availability, see Antihistamines group monograph.

Indications:

Treatment and prophylaxis (oral only) of motion sickness.

Administration and Dosage:

Oral: Adults – 25 to 50 mg 3 or 4 times daily.

Children > 20 lbs (9.1kg) – 12.5 to 25 mg 3 or 4 times daily (5 mg/kg/24 hrs, or 150 mg/m^2/24 hours. Do not exceed 300mg.

Give first dose 30 minutes before exposure to motion and repeat before meals and upon retiring for the duration of journey.

Parenteral: For use only when the oral form is impractical.

Adults – 10 to 50 mg IV or deep IM; 100 mg if required. Maximum daily dosage is 400 mg.

Children – 5 mg/kg/24 hrs or 150 mg/m^2/24 hrs, in 4 divided doses, IV or deep IM. Maximum daily dosage is 300 mg.

DIMENHYDRINATE

Tablets: 50 mg (*Rx*)	*Dimetabs* (Jones Medical)
Tablets: 50 mg (*otc*)	Various, *Calm-X* (Republic Drug), *Dramamine* (Upjohn), *Triptone Caplets* (Commerce)
Tablets, chewable: 50 mg (*otc*)	*Dramamine* (Upjohn)
Capsules: 50 mg (*otc*)	*Vertab* (UAD)
Injection: 50 mg per ml (*Rx*)	Various, *Dinate* (Seatrace), *Dramamine* (Pasadena), *Dymenate* (Keene), *Hydrate* (Hyrex)
Liquid: 12.5 mg per 4 ml (*otc*)	Various, *Dramamine* (Upjohn),
Liquid: 12.5 mg per 5 ml (*otc*)	*Children's Dramamine* (Upjohn)
Liquid: 15.62 mg per 5 ml (*Rx*)	*Dramamine* (Upjohn)

Actions:

Pharmacology: Dimenhydrinate consists of equimolar proportions of diphenhydramine and chlorotheophylline.

Pharmacokinetics: Dimenhydrinate has a depressant action on hyperstimulated labyrinthine function. The precise mode of action is not known. The antiemetic effects are believed to be due to the diphenhydramine, an antihistamine also used as an antiemetic agent.

Indications:

For the prevention and treatment of nausea, vomiting, dizziness or vertigo of motion sickness.

Contraindications:

Neonates; patients hypersensitive to dimenhydrinate or its components.

Note: Most IV products contain Benzyl Alcohol, which has been associated with a fatal "Gasping Syndrome" in premature infants and low birth weight infants.

Warnings:

Pregnancy: *Category B.*

Lactation: Small amounts of dimenhydrinate are excreted in breast milk. Because of the potential for adverse reactions in nursing infants, decide whether to discontinue nursing or to discontinue the drug, taking into account the importance of the drug to the mother.

Children: For infants and children especially, an overdose of antihistamines may cause hallucinations, convulsions or death. Mental alertness may be diminished. In the young child, dimenhydrinate may produce excitation. Do not give to children under 2 years of age unless directed by a physician.

Precautions:

Use with caution in conditions which might be aggravated by anticholinergic therapy (eg, prostatic hypertrophy, stenosing peptic ulcer, pyloroduodenal obstruction, bladder neck obstruction, narrow angle glaucoma, bronchial asthma, cardiac arrhythmias, etc).

Drug Interactions:

Drugs that may interact with dimenhydrinate may include: CNS depressants and antibiotics.

Adverse Reactions:

Adverse reactions may include: Drowsiness; confusion; nervousness; restlessness; headache; insomnia (especially in children); tingling, heaviness and weakness of hands; vertigo; dizziness; lassitude; excitation; nausea; vomiting; diarrhea; epigastric distress; constipation; anorexia; blurring of vision; diplopia; palpitations; hypotension; tachycardia; anaphylaxis; photosensitivity; urticaria; drug rash; hemolytic anemia; difficult or painful urination; nasal stuffiness; tightness of chest; wheezing; thickening of bronchial secretions; dryness of mouth, nose and throat.

Administration and Dosage:

Adults:

Oral – 50 to 100 mg every 4 to 6 hours. Do not exceed 400 mg in 24 hours.

IM – 50 mg, as needed.

IV – 50 mg in 10 ml Sodium Chloride Injection given over 2 minutes. Do not inject intra-arterially.

Children:

Oral (6 to 12 years) – 25 to 50 mg every 6 to 8 hours; do not exceed 150 mg in 24 hours.

Oral (2 to 6 years) – Up to 12.5 to 25 mg every 6 to 8 hours; do not exceed 75 mg in 24 hours.

IM – 1.25 mg/kg or 37.5 mg/m^2 4 times daily; do not exceed 300 mg daily.

Children (under 2 years): Only on advice of a physician.

TRIMETHOBENZAMIDE HCl

Capsules: 100 mg (*Rx*)	*Tigan* (Roberts), *Trimazide* (Major)
Capsules: 250 mg (*Rx*)	Various, *Tigan* (Roberts),
Pediatric Suppositories: 100 mg (*Rx*)	Various, *Pediatric Triban* (Great Southern), *Tebamide* (G&W Labs), *T-Gen* (Goldline), *Tigan* (Roberts), *Trimazide* (Major)
Suppositories: 200 mg (*Rx*)	Various, *Tebamide* (G&W), *T-Gen* (Goldline), *Tigan* (Roberts), *Triban* (Great Southern), *Trimazide* (Major),
Injection: 100 mg per ml (*Rx*)	Various, *Arrestin* (Vortech), *Pediatric Triban* (Great Southern), *Ticon* (Hauck), *Tigan* (Roberts)

Actions:

Pharmacokinetics: Mechanism is obscure, but may be mediated through the chemoreceptor trigger zone; direct impulses to vomiting center are not inhibited.

Indications:

Control of nausea and vomiting.

Contraindications:

Hypersensitivity to trimethobenzamide, benzocaine or similar local anesthetics; parenteral use in children; suppositories in premature infants or neonates.

Warnings:

Pregnancy: Safety for use has not been established.

Lactation: Safety for use in the nursing mother has not been established.

Precautions:

Encephalitides, gastroenteritis, dehydration, electrolyte imbalance (especially in children and the elderly or debilitated) and CNS reactions have occurred when used during acute febrile illness.

Exercise caution when giving the drug with alcohol and other CNS-acting agents such as phenothiazines, barbiturates and belladonna derivatives.

Adverse Reactions:

Adverse reactions may include: Hypersensitivity reactions; parkinson-like symptoms; hypotension or pain following IM injection; blood dyscrasias; blurred vision; coma; convulsions; depression; diarrhea; disorientation; dizziness; drowsiness; headache; jaundice; muscle cramps; opisthotonos; allergic-type skin reactions.

Administration and Dosage:

Oral: Adults — 250 mg, 3 or 4 times daily.

Children (30 to 90 lbs; 13.6 to 40.9 kg) – 100 to 200 mg, 3 or 4 times daily.

Rectal: Adults — 200 mg, 3 or 4 times daily.

Children (30 to 90 lbs; 13.6 to 40.9 kg) – 100 to 200 mg, 3 or 4 times daily.

(< 30 lbs) – 100 mg, 3 or 4 times daily. Do not use in premature or newborn infants.

Injection: For IM use only. *Adults* — 200 mg 3 or 4 times/day. Pain, stinging, burning, redness and swelling may develop at injection site.

DRONABINOL

Gelatin Capsules: 2.5, 5 and 10 mg *(c-II)*	*Marinol* (Roxane)

Actions:

Pharmacology: Dronabinol is the principal psychoactive substance present in Cannabis sativa L (marijuana). Nontherapeutic effects of dronabinol are identical to those of marijuana and other centrally active cannabinoids. The mechanism of action is unknown.

Cannabinoids have complex CNS effects, including central sympathomimetic activity. Cannabinoid receptors have been discovered in neural tissues. These receptors may play a role in mediating the effects of dronabinol. Patients may experience mood changes, decrements in cognitive performance and memory, a decreased ability to control drives and impulses, and alterations of reality.

Pharmacokinetics:

Absorption/Distribution – Following oral administration, dronabinol is almost completely absorbed (90% to 95%). It has a systemic bioavailability of 10% to 20%, an onset of action of ≈ 0.5 to 1 hour and peak effect at 2 to 4 hours. Duration for psychoactive effects is 4 to 6 hours, but the appetite stimulant effect may continue for ≥ 24 hours after administration. Dronabinol has a large apparent volume of distribution, ≈ 10 L/kg, because of its lipid solubility. The plasma protein binding of dronabinol and its metabolites is ≈ 97%.

Metabolism/Excretion – Dronabinol undergoes extensive first-pass hepatic metabolism, primarily by microsomal hydroxylation, yielding both active and inactive metabolites. Dronabinol and its principal active metabolite, 11-OH-delta-9-THC, are present in approximately equal concentrations in plasma. Concentrations of both parent drug and metabolite peak at ≈ 2 to 4 hours after oral dosing and decline over several days.

Biliary excretion is the major route of elimination. Within 72 hours following oral administration, ≈ 50% of the dose is recovered in feces; another 10% to 15% appears in the urine. Less than 5% is excreted unchanged in the urine. The elimination phase of dronabinol exhibits biphasic kinetics with an alpha half-life of 4 hours and a terminal half-life of 25 to 36 hours. Extended use at the recommended doses may cause accumulation of toxic amounts of dronabinol and its metabolites.

Indications:

Antiemetic: Treatment of nausea and vomiting associated with cancer chemotherapy in patients not responding adequately to conventional antiemetic treatment.

Appetite stimulation: Treating anorexia associated with weight loss in AIDS patients.

Contraindications:

Hypersensitivity to dronabinol, marijuana or sesame oil.

Warnings:

Tolerance: Following 12 days of dronabinol, tolerance to the cardiovascular and subjective effects developed at doses up to 210 mg/day. An initial tachycardia induced by dronabinol was replaced successively by normal sinus rhythm and then bradycardia. A fall in supine blood pressure, made worse by standing, was also observed initially. Within days, these effects disappeared, indicating development of tolerance. Tachyphylaxis and tolerance did not, however, appear to develop to the appetite stimulant effect. In AIDS patients, the appetite stimulant effect was sustained for up to 5 months at doses of 2.5 to 20 mg/day.

Patient supervision: Because of individual variation, determine clinically the period of patient supervision required. Closely observe patients within an inpatient setting, if possible. This is especially important during treatment of patients with no prior experience with cannabis or dronabinol. However, even patients experienced with these agents may have serious untoward responses not predicted by prior uneventful exposures. Closely observe any patient who has a psychotic experience with dronabinol until the mental state returns to normal. Do not give additional doses until the patient has been examined and the circumstances evaluated. If the situation warrants it, give a lower dose under very close supervision.

Elderly: Use caution because the elderly are generally more sensitive to the psychoactive effects. In antiemetic studies, no difference in tolerance or efficacy was apparent in patients > 55 years old.

Pregnancy: Category B.

Lactation: Dronabinol is concentrated and excreted in breast milk, and is absorbed by the nursing baby. Because the effects on the infant of chronic exposure to the drug and its metabolites are unknown, nursing mothers should not use dronabinol.

Children: Not recommended for AIDS-related anorexia in children because it has not been studied in this population. Dosage for chemotherapy-induced emesis is the same as in adults. Use caution in children because of the psychoactive effects.

Precautions:

Hypertension or heart disease: Use with caution since dronabinol may cause a general increase in central sympathomimetic activity.

Psychiatric patients: In manic, depressive or schizophrenic patients, symptoms of these disease states may be exacerbated by the use of cannabinoids.

Drug abuse and dependence: Dronabinol is highly abusable. Limit prescriptions to the amount necessary for a single cycle of chemotherapy.

It is not known what proportion of individuals exposed chronically to these drugs will develop either psychological or physical dependence. Long-term use of cannabinoids has been associated with disorders of motivation, judgment and cognition. It is not clear if this is a manifestation of the underlying personalities of chronic users of this class of drugs, or if cannabinoids are directly responsible.

A withdrawal syndrome consisting of irritability, insomnia and restlessness was observed in some subjects within 12 hours following abrupt withdrawal of dronabinol. The syndrome reached its peak intensity at 24 hours when subjects exhibited hot flashes, sweating, rhinorrhea, loose stools, hiccoughs and anorexia. The syndrome was essentially complete within 96 hours. EEG changes following discontinuation were consistent with a withdrawal syndrome. Several subjects reported impressions of disturbed sleep for several weeks after discontinuing high doses.

Hazardous tasks: Because of its profound effects on mental status, warn patients not to drive, operate complex machinery or engage in any activity requiring sound judgment and unimpaired coordination while receiving treatment. Effects may persist for a variable and unpredictable period of time. Dronabinol is highly lipid soluble, and its metabolites may persist in tissues, including plasma, for days.

Drug Interactions:

Drugs that may be affected by dronabinol include amphetamines, cocaine, sympathomimetics, anticholinergics, antihistamines, tricyclic antidepressants, alcohol, sedatives, hypnotics, psychomimetics, disulfiram, fluoxetine and theophylline.

Adverse Reactions:

Adverse reactions occurring in ≥ 3% of patients include euphoria, nausea, vomiting, dizziness, paranoid reaction and somnolence.

Administration and Dosage:

Antiemetic: Initially, give 5 mg/m^2 1 to 3 hours prior to the administration of chemotherapy, then every 2 to 4 hours after chemotherapy is given, for a total of 4 to 6 doses/day. If the 5 mg/m^2 dose is ineffective, and there are no significant side effects, increase the dose by 2.5 mg/m^2 increments to a maximum of 15 mg/m^2 per dose. Use caution, however, as the incidence of disturbing psychiatric symptoms increases significantly at this maximum dose. Administration with phenothiazines may improve efficacy (vs either drug alone) without additional toxicity.

Appetite stimulation: Initially, give 2.5 mg twice a day before lunch and supper. For patients who cannot tolerate 5 mg/day, reduce dosage to 2.5 mg/day as a single evening or bedtime dose. When adverse reactions are absent or minimal and further therapeutic effect is desired, increase to 2.5 mg before lunch and 5 mg before supper (or 5 mg at lunch and 5 mg after supper). Although most patients respond to 2.5 mg twice daily, 10 mg twice daily has been tolerated in about 50% of patients. The dosage may be increased to a maximum of 20 mg/day in divided doses. Use caution in escalating the dosage because of the increased frequency of dose-related adverse reactions at higher dosages.

ONDANSETRON HCl

Tablets: 4 and 8 mg (*Rx*)	*Zofran* (Cerenex)
Injection: 2 mg/ml and 32 mg/50 ml (premixed) (*Rx*)	

Actions:

Pharmacology: Ondansetron is a selective 5-HT$_3$ receptor antagonist used for prevention of nausea and vomiting associated with cancer chemotherapy. While its mechanism of action has not been fully characterized, it is not a dopamine receptor antagonist. It is not certain whether ondansetron's antiemetic action is mediated centrally, peripherally, or in both sites.

Pharmacokinetics: Ondansetron is extensively metabolized, with ≈ 5% of a dose recovered as the parent compound from the urine. The primary metabolic pathway is hydroxylation on the indole ring followed by glucuronide or sulfate conjugation.

Oral ondansetron is well absorbed and undergoes limited first-pass metabolism. Following a single 8 mg dose to healthy male volunteers, time to peak level is ≈ 1.7 hours, terminal elimination half-life is ≈ 3 hours, and bioavailability is ≈ 56%. Extent and rate of absorption is greater in women than men. Slower clearance in women, smaller apparent volume of distribution and higher absolute bioavailability resulted in higher plasma levels.

Plasma protein binding was 70% to 76%. Circulating drug also distributes into erythrocytes.

Indications:

Parenteral: Prevention of nausea and vomiting associated with initial and repeat courses of emetogenic cancer chemotherapy, including high-dose cisplatin.

Prevention of postoperative nausea or vomiting. Routine prophylaxis is not recommended for patients in whom there is little expectation that nausea or vomiting will occur postoperatively. In patients where nausea or vomiting must be avoided postoperatively, ondansetron is recommended even where the incidence of postoperative nausea or vomiting is low. For patients who have postoperative nausea or vomiting, ondansetron may be given to prevent further episodes.

Oral: Prevention of nausea and vomiting associated with initial and repeat courses of emetogenic cancer chemotherapy.

Prevention of nausea and vomiting associated with radiotherapy in patients receiving either total body irradiation, single high-dose fraction or daily fractions to the abdomen.

Prevention of postoperative nausea or vomiting.

Routine prophylaxis is not recommended for patients in whom there is little expectation that nausea or vomiting will occur postoperatively. In patients where nausea or vomiting must be avoided postoperatively, ondansetron is recommended even where the incidence of postoperative nausea or vomiting is low. For patients who have postoperative nausea or vomiting, ondansetron may be given to prevent further episodes.

Contraindications:

Hypersensitivity to the drug.

Warnings:

Peristalsis: Ondansetron does not stimulate gastric or intestinal peristasis. Do not use instead of nasogastric suction. Use in abdominal surgery may mask a progressive ileus or gastric distension.

Elderly: A reduction in clearance and increase in elimination half-life are seen in patients > 75 years old. Prevention of nausea and vomiting in elderly patients is no different than in younger age groups. No adjustment in dosage is recommended in the elderly.

Pregnancy: *Category B.*

Lactation: It is not known whether ondansetron is excreted in human breast milk.

Children: Patients aged 4 to 12 years generally showed higher clearance and somewhat larger volume of distribution than adults. Most pediatric cancer patients < 15 years of age had a shorter (2.4 hours) plasma half-life than patients > 15 years of age. It is not known whether these differences in plasma half-life may result in differences in efficacy between adults and some young children.

Little information is available about dosage in children ≤ 3 years of age. See Administration and Dosage section for use in children 4 to 18 years of age.

Drug Interactions:

Because ondansetron is metabolized by hepatic cytochrome P-450 drug metabolizing enzymes, inducers or inhibitors of these enzymes may change the clearance and, hence, the half-life of ondansetron. However, on the basis of available data, no dosage adjustment is recommended for patients on these drugs.

Drug/Food interactions: The extent of absorption of oral ondansetron is significantly increased (≈ 17%) by food. Peak plasma concentration and time to peak plasma concentration are not significantly affected. This is not believed to be clinically relevant.

Adverse Reactions:

Adverse reactions occurring in ≥ 3% of patients include diarrhea, headache, fever, constipation, dizziness, musculoskelatal pain, drowsiness/sedation, shivers, malaise/fatigue, injection site reaction, urinary retention, wound problem, hypoxia, pyrexia, gynecological disorder, bradycardia, hypotension, pruritus.

Administration and Dosage:

Prevention of nausea/vomiting associated with cancer chemotherapy:

Parenteral – Dilute in 50 ml of 5% Dextrose Injection or 0.9% Sodium Chloride Injection before administration. Do not mix with solutions for which compatibility have not been established; in particular, this applies to alkaline solutions since a precipitate may form.

The recommended IV dosage is three 0.15 mg/kg doses or a single 32 mg dose. With the 3 dose regimen, the first dose is infused over 15 minutes beginning 30 minutes before the start of emetogenic chemotherapy. Subsequent doses are administered 4 and 8 hours after the first dose. The single 32 mg dose is infused over 15 minutes beginning 30 minutes before the start of emetogenic chemotherapy.

Children: On the basis of the limited available information, the dosage in children 4 to 18 years of age should be three 0.15 mg/kg doses (see above). Little information is available about dosage in children ≤ 3 years of age.

Oral – Recommended dose is 8 mg twice daily. Administer the first dose 30 minutes before the start of emetogenic chemotherapy, with a subsequent dose 8 hours after the first dose. Administer 8 mg twice a day (every 12 hours) for 1 to 2 days after completion of chemotherapy.

Children: For patients ≥ 12 years of age, dosage is same as adults; for children 4 to 11 years, use 4 mg 3 times a day. Give the first dose 30 min before chemotherapy, with subsequent doses 4 and 8 hours after the first dose. Give 4 mg 3 times a day (every 8 hours) for 1 to 2 days after completion of chemotherapy.

Prevention of postoperative nausea or vomiting:

Parenteral – Immediately before induction of anesthesia, or postoperatively if the patient experiences nausea or vomiting occurring shortly after surgery, administer 4 mg undiluted IV in not less than 30 seconds, preferably over 2 to 5 minutes. Repeat dosing for patients who continue to experience nausea or vomiting postoperatively has not been studied.

Oral – 16 mg given as a single dose 1 hour before induction of anesthesia.

Children – There is no experience in children for this use.

Hepatic function impairment: Do not exceed an 8 mg oral dose. For IV use, a single maximum daily dose of 8 mg infused over 15 minutes beginning 30 minutes before the start of emetogenic chemotherapy is recommended.

GRANISETRON HCl

Injection: 1 mg/ml as free base (1.12 mg/ml as HCl) (*Rx*) *Kytril* (SK-Beecham Pharm)
Tablets: 1 mg (1.12 mg as HCl) (*Rx*)

Actions:

Pharmacology: Granisetron, an antinauseant and antiemetic agent, is a selective 5-hydroxytryptamine$_3$ (5-HT$_3$) receptor antagonist with little or no affinity for other serotonin, alpha- or beta-adrenergic, dopamine-D$_2$, histamine-H$_1$, benzodiazepine, picrotoxin or opioid receptors.

Serotonin receptors of the 5-HT$_3$ type are located peripherally on vagal nerve terminals and centrally in the chemoreceptor trigger zone. Granisetron blocks serotonin stimulation and subsequent vomiting after emetogenic stimuli such as cisplatin.

Pharmacokinetics: No difference in mean AUC was found between males and females, although males had a higher C_{max} generally.

Granisetron metabolism involves N-demethylation and aromatic ring oxidation followed by conjugation. Some of the metabolites may also have 5-HT$_3$ receptor antagonist activity.

Clearance is predominantly by hepatic metabolism, possibly mediated by the cytochrome P-450 3A subfamily. In healthy volunteers, ≈ 12% of the administered dose is eliminated unchanged in the urine in 48 hours. The remainder of the dose is excreted as metabolites, 49% in the urine and 34% in the feces.

Plasma protein binding is ≈ 65%; the drug distributes freely between plasma and red blood cells.

Indications:

Antiemetic: Prevention of nausea and vomiting associated with initial and repeat courses of emetogenic cancer therapy, including high-dose cisplatin.

Contraindications:

Hypersensitivity to the drug.

Warnings:

Hepatic function impairment: In patients with hepatic impairment due to neoplastic liver involvement, total clearance was approximately halved compared to patients without hepatic impairment. However, given the wide variability in pharmacokinetic parameters noted in patients and the good tolerance of doses well above the recommended 10 mcg/kg dose, dosage adjustment in patients with possible hepatic function impairment is not necessary.

Carcinogenesis/Mutagenesis: Granisetron produced a significant increase in UDS in HeLa cells in vitro and a significant increased incidence of cells with polyploidy in an in vitro human lymphocyte chromosomal aberration test.

Elderly: The pharmacokinetics in elderly volunteers (mean age, 71 years) given a single 40 mcg/kg IV dose were generally similar to those in younger healthy volunteers; mean values were lower for clearance and longer for half-life in the elderly.

Pregnancy: *Category B.*

Lactation: It is not known whether granisetron is excreted in breast milk.

Children: Safety and efficacy in children < 2 years of age have not been established. See Administration and Dosage for use in children 2 to 16 years of age. Safety and efficacy of the oral doseform in children has not been established.

Drug Interactions:

Because granisetron is metabolized by hepatic cytochrome P-450 drug-metabolizing enzymes, inducers or inhibitors of these enzymes may change the clearance and, hence, the half-life of granisetron.

Drug/Food interactions: When a single oral 10 mg dose was administered with food, AUC was decreased by 5% and C_{max} increased by 30% in non-fasted healthy volunteers.

Adverse Reactions:

Adverse reactions with granisetron may include headache, asthenia, somnolence, abdominal pain, nausea, vomiting, dizziness, insomnia, leukopenia, decreased appetite, anemia, alopecia, thrombocytopenia, fever, diarrhea, constipation and elevations of AST and ALT > 2 times the upper limit of normal.

Administration and Dosage:

IV: The recommended dosage is 10 mcg/kg infused IV over 5 minutes, beginning within 30 minutes before initiation of chemotherapy, and only on the day(s) chemotherapy is given.

Children – The recommended dose in children 2 to 16 years of age is 10 mcg/kg. Children < 2 years of age have not been studied.

Elderly, renal or hepatic function impairment – No dosage adjustment is recommended.

Infusion preparation – Dilute granisetron in 0.9% Sodium Chloride or 5% Dextrose to a total volume of 20 to 50 ml.

Admixture incompatibility – As a general precaution, granisetron injection should not be mixed in solution with other drugs.

Oral: 1 mg twice daily. Give the first dose up to 1 hour before chemotherapy and the second dose 12 hours after the first, only on the day(s) chemotherapy is given. Continued treatment while not on chemotherapy has not been found to be useful.

Children – Data not available.

Elderly, renal/hepatic function impairment – No dosage adjustment is recommended.

MEPROBAMATE

Tablets: 200, 400 and 600 mg (*c-iv*)	Various, *Equanil* (Wyeth-Ayerst), *Miltown* (Wallace)
Capsules, sustained release: 200 and 400 mg (*c-iv*)	*Merospan* (Wallace)

Actions:

Pharmacology: Meprobamate, an antianxiety agent, is a carbamate derivative that has selective effects at multiple sites in the CNS, including the thalamus and limbic system. It also appears to inhibit multineuronal spinal reflexes. Meprobamate is mildly tranquilizing, and has some anticonvulsant and muscle relaxant properties.

Pharmacokinetics:

Absorption/Distribution – Meprobamate is well absorbed from the GI tract; peak plasma concentrations are reached within 1 to 3 hours. During chronic administration of sedative doses, concentrations in blood range between 5 and 20 mcg/ml. Plasma protein binding is approximately 15%.

Metabolism/Excretion – The liver metabolizes 80% to 92% of the drug; the remainder is excreted unchanged in the urine. Following a single dose, the plasma half-life ranges from 6 to 17 hours, but during chronic administration, may be as long as 24 to 48 hours. Meprobamate can induce some hepatic microsomal enzymes, but it is not known whether it induces its own metabolism. Excretion is mainly renal (90%), with < 10% appearing in feces.

Indications:

Management of anxiety disorders or short-term relief of the symptoms of anxiety.

Contraindications:

Acute intermittent porphyria; allergic or idiosyncratic reactions to meprobamate or related compounds.

Warnings:

Drug dependence: Physical and psychological dependence and abuse may occur. Avoid prolonged use, especially in alcoholics and addiction prone persons. Consider possibility of suicide attempts. Carefully supervise dose and amounts prescribed; dispense least amount of drug feasible at any one time.

Abrupt discontinuation after prolonged and excessive use may precipitate a recurrence of pre-existing symptoms or withdrawal syndrome characterized by anxiety, anorexia, insomnia, vomiting, ataxia, tremors, muscle twitching, confusional states and hallucinations. Generalized seizures occur in about 10% of cases and are more likely to occur in persons with CNS damage or preexistent or latent convulsive disorders. Onset of withdrawal symptoms usually occurs within 12 to 48 hours after drug discontinuation; symptoms usually cease in the next 12 to 48 hours.

When excessive dosage has continued for weeks or months, reduce gradually over a period of 1 or 2 weeks rather than stopping abruptly.

Hypersensitivity: Usually seen between the first to fourth dose in patients having no previous exposure to the drug. Refer to Management of Acute Hypersensitivity Reactions.

Renal function impairment: Use with caution to avoid accumulation, since meprobamate is metabolized in the liver and excreted by the kidney.

Elderly: To avoid oversedation, use lowest effective dose.

Pregnancy: Category D. Meprobamate passes the placental barrier. It is present in umbilical cord blood, at or near maternal plasma levels. An increased risk of congenital malformations is associated with its use during the first trimester of pregnancy.

Lactation: Meprobamate is excreted into breast milk at concentrations 2 to 4 times that of maternal plasma.

Children: Do not administer to children < 6 years of age. The 600 mg tablet is not intended for use in children.

Precautions:

Epilepsy: May precipitate seizures in epileptic patients.

Hazardous tasks: May produce drowsiness, dizziness or blurred vision; patients should observe caution while driving or performing other tasks requiring alertness.

Drug Interactions:

Alcohol: Acute ingestion may result in a decreased clearance of meprobamate through inhibition of hepatic metabolic systems; enhanced CNS depressant effects may occur.

Adverse Reactions:

Adverse reactions may include: Drowsiness; ataxia; dizziness; slurred speech; headache; vertigo; weakness; impairment of visual accommodation; euphoria; overstimulation; paradoxical excitement; nausea; vomiting; diarrhea; palpitations; tachycardia; various arrhythmias; syncope; hypotensive crises; allergic/idiosyncratic reactions; leukopenia; acute nonthrombocytopenic purpura; petechiae; ecchymoses; eosinophilia; peripheral edema; fever; hyperpyrexia; chills; angioneurotic edema; bronchospasm; oliguria; anuria; anaphylaxis; erythema multiforme; exfoliative dermatitis; stomatitis; proctitis; Stevens-Johnson syndrome; bullous dermatitis; paresthesias; agranulocytosis; aplastic anemia; thrombocytopenic purpura.

Administration and Dosage:

Adults: 1.2 to 1.6 g/day in 3 to 4 divided doses; do not exceed 2.4 g/day.

Sustained release – 400 to 800 mg in the morning and at bedtime.

Children: 100 to 200 mg 2 or 3 times daily.

Sustained release – 200 mg in the morning and at bedtime.

BENZODIAZEPINES

OXAZEPAM	
Capsules: 10, 15 or 30 mg (*c-iv*)	Various, *Serax* (Weth-Ayerst)
Tablets: 15 mg (*c-iv*)	Various, *Serax* (Weth-Ayerst)
PRAZEPAM	
Capsules: 5, 10 or 20 mg (*c-iv*)	Various, *Centrax* (Parke-Davis)
Tablets: 5 or 10 mg (*c-iv*)	Various, *Centrax* (Parke-Davis)
LORAZEPAM	
Tablets: 0.5, 1 or 2 mg (*c-iv*)	Various, *Ativan* (Wyeth-Ayerst)
Concentrated oral solution: 2 mg/ml (*c-iv*)	*Lorazepam Intensol* (Roxane)
Injection: 2 or 4 mg/ml (*c-iv*)	Various, *Ativan* (Wyeth-Ayerst)
ALPRAZOLAM	
Tablets: 0.25, 0.5 1 or 2 mg (*c-iv*)	Various, *Xanax* (Upjohn)
Oral solution: 0.5 mg/5 ml (*c-iv*)	*Alprazolam* (Roxane)
Intensol solution: 1 mg/ml (*c-iv*)	*Alprazolam* (Roxane)
CHLORDIAZEPOXIDE	
Capsules: 5, 10 or 25 mg (*c-iv*)	Various, *Librium* (Roche)
Tablets: 10 or 25 mg (*c-iv*)	*Libritabs* (Roche)
Powder for Injection: 100 mg (*c-iv*)	*Librium* (Roche)
DIAZEPAM	
Tablets: 2, 5 or 10 mg (*c-iv*)	Various, *Valium* (Roche), *Dizac* (Ohmeda)
Oral solution: 5 mg/5 ml(*c-iv*)	Various
Oral solution, intensol: 5 mg/ml (*c-iv*)	*Diazepam Intensol* (Roxane)
Injection: 5 mg/ml (*c-iv*)	Various, *Valium* (Roche)
CLORAZEPATE DIPOTASSIUM	
Capsules: 3.75, 7.5 or 15 mg (*c-iv*)	Various
Tablets: 3.75, 7.5 or 15 mg (*c-iv*)	Various, *Tranxene* (Abbott)
Tablets: 11.25 or 22.5 mg (*c-iv*)	*Tranxene-SD Half Strength* (Abbott), *Tranxene-SD* (Abbott)

Actions:

Pharmacology: Benzodiazepines appear to potentiate the effects of gamma-aminobutyrate (GABA) (ie, they facilitate inhibitory GABA neurotransmission) and other inhibitory transmitters by binding to specific benzodiazepine receptor sites.

Pharmacokinetics:

Absorption – Benzodiazepines are readily absorbed following oral administration.

IM administration of chlordiazepoxide and diazepam results in slow erratic absorption and lower peak plasma levels than oral or IV administration. However, IM administration of diazepam into the deltoid muscle is more likely to be rapid and complete. Lorazepam IM is rapidly and completely absorbed.

Distribution – The highly lipid soluble benzodiazepines are widely distributed in the body tissues and highly bound to plasma proteins (70% to 99%).

Metabolism –

Benzodiazepine Metabolic Pathways

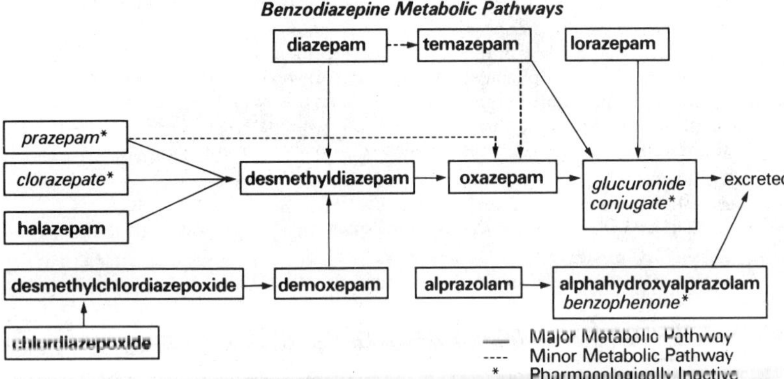

Excretion – Elimination – Most of the benzodiazepines are excreted almost entirely in the urine and in the form of oxidized and glucuronide-conjugated metabolites.

Benzodiazepine Pharmacokinetics

Drug	Dosage Range (mg/day)[1]	Peak Plasma Level (hrs)[1]	Elimination t½ (hrs.)	Metabolites	Speed of Onset[1]	Protein Binding
Alprazolam	0.75-4	1-2	6.3-26.9	Alpha-hydroxyalprazolam; Benzophenone	inter-mediate	80%
Chlordiazepoxide	15-100	0.5-4	5-30	Desmethyl-chlordiazepoxide[2]; Demoxepam; Desmethyldiazepam	inter-mediate	96%
Clonazepam	1.5-20	1-2	18-50	Inactive 7–amino or 7–acetylamino derivatives[2]	inter-mediate	97%
Clorazepate	15-60	1-2	40-50	Desmethyldiazepam	fast	97%-98%
Diazepam	4-40	0.5-2	20-80	Desmethyldiazepam[2]; nordiazepam	very fast	98%
Halazepam	60-160	1-3	14	Desmethyldiazepam[2]; 3-hydroxyhalazepam	slow	97%
Lorazepam	2-4	2-4	10-20	Inactive glucuronide conjugate	inter-mediate	85%
Oxazepam	30-120	2-4	5-20	Inactive glucuronide conjugate	slow	87%

[1] Oral administration.
[2] Major metabolite.
[3] Nordiazepam (active metabolite).

Indications:

Anxiety: For the management of anxiety disorders or for the short-term relief of the symptoms of anxiety. Anxiety or tension associated with the stress of everyday life usually does not require treatment with an antianxiety agent.

Unlabeled uses: Management of irritable bowel syndrome; panic attacks; depression; premenstrual syndrome; status epilepticus, chemotherapy-induced nausea and vomiting, acute alcohol withdrawal syndrome, psychogenic catatonia; chronic insomnia.

Contraindications:

Hypersensitivity to benzodiazepines; psychoses; acute narrow-angle glaucoma; patients with clinical or biochemical evidence of significant liver disease (clonazepam); intra-arterial use (lorazepam injection); children < 6 months, lactation (diazepam); coadministration with ketoconazole and itraconazole due to inhibition of cytochrome P450 3A.

Warnings:

Psychiatric disorders: These agents are not intended for use in patients with a primary depressive disorder or psychosis, nor in those psychiatric disorders in which anxiety is not a prominent feature.

Dependence: Prolonged use of therapeutic doses can lead to dependence. Withdrawal syndrome has occurred after as little as 4 to 6 weeks of treatment. It is more likely if the drug was short-acting (eg, alprazolam), if it was taken regularly for > 3 months and if it was abruptly discontinued. Higher dosages may not be a factor affecting withdrawal.

Parenteral administration – Parenteral (IM or IV) therapy is indicated primarily in acute states. Keep patients under observation, preferably in bed, for up to 3 hours.

Renal function impairment: Observe usual precautions in the presence of impaired renal or hepatic function to avoid accumulation of these agents.

Elderly: The initial dose should be small and dosage increments made gradually, in accordance with the response of the patient, to preclude ataxia or excessive sedation.

Pregnancy: *Category D.* Benzodiazepines and their metabolites freely cross the placenta and accumulate in the fetal circulation.

Lactation: Benzodiazepines are excreted in breast milk (**lorazepam** not known). Chronic **diazepam** use in nursing mothers reportedly caused infants to become lethargic and to lose weight; do not give to nursing mothers.

Children:

Chlordiazepoxide is not recommended in children < 6 years (oral) or 12 years (injectable).

Halazepam, prazepam, alprazolam – Safety and efficacy for use in patients < 18 years old have not been established.

Lorazepam – Do not use in patients < 18 years old (injection); safety and efficacy for use in patients < 12 years old are not established (oral).

Clorazepate – Not recommended for use in patients < 9 years old.

Diazepam – Not for use in children < 6 months old (oral); safety and efficacy have not been established in the neonate (≤ 30 days old; injectable).

Precautions:

Monitoring: Because of isolated reports of neutropenia and jaundice, perform periodic blood counts and liver function tests during long-term therapy.

Suicide: In those patients in whom depression accompanies anxiety, suicidal tendencies may be present, and protective measures may be required. Dispense the least amount of drug feasible to the patient.

Paradoxical reactions: Excitement, stimulation and acute rage have occurred in psychiatric patients and hyperactive aggressive children. These reactions may be secondary to relief of anxiety and usually appear in the first 2 weeks of therapy.

Multiple seizure type: When used in patients in whom several different types of seizure disorders coexist, **clonazepam** may increase the incidence or precipitate the onset of generalized tonic-clonic (grand mal) seizures.

Chronic respiratory disease: **Clonazepam** may produce an increase in salivation. Use with caution in patients if increased salivation causes respiratory difficulty.

Hazardous tasks: May produce drowsiness or dizziness; observe caution while driving or performing other tasks requiring alertness.

Drug Interactions:

Drugs that may affect benzodiazepines include cimetidine, oral contraceptives, disulfiram, fluoxetine, isoniazid, ketoconazole, metoprolol, propoxyphene, propranolol, valproic acid, alcohol, barbiturates, narcotics, antacide, probenecid, ranitidine, rifampin, scopolamine and theophyllines.

Drugs that may be affected by benzodiazepines include digoxin, levodopa, neuromuscular blocking agents and phenytoin.

Adverse Reactions:

CNS: Sedation and sleepiness; depression; lethargy; apathy; fatigue; hypoactivity; lightheadedness; memory impairment; disorientation; anterograde amnesia; restlessness; confusion; crying; sobbing; delirium; headache; slurred speech; stupor; seizures; coma; syncope; rigidity; tremor; vertigo; dizziness; euphoria; nervousness; irritability; difficulty in concentration; agitation; inability to perform complex mental functions; unsteadiness; ataxia; incoordination; weakness; vivid dreams.

Psychiatric: Behavior problems; hysteria; psychosis; suicidal tendencies.

GI: Constipation; diarrhea; dry mouth; sore gums; nausea; anorexia; change in appetite; vomiting; difficulty in swallowing; increased salivation; gastritis.

GU: Incontinence; changes in libido; urinary retention; menstrual irregularities.

Cardiovascular: Bradycardia; tachycardia; cardiovascular collapse; hypertension; hypotension; palpitations; edema.

Ophthalmic: Visual disturbances; diplopia; nystagmus.

Respiratory: Respiratory disturbances; nasal congestion.

Dermatologic: Urticaria; pruritus; skin rash; dermatitis; hair loss; hirsutism; ankle and facial edema.

Body as a whole: Depressed hearing; auditory disturbances; hiccoughs; fever; diaphoresis; paresthesias; muscular disturbance; gynecomastia; galactorrhea; leukopenia; blood dyscrasias including agranulocytosis; anemia; thrombocytopenia; eosinophilia; increase or decrease in body weight; dehydration; joint pain.

Administration and Dosage:

OXAZEPAM:

Mild to moderate anxiety, with associated tension, irritability, agitation or related symptoms of functional origin or secondary to organic disease – 10 to 15 mg 3 or 4 times daily.

Severe anxiety syndomrs, agitation or anxiety associated with depressioin – 15 to 30 mg 3 or 4 times daily.

Older patients with anxiety, tension, irritability and agitation – Initial dosage is 10 mg 3 times daily. If necessary, increase cautionsly to 15 mg 3 or 4 times daily.

Alcoholics with acute inebriation, tremulousness or anxiety on withdrawal – 15 to 30 mg 3 or 4 times daily.

Children (6 to 12 years) – Dosage is not established.

PRAZEPAM: The usual dose is 30 mg/day administered in divided doses. Adjust dosage gradually within the range of 20 to 60 mg/day.

Elderly – Initiate treatment at 10 to 15 mg/day in divided doses.

May also be administered as a single daily dose at bedtime. The starting dose is 20 mg/night. The optimum dose ranges from 20 to 40 mg.

LORAZEPAM:

Oral – 2 to 6 mg/day (varies from 1 to 10 mg/day) given in divided doses; take the largest dose before bedtime.

Anxiety: Initial dose, 2 to 3 mg/day given 2 or 3 times daily.

Insomnia due to anxiety or transient situational stress: 2 to 4 mg at bedtime.

Elderly or debilitated patients: Initial dose, 1 to 2 mg/day in divided doses.

IM – 0.05 mg/kg up to a maximum of 4 mg. For optimum effect, administer at least 2 hours before operative procedure.

IV – Initial dose is 2 mg total or 0.044 mg/kg (0.02 mg/lb), whichever is smaller. This will sedate most adults; ordinarily, do not exceed in patients > 50 years old. If a greater lack of recall would be beneficial, doses as high as 0.05 mg/kg up to a total of 4 mg may be given. For optimum effect, give 15 to 20 minutes before the procedure.

Children (< 18 years) – Parenteral use is not recommended.

ALPRAZOLAM: Reduce gradually when terminating or decreasing daily dose. Decrease by no more than 0.5 mg every 3 days.

Anxiety disorders – Initial dose is 0.25 to 0.5 mg 3 times/day. Titrate to max total dose of 4 mg/day in divided doses.

Elderly or debilitated patients – 0.25 mg, given 2 or 3 times daily. Gradually increase if needed and tolerated.

Panic disorder – Initial dose is 0.5 mg 3 times daily. Depending on response, increase dose at intervals of 3 to 4 days in increments of no more than 1 mg/day.

Successful treatment has required doses > 4 mg/day; in controlled studies, doses in the range of 1 to 10 mg/day were used.

CHLORDIAZEPOXIDE:

Oral –

Mild to moderate anxiety: 5 or 10 mg 3 or 4 times daily.

Severe anxiety: 20 or 25 mg 3 or 4 times daily.

Geriatric patients or patients with debilitating disease: 5 mg 2 to 4 times daily.

Preoperative apprehension and anxiety: On days preceding surgery, 5 to 10 mg 3 or 4 times daily.

Acute alcohol withdrawal: 50 to 100 mg; repeat as needed (up to 300 mg/day). Parenteral form usually used initially. Reduce to maintenance levels.

Children: Initially, 5 mg 2 to 4 times daily (may be increased in some children to 10 mg 2 or 3 times daily). Not recommended in children under 6 years of age.

A dosage of 0.5 mg/kg/day every 6 to 8 hours inchildren > 6 years of age has also been recommended.

Parenteral – Use lower doses (25 to 50 mg) for elderly or debilitated patients and for older children. A dosage of 0.5 mg/kg/day every 6 to 8 hours IM in children > 12 years of age has also been recommended. Acute symptoms may be rapidly controlled by parenteral administration; subsequent treatment, if necessary, may be given orally. While 300 mg may be given during a 6 hour period, do not exceed this dose in any 24 hour period. Not recommended in children < 12 years of age.

Acute alcohol withdrawal: 50 to 100 mg IM or IV initially; repeat in 2 to 4 hours if necessary.

Acute or severe anxiety: 50 to 100 mg IM or IV initially; then 25 to 50 mg 3 or 4 times daily if necessary.

Preoperative apprehension/anxiety: 50 to 100 mg IM 1 hour prior to surgery.

DIAZEPAM:

Oral –

Management of anxiety disorders and relief of symptoms of anxiety (depending upon severity of symptoms): 2 to 10 mg 2 to 4 times daily.

Acute alcohol withdrawal: 10 mg 3 or 4 times during the first 24 hours; reduce to 5 mg 3 or 4 times daily, as needed.

Adjunct in skeletal muscle spasm: 2 to 10 mg 3 or 4 times daily.

Adjunct in convulsive disorders: 2 to 10 mg 2 to 4 times daily.

Elderly patients or in the presence of debilitating disease: 2 to 2.5 mg 1 or 2 times daily initially; increase gradually as needed and tolerated.

Children: 1 to 2.5 mg 3 or 4 times daily initially; increase gradually as needed and tolerated. Not for use in children under 6 months. For sedation or muscle relaxation, a dosage of 0.12 to 0.8 mg/kg/24 hours divided 3 to 4 times a day has been recommended.

Oral, sustained release – Do not crush or chew sustained release formula

Whenever oral diazepam 5 mg 3 times a day would be considered appropriate dosage, one 15 mg sustained release capsule daily may be used.

Management of anxiety disorders and relief of symptoms of anxiety: 15 to 30 mg/day, depending upon severity of symptoms.

Adjunct in skeletal muscle spasm: 15 to 30 mg/day.

Oral, solution – Dosage same as oral tablets.

Intensol: The **Intensol** is a concentrated oral solution as compared to standard oral liquid medications. It is recommended that the **Intensol** be mixed with liquid or semisolid food such as water, juices, soda or soda-like beverages, applesauce and puddings. Use only the calibrated dropper provided with the product.

Parenteral –

Children: Administer slowly over 3 minutes. Do not exceed 0.25 mg/kg. After an interval of 15 to 30 minutes, the initial dose can be repeated.

Moderate anxiety disorders and symptoms of anxiety: 2 to 5 mg IM or IV. Repeat in 3 to 4 hours if necessary.

Severe anxiety disorders and symptoms of anxiety: 5 to 10 mg IM or IV. Repeat in 3 to 4 hours if necessary.

Acute alcohol withdrawal: 10 mg IM or IV initially; then 5 to 10 mg in 3 to 4 hours if necessary.

Endoscopic procedures:

IV – 10 mg or less is usually adequate; up to 20 mg may be used, especially when concomitant narcotics are omitted.

IM – 5 to 10 mg 30 minutes prior to procedure if IV route cannot be used.

Muscle spasm: 5 to 10 mg IM or IV initially; then 5 to 10 mg in 3 to 4 hours if necessary. Tetanus may require larger doses.

Status epilepticus and severe recurrent convulsive seizures: The IV route is preferred; administer slowly. Use the IM route if IV administration is impossible. Administer 5 to 10 mg initially; repeat if necessary at 10 to 15 minute intervals up to maximum dose of 30 mg. If necessary, repeat therapy in 2 to 4 hours. A dose of 0.2 to 0.5 mg/kg every 15 to 30 minutes for 2 to 3 doses (maximum dose, 30 mg).

Infants (over 30 days of age) and children (under 5 years): Inject 0.2 to 0.5 mg slowly every 2 to 5 minutes up to a maximum of 5 mg; 0.2 to 0.5 mg/kg/dose every 15 to 30 minutes for 2 to 3 doses (maximum dose, 5 mg) has been recommended.

Neonates: 0.5 to 1 mg/kg/dose every 15 to 30 minutes for 2 to 3 doses has been suggested.

Preoperative medication: 10 mg IM before surgery.

Cardioversion: 5 to 15 mg IV, 5 to 10 minutes prior to procedure.

Tetanus:

Infants (over 30 days of age) – 1 to 2 mg IM or IV slowly, repeated every 3 to 4 hours as necessary.

Children (5 years or older) – 5 to 10 mg repeated every 3 to 4 hours may be required.

Sedation or muscle relaxation:

Children – 0.04 to 0.2 mg/kg/dose every 2 to 4 hours, maximum of 0.6 mg/kg within an 8 hour period.

Adults – 2 to 10 mg/dose every 3 to 4 hours as needed.

HALAZEPAM: The usual dose is 20 to 40 mg 3 or 4 times a day. The optimal dosage usually ranges from 80 to 160 mg daily.

Elderly (≥ 70 years) or debilitated patients – 20 mg once or twice/day.

CHLORAZEPATE DIPOTASSIUM:

Symptomatic relief of anxiety – 30 mg/day in divided doses. Adjust gradually within the range of 15 to 60 mg/day. *Elderly or debilitated patients* — Initiate treatment at a dose of 7.5 to 15 mg/day.

Maintenance therapy: Give the 22.5 mg tablet in a single daily dose as an alternate dosage form for patients stabilized on 7.5 mg 3 times/day. Do not use to initiate therapy. The 11.25 mg tablet may be administered as a single dose every 24 hours.

Symptomatic relief of acute alcohol withdrawal –

Day 1: 30 mg initially, followed by 30 to 60 mg in divided doses.

Day 2: 45 to 90 mg in divided doses.

Day 3: 22.5 to 45 mg in divided doses.

Day 4: 15 to 30 mg in divided doses.

Thereafter, gradually reduce the dose to 7.5 to 15 mg once daily. Discontinue drug as soon as patient's condition is stable.

The maximum recommended total daily dose is 90 mg. Avoid excessive reductions in the totalk amount of drug administered on successive days.

BUSPIRONE HCl

Tablets: 5 and 10 mg (*Rx*)	*BuSpar* (Mead Johnson Pharm)

Actions:

Pharmacology: Mechanism of action is unknown. It differs from benzodiazepines in that it does not exert anticonvulsant or muscle relaxant effects. It also lacks prominent sedative effects associated with more typical anxiolytics. In vitro, buspirone has a high affinity for serotonin ($5\text{-}HT_1A$) receptors. Buspirone has moderate affinity for brain D_2-dopamine receptors and appears to act as a presynaptic dopamine agonist. It also increases norepinephrine metabolism in the locus ceruleus.

Pharmacokinetics:

Absorption – Buspirone is rapidly absorbed and undergoes extensive first-pass metabolism.

Distribution – Approximately 95% of buspirone is plasma protein bound.

Metabolism – Buspirone is metabolized primarily by oxidation, producing several hydroxylated derivatives and a pharmacologically active metabolite, 1-pyrimidinyl piperazine (1-PP).

Elimination: In a single dose study, 29% to 63% of the dose was excreted in the urine within 24 hours, primarily as metabolites; fecal excretion accounted for 18% to 38% of the dose. The average elimination half-life of unchanged buspirone after single doses of 10 to 40 mg is about 2 to 3 hours (range, 2 to 11 hours).

Indications:

Management of anxiety disorders or short-term relief of symptoms of anxiety.

Unlabeled uses: Buspirone may be useful in decreasing the symptoms of premenstrual syndrome.

Contraindications:

Hypersensitivity to buspirone HCl.

Warnings:

Renal/Hepatic function impairment: Since buspirone is metabolized by the liver and excreted by the kidneys, do not use in patients with severe hepatic or renal impairment.

Elderly: No unusual adverse age-related phenomena have been identified.

Pregnancy: Category B.

Lactation: The extent of the excretion in breast milk of buspirone or its metabolites is not known.

Children: Safety and efficacy for use in children < 18 years are not known.

Precautions:

Interference with cognitive and motor performance: Buspirone is less sedating than other anxiolytics and does not produce significant functional impairment. However, its CNS effect may not be predictable. Therefore, caution patients about driving or using complex machinery until they are certain that buspirone does not affect them adversely.

Withdrawal reactions: Withdraw patients from their prior treatment gradually before starting buspirone, especially patients who have been using a CNS depressant chronically.

Dopamine receptor binding: Buspirone can bind to central dopamine receptors.

Monitoring: Patients have been treated for several months without ill effect. If used for extended periods, periodically reassess the usefulness of the drug.

Drug Interactions:

Drugs that may interact with buspirone include alcohol, haloperidol, monoamine oxidase inhibitors and trazodone.

Drug/Food interactions: Administration with food may decrease the rate of absorption, but it may increase the bioavailability by decreasing the first-pass metabolism.

Adverse Reactions:

Adverse reactions occurring in ≥ 3% of patients include dizziness, drowsiness, nervousness, insomnia, lightheadedness, nausea, dry mouth, headache and fatigue.

Administration and Dosage:

Initial dose: 15 mg daily (5 mg 3 times a day).

To achieve an optimal therapeutic response, increase the dosage 5 mg/day, at intervals of 2 to 3 days, as needed. Do not exceed 60 mg/day. Divided doses of 20 to 30 mg/day have been commonly used.

HYDROXYZINE

Tablets: 10, 25, 50 and 100 mg (as HCl) (*Rx*)	Various, *Atarax* (Roerig)
Syrup: 10 mg per 5 ml (as HCl)	Various, *Atarax* (Roerig)
Capsules: 25, 50 and 100 mg (as pamoate equivalent to HCl)	Various, *Vistaril* (Pfizer)
Oral Suspension: 25 mg per 5 ml (as pamoate equiv. to HCl)	
Injection: 25 and 50 mg/ml (as HCl)	Various, *Vistaril* (Pfizer), *Hyzine-50* (Hyrex), *Quiess* (Forest)

Actions:

Pharmacology: Hydroxyzine is a piperazine antihistamine. It is not a cortical depressant; its action may be due to suppressing activity in subcortical areas of CNS.

Bronchodilator activity, antihistaminic and analgesic effects have been confirmed. Hydroxyzine has antispasmodic properties, apparently mediated through interference with the mechanism that responds to spasmogenic agents such as serotonin, acetylcholine and histamine. An antiemetic effect has been demonstrated.

Pharmacokinetics: Oral hydroxyzine is rapidly absorbed from the GI tract; clinical effects are usually noted within 15 to 30 minutes after administration. Mean elimination half-life is 3 hours; half-life may be longer in elderly patients. Hydroxyzine is mainly metabolized by the liver.

Indications:

Symptomatic relief of anxiety and tension associated with psychoneurosis and as an adjunct in organic disease states in which anxiety is manifest.

Management of pruritus due to allergic conditions such as chronic urticaria, atopic and contact dermatoses and in histamine-mediated pruritus.

As a sedative when used as premedication and following general anesthesia.

IM only: For the acutely disturbed or hysterical patient; the acute or chronic alcoholic with anxiety withdrawal symptoms or delirium tremens; as pre- and postoperative and pre- and postpartum adjunctive medication to permit reduction in narcotic dosage, allay anxiety and control emesis; adjunctive therapy in asthma.

Contraindications:

Hypersensitivity to hydroxyzine; early pregnancy, lactation.

Hydroxyzine injection is for IM use only. Do not inject SC, IV or intra-arterially.

Warnings:

Hypersensitivity reactions have occurred.

Pregnancy: Do not use in pregnancy.

Lactation: It is not known whether this drug is excreted in breast milk.

Precautions:

Potentially hazardous tasks: May produce drowsiness.

Drug Interactions:

Drugs that may interact with hydroxyzine include CNS depressants.

Adverse Reactions:

Adverse reactions may include Dry mouth; drowsiness; involuntary motor activity, including rare instances of tremor and convulsions; hypersensitivity reactions, including wheezing, dyspnea, chest tightness.

Administration and Dosage:

Start patients on IM therapy when indicated. Maintain on oral therapy whenever practicable. Adjust dosage according to patient's response.

Oral:

Symptomatic relief of anxiety – Adults: 50 to 100mg 4 times/day. Children (> 6): 50 to 100 mg/day in divided doses. Children (< 6): 50 mg/day in divided doses.

Management of pruritus – Adults: 25 mg 3 or 4 times daily. Children (> 6): 50 to 100 mg/day in divided doses. Children (< 6): 50 mg/day in divided doses.

Sedative (as premedication and following general anesthesia) – Adults: 50 to 100 mg. Children: 0.6 mg/kg.

IM: Inject well within the body of a relatively large muscle. In adults, the preferred site is the upper outer quadrant of the buttock or the midlateral thigh. In children, inject into the midlateral muscles of the thigh. In infants and small children, use the periphery of the upper outer quadrant of the gluteal region only when necessary, such as in burn patients, in order to minimuze the possibility of sciatic nerve damage.

Use the deltoid area only if well developed, and then only with caution to avoid radial nerve injury. Do not inject into the lower and mid-third of the upper arm.

For adult psychiatric and emotional emergencies, including acute alcoholism – 50 to 100 mg immediately and every 4 to 6 hours as needed.

Nausea and vomiting – Adults: 25 to 100 mg. Children: 1.1 mg/kg.

Pre- and postoperative adjunctive medication – Adults: 25 to 100 mg. Children: 1.1 mg/kg.

Pre- and postpartum adjunctive therapy – 25 to 100 mg.

DOXEPIN HCl

Doxepin is a tricyclic antidepressant which also has antianxiety effects. The following is an abbreviated monograph for doxepin. For complete information, refer to the Tricyclic Antidepressants monograph.

Indications:

For the treatment of psychoneurotic patients with depression or anxiety; depression or anxiety associated with alcoholism or organic disease; psychotic depressive disorders with associated anxiety including involutional depression and manic-depressive disorders.

The target symptoms of psychoneurosis that respond to doxepin include anxiety, tension, depression, somatic symptoms and concerns, insomnia, guilt, lack of energy, fear, apprehension and worry.

Administration and Dosage:

The total daily dosage may be given on a divided or once-a-day dosage schedule. If the once-a-day schedule is employed, the maximum recommended dose is 150 mg/day, given at bedtime.

Not recommended in children < 12 years old.

Mild to moderate severity: Start with 75 mg/day. The optimum dose range is 75 to 150 mg/day.

More severely ill: Gradual increase to 300 mg/day may be necessary. Additional therapeutic effect is rarely obtained by exceeding a dose of 300 mg/day.

Very mild symptoms or emotional symptoms accompanying organic disease: Some of these patients have been controlled on doses as low as 25 to 50 mg/day.

Dilute the oral concentrate with 120 ml of liquid (eg, water, milk and some fruit juices) just prior to administration; not compatible with a number of carbonated beverages. For patients on methadone maintenance taking oral doxepin, mix the concentrate with methadone and lemonade, orange juice, water, sugar water or powdered fruit drink. *Do not mix with grape juice*. Preparation and storage of bulk dilutions are not recommended.

ANTIDEPRESSANTS

Drugs with clinically useful antidepressant effects include the tricyclic antidepressants (TCAs), maprotiline, trazodone, bupropion, venlafaxine, nefazodone, selective serotonin reuptake inhibitors (SSRIs) and the monoamine oxidase inhibitors (MAOIs).

Mechanism of action: The emphasis of research has shifted from acute reuptake effects to the slower adaptive changes in norepinephrine and serotonin receptor systems induced by chronic antidepressant therapy. Postsynaptic receptors participate in nerve impulse neurotransmission while the presynaptic receptors regulate neurotransmitter release and reuptake, an important mechanism of neurotransmitter inactivation. Long-term antidepressant treatment produces complex changes in the sensitivities of both presynaptic and postsynaptic receptor sites. The available antidepressant agents may increase the sensitivity of postsynaptic alpha (α_1) adrenergic and serotonin receptors and may decrease the sensitivity of presynaptic receptor sites. The net effect is the correction (re-regulation) of an abnormal receptor-neurotransmitter relationship.

Drug selection: The non-MAOIs are used much more frequently than the MAOIs mainly because of (1) the perception that MAOIs are less effective than the non-MAOI antidepressants and (2) the risk of hypertensive crisis when the patient ingests foods containing tyramine or via drug interaction (eg, sympathomimetics) with the MAOIs. However, when MAOIs are used in therapeutic doses, they are probably equieffective to non-MAOIs for the treatment of depression. In general, MAOIs are used for atypical depression.

Base antidepressant drug selection on the patient's history of drug response (if any), the specific drug's side effect profile relative to patient medical conditions and other factors, and clinician familiarity with specific antidepressants. Trazodone has less anticholinergic activity than TCAs and causes fewer problems than TCAs when taken in overdose. SSRIs generally lack the adverse reactions (eg, sedation, anticholinergic effects) associated with TCAs, cause few cardiovascular side effects (including orthostasis), are associated with weight loss rather than weight gain as is the case with TCAs, and cause fewer problems than TCAs when taken in overdose. However, their use is associated with other side effects such as headache, nervousness and insomnia. Use maprotiline and bupropion only when other antidepressants have not proven effective. In cases of mild depression, drug therapy and psychotherapy appear to be equally effective.

Antidepressant Pharmacologic and Pharmacokinetic Parameters

0 -none + -slight ++ -moderate +++ -high ++++ -very high +++++ -highest	Major side effects			Amine uptake blocking activity					
	Anticholinergic	Sedation	Orthostatic hypotension	Norepinephrine	Serotonin	Half-life (hours)	Therapeutic plasma level (ng/ml)	Time to reach steady state (days)	Dose range (mg/day)
Tricyclics - Tertiary Amines									
Amitriptyline	++++	++++	++	++	++++	31-46	110-250[1]	4-10	50-300
Clomipramine	+++	+++	++	++	+++++	19-37	80-100	7-14	25-250
Doxepin	++	+++	++	+	++	8-24	100-200[1]	2-8	25-300
Imipramine	++	++	+++	++[2]	++++	11-25	200-350[1]	2-5	30-300
Trimipramine	++	+++	++	+	+	7-30	180[1]	2-6	50-300
Tricyclics - Secondary Amines									
Amoxapine[3]	+++	++	+	+++	++	8[4]	200-500	2-7	50-600
Desipramine	+	+	+	++++	++	12-24	125-300	2-11	25-300
Nortriptyline	++	++	+	++	+++	18-44	50-150	4-19	30-100
Protriptyline	+++	+	+	++++	++	67-89	100-200	14-19	15-60
Phenethylamine									

Antidepressant Pharmacologic and Pharmacokinetic Parameters

0 -none + -slight ++ -moderate +++ -high ++++ -very high +++++ -highest	Major side effects			Amine uptake blocking activity					
	Anticholinergic	Sedation	Orthostatic hypotension	Norepinephrine	Serotonin	Half-life (hours)	Therapeutic plasma level (ng/ml)	Time to reach steady state (days)	Dose range (mg/day)
Venlafaxine	0	0	0	+++	+++	5-11[1]	-	3-4	75-375
Tetracyclic									
Maprotiline	++	++	+	+++	0/+	21-25	200-300[1]	6-10	50-225
Triazolopyridine									
Trazodone	+	++	++	0	+++	4-9	800-1600	3-7	150-600
Aminoketone									
Bupropion[5]	++	++	+	0/+	0/+	8-24	-	1.5-5	200-450
Selective Serotonin Reuptake Inhibitors									
Fluoxetine	0/+	0/+	0/+	0/+	+++++	2-9 days[1]	-	2-4 weeks	20-80
Paroxetine	0	0/+	0	0/+	+++++	10-24	-	7-14	10-50
Sertraline	0	0/+	0	0/+	+++++	1-4[1]	-	7	50-200
Fluvoxamine	0/+	0/+	0	0/+	++++	15.6	-	3-8 hours	50-300
Monoamine Oxidase Inhibitors									
Tranylcypromine	+	+	0	-	-	2.4-2.8	-	-	30-60
Phenelzine	+	+	+	-	-	-	-	-	45-90
Miscellaneous									
Nefazodone	0/+	++	+	0/+	++++	2-4	-	4-5	200-600

[1] Parent compound plus active metabolite.
[2] Via desipramine, the major metabolite.
[3] Also blocks dopamine receptors.
[4] 30 hours for major metabolite 8-hydroxyamoxapine.
[5] Inhibits dopamine uptake.

TRICYCLIC COMPOUNDS

AMITRIPTYLINE	
Tablets: 10, 25, 50, 75, 100 and 150 mg (*Rx*)	Various, *Elavil* (Zeneca)
Injection: 10 mg/ml (*Rx*)	Various, *Elavil* (Zeneca)
NORTRIPTYLINE HCl	
Capsules: 10, 25, 50 and 75 mg (*Rx*)	Various, *Aventyl HCl Pulvules* (Lilly), *Pamelor* (Sandoz)
Solution: 10 mg/5 ml (*Rx*)	*Aventyl* (Lilly), *Pamelor* (Sandoz)
IMIPRAMINE HCl	
Tablets: 10, 25 and 50 mg (*Rx*)	Various, *Tofranil* (Geigy)
Injection: 25 mg/2 ml (*Rx*)	*Tofranil* (Geigy)
IMIPRAMINE PAMOATE	
Capsules: 75, 100, 125 and 150 mg (*Rx*)	*Tofranil-PM* (Geigy)
DOXEPIN HCl	
Capsules: 10, 25, 50, 100 and 150 mg (*Rx*)	Various, *Sinequan* (Roerig)
Oral concentrate: 10 mg/ml (*Rx*)	Various, *Sinequan* (Roerig)
TRIMIPRAMINE MALEATE	
Capsules: 25, 50 and 100 mg (*Rx*)	Various, *Surmontil* (Wyeth-Ayerst)
AMOXAPINE	

Tablets: 25, 50, 100 and 150 mg (*Rx*)	Various, *Asendin* (Lederle)
DESIPRAMINE HCl	
Tablets: 10, 25, 50, 75, 100 and 150 mg (*Rx*)	Various, *Norpramin* (Merrell Dow), *Pertofrane* (Rorer)
Capsules: 25 and 50 mg (*Rx*)	*Pertofrane* (Rorer)
PROTRIPTYLINE HCl	
Tablets: 5 and 10 mg (*Rx*)	*Vivactil* (Merck)
CLOMIPRAMINE HCl	
Capsules: 25, 50 and 75 mg (*Rx*)	*Anafranil* (Ciba)

Actions:

Pharmacology: The tricyclic antidepressants (TCAs), structurally related to the phenothiazine antipsychotic agents, possess three major pharmacologic actions in varying degrees: Blocking of the amine pump, sedation, and peripheral and central anticholinergic action. In contrast to phenothiazines, which act on dopamine recep- tors, TCAs inhibit reuptake of norepinephrine or serotonin (5-hydroxytryptamine, 5-HT) at the presynaptic neuron. Amoxapine, a metabolite of loxapine, retains some of the postsynaptic dopamine receptor-blocking action of neuroleptics.

Other pharmacological effects – Clinical effects, in addition to antidepressant effects, include sedation, anticholinergic effects, mild peripheral vasodilator effects and possible "quinidine-like" actions.

Pharmacokinetics:

Absorption/Distribution – The TCAs are well absorbed from the GI tract with peak plasma concentrations occurring in 2 to 4 hours; they undergo a significant first-pass effect. They are highly bound (> 90%) to plasma proteins, are lipid soluble and are widely distributed in tissues, including the CNS.

Metabolism/Excretion – Metabolism of TCAs occurs in the liver by demethylation, hydroxylation and glucuronidation, and it varies for each patient. Some intermediate active metabolites include:

Amitriptyline ➡nortriptyline
Amoxapine ➡7 hydroxy and 8 hydroxyamoxapine
Clomipramine ➡desmethylclomipramine
Doxepin ➡desmethyldoxepin
Imipramine ➡desipramine

Because of the long half-life, a single daily dose may be given. Up to 2 to 4 weeks may be required to achieve maximal clinical response.

Indications:

Relief of symptoms of depression (except clomipramine).

Agents with significant sedative action may be useful in depression associated with anxiety and sleep disturbances.

Doxepin: Anxiety.

Imipramine: Treatment of enuresis in children ≥ 6 years of age.

Clomipramine: Only for treatment of Obsessive-Compulsive Disorder (OCD).

Unlabeled uses:

Chronic pain(migraine, chronic tension headache, diabetic neuropathy, tic douloureux, cancer pain, peripheral neuropathy with pain, postherpetic neuralgia, arthritic pain) – Amitriptyline; doxepin; imipramine; clomipramine.

Pathologic laughing and weeping secondary to forebrain disease – Amitriptyline.

Obstructive sleep apnea – Protriptyline.

Peptic ulcer disease – Trimipramine; doxepin.

Facilitation of cocaine withdrawal – Desipramine.

Panic disorder – Imipramine; clomipramine; nortriptyline. Other antidepressants may also be used.

Eating disorders (effective in bulimia nervosa) – Imipramine; desipramine; amitriptyline.

Premenstrual depression – Nortriptyline.

Dermatologic disorders (chronic urticaria and angioedema, nocturnal pruritus in atopic eczema) – Doxepin; trimipramine; nortriptyline.

Contraindications:

Prior sensitivity to any tricyclic drug. Not recommended for use during the acute recovery phase following myocardial infarction. Concomitant use of monoamine oxidase inhibitors (MAOIs) is generally contraindicated.

Doxepin: Patients with glaucoma or a tendency for urinary retention.

Warnings:

Tardive dyskinesia a syndrome consisting of potentially irreversible, involuntary, dyskinetic movements may develop in patients treated with neuroleptics (eg, antipsychotics). Amoxapine is not an antipsychotic, but it has substantive neuroleptic activity.

Neuroleptic malignant syndrome (NMS) is a potentially fatal condition reported in association with antipsychotic drugs and with **amoxapine**.

Hyperthermia has occurred with **clomipramine;** most cases occurred when it was used with other drugs (eg, neuroleptics) and may be examples of an NMS.

Seizure disorders: Because TCAs lower the seizure threshold, use with caution in patients with a history of seizures. However, seizures have occurred both in patients with and without a history of seizure disorders. Seizure was identified as the most significant risk of **clomipramine** use.

Anticholinergic effects: Use with caution in patients with a history of urinary retention, urethral or ureteral spasm; angle-closure glaucoma or increased intraocular pressure.

Cardiovascular disorders: Use with extreme caution in patients with cardiovascular disorders (eg, severe coronary heart disease with ECG abnormalities, progressive heart failure, conduction disturbances, angina pectoris, paroxysmal tachycardia). In high doses, TCAs may produce arrhythmias, sinus tachycardia and prolong conduction time. Tachycardia and postural hypotension may occur more frequently with **protriptyline**.

Hyperthyroid patients: or those receiving thyroid medication require close supervision because of the possibility of cardiovascular toxicity, including arrhythmias.

Psychiatric patients: Schizophrenic or paranoid patients may exhibit a worsening of psychosis with TCA therapy, and manic-depressive patients may experience a shift to a hypomanic or manic phase; this may also occur when switching antidepressants and withdrawing them. In overactive or agitated patients, increased anxiety or agitation may occur. Paranoid delusions, with or without associated hostility, may be exaggerated. Reduction of TCA dosage and concomitant antipsychotic therapy may be necessary.

The possibility of suicide in depressed patients remains during treatment and until significant remission occurs. Patients should not have easy access to large quantities of the drug; prescribe small quantities of TCAs.

Renal/Hepatic function impairment: Use with caution and in reduced doses in patients with hepatic impairment; metabolism may be impaired, leading to drug accumulation. Use with caution in patients with significantly impaired renal function.

Pregnancy: (Category C - amoxapine, trimipramine; Category B - imipramine).

Lactation: These agents are excreted into breast milk in low concentrations (approximate milk:plasma ratio of 0.4 to 1.5).

Children: Not recommended for patients < 12 years of age. Safety and efficacy not established for **amoxapine** in children < 16 or **trazodone** or **clomipramine** in children < 10 years old. Safety and efficacy are not established in the pediatric age group for **trimipramine,nortriptyline** and **protriptyline**.

Do not exceed 2.5 mg/kg/day of **imipramine**.

Precautions:

Monitoring: Perform baseline and periodic leukocyte and differential counts and liver function studies. Fever or sore throat may signal serious neutrophil depression; discontinue therapy if there is evidence of pathological neutropenia.

Monitor ECG prior to initiation of large doses of TCAs and at appropriate intervals thereafter.

Electroconvulsive therapy: with coadministration of TCAs may increase the hazards of therapy.

Elective surgery: Discontinue therapy for as long as possible before elective surgery.

Elevated and lowered blood sugar levels have occurred.

Sexual dysfuntion was markedly increased in male patients with OCD taking clomipramine (42% ejaculatory failure, 20% impotence) compared to placebo.

Weight changes: Weight gain occurred in 18% of patients receiving **clomipramine**. Some patients had weight gain in excess of 25% of their initial body weight. Weight gain also occurs with other TCAs.

Hazardous tasks: May impair mental or physical abilities required for the performance of potentially hazardous tasks.

Photosensitivity: Photosensitization (photoallergy or phototoxicity) may occur.

Drug Interactions:

Drugs that may affect tricyclic compounds include barbiturates, charcoal, cimetidine, disulfiram, fluoxetine, haloperidol, oral contraceptives, phenothiazines and smoking.

Drugs that may be affected by tricyclic compounds include anticholinergics, clonidine, dicumarol, guanethidine, levodopa and MAOIs.

Adverse Reactions:

Sedation and anticholinergic effects are reported most frequently.

Withdrawal symptoms: Although not indicative of addiction, abrupt cessation after prolonged therapy may produce nausea, headache, vertigo, nightmares, malaise. Gradual dosage reduction may produce, within 2 weeks, transient symptoms including irritability, restlessness, dreams and sleep disturbance.

Enuretic children: Consider adverse reactions reported with adult use. Most common are nervousness, sleep disorders, tiredness and mild GI disturbances. These usually disappear with continued therapy or dosage reduction.

Cardiovascular: Orthostatic hypotension; hypertension; syncope; tachycardia; palpitations; myocardial infarction; arrhythmias; heart block; precipitation of CHF; stroke.

CNS: Confusion (especially in the elderly); disturbed concentration; hallucinations, disorientation; decrease in memory; feelings of unreality; delusions; anxiety; nervousness; restlessness; agitation; panic; insomnia; nightmares; hypomania; mania; exacerbation of psychosis; drowsiness; dizziness; weakness; fatigue; headache.

Miscellaneous: Nasal congestion; excessive appetite; weight gain or loss; increased perspiration; hyperthermia; flushing; chills; alopecia; tooth disorder, abnormal skin odor, chest pain, fever, halitosis, thirst, myalgia, back pain, arthralgia, muscle weakness **(clomipramine)**.

Hypersensitivity: Skin rash; pruritus; vasculitis; petechiae, urticaria; photosensitization; itching; edema (general or of face and tongue); drug fever.

Hematologic: Bone marrow depression including agranulocytosis; eosinophilia; purpura; thrombocytopenia; leukopenia.

GI: Nausea and vomiting; anorexia; epigastric distress; diarrhea; flatulence; dysphagia; increased salivation; stomatitis; glossitis; parotid swelling; abdominal cramps; pancreatitis; black tongue.

Endocrine: Gynecomastia and testicular swelling in the male; breast enlargement, menstrual irregularity and galactorrhea in the female; increased or decreased libido; painful ejaculation; impotence; nocturia; urinary frequency.

Special senses: Speech blockage; dysarthria; tinnitus; abnormal lacrimation.

Administration and Dosage:

Plasma levels: Determination of plasma levels may be useful in identifying patients who appear to have toxic effects and may have excessively high levels, or those in whom lack of absorption or noncompliance is suspected. Make adjustments in dosage according to patient's clinical response and not based on plasma levels.

AMITRIPTYLINE HCl:

Outpatients – 75 mg/day in divided doses. May increase to 150 mg/day. Alternatively, initiate therapy with 50 to 100 mg at bedtime. Increase by 25 to 50 mg as necessary, to a total of 150 mg/day.

Hospitalized patients may require 100 mg/day initially. Gradually increase to 200 to 300 mg, if necessary.

Adolescent and elderly patients – 10 mg 3 times a day with 20 mg at bedtime may be satisfactory in adolescent and elderly patients who cannot tolerate higher doses.

Maintenance – 40 to 100 mg/day. Total daily dosage may be given in a single dose, preferably at bedtime.

IM – Do not administer IV. Initially, 20 to 30 mg IM, 4 times a day. The effects may be more rapid with IM than with oral administration.

Children – Not recommended for children < 12 years.

NORTRIPTYLINE:

Adults – 25 mg 3 or 4 times daily; begin at a low level and increase as required. Doses above 100 mg/day are not recommended.

Elderly and adolescent patients – 30 to 50 mg daily in divided doses. Not recommended for use in children.

IMIPRAMINE HCl:

Depression – Use parenteral administration for starting therapy only in patients unable or unwilling to use oral medication. Do not administer IV. Initially, up to 100 mg/day IM in divided doses.

Hospitalized patients: Initially, 100 to 150 mg/day orally in divided doses; gradually increase to 200 mg/day, as required. If no response occurs after 2 weeks, increase to 250 to 300 mg/day. Administer the total daily dosage once daily at bedtime.

Outpatients: Initially, 75 mg/day, increased to 150 mg/day. Do not exceed 200 mg/day. Give once daily, preferably at bedtime. Maintenance: 50 to 150 mg/day.

Children: 1.5 mg/kg/day divided 3 times a day has been recommended, with increments of 1 to 1.5 mg/kg/day every 3 to 5 days. Maximum is 5 mg/kg/day.

Adolescent and elderly patients: Initially, 30 to 40 mg/day orally; it is generally not necessary to exceed 100 mg/day.

Childhood enuresis (≥ 5 years old) – Initially, 25 mg/day 1 hour before bedtime. If no satisfactory response in 1 week, increase up to 50 mg/night if < 12; up to 75 mg/night if >12. A dose > 75 mg/day does not enhance efficacy and increases side effects. Do not exceed 2.5 mg/kg/day. In early night bedwetters, it may be more effective given earlier and in divided amounts (25 mg midafternoon and bedtime).

DOXEPIN HCl: Not recommended for use in children < 12 years old.

Mild to moderate anxiety or depression – Initially, 75 mg/day. Usual optimum dosage is 75 to 150 mg/day. Alternatively, the total daily dosage, up to 150 mg, may be given at bedtime.

Mild symptomatology or emotional symptoms accompanying organic disease – 25 to 50 mg/day as often as effective.

More severe anxiety or depression – Higher doses (eg, 50 mg 3 times per day) may be required; if necessary, gradually increase to 300 mg/day.

Dilute oral concentrate with ≈ 120 ml of water, milk or fruit juice prior to administration.

TRIMIPRAMINE MALEATE: Not recommended for use in children.

Adult outpatients – Initially, 75 mg/day in divided doses; increase to 150 mg/day. Do not exceed 200 mg/day. The total dosage requirement may be given at bedtime.

Adult hospitalized patients – Initially, 100 mg/day in divided doses, increased gradually in a few days to 200 mg/day depending upon individual response and tolerance. If improvement does not occur in 2 to 3 weeks, increase to a maximum dose of 250 to 300 mg/day.

Adolescent and elderly patients – Initially, 50 mg/day, with gradual increments up to 100 mg/day.

Maintenance medication may be required at the lowest dose that will maintain remission (range 50 to 150 mg/day). Administer as a single bedtime dose.

AMOXAPINE: Amoxapine is not recommended for patients < 16 years old.

Usual effective dose range is 200 to 300 mg/day. If no response is seen at 300 mg, increase dosage, depending upon tolerance, to 400 mg/day. Hospitalized patients refractory to antidepressant therapy and who have no history of convulsive seizures may have dosage cautiously increased up to 600 mg/day in divided doses.

Adults – Initially, 50 mg 2 or 3 times daily. Depending upon tolerance, increase dosage to 100 mg 2 or 3 times daily by the end of the first week. Increase above 300 mg/day only if 300 mg/day has been ineffective for at least 2 weeks. Once an effective dosage is established, the drug may be given in a single bedtime dose (not to exceed 300 mg). If the total daily dosage exceeds 300 mg, give in divided doses.

Elderly patients – Initially, 25 mg 2 or 3 times a day. If tolerated, dosage may be increased by the end of the first week to 50 mg 2 or 3 times a day. Although 100 to 150 mg/day may be adequate for many elderly patients, some may require higher dosage; carefully increase up to 300 mg/day.

DESIPRAMINE HCl: Not recommended for use in children < 12 years of age.

Adults – 100 to 200 mg/day. Initial therapy may be given in divided doses or as a single daily dose. In more severely ill patients, gradually increase to 300 mg/day, if necessary. Do not exceed 300 mg/day.

Elderly and adolescents – 25 to 100 mg/day. Dosages > 150 mg not recommended.

PROTRIPTYLINE HCl: Not recommended for use in children.

Adults – 15 to 40 mg/day divided into 3 or 4 doses. May increase to 60 mg/day. Dosages above 60 mg/day are not recommended. Make any increases in the morning dose.

Adolescent and elderly patients – Initially, 5 mg 3 times/day; increase gradually, if necessary. In elderly patients, monitor the cardiovascular system closely if dose exceeds 20 mg/day.

CLOMIPRAMINE HCl: Administer in divided doses with meals to reduce GI side effects. After titration, the total daily dose may be given once daily at bedtime to minimize daytime sedation.

Adults – Initiate at 25 mg daily and gradually increase, as tolerated, to approximately 100 mg during the first 2 weeks. Thereafter, the dosage may be increased gradually over the next several weeks to a maximum of 250 mg/day.

Children and adolescents – Initiate at 25 mg daily and gradually increase during the first 2 weeks, as tolerated, to a daily maximum of 3 mg/kg or 100 mg, whichever is smaller. Thereafter, the dosage may be increased to a daily maximum of 3 mg/kg or 200 mg, whichever is smaller.

TETRACYCLIC COMPOUNDS

MAPROTILINE	
Tablets: 25, 50 and 75 mg (*Rx*)	Various, *Ludiomil* (Ciba)
MIRTAZAPINE	
Tablets: 15 and 30 mg	*Remeron* (Organon)

Actions:

Pharmacology: The mechanism of action is unknown. Tetracyclics enhance central noradrenergic and serotonergic activity.

Mirtazapine is a potent antagonist of 5–HT_2 and 5–HT_3 receptors. It is apotent antagonist of histamine (H_1) receptors, a property that may explain its prominent sedative effects. It is also a moderate antagonist at muscarinic receptors, a property that may explain the relatively low incidence of anticholinergic side effects.

Pharmacokinetics:

Maprotiline – The mean time to peak is 12 hours. The elimination half-life averages 61 hours.

Mirtazapine is rapidly and completely absorbed following oral administration and has a half-life of ≈ 20 to 40 hours, with females of all ages exhibiting significantly longer elimination half-lives than males (37 hours vs 26 hours). The presence of food in the stomach has a minimal effect on both the rate and extent of absorption and does not require a dosage adjustment. Steady-state plasma levels of mirtazapine are attained within 5 days. Mirtazapine is ≈ 85% bound to plasma protein.

Metabolism/Excretion: Major pathways of biotransformation are demethylation and hydroxylation followed by glucuronide conjugation. Mirtazapine has an absolute bioavailability of ≈ 50%. It is eliminated predominatnly via urine (75%) with 15% in feces.

Indications:

Depression: Treatment of depression.

Contraindications:

Hypersensitivity to maprotiline or mirtazapine; coadministration with monamine oxidase inhibitors (MAOIs).

Maprotiline: Known or suspected seizure disorders.

Warnings:

Anticholinergic properties: Maprotiline should be administered with caution in patients with increased intraocular pressure, history of urinary retention or history of marrow-angle glaucoma because of the drug's anticholinergic properties.

Monoamine oxidase inhibitors (MAOIs): Do not give tetracyclics with MAOIs. Allow a minimum of 14 days to elapse after discontinuation of MAOIs before starting a tetracyclic.

Seizures are rare. The risk of seizures may be increased when tetracyclics are taken concomitantly with phenothiazines, when the dosage of benzodiazepines is rapidly tapered in patients receiving tetracyclics or when the recommended dosage of the tetracyclic is exceeded.

Cardiovascular: Use with caution in patients with a history of myocardial infarction and angina because of the possibility of conduction defects, arrhythmia, myocardial infarction, strokes and tachycardia. Use with caution in patients predisposed to hypotension.

Electroshock therapy: Avoid concurrent administration of maprotiline with electroshock therapy because of the lack of experience in this area.

Agranulocytosis: In clinical trials, two patients treated with mirtazapine developed agranulocytosis (absolute neutorphil count [ANC]< 500/mm^3 with associated signs and symptoms, eg, fever infection) and a third patient developed severe neutropenia (ANC < 500/mm^3 without any associated symptoms). All three patients recovered after mirtazapine was stopped.

Renal/Hepatic function impairment: Use mirtazapine with caution in patients with impaired renal and hepatic function.

Elderly: Oral clearance was reduced in the elderly compared with the younger subjects. Caution is indicated in administering mirtazapine to elderly patients.

Pregnancy:

Maprotiline – *Category B.*

Mirtazapine – *Category C.*

Lactation:

Maprotiline is excreted in breast milk. At steady-state, the concentration in milk corresponds closely to the concentrations in whole blood.

Mirtazapine – It is not known if mirtazapine is excreted in breast milk.

Children: Safety and efficacy in children have not been established.

Precautions:

Somnolence was reported in 54% of patients treated with mirtazapine.

Dizziness was reported in 7% of patients treated with mirtazapine.

Increased appetite/Weight gain: Appetitie increase was reported in 17% of patients treated with mirtazapine. In some trials, weight gain of ≥ 7% of body weight occurred in 7.5% of patients treated.

Cholesterol/Triglycerides: Nonfasting cholesterol increases to ≥ 20% above the upper limits of normal and nonfasting triglyceride increases to ≥ 500 mg/dl were observed.

Mania/Hypomania: Use carefully in patients with a history of mania/hypomania.

Suicidal ideation: Closely supervise high-risk patients during initial drug therapy.

Transaminase elevations: Clinically significant ALT elevations (≥ 3 times the upper limit of the normal range) were observed in 2% of patients exposed to mirtazapine.

Orthostatic hypotension: Orthostatic hypotension was infrequently observed in clinical trials with depressed patients.

Drug Interactions:

Drugs that may affect maprotiline include thyroid hormones. Drugs that may be affected by maprotiline include anticholinergics, guanethidine and phenothiazines. Drugs that may be affected by mirtazapine include alcohol and diazepam.

Adverse Reactions:

Adverse reactions include: Asthenia; flu syndrome; dry mouth; constipation; increased appetite; weight gain; abnormal dreams; anxiety; dizziness; drowsiness; headache; nervousness; somnolence; abnormal thinking; tremor; weakness and fatigue; blurred vision.

Administration and Dosage:

MAPROTILINE HCl: May be given as a single daily dose or in divided doses. Therapeutic effects are sometimes seen within 3 to 7 days, although as long as 2 to 3 weeks are usually necessary before improvement is observed.

Initial adult dosage –

Mild to moderate depression: An initial dose of 75 mg/day is suggested for outpatients. In some patients, especially the elderly, an initial dose of 25 mg daily may be used. Because of the long half-life of maprotiline, maintain initial dosage for 2 weeks. The dosage may then be increased gradually in 25 mg increments, as required and tolerated. Most patients respond to a dose of 150 mg/day, but doses as high as 225 mg/day may be required.

Severe depression: Give hospitalized patients an initial daily dose of 100 to 150 mg, which may be gradually increased, as required and tolerated. Most hospitalized patients with moderate to severe depression respond to a daily dosage of 150 mg, although doses as high as 225 mg may be required. Do not exceed 225 mg/day.

Maintenance – Dosage may be reduced to 75 to 150 mg/day with adjustment depending on therapeutic response.

Elderly – In general, lower doses are recommended for patients > 60 years of age. Doses of 50 to 75 mg/day are satisfactory as maintenance therapy for elderly patients who do not tolerate higher amounts.

Maprotiline is not recommended for patients < 18 years of age.

MIRTAZAPINE:

Initial treatment – The recommended starting dose for mirtazapine is 15 mg/day administered in a single dose, preferably in the evening prior to sleep.

Maintenance/Extended treatment – Treatment for acute episodes of depression should continue for 6 months.

Switching to or from a monoamine oxidase inhibitor (MAOI) – At least 14 days should elapse between discontinuation of an MAOI and initiation of therapy with mirtazapine. In addition, allow at least 14 days after stopping mirtazapine before starting an MAOI.

TRAZODONE HCl

Tablets: 50 and 100 mg (*Rx*)	Various, *Desyrel* (Mead Johnson Pharm)
Tablets: 150 and 300 mg (*Rx*)	Various, *Desyrel Dividose* (Mead Johnson Pharm.)

Actions:

Pharmacology: The mechanism of antidepressant action is not fully understood. Trazodone is not a monoamine oxidase inhibitor and does not stimulate the CNS. In animals, it selectively inhibits serotonin uptake by brain synaptosomes and potentiates the behavioral changes induced by the serotonin precursor, 5–hydroxytryptophan.

Pharmacokinetics:

Absorption/Distribution – Trazodone is well absorbed after oral administration. Peak plasma levels occur in ≈ 1 hour when taken on an empty stomach or in 2 hours when taken with food.

Metabolism/Excretion – Trazodone is extensively metabolized in the liver; < 1% is excreted unchanged in the urine and feces. Elimination is biphasic, with a half-life of 3 to 6 hours and 5 to 9 hours, respectively, and is unaffected by food. The clearance of trazodone may be reduced in elderly male patients.

Indications:

Treatment of depression.

Unlabeled uses: May be useful for treatment of patients with panic disorder or agoraphobia with panic attacks.

Contraindications:

Hypersensitivity to trazodone.

Warnings:

Preexisting cardiac disease: Not recommended for use during the initial recovery phase of myocardial infarction. Trazodone may be arrhythmogenic in some patients. Arrhythmias identified include isolated PVCs, ventricular couplets and short episodes (3 to 4 beats) of ventricular tachycardia. Closely monitor patients with preexisting cardiac disease, particularly for cardiac arrhythmias.

Priapism: Patients with prolonged or inappropriate penile erection should discontinue use immediately and consult a physician.

Pregnancy: Category C.

Lactation: The drug may be excreted in breast milk.

Children: Safety and efficacy for use in children < 18 years of age are not established.

Precautions:

Suicide: The possibility of suicide in seriously depressed patients is inherent in the illness and may persist until significant remission occurs. Therefore, write prescriptions for the smallest number of tablets consistent with good patient management.

Hypotension, including orthostatic hypotension and syncope, has occurred.

Electroconvulsive therapy: Avoid concurrent administration with electroconvulsive therapy because of the absence of experience in this area.

Laboratory tests: Discontinue the drug in any patient whose white blood cell count or absolute neutrophil count falls below normal levels. White blood cell and differential counts are recommended for patients who develop fever and sore throat (or other signs of infection) during therapy.

Hazardous tasks: May produce drowsiness, dizziness or blurred vision.

Drug Interactions:

Drugs that may interact with trazodone include CNS depressants, digoxin, monoamine oxidase inhibitors, phenytoin and warfarin.

Adverse Reactions:

Adverse reactions may include: Allergic reaction; purpuric and maculopapular eruptions; rash; pruritis; urticaria; hematuria; delayed urine flow; increased urinary frequency; urinary incontinence/retention; decreased appetite; sweating; clamminess; weight gain or loss; malaise; nasal/sinus congestion; increased appetite; apnea; alopecia; edema; tinnitus; red eyes; diplopia; hypertension; hypotension; shortness of breath; tachycardia; palpitations; chest pain; ventricular tachycardia; vasodilation; bradycardia; atrial fibrillation; anger; hostility; nightmares/vivid dreams; confusion; disorientation; decreased concentration; lightheadedness; excitement; fatigue; headache; insomnia; impaired memory; nervousness; incoordination; paresthesia; tremors; hallucinations; psychosis; vertigo; hypomania; mania; impaired speech; akathisia; numbness; delusions; agitation; weakness; grand mal seizures; extrapyramidal symptoms; tardive dyskinesia; stupor; decreased/increased libido; impotence; retrograde ejaculation; early menses; missed periods; breast enlargement and engorgement; lactation; abdominal/gastric disorder; bad taste in mouth; dry mouth; nausea; vomiting; diarrhea; constipation; flatulence; hypersalivation; anemia; liver enzyme alterations; hyperbilirubinemia; jaundice; musculoskeletal aches and pains; muscle twitches; ataxia.

Administration and Dosage:

Initiate dosage at a low level and increase gradually. Drowsiness may require the administration of a major portion of the daily dose at bedtime or a reduced dosage. Take shortly after a meal or light snack.

Adults: An initial dose is 150 mg/day. This may be increased by 50 mg/day every 3 to 4 days. The maximum dose for outpatients usually should not exceed 400 mg/day in divided doses. Inpatients or more severely depressed subjects may be given up to, but not in excess of, 600 mg/day in divided doses.

Maintenance: Keep dosage at the lowest effective level. Once an adequate response has been achieved, dosage may be gradually reduced with subsequent adjustment depending on response.

BUPROPION HCl

Tablets: 75 and 100 mg (*Rx*)	*Wellbutrin* (Glaxo Wellcome)

Actions:

Pharmacology: The mechanism of the antidepressant effect of bupropion is not known. Bupropion does not inhibit monoamine oxidase. It is a weak blocker of the neuronal uptake of serotonin and norepinephrine; it also inhibits the neuronal reuptake of dopamine to some extent.

Pharmacokinetics:

Absorption/Distribution – Following oral administration, peak plasma concentrations are usually achieved within 2 hours, followed by a biphasic decline. The average half-life of the second (post-distributional) phase ranges 8 to 24 hours.

Metabolism/Excretion – Several of the metabolites of bupropion are pharmacologically active, but their potency and toxicity relative to bupropion have not been fully characterized. However, because of their longer elimination half-lives, the plasma concentrations of at least two of the known metabolites will be much higher than the plasma concentration of bupropion, especially in long-term use.

Indications:

Depression treatment: Effectiveness of bupropion in long-term use (> 6 weeks) has not been evaluated

Contraindications:

Hypersensitivity to the drug; seizure disorder; current or prior diagnosis of bulimia or anorexia nervosa (because of a higher incidence of seizures noted in such patients treated with bupropion); concurrent administration of a monoamine oxidase inhibitor (MAOI; at least 14 days should elapse between discontinuation of an MAOI and initiation of treatment with bupropion).

Warnings:

Seizures: Bupropion is associated with seizures in ≈ 0.4% of patients treated at doses up to 450 mg/day. The estimated seizure incidence increases almost 10–fold between 450 and 600 mg/day, which is twice the usually required daily dose (300 mg) and 1 ⅓ the maximum recommended daily dose (450 mg).

The risk of seizure appears strongly associated with dose and the presence of predisposing factors. A significant predisposing factor (eg, history of head trauma or prior seizure, CNS tumor, concomitant medications that lower seizure threshold) was present in approximately 50% of patients experiencing a seizure. Sudden and large increments in dose may also increase risk. While many seizures occurred early in the course of treatment, some seizures occurred after several weeks at fixed dose.

Recommendations for reducing seizure risk: (1) The total daily dose does not exceed 450 mg, (2) the daily dose is administered 3 times daily, with each single dose not to exceed 150 mg to avoid high peak concentrations of bupropion or its metabolites, and (3) the rate of incrementation of dose is very gradual.

Use extreme caution when: (1) Administered to patients with a history of seizure, cranial trauma, or other predisposition toward seizure, or (2) prescribed with other agents (eg, antipsychotics, other antidepressants) or treatment regimens (eg, abrupt discontinuation of a benzodiazepine) that lower seizure threshold.

Renal/Hepatic function impairment: Initiate treatment of patients with renal or hepatic impairment at reduced dosage. Closely monitor for possible toxic effects of elevated blood and tissue levels of drug and metabolites.

Half-lives of the metabolites are prolonged by cirrhosis and the metabolites accumulate to levels 2 to 3 times those in healthy individuals.

Pregnancy: Category B.

Lactation: Use only when clearly needed and when the potential benefits to the mother outweigh the possible risks to the infant.

Children: The safety and efficacy in individuals < 18 years old have not been established.

Precautions:

CNS symptoms: A substantial proportion of patients experience some degree of increased restlessness, agitation, anxiety and insomnia, especially shortly after initiation of treatment.

Neuropsychiatric phenomena: Patients have shown a variety of neuropsychiatric signs and symptoms including delusions, hallucinations, psychotic episodes, confusion and paranoia.

Activation of psychosis or mania: Antidepressants can precipitate manic episodes in Bipolar Manic Depressive patients during the depressed phase of their illness and may activate latent psychosis in other susceptible patients.

Altered appetite and weight: A weight loss of > 5 pounds occurred in 28% of patients. This incidence is approximately double that seen in comparable patients treated with tricyclic antidepressants or placebo. Furthermore, 34.5% of patients receiving tricyclic antidepressants gained weight, vs only 9.4% of bupropion patients.

Suicide: The possibility of a suicide attempt is inherent in depression and may persist until significant remission occurs. Accordingly, write prescriptions for the smallest number of tablets consistent with good patient management.

Heart disease: Exercise care in patients with a recent history of myocardial infarction or unstable heart disease.

Drug Interactions:

Drugs that may interact with bupropion include MAOIs and levodopa.

Bupropion may be an inducer of drug metabolizing enzymes. Exercise care when administering drugs known to affect hepatic drug metabolizing enzyme systems.

Use and cessation of use of alcohol may alter the seizure threshold; therefore, minimize the consuption of alcohol and, if possible, avoid completely.

Adverse Reactions:

Adverse reactions occurring in ≥ 3% of patients include: Constipation; nausea/vomiting; anorexia; diarrhea; appetite increase; dyspepsia; menstrual complaints; impotence; dry mouth; headache/migraine; excessive sweating; tremor; sedation; akinesia/bradykinesia; sensory disturbance; impaired sleep quality; increased salivary flow; auditory disturbance; blurred vision; gustatory disturbance; dizziness; tachycardia; cardiac arrythmias; hypertension; palpitations; rash; confusion; hostility; disturbed concentration; decreased libido; upper respiratory complaints; fatigue; arthritis; agitation; abnormalities in mental status.

Administration and Dosage:

General: Do not exceed dose increases of 100 mg/day in a 3 day period. No single dose of bupropion should exceed 150 mg. Administer 3 times daily, preferably with at least 6 hours between successive doses.

Adults: 300 mg/day, given 3 times daily. Begin dosing at 200 mg/day, given as 100 mg twice daily. Based on clinical response, this dose may be increased to 300 mg/day, given as 100 mg 3 times daily no sooner than 3 days after beginning therapy.

Bupropion Dosage Regimen

			Number of Tablets		
Treatment Day	Total Daily Dose	Tablet Strength	Morning	Midday	Evening
1	200 mg	100 mg	1	0	1
4	300 mg	100 mg	1	1	1

Increasing the dosage above 300 mg/day: An increase in dosage, up to a maximum of 450 mg/day, given in divided doses of not more than 150 mg each, may be considered for patients in whom no clinical improvement is noted after several weeks of treatment at 300 mg/day. Dosing above 300 mg/day may be accomplished using the 75 or 100 mg tablets. The 100 mg tablets must be administered 4 times daily with at least 4 hours between successive doses in order not to exceed the limit of 150 mg in a single dose. Discontinue in patients who do not demonstrate an adequate response after an appropriate period of 450 mg/day.

Maintenance: Use the lowest dose that maintains remission.

VENLAFAXINE

Tablets: 25, 37.5, 50, 75 and 100 mg (*Rx*)	*Effexor* (Wyeth-Ayerst)

Actions:

Pharmacology: Venlafaxine is chemically unrelated to other available antidepressant agents. Venlafaxine and its active metabolite, O-desmethylvenlafaxine (ODV), are potent inhibitors of neuronal serotonin and norepinephrine reuptake and weak inhibitors of dopamine reuptake.

Pharmacokinetics: Venlafaxine is well absorbed (at least 92%) and extensively metabolized in the liver. ODV is the only major active metabolite. Renal elimination of venlafaxine and its metabolites is the primary route of excretion.

Indications:

Treatment of depression.

Warnings:

MAO inhibitors: Because venlafaxine is an inhibitor of both norepinephrine and serotonin reuptake, it is recommended that venlafaxine not be used in combination with an MAOI. Based on the half-life of venlafaxine, allow at least 7 days after stopping venlafaxine before starting an MAOI.

Elderly: No overall differences in effectiveness, safety or response were observed between elderly and younger patients.

Pregnancy: Category C.

Lactation: It is not known whether venlafaxine or its metabolites are excreted in breast milk.

Children: Safety and efficacy in patients < 18 years old have not been established.

Precautions:

Long-term use: The effectiveness of venlafaxine in long-term use (ie, > 4 to 6 weeks) has not been evaluated.

Anxiety and insomnia: Anxiety, nervousness and insomnia were reported for venlafaxine-treated patients, and led to drug discontinuation.

Appetite/Weight changes: Anorexia was reported for venlafaxine-treated patients. A dose-dependent weight loss was often noted in patients treated for several weeks.

Mania/Hypomania: Hypomania or mania has occurred in patients treated with venlafaxine.

Seizures have been reported in venlafaxine-treated patients.

Suicide: The possibility of a suicide attempt is inherent in depression and may persist until significant remission occurs. Write prescriptions for the smallest quantity of tablets consistent with good patient management in order to reduce the risk of overdose.

Drug abuse and dependence: Carefully evaluate patients for history of drug abuse and follow such patients closely, observing them for signs of misuse or abuse of venlafaxine.

Drug Interactions:

Drugs that may interact with venlafaxine include cimetidine and MAOIs. Avoid alcohol.

Venlafaxine is metabolized to its active metabolite, ODV, by cytochrome P–450IID$_6$. Therefore, the potential exists for a drug interaction between venlafaxine and drugs that inhibit this isoenzyme.

Adverse Reactions:

Adverse reactions occurring in ≥ 3% of patients include Nausea; somnolence; insomnia; dizziness; abnormal ejaculation/orgasm; blurred vision; vasodilation; dry mouth; nervousness; anxiety; tremor; abnormal dreams; hypertonia; paresthesia; headache; asthenia; infection; chills; yawning; sweating; rash; constipation; anorexia; diarrhea; vomiting; dyspepsia; flatulence; impotence; urinary frequency; abdominal pain; abnormality of accomodation.

Administration and Dosage:

Initial treatment: The recommended starting dose is 75 mg/day, administered in 2 or 3 divided doses, taken with food. Depending on tolerability and the need for further clinical effect, the dose may be increased to 150 mg/day. If needed, further increase the dose up to 225 mg/day. When increasing the dose, make increments of up to 75 mg/day at intervals of ≥ 4 days. In outpatient settings there was no evidence of usefulness of doses > 225 mg day for moderately depressed patients, but more severely depressed inpatients responded to a mean dose of 350 mg/day. Certain patients, including more severely depressed patients, may therefore respond more to higher doses, up to a maximum of 375 mg/day, generally in 3 divided doses.

Renal/Hepatic function impairment: It is recommended that the total daily dose be reduced by 50% in patients with moderate hepatic impairmentand by 25% in patients with mild to moderate renal impairment. It is recommended that the total daily dose be reduced by 50% and the dose be withheld until the dialysis treatment is completed (4 hrs) in patients undergoing hemodialysis.

Elderly: No dose adjustment is recommended for elderly patients on the basis of age.

Discontinuing venlafaxine: When discontinuing venlafaxine after > 1 week of therapy, it is generally recommended that the dose be tapered to minimize the risk of discontinuation symptoms. Patients who have received venlafaxine for ≥ 6 weeks should have their dose tapered gradually over a 2 week period.

NEFAZODONE HCl

Tablets: 100, 150, 200 and 250 mg (*Rx*)	*Serzone* (Bristol-Myers Squibb)

Actions:

Pharmacology: Nefazodone is an antidepressant with a chemical structure unrelated to available antidepressant agents. The mechanism of action is unknown. Nefazodone inhibits neuronal uptake of serotonin and norepinephrine.

Pharmacokinetics:

Absorption/Distribution – Nefazodone is rapidly and completely absorbed, but is subject to extensive metabolism so that its absolute bioavailability is low (about 20%) and variable. Peak plasma concentrations occur at about 1 hour. Half-life is 2 to 4 hours. Nefazodone is widely distributed in body tissues, including the CNS. Volume of distribution ranges from 0.22 to 0.87 L/kg.

Metabolism/Excretion – Nefazodone is extensively metabolized after oral administration by < 1% is excreted unchanged in urine. Three active metabolites identified in plasma include hydroxynefazodone (HO-NEF), meta-chlorophenylpiperazine (mCPP) and a triazole-dione metabolite.

The mean half-life of nefazodone ranged between 11 and 24 hours. Approximately 55% was detected in urine and about 20% to 30% in feces. Nefazodone is extensively (> 99%) bound to human plasma proteins in vitro.

Indications:

Depression: Treatment of depression.

Contraindications:

Coadministration with terfenadine or astemizole; hypersensitivity to nefazodone or other phenylpiperazine antidepressants.

Warnings:

Long-term use: The effectiveness of nefazodone in long-term use (ie, for more than 6 to 8 weeks) has not been systematically evaluated.

MAO *inhibitors:* Because nefazodone is an inhibitor of both serotonin and norepinephrine reuptake, it is recommended that nefazodone not be used in combination with an MAOI, or within 14 days of discontinuing treatment with an MAOI. Allow at least 1 week after stopping nefazodone before starting an MAOI.

Pregnancy: Category C.

Lactation: It is not known whether nefazodone or its metabolites are excreted in breast milk.

Children: Safety and efficacy in individuals < 18 years old have not been established.

Precautions:

Postural hypotension: Use nefazodone with caution in patients with known cardiovascular or cerebrovascular disease that could be exacerbated by hypotension and conditions that would predispose patients to hypotension.

Mania/hypomania: As with all antidepressants, use nefazodone cautiously in patients with a history of mania.

Suicide: The possibility of a suicide attempt is inherent in depression and may persist until significant remission occurs. Closely supervise high-risk patients during initial therapy. Write prescriptions for the smallest quantity of nefazodone consistent with good patient management to reduce the risk of overdose.

Priapism: If patients present with prolonged or inappropriate erections, they should discontinue therapy immediately and consult their physicians.

Bradycardia: Sinus bradycardia was observed in nefazodone patients. Treat patients with a recent MI or unstable heart disease with caution.

Hepatic cirrhosis: In patients with cirrhosis of the liver, the AUC values of nefazodone and its metabolite HO-NEF were increased by ≈ 25%.

Drug abuse and dependence: Carefully evaluate patients for a history of drug abuse and follow such patients closely, observing them for signs of misuse or abuse of nefazodone.

Drug Interactions:

Drugs that may interact with nefazodone include: MAOIs, nonsedating antihistamines, benzodiazepines, digoxin, haloperidol and propranolol.

Potential interaction with drugs that inhibit or are metabolized by cytochrome P450 (IIIA4 and IID6) isozymes: Caution is indicated in the combined use of nefazodone with any drugs known to be metabolized by the IIIA4 isozyme (in particular, terfenadine or astemizole).

Drugs highly bound to plasma protein: Administration to a patient taking another drug that is highly protein bound may cause increased free concentrations of the other drug, potentially resulting in adverse events. Conversely, adverse effects could result from displacement of nefazodone by other highly bound drugs.

Drug/Food interactions: Food delays absorption of nefazodone and decreases the bioavailability by ≈ 20%.

Adverse Reactions:

Adverse reactions occurring in ≥ 3% of patients include nausea; headache; asthenia; flu syndrome; dry mouth; nausea; constipation; dyspepsia; diarrhea; increased appetite; peripheral edema; pharyngitis; cough; blurred vision; abnormal vision; somnolence; dizziness; insomnia; lightheadedness; confusion; memory impairment; paresthesia; vasodilation; concentration decreased; postural hypotension; tinnitus.

Administration and Dosage:

Initial treatment: Recommended starting dose is 200 mg/day, administered in two divided doses. In clinical trials, the effective dose range was generally 300 to 600 mg/day. Increase doses in increments of 100 to 200 mg/day, again on a twice daily schedule, at intervals of no less than 1 week.

Elderly/Debilitated patients: The recommended initial dose is 100 mg/day on a twice daily schedule.

SELECTIVE SEROTONIN REUPTAKE INHIBITORS

SERTRALINE HCl	
Tablets: 50 and 100 mg (*Rx*)	*Zoloft* (Roerig)
PAROXETINE HCl	
Tablets: 10, 20, 30 and 40 mg (*Rx*)	*Paxil* (SK-Beecham)
FLUOXETINE HCl	
Pulvules: 10 and 20 mg (*Rx*)	*Prozac* (Dista)
Liquid: 20 mg/5 ml (*Rx*)	*Prozac* (Dista)
FLUVOXAMINE MALEATE	
Tablets: 50 and 100 mg (*Rx*)	*Luvox* (Solvay)

Actions:

Pharmacology: The antidepressant action of the SSRIs is presumed to be linked to their inhibition of CNS neuronal uptake of serotonin (5HT). These agents are potent and selective inhibitors of neuronal serotonin reuptake and they also have a weak effect on norepinephrine and dopamine neuronal reuptake.

Pharmacokinetics:

SSRI Pharmacokinetics

SSRIs	Time to peak plasma concentration (hr)	Peak plasma concentration (ng/ml)	Half-life (hrs)	Protein binding (%)	Time to reach steady state (days)	Primary route of elimination	Bioavailability (%)
Fluoxetine	6-8	15-55	48-216[1]	94.5	28-35	hepatic	72
Fluvoxamine	3-8	88-546	13.6-15.6	77-80	7	renal	53
Paroxetine	5.2	61.7	21	93-95	≈10	64% renal, 36% hepatic	100

SSRI Pharmacokinetics							
SSRIs	Time to peak plasma concentration (hr)	Peak plasma concentration (ng/ml)	Half-life (hrs)	Protein binding (%)	Time to reach steady state (days)	Primary route of elimination	Bioavailability (%)
Sertraline	4.5-8.4	20-55	26-65[1]	98	7	40%-45% renal, 40%-45% hepatic	

[1] t½ includes the active metabolite.

Indications:

Depression: Fluoxetine, paroxetine, sertraline.

Obsessive-Compulsive disorder (OCD): Fluoxetine, fluvoxamine, sertraline, paroxetine-Treatment of obsessions and compulsions in patients with OCD, as defined in the DSM-III-R.

Bulimia nervosa: Fluoxetine - Treatment of binge-eating and vomiting behaviors in patients with moderate to severe bulimia nervosa.

Panic disorder: Paroxetine - Treatment of panic disorder, with or without agoraphobia, as defined in DSM-IV.

Unlabeled uses: Fluoxetine -Alcoholism; anorexia nervosa; attention-derficit hyperactivity disorder; bipolar II affective disorder; kleptomania; migraine, chronic daily headaches and tension-type headache; obesity; posttraumatic stress disorder; premenstrual syndrome; recurrent syncope; schizophrenia; tourette's syndrome; trichotilomania; levodopa-induced dyskinesia; social phobia.

Fluvoxamine is being investigated in the treatment of depression.

Paroxetine - Diabetic neuropathy (10 to 60 mg/day); headaches (10 to 50 mg/day); premature ejaculation (20 mg/day).

Sertraline may be effective in patients with obsessive-compulsive disorder.

Contraindications:

Hypersensitivity to SSRIs; in combination with an MAO inhibitor, or within 14 days of discontinuing an MAOI; coadministration of **fluvoxamine** with astemizole or terfenadine.

Warnings:

Long-term use: The effectiveness of long-term use of SSRIs (> 5 to 6 weeks for depression [sertraline >16 weeks]) (>13 weeks for OCD with **fluoxetine**), has not been systematically evaluated, except for paroxetine (the efficacy of **paroxetine** in maintaining an antidepressant response for up to 1 year was demonstrated in a placebo controlled trial).

MAO Inhibitors: It is recommended that SSRIs not be used in combination with an MAOI, or within 14 days of discontinuing treatment with an MAOI. Allow at least 2 weeks after stopping the SSRIs before starting an MAOI.

Altered platelet function or abnormal results from laboratory studies in patients taking **fluoxetine, paroxetine** or **sertraline** have occured.

Rash and accompanying events: Approximately 4% of patients taking **fluoxetine** have developed a rash or urticaria; ≈ 33% were withdrawn from treatment. Most patients improved promptly with discontinuation of fluoxetine or adjunctive treatment with antihistamines or steroids; all patients recovered completely. Several other patients have had systemic syndromes suggestive of serum sickness.

Systemic events, possibly related to vasculitis, have developed in patients with rash. Although rare, these events may be serious, involving lung, kidney or liver. Death has been associated with the events.

Renal function impairment: With chronic use, additional accumulation of fluoxetine or its metabolites may occur with severely impaired renal function; use a lower or less frequent dose.

Increased plasma concentrations of **paroxetine** occur in subjects with renal and hepatic impairment. Therefore, reduce the initial dosage of paroxetine in patients with severe renal impairment.

Since **sertraline** is extensively metabolized by the liver, excretion of unchanged drug in the urine is a minor route of elimination. However, use with caution in patients with severe renal impairment.

Hepatic function impairment: SSRIs are extensively metabolized by the liver. Use with caution in patients with severe liver impairment. Use a lower or less frequent dose of fluoxetine in patients with liver impairment. Slowly titrate **fluvoxamine** during initiation of treatment. Reduce the initial dosage of **paroxetine** in patients with severe hepatic impairment; upward titration, if necessary, should be at increased intervals. The clearance of **sertraline** is decreased in mild, stable cirrhotics. Give a lower or less frequent dose in patients with severe hepatic dysfunction.

Elderly: The disposition of single doses of **fluoxetine** in healthy elderly subjects (≥ 65 years of age) did not differ significantly from that in younger normal subjects. Clearance of **fluvoxamine** is decreased by ≈ 50% in elderly patients. Pharmacokinetic studies revealed a decreased clearance of paroxetine in the elderly, and a lower starting dose is recommended. Sertraline plasma clearance may be lower.

Pregnancy: Category B (**fluoxetine, paroxetine, sertraline**); Category C (**fluvoxamine**).

Lactation: **Fluoxetine, fluvoxamine** and **paroxetine** are excreted in breast milk. It is not known whether **sertraline** or its metabolites are excreted in breast milk.

Children: Safety and efficacy in children (**fluvoxamine**, children < 18 years of age) have not been established.

Precautions:

Anxiety, nervousness and insomnia occurred in 3% to 33% of patients treated with an SSRI. These side effects led to discontinuation of drug therapy in 1.1% to 5.3%.

Altered appetite and weight: Significant weight loss, especially in underweight depressed patients, has occurred. Approximately 3% to ≈ 9% of patients treated with an SSRI experienced anorexia.

Activation of mania/hypomania occurred infrequently in ≈ 0.1% to 2.2% of patients taking SSRIs. Use cautiously in patients with a history of mania.

Seizures have occurred with **fluoxetine** (0.2%), **fluvoxamine** (0.2%), **paroxetine** (0.1%) and **sertraline** (< 0.1%). These percentages appear similar to the rate associated with other antidepressants. Use with care in patients with history of seizures.

Suicide: The possibility of a suicide attempt is inherent in depression and may persist until significant remission occurs. Close supervision of high-risk patients should accompany initial drug therapy. Write prescriptions for the smallest quantity of tablets or capsules in order to reduce the risk of overdose.

Concomitant illness: Use caution in patients with diseases or conditions that could affect metabolism or hemodynamic responses.

Hyponatremia: Several cases of **fluoxetine**, **sertraline** and **paroxetine**-induced hyponatremia (some with serum sodium < 110 mmol/L) have occurred. The hyponatremia appeared to be reversible when fluoxetine or paroxetine were discontinued. The majority of these occurrences have been in older patients and in patients taking diuretics or who were otherwise volume-depleted.

Diabetes: **Fluoxetine** may alter glycemic control. Hypoglycemia has occurred during therapy, and hyperglycemia has developed following discontinuation of the drug. The dosage of insulin or the sulfonylurea may need to be adjusted when fluoxetine is started or discontinued.

Uricosuric effect: **Sertraline** is associated with a mean decrease in serum uric acid of ≈ 7%. The clinical significance of this weak uricosuric effect is unknown, and there have been no reports of acute renal failure with sertraline.

Drug abuse and dependence: Before staring an SSRI, carefully evaluate patients for history of drug abuse and follow such patients closely, observing them for signs of misuse or abuse.

Hazardous tasks: SSRIs may cause dizziness or drowsiness. Patients should be instructed to observe caution while driving or performing tasks requiring alertness, coordination or physical dexterity.

Photosensitivity: Photosensitization may occur.

Drug Interactions:

Drugs highly bound to plasma protein: Because **paroxetine** and **sertraline** are highly bound to plasma protein, administration to a patient taking another drug that is highly protein-bound may cause increased free concentrations of the other drug, potentially resulting in adverse events. Conversely, adverse effects could result from displacement of paroxetine or sertraline by other highly bound drugs.

Microsomal enzyme induction: Concomitant use of **paroxetine** with drugs metabolized by cytochrome $P450IID_6$ may require lower doses than usually prescribed for either paroxetine or the other drug since paroxetine may significantly inhibit the activity of this isozyme.

Drugs that may affect selective serotonin reuptake inhibitors include cimetidine, cyproheptadine, dextromethorphan, lithium, MAO inhibitors, phenobarbital, phenytoin, smoking and L-tryptophan.

Drugs that may be affected by selective serotonin reuptake inhibitors include phenytoin, alcohol, triclic antidepressants, nonsedating antihistamines, cyclosporine, haloperidol, phentermine, pimozide, sumatripten, benzodiazepines, beta blockers, buspirone, carbamazepine, clozapine, diltiazem, digoxin, lithium, methadone, procyclidine, theophylline, tolbutamide and warfarin.

Drug/Food interactions: In one study following a single dose of **sertraline** with and without food, sertraline AUC was slightly increased and C_{max} was 25% greater. Time to reach peak plasma level decreased from 8 hours post dosing to 5.5 hours.

Food does not appear to affect systemic bioavailability of **fluoxetine** although it may delay absorption. **Fluvoxamine** bioavailability is not affected by food. Thus, fluoxetine and fluvoxamine may be given with or without food.

Adverse Reactions:

Commonly observed:

SSRIs Adverse Reactions (%) (≥ 3% in at least one agent)				
Adverse reaction	Fluoxetine	Fluvoxamine	Paroxetine	Sertraline
Body as a whole				
Headache	21	22	18	20
Asthenia	12	14	15	1
Abdominal pain	3.4	—	3.1	2.4
Infection, viral or bacterial	3.4	—	—	—
Influenza/Flu syndrome	5	3	—	—
Accidental injury	4	≥ 1	—	—
Cardiovascular				
Palpitations	2	3	3	4
Vasodilation	3	3	3	—
Chest pain	1.3	—	3	3
CNS				
Insomnia	20	21	13	16
Somnolence	13	22	23	13
Nervousness	13	12	5	3
Anxiety	13	5	5	3
Dizziness	10	11	13	12
Tremor	10	5	8	11
Libido decreased/ sexual dysfunction	4	2	3	2 (female) 16 (male)
Agitation	≥ 1	2	5	6
Paresthesia	—	—	4	3
Drowsiness	11.6	—	—	—
Fatigue /Malaise	4.2	≥ 1	—	11
Sedation	1.9	—	—	—

SSRIs Adverse Reactions (%) (≥ 3% in at least one agent)				
Adverse reaction	Fluoxetine	Fluvoxamine	Paroxetine	Sertraline
Abnormal dreams	5	—	4	0.1-1
Abnormal thinking	4	—	0.1-1	0.1-1
Sleep disorder	3	—	—	—
Depersonalization	0.1-1	0.1-1	3	3
GI				
Nausea	23	40	26	26
Vomiting	3	5	—	4
Diarrhea/loose stools	12	11	12	18
Dyspepsia	8	10	2	6
Dry mouth	10	14	18	16
Anorexia	11	6	6	3
Constipation	4.5	10	14	8
Abdominal pain	3.4	—	4	—
Flatulence	3	4	4	4
Tooth disorder/caries	—	3	< 0.1	—
Increased appetite	≥ 1	—	3	3
Tooth disorder/caries	—	3	< 0.1	—
GI disorder	6	—	—	—
Musculoskeletal				
Myalgia	5	—	2	1.7
Arthralgia	3	0.1-1	0.1-1	0.1-1
Respiratory				
Upper respiratory infection	7.6	9	—	—
Pharyngitis	5	—	—	4
Rhinitis	≥ 1	—	3	2
Yawn	3	2	4	2
Respiratory disorder	—	—	5.9	—
Skin				
Sweating, excessive	8	7	11	8
Rash	4	—	2	2
Pruritus	3	—	1	0.1-1
Special senses				
Vision disturbances/ blurred vision	3	—	4	4
Taste perversion/change	1	3	2	3
Amblyopia	3	3	—	—
GU				
Sexual dysfunction/ impotence/anorgasmia	1.9	2	6.5	16
Urinary frequency	1	3	3	2
Abnormal ejaculation	—	8	13	17
Male genital disorders, others	—	—	10	—
Urination disorder/ retention	—	1	3	Rare

Administration and Dosage:

SERTRALINE HCl:

Initial treatment – 50 mg once daily, either in the morning or evening. While a relationship between dose and antidepressant effect has not been established, patients were dosed in a range of 50 to 200 mg/day in the clinical trials. Consequently, patients not responding to a 50 mg dose may benefit from dose increases up to a maximum of 200 mgday. Given the 24 hour elimination half-life of sertraline, dose changes should not occur at intervals of < 1 week.

Hepatic/Renal function impairment – Give a lower or less frequent dosage in patients with hepatic or renal impairment.

Maintenance/Continuation/Extended treatment – There is evidence to suggest that depressed patients responding during an initial 8 week treatment phase will continue to benefit during an additional 8 weeks of treatment. While there are insufficient data regarding any benefits from treatment beyond 16 weeks, it is generally agreed among expert psychopharmacologists that acute episodes of depression require several months or longer of sustained pharmacological therapy.

PAROXETINE HCl:

Depression –

Initial dose: 20 mg/day. Administer as a single daily dose, usually in the morning. Usual range is 20 to 50 mg/day. Some patients not responding to a 20 mg dose may benefit from dose increases, in 10 mg/day increments, up to a maximum of 50 mg/day. Dose changes should occur at intervals of at least 1 week.

Maintenace therapy: It is generally agreed that acute episodes of depression require several months or longer of sustained pharmacologic therapy. Efficacy has been maintained for period up to 1 year with doses that averaged about 30 mg.

OCD –

Initial: 40 mg/day. Administer as a single daily dose, usually in the morning. Start with 20 mg/day and may be increased in 10 mg/day increments. Dose changes should occur at intervals of at least 1 week. Usual range is 20 to 60 mg/day. The maximum dosage should not exceed 60 mg/day.

Maintenance therapy: Patients have been continued on therapy for 6 months without loss of benefit. However, make dosage adjustments to maintain the patient on the lowest effective dosage, and periodically reassess the patient to determine the need for treatment.

Panic disorder –

Initial: 40 mg/day. Administer as a single daily dose, usually in the morning. Start with 10 mg/day and may be increased in 10 mg/day increments. Dose changes should occur at intervals of at least 1 week. Usual range is 10 to 60 mg/day. The maximum dosage should not exceed 60 mg/day.

Maintenance therapy: Long-term maintenance of efficacy has been demonstrated for 3 months. Make dosage adjustments to maintain the patient on the lowest effective dosage, and reassess the patients periodically to determine the need for continued treatment.

FLUOXETINE HCl:

Depression –

Initial: 20 mg/day in the morning. Consider a dose increase after several weeks if no clinical improvement is observed. Administer doses > 20 mg/day on a once (morning) or twice (eg, morning and noon) daily schedule. Do not exceed a maximum dose of 80 mg/day.

Maintenance: Optimal duration of fluoxetine therapy remains speculative. Acute episodes of depression generally require several months or longer of sustained pharmacological therapy.

Obsessive-Compulsive disorder –

Initial: 20 mg/day in the morning. Consider a dose increase after several weeks if insufficient clinical improvement is observed. Administer doses > 20 mg/day on a once (morning) or twice (morning and noon) daily schedule. A dose range of 20 to 60 mg/day is recommended; however, doses of up to 80 mg/day have been well tolerated. Do not exceed 80 mg/day.

Maintenance: Patients have been continued on therapy for an additional 6 months without loss of benefit.

Bulimia nervosa –

Initial: The recommended dose is 60 mg/day, administered in the morning. For some patients it may be advisable to titrate up to this target dose over several days. Fluoxetine doses > 60 mg/day have not been systematically studied in patients with bulimia.

Maintenance: Patients have been continued on therapy for an additional 6 months without loss of benefit. However, make dosage adjustments to maintain the patient on the lowest effective dosage, and periodically reasses the patient to determine the need for treatment.

Renal/Hepatic function impairment – Use a lower or less frequent dosage.

Special risk patients – Consider a lower or less frequent dosage for patients, such as the elderly, with concurrent disease or on multiple medications.

FLUVOXAMINE MALEATE:

Initial therapy – Recommended starting dose is 50 mg as a single bedtime dose. In trials, patients were titrated within a range of 100 to 300 mg/day. Increase dose in 50 mg increments every 4 to 7 days, as tolerated, until maximum therapeutic benefit is achieved, not to exceed 300 mg/day. It is advisable to give total daily doses > 100 mg in two divided doses; if doses are unequal, give larger dose at bedtime.

Maintenance therapy – Although efficacy has not been documented > 10 weeks in controlled trials, OCD is a chronic condition; it is reasonable to consider continuation for a responding patient.

Elderly/Hepatic function impairment – These patients have been observed to have decreased fluvoxamine clearance. It may be appropriate to modify initial dose and subsequent titration.

MONOAMINE OXIDASE INHIBITORS

PHENELZINE	
Tablets: 15 mg (as sulfate) (Rx)	*Nardil* (Parke-Davis)
TRANYLCYPROMINE	
Tablets: 10 mg (as sulfate) (Rx)	*Parnate* (SK-Beecham)

Actions:

Pharmacology: Drugs that inhibit this enzyme system (MAOIs) cause an increase in the concentration of endogenous epinephrine, norepinephrine and serotonin (5HT) in storage sites throughout the nervous system. The increase in the concentration of monoamines in the CNS is the basis for the antidepressant activity of these agents.

Pharmacokinetics: Phenelzine and tranylcypromine are well absorbed orally. The clinical effects of phenelzine may continue for up to 2 weeks after discontinuation of therapy. When tranylcypromine is withdrawn, MAO activity is recovered in 3 to 5 days (possibly up to 10 days), although the drug is excreted in 24 hours.

Indications:

Depression: In general, the MAOIs appear to be indicated in patients with atypical (exogenous) depression, and in some patients unresponsive to other antidepressive therapy. They are rarely a drug of first choice.

Unlabeled uses: MAOIs have shown promise in the treatment of bulimia. Phenelzine has been investigated in the treatment of cocaine addiction as a deterrent; careful supervision is required. Anecdotal cases and small studies indicate beneficial effects of phenelzine in patients with night terrors; post-traumatic stress disorder; some migraines resistant to other therapies; likewise, with tranylcypromine in Binswanger's encephalopathy; seasonal affective disorder; and subjective symptoms in multiple sclerosis patients. MAOIs have also been used in the treatment of panic disorder with associated agoraphobia and globus hystericus syndrome.

Contraindications:

Hypersensitivity to these agents; pheochromocytoma; congestive heart failure; a history of liver disease or abnormal liver function tests; severe impairment of renal function; confirmed or suspected cerebrovascular defect; cardiovascular disease; hypertension; history of headache; in patients over 60 because of the possibility of existing cerebral sclerosis with damaged vessels.

Warnings:

Hypertensive crises: The most serious reactions involve changes in blood pressure; it is inadvisable to use these drugs in elderly or debilitated patients or in the presence of hypertension, cardiovascular or cerebrovascular disease. Not recommended in patients with frequent or severe headaches because headache during therapy may be the first symptom of a hypertensive reaction.

Warning to the patient – Warn all patients against eating foods with high tyramine or tryptophan content (see table) and for 2 weeks after discontinuing MAOIs. Also warn patients against drinking alcoholic beverages and against self-medication with certain proprietary agents such as cold, hay fever or weight reduction preparations containing sympathomimetic amines while undergoing therapy. Instruct patients not to consume excessive amounts of caffeine in any form and to report promptly the occurrence of headache or other unusual symptoms.

Tyramine-Containing Foods[1]		
Cheese/Dairy Products		
American, processed Blue Boursault[2] Brick, natural Brie	Camembert[2] Cheddar[2] Emmenthaler[2] Gruyere Mozzarella Parmesan	Romano Roquefort Sour cream Stilton[2] Yogurt
Meat/Fish		
Beef or chicken liver, other meats, fish (unrefrigerated, fermented) Meats prepared with tenderizer	Fermented sausages (bologna, pepperoni, salami, summer sausage)[2] Game meat Meat extracts	Caviar Dried fish (salted herring) Herring, pickled, spoiled[2] Shrimp paste
Alcoholic Beverages (Undistilled)		
Beer and ale (imports, some nonalcoholic)	Red wine (especially Chianti)	Sherry
Fruit/Vegetables		
Avocados (especially overripe) Yeast extracts (Marmite, etc.)[2]	Bananas Figs, canned (overripe) Raisins Sauerkraut	Soy sauce Miso soup Bean curd
Foods Containing Other Vasopressors		
Fava beans (overripe) – dopamine	Caffeine (eg, coffee, tea, colas)	Chocolate – phenylethylamine Ginseng

[1] Tyramine contents are not predictable and may vary. The amounts of tyramine are estimated from low to very high.
[2] Contains high to very high amounts of tyramine.

Suicidal risks: In patients who may be suicidal risks, no single form of treatment, such as MAOIs, electroconvulsive or other therapy should be relied upon as a sole therapeutic measure.

Concomitant antidepressants: In patients receiving a selective serotonin reuptake inhibitor (SSRIs) in combination with an MAOI, there have been reports of serious, sometimes fatal, reactions including hyperthermia, rigidity, myoclonus, autonomic instability with possible rapid fluctuations of vital signs, and mental status changes that include extreme agitation progressing to delirium and coma. It is recommended that SSRIs not be used in combination with an MAOI, or within 14 days of an MAOI. Allow at least 2 weeks after stopping the SSRIs before starting an MAOI.

MAOIs should not be administered together with or immediately following tricyclic antidepressants (TCAs). At least 14 days should elapse between the discontinuation of the MAOIs and the institution of a TCA. Some TCAs have been used safely and successfully in combination with MAOIs.

Withdrawal may be associated with nausea, vomiting and malaise.

Coexisting symptoms: **Tranylcypromine** may aggravate coexisting symptoms in depression, such as anxiety and agitation.

Renal function impairment: Observe caution in patients with impaired renal function because there is a possibility of cumulative effects in such patients.

Elderly: Older patients may suffer more morbidity than younger patients during and following an episode of hypertension or malignant hyperthermia with MAOI use. Older patients have less compensatory reserve to cope with any serious adverse reactions. Therefore, use tranylcypromine with caution in the elderly.

Pregnancy: Category C.

Lactation: Safety for use during lactation has not been established. **Tranylcypromine** is excreted in breast milk.

Children: Not recommended for patients < 16 years of age.

Precautions:

Hypotension: Follow all patients for symptoms of postural hypotension. Blood pressure usually returns to pretreatment levels rapidly when the drug is discontinued or the dosage is reduced.

Hypomania: Hypomania has been the most common severe psychiatric side effect reported. This has been largely limited to patients in whom disorders characterized by hyperkinetic symptoms coexist with, but are obscured by, depressive affect.

Diabetes: There is conflicting evidence as to whether MAOIs affect glucose metabolism or potentiate hypoglycemic agents. Consider this if used in diabetics.

Epilepsy: The effect of MAOIs on the convulsive threshold may vary; take adequate precautions when treating epileptic patients.

Hepatic complications. Perform periodic liver function tests, such as bilirubins, alkaline phosphatase or transaminases during therapy; discontinue at the first sign of hepatic dysfunction or jaundice.

Myocardial ischemia: MAO inhibitors may suppress anginal pain that would otherwise serve as a warning of myocardial ischemia, apparently due to their peripheral vasodilatory, postural hypotensive actions.

Hyperthyroid patients: Use **tranylcypromine** cautiously because of increased sensitivity to pressor amines.

Pyridoxine deficiency has occurred in **phenelzine** patients.

Switching MAOIs: In several case reports, hypertensive crisis, cerebral hemorrhage and death have possibly resulted from switching from one MAOI to another without a waiting period. However, in other patients no adverse reactions occurred. Nevertheless, a waiting period of 10 to 14 days is recommended when switching from one MAOI to another.

Drug abuse and dependence: There have been reports of drug dependency in patients using doses of **tranylcypromine** significantly in excess of the therapeutic range.

Drug Interactions:

Drugs that may affect MAOIs include dibenzazepine-related entities, disulfiram, methylphenidate, metrizamide and sulfonamide.

Drugs that may be affected by MAOIs include anesthetics, antidepressants, antidiabetic agents, barbiturates, beta blockers, dextromethorphan, guanethidine, levodopa, meperidine, methyldopa, rauwolfia alkaloids, sulfonamide, sumatriptan, sympathomimetics, thiazide diuretics and L-tryptophan.

Drug/Food interactions: Warn all patients against eating foods with a high **tyramine** content. Hypertensive crisis may result (see Warnings).

Adverse Reactions:

Common:

Cardiovascular – Orthostatic hypotension, associated in some patients with falling; disturbances in cardiac rate and rhythm.

CNS – Dizziness; vertigo; headache; overactivity; hyperreflexia; tremors; muscle twitching; mania; hypomania; jitteriness; confusion; memory impairment; sleep disturbances including hypersomnia and insomnia; weakness; myoclonic movements; fatigue; drowsiness; restlessness; overstimulation including increased anxiety, agitation and manic symptoms.

GI – Constipation; nausea; diarrhea; abdominal pain.

Miscellaneous – Edema; dry mouth; blurred vision; hyperhidrosis; elevated serum transaminases; minor skin reactions such as skin rashes; anorexia; weight changes. Weight gain appears to be most common with phenelzine, least likely with tranylcypromine.

Administration and Dosage:

PHENELZINE:

Initial dose – 15 mg 3 times a day.

Early phase treatment – Increase dosage to at least 60 mg/day at a fairly rapid pace consistent with patient tolerance. It may be necessary to increase dosage up to 90 mg/day to obtain sufficient MAO inhibition.

Maintenance dose – After maximum benefit is achieved, reduce dosage slowly over several weeks. Maintenance dose may be as sow as 15 mg/day or every other day; continue for as long as required.

TRANYLCYPROMINE: The usual effective dosage is 30 mg/day in divided doses. If there is no improvement after 2 weeks, increase dosage in 10 mg/day increments of 1 to 3 weeks. Dosage range may be extended to a maximum of 60 mg/day from the usual 30 mg/day. Withdrawal from tranylcypromine should be gradual.

ANTIPSYCHOTIC AGENTS

Actions:

Pharmacology:

Select Dosage and Pharmacologic Parameters of Antipsychotics

Incidence of Side Effects: +++ = High, ++ = Moderate, + = Low Antipsychotic agent	Approx. equiv. dose (mg)	Adult daily dosage range (mg)	Sedation	Extrapyramidal symptoms	Anticholinergic effects	Orthostatic hypotension	Therapeutic plasma concentration (ng/ml)
Phenothiazines: Aliphatic							
Chlorpromazine	100	30-800	+++	++	++	+++	30-500
Promazine	200	40-1200	++	++	+++	++	
Triflupromazine	25	60-150	+++	++	+++	++	
Phenothiazines: Piperidine							
Thioridazine	100	150-800	+++	+	+++	+++	
Mesoridazine	50	30-400	+++	+	+++	++	
Phenothiazines: Piperazine							
Acetophenazine	20	60-120	++	+++	+	+	
Perphenazine	10	12-64	+	+++	+	+	0.8-1.2
Prochlorperazine	15	15-150	++	+++	+	+	
Fluphenazine	2	0.5-40	+	+++	+	+	0.13-2.8
Trifluoperazine	5	2-40	+	+++	+	+	
Thioxanthenes							
Chlorprothixene	100	75-600	+++	++	++	++	
Thiothixene	4	8-30	+	+++	+	+	2-57
Butyrophenone							
Haloperidol	2	1-15	+	+++	+	+	5-20
Dihydroindolone							
Molindone	10	15-225	+	+++	+	+	
Dibenzoxazepine							
Loxapine	15	20-250	++	+++	+	++	
Dibenzodiazepine							
Clozapine	50	300-900	+++	+	+++	+++	
Benzisoxazole							
Risperidone		4-16	+	0/+	+	+	
Diphenylbutylpiperidine							
Pimozide	0.3-0.5	1-10	++	+++	++	+	

The exact mode of action is not fully understood. Antipsychotics block postsynaptic dopamine receptors in the basal ganglia, hypothalamus, limbic system, brain stem and medulla. Inhibition or alteration of dopamine release, an increased neuronal cell firing rate in the midbrain and an increased turnover rate of dopamine in the forebrain have been noted. These observations support the theory that antipsychotics interfere with dopamine, but do not prove that dopaminolytic activity is sufficient for antipsychotic efficacy.

There is little evidence of clinical differences in efficacy among these agents (except clozapine) when used in equitherapeutic dosages; however, a patient who fails to respond to one agent may respond to another and agents are not necessarily interchangeable. Clozapine is used for severely ill schizophrenic patients who fail to respond adequately to standard antipsychotic treatment.

The principal differences between antipsychotic agents are the type and severity of side effects which include: Sedation, extrapyramidal effects. Coadministration of two or more antipsychotics does not improve clinical response and may increase the potential for adverse effects.

In chronic therapy, full clinical effects may not be achieved for ≥ 6 weeks. Approximately 4 to 7 days are required to achieve steady-state plasma levels; therefore, do not make more than weekly dosage adjustments in chronic therapy.

Since plasma concentrations of antipsychotics are highly variable from patient to patient, plasma monitoring of these agents may not be useful for determining therapeutic response.

Pharmacokinetics:

Absorption – Oral absorption tends to be erratic and variable. Peak plasma levels are seen 2 to 4 hours after oral use.

Distribution – These agents are widely distributed in tissues; CNS concentrations exceed those in plasma. They are highly bound to plasma proteins (91% to 99%). Because they are highly lipophilic, the antipsychotics and metabolites accumulate in the brain, lungs and other tissues with high blood supply. They are stored in these tissues and may be found in urine for up to 6 months after the last dose.

Metabolism – Extensive biotransformation occurs in the liver. Numerous active metabolites, which persist for prolonged periods, have important side effects and contribute to the biological activity of the parent drug.

Excretion – One-half of the excretion of these agents occurs via the kidneys and the other half occurs through enterohepatic circulation. Elimination half-lives range from 10 to 20 hours. Less than 1% is excreted as unchanged drug.

Indications:

Management of psychotic disorders.

Some of these agents are used as antiemetics (refer to Antiemetic/Antivertigo Agents).

Unlabeled uses: Chlorpromazine and haloperidol are effective in the treatment of phencyclidine (PCP) psychosis; coadministration of ascorbic acid with haloperidol may be more effective than haloperidol alone.

IV or IM chlorpromazine may be beneficial for migraine headaches; IV prochlorperazine may be effective in treating severe vascular or tension headaches.

Neuroleptics appear useful for the treatment of Tourette's syndrome.

Neuroleptics are effective in control of acute agitation in the elderly. May also be useful in treating some symptoms of dementia including agitation, hyperactivity, hallucinations, suspiciousness, hostility and uncooperativeness; however, they do not improve memory loss and may impair cognitive function.

Other potential uses include treatment of: Huntington's chorea (chlorpromazine, fluphenazine, haloperidol); hemiballismus (perphenazine, haloperidol); chorea associated with rheumatic fever or SLE, spasmodic torticollis and Meige's syndrome (haloperidol).

Contraindications:

Comatose or severely depressed states; hypersensitivity (cross sensitivity between phenothiazines may occur); presence of large amounts of other CNS depressants; bone marrow depression; blood dyscrasias; circulatory collapse (thioxanthenes); subcortical brain damage; Parkinson's disease (haloperidol); liver damage; cerebral arteriosclerosis; coronary artery disease; severe hypotension or hypertension; pediatric surgery (prochlorperazine).

Warnings:

Tardive dyskinesia (TD), a syndrome consisting of potentially irreversible, involuntary dyskinetic movements, may develop in patients treated with neuroleptic drugs. Both the risk of developing TD and the likelihood that it will become irreversible are increased as duration of treatment and total cumulative dose administered increase.

Neuroleptic malignant syndrome (NMS) is a rare idiosyncratic combination of EPS, hyperthermia and autonomic disturbance. Onset may be hours to months after drug initiation, but once started, proceeds rapidly over 24 to 72 hours. It is most commonly associated with **haloperidol** and depot **fluphenazines**, but has occurred with **thiothixene** and **thioridazine** and may occur with other agents. NMS is potentially fatal, and requires intensive symptomatic treatment and immediate discontinuation of neuroleptic treatment.

CNS effects: These agents may impair mental or physical abilities, especially during the first few days. Drowsiness may occur during the first or second week, after which it generally disappears. If troublesome, lower the dosage. Caution patients against activities requiring alertness (eg, operating vehicles or machinery).

Antiemetic effects: Drugs with antiemetic effect can obscure signs of toxicity of other drugs, or mask symptoms of disease (eg, brain tumor, intestinal obstruction, Reye's syndrome). They can suppress the cough reflex; aspiration of vomitus is possible.

Decreased serum cholesterol occurs. **Chlorpromazine** may raise plasma cholesterol.

Cardiovascular: Use with caution in patients with cardiovascular disease or mitral insufficiency. Increased pulse rates occur in most patients.

Hypotension – Carefully watch patients who are undergoing surgery, and who are on large doses of phenothiazines, for hypotensive phenomena. The hypotensive effects may occur after the first injection of the antipsychotic, occasionally after subsequent injections, and rarely after the first oral dose. Recovery is usually spontaneous and symptoms disappear within 0.5 to 2 hours.

Ophthalmic: Use with caution in patients with a history of glaucoma. During prolonged therapy, ocular changes may occur; these include particle deposition in the cornea and lens, progressing in more severe cases to star-shaped lenticular opacities. Pigmentary retinopathy occurs most frequently in patients receiving **thioridazine** dosages > 1 g/day.

Seizure disorders: These drugs can lower the convulsive threshold and may precipitate seizures. Use cautiously in patients with a history of epilepsy and only when absolutely necessary.

Adynamic ileus occasionally occurs with phenothiazine therapy and, if severe, can result in complications and death.

Sudden death: Previous brain damage or seizures may be predisposing factors; avoid high doses in known seizure patients.

Hepatic effects: Jaundice usually occurs between the second and fourth weeks of treatment and is regarded as a hypersensitivity reaction.

Renal function impairment: Administer cautiously to those with diminished renal function.

Hepatic function impairment: Use with caution in patients with impaired hepatic function. Patients with a history of hepatic encephalopathy due to cirrhosis have increased sensitivity to the CNS effects of antipsychotic drugs (ie, impaired cerebration and abnormal slowing of the EEG).

Carcinogenesis: Neuroleptic drugs (except promazine) elevate prolactin levels which persist during chronic use. Tissue culture experiments indicate ≈⅓ of human breast cancers are prolactin-dependent in vitro, a factor of potential importance if use of these drugs is contemplated in a patient with previously detected breast cancer.

Elderly: Dosages in the lower range are sufficient for most elderly patients. Monitor response and adjust dosage accordingly. Increase dosage gradually in elderly patients.

Pregnancy: Safety for use during pregnancy has not been established. Phenothiazines readily cross the placenta.

Lactation: **Chlorpromazine** and **haloperidol** have been detected in breast milk. Although few cases are documented, a milk:plasma ratio of 0.5 to 0.7 or less is reported, representing a milk drug level of 290 ng/ml and 2 to 23.5 ng/ml, respectively. Safety for use in the nursing mother has not been established.

Children: In general, these products are not recommended for children < 12 years old. Loxapine is not recommended in children < 16 years old.

Precautions:

Concomitant conditions: Use with caution in patients: Exposed to extreme heat or phosphorus insecticides; in a state of alcohol withdrawal; with dermatoses or other allergic reactions to phenothiazine derivatives because of the possibility of cross-sensitivity; who have exhibited idiosyncrasy to other centrally-acting drugs.

Hematologic: Various blood dyscrasias have occurred.

Myelography: Discontinue phenothiazines at least 48 hours before myelography due to the possibility of seizures; do not resume therapy for at least 24 hours postprocedure.

Thyroid: Severe neurotoxicity (rigidity, inability to walk or talk) may occur in patients with thyrotoxicosis who are also receiving antipsychotics.

Hyperpyrexia: A significant, not otherwise explained rise in body temperature may indicate intolerance to antipsychotics.

ECT: Reserve concurrent use with electroconvulsive treatment for those patients for whom it is essential; the hazards may be increased.

Abrupt withdrawal: These drugs are not known to cause psychic dependence and do not produce tolerance or addiction. However, following abrupt withdrawal of high dose therapy, symptoms such as gastritis, nausea, vomiting, dizziness, headache, tachycardia, insomnia and tremulousness have occurred. These symptoms can be reduced by gradual reduction of the dosage (one suggestion is 10% to 25% every 2 weeks) or by continuing antiparkinson agents for several weeks after the antipsychotic is withdrawn.

Suicide possibility in depressed patients remains during treatment and until significant remission occurs. This type of patient should not have access to large quantities of the drug.

Cutaneous pigmentation changes/photosensitivity: Rare instances of skin pigmentation have occurred, primarily in females on long-term, high dose therapy. Photosensitization may occur; caution patients against exposure to ultraviolet light or undue exposure to sunlight during phenothiazine therapy. These effects occur most commonly with **chlorpromazine** (3%).

Drug Interactions:

Drugs that may affect phenothiazines include alcohol, aluminum salts, anorexiants, anticholinergics, barbiturates, carbamazepine, charcoal, fluoxetine, lithium, meperidine, methyldopa, metrizamide and propranolol. Drugs that may be affected by phenothiazine include barbiturate anesthetics, bromocriptine, norepinephrine and epinephrine, guanethidine, phenytoin, propranolol, TCAs and valproic acid.

Drug/Lab test interactions: An increase in **cephalin flocculation** sometimes accompanied by alterations in other **liver function tests** has occurred in patients receiving fluphenazine enanthate who have had no clinical evidence of liver damage.

Phenothiazines may discolor the urine pink to red-brown.

False-positive **pregnancy tests** have occurred, but are less likely to occur when a serum test is used.

An increase in **protein bound iodine**, not attributable to an increase in thyroxine, has been noted.

Adverse Reactions:

CNS effects: Headache; weakness; tremor; staggering gait; twitching; tension; jitteriness; fatigue; slurring; insomnia; vertigo; drowsiness (80%, usually lasts 1 week). Exacerbation of psychotic symptoms including hallucinations; catatonic-like states; lethargy; restlessness; hyperactivity; agitation; nocturnal confusion; toxic confusional states; bizarre dreams; depression; euphoria; excitement; paranoid reactions.

Autonomic: Dry mouth; nasal congestion; nausea; vomiting; paresthesia; anorexia; pallor; flushed facies; salivation; perspiration; constipation; fecal impaction; diarrhea; urinary retention, frequency or incontinence; polyuria; enuresis; priapism; ejaculation inhibition; male impotence (not reported with **molindone**).

Heatstroke/Hyperpyrexia induced by neuroleptics has occurred.

Extrapyramidal: These are usually dose-related and take three forms: Pseudoparkinsonism (4% to 40%); akathisia (7% to 20%); dystonias (2% to 50%).

Hepatic: Jaundice usually occurs between the second and fourth weeks of therapy and is regarded as a hypersensitivity reaction.

Hematologic: Eosinophilia; leukopenia; leukocytosis; anemia; tendency toward lymphomonocytosis; thrombocytopenia; granulocytopenia; aplastic anemia; hemolytic anemia; thrombocytopenic or nonthrombocytopenic purpura; agranulocytosis; pancytopenia.

Cardiovascular: Hypotension; postural hypotension; hypertension; tachycardia (especially with rapid increase in dosage); bradycardia; cardiac arrest; circulatory collapse; syncope; lightheadedness; faintness; dizziness.

Cardiovascular effects are generally attributable to the piperidine phenothiazines > aliphatic > piperazines (see table).

Hypersensitivity: Urticarial (5%), maculopapular hypersensitivity reactions; pruritus; dry skin; erythema; photosensitivity; eczema; asthma; rashes, including acneiform; hair loss; exfoliative dermatitis.

Endocrine: Lactation and moderate breast engorgement in females; galactorrhea; mastalgia; amenorrhea; menstrual irregularities; changes in libido; hyperglycemia or hypoglycemia; hyponatremia; glycosuria; raised plasma cholesterol levels. Resumption of menses in previously amenorrheic women has been reported with **molindone**. Initially, heavy menses may occur.

Ophthalmic: Glaucoma; photophobia; blurred vision; miosis; mydriasis; ptosis; star-shaped lenticular opacities; pigmentary retinopathy.

Respiratory: Laryngospasm; bronchospasm; increased depth of respiration; dyspnea.

Miscellaneous: Increases in appetite and weight (excessive weight gain has not occurred with **molindone**); dyspepsia, peripheral or facial edema; suppression of cough reflex (with potential for aspiration or asphyxia).

OLANZAPINE

Tablets: 5, 7.5 and 10 mg	*Zyprexa* (Eli Lilly)

Actions:

Pharmacology: The mechanism of action of olanzapine, a thienbenzodiazepine, is unknown. However, it has been proposed that this drug's antipsychotic activity is mediated through a combination of dopamine and serotonin type 2 ($5HT_2$) antagonism. Antagonism at receptors other than dopamine and $5HT_2$ with similar receptor affinities may explain some of the other therapeutic and side effects of olanzapine. Olanzapine's antagonism of muscarinic M_{1-5} receptors may explain its anticholinergic effects, with somnolence and orthostatic hypotension resulting from antagonism of histaminic H_1 and alpha$_1$ adrenergic receptors, respectively.

Pharmacokinetics:

Absorption/Distribution – Olanzapine is well absorbed and reaches peak concentrations in ≈ 6 hours following an oral dose. It is eliminated extensively by first pass metabolism, with ≈ 40% of the dose metabolized before reaching the systemic circulation. Food does not affect the rate or extent of olanzapine absorption.

Its half-life ranges from 21 to 54 hours (mean, 30 hr), and apparent plasma clearance ranges from 12 to 47 L/hr (mean, 25 L/hr).

Administration of olanzapine once daily leads to steady-state concentrations in ≈ 1 that are ≈ twice the concentrations after single doses.

Olanzapine in extensively distributed throughout the body, with a volume of distribution of ≈ 1000 L. It is 93% bound to plasma proteins over the concentration range of 7 to 1100 ng/ml, binding primarily to albumin and alpha$_1$-acid glycoprotein.

Metabolism/Excretion – Olanzapine is highly metabolized. Approximately 57% and 30% of the dose was recovered in the urine and feces, respectively.

Direct glucuronidation and cytochrome P450 (CYP) mediated oxidation are the primary metabolic pathways for olanzapine.

Gender: Clearance of olanzapine is ≈ 30% lower in women than in men. There were, however, no apparent differences between men and women in effectiveness or adverse effects. Dosage modifications based on gender should not be needed.

Smoking: Olanzapine clearance is ≈ 40% higher in smokers than in non-smokers, although dosage modifications are not routinely recommended.

Indications:

Psychotic disorders: Management of the manifestations of psychotic disorders.

Contraindications:

Hypersensitivity to the product.

Warnings:

Neuroleptic Malignant Syndrome (NMS): A potentially fatal symptom complex somtimes referred to as Neuroleptic Malignant Syndrom (NMS) has been reported in association with administration of antipsychotic drugs.

Tardive dyskinesia may develop in patients treated with antipsychotic drugs.

Tachycardia: Olanzapine use was associated with a mean increase in heart rate of 2.4 beats/minute compared with no change among placebo patients. This slight tendency to tachycardia may be related to olanzapine's potential for inducing orthostatic changes (see Precautions).

Hepatic function impairment: Use caution in patients with signs and symptoms of hepatic impairment, in patients with pre-existing conditions associated with limited hepatic functional reserve, and in patients who are being teated with potentially hepatotoxic drugs.

Elderly: The mean elimination half-life of olanzapine may be ≈ 1.5 times greater in elderly (> 65 years of age) than in non-elderly subjects (≤ 65 years of age). Use caution in dosing the elderly. In general, there was no indication of any different tolerability of olanzapine in the elderly compared with younger adults.

Pregnancy: Category C.

Lactation: It is not known if olanzapine is excreted in breast milk. Advise patients not to breastfeed an infant if they are taking olanzapine.

Children: Safely and effectiveness in pediatric patients < 18 years of age have not been established.

Precautions:

Monitoring: Periodic assessment of transaminases is recommended in patients with significant hepatic disease.

Orthostatic hypotension: Olanzapine may induce orthostatic hypotension associated with dizziness, tachycardia, and in some patients, syncope, especially during the intial dose-titration period. The risk of orthostatic hypotension and syncope may be minimized by initiating therapy with 5 mg once daily. Use olanzapine with caution in patients with known cardiovascular disease, cerebrovascular disease and conditions which would predispose patients to hypotension.

Seizures: Seizures occurred in 0.9% of olanzapine-treated patients. Use olanzapine with cuation in patients with a history of seizures in many of these cases. Use olanzapine with caution in patients with a history of seizures or with conditions that potentially lower the seizure threshold.

Hyperprolactinemia: As with other drugs that antagonize dopamine D_2 receptors, olanzapine elevates prolactin levels and and a modest elevation persists during chronic administration.

Transaminase elevations: Clinically significant ALT elevations (≥ 3 times the upper limit of the normal range) were observed in 2% of patients. No patients experienced jaundice. In two patients, liver enzymes decreased toward normal despite continued treatment and in two others, enzymes decreased upon discontinuation of olanzapine.

About 1% of patients discontinued treatment due to transaminase increases. Periodic assessment of transaminases is recommended in patients with significant hepatic disease.

Potential for cognitive and motor impairment: Somnolence was a commonly reported adverse event associated with olanzapine treatment, occurring in 26% of olanzapine patients. This adverse even was also dose related. Somnolence led to discontinuation in 0.4% of patients.

Body temperature regulation: Disruption of the body's ability to reduce core body temperature has been attributed to antipsychotic agents.

Dysphagia: Esophageal dysmotility and aspiration have been associated with antipsychotic drug use.

Suicide: The possibility of a suicide attempt is inherent in schizophrenia, and close supervision of high-risk patients should accompany drug therapy.

Anticholinergic effects: Olanzapine exhibits in vitro muscarinic receptor affinity. Olanzapine was associated with constipation, dry mouth and tachycardia, all adverse events possibly related to cholinergic antagonism. Use caution in patients with clinically significant prostatic hypertrophy, narrow-angle glaucoma or a history of paralytic ileus.

Drug Interactions:

Agents that induce CYP1A2 or glucuronyl transferase enzymes, such as omeprazole and rifampin, may cause an increase in olanzapine clearance. Inhibitors of CYP1A2 (eg, fluvoxamine) could potentially inhibit olanzapine elimination.

Drugs that may affect olanzapine include carbamazapine. Drugs that may be affected by olanzapine include antihypertensive agents, CNS acting drugs (eg, alcohol) and levodopa and dopamine agonists.

Adverse Reactions:

Adverse reactions occurring in ≥ 3% of patients include: Headache; fever; abdominal pain; back pain; chest pain; postural hypotension; tachycardia; constipation; dry mouth; weight gain; join pain; extremity pain (other than joint); somnolence; agitation; insomnia; nervousness; hostility; dizziness; anxiety; personality disorder; akathisia; hypertonia; tremor; rhinitis; cough increased; pharyngitis; amblyopia.

Administration and Dosage:

Usual dose: Administer olanzapine on a once-a-day schedule without regard to meals, generally beginning with 5 to 10 mg initially, with a target dose of 10 mg/day within several days. Further dosage adjustments, if indicated, should generally occur at intervals of not < 1 week, because steady-state for olanzapine would not be achieved for ≈ 1 week in the typical patient. When dosage adjustments are necessary, dose increments/decrements of 5 mg once daily are recommended.

Antipsychotic efficacy was demonstrated in a dose range of 10 to 15 mg/day in the clinical trials. However, increases in efficacy were not demonstrated in doses above 10 mg/day. An increase to a dose greater than the target dose of 10 mg/day is recommended only after clinical assessment. The safety of doses > 20 mg/day has not been evaluated in clinical trials.

Dosing in special populations: The recommended starting dose is 5 mg in patients who are debilitated, who have a predisposition to hypotensive reasctions, who otherwise exhibit a combination of factors that may result in slower metabolism of olanzapine (eg, nonsmoking female patients ≥ 65 years of age), or who may be more pharmacodynamically sensitive to olanzapine.

When indicated, use caution with dose escalation.

Maintenance treatment: While there is no body of evidence available to answer the question of how long the patient treated with olanzapine should remain on it, the effectiveness of maintenance treatment is well established for many other antipsychotic drugs. It is recommended that responding patients be continued on olanzapine, but at the lowest dose needed to maintain remission. Periodically reassess patients to determine the need for maintenance treatment.

PHENOTHIAZINE AND THIOXANTHENE DERIVATIVES

PHENOTHIAZINE DERIVATIVES	
CHLORPROMAZINE HCl	
Tablets: 10, 25, 50, 100 and 200 mg (*Rx*)	Various, *Thorazine* (SK-Beecham)
Capsules, sustained release: 30, 75, 150, 200 and 300 mg (*Rx*)	*Thorazine Spansules* (SK-Beecham)
Syrup: 10 mg/5 ml (*Rx*)	*Thorazine* (SK-Beecham)
Concentrate: 30 mg/ml and 100 mg/ml (*Rx*)	Various, *Thorazine* (SK-Beecham)
Suppositores (as base): 25 and 100 mg (*Rx*)	*Thorazine* (SK-Beecham)
Injection: 25 mg/ml (*Rx*)	Various, *Thorazine* (SK-Beecham)
FLUPHENAZINE	
Tablets: 1, 2.5, 5 and 10 mg (*Rx*)	Various, *Permitil* (Schering), *Prolixin* (Princeton)
Elixir: 2.5 mg/5 ml (*Rx*)	*Prolixin* (Princeton)
Concentrate: 5 mg/ml (*Rx*)	*Prolixin* (Princeton)
Injection: 2.5 mg/ml (*Rx*)	Various, *Prolixin* (Princeton)
FLUPHENAZINE ENANTHATE AND DECANOATE	
Injection: 25 mg/ml (*Rx*)	Various, *Prolixin Decanoate* (Princeton), *Prolixin Enanthate* (Princeton)
MESORIDAZINE	
Tablets: 10, 25, 50 and 100 mg (*Rx*)	*Serentil* (Boehringer Ingelheim)
Concentrate: 25 mg/ml (*Rx*)	*Serentil* (Boehringer Ingelheim)
Injection: 25 mg/ml (*Rx*)	*Serentil* (Boehringer Ingelheim)
PERPHENAZINE	
Tablets: 2, 4, 8 and 16 mg (*Rx*)	Various, *Trilafon* (Schering)
Concentrate: 16 mg/5 ml (*Rx*)	*Trilafon* (Schering)
Injection: 5 mg/ml (*Rx*)	*Trilafon* (Schering)
PROCHLORPERAZINE	
Tablets: 5, 10 and 25 mg (*Rx*)	Various, *Compazine* (SK-Beecham)
Capsules, sustained release: 10, 15 and 30 mg (*Rx*)	*Compazine Spansules* (SK-Beecham)
Suppositories: 2.5, 5 and 25 mg (*Rx*)	*Compazine* (SK-Beecham)
Syrup: 5 mg/5 ml (*Rx*)	*Compazine* (SK-Beecham)
Injection: 5 mg/ml (*Rx*)	Various, *Compazine* (SK-Beecham)
PROMAZINE HCl	
Tablets: 25, 50 and 100 mg (*Rx*)	Various, *Sparine* (Wyeth-Ayerst)
Injection: 50 mg/ml (*Rx*)	Various, *Sparine* (Wyeth-Ayerst)
TRIFLUPROMAZINE HCl	
Injection: 10 mg/ml or 20 mg/ml (*Rx*)	*Vesprin* (Princeton)
THIORIDAZINE HCl	
Tablets: 10, 15, 25, 50, 100, 150 and 200 mg (*Rx*)	Various, *Mellaril* (Sandoz)
Concentrate: 30 mg/ml and 100 mg/ml (*Rx*)	Various, *Mellaril* (Sandoz)
Suspension: 25 mg/5 ml and 100 mg/5 ml (*Rx*)	*Mellaril-S* (Sandoz)
TRIFLUOPERAZINE	
Tablets: 1, 2, 5 and 10 mg (*Rx*)	Various, *Stelazine* (SK-Beecham)
Concentrate: 10 mg/ml (*Rx*)	Various, *Stelazine* (SK-Beecham)
Injection: 2 mg/ml (*Rx*)	Various, *Stelazine* (SK-Beecham)
THIOXANTHENE DERIVATIVES	
THIOTHIXENE	
Capsules: 1, 2, 5, 10 and 20 mg (*Rx*)	Various, *Navane* (Roerig)
Concentrate: 5 mg/ml (*Rx*)	Various, *Navane* (Roerig)
IM solution: 2 mg/ml (*Rx*)	*Navane* (Roerig)
Powder for Injection: 5 mg/ml when reconstituted (*Rx*)	*Navane* (Roerig)

CHLORPROMAZINE:

Adults:

Concentrate – Add desired dosage to ≥ 60 ml of diluent just prior to administration. Suggested vehicles are tomato or fruit juice, milk, simple syrup, orange syrup, carbonated beverages, coffee, tea or water. Semisolid foods (eg, soups, puddings) may also be used.

Sustained release capsules – Do not crush or chew. Swallow whole.

Injection – Do not inject SC. Inject IM slowly, deep into upper outer quadrant of buttock. Use the IV route only for severe hiccoughs, surgery and tetanus.

Outpatients – For prompt control of severe symptoms 25 mg IM; if necessary, repeat in 1 hour. Give subsequent oral doses of 25 to 50 mg 3 times daily.

The usual initial oral dose is 10 mg 3 or 4 times daily or 25 mg 2 or 3 times daily. For more serious cases, give 25 mg 3 times/day. After 1 or 2 days, increase daily dosage by 20 to 50 mg semiweekly, until patient becomes calm and cooperative. Continue optimum dosage for 2 weeks, then gradually reduce to maintenance level; 200 mg per day is not unusual.

Surgery –

Preoperative: 25 to 50 mg orally 2 to 3 hours before surgery or 12.5 to 25 mg IM 1 to 2 hours before surgery.

Intraoperative (to control acute nausea and vomiting):

IM – 12.5 mg. Repeat in hour if necessary and if no hypotension occurs.

IV – 2 mg per fractional injection at 2 minute intervals. Do not exceed 25 mg (dilute to 1 mg/ml with saline).

Acute intermittent porphyria – 25 to 50 mg orally or 25 mg IM 3 or 4 times daily until patient can take oral therapy.

Tetanus – 25 to 50 mg IM 3 or 4 times daily, usually with barbiturates. For IV use, 25 to 50 mg diluted to at least 1 mg/ml and administered at a rate of 1 mg/minute.

Psychiatry, hospitalized patients (acutely manic or disturbed) –

IM: 25 mg initially. If necessary, give an additional 25 to 50 mg injection in 1 hour. Increase gradually over several days (up to 400 mg every 4 to 6 hours in severe cases) until patient is controlled. Substitute oral dosage and increase until the patient is calm; 500 mg/day is usually sufficient.

Psychiatry, hospitalized patients (less acutely disturbed) –

Oral: 25 mg 3 times daily. Increase gradually until effective dose is reached, usually 400 mg/day.

Children: Chlorpromazine should generally not be used in children < 6 months old except where potentially lifesaving.

Psychiatric outpatients –

Oral: 0.5 mg/kg every 4 to 6 hours, as needed.

Rectal: 1 mg/kg every 6 to 8 hours, as needed.

IM: 0.5 mg/kg every 6 to 8 hours, as needed.

Surgery –

Preoperative: 0.5 mg/kg orally 2 to 3 hours before operation or 0.5 mg/kg IM 1 to 2 hours before operation.

Intraoperative (administer only to control acute nausea and vomiting):

IM – 0.25 mg/kg; repeat in hour if needed, and if no hypotension occurs.

IV – 1 mg per fractional injection at 2 minute intervals; do not exceed IM dosage. Always dilute to 1 mg/ml with saline.

Psychiatry, hospitalized patients –

Oral: In severe behavior disorders or psychotic conditions, 50 to 100 mg daily, or in older children, 200 mg or more daily may be necessary.

IM: Up to 5 years: Do not exceed 40 mg/day. *5 to 12 years old* — Do not exceed 75 mg/day, except in unmanageable cases.

Tetanus (IM or IV) – 0.5 mg/kg every 6 to 8 hours. When given IV, dilute to at least 1 mg/ml and administer at a rate of 1 mg per 2 minutes. In children up to 23 kg (50 lbs), do not exceed 40 mg daily; 23 to 45 kg (50 to 100 lbs), do not exceed 75 mg/day, except in severe cases.

FLUPHENAZINE HCl:

Oral:

Adults – Initially 0.5 to 10 mg/day in divided doses administered at 6 to 8 hour intervals. In general, a daily dose in excess of 3 mg is rarely necessary. Use doses in excess of 20 mg with caution. When symptoms are controlled, reduce dosage gradually to daily maintenance doses of 1 to 5 mg, often given as a single daily dose.

Geriatric patients: Starting dose is 1 to 2.5 mg/day, adjusted according to response.

IM: The average starting dose is 1.25 mg IM. The initial total daily dosage may range from 2.5 to 10 mg, divided and given at 6 to 8 hour intervals. In general, the parenteral dose is approximately ⅓ to ½ the oral dose. Use dosages exceeding 10 mg/day IM with caution.

FLUPHENAZINE ENANTHATE AND DECANOATE: Administer IM or SC. Initiate with 12.5 to 25 mg. Determine subsequent injections and dosage interval in accordance with patient response. Do not exceed 100 mg. If doses > 50 mg are needed, increase succeeding doses cautiously in 12.5 mg increments.

Initially, treat patients who have never taken phenothiazines with a shorter-acting form of the drug before administering the enanthate or decanoate. This helps to determine the response to fluphenazine and to establish appropriate dosage.

Severely agitated patients: Treat initially with a rapid-acting phenothiazine such as fluphenazine HCl injection. When acute symptoms have subsided, administer 25 mg of the enanthate or decanoate; adjust subsequent dosage as necessary.

MESORIDAZINE:

Mesoridazine Dosage Guidelines

Disease state	Initial oral dose	Optimum total dosage range (mg/day)
Schizophrenia	50 mg tid	100-400
Behavior problems in mental deficiency and chronic brain syndrome	25 mg tid	75-300
Alcoholism	25 mg bid	50-200
Psychoneurotic manifestations	10 mg tid	30-150

IM administration: For most patients, 25 mg initially. May repeat dose in 30 to 60 minutes, if necessary. The usual optimum dosage range is 25 to 200 mg/day.

PERPHENAZINE:

Oral: Moderately disturbed nonhospitalized patients: 4 to 8 mg 3 times/day; reduce as soon as possible to minimum effective dosage.

Hospitalized patients: 8 to 16 mg 2 to 4 times/day; avoid dosages > 64 mg/day.

IM:

Initial dose – 5 mg every 6 hours. The total daily dosage should not exceed 15 mg in ambulatory patients or 30 mg in hospitalized patients.

Psychotic conditions – While 5 mg IM has a definite tranquilizing effect, it may be necessary to use 10 mg to initiate therapy in severely agitated states. Most patients are controlled and oral therapy can be instituted within a maximum of 24 to 48 hours.

Children: Pediatric dosage has not been established. Children > 12 years of age may receive the lowest limit of the adult dosage.

Elderly: Administer one-third to one-half the adult dose.

PROCHLORPERAZINE:

Adults: Administration SC is not advisable because of local irritation.

Elderly – Lower doses are sufficient for most elderly patients.

Nonpsychotic anxiety –

Oral: 5 mg 3 or 4 times daily; 15 mg (sustained release) on arising, or 10 mg (sustained release) every 12 hours. Do not administer > 20 mg/day or for > 12 weeks.

Psychiatry –

Oral: In mild conditions, give 5 or 10 mg 3 or 4 times daily. In moderate to severe conditions, for hospitalized or adequately supervised patients, give 10 mg 3 or 4 times daily. Increase dosage gradually until symptoms are controlled or side effects become bothersome. Some patients respond to 50 to 75 mg/day. In more severe disturbances, optimum dosage is 100 to 150 mg/day.

IM: For immediate control of severely disturbed adults, inject an initial dose of 10 to 20 mg deeply into the upper outer quadrant of the buttock. Many patients respond shortly after the first injection. If necessary, repeat every 2 to 4 hours (or in resistant cases, every hour) to gain control. More than 3 or 4 doses are seldom necessary.

Children: Do not use in children < 9.1 kg or < 2 years of age. Do not use in pediatric surgery. Children seem more prone to develop extrapyramidal reactions, even on moderate doses.

Oral or rectal –

Children 2 to 12 years: 2.5 mg 2 or 3 times daily. Do not give > 10 mg on first day.

Children 2 to 5 years: Do not exceed 20 mg total daily dose.

Children 6 to 12 years: Do not exceed 25 mg total daily dose.

IM –

Children < 12 years: 0.03 mg/kg by deep IM injection. After control is achieved, usually after 1 dose, switch to oral form at same dosage level or higher.

PROMAZINE: Injection IM is preferred. Give IM injections deep into large muscle masses (eg, gluteal region). IV administration is not recommended.

Adults: In the management of severely agitated patients, administer initial doses of 50 to 150 mg IM, depending on the degree of excitation. Once control is obtained, administer orally. The oral or IM dose is 10 to 200 mg at 4 to 6 hour intervals. Maintenance dosage may range from 10 to 200 mg given at 4 to 6 hour intervals.

Do not exceed a total daily dose of 1000 mg, since higher doses have not yielded greater results.

Children (> 12 years of age): In acute episodes of chronic psychotic disease, 10 to 25 mg may be given every 4 to 6 hours.

THIORIDAZINE:

Psychotic manifestations: Usual initial dose is 50 to 100 mg 3 times daily; increase gradually to a maximum of 800 mg/day, if necessary, to control symptoms; then reduce gradually to the minimum maintenance dose. Total daily dosage ranges from 200 to 800 mg divided into 2 to 4 doses.

Short-term treatment of moderate to marked depression with variable degrees of anxiety, and treatment of multiple symptoms such as agitation, anxiety, depressed mood, tension, sleep disturbances and fears in geriatric patients: Usual initial dose is 25 mg 3 times daily. Dosage ranges from 10 mg 2 to 4 times daily in milder cases, to 50 mg 3 or 4 times daily for more severely disturbed patients. Total daily dosage ranges from 20 to 200 mg.

Children: Not recommended for children < 2 years of age. For children aged 2 to 12, the dosage ranges from 0.5 mg to a maximum of 3 mg/kg/day.

Moderate disorders – 10 mg 2 or 3 times daily is the usual starting dose.

Hospitalized, severely disturbed or psychotic children – 25 mg 2 or 3 times daily.

TRIFLUPROMAZINE:

Psychotic disorders: 60 mg IM, up to a maximum of 150 mg/day.

Children – The recommended IM dosage range is 0.2 to 0.25 mg/kg, up to a maximum total dose of 10 mg/day. Do not administer to children < 2 years of age.

TRIFLUOPERAZINE:

Psychotic disorders: 2 to 5 mg orally twice daily. Most patients will show optimum response with 15 or 20 mg/day, although a few may require ≥ 40 mg/day. Optimum therapeutic dosage levels should be reached within 2 or 3 weeks.

IM (for prompt control of severe symptoms): 1 to 2 mg by deep injection every 4 to 6 hours, as needed. More than 6 mg/24 hours is rarely necessary.

Children: Adjust dosage to the weight of the child and severity of symptoms. These dosages are for children, aged 6 ro 12, who are hospitalized or under close supervision.

Oral – Initial dose is 1 mg once or twice daily. While it is usually not necessary to exceed 15 mg/day, older children with severe symptoms may require higher doses.

IM – There has been little experience in children. However, if it is necessary to achieve rapid control of severe symptoms, administer 1 mg once or twice a day.

Elderly patients: Usually, lower dosages are sufficient.

Treatment of nonpsychotic anxiety: 1 or 2 mg twice daily. Do not administer > 6 mg per day or for > 12 weeks.

THIOTHIXENE:

Oral:

Mild conditions – Not recommended in children < 12 years of age.

Initially 2 mg 3 times daily. If indicated, an increase to 15 mg/day is often effective.

Severe conditions – Initially 5 mg twice/day. Optimal is 20 to 30 mg/day. If indicated, 60 mg/day is often effective. Exceeding 60 mg/day rarely increases response.

IM: 4 mg 2 to 4 times daily. Most patients are controlled on 16 to 20 mg/day (maximum 30 mg/day).

HALOPERIDOL

Tablets: 0.5, 1, 2, 5, 10 and 20 mg (*Rx*)	Various, *Haldol* (McNeil-CPC)
Concentrate: 2 mg/ml (*Rx*)	Various, *Haldol* (McNeil-CPC)
Injection: 5 mg/ml, 50 mg/ml, 100 mg/ml (*Rx*)	Various, *Haldol* (McNeil-CPC), *Haldol Decanoate 50* (McNeil-CPC), *Haldol Decanoate 100* (McNeil-CPC)

Actions:

Pharmacology: An antipsychotic agent with pharmacologic effects similar to piperazine phenothiazines.

Pharmacokinetics: Haloperidol is 60% and 75% absorbed via the oral and IM route, respectively. Protein binding is 90% to 92%. It is metabolized by the liver, and 40% is excreted in the urine and 15% in the bile.

Indications:

Psychotic disorder management.

Tourette's disorder in children and adults for the control of tics and vocal utterances.

Severe behavioral problems in children with combative, explosive hyperexcitability which cannot be accounted for by immediate provocation.

Hyperactive children (short-term treatment) who show excessive motor activity with accompanying conduct disorders consisting of impulsivity, difficulty sustaining attention, aggression, mood lability or poor frustration tolerance.

Prolonged parenteral neuroleptic therapy (eg, chronic schizophrenia): Haloperidol decanoate is a long-acting parenteral antipsychotic for patients requiring such therapy.

Unlabeled uses: Haloperidol is an effective antiemetic in small doses. It has been given IV for acute psychiatric situations. It is effective in the treatment of phencyclidine (PCP) psychosis (possibly more effective with concurrent ascorbic acid).

Administration and Dosage:

Individualize dosage. Children, debilitated or geriatric patients and those with a history of adverse reactions to neuroleptic drugs may require less haloperidol.

Adults: Initial dosage range: Moderate symptoms or geriatric or debilitated patients: 0.5 to 2 mg 2 or 3 times daily; severe symptoms or chronic or resistant patients: 3 to 5 mg 2 or 3 times daily.

Patients who remain severely disturbed or inadequately controlled may require dosage adjustment. Daily dosages up to 100mg may be necessary. Infrequently, doses >100 mg have been used for severely resistant patients.

Children: Do not use in children < 3 years of age. Initial dose is 0.5 mg/day. If required, increase in 0.5mg increments each 5 to 7 days until therapeutic effect is obtained. Total dose may be divided and given 2 or 3 times daily.

Psychotic disorders – 0.05 to 0.15 mg/kg/day.

Nonpsychotic behavior disorders; Tourette's disorder: 0.05 to 0.075 mg/kg/day.

Severely disturbed psychotic children may require higher doses.

Other suggested doses for children 3 to 6 years old include: Agitation and hyperkinesia – 0.01 to 0.03 mg/kg/day orally; infantile autism – 0.5 to 4 mg/day.

Maintenance dosage – Upon achieving a satisfactory therapeutic response, gradually reduce dosage to the lowest effective maintenance level.

Adults: IM administration: 2 to 5 mg for prompt control of the acutely agitated patient with moderately severe to very severe symptoms. Depending on response, administer subsequent doses as often as every 60 minutes, although 4 to 8 hour intervals may be satisfactory.

The oral form should replace the injectable as soon as feasible. For an approximation of the total daily dose required, use the parenteral dose administered in the preceding 24 hours. Give the first oral dose within 12 to 24 hours following the last parenteral dose.

Haloperidol decanoate injection – Administer by deep IM injection. The maximum volume per injection site should not exceed 3 ml. The recommended interval between doses is 4 weeks. Do not administer IV.

For patients previously maintained on low doses of antipsychotics (eg, up to the equivalent of 10 mg/day oral haloperidol), it is recommended that the initial dose of haloperidol decanoate be 10 to 15 times the previous daily dose in oral haloperidol equivalents; limited clinical experience suggests that lower initial doses may be adequate. The initial dose of haloperidol decanoate should not exceed 100 mg regardless of previous antipsychotic dose requirements. Haloperidol decanoate has been effectively administered at monthly intervals in several clinical studies.

Elderly/Debilitated – Lower initial doses and more gradual adjustment are recommended.

MOLINDONE HCl

Tablets: 5, 10, 25, 50 and 100 mg (*Rx*)	*Moban* (DuPont)
Concentrate: 20 mg/ml (*Rx*)	

Actions:

Pharmacology: Molindone is structurally unrelated to the phenothiazines, butyrophenones or thioxanthenes, but it resembles the piperazine phenothiazines in its clinical action.

Pharmacokinetics: Molindone is rapidly absorbed and metabolized. Unmetabolized drug reaches peak blood levels at 1.5 hours. Effects from a single oral dose persist for 24 to 36 hours. Less than 2% to 3% is excreted unmetabolized in urine and feces.

Indications:

Management of manifestations of psychotic disorders.

Drug Interactions:

Tablets contain calcium sulfate as an excipient; calcium ions may interfere with the absorption of drugs such as phenytoin sodium or tetracyclines.

Administration and Dosage:

Initial dosage: 50 to 75 mg/day, increased to 100 mg/day in 3 or 4 days. Individualize dosage; patients with severe symptoms may require up to 225 mg/day.

Start elderly and debilitated patients on lower dosage.

Maintenance therapy:

Mild – 5 to 15 mg 3 or 4 times daily;
Moderate – 10 to 25 mg 3 or 4 times daily;
Severe – 225 mg/day may be required.

LOXAPINE

Capsules: 5, 10, 25 and 50 mg (*Rx*)	Various, *Loxitane* (Lederle)
Concentrate: 25 mg/ml (*Rx*)	*Loxitane* C (Lederle)
Injection: 50 mg/ml (*Rx*)	*Loxitane* IM (Lederle)

Complete prescribing information for these products begins on page 265.

Actions:

Pharmacology: Loxapine is chemically distinct from the thioxanthenes, butyrophenones and phenothiazines. No clear advantages over other antipsychotic agents are established.

Pharmacokinetics: Loxapine is metabolized extensively and is excreted within the first 24 hours. Metabolites are excreted in the urine as conjugates and in the feces unconjugated. Signs of sedation are usually seen within 20 to 30 minutes after administration, are most pronounced within 1.5 to 3 hours and last approximately 12 hours.

Indications:

Management of the manifestations of psychotic disorders.

Administration and Dosage:

Oral: Individualize dosage. Administer in divided doses, 2 to 4 times daily.

Initial dosage – 10 mg twice daily. In severely disturbed patients, up to 50 mg/day may be desirable. Increase dosage fairly rapidly over the first 7 to 10 days until psychotic symptoms are controlled. The usual range is 60 to 100 mg/day. Dosage > 250 mg/day is not recommended.

Maintenance therapy – Reduce dosage to the lowest level compatible with control of symptoms; usual range is 20 to 60 mg/day.

Mix the concentrate with orange or grapefruit juice shortly before use.

IM – For prompt symptomatic control in the acutely agitated patient and in patients whose symptoms render oral medication temporarily impractical.

Administer IM (not IV) in 12.5 to 50 mg doses at intervals of 4 to 6 hours or longer. Many patients respond satisfactorily to twice daily dosage. Once control is achieved, institute oral medication, usually within 5 days.

CLOZAPINE

Tablets: 25 and 100 mg (*Rx*) — *Clozaril* (Sandoz)

Warning:

Because of the significant risk of agranulocytosis, a potentially life-threatening adverse event, reserve clozapine for use in the treatment of severely ill schizophrenic patients who fail to show an acceptable response to adequate courses of standard antipsychotic drug treatment, either because of insufficient effectiveness or the inability to achieve an effective dose due to intolerable adverse effects from those drugs. Consequently, before initiating treatment with clozapine, it is strongly recommended that a patient be given at least two trials, each with a different standard antipsychotic drug product, at an adequate dose and for an adequate duration. Patients who are being treated with clozapine must have a baseline white blood cell (WBC) and differential count before initiation of treatment, and a WBC count every week throughout treatment and for 4 weeks after the discontinuation of clozapine.

Actions:

Pharmacology: Clozapine is a tricyclic dibenzodiazepine derivative with a profile of binding to dopamine receptors. Although clozapine does interfere with the binding of dopamine at both D-1 and D-2 receptors, it does not induce catalepsy nor inhibit apomorphine-induced stereotypy. This evidence, consistent with the view that clozapine is preferentially more active at limbic than at striatal dopamine receptors, may explain clozapine's relative freedom from extrapyramidal side effects. Clozapine also acts as an antagonist at adrenergic, cholinergic, histaminergic and serotonergic receptors. In contrast to more typical antipsychotic drugs, clozapine therapy produces little or no prolactin elevation.

As is true of more typical antipsychotic drugs, clozapine increases delta and theta activity and slows dominant alpha frequencies of the EEG. Enhanced synchronization occurs, and sharp wave activity and spike and wave complexes may also develop. Patients rarely may report intensification of dream activity. REM sleep was increased to 85% of the total sleep time. In these patients, the onset of REM sleep occurred almost immediately after falling asleep.

Pharmacokinetics:

Absorption/Distribution – Clozapine tablets are equally bioavailable relative to a clozapine solution. Following a dosage of 100 mg twice daily, the average steady-state peak plasma concentration was 319 ng/ml (range: 102 to 771 ng/ml), occurring at an average of 2.5 hours (range: 1 to 6 hours) after dosing. The average minimum concentration at steady state was 122 ng/ml (range: 41 to 343 ng/ml) after 100 mg twice daily dosing.

Clozapine is approximately 95% bound to serum proteins. The interaction between clozapine and other highly protein-bound drugs has not been fully evaluated but may be important.

Metabolism/Excretion – Clozapine is almost completely metabolized prior to excretion and only trace amounts of unchanged drug are detected in the urine and feces.

The mean elimination half-life of clozapine after a single 75 mg dose was 8 hours, compared to a mean elimination half-life of 12 hours after achieving steady state with 100 mg twice daily dosing. In comparisons of single and multiple dose administration of clozapine, the elimination half-life increased significantly after multiple dosing relative to that after single dose administration, suggesting concentration dependent pharmacokinetics.

Indications:

Management of severely ill schizophrenic patients who fail to respond adequately to standard antipsychotic drug treatment.

Contraindications:

Myeloproliferative disorders; history of clozapine-induced agranulocytosis or severe granulocytopenia; simultaneous administration with other agents having a well-known potential to suppress bone marrow function; severe CNS depression or comatose states from any cause.

Warnings:

Agranulocytosis, defined as a granulocyte count of < 500/mm³, occurs in association with clozapine use at a cumulative incidence at 1 year ≈ 1.3%. This occurred when the need for close monitoring of WBC counts was already recognized. The reaction could prove fatal if not detected early and therapy interrupted. Of the 112 cases of agranulocytosis reported worldwide in association with clozapine use as of December 31, 1986, 35% were fatal. However, few of these deaths occurred since 1977, when knowledge of clozapine-induced agranulocytosis became more widespread, and close monitoring of WBC counts more widely practiced.

Patients must have a blood sample drawn for a WBC count before initiation of treatment with clozapine, and must have subsequent WBC counts done at least weekly for the duration of therapy, as well as for 4 weeks thereafter. The distribution of clozapine is contingent upon performance of the required blood tests.

Clozapine Therapy Guidelines Based on WBC and Granulocyte Count

WBC Count (mm³)	Granulocyte Count (mm³)	Guidelines
< 3500, or history of myeloproliferative disorder, or previous clozapine-induced agranulocytosis or granulocytopenia		Do not initiate treatment.
< 3500, or > 3500 with a substantial drop from baseline, following initiation of treatment		Repeat WBC and differential counts. Symptoms of infection: Lethargy, weakness, fever, sore throat.
3000 to 3500 on subsequent counts	> 1500	Perform twice weekly WBC and differential counts.
< 3000	< 1500	Interrupt therapy, monitor for flu-like symptoms or other symptoms of infection. May resume therapy if no signs of infection develop, WBC count > 3000 and granulocyte count > 1500. However, continue twice weekly WBC and differential counts until WBC returns to 3500.
< 2000	<1000	Consider bone marrow aspiration to ascertain granulopoietic status. If granulopoiesis is deficient, consider protective isolation. If infection develops, perform cultures and institute antibiotics. Do not rechallenge with clozapine since agranu locytosis may develop with a shorter latency.

To reduce the risk of agranulocytosis developing undetected, clozapine will be dispensed only within the clozapine Patient Management System.

Seizure occurs in association with clozapine use at a cumulative incidence at 1 year of ≈ 5%. Dose appears to be an important predictor of seizure, with a greater likelihood of seizure at the higher clozapine doses used.

Use caution when administering to patients with history of seizures or other predisposing factors. Advise patients not to engage in any activity where sudden loss of consciousness could cause serious risk to themselves or others.

Orthostatic hypotension can occur, especially during initial titration in association with rapid dose escalation, and may represent a continuing risk in some patients.

Tachycardia, which may be sustained, has also been observed in approximately 25% of patients, with patients having an average increase in pulse rate of 10 to 15 bpm.

The sustained tachycardia is not simply a reflex response to hypotension, and is present in all positions monitored.

Either tachycardia or hypotension may pose a serious risk for an individual with compromised cardiovascular function.

ECG Changes: A minority of patients experience ECG repolarization changes similar to those seen with other antipsychotic drugs, including S-T segment depression and flattening or inversion of T waves, which all normalize after discontinuation of clozapine. Several patients have experienced significant cardiac events, including ischemic changes, myocardial infarction, nonfatal arrhythmias and sudden unexplained death.

Neuroleptic Malignant Syndrome (NMS), a potentially fatal symptom complex, has occurred in association with antipsychotic drugs.

There is no general agreement about specific pharmacological treatment regimens for uncomplicated NMS, but management of NMS should begin immediately.

No cases of NMS have been attributed to clozapine alone. However, there have been several reported cases of NMS in patients treated concomitantly with lithium or other CNS-active agents.

Tardive dyskinesia, There have been no confirmed cases of tardive dyskinesia developing in association with clozapine use. Nevertheless, it cannot yet be concluded that clozapine is incapable of inducing this syndrome. If signs and symptoms of tardive dyskinesia appear in a patient on clozapine, consider drug discontinuation.

Pregnancy: Category B.

Lactation: Women taking clozapine should not nurse.

Children: Safety and efficacy in children < 16 years old have not been established.

Precautions:

Fever: Patients may experience transient temperature elevations > 100.4°F (38°C), with the peak incidence within the first 3 weeks of treatment.

Anticholinergic effects of clozapine are very potent; exercise great care in using this drug in the presence of prostatic enlargement or narrow angle glaucoma.

Interference with cognitive and motor performance: Because of initial sedation, clozapine may impair mental or physical abilities, especially during the first few days of therapy. Carefully adhere to the recommendations for gradual dose escalation, and caution patients about activities requiring alertness.

Concomitant illness: Caution is advisable when using clozapine in patients with hepatic, renal or cardiac disease.

Drug Interactions:

Anticholinergics: The anticholinergic effects may be potentiated by clozapine.

Antihypertensives: The hypotensive effects may be potentiated by clozapine.

CNS drugs: Given the primary CNS effects of clozapine, caution is advised in using it concomitantly with other CNS-active drugs.

Agents that suppress bone marrow function: Do not use with other agents that suppress bone marrow function.

Protein binding: Because clozapine is highly bound to serum protein, the administration of clozapine to a patient taking another drug which is highly bound to protein may cause an increase in plasma concentrations of these drugs, potentially resulting in adverse effects. Conversely, adverse effects may result from displacement of protein-bound clozapine by other highly bound drugs.

Adverse Reactions:

Adverse reactions may include: Drowsiness; sedation; seizures; dizziness; syncope; fever; vertigo; headache; tremor; disturbed sleep; nightmares; restlessness; confusion; agitation; convulsions; hypokinesia; akinesia; tachycardia; hypotention; hypertension; ECG changes; nausea; vomiting; constipation; abdominal discomfort; leukopenia; granulocytopenia; agranulocytosis; rigidity; akathisia; salivation; sweating; dry mouth; visual disturbances; heartburn; weight gain.

Administration and Dosage:

Initial: 25 mg once or twice daily, and then continued with daily dosage increments of 25 to 50 mg/day, if well tolerated, to achieve a target dose of 300 to 450 mg/day by the end of 2 weeks. Make subsequent dosage increments no more than once or twice weekly, in increments not to exceed 100 mg. Cautious titration and a divided dosage schedule are necessary to minimize the risks of hypotension, seizure and sedation.

Dose adjustment: Continue daily dosing on a divided basis to an effective and tolerable dose level. While many patients may respond adequately at doses between 300 to 600 mg/day, it may be necessary to raise the dose to the 600 to 900 mg/day range. Do not exceed 900 mg/day. The mean and median clozapine doses are approximately 600 mg/day.

Because of the possibility of increased adverse reactions at higher doses, particularly seizures, give patients adequate time to respond to a given dose level before escalation to a higher dose.

Because of the significant risk of agranulocytosis and seizure, events which both present a continuing risk over time, avoid the extended treatment of patients failing to show an acceptable level of clinical response.

Maintenance: Continue clozapine at the lowest level needed to maintain remission. Periodically reassess patients to determine the need for maintenance treatment.

Discontinuation: In the event of planned termination of clozapine therapy, gradual reduction in dose is recommended over a 1 to 2 week period. However, should a patient's medical condition require abrupt discontinuation (eg, leukopenia), carefully observe the patient for the recurrence of psychotic symptoms.

Reinitiation of treatment: Follow the original dosage build-up guidelines. However, certain additional precautions seem prudent. Reexposure of a patient might enhance the risk of an untoward event's occurrence and increase its severity. Patients discontinued for WBC counts < 2000 per mm^3 or a granulocyte count < 1000 per mm^3 must not be restarted on clozapine. (See Warnings.)

Clozapine is available only through the *Clozaril* Patient Management System, a program that combines WBC testing, patient monitoring, pharmacy, and drug distribution services, all linked to compliance with required safety monitoring. Do not dispense more than a 1 week supply.

RISPERIDONE

Tablets: 1, 2, 3 and 4 mg (*Rx*)	*Risperdal* (Janssen)

Actions:

Pharmacology: Risperidone is an antipsychotic agent belonging to the benzisoxazole derivatives class. The mechanism of action is unknown. However, antipsychotic activity may be mediated through a combination of dopamine (D_2 and serotonin $5HT_2$) antagonism. Antagonism at receptors other than D_2 and serotonin $5HT_2$ may explain some of the other effects of risperidone. Risperidone is a selective monoaminergic antagonist that also has high affinity for the α_1, α_2 and H_1 histaminergic receptors. Risperidone antagonizes other receptors, but with lower potency.

Pharmacokinetics: Risperidone is well absorbed. It is extensively metabolized in the liver to a major active metabolite, 9-hydroxyrisperidone. Plasma concentrations of risperidone and 9-hydroxyrisperidone are dose-proportional over the dosing range of 1 to 16 mg daily. The absolute oral bioavailability of risperidone is 70%.

Following oral administration, mean peak plasma concentrations occurred at about 1 hour. The apparent half-life of risperidone and 9-OH-RISP was 3 hours and 21 hours, repectively, in extensive metabolizers and 20 and 30 hours in poor metabolizers, respectively. Steady-state concentrations of risperidone are reached in 1 day in extensive metabolizers and would be expected to reach steady-state in about 5 days in poor metabolizers.

The plasma protein binding of risperidone and was about 90%.

Indications:

Management of the manifestations of psychotic disorders.

Contraindications:

Hypersensitivity to risperidone.

Warnings:

Long-term use: The effectiveness of risperidone in long-term use (eg, > 6 to 8 weeks) has not been systematically evaluated. Therefore, periodically re-evaluate the long-term usefulness of the drug for the individual patient.

Neuroleptic malignant syndrome (NMS): A potentially fatal symptom complex sometimes referred to as NMS has occurred with antipsychotic drugs.

There is no general agreement about specific pharmacological treatment regimens for uncomplicated NMS, but management of NMS should begin immediately. If a patient requires antipsychotic drug treatment after recovery from NMS, carefully consider the potential reintroduction of drug therapy. Carefully monitor the patient since recurrences of NMS have been reported.

Tardive dyskinesia: A syndrome of potentially irreversible, involuntary, dyskinetic movements may develop in patients treated with antipsychotic drugs.

Prescribe risperidone in a manner that is most likely to minimize the occurrence of tardive dyskinesia. Generally reserve chronic treatment for patients who suffer from a chronic illness that (1) is known to respond to antipsychotic drugs, and (2) for whom alternative, equally effective, but potentially less harmful treatments are not available or appropriate. In patients who do require chronic treatment, seek the smallest dose and the shortest duration of treatment producing a satisfactory clinical response. Periodically reassess the need for continued treatment. If signs and symptoms of tardive dyskinesia appear, consider drug discontinuation. However, some patients may require treatment with risperidone despite the presence of the syndrome.

Cardiac effects:

Proarrhythmic effects – Risperidone or 9-hydroxyrisperidone appear to lengthen the QT interval in some patients. Other drugs that prolong the QT interval have been associated with the occurrence of torsade de pointes, a life-threatening arrhythmia. Bradycardia, electrolyte imbalance, concomitant use with other drugs that prolong QT or the presence of congenital prolongation in QT can increase the risk.

Orthostatic hypotension – Risperidone may induce orthostatic hypotension associated with dizziness, tachycardia, and in some patients, syncope, especially during the initial dose-titration period, probably reflecting its alpha-adrenergic antagonistic properties. Syncope was reported in 0.2%. Risk may be minimized by limiting the initial dose to 1 mg twice daily in healthy adults and 0.5 mg twice daily in the elderly and patients with renal or hepatic impairment.

Cardiac patients – Because of the risks of orthostatic hypotension and QT prolongation, observe caution in cardiac patients.

Renal/Hepatic function impairment:

Renal impairment – In patients with moderate to severe renal disease, clearance of the sum of risperidone and its active metabolite decreased by 60% compared to young healthy subjects. Reduce doses in patients with renal disease.

Hepatic impairment – While the pharmacokinetics of risperidone in subjects with liver disease were comparable to those in young healthy subjects, the mean free fraction of risperidone in plasma was increased by about 35% because of the diminished concentration of both albumin and α_1-acid glycoprotein. Reduce doses in patients with liver disease.

Elderly: In general, a lower starting dose is recommended for an elderly patient, reflecting a decreased pharmacokinetic clearance as well as a greater frequency of decreased hepatic, renal or cardiac function, and a greater tendency to postural hypotension (see Administration and Dosage).

Pregnancy: Category C.

Lactation: It is not known whether risperidone is excreted in breast milk. Women receiving risperidone should not breastfeed.

Children: Safety and efficacy in children have not been established.

Precautions:

Seizures occurred in 0.3% of patients, two in association with hyponatremia. Use cautiously in patients with a history of seizures.

Hyperprolactinemia: As with other drugs that antagonize dopamine D_2 receptors, risperidone elevates prolactin levels and the elevation persists during chronic administration. Approximately 33% of human breast cancers are prolactin-dependent in vitro, a factor of potential importance if use of these drugs is contemplated in a patient with previously detected breast cancer. Although disturbances such as galactorrhea, amenorrhea, gynecomastia and impotence have occurred with prolactin-elevating compounds, the clinical significance of elevated serum prolactin levels is unknown for most patients.

Cognitive/Motor impairment: Somnolence was a commonly reported adverse event. This reaction is dose-related.

Antiemetic effect: Risperidone has an antiemetic effect in animals which may also occur in humans, and may mask signs and symptoms of overdosage with certain drugs or of conditions such as intestinal obstruction, Reye's syndrome and brain tumor.

Body temperature regulation: Disruption of body temperature regulation has been attributed to other antipsychotic agents. Caution is advised when prescribing for patients who will be exposed to extreme heat.

Suicide: The possibility of a suicide attempt is inherent in schizophrenia, and close supervision of high-risk patients should accompany drug therapy. Write prescriptions for the smallest quantity of tablets consistent with good patient management, in order to reduce the risk of overdose.

Drug abuse and dependence: Evaluate patients for a history of drug abuse, and observe such patients closely for signs of risperidone misuse or abuse (eg, development of tolerance, increases in dose, drug-seeking behavior).

Photosensitivity: Photosensitization may occur; therefore, caution patients to take protective measures against exposure to ultraviolet light or sunlight until tolerance is determined.

Drug Interactions:

Drugs that may interact with risperidone include levodopa, carbamazepine and clozapine.

Adverse Reactions:

Adverse reactions in ≥ 3% include: Insomnia; agitation; anxiety; somnolence; aggressive reaction; extrapyramidal symptoms; headache, dizziness; constipation; nausea; dyspepsia; vomiting; abdominal pain; rhinitis; coughing; upper respiratory infection; pharyngitis; tachycardia; arthralgia; chest pain; fever; rash; dry skin; hyperkinesia; somnolence; nausea; weight gain.

Administration and Dosage:

Usual initial dose: Administer on a twice-daily schedule, generally beginning with 1 mg twice daily, with increases in increments of 1 mg twice daily on the second and third day, as tolerated, to a target dose of 3 mg twice daily by the third day. Further dosage adjustments, if indicated, should generally occur at intervals of ≥ 1 week, since steady state for the active metabolite would not be achieved for ≈ 1 week in the typical patient. When dosage adjustments are necessary, small dose increments/decrements of 1 mg twice daily are recommended.

Antipsychotic efficacy was demonstrated in a dose range of 4 to 16 mg/day; however, maximal effect was generally seen in a range of 4 to 6 mg/day. Doses > 6 mg/day were not demonstrated to be more efficacious than lower doses, were associated with more extrapyramidal symptoms and other adverse effects, and are not generally recommended. Safety of doses > 16 mg/day has not been evaluated.

Special populations: The recommended initial dose is 0.5 mg twice daily in patients who are elderly or debilitated, patients with severe renal or hepatic impairment, and patients either predisposed to hypotension or for whom hypotension would pose a risk. Use dosage increases in these patients in increments of 0.5 mg twice daily. Dosage increases above 1.5 mg twice daily should generally occur at intervals of ≥ 1 week.

Maintenance therapy: It is recommended that responding patients be continued on risperidone, but at the lowest dose needed to maintain remission. Periodically reassess patients to determine the need for maintenance treatment.

Reinitiation of treatment: When restarting patients who have had an interval off risperidone, follow the initial 3-day dose titration schedule.

Switching from other antipsychotics: When switching from other antipsychotics to risperidone, immediate discontinuation of the previous antipsychotic treatment upon initiation of risperidone therapy is recommended when medically appropriate. In all cases, minimize the period of overlapping antipsychotic administration. When switching patients from depot antipsychotic, initiate risperidone therapy in place of the next scheduled injection. Periodically reevaluate the need for continuing existing EPS medications.

PIMOZIDE

Tablets: 2 mg (*Rx*)	*Orap* (Lemmon)

Actions:

Pharmacology: Pimozide is a neuroleptic which blocks CNS dopaminergic receptors. It has no effect on norepinephrine receptors.

Pharmacokinetics: More than 50% of a dose of pimozide is absorbed after oral administration. Peak serum levels occur 6 to 8 hours (range 4 to 12 hours) after dosing. There are few correlations between plasma levels and clinical findings. Pimozide is extensively metabolized in the liver; mean elimination half-life in schizophrenic patients is ≈ 55 hours. Two major metabolites with undetermined neuroleptic activity have been identified. The major route of elimination is via the kidney; 38% to 45% of the dose is recovered in the urine, mostly as metabolites.

Indications:

For the suppression of severely compromising motor and phonic tics in patients with Tourette's Disorder who have failed to respond satisfactorily to standard treatment.

Contraindications:

Treatment of simple tics or tics other than those associated with Tourette's Disorder.

Drug-induced motor and phonic tics until it is determined whether the tics are caused by drugs or Tourette's Disorder.

Patients with congenital long QT syndrome or history of cardiac arrhythmias.

Administration with other drugs that prolong the QT interval.

Severe toxic CNS depression or comatose states from any cause.

Hypersensitivity to pimozide. It is not known whether cross-sensitivity exists among anti-psychotics. Use pimozide with caution in patients hypersensitive to other antipsychotics.

Warnings:

Persistent tardive dyskinesia may appear on long-term therapy or after drug therapy has been discontinued. The risk appears to be greater in elderly patients on high-dose therapy, especially females. The symptoms are persistent, and in some patients appear irreversible. The risk of developing tardive dyskinesia and the likelihood that it will become irreversible are believed to increase as treatment duration and total cumulative dose increase. However, the syndrome can develop after relatively brief treatment periods at low doses. Fine vermicular movement of the tongue may be an early sign of the syndrome; if the medication is stopped at this time, the syndrome may not develop. There is no known treatment for established cases of tardive dyskinesia, although the syndrome may remit, partially or completely, if antipsychotics are withdrawn. However, antipsychotic drugs may suppress signs and symptoms of the syndrome, possibly masking the underlying process. The effect of symptomatic suppression on the long-term course of the syndrome is unknown.

Prolongation of QT interval: Sudden death has occurred in conditions other than Tourette's Disorder in patients receiving dosages of ≈ 1 mg/kg. Perform an ECG before treatment is initiated and periodically thereafter, especially during dose adjustment. If the QT interval is prolonged beyond a limit of 0.47 seconds (children) or 0.52 seconds (adults), or more than 25% above the patient's original baseline, stop further dose increase and consider a lower dose.

Tumorigenicity: Pimozide may be tumorigenic. Consider this effect, especially in young patients and when chronic use is anticipated.

Neuroleptic malignant syndrome (NMS) is a potentially fatal symptom complex that has been associated with antipsychotic drugs.

There is no general agreement about treatment regimens for uncomplicated NMS, but management of NMS should begin immediately.

If a patient requires antipsychotic drug treatment after recovery from NMS, carefully consider the potential reintroduction of drug therapy. Monitor the patient carefully, since recurrences of NMS have been reported.

Pregnancy: Category C.

Lactation: Women taking pimozide should not breastfeed.

Children: Although Tourette's Disorder often has its onset between the ages of 2 and 15 years, the use of pimozide in patients less than 12 years is limited. Pimozide is not recommended for any childhood condition other than Tourette's Disorder.

Precautions:

Hypokalemia has been associated with ventricular arrhythmias. Correct potassium insufficiency secondary to diuretics, diarrhea or any other cause before initiating therapy; maintain normal potassium during therapy.

Anticholinergic side effects are produced by pimozide; use with caution in individuals whose conditions may be aggravated by anticholinergic activity.

Hepatic or renal function impairment: Use with caution since pimozide is metabolized by the liver and excreted by the kidney.

Hazardous tasks: May produce drowsiness or blurred vision; patients should observe caution while driving or performing other tasks requiring alertness.

Drug Interactions:

Drugs that may interact with pimozide include anticonvulsants, phenothiazines, tricyclic antidepressants, antiarrhythmic agents and CNS depressants.

Adverse Reactions:

Adverse reactions occurring in ≥ 3% of patients include: Extrapyramidal reactions; withdrawal emergent neurological signs; persistent tardive dyskinesia; neuroleptic malignant syndrome; ECG changes; visual disturbance; taste change; sensitivity of eyes to light; decreased accommodation; blurred vision; spots before eyes; cataracts; impotence; nocturia; urinary frequency; postural hypotension; hypotension; hypertension; tachycardia; palpitations; chest pain; hyperpyrexia; dry mouth; diarrhea; constipation; thirst; appetite increase; belching; increased salivation; nausea; vomiting; anorexia; GI distress; muscle tightness; muscle cramps; asthenia; stooped posture; headache; drowsiness; sedation; insomnia; rigidity; speech disorder; handwriting change; akinesia; dizziness; tremor; fainting; dyskinesia; akathesia; depression; excitement; nervousness; adverse behavior effect; parkinsonism; rash; sweating; skin irritation; weight gain; weight loss; periorbital edema; loss of libido; menstrual disorder and breast secretions.

Administration and Dosage:

Introduce the drug slowly and gradually. Perform ECG at baseline and periodically thereafter, especially during dosage adjustment.

Initial dose: 1 to 2 mg/day in divided doses. Thereafter, increase dose every other day.

Maintenance dose: < 0.2 mg/kg/day or 10 mg/day, whichever is less. Do not exceed 0.2 mg/kg/day or 10 mg/day.

Gradual withdrawal: Periodically attempt to reduce dosage to see if tics persist. Increases of tic intensity and frequency may represent a transient, withdrawal-related phenomenon rather than a return of symptoms. Allow 1 or 2 weeks to elapse before concluding that an increase in tic manifestations is due to the underlying disease rather than drug withdrawal.

LITHIUM

Capsules: 150 mg lithium carbonate (4.06 mEq lithium) (*Rx*)	*Lithium Carbonate* (Roxane)
Capsules: 300 mg lithium carbonate (8.12 mEq lithium) (*Rx*)	Various, *Eskalith* (SKF), *Lithonate* (Solvay Pharm.)
Capsules: 600 mg lithium carbonate (16.24 mEq lithium) (*Rx*)	*Lithium Carbonate* (Roxane)
Tablets: 300 mg lithium carbonate (8.12 mEq lithium) (*Rx*)	Various, *Eskalith* (SK-Beecham), *Lithane* (Miles Pharm.), *Lithotabs* (Solvay Pharm.)
Tablets, slow release: 300 mg lithium carbonate (8.12 mEq lithium) (*Rx*)	*Lithobid* (Ciba)
Tablets, controlled release: 450 mg lithium carbonate (12.18 mEq lithium) (*Rx*)	*Eskalith* CR (SK-Beecham)
Syrup: 8 mEq lithium (as citrate equivalent to 300 mg lithium carbonate) per 5 ml (*Rx*)	Various

Warning:

Toxicity is closely related to serum lithium levels and can occur at therapeutic doses. Facilities for serum lithium determinations are required to monitor therapy.

Actions:

Pharmacology: Lithium alters sodium transport in nerve and muscle cells, and effects a shift toward intraneuronal catecholamine metabolism. The specific mechanism in mania is unknown, but it affects neurotransmitters associated with affective disorders. Its antimanic effects may be the result of increases in norepinephrine reuptake and increased serotonin receptor sensitivity.

Pharmacokinetics:

Absorption/Distribution – Lithium is readily absorbed from the GI tract. Peak serum levels occur in 1 to 4 hours and absorption is complete within 8 hours. Onset of action is slow (5 to 14 days). Until the desired therapeutic effect is attained, maintain a steady-state serum level of 0.8 to 1.4 mEq/L, then slowly decrease the lithium dose to a maintenance level. The therapeutic serum level range is from 0.4 to 1 mEq/L.

Distribution approximates total body water. Lithium is not protein bound. Although distribution across the blood-brain barrier is slow, the cerebrospinal fluid lithium level is about 40% of the plasma concentration.

Excretion – About 95% of the lithium dose is eliminated by the kidney. Renal clearance is 20% of creatinine clearance (15 to 30ml/min). It varies with the age and renal status of the patient. In the elderly, and in patients with renal impairment, clearance will be low; in younger patients, it will be higher. The average elimination half-life is 24 hours (range, 17 to 36 hours); steady state is reached in 5 to 7 days.

In the kidneys, 80% of lithium is reabsorbed. Lithium and sodium compete for reabsorption in the proximal renal tubule. During periods of sodium depletion, the kidney will try to conserve sodium and lithium by reabsorbing > 80% from the proximal tubule. The increased reabsorption causes the lithium serum level to rise, possibly leading to toxicity. Sodium loading will cause increased lithium excretion and the serum levels will decrease.

Indications:

For the treatment of manic episodes of manic-depressive illness. Maintenance therapy prevents or diminishes the frequency and intensity of subsequent manic episodes in those manic-depressive patients with a history of mania.

Unlabeled uses: Improved the neutrophil count in patients with cancer chemotherapy-induced neutropenia, in children with chronic neutropenia and in AIDS patients receiving zidovudine; prophylaxis of cluster headache; premenstrual tension; bulimia; alcoholism; syndrome of inappropriate secretion of ADH; tardive dyskinesia; hyperthyroidism; postpartum affective psychosis; corticosteroid-induced psychosis.

Warnings:

High-risk patients: The risk of lithium toxicity is very high in patients with significant renal or cardiovascular disease, severe debilitation, dehydration or sodium depletion, or in patients receiving diuretics. Undertake treatment with extreme caution.

Encephalopathic syndrome has occurred in a few patients given lithium plus a neuroleptic. In some instances, irreversible brain damage occurred. Monitor closely for evidence of neurologic toxicity.

Renal function impairment: Morphologic changes with glomerular and interstitial fibrosis and nephron atrophy have occurred in patients on chronic lithium therapy. The relationship between such changes and renal function has not been established.

Acquired nephrogenic diabetes insipidus unresponsive to vasopressin has been associated with chronic lithium administration. Polydipsia and polyuria occur frequently. The mechanism is thought to be the decreased response of the renal tubules to the antidiuretic hormone causing decreased reabsorption of water. Impairment of the concentrating ability of the kidneys is reversed when lithium therapy is discontinued. Management may involve decreasing the dose, discontinuing lithium, or the cautious use of a thiazide diuretic or amiloride. Monitor the patient's renal status.

Elderly: The decreased rate of excretion in the elderly contributes to a high incidence of toxic effects. Use lower doses and more frequent monitoring.

Pregnancy: *Category D.*

Lactation: Do not nurse during lithium therapy.

Children: Safety and efficacy for use in children < 12 years old have not been established.

Precautions:

Concomitant infection with elevated temperature may necessitate a temporary reduction or cessation of medication.

Potentially hazardous tasks: Observe caution while driving or performing other tasks requiring alertness.

Tolerance of lithium is greater during the acute manic phase and decreases when manic symptoms subside.

Hypothyroidism may occur with long-term lithium administration. Patients may develop enlargement of the thyroid gland and increased thyroid-stimulating hormone levels.

Sodium depletion: Lithium decreases renal sodium reabsorption, which could lead to sodium depletion. Therefore, the patient must maintain a normal diet (including salt) and an adequate fluid intake (2500 to 3000 ml).

Parameters to monitor: Perform the following laboratory tests prior to and periodically during lithium therapy: Serum creatinine; complete blood count; urinalysis; sodium and potassium; fasting glucose; electrocardiogram; and thyroid function tests. Check lithium serum levels twice weekly until dosage is stabilized. Once steady state has been reached, monitor the level weekly. Once the patient is on maintenance therapy, the level may be checked every 2 to 3 months.

Drug Interactions:

Drugs that may affect lithium include acetazolamide, carbamazepine, fluoxetine, haloperidol, loop diuretics, methyldopa, NSAIDS, osmotic diuretics, theophyllines, thiazide diuretics, urinary alkalinizers and verapamil.

Drugs that may be affected by lithium include phenothiazines, sympathomimetics and tricyclic antidepressants.

Adverse Reactions:

Adverse reactions may include: Arrhythmia; hypotension; peripheral circulatory collapse; bradycardia; sinus node dysfunction with severe bradycardia; ECG changes; tremor; muscle hyperirritability; ataxia; choreoathetotic movements; hyperactive deep tendon reflexes; pseudotumor cerebri; euthyroid goiter; hypothyroidism; EEG changes; blackout spells; epileptiform seizures; slurred speech; dizziness; vertigo; incontinence of urine or feces; somnolence; psychomotor retardation; restlessness; confusion; stupor; coma; acute dystonia; downbeat nystagmus; blurred vision; startled response; hypertonicity; slowed intellectual functioning; hallucinations; poor memory; tongue movements; tics; tinnitus; cog wheel rigidity; anorexia; nausea; vomiting; diarrhea; dry mouth; gastritis; salivary gland swelling; abdominal pain; excessive salivation; flatulence; indigestion; albuminuria; oliguria; glycosuria; decreased creatinine clearance; symptoms of nephrogenic diabetes; drying and thinning of hair; anesthesia of skin; chronic folliculitis; xerosis cutis; alopecia; exacerbation of psoriasis; acne; angioedema; fatigue; lethargy; sleepiness; dehydration; weight loss; transient scotomata; impotence; sexual dysfunction; dysgeusia; taste distortion; tightness in chest; hypercalcemia; hyperparathyroidism; salty taste; swollen lips; swollen, painful joints; fever; polyarthralgia; dental caries; leukocytosis; headache; transient hyperglycemia; generalized pruritis with or without rash; cutaneous ulcers; worsening of organic brain syndromes; excessive weight gain; edematous swelling of ankles or wrists; thirst or polyuria, sometimes resembling diabetes insipidus; metallic taste; painful discoloration of fingers and toes and coldness of the extremities.

Administration and Dosage:

Individualize dosage according to both serum levels and clinical response.

Serum lithium levels: Draw blood samples immediately prior to the next dose (8 to 12 hours after the previous dose) when lithium concentrations are relatively stable. Do not rely on serum levels alone.

Acute mania: Optimal patient response is usually established and maintained with 600 mg 3 times daily or 900 mg twice daily for the slow release form. Such doses normally produce an effective serum lithium level ranging between 1 and 1.5 mEq/L.

Determine serum levels twice weekly during the acute phase, and until the serum level and clinical condition of the patient have been stabilized.

Long-term use: The desirable serum levels are 0.6 to 1.2 mEq/L. Dosage will vary, but 300 mg 3 to 4 times/day will usually maintain this level. Monitor serum levels in uncomplicated cases on maintenance therapy during remission every 2 to 3 months.

METHYLPHENIDATE HCl

Tablets: 5, 10, 20 and mg	Various, *Ritalin* (Ciba-Geigy)
Tablets, sustained release: 20 mg	Various, *Ritalin-SR* (Ciba-Geigy)

Actions:

Pharmacology: A mild cortical stimulant with CNS actions similar to the amphetamines. The exact mechanism of action is not fully understood.

Pharmacokinetics: Rapidly and well absorbed from the GI tract, methylphenidate achieves peak blood levels in 1 to 3 hours. Peak plasma levels occur in children in 4.7 hours for the sustained release (SR) tablets and 1.9 hours for the regular tablets. Plasma half-life ranges from 1 to 3 hours, but pharmacologic effects persist up to 4 to 6 hours.

Indications:

Attention deficit disorders: As part of a total treatment program in children with a behavioral syndrome characterized by moderate to severe distractibility, short attention span, hyperactivity, emotional lability and impulsivity.

Narcolepsy.

Unlabeled uses: Some success has been reported in the treatment of depression in elderly, cancer, post-stroke patients and in anesthesia-related hiccups.

Contraindications:

Marked anxiety, tension and agitation, since the drug may aggravate these symptoms; hypersensitivity to methylphenidate; glaucoma.

Patients with motor tics or with a family history or diagnosis of Tourette's syndrome.

Severe depression of either exogenous or endogenous origin; for the prevention or treatment of normal fatigue states.

Warnings:

Do not use for severe depression of either exogenous or endogenous origin. Do not use for the prevention or treatment of normal fatigue states.

Seizure disorders: Methylphenidate may lower the seizure threshold in patients with history of seizures, with prior EEG abnormalities in absence of seizures and, very rarely, in the absence of history of seizures and no prior EEG evidence of seizures.

Hypertension: Use cautiously; monitor blood pressure in all patients, especially those with hypertension.

Visual disturbances have been encountered rarely. Difficulties with accommodation and blurring of vision have been reported.

Pregnancy: Category C.

Lactation: The amount of methylphenidate excreted in breast milk is unknown.

Children: Do not use in children under 6 years, since safety and efficacy have not been established. In psychotic children, the drug may exacerbate symptoms of behavior disturbance and thought disorder. Precipitation of Tourette's syndrome has been reported following.

Safety and efficacy of long-term use in children are not established.

Precautions:

Patients with an element of agitation may react adversely; discontinue therapy if necessary.

Perform periodic CBC, differential and platelet counts during prolonged therapy.

Drug abuse and dependence: Give cautiously to emotionally unstable patients, such as those with a history of drug dependence or alcoholism, because such patients may increase dosage on their own initiative.

Drug Interactions:

Drugs that may affect methyphenidate include MAOIs. Drugs that may be affected by methylphenidate HCl include guanethidine, phenytoin and TCAs.

Adverse Reactions:

Adverse reactions may include: Skin rash; urticaria; fever; arthralgia; exfoliative dermatitis; erythema multiforme with necrotizing vasculitis; thrombocytopenic purpura; Dizziness; headache; dyskinesia; drowsiness; Tourette's syndrome; toxic psychosis; blood pressure and pulse changes; tachycardia; angina; cardiac arrhythmias; palpitations; anorexia; nausea; abdominal pain; weight loss; nervousness; insomnia; leukopenia; anemia; hair loss; loss of appetite and abdominal pain.

Administration and Dosage:

Adults: Individualize dosage. Administer in divided doses 2 or 3 times daily, preferably 30 to 45 minutes before meals. Average dose is 20 to 30 mg/day. Dosage ranges from 10 to 15 mg/day up to 40 to 60 mg/day. In patients who are unable to sleep if medication is taken late in the day, take the last dose before 6 pm.

All patients: *Timed release tablets* have a duration of approximately 8 hours and may be used in place of regular tablets when the 8 hour dosage of the timed release tablets corresponds to the titrated 8 hour dosage of the regular tablets. Timed release tablets must be swallowed whole, never crushed or chewed.

Children (≥ 6): Start with small doses (eg, 5 mg before breakfast and lunch) with gradual increments of 5 to 10 mg weekly. Daily dosage above 60 mg is not recommended. If improvement is not observed after dosage adjustment over 1 month, discontinue use. If paradoxical aggravation of symptoms or other adverse effects occurs, reduce dosage or discontinue the drug.

Discontinue periodically to assess condition. Improvement may be sustained when the drug is either temporarily or permanently discontinued. Drug treatment should not be indefinite and usually may be discontinued after puberty.

TACRINE HCl (Tetrahydroaminoacridine; THA)

Capsules: 10, 20, 30 and 40 mg (*Rx*)	*Cognex* (Parke-Davis)

Actions:

Pharmacology: Tacrine is a centrally acting reversible cholinesterase inhibitor, commonly referred to as THA.

Pharmacokinetics:

Absorption – Maximal plasma concentrations occur within 1 to 2 hours. Absolute bioavailability of tacrine is ≈ 17%.

Distribution – Mean volume of distribution of tacrine is ≈ 349 L. Tacrine is about 55% bound to plasma proteins.

Metabolism – Tacrine is extensively metabolized by the cytochrome P450 system to multiple metabolites, not all of which have been identified. Cytochrome P450 IA2 is the principal isozyme involved in metabolism.

Excretion – Tacrine undergoes first-pass metabolism, the extent of which depends on the dose administered. Elimination of tacrine from the plasma is not dose-dependent. The elimination half-life is ≈ 2 to 4 hours. Following initiation of therapy or a change in daily dose, steady-state plasma concentrations should be attained within 24 to 36 hours.

Special populations:

Smoking – Mean plasma tacrine concentrations in current smokers are ≈ ⅓ the concentrations in nonsmokers.

Indications:

Alzheimer's disease: Treatment of mild to moderate dementia of the Alzheimer's type.

Contraindications:

Hypersensitivity to tacrine or acridine derivatives; patients previously treated with tacrine who developed treatment-associated jaundice confirmed by elevated total bilirubin > 3 mg/dl.

Warnings:

Anesthesia: Tacrine is likely to exaggerate succinylcholine-type muscle relaxation during anesthesia.

Cardiovascular conditions: Because of its cholinomimetic action, tacrine may have vagotonic effects on the heart rate. This action may be particularly important to patients with a 'sick sinus syndrome'.

GI disease/dysfunction: Tacrine is an inhibitor of cholinesterase and may be expected to increase gastric acid secretion due to increased cholinergic activity. Therefore, closely monitor patients at increased risk for developing ulcers for symptoms of active or occult GI bleeding.

Hepatic effects: Prescribe with care in patients with current evidence or history of abnormal liver function indicated by significant abnormalities in serum transaminase, bilirubin and gamma-glutamyl transpeptidase levels.

The incidence of transaminase elevations is higher among females. There are no other known predictors of the risk of hepatocellular injury.

GU effects: Cholinomimetics may cause bladder outflow obstruction.

Neurological conditions:

Seizures – Cholinomimetics are believed to have some potential to cause generalized convulsions; seizure activity may, however, also be a manifestation of Alzheimer's disease.

Worsening of cognitive function has been reported following abrupt discontinuation of tacrine or after a large reduction in total daily dose (≥ 80 mg/day).

Pulmonary conditions: Because of its cholinomimetic action, use tacrine with care in patients with a history of asthma.

Hepatic disease: Although studies in patients with liver disease have not been done, it is likely that functional hepatic impairment will reduce the clearance of tacrine and its metabolites.

Pregnancy: Category C.

Lactation: It is not known whether this drug is excreted in breast milk.

Children: There are no adequate and well controlled trials to document the safety and efficacy of tacrine in any dementing illness occurring in children.

Precautions:

Hematology: Decreased absolute neutrophil counts (ANC) < 500 to 1500/mcl has been reported rarely. The total clinical experience in > 8000 patients does not indicate a clear association between tacrine treatment and serious white blood cell abnormalities.

Drug Interactions:

Drugs that may be affected by tacrine include anticholinergics, cholinomimetics, cholinesterase inhibitors and theophylline.

Drugs that may affect tacrine include cimetidine.

Tacrine is primarily eliminated by hepatic metabolism via cytochrome P450 drug metabolizing enzymes. Drug interactions may occur when it is given concurrently with agents such as theophylline that undergo extensive metabolism via cytochrome P450 IA2.

Adverse Reactions:

Adverse reactions occurring in ≥ 3% of patients include: Elevated transaminases; nausea; vomiting; diarrhea; dyspepsia; myalgia; anorexia; ataxia; headache; fatigue; chest pain; weight decrease; agitation; depression; abnormal thinking; anxiety; anorexia; abdominal pain; flatulence; constipation; dizziness; confusion; ataxia; insomnia; somnolence; myalgia; elevated transaminase; urinary incontinence; urinary tract infection; urination frequency; rash; facial flushing; coughing; upper respiratory infection and rhinitis.

Administration and Dosage:

The rate of dose escalation may be slowed if a patient is intolerant to the recommended titration schedule. It is not advisable, however, to accelerate the dose incrementation plan. Following initiation of therapy, or any dosage increase, observe patients carefully for adverse effects. Take between meals whenever possible; however, if minor GI upset occurs, take with meals to improve tolerability. Taking tacrine with meals can be expected to reduce plasma levels ≈ 30% to 40%.

Initiation of treatment: The initial dose of tacrine is 40 mg/day (10 mg 4 times daily). Maintain this dose for a minimum of 6 weeks with weekly monitoring of transaminase levels. It is important that the dose not be increased during this period because of the potential for delayed onset of transaminase elevations.

Dose titration: Following 6 weeks of treatment at 40 mg/day, increase the dose to 80 mg/day (20 mg 4 times daily), providing there are no significant transaminase elevations and the patient is tolerating treatment. Titrate patients to higher doses (120 and 160 mg/day, in divided doses on a 4 times daily schedule) at 6 week intervals on the basis of tolerance.

Dose adjustment: Monitor serum transaminase levels (specifically ALT) every other week for at least the first 16 weeks following initiation of treatment, after which monitoring may be decreased to monthly for 2 months and every 3 months, thereafter. Resume weekly monitoring for a minimum of 6 weeks. Repeat a full monitoring sequence in the event that a patient suspends treatment with tacrine for > 4 weeks. If transaminase elevations occur, modify the dose according to the following table.

Recommended Tacrine Dose Modification in Response to Transaminase Elevations

Transaminase levels	Treatment regimen
≤ 2 x ULN	Continue treatment according to recommended titration and monitoring schedule.
> 2 to ≤ 3 x ULN	Continue treatment according to recommended titration. Monitor transaminase levels weekly until levels return to normal limits.
> 3 to ≤ 5 x ULN	Reduce the daily dose by 40 mg/day. Resume dose titration and every other week monitoring when transaminases return to within normal limits.
> 5 x ULN	Stop treatment. Monitor transaminase levels until within normal limits (see Rechallenge section).

Experience is limited with patients with ALT > 10 x ULN. The risk of rechallenge must be considered against demonstrated clinical benefit. Patients with clinical jaundice confirmed by a significant elevation in total bilirubin (> 3 mg/dl) should permanently discontinue tacrine and not be rechallenged.

Rechallenge: Patients who are required to discontinue treatment because of transaminase elevations may be rechallenged once transaminase levels return to within normal limits. Rechallenge of patients exposed to transaminase elevations < 10 x ULN has not resulted in serious liver injury. However, because experience in the rechallenge of patients who had elevations > 10 x ULN is limited, the risks associated with the rechallenge of these patients are not well characterized. Careful, frequent (weekly) monitoring of serum ALT should be undertaken when rechallenging such patients. If rechallenged, give patients an initial dose of 40 mg/day (10 mg 4 times daily) and monitor transaminase levels weekly. If, after 6 weeks on 40 mg/day, the patient is tolerating the dosage with no unacceptable elevations in transaminases, recommended dose titration and transaminase monitoring may be resumed.

DONEPEZIL HCl

Tablets: 5 and 10 mg	*Aricept* (Eisai/Pfizer)

Actions:

Pharmacology: Donepezil is postulated to exert its therapeutic effect by enhancing cholinergic function. This increase in cholinergic function is accomplished by increasing the concentration of acetylcholine through reversible inhibition of its hydrolysis by acetylcholinesterase (AChE). If this proposed mechanism of action is correct, donepezil's effect may lessen as the disease process advances and fewer cholinergic neurons remain functionally intact. There is no evidence that donepezil alters the course of the underlying dementing process.

Pharmacokinetics:

Absorption – Donepezil is well absorbed with a relative oral bioavailability of 100% and reaches peak plasma concentrations in 3 to 4 hours. Neigher food nor time of administration (morning vs evening dose) influences the rate or extent of absorption.

Distribution – Following multiple dose administration, steady-state is reached within 15 days. The steady-state volume of distribution is 12 L/kg. Donepezil is ≈ 96% bound to human plasma proteins.

Metabolism – Donepezil is both excreted in the urine intact and extensively metabolized to four major metabolites, two of which are known to be active. Donepezil is metabolized by CYP 450 isoenzyme 2D6 and 3A4 and undergoes glucuronidation.

Excretion – The elimination half-life of donepezil is ≈ 70 hours and the mean apparent plasma clearance is 0.13 L/hr/kg.

Approximately 57% and 15% of the total dose was recovered in urine and feces, respectively, over a period of 10 days, while 28% remained unrecovered, with ≈ 17% of the donepezil dose recovered in the urine as unchanged drug.

Indications:

Alzheimer's disease: The treatment of mild to moderate dementia of the Alzheimer's type.

Contraindications:

Hypersensitivity to donepezil or to piperidine derivatives.

Warnings:

Anesthesia: Donepezil, as a cholinesterase inhibitor, is likely to exaggerate succinylcholine-type muscle relaxation during anesthesia.

Cardiovascular: Cholinesterase inhibitors may have vagotonic effects on heart rate (eg, bradycardia). The potential for this action may be particularly important to patients with "sick sinus syndrome" or other supraventricular cardiac conduction conditions. Syncopal episodes have been reported in association with the use of donepezil.

GI: Through their primary action, cholinesterase inhibitors may be expected to increase gastric acid secretion because of increased cholinergic activity. Therefore, monitor patients closely for symptoms of active or occult GI bleeding, especially those at increased risk for developing ulcers.

Donepezil has been shown to produce diarrhea, nausea and vomiting. These effects, when they occur, appear more frequently with the 10 mg/day dose than with the 5 mg/day dose. In most cases, these effects have been mild and transient, sometimes lasting 1 to 3 weeks, and have resolved during continued use of donepezil.

GU: Cholinomimetics may cause bladder outflow obstruction.

Seizures: Cholinomimetics are believed to have some potential to cause generalized convulsions. However, seizure activity also may be a manifestation of Alzheimer's disease.

Pulmonary: Prescribe cholinesterase inhibitors with care for patients with a history of asthma or obstructive pulmonary disease.

Pregnancy: Category C.

Lactation: It is not known whether donepezil is excreted in breast milk.

Children: There are no adequate and well controlled tirals to document the safety and efficacy of donepezil in any illness occurring in children.

Drug Interactions:

Drugs that may affect donepezil are ketoconazole and quinidine. Drugs that may be affected by donepezil include anticholinergics, cholinometics/cholinesterase inhibitors, NSAIDs, furosemide, digoxin, warfarin, theophylline and cimetidine.

Adverse Reactions:

Adverse reactions that may occur in ≥ 3% of patients include: Headache, whole body pain, fatigue, nausea, diarrhea, vomiting, anorexia, muscle cramps, insomnia, dizziness, depression, abnormal dreams, ecchymosis and weight decrease.

Administration and Dosage:

The dosages of donepezil are 5 and 10 mg once per day in the evening, just prior to retiring.

The higher dose of 10 mg did not provide a statistically significant clinical benefit greater than that of 5 mg. Do not increase to 10 mg until patients have been on a daily dose of 5 mg for 4 to 6 weeks.

Donepezil may be taken with or without food.

AMPHETAMINES

Amphetamine, dextroamphetamine and methamphetamine are also indicated for attention deficit disorders in children, as part of a total treatment program.

For complete prescribing information on the amphetamines for this and other uses, consult the general amphetamine monograph.

ERGOLOID MESYLATES (Dihydrogenated Ergot Alkaloids, Dihydroergotoxine)

Tablets, sublingual: 0.5 mg (Rx)	Various, *Gerimal* (Rugby), *Hydergine* (Sandoz)
Tablets, oral: 0.5 mg (Rx)	Various
Tablets, sublingual: 1 mg (Rx)	Various, *Gerimal* (Rugby), *Hydergine* (Sandoz)
Tablets, oral: 1 mg (Rx)	Various, *Gerimal* (Rugby), *Hydergine* (Sandoz)
Capsules, liquid: 1 mg	*Hydergine LC* (Sandoz)
Liquid: 1 mg per ml	*Hydergine* (Sandoz)

Actions:

Pharmacology: Ergoloid mesylates contain equal proportions of dihydroergocornine mesylate, dihydroergocristine mesylate and dihydroergocryptine mesylate.

The mechanism by which ergoloid mesylates produce mental effects is unknown. There is no conclusive evidence they directly affect cerebral arteriosclerosis or cerebrovascular insufficiency. Formerly, it was believed this drug caused cerebral vasodilation by alpha-adrenergic blockade; recent evidence suggests it may act primarily to increase brain metabolism, possibly increasing cerebral blood flow. It does not possess the vasoconstrictor properties of the natural ergot alkaloids.

Pharmacokinetics: Ergoloid mesylates are rapidly absorbed from the GI tract; peak plasma concentrations are achieved within 0.6 to 3 hours. The drug undergoes rapid first-pass biotransformation in the liver. Systemic bioavailability is ≈ 6% to 25%. The liquid capsule has a 12% greater bioavailability than the oral tablet. The mean half-life of unchanged ergoloid in plasma is about 2.6 to 5.1 hours.

Indications:

Age-related mental capacity decline: Individuals over 60 years of age who manifest signs and symptoms of an idiopathic decline in mental capacity. Patients who respond suffer from some process related to aging or have some underlying dementing condition.

Contraindications:

Hypersensitivity to ergoloid mesylates.

Acute or chronic psychosis, regardless of etiology.

Precautions:

Before prescribing ergoloid mesylates, exclude the possibility that the patient's signs and symptoms arise from a potentially reversible and treatable condition. Exclude delirium and dementiform illness secondary to systemic disease, primary neurological disease or primary disturbance of mood.

Periodically reassess the diagnosis and the benefit of current therapy to the patient.

Adverse Reactions:

Adverse reactions may include: Sublingual irritation; transient nausea and GI disturbances.

Administration and Dosage:

The usual starting dose is 1 mg 3 times daily. Alleviation of symptoms is usually gradual; results may not be observed for 3 to 4 weeks. Doses up to 4.5 to 12 mg/day have been used. Up to 6 months of treatment may be necessary to determine efficacy, using doses of at least 6 mg/day. Do not chew or crush sublingual tablets.

SEDATIVE/HYPNOTICS, NONBARBITURATE

To facilitate comparison, the products are divided into two groups: The miscellaneous nonbarbiturates and the benzodiazepines. Although sedative doses can be given, these agents are primarily intended to be hypnotics.

In the table below, some pharmacokinetic properties of the nonbarbiturate sedative/hypnotics are compared. Do not use this table to predict exact duration of effect, but use as a guide in drug selection.

Nonbarbiturate Sedative/Hypnotics Pharmacokinetic Parameters

Drug	Adult oral dose		Onset (min)	Duration of action (hrs)	Half-life (hrs)	Protein binding (%)	Urinary excretion, unchanged (%)
	Hypnotic	Sedative					
Miscellaneous nonbarbiturates							
Chloral hydrate	0.5-1 g	250 mg tid pc	30	nd	7-10[1]	35-41	nd
Ethchlorvynol	500 mg	100-200 mg bid or tid	15-60	5	10-20[2]	nd	40[3]
Paraldehyde	10-30 ml	5-10 ml	10-15	8-12	3.4-9.8	nd	small
Propiomazine	nd	10-20 mg	nd	nd	nd	nd	nd
Benzodiazepines							
Estazolam	1-2 mg	na	nd	nd	10-24	93	< 5
Flurazepam	15-30 mg	na	17	7-8	150-100[4]	97	< 1[4]
Quazepam	15 mg	na	nd	nd	25-41	> 95>	trace
Temazepam	15-30 mg	na	nd	nd	10-17	98	1.5
Triazolam	0.125-0.5 mg	na	nd	nd	1.5-5.5	90	2

na = Not applicable. nd = No data.

[1] Trichloroethanol, the principal metabolite.

[2] In acute use, half-life of the distribution phase (1 to 3 hours) is more appropriate.

[3] Free and conjugated forms of the major metabolite, secondary alcohol of ethchlorvynol.

[4] Active metabolite, desalkylflurazepam.

ZOLPIDEM TARTRATE

Tablets: 5 and 10 mg (*c-iv*) *Ambien* (Searle)

Actions:

Pharmacology: Zolpidem is a non-benzodiazepine hypnotic of the imidazopyridine class. While zolpidem is a hypnotic agent with a chemical structure unrelated to benzodiazepines, barbiturates or other drugs with known hypnotic properties, it interacts with a GABA-BZ receptor complex and shares some of the pharmacological properties of the benzodiazepines. Zolpidem in vitro binds the omega$_1$ receptor preferentially. This selective binding of zolpidem on the omega$_1$ receptor is not absolute, but it may explain the relative absence of myorelaxant and anticonvulsant effects, as well as the preservation of deep sleep at hypnotic doses.

Pharmacokinetics: The pharmacokinetic profile is characterized by rapid absorption from the GI tract and a short elimination half-life. Zolpidem is converted to inactive metabolites that are eliminated primarily by renal excretion.

Indications:

Insomnia: Short-term treatment.

Warnings:

Duration of therapy: Generally limit hypnotics to 7 to 10 days of use; re-evaluate the patient if they are to be taken for > 2 to 3 weeks. Do not prescribe in quantities exceeding a 1 month supply.

Psychiatric/physical disorder: Since sleep disturbances may be the presenting manifestation of a physical or psychiatric disorder, initiate symptomatic treatment of insomnia only after a careful evaluation of the patient. The failure of insomnia to remit after

7 to 10 days of treatment may indicate the presence of a primary psychiatric or medical illness which should be evaluated.

Abrupt discontinuation: Following the rapid dose decrease or abrupt discontinuation of sedative/hypnotics, signs and symptoms similar to those associated with withdrawal from other CNS-depressant drugs have occurred.

CNS-depressant effects: Zolpidem, like other sedative/hypnotic drugs, has CNS-depressant effects. Due to the rapid onset of action, only ingest immediately prior to going to bed. Zolpidem had additive effects when combined with alcohol; therefore, do not take with alcohol.

Renal function impairment: Data in end stage renal failure patients repeatedly treated with zolpidem did not demonstrate drug accumulation or alterations in pharmacokinetic parameters. No dosage adjustment in renally impaired patients is required; however, closely monitor these patients.

Hepatic function impairment: Modify dosing accordingly in patients with hepatic insufficiency.

Elderly: Closely monitor these patients. Impaired motor or cognitive performance after repeated exposure or unusual sensitivity to sedative/hypnotic drugs is a concern in the treatment of elderly or debilitated patients.

Pregnancy: Category B.

Lactation: The use of zolpidem in nursing mothers is not recommended.

Children: Safety and efficacy in children < 18 years of age have not been established.

Precautions:

Respiratory depression: Although preliminary studies did not reveal respiratory depressant effects at hypnotic doses in healthy individuals, observe caution if zolpidem is prescribed to patients with compromised respiratory function, since sedative/hypnotics have the capacity to depress respiratory drive.

Depression: As with other sedative/hypnotic drugs, administer zolpidem with caution to patients exhibiting signs or symptoms of depression. Suicidal tendencies may be present in such patients and protective measures may be required. Intentional overdosage is more common in this group of patients; therefore, prescribe the least amount of drug that is feasible for the patient at any one time.

Drug abuse and dependence: Sedative/hypnotics have produced withdrawal signs and symptoms following abrupt discontinuation. These reported symptoms range from mild dysphoria and insomnia to a withdrawal syndrome that may include abdominal and muscle cramps, vomiting, sweating, tremors and convulsions. Zolpidem does not reveal any clear evidence for withdrawal syndrome.

Because individuals with a history of addiction to, or abuse of, drugs or alcohol are at risk of habituation and dependence, they should be under careful surveillance when receiving zolpidem or any other hypnotic.

Drug Interactions:

Drug/Food interactions: For faster sleep onset, do not administer with or immediately after a meal.

Adverse Reactions:

Adverse reactions occurring in ≥ 3% of patients include: Dizziness; drugged feelings; headache; allergy; back pain; headache; drowsiness; dizziness; lethargy; nausea; dyspepsia; diarrhea; myalgia; arthralgia; upper respiratory infection; sinusitis; pharyngitis and dry mouth.

Administration and Dosage:

Adults: Individualize dosage. Usual dose is 10 mg immediately before bedtime.

Downward dosage adjustment may be necessary when given with agents having known CNS depressant effects because of the potentially additive effects.

Elderly or debilitated patients may be especially sensitive to the effects of zolpidem. Patients with hepatic insufficiency do not clear the drug as rapidly as healthy individuals. An initial 5 mg dose is recommended in these patients.

Maximum dose: The total dose should not exceed 10 mg.

BENZODIAZEPINES

ESTAZOLAM	
Tablets: 1 and 2 mg (*c-iv*)	*ProSom* (Abbott)
FLURAZEPAM HCl	
Capsules: 15 and 30 mg (*c-iv*)	Various, *Dalmane* (Roche)
QUAZEPAM	
Tablets: 7.5 and 15 mg (*c-iv*)	*Doral* (Wallace)
TEMAZEPAM	
Capsules: 7.5, 15 and 30 mg (*c-iv*)	Various, *Restoril* (Sandoz)
TRIAZOLAM	
0.125 and 0.25 mg (*c-iv*)	Various, *Halcion* (Upjohn)

Actions:

Pharmacology: Estazolam, flurazepam, quazepam, temazepam and triazolam are benzodiazepine derivatives useful as hypnotics. Benzodiazepines are believed to potentiate gamma aminobutyric acid (GABA) neuronal inhibition.

Pharmacokinetics:

Absorption – These agents are rapidly and completely absorbed within 1 to 3 hours of oral administration. Times to peak plasma concentration range from 0.5 to 2 hours for parent compounds. The major active metabolite of flurazepam reaches peak plasma levels in ≈ 10 hours.

Distribution – Plasma protein binding ranges from 70% to 99% with free-drug concentrations closely approximating CSF levels. IV and rapidly absorbed oral benzodiazepines are rapidly taken into the brain and other highly perfused organs. They also cross the placenta and are secreted in breast milk.

Metabolism – Benzodiazepines are extensively metabolized in the liver. Biotransformation to active metabolites is an important factor in product selection especially in the elderly or patients with severe liver disease. Temazepam, estazolam and triazolam do not form active long-acting metabolites.

Select Benzodiazepine (Hypnotic) Pharmacokinetic Parameters					
Drug	Usual adult oral dose (mg)	Time to peak plasma levels (hrs)	Half-life (hrs)	Protein binding (%)	Urinary excretion, unchanged (%)
Estazolam	1-2	2	8-28	93	< 5
Flurazepam	15-30	0.5-1 (7.6-13.6)[1]	2-3 (47-100)[1]	97	< 1
Quazepam	7.5-15	2 (1-2)	41 (47-100)[1]	> 95	trace
Temazepam	15-30	1.2-1.6	3.5-18.4 (9-15)	96	0.2
Triazolam	0.125-0.5	1-2	1.5-5.5	78-89	2

[1] N-desalkylflurazepam, active metabolite.

Indications:

Insomnia characterized by difficulty in falling asleep, frequent nocturnal awakenings or early morning awakening. Can be used for recurring insomnia or poor sleeping habits, and in acute or chronic medical situations requiring restful sleep.

Contraindications:

Hypersensitivity to other benzodiazepines; pregnancy (see Warnings); established or suspected sleep apnea (quazepam).

Concurrent use with ketoconazole, itraconazole and nefazodone, medications that significantly impair the oxidative metabolism of **triazolam** mediated by cytochrome P450 3A (CYP3A).

Warnings:

Anterograde amnesia of varying severity and paradoxical reactions has occurred following therapeutic doses of **triazolam**. Although this effect generally occurred with a dose of 0.5 mg, it has also been reported with 0.125 and 0.25 mg doses. This effect may occur with some other benzodiazepines, but data suggest that it may occur at a higher rate with triazolam. Cases of "traveler's amnesia" have been reported by individuals who have taken triazolam to induce sleep while traveling.

Renal/Hepatic function impairment: Observe usual precautions under these conditions.

Abnormal liver function tests as well as blood dyscrasias have been reported with benzodiazepines.

Elderly: The risk of developing oversedation, dizziness, confusion or ataxia increases substantially with larger doses of benzodiazepines in elderly and debilitated patients. Initiate with lowest effective dose.

Pregnancy: *Category X* (estazolam, quazepam, temazepam, triazolam, flurazepam). Benzodiazepines may cause fetal damage when administered during pregnancy.

If there is a likelihood of the patient becoming pregnant while receiving benzodiazepines, warn of the potential risk to the fetus. Instruct patients to discontinue the drug prior to becoming pregnant.

Lactation: Safety for use in the nursing mother has not been established. Benzodiazepines are excreted in breast milk. Therefore, administration to nursing mothers is not recommended.

Children:

Flurazepam – Not for use in children < 15 years of age.

Estazolam, quazepam, temazepam, triazolam – Not for use in children < 18 years old.

Precautions:

Monitoring: When triazolam or estazolam treatment is protracted, obtain periodic blood counts, urinalysis and blood chemistry analyses.

Depression: Administer with caution in severely depressed patients or in those in whom there is evidence of latent depression or suicidal tendencies. Signs or symptoms of depression may be intensified by hypnotic drugs.

Rebound sleep disorder, which is characterized by recurrence of insomnia to levels worse than before treatment began, may occur following abrupt withdrawal of triazolam, usually during the first 1 to 3 nights. Gradual rather than abrupt discontinuation of the drug may help avoid this syndrome.

Disturbed nocturnal sleep may occur for the first or second night after discontinuing use.

Early morning insomnia, or early morning awakenings, appears to be more common with the use of short half-life agents (temazepam, triazolam) than agents with intermediate or long half-lives (estazolam, flurazepam, quazepam). However, daytime sleepiness appears to be more prevalent with the long half-life agents.

Respiratory depression and sleep apnea: Observe caution. In patients with compromised respiratory function, respiratory depression and sleep apnea have occurred.

Drug abuse and dependence: Withdrawal symptoms following abrupt discontinuation of benzodiazepines have occurred in patients receiving excessive doses over extended periods of time. Gradual withdrawal is preferred.

Hazardous tasks: Observe caution while driving or performing tasks requiring alertness.

Drug Interactions:

Drugs that may affect benzodiazepines include alcohol/CNS dpressants, cimetidine, oral contraceptives, disulfiram, isoniazid, probenecid, rifampin, smoking, theophyllines and macrolides.

Drugs that may be affected by benzodiazepines include digoxin, neuromuscular blocking agents (nondepolarizing) and phenytoin.

Adverse Reactions:

Estazolam: Other adverse reactions reported only for estazolam include the following: Somnolence (42%); asthenia (11%); hypokinesia (8%); hangover (3%); cold symptoms, lower extremity/back/abdominal pain (1% to 3%).

CNS: Headache; nervousness; apprehension; irritability; confusion; euphoria; relaxed feeling; weakness; tremor; lack of concentration; coordination disorders; confusional states/memory impairment; depression; dreaming/nightmares; insomnia; paresthesia; restlessness; tiredness; dysesthesia.

GI: Heartburn; nausea; vomiting; diarrhea; constipation; GI pain; anorexia; taste alterations; dry mouth.

Cardiovascular: Palpitations; chest pains; tachycardia.

Miscellaneous: Body/joint pain; tinnitus; GU complaints; cramps/pain; congestion.

Administration and Dosage:

ESTAZOLAM:

Adults – 1 mg at bedtime; however, some patients may need a 2 mg dose.

Elderly – If healthy, 1 mg at bedtime; initiate increases with particular care.

Debilitated or small elderly patients – Consider a starting dose of 0.5 mg, although this is only marginally effective in the overall elderly population.

FLURAZEPAM:

Adults – 30 mg before bedtime. In some patients, 15 mg may suffice.

Elderly or debilitated – Initiate with 15 mg until individual response is determined.

QUAZEPAM:

Adults – Initiate at 15 mg until individual responses are determined; may reduce to 7.5 mg in some patients.

Elderly or debilitated – Attempt to reduce nightly dosage after the first 1 or 2 nights.

TEMAZEPAM:

Adults – Give 15 to 30 mg before bedtime.

Elderly or debilitated – Initiate with 15 mg until individual response is determined.

TRIAZOLAM:

Adults – 0.125 to 0.5 mg before bedtime.

Elderly or debilitated – 0.125 to 0.25 mg. Initiate with 0.125 mg until individual response is determined.

SEDATIVES AND HYPNOTICS, BARBITURATES

AMOBARBITAL SODIUM	
Powder for Injection *(c-ii)*	*Amytal Sodium* (Lilly)
APROBARBITAL	
Elixir: 40 mg/5 ml *(c-iii)*	*Alurate* (Roche)
BUTABARBITAL SODIUM	
Tablets: 15, 30, 50 and 100 mg *(c-iii)*	Various, *Butisol Sodium* (Wallace)
Elixir: 30 mg/5 ml *(c-iii)*	Various, *Butisol Sodium* (Wallace)
MEPHOBARBITAL	
Tablets: 32, 50 and 100 mg *(c-iv)*	*Mebaral* (Sanofi Winthrop)
PENTOBARBITAL SODIUM	
Capsules: 50, 100 mg *(c-ii)*	Various, *Nembutal Sodium* (Abbott)
Suppositories: 30, 60, 120 and 200 mg *(c-iii)*	*Nembutal Sodium* (Abbott)
Injection: 50 mg/ml *(c-ii)*	*Pentobarbital Sodium* (Wyeth-Ayerst), *Nembutal Sodium* (Abbott)
PHENOBARBITAL	
Tablets: 15, 16, 30, 60, 100 mg *(c-iv)*	Various, *Solfoton* (ECR Pharm.)
Capsules: 16 mg *(c-iv)*	*Solfoton* (ECR Pharm.)
Elixir: 15 mg/5 ml and 20 mg/5 ml *(c-iv)*	Various
Injection: 30 mg/ml, 60 mg/ml, 65 mg/ml, 130 mg/ml *(c-iv)*	Various, *Luminal Sodium* (Sanofi Winthrop)
SECOBARBITAL SODIUM	
Capsules: 100 mg *(c-ii)*	Various, *Seconal Sodium Pulvules* (Lilly)
Injection: 50 mg/ml *(c-ii)*	*Secobarbital Sodium* (Wyeth-Ayerst)
ORAL COMBINATIONS	
Capsules: 50 mg amobarbital sodium and 50 mg secobarbital sodium; 100 mg amobarbital sodium and 100 mg secobarbital sodium *(c-ii)*	*Tuinal 100 mg Pulvules* (Lilly), *Tuinal 200 mg Pulvules* (Lilly)

The following general discussion of the barbiturates refers to their use as sedative-hypnotic agents and as anticonvulsants.

Actions:

Pharmacology: Barbiturates can produce all levels of CNS mood alteration from excitation to mild sedation, hypnosis and deep coma. In sufficiently high therapeutic doses, barbiturates induce anesthesia. Overdosage can produce death.

These agents depress the sensory cortex, decrease motor activity, alter cerebellar function and produce drowsiness, sedation and hypnosis.

Barbiturates have little analgesic action at subanesthetic doses and may increase the reaction to painful stimuli. All barbiturates exhibit anticonvulsant activity in anesthetic doses. However, only phenobarbital and mephobarbital are effective as oral anticonvulsants in subhypnotic doses.

Barbiturates are respiratory depressants; the degree of respiratory depression is dose-dependent.

Pharmacokinetics:

Absorption – Barbiturates are absorbed in varying degrees following oral, rectal or parenteral administration. The salts are more rapidly absorbed than the acids. The rate of absorption is increased if the sodium salt is ingested as a dilute solution or taken on an empty stomach.

Onset of action for oral or rectal administration varies from 20 to 60 minutes. For IM administration, onset is slightly faster than the oral route. Following IV administration, onset ranges from almost immediate for pentobarbital sodium and secobarbital to 5 minutes for phenobarbital sodium. Maximal CNS depression may not occur for ≥ 15 minutes after IV administration of phenobarbital sodium.

Pharmacokinetics of Sedatives and Hypnotic Barbiturates							
		Half-Life (hrs)		Oral dosage range (mg)		Onset	Duration
	Barbiturate	Range	Mean	Sedative[1]	Hypnotic	(minutes)	(hours)
Long-Acting	Phenobarbital	53 – 118	79	30 – 120	100 – 320	≥ 30	10 – 16
	Mephobarbital	11 – 67	34	32 – 200	—		
Intermediate	Amobarbital[2]	16 – 40	25	—	—	45 – 60	6 – 8
	Aprobarbital	14 – 34	24	120	40 – 160		
	Butabarbital	66 – 140	100	45 – 120	50 – 100		
Short-Acting	Secobarbital	15 – 40	28	—	100	10 – 15	3 – 4
	Pentobarbital	15 – 50	†[3]	40 – 120	100		

[1] Total daily dose; administered in 2 to 4 divided doses.
[2] Available as injection only.
[3] May follow dose-dependent kinetics. Mean t½ is 50 hrs for 50 mg and 22 hrs for 100 mg.

Distribution – Barbiturates are weak acids that are rapidly distributed to all tissues and fluids with high concentrations in the brain, liver and kidneys. Barbiturates are bound to plasma and tissue proteins; the degree of binding increases directly as a function of lipid solubility.

Excretion – Barbiturates are metabolized primarily by the hepatic microsomal enzyme system, and the metabolic products are excreted in the urine, and less commonly, in the feces. Approximately 25% to 50% of a phenobarbital dose and 13% to 24% of an aprobarbital dose is eliminated unchanged in the urine, whereas the amount of other barbiturates excreted unchanged in the urine is negligible. The excretion of unmetabolized barbiturate is one feature that distinguishes the long-acting agents.

Indications:

Sedation: Although traditionally used as nonspecific CNS depressants for daytime sedation, the barbiturates have generally been replaced by the benzodiazepines.

Hypnotic: Short-term treatment of insomnia, since barbiturates appear to lose their effectiveness in sleep induction and maintenance after 2 weeks. If insomnia persists, seek alternative therapy (including nondrug) for chronic insomnia.

Preanesthetic: Used as preanesthetic sedatives.

Anticonvulsant (**mephobarbital, phenobarbital**): Treatment of partial and generalized tonic-clonic and cortical focal seizures.

Acute convulsive episodes: Emergency control of certain acute convulsive episodes (eg, those associated with status epilepticus, cholera, eclampsia, meningitis, tetanus and toxic reactions to strychnine or local anesthetics).

Contraindications:

Barbiturate sensitivity; manifest or latent porphyria; marked impairment of liver function; severe respiratory disease when dyspnea or obstruction is evident; nephritic patients; patients with respiratory disease where dyspnea or obstruction is present; intra-arterial administration; SC administration; previous addiction to the sedative/hypnotic group.

Warnings:

Habit forming: Tolerance or psychological and physical dependence may occur with continued use. Administer with caution, if at all, to patients who are mentally depressed, have suicidal tendencies or a history of drug abuse. Limit prescribing and dispensing to the amount required for the interval until the next appointment.

Withdrawal symptoms can be severe and may cause death.

Treatment of dependence consists of cautions and gradual withdrawal of the drug which takes an extended period of time.

IV administration: Too rapid administration may cause respiratory depression, apnea, laryngospasm or vasodilation with fall in blood pressure. Parenteral solutions of barbiturates are highly alkaline. Therefore, use extreme care to avoid perivascular extravasation or intra-arterial injection.

Phenobarbital sodium may be administered IM or IV as an anticonvulsant for emergency use. When administered IV, it may require ≥ 15 minutes before reaching peak concentrations in the brain.

Pain: Exercise caution when administering to patients with acute or chronic pain, because paradoxical excitement could be induced or important symptoms could be masked.

Seizure disorders: Status epilepticus may result from abrupt discontinuation, even when administered in small daily doses in the treatment of epilepsy.

Effects on vitamin D: Barbiturates may increase vitamin D requirements, possibly by increasing the metabolism of vitamin D via enzyme induction.

Renal function impairment: Barbiturates are excreted either partially or completely unchanged in the urine and are contraindicated in patients with impaired renal function.

Hepatic function impairment: Barbiturates are metabolized primarily by hepatic microsomal enzymes. Administer with caution and initially in reduced doses.

Elderly: May produce marked excitement, depression and confusion.

Pregnancy: Category D.

Lactation: Exercise caution when administering to the nursing mother, since small amounts are excreted in breast milk. Drowsiness in the nursing infant has been reported.

Children: In some persons, especially children, barbiturates repeatedly produce excitement rather than depression. Barbiturates may produce irritability, excitability, inappropriate tearfulness and aggression in children. Safety and efficacy of amobarbital (children < 6 years of age) and aprobarbital have not been established.

Precautions:

Monitoring: During prolonged therapy, perform periodic laboratory evaluation of organ systems, including hematopoietic, renal and hepatic systems.

Special risk patients: Untoward reactions may occur in the presence of fever, hyperthyroidism, diabetes mellitus and severe anemia. Use with caution.

Use **mephobarbital** with caution in patients with myasthenia gravis and myxedema.

Drug Interactions:

Drugs that may affect barbiturates include alcohol, charcoal, chloramphenicol, MAO inhibitors, rifampin and valproic acid. Drugs that may be affected by barbiturates include acetaminophen, anticoagulants, beta blodkers, carbamazepine, chloramphenicol, clonazepam, oral contraceptives, corticosteroids, digitoxin, doxorubicin, doxycycline, felodipine, fenoprofen, griseofulvin, hydantoins, methoxyflurane, metronidazole, narcotics, phenmetrazine, phenylbutazone, quinidine, theophylline and verapamil.

Adverse Reactions:

Adverse reactions may include: Somnolence; agitation; confusion; hyperkinesia; ataxia; CNS depression; nightmares; nervousness; psychiatric disturbance; hallucinations; insomnia; anxiety; dizziness; abnormal thinking; headache; fever (especially with chronic phenobarbital use); hypoventilation; apnea; bradycardia; hypotension; syncope; nausea; vomiting; constipation; liver damage, particularly with chronic phenobarbital use; skin rashes; angioedema (particularly following chronic phenobarbital use).

Administration and Dosage:

IM injection of the sodium salts should be made deeply into a large muscle. Do not exceed 5 ml at any one site because of possible tissue irritation. Monitor patient's vital signs.

IV: Restrict to conditions in which other routes are not feasible, either because the patient is unconscious, or because the patient resists, or because prompt action is imperative. Slow IV injection is essential; observe patients carefully during administration.

Rectal administration: Rectally administered barbiturates are absorbed from the colon and are used occasionally in infants for prolonged convulsive states, or when oral or parenteral administration may be undesirable.

Elderly/Debilitated: Reduce dosage because these patients may be more sensitive to barbiturates.

Hepatic/Renal function impairment: Reduce dosage.

MEPHOBARBITAL:

Sedative –

Adults: 32 to 100 mg 3 or 4 times a day. Optimum dose is 50 mg 3 or 4 times/day.

Children: 16 to 32 mg 3 or 4 times per day.

Epilepsy –

Aduls: Average dose is 400 to 600 mg daily.

Children (< 5 years of age): 16 to 32 mg 3 or 4 times per day.

Children (> 5 years of age): 32 to 64 mg 3 or 4 times per day.

Take at bedtime if seizures generally occur at night, and during the day if attacks are diurnal. Start treatment with a small dose and gradually increase over 4 or 5 days until optimum dosage is determined.

Combination drug therapy – May be used in combination with phenobarbital, in alternating courses or concurrently. When the two are used at the same time, the dose should be about one-half the amount of each used alone. The average daily dose for an adult is 50 to 100 mg phenobarbital and 200 to 300 mg mephobarbital. May also be used with phenytoin. When used concurrently, a reduced dose of phenytoin is advisable, but the full dose of mephobarbital may be given. Satisfactory results have been obtained with an average daily dose of 230 mg phenytoin plus about 600 mg mephobarbital.

AMOBARBITAL SODIUM: The maximum single dose for an adult is 1 g.

Sedative – The usual adult dosage is 30 to 50 mg, 2 or 3 times per day.

Hypnotic – The usual adult dose is 65 to 200 mg.

IM – The aver age IM dose ranges from 65 to 500 mg.

IV – Do not exceed the rate of 50 mg/min. Ordinarily, 65 to 500 mg may be given to a child 6 to 12 years of age.

APROBARBITAL:

Sedative – 40 mg, 3 times per day.

Mild insomnia – 40 to 80 mg before retiring.

Pronounced insomnia – 80 to 160 mg before retiring.

BUTABARBITAL SODIUM:

Adults –

Daytime sedation: 15 to 30 mg, 3 or 4 times daily.

Bedtime hypnotic: 50 to 100 mg

Preoperative sedation: 50 to 100 mg, 60 to 90 minutes before surgery.

Children –

Preoperative sedation: 2 to 6 mg/kg/day (maximum 100 mg).

PENTOBARBITAL SODIUM:

Oral –

Adults:

Sedation – 20 mg 3 or 4 times per day.

Hypnotic – 100 mg at bedtime.

Children:

Sedation/Preanesthetic – 2 to 6 mg/kg/day (max. 100 mg), depending on age, weight and degree of sedation desired.

Hypnotic – Base dosage on age and weight.

Rectal – Do not divide suppositories.

Adults: 120 to 200 mg.

Children:

12 to 14 years (36.4 to 50 kg; 80 to 110 lbs) – 60 or 120 mg.

5 to 12 years (18.2 to 36.4 kg; 40 to 80 lbs) – 60 mg.

1 to 4 years (9 to 18.2 kg; 20 to 40 lbs) – 30 or 60 mg.

2 months to 1 year (4.5 to 9 kg; 10 to 20 lbs) – 30 mg.

Parenteral –

IV: Initially administer 100 mg in the 70 kg adult. Reduce dosage proportionally for pediatric or debilitated patients. At least 1 minute is necessary to determine the full effect. If needed, additional small increments of the drug may be given to a total of 200 to 500 mg for healthy adults.

IM: The usual adult dosage is 150 to 200 mg; children's dosage frequently ranges from 2 to 6 mg/kg as a single IM injection, not to exceed 100 mg.

PHENOBARBITAL:

Anticonvulsant – In infants and children, a loading dose of 15 to 20 mg/kg produces blood levels of ≈ 20 mcg/ml shortly after administration.

Oral –

Adults:

Sedation – 30 to 120 mg/day in 2 to 3 divided doses. A single dose of 30 to 120 mg may be given at intervals; frequency is determined by response. It is generally considered that no more than 400 mg should be given during a 24 hour period.

Hypnotic – 100 to 200 mg.

Anticonvulsant – 60 to 100 mg/day.

Children:

Anticonvulsant – 3 to 6 mg/kg/day.

Sedation – 8 to 32 mg.

Hypnotic – Determined by age and weight.

Parenteral –

Adults:

Sedation – 30 to 120 mg/day IM or IV in 2 to 3 divided doses.

Preoperative sedation – 100 to 200 mg, IM only, 60 to 90 min before surgery.

Hypnotic – 100 to 320 mg IM or IV.

Acute convulsions – 200 to 320 mg IM or IV, repeated in 6 hours as necessary.

Children:

Preoperative sedation – 1 to 3 mg/kg IM or IV.

Anticonvulsant – 4 to 6 mg/kg/day for 7 to 10 days to blood level of 10 to 15 mcg/ml, or 10 to 15 mg/kg/day, IV or IM.

Status epilepticus – 15 to 20 mg/kg IV over 10 to 15 minutes. It is imperative to achieve therapeutic levels as rapidly as possible. When given IV, it may require ≥ 15 minutes to attain peak levels in the brain.

SECOBARBITAL SODIUM:

Oral –

Adults:

Preoperative sedation – 200 to 300 mg 1 to 2 hours before surgery.

Bedtime hypnotic – 100 mg.

Children: For preoperative sedation, 2 to 6 mg/kg (max. 100 mg).

Parenteral –

Adults:

Hypnotic – Usual dose is 100 to 200 mg IM or 50 to 250 mg IV.

Preoperative sedation – For light sedation, 1 mg/kg (0.5 to 0.75 mg/lb) IM, 10 to 15 minutes before procedure.

Dentistry – In patients who are to receive nerve blocks, 100 to 150 mg IV.

Children:

Preoperative sedation – 4 to 5 mg/kg IM.

Status epilepticus – 15 to 20 mg/kg IV over 15 minutes.

ANTICONVULSANTS

Anticonvulsants: Indications and Pharmacokinetics						
	Drug	Labeled indications	Protein binding (%)	Metabolism/ Excretion	t½ (hrs)	Therapeutic serum levels (mcg/ml)
Barbiturates	Phenobarbital[1] (PB)	Status epilepticus Epilepsy, all forms Tonic-clonic	40-60	Liver; 25% eliminated unchanged in urine	53-140	15-40
Hydantoins	Phenytoin	Tonic-clonic Psychomotor	≈90	Liver; renal excretion. < 5% excreted unchanged	Dose-dependent[2]	5-20
	Mephenytoin	Tonic-clonic Psychomotor Focal Jacksonian	nd	Liver	95 (active metabolite)	nd
	Ethotoin	Tonic-clonic Psychomotor	nd	Liver; renal excretion of metabolites	3-9[3]	15-50
Succinimides	Ethosuximide	Absence	0	Liver; 25% excreted unchanged in urine	30 (children 7-9 yrs) 40-60 (adults)	40-100
	Methsuximide	Absence	nd	Liver; < 1% excreted unchanged in urine	<2 (40, active metabolite)	nd
	Phensuximide	Absence	nd	Urine, bile	8 (active metabolite)	nd
Oxazolidinediones	Paramethadione	Absence	nd	Demethylated to active metabolite; excreted in urine	nd	nd
	Trimethadione	Absence	0	Demethylated to dimethadione; 3% excreted unchanged	6-13 days (dimethadione)	≥700 (dimethadione)
Benzodiazepines	Clonazepam	Absence Myoclonic Akinetic	50-85	5 metabolites identified; urine is major excretion route	18-60	20-80 ng/ml
	Clorazepate	Partial[4]	97	Hydrolyzed in stomach to desmethyldiazepam (active); metabolized in liver, renally excreted	30-100	nd
	Diazepam	Status epilepticus[4] Epilepsy, all forms[4]	97-99	Liver, active metabolites	20-50	nd
Miscellaneous	Primidone	Tonic-clonic Psychomotor Focal	20-25	Metabolized to PB and PEMA, both active	5-15 (primidone) 10-18 (PEMA) 53-140 (PB)	5-12 (primidone) 15-40 (PB)
	Valproic acid	Absence	80-94	Liver; excreted in urine	5-20	50-150
	Carbamazepine	Tonic-clonic Mixed Psychomotor	≈75	Liver to active 10, 11–epoxide. 72% excreted in urine, 28% in feces	18-54 (initial) 10-20[5] ≈ 6 (10, 11-epoxide)	4-12
	Phenacemide	Severe mixed psychomotor	nd	Liver	nd	nd
	Felbamate	Partial (adults) Partial/generalized assoc. with Lennox-Gastaut syndrome (children	22-25	40% to 50% unchanged in urine, 40% as unidentified metabolites and conjugates	20-23	nd[6]

[1] Other barbiturates are also used as anticonvulsants. See Sedatives/Hypnotics section.
[2] Exhibits dose-dependent, nonlinear pharmacokinetics.
[3] Below 8 mcg/ml; > 8 mcg/ml, t½ not defined due to dose-dependent, nonlinear pharmacokinetics.
[4] Recommended for adjunctive use.
[5] Undergoes autoinduction. Half-life after repeated doses.
[6] Value of monitoring blood levels not established.

HYDANTOINS

PHENYTOIN SODIUM, PARENTERAL	
Injection: 50 mg/ml (*Rx*)	Various, *Dilantin* (Parke-Davis)
PHENYTOIN, ORAL	
Tablets, chewable: 50 mg (*Rx*)	*Dilantin Infatab* (Parke-Davis)
Oral suspension: 30 or 125 mg/ 5 ml (*Rx*)	*Dilantin-30 or -125* (Parke-Davis)
PHENYTOIN SODIUM, ORAL, PROMPT	
Capsules: 30 or 100 mg (*Rx*)	Various, *Diphenylan Sodium* (Lannett)
PHENYTOIN SODIUM, EXTENDED	
Capsules: 30 or 100 mg (*Rx*)	*Dilantin Kapseals* (Parke-Davis)
PHENYTION SODIUM WITH PHENOBARBITAL	
Capsules: 100 mg/16 or 32 mg (*Rx*)	*Dilantin with Phenobarbital Kapseals* (Parke-Davis)
MEPHENYTOIN	
Tablets: 100 mg (*Rx*)	*Mesantoin* (Sandoz)
ETHOTOIN	
Tablets: 250 or 500 mg (*Rx*)	*Peganone* (Abbott)
FOSPHENYTOIN SODIUM	
Injection: 150 mg (100 mg phenytoin), 750 mg (500 mg phenytoin)	*Cerebyx* (Parke-Davis)

Actions:

Pharmacology: The primary site of action of the hydantoins appears to be the motor cortex, where the spread of seizure activity is inhibited. Possibly by promoting sodium efflux from neurons, hydantoins tend to stabilize the threshold against hyperexcitability.

Pharmacokinetics:

Absorption/Distribution – Phenytoin is slowly absorbed from the small intestine. Rate and extent of absorption varies and is dependent on the product formulation. Bioavailability may differ among products of different manufacturers. Administration IM results in precipitation of phenytoin at the injection site, resulting in slow and erratic absorption, which may continue for up to 5 days or more; 50% to 75% of an IM dose is absorbed within 24 hours. Plasma levels vary and are significantly lower than those achieved with an equal oral dose. Plasma protein binding is 87% to 93% and is lower in uremic patients and neonates. Volume of distribution averages 0.6 L/kg.

Phenytoin's therapeutic plasma concentration is 10 to 20 mcg/ml, although many patients achieve complete seizure control at lower serum concentrations.

Metabolism/Excretion – Phenytoin is metabolized in the liver to inactive hydroxylated metabolites and excreted in the urine by tubular secretion. The metabolism of phenytoin is capacity-limited and shows saturability. The major metabolite is 5–(p–hydroxyphenyl)-5–phenylhydantoin (p–HPPH); 1% to 5% is excreted unchanged. Elimination is exponential (first-order) at plasma concentrations < 10 mcg/ml, and plasma half-life ranges from 6 to 24 hours. Good correlation is generally seen between total phenytoin plasma concentration and therapeutic effects.

Indications:

Control of grand mal and psychomotor seizures.

Phenytoin: To prevent and treat seizures occurring during or following neurosurgery.

Parenteral – For the control of status epilepticus of the grand mal type.

Mephenytoin: For patients refractory to less toxic anticonvulsants; focal and Jacksonian seizures.

Unlabeled uses: Phenytoin is useful as an antiarrhythmic agent, particularly in cardiac glycoside-induced arrhythmias.

Phenytoin has been used as an alternative to magnesium sulfate for severe preeclampsia.

Phenytoin has been used in the treatment of trigeminal neuralgia (tic douloureux), recessive dystrophic epidermolysis bullosa and junctional epidermolysis bullosa.

Contraindications:

Hypersensitivity to hydantoins.

Ethotoin: Hepatic abnormalities or hematologic disorders.

Phenytoin: Because of its effect on ventricular automaticity, do not use phenytoin in sinus bradycardia, sino-atrial block, second and third degree AV block or in patients with Adams-Stokes syndrome.

Warnings:

Abrupt withdrawal in epileptic patients may precipitate status epilepticus.

Other seizures: Hydantoins are not indicated in seizures due to hypoglycemia or other metabolic causes.

Mephenytoin: Use only if safer anticonvulsants have failed after an adequate trial.

Phenytoin: Use with caution in hypotension and severe myocardial insufficiency.

Hepatic function impairment: Biotransformation of hydantoins occurs in the liver; elderly patients or those with impaired liver function or severe illness may show early signs of toxicity.

Induced abnormalities – Phenytoin-induced hepatitis is one of the more commonly reported hypersensitivity syndromes.

Pregnancy: There is an association between use of anticonvulsant drugs by women with epilepsy and an elevated incidence of birth defects in children born to these women. The greatmejority of mothers receiving anticonvulsant medication deliver normal infants.

Lactation: These drugs are excreted in breast milk.

Precautions:

Hematologic effects: Perform blood counts and urinalyses when therapy is begun and at monthly intervals for several months thereafter. Blood dyscrasias have occurred.

Dermatologic effects: Discontinue these drugs if a skin rash appears. If the rash is exfoliative, purpuric or bullous, do not resume use.

Lymph node hyperplasia has been associated with hydantoins, and may represent a hypersensitivity reaction.

Hypersensitivity: Phenytoin hypersensitivity reactions are not typical; they may present as one of many different syndromes (eg, lymphoma, hepatitis, Stevens-Johnson syndrome) and may include such symptoms as fever, rash, arthralgias or lymphadenopathy.

Hyperglycemia, resulting from the drug's inhibitory effect on insulin release, has occurred. Hydantoins may also raise blood sugar levels in hyperglycemic persons.

Cardiovascular: Death from cardiac arrest has occurred after too-rapid IV administration, sometimes preceded by marked QRS widening. Administer cautiously in the presence of advanced AV block. Do not exceed an IV infusion rate of 50 mg/minute.

Osteomalacia has been associated with phenytoin therapy.

Acute intermittent porphyria: Administer hydantoins cautiously to patients with acute intermittent porphyria.

Drug Interactions:

Increased hydantoin effects:

Hydantoin Drug Interactions: Increased Hydantoin Effects			
Inhibit metabolism		Displace anticonvulsant	Unknown
Amiodarone	Metronidazole	Salicylates	Chlorpheniramine
Benzodiazepines	Miconazole	Tricyclic antidepressants	Ibuprofen
Chloramphenicol	Omeprazole	Valproic acid	Phenothiazines
Cimetidine	Phenacemide		
Disulfiram	Phenylbutazone		
Ethanol (acute ingestion)	Succinimides		
Fluconazole	Sulfonamides		
Isoniazid	Trimethoprim		
	Valproic acid		

Decreased hydantoin effects:

Hydantoin Drug Interactions: Decreased Hydantoin Effects		
Increase metabolism	Decrease absorption	Unknown
Barbiturates Carbamazepine Diazoxide Ethanol (chronic ingestion) Rifampin Theophylline	Antacids Charcoal Sucralfate	Antineoplastics Folic acid Influenza virus vaccine Loxapine Nitrofurantoin Pyridoxine

Hydantoin Drug Interactions: Decreased Effects of Other Drugs		
Increased metabolism by phenytoin		Other
Acetaminophen Amiodarone Carbamazepine Cardiac glycosides Corticosteroids Dicumarol Disopyramide Doxycycline Estrogens	Haloperidol Methadone Metyrapone Mexiletine Oral contraceptives Quinidine Theophylline Valproic acid	Cyclosporine Dopamine Furosemide Levodopa Levonorgestrel Mebendazole Nondepolarizing muscle relaxants Phenothiazines Sulfonylureas

Drugs that may be affected by hydantoins include corticosteroids, dopamine, lithium, meperidine, primidone and warfarin.

Drug/Lab test interactions: Phenytoin may interfere with the **metyrapone** and the 1 mg **dexamethasone** tests.

Drug/Food interactions: Several case reports and single-dose studies suggest that enteral nutritional therapy may decrease phenytoin concentrations; however, this has not been substantiated.

Adverse Reactions:

CNS: Nystagmus; ataxia; dysarthria; slurred speech; mental confusion; dizziness; insomnia; transient nervousness; motor twitchings; diplopia; fatigue; irritability; drowsiness; depression; numbness; tremor; headache.

Cardiovascular: Phenytoin IV-Cardiovascular collapse; CNS depression; hypotension (when the drug is administered rapidly IV).

GI: Nausea; vomiting; diarrhea; constipation.

Gingival hyperplasia occurs frequently with phenytoin.

Connective tissue system: Coarsening of the facial features; enlargement of the lips; Peyronie's disease.

Dermatologic: manifestations sometimes accompanied by fever have included scarlatiniform, morbilliform, maculopapular, urticarial and nonspecific rashes; a morbilliform rash is the most common. Rashes are more frequent in children and young adults. Serious forms which may be fatal include bullous, exfoliative or purpuric dermatitis, lupus erythematosus syndrome, Stevens-Johnson syndrome and toxic epidermal necrolysis.

Endocrine: Diabetes insipidus; hyperglycemia.

GU: Urinary retention; oliguria; dysuria; vaginitis; albuminuria; genital edema; kidney failure; polyuria; urethral pain; urinary incontinence; vaginal moniliasis.

Hematologic: Hematopoietic complications, some fatal, include thrombocytopenia, leukopenia, granulocytopenia, agranulocytosis and pancytopenia. Macrocytosis and megaloblastic anemia usually respond to folic acid therapy. Eosinophilia; monocytosis; leukocytosis; simple anemia; hemolytic anemia; aplastic anemia; ecchymosis.

Respiratory: Pneumonia; pharngitis; sinusitis; hyperventilation; rhinitis; apnea; aspiration pneumonia; asthma; dyspnea; atelectasis; increased chough/sputum; epistaxis; hypoxia; pneumothorax; hemoptysis; bronchitis; chest pain; pulmonary fibrosis.

Special senses: Tinnitus; diplopia; tast perversion; amblyopia; deafness; visual field; defect; eye pain; conjunctivitis; photophobia; hyperacusis; mydriasis; parosmia; ear pain; taste loss.

Body as a whole: Polyarthropathy; hyperglycemia; weight gain; chest pain; edema; fever; photophobia; conjunctivitis; gynecomastia.

Lab test abnormalities: Phenytoin may decrease serum thyroxine and free thyroxine concentrations.

Administration and Dosage:

PHENYTOIN SODIUM, PARENTERAL:

Status epilepticus – In adults, administer loading dose of 10 to 15 mg/kg slowly. Follow by maintenance doses of 100 mg orally or IV every 6 to 8 hours. For neonates and children, oral absorption of phenytoin is unreliable; IV loading dose is 15 to 20 mg/kg in divided doses of 5 to 10 mg/kg.

Neurosurgery (prophylactic dosage) – 100 to 200 mg IM at ≈ 4 hour intervals during surgery and the postoperative period.

PHENYTOIN AND PHENYTOIN SODIUM, ORAL: Phenytoin sodium contains 92% pehnytoin. Phenytoin and phenytoin sodium prompt are not for once-a-day dosing. Phenytoin sodium extended may be used for once daily dosing.

Loading dose – An oral loading dose of phenytoin may be used in adults who require rapid steady-state serum levels and where IV administration is not possible.

Initially, 1 g of phenytoin capsules is divided into 3 doses (400 mg, 300 mg, 300 mg) and administered at intervals of 2 hours. Normal maintenance dosage is then instituted 24 hours after the loading dose, with frequent serum level determinations.

Adults who have recieved no previous treatment may be started on 100 mg (125 mg suspension) 3 times daily. Satisfactory maintenance dosage — 300 to 400 mg/day. An increase to 600 mg/day (625 mg/day syspension) may be necessary.

Pediatric – Initially, 5 mg/kg/day in 2 or 3 equally divided doses with subsequent dosage individualized to a maximum of 300 mg/day. Daily maintenance dosage — 4 to 8 mg/kg. Children over 6 years may require the minimum adult dose (300 mg/day). If the daily dosage cannot be divided equally, the larger dose should be given before retiring.

Single daily dosage – In adults, if seizure control is established with divided doses of three 100 mg extended phenytoin sodium capsules daily, once-a-day dosage with 300 mg may be considered; patient compliance is essntial on a once-a-day regimen. Only extended phenytoin sodium capsules are recommended once-a-day.

Bioavailability – Because of the potential bioavailability differences between products, brand interchange is not recommended. Dosage adjustments may be required when switching from the extended to the prompt products.

MEPHENYTOIN: Start with 50 or 100 mg/day during the first week and therafter increase the daily dose by 50 or 100 mg at weekly intervals.

Adults – The average dose ranges from 200 to 600 mg/day. In some instances, as much as 800 mg/day may be required to obtain full seizure control.

Children usually require from 100 to 400 mg/day.

ETHOTOIN: Administer in 4 to 6 divided doses daily. Take after food; space doses as evenly as practical.

Adults – The initial daily dose should be ≤ 1 g, with subsequent gradual dosage increases over several days. The usual adult maintenance dose is 2 to 3 g/day; < 2 g/day is ineffective in most adults.

Pediatric – Initial dose should not exceed 750 mg/day. The usual maintenance dose in children ranges from 500 mg to 1 g/day, although occasionally 2 g or rarely 3 g daily may be necessary.

FOSPHENYTOIN: The dose, concentration in dosing solutions and infusion rate of IV fosphenytoin is expressed as phenytoin sodium equivalents (PE) to avoid the need to perform molecular weight-based adjustments when coverting between fosphenytoin and phenytoin sodium doses. Prescribe and dipense fosphenytoin in phenytoin sodium equivalent units (PE). Fosphenytoin has important differences in administration from those for parenteral phenytoin sodium.

Dilute fosphenytin in 5% Dextrose or 0.9% Saline Solution for Injection to a concentration rangeing from 1.5 to 25 mg PE/ml.

Status epilepticus – The loading dose 15 to 20 mg PE/kg administered at 100 to 150 mg PE/min.

Because the full antiepileptic effect of phenytoin, whether given as fosphenytoin or parenteral phenytoin, is not immediate, other measures, including concomitant administration of an IV benzodiazepine, will usually be necessary for control of status epilepticus.

Nonemergent and maintenance dosing –

Loading dose: 10 to 20 mg PE/kg given IV or IM.

Maintenance dose: 4 to 6 mg PE/kg/day.

Because if the risk of hypotension, administer at a rate of ≤ 150 mg PE/min.

Continuously monitor the electrocardiogram, blood pressure and respiratory function and observe the patient throughout the period of maximal serum phenytoin concentrations, ≈ 10 to 20 min after the end of the infusion.

Renal/Hepatic funciton impairment – Due to an increased fraction of unbound phenytoin in patients with renal or hepatic disease, or in those with hypoalbuminemia, interpret total phenytoin plasma concentrations with caution. Unbound phenytoin concentrations may be more useful in these patients. After IV administration, fosphenytoin clearance to phenytoin may be increased without a similar increase in phenytoin clearance. This has the potential to increase the frequency and severity of adverse events.

Elderly – Age does not have a significant impact on the pharmacokinetics of fosphenytoin following administration. Phenytoin clearance is decreased slightly in elderly patients and lower or less frequent dosing may be required.

CLONAZEPAM

Tablets: 0.5, 1 or 2 mg (*c-iv*)	*Klonopin* (Roche)

For complete prescribing information, refer to the Benzodiazepine monograph in the Antianxiety Agents section.

Indications:

Used alone or as adjunctive treatment of the Lennox-Gastaut syndrome (petit mal variant), akinetic and myoclonic seizures. It may be useful in patients with absence (petit mal) seizures who have failed to respond to succinimides.

Administration and Dosage:

Adults: Initial dose should not exceed 1.5 mg/day in 3 divided doses. Increase in increments of 0.5 to 1 mg every 3 days until seizures are adequately controlled or until side effects preclude any further increase. Individualize maintenance dosage. Maximum recommended dosage is 20 mg/day.

Infants and children (up to 10 years or 30 kg): To minimize drowsiness, the initial dose should be between 0.01 to 0.03 mg/kg/day, not to exceed 0.05 mg/kg/day, given in 2 or 3 divided doses. Increase dosage by not more than 0.25 to 0.5 mg every third day until a daily maintenance dose of 0.1 to 0.2 mg/kg has been reached, unless seizures are controlled or side effects preclude further increase. When possible, divide the daily dose into 3 equal doses. If doses are not equally divided, give the largest dose at bedtime.

CLORAZEPATE DIPOTASSIUM

Tablets: 3.75, 7.5, 11.25, 15 or 22.5 mg (*c-iv*)	Various, *Tranxene-T* (Abbott)

For complete prescribing information, refer to the Benzodiazepine monograph in the Antianxiety Agents section.

Indications:

Partial seizures: As adjunctive therapy in the management of partial seizures.

Alcohol withdrawal: Symptomatic relief of anxiety and for the symptomatic relief of acute alcohol withdrawal (see monograph in the Antianxiety Agents section).

Administration and Dosage:

Adults and children (> 12 years): The maximum initial dose is 7.5 mg 3 times daily. Increase dosage by no more than 7.5 mg every week and do not exceed 90 mg/day.

Children: Maximum initial dose is 7.5 mg 2 times/day. Increase by ≤ 7.5 mg every week; do not exceed 60 mg/day. Not recommended in patients < 9 years old.

DIAZEPAM

Tablets: 2, 5 or 10 mg (*c-iv*)	Various, *Valium* (Roche)
Solution (intensol): 5 mg/ml (*c-iv*)	*Diazepam Intensol* (Roxane)
Solution: 5 mg/5 ml (*c-iv*)	*Diazepam* (Roxane)
Injection: 5 mg/ml (*c-iv*)	Various, *Valium* (Roche), *Dizac Emulsified* (Ohmeda)

For complete prescribing information, refer to the Benzodiazepine monograph in the Antianxiety Agents section.

Indications:

Oral: May be used adjunctively in convulsive disorders; it is not proven useful as sole therapy.

Parenteral: Adjunct in status epilepticus and severe recurrent convulsive seizures.

Administration and Dosage:

Oral (tablets, oral solution and Intensol): Adults – 2 to 10 mg 2 to 4 times daily.

Elderly or debilitated patients – 2 to 2.5 mg once or twice daily initially.

Children – Not for use in children < 6 months of age. Give 1 to 2.5 mg 3 or 4 times daily initially; increase gradually as needed and tolerated.

Intensol preparation: Mix with liquid or semi-solid food such as water, juices, soda or soda-like beverages, applesauce and puddings. Consume the entire amount immediately. Do not store.

Parenteral:

Adults – 5 to 10 mg initially. May be repeated at 10 to 15 minute intervals up to a maximum dose of 30 mg if necessary. Therapy may be repeated in 2 to 4 hours; however, residual active metabolites may persist.

Children ≥ 5 years – 1 mg every 2 to 5 minutes up to a maximum of 10 mg. Repeat in 2 to 4 hours if necessary.

Infants > 30 days of age and children < 5 years – 0.2 to 0.5 mg slowly every 2 to 5 minutes up to a maximum of 5 mg.

Safety and efficacy of parenteral diazepam has not been established in the neonate (≤ 30 days of age).

LAMOTRIGINE

Tablets: 25, 100, 150 and 200 mg (*Rx*)	*Lamictal* (Glaxo Wellcome)

Actions:

Pharmacology: Lamotrigine is chemically unrelated to existing antiepileptic drugs AEDs. The precise mechanism(s) by which lamotrigine exerts its anticonvulsant action are unknown. In vitro studies suggest that it inhibits voltage-sensitive sodium channels thereby stabilizing neuronal membranes and consequently modulating presynaptic transmitter release of excitatory amino acids.

Pharmacokinetics:

Absorption/Distribution – Lamotrigine is rapidly and completely absorbed after oral administration with negligible first-pass metabolism (absolute bioavailability is 98%). The bioavailability is not affected by food.

Metabolism/Excretion – The clearance of lamotrigine is affected by the coadministration of antiepileptic drugs. Lamotrigine is eliminated more rapidly in patients who have been taking hepatic enzyme-inducing antiepileptic drugs. In vitro, lamotrigine is ≈ 55% bound to human plasma proteins.

Indications:

Epilepsy: Adjunctive therapy in the treatment of partial seizures in adults with epilepsy.

Unlabeled uses: Lamotrigine may be useful in adults with generalized tonic-clonic, absence, atypical absence and myoclonic seizures.

Lamotrigine may be beneficial in infants and children with Lennox-Gastaut syndrome.

Contraindications:

Hypersensitivity to the drug or its components.

Warnings:

Dermatologic: Approximately 10% of all lamotrigine exposed individuals develop a rash. Typically, rash occurs in the first 4 to 6 weeks of treatment initiation.

Serious rash leading to hospitalization – Among the rashes leading to hospitalization were Stevens-Johnson syndrome, toxic epidermal necrolysis, angioedema and a rash associated with a variable number of the following systemic manifestations: Fever, lymphadenopathy, facial swelling, hematologic and hepatologic abnormalities.

Withdrawal seizures: AEDs should not be abruptly discontinued because of the possibility of increasing seizure frequency. Unless safety concerns require a more rapid withdrawal, taper the dose of lamotrigine over a period of at least 2 weeks.

Pregnancy: Category C.

Lactation: Preliminary data indicate that lamotrigine passes into breast milk.

Children: Safety and efficacy in children < 16 years of age have not been established.

Precautions:

Monitoring: The value of monitoring plasma concentrations of lamotrigine has not been established. Because of the possible pharmacokinetic interactions between lamotrigine and other AEDs being taken concomitantly, monitoring of the plasma levels of lamotrigine and concomitant AEDs may be indicated, particularly during dosage adjustments.

Special risk patients: Caution is advised when using lamotrigine in patients with renal, hepatic function or cardiac function impairment.

Melanin-containing tissues: Lamotrigine binds to melanin and may cause toxicity in these tissues after extended use. Be aware of the possibility of long-term ophthalmologic effects.

Drug Interactions:

Drugs that may affect lamotrigine include carbamazepine, phenobarbital, primidone, phenytoin and valproic acid.

Drugs that may be affected by lamotrigine include carbamazepine and valproic acid.

Adverse Reactions:

Adverse reactions occurring in ≥ 3% of patients include rash, ataxia, blurred vision, diplopia, dizziness, nausea, vomiting, headache, fever, abdominal pain, infection, diarrhea, dyspepsia, constipation, somnolence, incoordination, insomnia, tremor, depression, anxiety, conbulsion, irritability, rhinitis, pharyngitis, cough increased, pruritus, vision abnormality, dysmenorrhea and vaginitis. Photosensitization (photoallergy or phototoxicity) may occur.

Administration and Dosage:

Adults (> 16 years of age): Recommended as add-on therapy in patients > 16 years of age.

Lamotrigine Dose Recommendations (mg/day) for Adults (> 16 years of age)			
Lamotrigine plus:	Weeks 1 and 2	Weeks 3 and 4	Usual maintenance dose
Enzyme-inducing AEDs and *no* valproic acid	50 mg (once a day)	100 mg (two divided doses)	300 to 500 mg/day (two divided doses). Escalate dose by 100 mg/day every week.
Enzyme-inducing AEDs *plus* valproic acid	25 mg (every other day)	25 mg (once a day)	100 to 150 mg/day (two divided doses). Escalate dose by 25 to 50 mg/day every 1 to 2 weeks.

In patients receiving multi-drug regimens employing enzyme-inducing AEDs without valproic acid, maintenance doses of lamotrigine as high as 700 mg/day have been used. In patients receiving multi-drug regimens using enzyme-inducing AEDs with valproic acid, maintenance doses of lamotrigine as high as 200 mg/day have been used. The advantage of using doses above those recommended in the table above have not been established.

The efficacy of add-on lamotrigine in patients taking valproic acid alone has not been evaluated in controlled trials although it has been used in some patients. Consequently, an effective and safe dosing recommendation for the use of lamotrigine and valproic acid as a two-drug regimen cannot be offered. If this regimen is nonetheless used, note that blood concentrations of lamotrigine appear to be twice those associated with the use of lamotrigine in a regimen containing both enzyme-inducing AEDs and valproic acid.

Renal function impairment: Base initial doses on patients AED regimen (see above); reduced maintenance doses may be effective for patients with significant renal functional impairment.

Discontinuation strategy: If a decision is made to discontinue therapy with lamotrigine, a stepwise reduction of dose over at least 2 weeks (≈ 50% per week) is recommended unless safety concerns require a more rapid withdrawal.

Discontinuing an enzyme-inducing AED should prolong the half-life of lamotrigine; discontinuing valproic acid should shorten the half-life of lamotrigine.

Target plasma levels: A therapeutic plasma concentration range has not been established for lamotrigine. Base dosing of lamotrigine on therapeutic response.

PRIMIDONE

Tablets: 50 mg (*Rx*)	*Mysoline* (Wyeth-Ayerst)
Tablets: 250 mg (*Rx*)	Various, *Mysoline* (Wyeth-Ayerst)
Oral Suspension: 250 mg per 5 ml (*Rx*)	*Mysoline* (Wyeth-Ayerst)

Actions:

Pharmacology: Primidone's mechanism of antiepileptic action is not known.

Primidone and its two metabolites, phenobarbital and phenylethylmalonamide (PEMA) have anticonvulsant activity.

Pharmacokinetics:

Absorption/Distribution – Primidone is readily absorbed from the GI tract. Phenobarbital appears in plasma after several days of continuous therapy. Monitoring of primidone therapy should include plasma level determinations of both primidone and phenobarbital. Therapeutic plasma concentrations are 5 to 12 mcg/ml for primidone and 15 to 40 mcg/ml for phenobarbital.

Metabolism/Excretion – The plasma half-life of primidone is 5 to 15 hours. PEMA and phenobarbital have longer half-lives (10 to 18 hrs and 53 to 140 hrs, respectively) and accumulate with chronic use. About 40% of primidone is excreted unchanged in the urine.

Indications:

Epilepsy: For control of grand mal, psychomotor or focal epileptic seizures, either alone or with other anitconvulsants. It may control grand mal seizures refractory to other anticonvulsants.

Unlabeled uses: Benign familial tremor (essential tremor, 750 mg/day).

Contraindications:

Porphyria; hypersensitivity to phenobarbital.

Warnings:

Status epilepticus: Abrupt withdrawal of antiepileptic medication may precipitate status epilepticus.

Therapeutic efficacy of a dosage regimen takes several weeks to assess.

Pregnancy: The effects of primidone in pregnancy are unknown.

Lactation: Primidone appears in breast milk in substantial quantities.

Precautions:

Monitoring: Since therapy generally extends over prolonged periods, perform complete blood counts and a sequential multiple analysis test every 6 months.

Hazardous tasks: Patients should use caution while driving or performing other tasks requiring alertness, coordination or physical dexterity.

Drug Interactions:

Drugs that may affect primidone include acetazolamide, carbamazepine, hydantoins, isoniazid, nicotinamide and succinimides.

Drugs that may be affected by primidone include carbamazepine.

Adverse Reactions:

Adverse reactions may include: Ataxia, vertigo, fatigue, hyperirritability, emotional disturbances, diplopia, nystagmus, drowsiness, personality deterioration with mood changes, paranoia, nausea, anorexia, vomiting, megaloblastic anemia, thrombocytopenia, impotence, morbilliform, maculopapular skin eruptions and crystalluria.

Administration and Dosage:

Individualize dosage.

Adults and children (> 8 years of age): Patients who have received no previous treatment may be started on primidone according to the following regimen:

Days 1 to 3 – 100 to 125 mg at bedtime.

Days 4 to 6 – 100 to 125 mg twice daily.

Days 7 to 9 – 100 to 125 mg 3 times daily.

Day 10 – maintenance – 250 mg 3 to 4 times daily. If required, increase dose to 250 mg 5 to 6 times daily, but do not exceed doses of 500 mg 4 times daily (2 g/day).

Children (< 8 years): The following regimen may be used to initiate therapy:

Days 1 to 3 – 50 mg at bedtime.

Days 4 to 6 – 50 mg twice daily.

Days 7 to 9 – 100 mg twice daily.

Day 10 – maintenance – 125 to 250 mg 3 times daily, or 10 to 25 mg/kg/day in divided doses.

Patients already receiving other anticonvulsants: Start primidone at 100 to 125 mg at bedtime; gradually increase to maintenance level as the other drug is gradually decreased. When therapy with primidone alone is the objective, the transition should not be completed in < 2 weeks.

Bioequivalence problems have been documented for primidone products marketed by different manufacturers. Brand interchange is not recommended unless comparative bioavailability data are available.

VALPROIC ACID and DERIVATIVES

Capsules: 250 mg (valproic acid) (*Rx*)	Various, *Depakene* (Abbott)
Syrup: 250 mg (as sodium valproate)/5 ml (*Rx*)	Various, *Depakene* (Abbott)
Tablets, delayed release: 125, 250 and 500 mg (as divalproex sodium) (*Rx*)	*Depakote* (Abbott)
Capsules, sprinkle: 125 mg (as divalproex sodium) (*Rx*)	*Depakote* (Abbott)

This group includes valproic acid, sodium valproate (the sodium salt) and divalproex sodium, a stable coordination compound containing equal proportions of valproic acid and sodium valproate. Regardless of form, dosage is expressed as valproic acid equivalents.

Warning:

Hepatic failure resulting in fatalities has occurred in patients receiving valproic acid and its derivatives. Children < 2 years of age are at a considerably increased risk of developing fatal hepatotoxicity, especially those on multiple anticonvulsants, those with congenital metabolic disorders, those with severe seizure disorders accompanied by mental retardation and those with organic brain disease. In this patient group, use with extreme caution and as a sole agent. Weigh benefits of seizure control against risks. Above this age group, the incidence of fatal hepatotoxicity decreases considerably in progressively older patient groups. Perform liver function tests prior to therapy and at frequent intervals thereafter, especially during first 6 months; however, serum biochemistry tests may not be abnormal. Also perform a careful interim medical history and physical examination.

Actions:

Pharmacology: Valproic acid is chemically unrelated to other drugs used to treat seizure disorders. Although the mechanism of action is not established, its activity may be related to increased brain levels of gamma-aminobutyric acid (GABA). This may also account for its prolactin-lowering effects.

Pharmacokinetics:

Absorption – Valproic acid is rapidly absorbed orally. Absorption of enteric coated divalproex is delayed 1 hour; thereafter, the enteric coated form is uniformly and reliably absorbed. Peak serum levels occur approximately 1 to 4 hours after a single oral dose. Absorption is more rapid from the syrup (sodium valproate), with peak levels reached in 15 minutes to 2 hours. A slight delay in absorption occurs when administered with meals, but this does not affect the bioavailability. Equivalent oral doses of divalproex sodium and valproic acid deliver equivalent quantities of valproate ion systemically.

Distribution – Valproic acid is rapidly distributed and is highly bound (90%) to plasma proteins, primarily albumin. Increases in dose may decrease protein binding. Although optimum serum levels have not been clearly defined, a therapeutic range of 50 to 100 mcg/ml is suggested.

Metabolism/Excretion – Primarily metabolized in liver and excreted as glucuronide. Elimination of valproic acid and its metabolites occurs principally in urine. Very little unmetabolized drug is excreted in urine and feces.

The serum half-life is in the range of 9 to 16 hours. Half-life in children < 10 days of age ranges from 10 to 67 hrs compared with a range of 7 to 13 hours in children > 2 months and up to 18 hours in patients with cirrhosis or acute hepatitis.

Indications:

Epilepsy: As monotherapy and adjunctive therapy in the treatment of patients with complex partial seizures that occur either in isolation or in association with other types of seizures. As sole and adjunctive therapy in simple (petit mal) and complex absence seizures. Adjunctively in patients with multiple seizure types including absence seizures.

Mania (divalproex sodium): Manic episodes associated with bipolar disorder.

Migraine: As prophylaxis of migraine headaches.

Unlabeled uses: May be effective alone or in combination in the treatment of atypical absence, myoclonic and grand mal seizures, and possibly effective against atonic, complex partial, elementary partial and infantile spasm seizures. It may also be effective in patients with intractable status epilepticus who have not responded to other therapies.

To prevent recurrent febrile seizures in children.

Subchronic administration may possibly be effective in treating minor incontinence after ileoanal anastomosis.

Migraine prophylaxis.

Management of anxiety disorders/panic attacks.

Contraindications:

Hepatic disease or significant hepatic dysfunction; hypersensitivity to valproic acid.

Warnings:

Discontinuation: Do not abruptly discontinue in patients in whom the drug is administered to prevent major seizures because of the strong possibility of precipitating status epilepticus with attendant hypoxia and threat to life.

Pregnancy: Category D.

Lactation: Concentrations of valproic acid in breast milk are 1% to 10% of serum concentrations.

Children: The safety and efficacy of divalproex sodium for the treatment of acute mania has not been studied in individuals < 18 years of age.

Migraine – The safety and effectiveness of divalproex sodium for the prophylaxis of migraines has not been studied in individuals < 16 years of age.

Precautions:

Hematologic effects: Thrombocytopenia, inhibition of the secondary phase of platelet aggregation and abnormal coagulation parameters have occurred; determine platelet counts and bleeding time before initiating therapy, at periodic intervals and prior to surgery.

Hyperammonemia, with or without lethargy or coma, may occur in the absence of abnormal liver function tests.

Suicidal ideation may be a manifestation of certain psychiatric disorders, and may persist until significant remission of symptoms occurs.

Hazardous tasks: Patients should use caution while driving or performing other tasks requiring alertness, coordination or physical dexterity.

Drug Interactions:

Drugs that may affect valproic acid include charcoal, chlorpromazine, cimetidine, felbamate, rifampin, salicylates, carbamazepine, erythromycin and phenytoin. Drugs that may be affected by valproic acid include alcohol and other CNS depressants, benzodiazepines, carbamazepine, clonazepam, clozapine, ethosuximide, diazepam, lamotrigine, phenytoin, phenobarbital, primidone, tolbutamide, warfarin and zidovudine.

Drug/Lab test interactions: Valproic acid is partially eliminated in the urine as a keto-metabolite which may lead to a false interpretation of the urine ketone test. There have been reports of altered thyroid function tests associated with valproic acid.

Drug/Food interactions: A slight delay in the absorption of valproic acid may occur when administered with meals, but this does not affect the bioavailability.

Adverse Reactions:

Adverse reactions may include nausea; vomiting; indigestion; diarrhea; abdominal cramps; dyspepsia; constipation; anorexia with weight loss; increased appetite with weight gain; sedation; somnolence; asthenia; tremor; ataxia; headache; nystagmus; diplopia; "spots before eyes"; dizziness; incoordination; emotional upset; depression; psychosis; aggression; hyperactivity; behavioral deterioration; transient hair loss; skin rash; petechiae; erythema multiforme; photosensitivity; generalized pruritis; Stevens-Johnson syndrome; thrombocytopenia; bruising; hematoma formation; frank hemorrhage; leukopenia; eosinophilia; anemia; bone marrow suppression or toxicity; acute intermittent porphyria; Minor elevations of AST, ALT and LDH; increases in serum bilirubin; irregular menses; secondary amenorrhea; parotid gland swelling; breast enlargement; galactorrhea; hyperammonemia; hyponatremia; inappropriate ADH secretion; edema of extremities; weakness; acute pancreatitis; lupus erythematosus; fever; enuresis; hearing loss.

Administration and Dosage:

Bedtime administration may minimize effects of CNS depression. GI irritation may be minimized by taking with food, or by slowly increasing the dose.

Sprinkle capsules: May swallow whole or open capsule and sprinkle entire contents on a small amount (teaspoonful) of soft food such as applesauce or pudding. Swallow drug/food mixture immediately; do not chew. Do not store for future use.

Younger children, especially those receiving enzyme-inducing drugs, will require larger maintenance doses to attain targeted total and unbound valproic acid concentrations.

Elderly: Due to a decrease in unbound clearance of valproate, reduce the starting dose; base therapeutic dose on clinical responase.

Epilepsy:

Complex partial seizures – Adults and children ≥ 10 years of age.

10 to 15 mg/kg/day; increase at 1 week intervals by 5 to 10 mg/kg/day until seizures are controlled or side effects preclude further increases. Maximum recommended dosage: 60 mg/kg/day. If total dose is > 250 mg/day, give in divided doses.

Conversion to monotherapy – Concomitant antiepilepsy drug (AED) dosage can ordinarily be reduced by ≈ 25% every 2 weeks. This reduction may be started at initiation of therapy, or delayed by 1 to 2 weeks. This reduction may be started at initiation of therapy, or delayed by 1 to 2 weeks if there is a concern that seizures are likely to occur with a reduction. The speed and duration of withdrawal of the concomitant AED can be highly variable; monitor patients closely during this period for increased seizure frequency.

Conversion from valproic acid to divalproex sodium – In patients previously receiving valproic acid, initiate divalproex sodium at the same total daily dose and dosing schedule.

Mania (divalproex sodium): 750 mg daily in divided doses; increase as rapidly as possible to achieve the lowest therapeutic dose that produces the desired clinical effect. Maximum recommended dosage is 60 mg/kg/day.

Migraine: 250 mg orally twice daily. Some patients may benefit from doses up to 1000 mg/day. There is no evidence that higher doses lead to greater efficacy.

CARBAMAZEPINE

Tablets, chewable: 100 mg (*Rx*)	Various, *Tegretol* (Geigy)
Tablets: 200 mg (*Rx*)	Various, *Epitol* (Lemmon), *Tegretol* (Geigy)
Suspension: 100 mg/5 ml (*Rx*)	*Tegretol* (Geigy)

Warning:

Aplastic anemia and agranulocytosis have been reported in association with carbamazepine therapy. The risk of developing these reactions is 5 to 8 times greater than in the general population. Consider discontinuation of the drug if any evidence of significant bone marrow depression develops.

Actions:

Pharmacology: Carbamazepine's mechanism of action is unknown. It appears to act by reducing polysynaptic responses and blocking the post-tetanic potentiation.

Pharmacokinetics:

Absorption/Distribution – Both the suspension and tablet deliver equivalent amounts of drug to the systemic circulation; however, the suspension is absorbed somewhat faster than the tablet. Carbamazepine is 76% bound to plasma proteins.

Metabolism/Excretion – Carbamazepine is metabolized in the liver to the 10,11–epoxide, which also has anticonvulsant activity. It may induce its own metabolism. Initial half-life ranges from 25 to 65 hours, and decreases to 12 to 17 hours with repeated doses.

Indications:

Epilepsy: Partial seizures with complex symptoms. Patients with these seizures appear to show greatest improvement. Generalized tonic-clonic seizures; mixed seizure patterns or other partial or generalized seizures.

Reserve carbamazepine for patients who have not responded satisfactorily to other agents such as phenytoin, phenobarbital or primidone, whose seizures are difficult to control or patients experiencing marked side effects.

Trigeminal neuralgia: Treatment of pain associated with true trigeminal neuralgia and glossopharyngeal neuralgia.

Unlabeled uses: Neurogenic diabetes insipidus.

Certain psychiatric disorders, including bipolar disorders, schizoaffective illness, resistant schizophrenia and dyscontrol syndrome associated with limbic system dysfunction.

Management of alcohol withdrawal.

Restless legs syndrome (100 to 300 mg at bedtime).

Contraindications:

History of bone marrow depression; hypersensitivity to carbamazepine and tricyclic antidepressants; concomitant use of monoamine oxidase (MAO) inhibitors. Discontinue MAO inhibitors for a minimum of 14 days before carbamazepine administration.

Warnings:

This drug is not a simple analgesic. Do not use for the relief of minor aches or pains.

Hematologic: Patients with a history of adverse hematologic reaction to any drug may be particularly at risk.

Glaucoma: Carbamazepine has shown mild anticholinergic activity; therefore, use with caution in patients with increased intraocular pressure.

CNS effects: Because of the drug's relationship to other tricyclic compounds, the possibility of activating latent psychosis, or confusion or agitation in elderly patients may occur.

Pregnancy: Category C.

Lactation: Concentration of carbamazepine in milk is approximately 60% of the maternal plasma concentration.

Children: Safety and efficacy for use in children below the age of 6 years have not been established.

Precautions:

Absence seizures (petit mal) do not appear to be controlled by carbamazepine.

Special risk patients: Prescribe carbamazepine only after benefit-to-risk appraisal in patients with a history of: Cardiac, hepatic or renal damage; adverse hematologic reaction to other drugs; interrupted courses of therapy with the drug.

Laboratory tests: Perform baseline liver function tests and periodic evaluations. Obtain baseline and periodic eye examinations (slit lamp, funduscopy and tonometry), urinalysis and BUN determinations.

Obtain complete pretreatment hematological testing as a baseline. Repeat these tests at monthly intervals during the first 2 months and thereafter obtain yearly or every other year CBC, white cell differential and platelet count.

Hazardous tasks: May produce drowsiness, dizziness or blurred vision; patients should observe caution while driving or performing other tasks requiring alertness.

Drug Interactions:

Drugs that may interact with carbamazepine include cimetidine, danazol, diltiazem, erythromycin, isoniazid, nicotinamide, propoxyphene, troleandomycin, verapamil, acetaminophen, oral anticoagulants, barbiturates, primidone, charcoal, doxycycline, haloperidol, hydantoins, lithium, nondepolarizing muscle relaxants, theophylline and valproic acid.

Adverse Reactions:

Adverse reactions may include: Dizziness; drowsiness; unsteadiness; nausea; vomiting; aplastic anemia; leukopenia; agranulocytosis; eosinophilia; leukocytosis; thrombocytopenia; pancytopenia; bone marrow depression; fever and chills; dyspnea; pneumonitis; pneumonia; pulmonary eosinophilia; asthma; abnormal liver function tests; cholestatic/hepatocellular jaundice; hepatitis; urinary frequency; acute urinary retention; oliguria with hypertension; renal failure; azotemia; impotence; albuminuria; glycosuria; elevated BUN; microscopic deposits in urine; disturbances of coordination; confusion; headache; fatigue; blurred vision; visual hallucinations; speech disturbances; abnormal involuntary movements; peripheral neuritis and paresthesias; depression with agitation; talkativeness; tinnitus; hyperacusis; behavioral changes in children; paralysis; cerebral arterial insufficiency; pruritic and erythematous rashes; urticaria; Stevens-Johnson syndrome; photosensitivity reactions; alterations in pigmentation; exfoliative dermatitis; alopecia; diaphoresis; erythema multiforme and nodosum; purpura; aggravation of disseminated lupus erythematosus; toxic epidermal necrolysis; gastric distress; abdominal pain; diarrhea; constipation; anorexia; dryness of mouth or pharynx; glossitis and stomatitis; congestive heart failure; hypotension; syncope and collapse; edema; primary thrombophlebitis; recurrence of thrombophlebitis; aggravation of coronary artery disease; arrhythmias; AV block; adenopathy or lymphadenopathy; cardiovascular complications which have resulted in fatalities; transient diplopia; oculomotor disturbances; nystagmus; scattered; punctate cortical lens opacities; conjunctivitis; aching joints; muscles; leg cramps; inappropriate antidiuretic hormone secretion syndrome (SIADH).

Administration and Dosage:

Individualize dosage. A low initial daily dosage with gradual increase is advised. As soon as adequate control is achieved, reduce dosage gradually to the minimum effective level. Take with meals.

Epilepsy:

Adults and children over 12 years –

Initial dose is 200 mg twice daily (100 mg 4 times daily of suspension). Increase at weekly intervals by up to 200 mg/day using a 3 or 4 times per day regimen until the best response is obtained. Do not exceed 1000 mg/day in children 12 to 15 years or 1200 mg/day in patients over 15 years. In rare instances, doses up to 1600 mg/day have been used in adults.

Maintenance: Adjust to minimum effective level, usually 800 to 1200 mg daily.

Children 6 to 12 years –

Initial dose is 100 mg twice daily (50 mg 4 times daily of suspension). Increase at weekly intervals gradually by adding 100 mg/day using a 3 or 4 times per day regimen until the best response is obtained. Do not exceed 1000 mg daily. May also be calculated on basis of 20 to 30 mg/kg/day, in divided doses 3 or 4 times a day.

Maintenance: Adjust to minimum effective level, usually 400 to 800 mg daily.

Combination therapy – When added to existing anticonvulsant therapy, do so gradually while other anticonvulsants are maintained or gradually decreased, except phenytoin which may have to be increased.

Trigeminal neuralgia:

Initial – 100 mg twice daily on the first day (50 mg 4 times daily of suspension). May increase by up to 200 mg/day using 100 mg increments every 12 hours (50 mg 4 times daily of suspension) as needed. Do not exceed 1200 mg daily.

Maintenance – Control of pain can usually be maintained with 400 to 800 mg daily (range 200 to 1200 mg/day). Attempt to reduce the dose to the minimum effective level or to discontinue the drug at least once every 3 months.

FELBAMATE

Tablets: 400 and 600 mg (*Rx*) — *Felbatol* (Wallace Labs)
Suspension: 600 mg/5 ml (*Rx*)

Warning:

There have been reports of 21 cases (including 3 deaths) of aplastic anemia (pancytopenia in the presence of a bone marrow largely depleted of myeloid and erythroid precursors) in association with the use of felbamate. Time to onset in these cases from time of treatment initiation ranged from 5 to 30 weeks; mean time to onset was 128 days. How long the risk persists and whether its magnitude changes with time are not known.

In addition to aplastic anemia, eight cases of acute liver failure have occurred, including four deaths, in association with the use of felbamate. One of the four survivors received a liver transplant. The number of cases reported greatly exceeds the number that is expected based on the annual incidence of acute liver failure in the US (about 2000 per year). In several cases there were nonspecific premonitory signs, but in others the patients were already in frank liver failure at the time the illness was detected. Time between initiation of treatment and diagnosis of these cases ranged from 14 to 257 days.

An FDA advisory committee has recommended that felbamate be used as a second-line therapy only. For further information, contact Wallace Labs at 800–526–3840.

Actions:

Pharmacology: Felbamate is an oral antiepileptic agent. The mechanism by which it exerts its anticonvulsant activity is unknown.

Pharmacokinetics:

Absorption/Distribution – Felbamate is well absorbed after oral administration.

Metabolism/Excretion – Following oral administration, felbamate is the predominant plasma species (about 90%). About 40% to 50% of absorbed dose appears unchanged in urine and an additional 40% is present as unidentified metabolites and conjugates.

Indications:

Partial seizures: Monotherapy and adjunctive therapy in the treatment of partial seizures with and without generalization in adults with epilepsy.

Lennox-Gastaut syndrome: Adjunctive therapy in the treatment of partial and generalized seizures associated with Lennox-Gastaut syndrome in children.

Contraindications:

Hypersensitivity to felbamate or ingredients of the product. Use cautiously in those who have demonstrated hypersensitivity reactions to other carbamates.

Warnings:

Aplastic anemia: There have been reports of 21 cases of aplastic anemia (including 3 deaths) in association with the use of felbamate.

Hepatic failure: There have been eight cases of acute liver failure (including four deaths) in association with the use of felbamate.

Discontinuation: Antiepileptic drugs should not be suddenly discontinued because of the possibility of increasing seizure frequency.

Elderly: In general, dosage selection for an elderly patient should be cautious, usually starting at the low end of the dosing range, reflecting the greater frequency of decreased hepatic, renal or cardiac function and of concomitant disease or other drug therapy.

Pregnancy: Category C.

Lactation: Felbamate has been detected in breast milk.

Children: Safety and efficacy in children, other than those with Lennox-Gastaut syndrome, have not been established.

Precautions:

Monitoring: Because of the effect of felbamate on the plasma levels of other AEDs being taken concomitantly, monitoring of the plasma concentrations of these AEDs may be indicated.

Photosensitivity: Photosensitization (photoallergy or phototoxicity) may occur; therefore, caution patients to take protective measures against exposure to ultraviolet light or sunlight (ie, sunscreens, protective clothing) until tolerance is determined.

Drug Interactions:

Drugs that may affect felbamate include phenytoin and carbamazepine.

Drugs that may be affected by felbamate include phenytoin, carbamazepine and valproic acid.

Adverse Reactions:

Adverse reactions occurring in ≥ 3% of patients include fatigue; weight decrease; facial edema; fever; pain; insomnia; headache; anxiety; somnolence; dizziness; nervousness; tremor; abnormal gait; depression; paresthesia; ataxia; thinking abnormal; emotional lability; moisis; acne; rash; dyspepsia; vomiting; constipation; diarrhea; AKT increased; nausea; anorexia; abdominal pain; hiccups; upper respiratory tract infection; rhinitis; sinustis; pharyngitis; coughing; diplopia; otitis media; taste perversion; vision abnormal; urinary incontinence; intramenstrual bleeding; UTI; purpura; leukopenia and hypophosphatemia.

Administration and Dosage:

Discontinuation of therapy: Because of reports of aplastic anemia in association with felbamate, it has been recommended to discontinue use of the drug unless the physician decides that withdrawal would pose an even greater risk to the patient.

Patients should not discontinue the drug on their own. If the decision is made to discontinue therapy, felbamate may be discontinued by reducing the dosage by one-third increments every 4 to 5 days. As with any antiepileptic, abrupt discontinuation may result in an increase in seizure frequency; however, if it is necessary to discontinue felbamate abruptly, it may be stopped without tapering as long as the patient is covered by adequate dosages of other antiepileptics.

Adults (≥ 14 years of age): Most of the patients received 3600 mg/day in clinical trials.

Monotherapy (initial therapy) – Felbamate has not been systematically evaluated as initial monotherapy. Initiate at 1200 mg/day in divided doses 3 or 4 times daily. Titrate previously untreated patients under close clinical supervision, increasing the dosage in 600 mg increments every 2 weeks to 2400 mg/day based on clinical response and thereafter to 3600 mg/day if clinically indicated.

Conversion to monotherapy – Initiate at 1200 mg/day in divided doses 3 or 4 times daily. Reduce the dosage of concomitant AEDs by one-third at initiation of felbamate therapy. At week 2, increase the felbamate dosage to 2400 mg/day while reducing the dosage of other AEDs up to an additional one-third of their original dosage. At week 3, increase the felbamate dosage up to 3600 mg/day and continue to reduce the dosage of other AEDs as clinically indicated.

Adjunctive therapy – Add felbamate at 1200 mg/day in divided doses 3 or 4 times daily while reducing present AEDs by 20% in order to control plasma concentrations of concurrent phenytoin, valproic acid and carbamazepine (and its metabolites). Further reductions of the concomitant AED dosage may be necessary to minimize side effects due to drug interactions. Increase the dosage of felbamate by 1200 mg/day increments at weekly intervals to 3600 mg/day. Most side effects seen during adjunctive therapy resolve as the dosage of concomitant AEDs is decreased.

While the previous conversion guidelines may result in a felbamate 3600 mg/day dose within 3 weeks, in some patients titration to 3600 mg/day has been achieved in as little as 3 days with appropriate adjustment of other AEDs.

Children with Lennox-Gastaut syndrome (ages 2 to 14 years):

Adjunctive therapy – Add felbamate at 15 mg/kg/day in divided doses 3 or 4 times daily while reducing present AEDs by 20% in order to control plasma levels of concurrent phenytoin, valproic acid and carbamazepine (and its metabolites). Further reductions of the concomitant AED dosage may be necessary to minimize side effects due to drug interactions. Increase the dosage of felbamate by 15 mg/kg/day increments at weekly intervals to 45 mg/kg/day. Most side effects seen during adjunctive therapy resolve as the dosage of concomitant AEDs is decreased.

GABAPENTIN

Capsules: 100, 300 and 400 mg (*Rx*)	*Neurontin* (Parke-Davis)

Actions:

Pharmacology: Gabapentin is an oral antiepileptic agent. The mechanism by which it exerts its anticonvulsant action is unknown.

Pharmacokinetics:

Absorption – Gabapentin bioavailability is not dose-proportional.

Distribution – Gabapentin circulates largely unbound (< 3%) to plasma protein.

Metabolism/Excretion – Gabapentin is eliminated from the systemic circulation by renal excretion as unchanged drug; it is not appreciably metabolized.

Special populations:

Renal insufficiency – Dosage adustment in patients with compromised renal function is necessary.

Hemodialysis – Hemodialysis has a significant effect on gabapentin elimination in anuric subjects. Dosage adjustment in patients undergoing hemodialysis is necessary.

Indications:

Adjunctive therapy in the treatment of partial seizures with and without secondary generalization in adults with epilepsy.

Contraindications:

Hypersensitivity to the drug or its ingredients.

Warnings:

Withdrawal-precipitated seizure: Antiepileptic drugs should not be abruptly discontinued because of the possibility of increasing seizure frequency.

Status epilepticus: In the placebo controlled studies, the incidence of status epilepticus in patients receiving gabapentin was 0.6% vs 0.5% with placebo. Among the 2074 patients treated with gabapentin across all studies, 31 (1.5%) had status epilepticus.

Sudden and unexplained deaths: During the course of premarketing development of gabapentin, eight sudden and unexplained deaths were recorded among 2203 patients.

Elderly: No systematic studies in geriatric patients have been conducted. Adverse clinical events reported among 59 gabapentin-exposed patients over age 65 did not differ in kind from those reported for younger individuals.

Pregnancy: Category C.

Lactation: It is not known if gabapentin is excreted in breast milk.

Children: Safety and efficacy in children < 12 years of age have not been established.

Precautions:

Monitoring: Clinical trials data do not indicate that routine monitoring of clinical laboratory parameters is necessary for the safe use of gabapentin.

Drug Interactions:

Drugs that may affect gabapentin include antacids and cimetidine. Drugs that may be affected by gabapentin include oral contraceptives.

Drug/Lab test interactions: Because false positive readings were reported with the *Ames N-Multistix* SG dipstick test for urinary protein when gabapentin was added to other antiepileptic drugs, the more specific sulfosalicylic acid precipitation procedure is recommended to determine the presence of urine protein.

Adverse Reactions:

Adverse reactions occurring in ≥ 3% of patients include somnolence, dizziness, ataxia, fatigue, nystagmus, rhinitis, diplopia, amblyopia and tremor.

Administration and Dosage:

Recommended for add-on therapy in patients > 12 years of age, taken with or without food.

The effective dose is 900 to 1800 mg/day in divided doses (3 times a day). Titration to an effective dose can take place rapidly, over a few days, giving 300 mg on day 1; 300 mg twice a day on day 2 and 300 mg 3 times a day on day 3. To minimize potential side effects, especially somnolence, dizziness, fatigue and ataxia, the first dose on day 1 may be administered at bedtime. If necessary, the dose may be increased by using 300 or 400 mg 3 times a day up to 1800 mg/day. Dosages up to 2400 to 3600 mg/day bave been well tolerated. The maximum time between doses in the 3 times daily schedule should not exceed 12 hours.

It is not necessary to monitor gabapentin plasma concentrations to optimize therapy. Further, because there are no significant pharmacokinetic interactions with other commonly used anti-epileptic drugs, the addition of gabapentin does not alter the plasma levels of these drugs appreciably.

If gabapentin is discontinued or an alternate anticonvulsant medication is added to the therapy, this should be done gradually over a minimum of 1 week.

Renal function impairment:

Gabapentin Dosage Based on Renal Function		
Creatinine clearance (ml/min)	Total daily dose (mg/day)	Dose regimen (mg)
> 60	1200	400 tid
30 to 60	600	300 bid
15 to 30	300	300 qd
< 15	150	300 qod[1]
Hemodialysis	—	200 to 300[2]

[1] Every other day.

[2] Loading dose of 300 to 400 mg in patients who have never received gabapentin, then 200 to 300 mg gabapentin following each 4 hours of hemodialysis.

MAGNESIUM SULFATE

Injection: 12.5% (1 mEq/ml) and 50% (4 mEq/ml) (*Rx*) Various

Actions:

Pharmacology: Magnesium prevents or controls convulsions by blocking neuromuscular transmission and decreasing the amount of acetylcholine liberated at the end plate by the motor nerve impulse. Magnesium has a CNS depressant effect. Normal plasma magnesium levels range from 1.5 to 3 mEq/L.

One gram of magnesium sulfate provides 8.12 mEq of magnesium.

Pharmacokinetics: With IV use, the onset of anticonvulsant action is immediate and lasts about 30 minutes. With IM use, onset occurs in 1 hour and persists for 3 to 4 hours. Effective anticonvulsant serum levels range from 2.5 or 3 to 7.5 mEq/L. Magnesium is excreted by the kidney.

Indications:

Seizure prevention and control in severe pre-eclampsia or eclampsia without producing deleterious CNS depression in the mother or infant, and in convulsions associated with abnormally low levels of plasma magnesium as a contributing factor.

Acute nephritis in children to control hypertension, encephalopathy and convulsions.

Hypomagnesemia: Magnesium deficiency, prevention and correction in total parenteral nutrition.

Unlabeled uses: Magnesium has demonstrated some effectiveness as an agent to inhibit premature labor (tocolytic); however, it is not a first-line agent. It also appears to be beneficial when added to ritodrine therapy, although efficacy has been questioned and an increase in adverse reactions has been observed.

In asthmatic patients who respond poorly to β-agonists, IV magnesium sulfate (1.2 g) may be a beneficial adjunct for treatment of acute exacerbations of moderate to severe asthma.

The use of IV magnesium sulfate appears to be effective in reducing early mortality in patients with acute myocardial infarction when given as soon as possible after the MI and continued for 24 to 48 hours.

Contraindications:

Do not give in toxemia of pregnancy during the 2 hours preceding delivery.

Warnings:

IV use in eclampsia is reserved for immediate control of life-threatening convulsions.

Renal function impairment: Because magnesium is excreted by the kidneys, parenteral use in the presence of renal insufficiency may lead to magnesium intoxication. Use with caution.

Pregnancy: *Category* A. When administered by continuous IV infusion (especially for > 24 hours preceding delivery) to control convulsions in toxemic mothers, the newborn may show signs of magnesium toxicity, including neuromuscular or respiratory depression.

Precautions:

Monitoring: Monitor serum magnesium levels and clinical status to avoid overdosage.

Urine output: Maintain at a level of 100 ml every 4 hours.

Drug Interactions:

Drugs that may interact with magnesium sulfate include neuromuscular blockers.

Adverse Reactions:

Adverse reactions may include: Magnesium intoxication; flushing; sweating; hypotension; depressed reflexes; flaccid paralysis; hypothermia; circulatory collapse; cardiac depression; CNS depression; respiratory paralysis; hypocalcemia and tetany.

Administration and Dosage:

Individualize dosage. Monitor the patient's clinical status to avoid toxicity. Discontinue as soon as the desired effect is obtained. Repeat doses are dependent on continuing presence of the patellar reflex and adequate respiratory function.

IM: 4 to 5 g of a 50% solution every 4 hours as necessary.

IV: 4 g of a 10% to 20% solution, not exceeding 1.5 ml/min of a 10% solution.

IV infusion: 4 to 5 g in 250 ml of 5% Dextrose or Sodium Chloride, not exceeding 3 ml/min.

Pediatric: IM - 20 to 40 mg/kg in a 20% solution; repeat as necessary.

CYCLOBENZAPRINE HCl

Tablets: 10 mg (*Rx*)	Various, *Flexeril* (Merck)

Actions:

Pharmacology: Cyclobenzaprine, structurally related to the tricyclic antidepressants (TCAs), relieves skeletal muscle spasm of local origin without interfering with muscle function. It is ineffective in muscle spasm due to CNS disease. The net effect is a reduction of tonic somatic motor activity, influencing both gamma and alpha motor systems.

Pharmacokinetics: Cyclobenzaprine is well absorbed after oral administration, but there is a large intersubject variation in plasma levels. Peak plasma levels are reached in 4 to 6 hours. The onset of action occurs in 1 hour with a duration of 12 to 24 hours. It is highly bound to plasma proteins, extensively metabolized primarily to glucuronide-like conjugates and excreted primarily via the kidneys. Elimination half-life is 1 to 3 days.

Indications:

Musculoskeletal conditions: Adjunct to rest and physical therapy for relief of muscle spasm associated with acute painful musculoskeletal conditions.

Unlabeled uses: Cyclobenzaprine (10 to 40 mg/day) appears to be a useful adjunct in the management of the fibrositis syndrome.

Contraindications:

Hypersensitivity to cyclobenzaprine; concomitant use of monoamine oxidase (MAO) inhibitors or within 14 days after their discontinuation; acute recovery phase of myocardial infarction and in patients with arrhythmias, heart block or conduction disturbances or congestive heart failure; hyperthyroidism.

Warnings:

Spasticity: Cyclobenzaprine is not effective in the treatment of spasticity associated with cerebral or spinal cord disease, or in children with cerebral palsy.

Duration: Use only for short periods (up to 2 or 3 weeks); effectiveness for more prolonged use is not proven.

Similarity to TCAs: Cyclobenzaprine is closely related to the TCAs. In short-term studies for indications other than muscle spasm associated with acute musculoskeletal conditions, and usually at doses greater than those recommended, some of the more serious CNS reactions noted with the TCAs have occurred.

Pregnancy: Category B.

Lactation: It is not known whether cyclobenzaprine is excreted in breast milk.

Children: Safety and efficacy in children < 15 years of age have not been established.

Precautions:

Anticholinergic effects: Because of its anticholinergic action, use with caution in patients with a history of urinary retention, angle-closure glaucoma and increased intraocular pressure.

Hazardous tasks: May impair mental or physical abilities required for performance of hazardous tasks; patients should observe caution while driving or performing other tasks requiring alertness, coordination and physical dexterity.

Drug Interactions:

Drugs that may interact with cyclobenzaprine HCl include MAO inhibitors and TCAs.

Adverse Reactions:

Adverse reactions occurring in ≥ 3% of patients include drowsiness, dizziness, fatigue, tiredness, asthenia, blurred vision, headache, nervousness, confusion, dry mouth, nausea, constipation, dyspepsia, unpleasant taste, purpura, bone marrow depression, leukopenia, eosinophilia, thrombocytopenia, elevation and lowering of blood sugar levels and weight gain or loss.

Administration and Dosage:

Give 10 mg 3 times daily (range, 20 to 40 mg daily in divided doses). Do not exceed 60 mg/day. Do not use longer than 2 or 3 weeks.

DIAZEPAM

The following is an abbreviated monograph. For complete prescribing information, refer to the monograph in the Antianxiety Agents section.

Tablets: 2, 5 and 10 mg (c-iv)	Various, *Valium* (Roche)
Oral Solution: 5 mg/5 ml (c-iv)	*Diazepam* (Roxane)
Concentrated Oral Solution: 5 mg/ml (c-iv)	*Diazepam Intensol* (Roxane)
Injection: 5 mg/ml (c-iv)	Various, *Valium* (Roche), *Zetran* (Hauck), *Dizac* (Ohmeda)

Actions:

Pharmacology: Major muscle relaxant actions occur in two proposed sites: At the spinal level resulting in enhancement of GABA-mediated presynaptic inhibition, and at supraspinal sites, probably in the brain stem reticular formation.

Indications:

An adjunct for the relief of skeletal muscle spasm due to reflex spasm to local pathology (such as inflammation of the muscles or joints, or secondary to trauma); spasticity caused by upper motor neuron disorders; athetosis; stiff-man syndrome. Injectable diazepam may also be used as an adjunct in tetanus.

Also used as an antianxiety agent and an anticonvulsant.

Administration and Dosage:

Oral: Individualize dosage for maximum beneficial effect.

Adults – 2 to 10 mg 3 or 4 times daily.

Geriatric or debilitated patients – 2 to 2.5 mg 1 or 2 times daily initially, increasing as needed and tolerated.

Children – 1 to 2.5 mg 3 or 4 times daily initially, increasing as needed and tolerated (not for use in children > 6 months of age).

Intensol – Dosages are same as those listed above. Mix with liquid or semi-solid food such as water, juices, soda or soda-like beverages, applesauce and puddings. Stir in gently. Consume the entire mixture immediately. Do not store for future use.

Sustained release – 15 to 30 mg once daily.

Parenteral: Use lower doses (2 to 5 mg) and slow dosage increases for elderly or debilitated patients and when other sedatives are given. When acute symptoms are controlled with the injectable form, administer oral therapy if further treatment is required.

Neonates (≤ 30 days of age) – Safety and efficacy have not been established. Prolonged CNS depression has been observed in neonates, apparently due to inability to biotransform diazepam into inactive metabolites.

Children – Give slowly over 3 minutes in a dosage not to exceed 0.25 mg/kg. After a 15 to 30 minute interval, the initial dosage can be safely repeated. If relief is not obtained after a third administration, begin adjunctive therapy appropriate to the condition being treated.

IM: Inject deeply into the muscle.

IV: Inject slowly, taking at least 1 minute for each 5 mg (1 ml). Do not use small veins (ie, dorsum of hand or wrist). Avoid intra-arterial administration or extravasation. Do not mix or dilute with other solutions or drugs.

Adults – 5 to 10 mg, IM or IV initially, then 5 to 10 mg in 3 to 4 hours, if necessary. For tetanus, larger doses may be required.

Children – For tetanus in infants > 30 days of age, 1 to 2 mg IM or IV slowly; repeat every 3 to 4 hours as necessary. In children ≥ 5 years of age, 5 to 10 mg. Repeat every 3 to 4 hours if necessary to control tetanus spasms. Have respiratory assistance available.

BACLOFEN

Tablets: 10 mg, 20 mg (*Rx*)	Various, *Lioresal* (Geigy)
Intrathecal: 10 mg/20 ml (500 mcg/ml) and 10 mg/5 ml (2000 mcg/ml) (*Rx*)	*Lioresal* (Medtronic)

Actions:

Pharmacology: The precise mechanism of action is not known. Baclofen can inhibit both monosynaptic and polysynaptic reflexes at the spinal level, possibly by hyperpolarization of afferent terminals, although actions at supraspinal sites may also contribute to its clinical effect. Baclofen has CNS depressant properties.

When introduced directly into the intrathecal space, effective CSF concentrations are achieved with resultant plasma concentrations 100 times less than those occurring with oral administration.

Pharmacokinetics:

Oral – Baclofen is rapidly and extensively absorbed. Absorption may be dose-dependent, being reduced with increasing doses. Peak serum levels are reached in approximately 2 hours; half-life is 3 to 4 hours. It is excreted primarily by the kidney in unchanged form with intersubject variation in absorption or elimination.

Intrathecal –

Bolus: The onset of action is generally 0.5 to 1 hour after an intrathecal bolus dose. Peak spasmolytic effect is seen at approximately 4 hours after dosing and effects may last 4 to 8 hours. Onset, peak response, and duration of action may vary with individual patients depending on the dose and severity of symptoms. After a bolus lumbar injection of 50 or 100 mcg in seven patients, the average CSF elimination half-life was 1.51 hours over the first 4 hours and the average CSF clearance was ≈ 30 ml/hour.

Continuous infusion: The antispastic action is first seen at 6 to 8 hours after initiation of continuous infusion. Maximum activity is observed in 24 to 48 hours. The mean CSF clearance was approximately 30 ml/hour in ten patients on continuous intrathecal infusion.

Indications:

Oral: For the alleviation of signs and symptoms of spasticity resulting from multiple sclerosis, particularly for the relief of flexor spasms and concomitant pain, clonus and muscular rigidity. Patients should have reversible spasticity so that treatment will aid in restoring residual function.

May be of some value in patients with spinal cord injuries and other spinal cord diseases.

Intrathecal: Management of severe spasticity of spinal cord origin in patients who are unresponsive to oral baclofen therapy or experience intolerable CNS side effects at effective doses. Intended for use by the intrathecal route in single bolus test doses (via spinal catheter or lumbar puncture) and, for chronic use, only in implantable pumps approved by the FDA specifically for the administration of baclofen into the intrathecal space.

Intrathecal therapy may be considered an alternative to destructive neurosurgical procedures. Prior to implantation of a device for chronic intrathecal infusion, patients must show a response in a screening trial.

The efficacy as a treatment for spasticity of cerebral origin is not established.

Unlabeled uses:

Oral – Treatment of trigeminal neuralgia (50 to 60 mg/day).

Treatment of tardive dyskinesia in combination with neuroleptics.

Intrathecal – 25, 50 or 100 mcg appears to be beneficial in children for reducing spasticity in cerebral palsy.

Contraindications:

Hypersensitivity to baclofen.

Oral: Treatment of skeletal muscle spasm resulting from rheumatic disorders; stroke, cerebral palsy and Parkinson's disease.

Intrathecal: IV, IM, SC or epidural administration.

Warnings:

Intrathecal administration: Because of the possibility of potentially life-threatening CNS depression, cardiovascular collapse or respiratory failure, physicians must be adequately trained and educated in chronic intrathecal infusion therapy.

Infection: Patients should be infection-free prior to the screening trial with baclofen injection because the presence of a systemic infection may interfere with an assessment of the patient's response.

Patients should be infection-free prior to pump implantation because the presence of infection may increase the risk of surgical complications. Moreover, a systemic infection may complicate attempts to adjust the pump's dosing rate.

Abrupt drug withdrawal: Hallucinations and seizures have occurred on abrupt withdrawal. An isolated case of manic psychosis has been reported. Except in cases of serious adverse reactions, reduce dose slowly when drug is discontinued.

Stroke: Baclofen has not significantly benefited patients with stroke; they also have poor drug tolerance.

Renal function impairment: Because baclofen is primarily excreted unchanged through the kidneys, administer with caution to patients with impaired renal function. Dosage reduction may be necessary.

Pregnancy: Category C.

Lactation: In mothers treated with oral baclofen in therapeutic doses, the active substance passes into the breast milk. It is not known whether detectable levels of drug are present in breast milk of nursing mothers receiving intrathecal baclofen.

Children:

Oral – Safety for use in children < 12 years of age has not been established. Oral baclofen is not recommended for use in children.

Intrathecal – Safety in children < 4 years of age has not been established.

Precautions:

Epilepsy: Monitor the clinical state and EEG at regular intervals, since deterioration in seizure control and EEG changes have occurred in patients taking this drug.

Need for spasticity: Use with caution where spasticity is utilized to sustain upright posture and balance in locomotion, or whenever spasticity is utilized to obtain increased function.

Ovarian cysts have been found by palpation in about 4% of multiple sclerosis patients treated with baclofen for up to 1 year. In most cases, these cysts disappeared spontaneously while patients continued to receive the drug. Ovarian cysts are estimated to occur spontaneously in approximately 1% to 5% of the normal female population.

Psychotic disorders: Cautiously treat patients suffering from psychotic disorders, schizophrenia, or confusional states and keep under careful surveillance, because exacerbations of these conditions have been observed with oral administration.

Autonomic dysreflexia: Use with caution in patients with a history of autonomic dysreflexia. The presence of nociceptive stimuli or abrupt withdrawl may cause an autonomic dysreflexic episode.

Hazardous tasks: Because of the possibility of sedation, patients should observe caution while driving or performing other tasks requiring alertness, coordination or physical dexterity.

Adverse Reactions:

Adverse reactions occurring in ≥ 3% of patients include drowsiness, weakness of extremities, dizziness/lightheadedness, seizures, headache, nausea/vomiting, numbness/itching/tingling, hypotension, blurred vision, constipation, hypotonia, slurred speech, coma, lethargy/fatigue, confusion, insomnia and urinary frequency.

Administration and Dosage:

Oral: Individualize dosage. Start at a low dosage and increase gradually until the optimum effect is achieved (usually 40 to 80 mg daily).

The following dosage schedule is suggested: 5 mg 3 times daily for 3 days; 10 mg 3 times daily for 3 days; 15 mg 3 times daily for 3 days; 20 mg 3 times daily for 3 days. Thereafter, additional increases may be necessary, but the total daily dose should not exceed 80 mg daily (20 mg 4 times daily).

The lowest effective dose is recommended. If benefits are not evident after a reasonable trial period, withdraw the drug slowly.

Intrathecal: Refer to the manufacturer's manual for the implantable intrathecal infusion pump for specific instructions and precautions for programming the pump or refilling the reservoir.

Consult complete Drug Facts and Comparisons monograph and/or manufacturer product information for full intrathecal dosing information.

Dilution instructions –

Screening: Both strengths (10 mg/5 ml and 10 mg/20 ml) must be diluted with sterile preservative free Sodium Chloride for Injection, USP to a 50 mcg/ml concentration for bolus injection into the subarachnoid space.

Maintenance: For patients who require concentrations other than 500 or 2000 mcg/ml, baclofen intrathecal must be diluted with sterile, preservative free Sodium Chloride for Injection, USP.

Delivery regimen – Baclofen intrathecal is most often administered in a continuous infusion mode immediately following implant. For those patients implanted with programmable pumps who have achieved relatively satisfactory control on continuous infusion, further benefit may be attained using more complex schedules of delivery.

DANTROLENE SODIUM

Capsules: 25, 50 and 100 mg (*Rx*)	*Dantrium* (Procter & Gamble Pharm.)
Powder for Injection: 20 mg/vial. Concentration following reconstitution is ≈ 0.32 mg/ml. In 70 ml vials. (*Rx*)	*Dantrium Intravenous* (Procter & Gamble Pharm.)

Warning:

Dantrolene has a potential for hepatotoxicity. Do not use in conditions other than those recommended. The incidence of symptomatic hepatitis (fatal and nonfatal) reported in patients taking up to 400 mg/day is much lower than in those taking ≥ 800 mg/day. Even sporadic short courses of these higher dose levels within a treatment regimen markedly increased the risk of serious hepatic injury. Liver dysfunction, as evidenced by liver enzyme elevations, has been observed in patients exposed to the drug for varying periods of time. Overt hepatitis has been most frequently observed between the third and twelfth months of therapy. Risk of hepatic injury appears to be greater in females, in patients > 35 years of age and in patients taking other medications in addition to dantrolene.

Monitor hepatic function, including frequent determinations of AST or ALT. If no observable benefit is derived from therapy after 45 days, discontinue use.

Use the lowest possible effective dose for each patient.

Actions:

Pharmacology: In isolated nerve-muscle preparation, dantrolene produced relaxation by affecting contractile response of the skeletal muscle at a site beyond the myoneural junction and directly on the muscle itself. In skeletal muscle, the drug dissociates the excitation-contraction coupling, probably by interfering with the release of calcium from the sarcoplasmic reticulum. A CNS effect occurs, with drowsiness, dizziness and generalized weakness occasionally present.

Malignant hyperthermia – Dantrolene may prevent changes within the muscle cell which result in malignant hyperthermia syndrome by interfering with calcium release from the sarcoplasmic reticulum to the myoplasm. Administration of IV dantrolene, combined with supportive measures, is effective in reversing the hypermetabolic process of malignant hyperthermia.

Pharmacokinetics:

Absorption/Distribution – Absorbtion after oral administration is incomplete (≈ 70%) and slow but consistent, and dose-related blood levels are obtained. Peak plasma concentrations of approximately 1mg/ L are attained within 4 to 6 hours after a single 100 mg dose.

Metabolism – Metabolic patterns are similar in adults and children. Dantrolene is found in measurable amounts in blood and urine; the major metabolites noted are the 5-hydroxy analog and the acetamido analog. Mean half-life in adults is 9 hours after a 100 mg oral dose and 4 to 8 hours after IV administration. Since it is probably metabolized by hepatic microsomal enzymes, metabolism enhancement by other drugs is possible.

Indications:

Spasticity:

Oral – For the control of clinical spasticity resulting from upper motor neuron disorders such as spinal cord injury, stroke, cerebral palsy or multiple sclerosis. It is of particular benefit to the patient whose functional rehabilitation has been retarded by the sequelae of spasticity. Such patients must have presumably reversible spasticity where relief of spasticity will aid in restoring residual function.

Malignant hyperthermia:

IV – Management of the fulminant hypermetabolism of skeletal muscle characteristic of malignant hyperthermia crisis, along with appropriate supportive measures.

Preoperatively, and sometimes postoperatively, to prevent or attenuate the development of clinical and laboratory signs of malignant hyperthermia in individuals judged to be susceptible to malignant hyperthermia.

Oral – Preoperatively to prevent or attenuate the development of signs of malignant hyperthermia in susceptible patients who require anesthesia or surgery. Currently accepted clinical practices in the management of such patients must still be adhered to (careful monitoring for early signs of malignant hyperthermia, minimizing exposure to triggering mechanisms and prompt use of IV dantrolene and indicated supportive measures if signs of malignant hyperthermia appear).

Following a malignant hyperthermia crisis to prevent recurrence of malignant hyperthermia.

Unlabeled uses: Exercise-induced muscle pain; neuroleptic malignant syndrome; heat stroke.

Contraindications:

Oral: Active hepatic disease, such as hepatitis and cirrhosis; where spasticity is utilized to sustain upright posture and balance in locomotion or to obtain or maintain increased function; treatment of skeletal muscle spasm resulting from rheumatic disorders.

Warnings:

Hepatic effects: Fatal and nonfatal liver disorders of an idiosyncratic or hypersensitivity type may occur. At the start of therapy, perform baseline liver function studies. If abnormalities exist, the potential for hepatotoxicity could be enhanced.

Perform liver function studies at appropriate intervals during therapy. If such studies reveal abnormal values, generally discontinue therapy. Some laboratory values may return to normal with continued therapy; others may not.

If symptoms of hepatitis accompanied by liver function test abnormalities or jaundice appear, discontinue therapy. If caused by dantrolene and detected early, abnormalities may revert to normal when the drug is discontinued.

Use with caution in females and in patients > 35 years of age; there is a greater likelihood of drug-induced, potentially fatal hepatocellular disease in these populations.

Long-term use: Safety and efficacy have not been established.

Continued long-term administration is justified if use of the drug: Significantly reduces painful or disabling spasticity such as clonus; significantly reduces the intensity or degree of nursing care required; rids the patient of any annoying manifestation of spasticity considered important by the patient.

Brief withdrawal for 2 to 4 days will frequently demonstrate exacerbation of the manifestations of spasticity and may serve to confirm a clinical impression.

In view of the potential for liver damage in long-term use, discontinue therapy if benefits are not evident within 45 days.

Malignant hyperthermia (MH): IV use is not a substitute for previously known supportive measures. These measures include discontinuing the suspect triggering agents, attending to increased oxygen requirements, managing the metabolic acidosis, instituting cooling when necessary, attending to urinary output and monitoring electrolyte imbalance.

Pregnancy: Category C (parenteral).

Labor and delivery – In one uncontrolled study, 100 mg/day of prophylactic oral dantrolene was administered to term pregnant patients awaiting labor and delivery. Dantrolene readily crossed the placenta, with maternal and fetal whole blood levels approximately equal at delivery; neonatal levels then fell approximately 50% per day for 2 days before declining sharply. No neonatal respiratory and neuromuscular side effects were detected at low dose.

One patient developed postpartum uterine atony following dantrolene administration after a cesarean section.

Lactation: Do not use in nursing women.

Children: Safety for use in children < 5 years of age has not been established.

Precautions:

Special risk patients: Use with caution in patients with impaired pulmonary function, particularly those with obstructive pulmonary disease; severely impaired cardiac function due to myocardial disease; a history of previous liver disease or dysfunction.

Extravasation: Because of the high pH of the IV formulation, prevent extravasation into the surrounding tissues.

Hazardous tasks: Patients should use caution while driving or performing other tasks requiring alertness, coordination or physical dexterity.

Photosensitivity: Photosensitization may occur; therefore, caution patients to take protective measures against exposure to ultraviolet light or sunlight until tolerance is determined.

Drug Interactions:

Drugs that may interact with dantrolene include: Clofibrate, estrogens, warfarin and verapamil.

Avoid alcohol and other CNS depressants.

Adverse Reactions:

Adverse reactions may include: Drowsiness; dizziness; weakness; general malaise; fatigue; diarrhea; constipation; GI bleeding; anorexia; dysphagia; gastric irritation; abdominal cramps; hepatitis; speech disturbance; seizure; headache; lightheadedness; visual disturbance; diplopia; alteration of taste; insomnia; mental depression; confusion; increased nervousness; tachycardia; erratic blood pressure; phlebitis; increased urinary frequency; hematuria; crystalluria; difficult erection; urinary incontinence; nocturia; dysuria; urinary retention; abnormal hair growth; acne-like rash; pruritus; urticaria; eczematoid eruption; sweating; myalgia; backache; chills; fever; feeling of suffocation; excessive tearing; pleural effusion with pericarditis; severity: pulmonary edema developing during treatment of MH crisis; thrombophlebitis following IV dantrolene; urticaria; erythema; hepatitis; seizures; pleural effusion with pericarditis.

Administration and Dosage:

Exercise caution at meals on the day of administration becaus difficulty swallowing and choking has been reported.

Chronic spasticity: Titrate and individualize dosage. In view of the potential for liver damage in long-term use, discontinue therapy if benefits are not evident within 45 days.

Adults – Begin with 25 mg once daily; increase to 25 mg, 2 to 4 times daily; then by increments of 25 mg up to as high as 100 mg, 2 to 4 times daily if necessary. As most patients will respond to 400 mg/day or less, higher doses are rarely needed. Maintain each dosage level for 4 to 7 days to determine response. Adjust dosage to achieve maximal benefit without adverse effects.

Children – Use a similar approach. Start with 0.5 mg/kg twice daily; increase to 0.5 mg/kg, 3 or 4 times daily; then by increments of 0.5 mg/kg, up to 3mg/kg, 2 to 4 times daily if necessary. Do not exceed doses higher than 100mg 4 times daily.

Malignant hyperthermia:

Preoperative prophylaxis – Dantrolene may be given orally or IV to patients judged susceptible to malignant hyperthermia as part of the overall patient management to prevent or attenuate development of clinical and laboratory signs of MH.

Oral – Give 4 to 8 mg/kg/day orally in 3 or 4 divided doses for 1 or 2 days prior to surgery, with last dose given ≈ 3 to 4 hours before scheduled surgery with a minimum of water. This dosage will usually be associated with skeletal muscle weakness and sedation (sleepiness or drowsiness) or excessive GI irritation (nausea or vomiting); adjust within the recommended dosage range to avoid incapacitation or excessive GI irritation.

IV – Dantrolene IV may decrease the grip strength and increase weakness of leg muscles, especially walking down stairs.

Treatment – As soon as the malignant hyperthermia reaction is recognized, discontinue all anesthetic agents. Use of 100% oxygen is recommended. Administer dantrolene by continuous rapid IV push beginning at a minimum dose of 1 mg/kg, and continuing until symptoms subside or a maximum cumulative dose of 10 mg/kg has been reached. If the physiologic and metabolic abnormalities reappear, repeat the regimen. Administration should be continuous until symptoms subside.

Children – Dose is the same as for adults.

Post-crisis follow-up – Following a malignant hyperthermia crisis, give 4 to 8 mg/kg/day orally, in 4 divided doses for 1 to 3 days to prevent recurrence. IV dantrolene may be used when oral administration is not practical. The IV dose must be individualized, starting with 1mg/kg or more as the clinical situation dictates.

PARKINSON'S DISEASE

Parkinsonism is a neurological disease with a variety of origins characterized by tremor, rigidity, akinesia, and disorders of posture and equilibrium. The onset is slow and progressive with symptoms advancing over months to years.

Drug Therapy for Parkinsonism

Drugs	Indications					Usual daily dose range (mg)
	Post-encephalitic	Arterio-sclerotic	Idiopathic	Drug/ chemical induced	Adjunct to Levodopa/ Carbidopa	
Anticholinergics						
Procyclidine	✓	✓	✓	✓		7.5-20
Trihexyphenidyl	✓	✓	✓	✓	✓	1-15
Benztropine	✓	✓	✓	✓		0.5-6.5
Biperiden	✓	✓	✓	✓		2-8
Ethopropazine	✓	✓	✓	✓		50-600
Diphenhydramine	✓	✓	✓	✓		10-400
Dopaminergic Agents						
Levodopa	✓	✓	✓	✓[1]		500-8000
Carbidopa/ levodopa	✓		✓	✓[1]		10/100-200/2000
Amantadine	✓	✓	✓	✓		200-400
Bromocriptine	✓		✓			12.5-100
Pergolide					✓	1-5
Selegiline					✓	10

[1] Not effective in drug-induced extrapyramidal symptoms.

ANTICHOLINERGICS

PROCYCLIDINE	
Tablets: 5 mg (*Rx*)	*Kemadrin* (Glaxo Wellcome)
TRIHEXYPHENIDYL HCl	
Tablets: 2 and 5 mg (*Rx*)	Various, *Artane* (Lederle)
Capsules, sustained release: 5 mg (*Rx*)	*Artane Sequels* (Lederle)
Elixir: 2 mg/5 ml (*Rx*)	*Artane* (Lederle)
BENZTROPINE MESYLATE	
Tablets: 0.5, 1 and 2 mg (*Rx*)	Various, *Cogentin* (Merck)
Injection: 1 mg/ml (*Rx*)	*Cogentin* (Merck)
BIPERIDEN	
Tablets: 2 mg (*Rx*)	*Akineton* (Knoll)
Injection: 5 mg/ml (*Rx*)	*Akineton* (Knoll)
ETHOPROPAZINE HCl	
Tablets: 10 and 50 mg (*Rx*)	*Parsidol* (Parke-Davis)

Actions:

Pharmacology: The anticholinergic agents, although generally less effective than levodopa, are useful in the treatment of all forms of parkinsonism. They reduce the incidence and severity of akinesia, rigidity and tremor by about 20%; secondary symptoms such as drooling are also reduced. In addition to suppressing central cholinergic activity, these agents may also inhibit the reuptake and storage of dopamine at central dopamine receptors, thereby prolonging the action of dopamine.

Pharmacokinetics:

Various Antiparkinson Anticholinergic Pharmacokinetic Parameters				
Anticholinergic	Time to peak concentration (hrs)	Peak concentration (mcg/L)	Half-life (hrs)	Oral bioavailability (%)
Benztropine[1]				
Biperiden	1-1.5	4-5	18.4-24.3	29
Diphenhydramine	2-4	65-90	4-15	50-72
Ethopropazine[1]				
Procyclidine	1.1-2	80	11.5-12.6	52-97
Trihexyphenidyl	1-1.3	87.2	5.6-10.2	≈ 100

[1] No data available.

Indications:

Adjunctive therapy in all forms of parkinsonism (postencephalitic, arteriosclerotic and idiopathic) and in the control of drug-induced extrapyramidal disorders.

Contraindications:

Hypersensitivity to any component; glaucoma, particularly angle-closure glaucoma; pyloric or duodenal obstruction; stenosing peptic ulcers; prostatic hypertrophy or bladder neck obstructions; achalasia (megaesophagus); myasthenia gravis; megacolon.

Benztropine: Children < 3 years of age; use with caution in older children.

Warnings:

Ophthalmic: Incipient narrow-angle glaucoma may be precipitated by these drugs.

Elderly: Geriatric patients, particularly > 60 years of age, frequently develop increased sensitivity to anticholinergic drugs and require strict dosage regulation. Occasionally, mental confusion and disorientation may occur; agitation, hallucinations and psychotic-like symptoms may develop.

Pregnancy: Category C.

Lactation: An inhibitory effect on lactation may occur.

Children: Safety and efficacy for use in children have not been established.

Precautions:

Concomitant conditions: Use caution in patients with tachycardia, cardiac arrhythmias, hypertension, hypotension, prostatic hypertrophy (particularly in the elderly), or any tendency toward urinary retention, liver or kidney disorders, and obstructive disease of the GI or GU tract.

CNS: When used to treat extrapyramidal reactions resulting from phenothiazines in psychiatric patients, antiparkinson agents may exacerbate mental symptoms and precipitate a toxic psychosis.

In addition, 19% to 30% of patients given anticholinergics develop depression, confusion, delusions or hallucinations.

Tardive dyskinesia may appear in some patients on long-term therapy with phenothiazines and related agents, or may occur after therapy has been discontinued.

Dry mouth: If dry mouth is so severe that swallowing or speaking is difficult, or if loss of appetite and weight occurs, reduce dosage or discontinue drug temporarily.

Abuse potential: Some patients may use these agents for mood elevations or psychedelic experiences. Cannabinoids, barbiturates, opiates and alcohol may have additive effects with anticholinergics.

Hazardous tasks: May impair mental or physical abilities; patients should observe caution while driving or performing other tasks requiring alertness.

Drug Interactions:

Drugs that may interact with anticholinergic antiparkinson agents include amantadine, digoxin, haloperidol, levodopa and phenothiazines.

Adverse Reactions:

Hypersensitivity: Skin rash; urticaria; other dermatoses.

CNS: Disorientation; confusion; memory loss; hallucinations; psychoses; agitation; nervousness; delusions; delirium; paranoia; euphoria; excitement; lightheadedness; dizziness; headache; listlessness; depression; drowsiness; weakness; giddiness; paresthesia; heaviness of the limbs.

Cardiovascular: Tachycardia; palpitations; hypotension.

GI: Dry mouth; nausea; vomiting; epigastric distress; constipation; development of duodenal ulcer.

Ophthalmic: Blurred vision; mydriasis; diplopia; increased intraocular tension; angle-closure glaucoma; dilation of pupils.

Renal: Urinary retention; urinary hesitancy; dysuria.

Musculoskeletal: Muscular weakness; muscular cramping.

Miscellaneous: Elevated temperature; flushing; numbness of fingers; decreased sweating, hyperthermia, heat stroke; difficulty in achieving or maintaining an erection.

Administration and Dosage:

Give before or after meals, as determined by patient's reaction. Postencephalitic patients (more prone to excessive salivation) may prefer to take it after meals and may, in addition, require small amounts of atropine. If the mouth dries excessively, take before meals, unless it causes nausea. If taken after meals, thirst can be allayed by mint candies, chewing gum or water.

PROCYCLIDINE:

Parkinsonism (for patients who have received no other therapy) Initially, 2.5 mg 3 times daily after meals. If well tolerated, gradually increase dose to 5 mg; administer 3 times daily, and occasionally before retiring, if necessary. In some cases, smaller doses may be effective.

For drug-induced extrapyramidal symptoms – Begin with 2.5 mg 3 times daily; increase by 2.5 mg daily increments until the patient obtains relief of symptoms. Individualize dosage. In most cases, results will be obtained with 10 to 20 mg daily.

TRIHEXYPHENIDYL HCl:

Parkinsonism – Initially, administer 1 to 2 mg the first day; increase by 2 mg increments at intervals of 3 to 5 days, until a total of 6 to 10 mg is given daily. Many patients derive maximum benefit from a total daily dose of 6 to 10 mg; however, postencephalitic patients may require a total daily dose of 12 to 15 mg. Trihexyphenidyl is tolerated best if divided into 3 doses and taken at mealtimes. High doses may be divided into 4 parts, administered at mealtimes and at bedtime.

Concomitant use with levodopa: Trihexyphenidyl 3 to 6 mg/day in divided doses is usually adequate.

Drug-induced extrpyramidal disorders – Start with a single 1 mg dose. Daily dosage usually ranges between 5 to 15 mg, although reactions have been controlled on as little as 1 mg/day.

Sustained release – Do not use for initial therapy. Once patients are stabilized on conventional dosage forms, they may be switched to sustained release capsules on a milligram per milligram of total daily dose basis. Administer as a single dose after breakfast or in 2 divided doses 12 hours apart.

BENZTROPINE MESYLATE: Because there is not significant difference in onset of action after IV or IM injection, there is usually no need to use the IV route. In emergency situations, when the condition of the patients is alarmine, 1 to 2 ml will normally provide quick relief.

Dosage titration – Because of cumulative action, initiate therapy with a low dose, increase in increments of 0.5 mg gradually at 5 or 6 day intervals to the smallest amount necessary for optimal relief. Maximum daily dose is 6 mg.

Dose intervals – Some patients experience greatest relief by taking the entire dose at bedtime; others react more favoably to divided doses, 2 to 4 times a day.

Pakinsonism – 1 to 2 mg/day, with a range of 0.5 to 6 mg/day, orally or parenterally.

Idiopathic parkinsonism: Start with 0.5 to 1 mg at bedtime; 4 to 6 mg per day may be required.

Postencephalitic parkinsonism: 2 mg per day in one or more doses. In highly sensitive patients, begin therapy with 0.5 mg at bedtime; increase as necessary.

Drug-induced extrapyramidal disorders – Administer 1 to 4 mg once or twice daily.

Acute dystonic reactions: 1 to 2 ml IM or IV usually relieves the condition quickly. After that, 1 to 2 ml orally 2 times daily usually prevents recurrence.

Estrapyramidal disorders which develop soon after initiating treatment with neuroleptic drugs are likely to be transient. A dosage of 1 to 2 mg orally 2 or 3 times a day usually provides relief within 1 or 2 days. After 1 or 2 weeks, withdraw drug to determine its continued need. If such disorders recur, reinstitute benztropine.

BIPERIDEN:

Parkinsonism – 2 mg 3 or 4 times daily, orally. Individualize dosage with dosing titrated to a maximum of 16 mg/224 hours.

Drug-induced extrapyramidal disorders –

Oral: 2 mg 1 to 3 times daily.

Parenteral: 2 mg IM or IV. Repeat every half-hour until symptoms are resolved, but do not give more than 4 consecutive doses per 24 hours.

ETHOPROPAZINE:

Initially – 50 mg once or twice daily; increase gradually, if necessary.

Mild to moderate symptoms – 100 to 400 mg daily.

Severe cases – Gradually increase to 500 or 600 mg or more daily.

DIPHENYDRAMINE:

Oral –

Adults: 25 to 50 mg 3 to 4 times daily.

Children > 20 lbs (9 kg): 12.5 to 25 mg 3 or 4 times daily or 5 mg/kg/day. Do not exceed 300 mg/day or 150 mg/m^2/day.

Parenteral – Administer IV or deeply IM.

Adults: 10 to 50 mg; 100 mg if required. Maximum daily dosage is 400 mg.

Children: 5 mg/kg/day or 150 mg/m^2/day.

LEVODOPA AND CARBIDOPA

Tablets: 10 mg carbidopa and 100 mg levodopa, 25 mg carbidopa and 100 mg levodopa, 25 mg carbidopa and 250 mg levodopa (*Rx*)	Various, *Sinemet* (DuPont Pharm)
Tablets, sustained release: 50 mg carbidopa and 200 mg levodopa, 25 mg carbidopa and 100 mg levodopa (*Rx*)	*Sinemet* CR (DuPont Pharm)

Actions:

Pharmacology: These agents are used in combination since carbidopa inhibits decarboxylation of levodopa and makes more levodopa available for transport to the brain. The sustained release formulation is designed to release the ingredients over a 4 to 6 hour period. There is less variation in plasma levodopa levels than with the conventional formulation. However, the sustained release form is less systemically bioavailable (70% to 75%) and may require increased daily doses to achieve the same level of symptomatic relief.

Pharmacokinetics: The half-life of levodopa may be prolonged following the sustained release form because of continuous absorption. In elderly subjects, the mean time to peak levodopa concentration was 2 hours for sustained release vs 0.5 hours for conventional. The maximum concentration following the sustained release form was about 35% of the conventional form.

Indications:

Treatment of symptoms of idiopathic Parkinson's disease (paralysis agitans), postencephalitic parkinsonism and sympathetic parkinsonism which may follow injury to the nervous system by carbon monoxide and manganese intoxication.

Warnings:

CNS effects: Certain adverse CNS effects (eg, dyskinesias) will occur at lower dosages and sooner during therapy with the sustained release form.

Drug Interactions:

Drug/Food interactions: Administration of a single dose of the sustained release form with food increased the extent of levodopa availability by 50% and increased peak levodopa concentrations by 25%.

Adverse Reactions:

In clinical trials, the adverse reaction profile of the sustained release form did not differ substantially from that of the conventional form.

Administration and Dosage:

Patients not receiving levodopa:

Sinemet – 1 tablet of 25 mg carbidopa/100 mg levodopa 3 times daily or 10 mg carbidopa/100 mg levodopa 3 or 4 times daily. Dosage may be increased by 1 tablet every day or every other day, as necessary, until a dosage of 8 tablets a day is reached.

Tablets of the two ratios (eg, 1:4, 25/100 or 1:10, 10/100 and 25/250) may be given separately or combined as needed to provide the optimum dosage.

Provide at least 70 to 100 mg carbidopa per day. When more carbidopa is required, substitute one 25/100 tablet for each 10/100 tablet. When more levodopa is required, substitute the 25/250 tablet for the 25/100 or 10/100 tablet.

Sinemet CR – 1 tablet twice daily at intervals of not less than 6 hours. Doses and dosing intervals may be increased or decreased based on response. Most patients have been adequately treated with 2 to 8 tablets per day (divided doses) at intervals of 4 to 8 hours while awake. Higher doses (≥ 12 tablets per day) and intervals < 4 hours have been used but are not usually recommended. If an interval of < 4 hours is used or if the divided doses are not equal, give the smaller doses at the end of the day.

Sinemet CR may be administered as whole or half tablets which should not be crushed or chewed.

Patients currently treated with levodopa: Levodopa must be discontinued at least 8 hours before therapy with levodopa/carbidopa. Substitute the combination drug at a dosage that will provide ≈ 25% of the previous levodopa dosage.

Sinemet – Suggested starting dosage is 1 tablet of 25 mg carbidopa/250 mg levodopa 3 or 4 times a day for patients taking > 1500 mg levodopa or 25 mg carbidopa/100 mg levodopa for patients taking < 1500 mg levodopa.

Sinemet CR – Usually 1 tablet twice daily.

Patients currently treated with conventional carbidopa/levodopa preparations: Substitute dosage with *Sinemet CR* at an amount that provides ≈ 10% more levodopa per day, although this may need to be increased to a dosage that provides up to 30% more levodopa per day. Use intervals of 4 to 8 hours while awake.

Guidelines for Initial Conversion from *Sinemet* to *Sinemet CR*	
Sinemet Total daily levodopa dose (mg)	*Sinemet CR* Suggested dosage regimen
300 to 400	1 tablet twice daily
500 to 600	1½ tablets twice daily or 1 tablet 3 times daily
700 to 800	Total of 4 tablets in ≥ 3 divided doses (eg, 1½ tablets am, 1½ tablets early pm, 1 tablet later pm)
900 to 1000	Total of 5 tablets in ≥ 3 divided doses (eg, 2 tablets am, 2 tablets early pm, 1 tablet later pm)

Combination therapy: Other antiparkinson drugs can be given concurrently; dosage adjustment may be necessary.

Sinemet (25/100 or 10/100) can be added to the dosage regimen of *Sinemet CR* in selected patients with advanced disease who need additional levodopa.

AMANTADINE HCl

Capsules: 100 mg (*Rx*)	Various, *Symadine* (Solvay), *Symmetrel* (DuPont)
Syrup: 50 mg/5 ml (*Rx*)	*Symmetrel* (DuPont)

This is an abbreviated monograph. For full prescribing information, refer to the Antiviral Agents monograph.

Actions:

Pharmacology: The exact mechanism of action is unknown, but amantadine is thought to release dopamine from intact dopaminergic terminals that remain in the substantia nigra of parkinson patients.

Amantadine is less effective than levodopa in the treatment of Parkinson's disease, but slightly more effective than anticholinergic agents.

Indications:

Parkinson's disease/syndrome and drug-induced extrapyramidal reactions: Idiopathic Parkinson's disease (paralysis agitans); postencephalitic parkinsonism; arteriosclerotic parkinsonism; drug-induced extrapyramidal reactions; symptomatic parkinsonism following injury to the nervous system by carbon monoxide intoxication.

Administration and Dosage:

Parkinson's disease: 100 mg twice/day when used alone. Onset of action is usually within 48 hrs. Initial dose is 100 mg/day for patients with serious associated medical illnesses or those receiving high doses of other antiparkinson drugs. After one to several weeks at 100 mg once/day, increase to 100 mg twice/day, if necessary. Patients whose responses are not optimal at 200 mg/day may occasionally benefit from an increase up to 400 mg/day in divided doses; supervise closely. Patients initially benefiting from amantadine often experience decreased efficacy after a few months. Benefit may be regained by increasing to 300 mg/day, or by temporary discontinuation for several weeks. Other antiparkinson drugs may be necessary.

Concomitant therapy – When amantadine and levodopa are initiated concurrently, the patient can exhibit rapid therapeutic benefits. Maintain the dose at 100 mg/day or twice/day, while levodopa is gradually increased to optimal benefit.

Renal function impairment: The following table is designed to yield steady-state plasma concentrations of 0.7 to 1 mcg/ml.

Suggested Dosage Guidelines for Amantadine in Impaired Renal Function		
Creatinine clearance (ml/min/1.73 m^2)	Estimated half-life (hours)	Suggested maintenance regimen[1]
100	11	100 mg twice a day or 200 mg daily
80	14	100 mg twice a day
60	19	200 mg alternated with 100 mg daily
50	23	100 mg daily
40	29	100 mg daily
30	40	200 mg twice weekly
20	66	100 mg three times weekly
10	178	200 mg alternated with 100 mg every 7 days
Three times weekly chronic hemodialysis	199	200 mg alternated with 100 mg every 7 days

[1] Loading dose on first day of 200 mg.

Reproduced with permission from Horadam VW, Sharp JG, Smilack JD, et al. Pharmacokinetics of amantadine HCl in subjects with normal and impaired renal function. *Ann Intern Med* 1981;94 (Part 1):454-58.

Drug-induced extrapyramidal reactions: 100 mg twice/day. Patients with suboptimal responses may benefit from 300 mg/day in divided doses.

BROMOCRIPTINE MESYLATE

Tablets: 2.5 mg (*Rx*)	*Parlodel SnapTabs* (Sandoz)
Capsules: 5 mg (*Rx*)	*Parlodel* (Sandoz)

Actions:

Pharmacology: Bromocriptine, a dopamine agonist, may relieve akinesia, rigidity and tremor in patients with Parkinson's disease. It produces its therapeutic effect by directly stimulating the dopamine receptors in the corpus striatum.

Indications:

Parkinson's disease: In the treatment of idiopathic or postencephalitic Parkinson's disease.

Administration and Dosage:

Parkinson's disease: Initiate treatment at a low dosage and individualize; increase the daily dosage slowly until a maximum therapeutic response is achieved. If possible, maintain the dosage of levodopa during this introductory period.

Initially, use 1.25 mg (one-half of a 2.5 mg tablet) twice daily with meals. Assess dosage titrations every 2 weeks to ensure that the lowest dosage producing an optimal therapeutic response is not exceeded. If necessary, increase the dosage every 2 to 4 weeks by 2.5 mg/day with meals. If it is necessary to reduce the dose because of adverse reactions, reduce dose gradually in 2.5 mg increments. Usual range is 10 to 40 mg/day.

The safety of bromocriptine has not been demonstrated in dosages exceeding 100 mg/day.

SELEGILINE HCl (L-Deprenyl)

Tablets: 5 mg (*Rx*)	*Eldepryl* (Somerset)

Actions:

Pharmacology: Selegiline hydrochloride is a levorotatory acetylenic derivative of phenethylamine. Although the mechanism of action is not fully understood, inhibition of monoamine oxidase (MAO) type B activity is of primary importance and selegiline may act through other mechanisms to increase dopaminergic activity.

Pharmacokinetics:

Absorption/Distribution – Selegiline is rapidly absorbed; ≈ 73% of a dose is absorbed; maximum plasma concentration occurs 0.5 to 2 hours following administration.

Metabolism/Excretion – The drug is rapidly metabolized. Three metabolites, N-desmethyldeprenyl, amphetamine and methamphetamine, were found in serum and urine. Over 48 hours, 45% of the dose appeared in the urine as these 3 metabolites. Unchanged selegiline is not detected in urine.

Indications:

Parkinson's disease: Adjunct in the management of Parkinsonian patients being treated with levodopa/carbidopa who exhibit deterioration in the quality of their response to this therapy.

Contraindications:

Hypersensitivity to the drug; use with meperidine.

Warnings:

Maximum dose: Do not use at daily doses exceeding those recommended (10 mg/day) because of the risks associated with nonselective inhibition of MAO.

Pregnancy: Category C.

Lactation: It is not known whether selegiline is excreted in breast milk.

Children: The effects of selegiline in children have not been evaluated.

Precautions:

Hypertensive crisis: In theory, because MAO-A of the gut is not inhibited, patients treated with selegiline at a dose of 10 mg/day can take medications containing pharmacologically active amines and consume tyramine-containing foods without risk of uncontrolled hypertension.

Levodopa side effects: Some patients given selegiline may experience an exacerbation of levodopa-associated side effects, presumably due to the increased amounts of dopamine reacting with supersensitive post-synaptic receptors.

Drug Interactions:

Drugs that may interact with selegiline include fluoxetine and meperidine.

Adverse Reactions:

Adverse reactions occurring in ≥ 3% of patients include nausea, dizziness, lightheadedness, fainting, abdominal pain, confusion, hallucinations, depression, loss of balance, insomnia, orthostatic hypotension, increased akinetic involuntary movements, agitation, arrhythmias, bradykinesia, chorea, delusions, hypertension, new or increased angina pectoris, syncope and dry mouth.

Administration and Dosage:

Parkinsonian patients receiving levodopa/carbidopa therapy who demonstrate a deteriorating response to this treatment: 10 mg per day administered as divided doses of 5 mg each taken at breakfast and lunch. There is no evidence that additional benefit will be obtained from the administration of higher doses.

After 2 to 3 days of treatment, attempt to reduce the dose of levodopa/carbidopa. A reduction of 10% to 30% appears typical. Further reductions of levodopa/carbidopa may be possible during continued selegiline therapy.

PERGOLIDE MESYLATE

Tablets: 0.05, 0.25 and 1 mg (*Rx*)	*Permax* (Athena Neurosciences)

Actions:

Pharmacology: Pergolide mesylate is a potent dopamine receptor agonist at both D_1 and D_2 receptor sites. In Parkinson's disease, pergolide is believed to exert its therapeutic effect by directly stimulating postsynaptic dopamine receptors in the nigrostriatal system.

Pharmacokinetics:

Absorption/Distribution – Following oral administration, ≈ 55% of the dose can be recovered from the urine and 5% from expired CO_2, suggesting that a significant fraction is absorbed. Pergolide is ≈ 90% bound to plasma proteins.

Metabolism/Excretion – At least 10 metabolites have been detected. It is not known whether any other metabolites are active. The major route of excretion is via the kidney.

Indications:

Parkinson's disease: Adjunctive treatment to levodopa/carbidopa in the management of the signs and symptoms of Parkinson's disease.

Contraindications:

Hypersensitivity to pergolide or other ergot derivatives.

Warnings:

Symptomatic hypotension: In clinical trials, ≈ 10% of patients taking pergolide with levodopa vs 7% taking placebo with levodopa experienced symptomatic orthostatic or sustained hypotension, especially during initial treatment. Increase the dosage in carefully adjusted increments over a period of 3 to 4 weeks.

Hallucinosis: Pergolide with levodopa caused hallucinosis in ≈ 14% of patients as opposed to 3% taking placebo with levodopa.

Pregnancy: Category B.

Lactation: It is not known whether this drug is excreted in breast milk.

Children: Safety and efficacy for use in children have not been established.

Precautions:

Cardiac dysrhythmias: Exercise caution in patients prone to cardiac dysrhythmias. In a study comparing pergolide and placebo, patients on pergolide had significantly more episodes of atrial premature contractions and sinus tachycardia.

The use of pergolide in patients on levodopa may cause or exacerbate preexisting states of confusion and hallucinations or preexisting dyskinesia.

Drug Interactions:

Drugs that may interact with pergolide mesylate include dopamine antagonists, metoclopramide and drugs known to affect protein binding.

Adverse Reactions:

Adverse reactions occucrring in ≥ 3% of patients include pain, abdominal pain, injury, accident, headache, asthenia, chest pain, flu syndrome, postural hypotension, vasodilation, nausea, constipation, diarrhea, dyspepsia, anorexia, dry mouth, dyskinesia, dizziness, hallucinations, dystonia, confusion, somnolence, insomnia, anxiety, tremor, depression, rhinitis, dyspnea, rash, abnormal vision, peripheral edema, hallucinations and confusion.

Administration and Dosage:

Initiate with a daily dose of 0.05 mg for the first 2 days. Gradually increase the dosage by 0.1 or 0.15 mg/day every third day over the next 12 days of therapy. The dosage may then be increased by 0.25 mg/day every third day until an optimal therapeutic dosage is achieved.

Pergolide is usually administered in divided doses 3 times per day. During dosage titration, the dosage of concurrent levodopa/carbidopa may be cautiously decreased.

In clinical studies, the mean therapeutic daily dosage of pergolide was 3mg/day. The average concurrent daily dosage of levodopa/carbidopa (expressed as levodopa) was ≈ 650 mg/day. The efficacy of pergolide at doses above 5mg/day has not been systematically evaluated.

Chapter 7
GASTROINTESTINALS

ANTACIDS

MAGNESIA (Magnesium Hydroxide)	
Tablets, chewable: 311 mg (*otc*)	*Phillips' Chewable* (Sterling Health)
Liquid: 400 mg/5 ml, 800 mg/5 ml (*otc*)	Various, *Phillips' Milk of Magnesia* (Sterling Health), *Phillips' Concentrated Milk of Magnesia* (*Sterling Health*)
ALUMINUM HYDROXIDE GEL	
Tablets: 300, 500, 600 mg (*otc*)	*Amphojel* (Wyeth-Ayerst), *Alu-Tab* (3M Pharm)
Capsules: 400, 500 mg (*otc*)	*Alu-Cap* (3M Pharm), *Dialume* (RPR)
Suspension: 320 mg/5ml, 450 mg/5 ml, 675 mg/5 ml (*otc*)	Various, *Amphojel* (Wyeth-Ayerst)
Liquid: 600 mg/5 ml (*otc*)	Various, *AlternaGEL* (J & J-Merck)
ALUMINUM CARBONATE GEL, BASIC	
Tablets: Equiv. to 608 mg dried aluminum hydroxide gel or 500 mg aluminum hydroxide (*otc*)	*Basaljel* (Wyeth-Ayerst)
Capsules: Equiv. to 608 mg dried aluminum hydroxide gel or 500 mg aluminum hydroxide (*otc*)	*Basaljel* (Wyeth-Ayerst)
Suspension: Equiv. to 400 mg aluminum hydroxide/5 ml (*otc*)	*Basaljel* (Wyeth-Ayerst)
CALCIUM CARBONATE	
Tablets, chewable: 350, 420, 750, 850, 1000 mg (*otc*)	*Amitone* (Menley & James), *Mallamint* (Roberts), *Extra Strength Tums E-X* (SmithKline-Beecham), *Alka-Mints* (Bayer), *Tums Ultra* (SmithKline-Beecham), *Extra Strength Alkets Antacid* (Roberts Pharm), *Dicarbosil* (BIRA)
Tablets: 500, 600, 650, 1000, 1250 mg (*otc*)	Various, *Maalox Antacid Caplets* (RPR)
Gum tablets: 500 mg (*otc*)	*Chooz* (Schering-Plough)
Suspension: 1250 mg/5 ml (*otc*)	Various
Lozenges: 600 mg (*otc*)	*Mylanta* (J&J-Merck)
MAGNESIUM OXIDE	
Tablets: 400, 420, 500 mg (*otc*)	Various, *Mag-Ox 400* (Blaine), *Maox 420* (Kenneth A. Manne)
Capsules: 140 mg (*otc*)	*Uro-Mag* (Blaine)
MAGALDRATE	
Suspension: 540 mg/5 ml (*otc*)	*Riopan* (Whitehall)
Liquid: 540 mg/5 ml (*otc*)	Various, *Iosopan* (Goldline)
SODIUM BICARBONATE	
Tablets: 325, 520, 650 mg (*otc*)	Various, *Bell/ans* (C.S. Dent)
SODIUM CITRATE	
Solution: 450 mg (*otc*)	*Citra pH* (ValMed)

Actions:

Pharmacology: Antacids neutralize gastric acidity, resulting in an increase in the pH of the stomach and duodenal bulb. Additionally, by increasing the gastric pH above 4, they inhibit the proteolytic activity of pepsin. Antacids do not "coat" the mucosal lining, but may have a local astringent effect. Antacids also increase the lower esophageal sphincter tone. Aluminum ions inhibit smooth muscle contraction, thus inhibiting gastric emptying.

Acid neutralizing capacity (ANC) is a consideration in selecting an antacid. It varies for commercial antacid preparations and is expressed as mEq/ml. Milliequivalents of ANC is defined by the mEq of HCl required to keep an antacid suspension at pH 3.5 for 10 minutes in vitro. An antacid must neutralize at least 5 mEq/dose. Also, any ingredient must contribute at least 25% of the total ANC of a given product to be considered an antacid.

Aluminum hydroxide and calcium-containing antacids may reduce LDL cholesterol and increase the HDL/LDL ratio.

Indications:

Hyperacidity: Symptomatic relief of upset stomach associated with hyperacidity (heartburn, gastroesophageal reflux, acid indigestion and sour stomach); hyperacidity associated with peptic ulcer and gastric hyperacidity.

Aluminum carbonate: Treatment, control or management of hyperphosphatemia or for use with a low phosphate diet.

Calcium carbonate: Treating calcium deficiency states.

Magnesium oxide: Treatment of magnesium deficiencies or magnesium depletion.

Unlabeled uses: Antacids with aluminum and magnesium hydroxides or aluminum hydroxide alone effectively prevent significant stress ulcer bleeding. Antacids are also effective in treatment and maintenance of duodenal ulcer, and may be effective in treating gastric ulcer. Antacids are also recommended, initially, for gastroesophageal reflux disease.

Aluminum hydroxide has been used to reduce phosphate absorption in hyperphosphatemia in patients with chronic renal failure.

Calcium carbonate may also be used to bind phosphate.

Warnings:

Sodium content of antacids may be significant. Patients with hypertension, CHF, marked renal failure or those on restricted or low-sodium diets should use a low sodium preparation.

"Acid rebound": Antacids may cause dose-related rebound hyperacidity since they may increase gastric secretion or serum gastrin levels.

Milk-alkali syndrome, an acute illness with symptoms of headache, nausea, irritability and weakness, or a chronic illness with alkalosis, hypercalcemia and possibly, renal impairment, has occurred following the concurrent use of high dose calcium carbonate and sodium bicarbonate.

Hypophosphatemia: Prolonged use of aluminum containing antacids may result in hypophosphatemia in normophosphatemic patients if phosphate intake is not adequate.

Renal function impairment: Use magnesium-containing products with caution, particularly when > 50 mEq magnesium is given daily. Hypermagnesemia and toxicity may occur due to decreased clearance of the magnesium ion.

Prolonged use of aluminum-containing antacids in patients with renal failure may result in or worsen dialysis osteomalacia.

Pregnancy: A pregnant woman should consult a physician before using.

Precautions:

GI hemorrhage: Use aluminum hydroxide with care in patients who have recently suffered massive upper GI hemorrhage.

Drug Interactions:

Drugs that may be affected by antacids include allopurinol, amphetamines, benzodiazepines, captopril, chloroquine, corticosteroids, dicumarol, diflunisal, digoxin, ethambutol, flecainide, fluoroquinolones, histamine H_2 antagonists, hydantoins, iron salts, isoniazid, ketoconazole, levodopa, lithium, methenamine, methotrexate, nitrofurantoin, penicillamine, phenothiazines, quinidine, salicylates, sodium polystyrene sulfonate, sulfonylureas, sympathomimetics, tetracyclines, thyroid hormones, ticlopidine, valproic acid.

Adverse Reactions:

Magnesium-containing antacids: Laxative effect as saline cathartic, may cause diarrhea; hypermagnesemia in renal failure patients.

Aluminum-containing antacids: Constipation (may lead to intestinal obstruction); aluminum-intoxication; osteomalacia and hypophosphatemia; accumulation of aluminum in serum, bone and the CNS (aluminum accumulation may be neurotoxic); encephalopathy.

Antacids: Dose-dependent rebound hyperacidity and milk-alkali syndrome.

Administration and Dosage:

MAGNESIA (*Magnesium Hydroxide*):

Antacid dose, adults and children over 12 –

Liquid: 5 to 15 ml up to 4 times daily with water.

Liquid, concentrated: 2.5 to 7.5 ml up to 4 times daily with water.

Tablets: 622 mg to 1244 mg up to 4 times daily.

ALUMINUM HYDROXIDE GEL:

Tablets/Capsules – 500 to 1500 mg 3 to 6 times daily, between meals and at bedtime.

Suspension – 5 to 30 ml as needed between meals and at bedtime or as directed.

ALUMINUM CARBONATE GEL, BASIC:

Antacid – 2 capsules or tablets or 10 ml of regular suspension (in water or fruit juice) as often as every 2 hours, up to 12 times daily.

CALCIUM CARBONATE: 0.5 to 1.5 g, as needed.

MAGNESIUM OXIDE:

Capsules – 140 mg 3 to 4 times daily.

Tablets – 400 to 800 mg/day.

MAGALDRATE (*Aluminum Magnesium Hydroxide Sulfate*):

Suspension/Liquid – 5 to 10 ml between meals and at bedtime.

SODIUM BICARBONATE: 0.3 to 2 g 1 to 4 times daily.

SODIUM CITRATE: 30 ml daily.

SUCRALFATE

Tablets: 1 g (*Rx*) — *Carafate* (Hoechst-Marion Roussel)
Suspension: 1 g per 10 ml (*Rx*)

Actions:

Pharmacology: Sucralfate, a basic aluminum salt of sulfated sucrose, is a polysaccharide with antipeptic activity. In the acidic medium of gastric juice, the aluminum ion splits off, leaving a highly polar anion which is essentially nonabsorbable. It exerts a local rather than systemic action. Sucralfate forms an ulcer-adherent complex with proteinaceous exudate. The ulcer-adherent complex covers the ulcer site and protects it against acid, pepsin and bile salts. Sucralfate has minimal acid neutralizing capacity.

Pharmacokinetics: Sucralfate is minimally absorbed (3% to 5%) from the GI tract. Approximately 90% is excreted in the stool. The small amounts of the sulfated disaccharide absorbed are excreted primarily in the urine.

Indications:

Duodenal ulcer: Short-term treatment (up to 8 weeks) of active duodenal ulcer.

Tablets: Maintenance therapy for duodenal ulcer patients at reduced dosage after healing of acute ulcers.

Unlabeled uses: Sucralfate has been used in the following conditions: Accelerating healing of gastric ulcers; long-term treatment of gastric ulcers; treatment of reflux and peptic esophagitis; treatment of NSAID- and aspirin induced GI symptoms and mucosal damage; prevention of stress ulcers and GI bleeding in critically ill patients. Since increased gastric pH may be implicated in causing nosocomial infections in critically ill patients, sucralfate may offer an advantage over antacids and histamine H_2 antagonists in stress ulcer prophylaxis.

Sucralfate in suspension has also been used in treatment of oral and esophageal ulcers due to radiation, chemotherapy and sclerotherapy.

Warnings:

Chronic renal failure/dialysis: During sucralfate administration, small amounts of aluminum are absorbed from the GI tract. Concomitant use with other aluminum-containing products may increase the total body burden of aluminum. Patients with normal renal function receiving these agents concomitantly adequately excrete aluminum in the urine. However, patients with chronic renal failure or receiving dialysis have impaired excretion of absorbed aluminum, and aluminum does not cross dialysis membranes. Aluminum accumulation and toxicity have occurred.

Pregnancy: Category B.

Lactation: It is not known whether this drug is excreted in breast milk.

Children: Safety and efficacy in children have not been established.

Drug Interactions:

Drugs that may interact include aluminum-containing antacids, anticoagulants, digoxin, hydantoins, ketoconazole, quinidine and quinolones.

Adverse Reactions:

Adverse reactions in clinical trials were minor and rarely led to drug discontinuation. Constipation was the most frequent complaint (2%).

Administration and Dosage:

Active duodenal ulcer: Adults- 1 g 4 times a day on an empty stomach (1 hour before meals and at bedtime).

Take antacids as needed for pain relief, but not within ½ hour before or after sucralfate.

While healing with sucralfate may occur within the first 2 weeks, continue treatment for 4 to 8 weeks unless healing is demonstrated by X-ray or endoscopic examination

Adults –

*Maintenance therapy (tablets only): Adults-*1 g twice daily.

GASTROINTESTINAL ANTICHOLINERGICS/ANTISPASMODICS

ANISOTROPINE METHYLBROMIDE	
Tablets: 50 mg (*Rx*)	Various
ATROPINE SULFATE	
Injection: 0.05 mg/ml, 0.1 mg/ml, 0.3 mg/ml, 0.4 mg/ml, 0.5 mg/ml, 0.8 mg/ml, 1 mg/ml (*Rx*)	Various
Tablets: 0.4 mg (*Rx*)	*Atropine Sulfate* (Lilly), *Sal-Tropine* (Hope)
Tablets, soluble: 0.4 and 0.6 mg (*Rx*)	*Atropine Sulfate* (Lilly)
BELLADONNA	
Liquids: 27 to 33 mg belladonna alkaloids/100 ml (*Rx*)	Various
CLIDINIUM BROMIDE	
Capsules: 2.5, 5 mg (*Rx*)	*Quarzan* (Roche)
DICYCLOMINE HCl	
Capsules: 10, 20 mg (*Rx*)	Various, *Bentyl* (Lakeside Pharm.)
Tablets: 20 mg (*Rx*)	Various, *Bentyl* (Lakeside Pharm.)
Syrup: 10 mg/5 ml (*Rx*)	Various, *Bentyl* (Lakeside Pharm.)
Injection: 10 mg/ml (*Rx*)	Various, *Bentyl* (Lakeside Pharm.)
GLYCOPYRROLATE	
Tablets: 1, 2 mg (*Rx*)	*Robinul* (Robins)
Injection: 0.2 mg/ml (*Rx*)	Various, *Robinul* (Robins)
LEVOROTATORY ALKALOIDS OF BELLADONNA	
Tablets: 0.25 mg (*Rx*)	*Bellafoline* (Sandoz)
L-HYOSCYAMINE SULFATE	
Tablets: 0.125, 0.15 mg (*Rx*)	*Levsin* (Schwarz Pharma), *Gastrosed* (Roberts/Hauck), *Cystospaz* (PolyMedica), *Donnamar* (Marnel), *ED-SPAZ* (Edwards)
Tablets, sublingual: 0.125 mg (*Rx*)	*Levsin/SL* (Schwarz Pharma), *A-Spas S/L* (Hyrex)
Tablets, extended release: 0.375 mg (*Rx*)	*Levbid* (Schwarz Pharma)
Capsules, timed release: 0.375 mg (*Rx*)	Various, *Cystospaz-M* (PolyMedica), *Levsinex Timecaps* (Schwarz Pharma)
Solution: 0.125 mg/ml (*Rx*)	*Levsin Drops* (Schwarz Pharma), *Gastrosed* (Roberts Hauck)
Elixir: 0.125 mg/5 ml (*Rx*)	*Levsin* (Schwarz Pharma)
Injection: 0.5 mg/ml (*Rx*)	*Levsin* (Schwarz Pharma)
METHSCOPOLAMINE BROMIDE	
Tablets: 2.5 mg (*Rx*)	*Pamine* (Kenwood/Bradley)
MEPENZOLATE BROMIDE	
Tablets: 25 mg (*Rx*)	*Cantil* (Hoechst-Marion Roussel)
METHANTHELINE BROMIDE	
Tablets: 50 mg (*Rx*)	*Banthine* (Schiapparelli Searle)
OXYPHENCYCLIMINE HCl	
Tablets: 10 mg (*Rx*)	*Daricon* (SK-Beecham)
PROPANTHELINE BROMIDE	
Tablets: 7.5, 15 mg (*Rx*)	Various, *Pro-Banthine* (Schiapparelli Searle)
SCOPOLAMINE HBr (Hyoscine HBr)	
Injection: 0.3 mg/ml, 0.4 mg/ml, 0.86 mg/ml, 1 mg/ml (*Rx*)	Various
TRIDIHEXETHYL CHLORIDE	
Tablets: 25 mg (*Rx*)	*Pathilon* (Lederle)

Actions:

Pharmacology: GI anticholinergics are used primarily to decrease motility (smooth muscle tone) in GI, biliary and urinary tracts and for antisecretory effects. Antispasmodics, related compounds, decrease GI motility by acting on smooth muscle.

These agents inhibit the muscarinic actions of acetylcholine at postganglionic parasympathetic neuroeffector sites including smooth muscle, secretory glands and CNS sites. Large doses may block nicotinic receptors at the autonomic ganglia and at the neuromuscular junction.

Pharmacokinetics:

Belladonna alkaloids are rapidly absorbed after oral use. They readily cross blood-brain barrier, and affect the CNS.

Atropine has a half-life of about 2.5 hours; 94% of a dose is eliminated through the urine in 24 hours.

Quaternary anticholinergics – Synthetic or semisynthetic derivatives structurally related to the belladonna alkaloids, they are poorly and unreliably absorbed orally. Since they do not cross the blood-brain barrier, CNS effects are negligible. Duration of action is more prolonged than alkaloids.

Indications:

Peptic ulcer: Adjunctive therapy for peptic ulcer. These agents suppress gastric acid secretion.

Other GI conditions: Functional GI disorders (diarrhea, pylorospasm, hypermotility, neurogenic colon), irritable bowel syndrome (spastic colon, mucous colitis), acute enterocolitis, ulcerative colitis, diverticulitis, mild dysenteries, pancreatitis, splenic flexure syndrome and infant colic.

Biliary tract: For spastic disorders of the biliary tract. Given in conjunction with a narcotic analgesic.

Urogenital tract: Uninhibited hypertonic neurogenic bladder.

Bradycardia: Atropine is used in the suppression of vagally-mediated bradycardias.

Preoperative medication: Atropine, scopolamine, hyoscyamine and glycopyrrolate are used as preanesthetic medication to control bronchial, nasal, pharyngeal and salivary secretions; and to block cardiac vagal inhibitory reflexes during induction of anesthesia and intubation. Scopolamine is used for preanesthetic sedation and for obstetric amnesia.

Antidotes for poisoning by cholinergic drugs: Atropine is used for poisoning by organophosphorous insecticides, chemical warfare nerve gases and as an antidote for mushroom poisoning due to muscarine in certain species such as Amanita muscaria.

Miscellaneous uses: Calming delirium; motion sickness (scopolamine), parkinsonism.

Unlabeled uses:

Bronchial asthma – Atropine and related agents are effective in some patients with cholinergic-mediated bronchospasm.

Glycopyrrolate may be effective in the treatment of bronchial asthma.

Contraindications:

Hypersensitivity to anticholinergic drugs. Patients hypersensitive to belladonna or to barbiturates may be hypersensitive to **scopolamine.**

Ocular: Narrow-angle glaucoma; adhesions (synechiae) between the iris and lens.

Cardiovascular: Tachycardia; unstable cardiovascular status in acute hemorrhage; myocardial ischemia.

GI: Obstructive disease (eg, achalasia, pyloroduodenal stenosis or pyloric obstruction, cardiospasm); paralytic ileus; intestinal atony of the elderly or debilitated; severe ulcerative colitis; toxic megacolon complicating ulcerative colitis; hepatic disease.

GU: Obstructive uropathy (eg, bladder neck obstruction due to prostatic hypertrophy); renal disease.

Musculoskeletal: Myasthenia gravis.

Atropine is contraindicated in asthma patients.

Dicyclomine: Infants < 6 months of age.

Warnings:

Heat prostration can occur with anticholinergic drug use (fever and heat stroke due to decreased sweating) in the presence of a high environmental temperature.

Diarrhea may be an early symptom of incomplete intestinal obstruction, especially in patients with ileostomy or colostomy. Treatment of diarrhea with these drugs is inappropriate and possibly harmful.

Anticholinergic psychosis has been reported in sensitive individuals given anticholinergic drugs.

Gastric ulcer may produce a delay in gastric emptying time and may complicate therapy (antral stasis).

Elderly: Elderly patients may react with excitement, agitation, drowsiness and other untoward manifestations to even small doses of anticholinergic drugs.

Pregnancy: Category B (glycopyrrolate, parenteral); *Category* C (hyoscyamine, atropine, scopolamine, propantheline, methantheline). Hyoscyamine crosses the placenta; atropine and scopolamine cross the placenta rapidly after IV use. Effects on the fetus depend on maturity of its parasympathetic nervous system.

Lactation: Hyoscyamine is excreted in breast milk; other anticholinergics (especially atropine) may be excreted in milk, causing infant toxicity, and may reduce milk production.

Children: Safety and efficacy are not established. Hyoscyamine has been used in infant colic. Safety and efficacy of **glycopyrrolate** in children < 12 are not established for peptic ulcer. Dicyclomine is contraindicated in infants < 6 months old.

Precautions:

Use with caution in:

Ocular – Glaucoma; light irides. Use caution in the elderly because of increased incidence of glaucoma.

GI – Hepatic disease; early evidence of ileus, as in peritonitis; ulcerative colitis; hiatal hernia associated with reflux esophagitis.

GU – Renal disease; prostatic hypertrophy.

Cardiovascular – Coronary heart disease; CHF; cardiac arrhythmias; tachycardia; hypertension.

Pulmonary – Debilitated patients with chronic lung disease; reduction in bronchial secretions can lead to inspissation and formation of bronchial plugs.

Miscellaneous: Autonomic neuropathy; hyperthyroidism.

Special risk patients: Use cautiously in infants, small children and persons with Down's syndrome, brain damage or spastic paralysis.

Hazardous tasks: May produce drowsiness, dizziness or blurred vision; observe caution while driving or performing other tasks requiring alertness.

Drug Interactions:

Drugs that may interact with GI anticholinergics include amantadine, atenolol, digoin, phenothiazines and tricyclic antidepressants.

Adverse Reactions:

Xerostomia; altered taste perception; nausea; vomiting; dysphagia; heartburn; constipation; bloated feeling; paralytic ileus; urinary hesitancy and retention; impotence; blurred vision; mydriasis; photophobia; cycloplegia; increased intraocular pressure; dilated pupils; palpitations; tachycardia (after higher doses); headache; flushing; nervousness; drowsiness; weakness; dizziness; confusion; insomnia; fever (especially in children); mental confusion or excitement; CNS stimulation (restlessness, tremor with large doses); severe allergic reactions including anaphylaxis, urticaria and other dermal manifestations; nasal congestion; decreased sweating.

Administration and Dosage:

ANISOTROPINE METHYLBROMIDE: 50 mg 3 times daily.

ATROPINE SULFATE:

Adults – 0.4 to 0.6 m.

Children –

Atropine Dosage Recommendations in Children		
Weight		Dose
lb	kg	mg
7 to 16	3.2 to 7.3	0.1
16 to 24	7.3 to 10.9	0.15
24 to 40	10.9 to 18.1	0.2
40 to 65	18.1 to 29.5	0.3
65 to 90	29.5 to 40.8	0.4
> 90	40.8	0.4 to 0.6

Hypotonic radiography – 1 mg IM.

Surgery – Give SC, IM or IV. The average adult dose is 0.5 mg (range 0.4 to 0.6 mg). In children, it has been suggested to use a dose of 0.01 mg/kg to a maximum of 0.4 mg, repeated every 4 to 6 hours as needed. A recommended infant dose is 0.04 mg/kg (infants < 5 kg) or 0.03 mg/kg (infants > 5 kg), repeated every 4 to 6 hours as needed.

Bradyarrhythmias – The usual IV adult dosage ranges from 0.4 to 1 mg every 1 to 2 hours as needed; larger doses, up to a maximum of 2 mg, may be required. In children, IV dosage ranges from 0.01 to 0.03 mg/kg.

Poisoning – In anticholinesterase poisoning from exposure to insecticides, give large doses of at least 2 to 3 mg parenterally; repeat until signs of atropine intoxication appear.

BELLADONNA:

Belladonna tincture –

Adults: 0.6 to 1 ml, 3 to 4 times daily.

Children: 0.03 ml/kg (0.8 ml/m^2) 3 times daily.

CLIDINIUM BROMIDE:

Adults – 2.5 to 5 mg, 3 or 4 times daily before meals and at bedtime.

Geriatric or debilitated patients – 2.5 mg, 3 times daily before meals.

DICYCLOMINE HCl:

Oral –

Adults: The only oral dose shown to be effective is 160 mg/day in 4 equally divided doses. However, because of side effects, begin with 80 mg/day (in 4 equally divided doses). Increase dose to 160 mg/day unless side effects limit dosage.

Parenteral – IM only. Not for IV use.

Adults: 80 mg/day in 4 divided doses.

GLYCOPYRROLATE: Not recommended for children under age 12 for the management of peptic ulcer.

Oral – 1 mg 3 times daily or 2 mg 2 to 3 times daily.

Maintenance: 1 mg 2 times daily.

Parenteral –

Peptic ulcer: 0.1 to 0.2 mg IM or IV 3 or 4 times daily.

Preanesthetic medication: 0.002 mg/lb (0.004 mg/kg) IM, 30 minutes to 1 hour prior to anesthesia. Children less than 2 years of age may require up to 0.004 mg/lb. Children under 12, give 0.002 to 0.004 mg/lb IM.

Intraoperative medication: Adults, 0.1 mg IV. Repeat as needed at 2 to 3 minute intervals. Children, give 0.002 mg/lb (0.004 mg/kg) IV, not to exceed 0.1 mg in a single dose; may be repeated at 2 to 3 minute intervals.

Reversal of neuromuscular blockade: Adults and children, 0.2 mg for each 1 mg neostigmine or 5 mg pyridostigmine. Administer IV simultaneously.

L-HYOSCYAMINE SULFATE:

Oral –

Adults: 0.125 to 0.25 mg, 3 or 4 times/day orally or sublingually; or 0.375 to 0.75 mg in sustained release form every 12 hours.

Children: Individualize dosage according to weight.

Parenteral – 0.25 to 0.5 mg SC, IM or IV, 2 to 4 times daily, as needed.

LEVOROTATORY ALKALOIDS OF BELLADONNA:

Oral –

Adults: 0.25 to 0.5 mg, 3 times daily.

Children (over 6 years): 0.125 to 0.25 mg, 3 times daily.

METHSCOPOLAMINE BROMIDE: 2.5 mg 30 minutes before meals and 2.5 to 5 mg at bedtime.

MEPENZOLATE BROMIDE:

Adults – 25 to 50 mg 4 times daily with meals and at bedtime.

Children – Safety and efficacy have not been establlished.

METHANTHELINE BROMIDE:

Adults – 50 to 100 mg every 6 hours.

Pediatric –

Newborns: 12.5 mg 2 times daily, then 12.5 mg 3 times daily.

Infants (1 to 12 months): 12.5 mg 4 times daily, increased to 25 mg 4 times daily.

Children (> 1 year): 12.5 to 50 mg 4 times daily.

OXPHENCYCLIMINE HCl:

Adults – 5 to 10 mg 2 or 3 times daily, preferably in the morning and at bedtime. Some respond to 5 mg 2 times day, while some may require higher dosage 3 times day.

Children – Not for use in children less than 12 years of age.

PROPANTHELINE BROMIDE:

Adults – 15 mg 30 minutes before meals and 30 mg at bedtime. For patients with mild manifestations, geriatric patients or those of small stature, take 7.5 mg, 3 times daily.

Children –

Peptic ulcer: Safety and efficacy have not been established.

Antisecretory: 1.5 mg/kg/day divided 3 to 4 times daily.

Antispasmodic: 2 to 3 mg/kg/day divided every 4 to 6 hours and at bedtime.

SCOPOLAMINE HBr (Hyoscine HBr): Give SC or IM; may giv IV after dilution with Sterile Water for Injection

Adults – 0.32 to 0.65 mg.

Children – 0.006 mg/kg. Maximum dosage, 0.3 mg.

TRIDIHEXETHYL CHLORIDE: 25 to 50 mg 3 or 4 times daily before meals and at bedtime. Bedtime dose: 50 mg.

HISTAMINE H_2 ANTAGONISTS

CIMETIDINE	
Tablets: 100 mg (*otc*)	*Tagamet HB* (SK-Beecham)
Tablets: 200, 300, 400, 800 mg (*Rx*)	Various, *Tagamet* (SK-Beecham)
Liquid: 300 mg (as HCl) per 5 ml (*Rx*)	*Cimetidine Oral Solution* (Barre-National), *Tagamet* (SK-Beecham)
Injection: 300 mg (as HCl) per 2 ml (*Rx*)	*Cimetidine* (Endo), *Tagamet* (SK-Beecham)
Injection, premixed: 300 mg (as HCl) in 50 ml 0.9% sodium chloride (*Rx*)	*Tagamet* (SK-Beecham)
FAMOTIDINE	
Tablets: 10 mg (*otc*)	*Pepcid AC Acid Controller* (J & J Merck)
Tablets: 20, 40 mg (*Rx*)	*Pepcid* (J & J Merck)
Powder for Oral Suspension: 40 mg per 5 ml when reconstituted (*Rx*)	
Injection: 10 mg per ml (*Rx*)	
Injection, premixed: 20 mg per 50 ml in 0.9% HCl (*Rx*)	
NIZATIDINE	
Capsules: 150, 300 mg (*Rx*)	*Axid Pulvules* (Lilly)
RANITIDINE	
Tablets: 75 mg (*otc*)	*Zantac 75* (Glaxo Wellcome)
Tablets: 150, 300 mg (as HCl) (*Rx*)	*Zantac* (Glaxo Wellcome)
Tablets, effervescent: 150 mg (*Rx*)	*Zantac EFFERdose* (Glaxo Wellcome)
Capsules: 150, 300 mg (*Rx*)	*Zantac GELdose* (Glaxo Wellcome)
Syrup: 15 mg (as HCl) per ml (*Rx*)	*Ranitidine HCl* (UDL), *Zantac* (Glaxo Wellcome)
Granules, effervescent: 150 mg (*Rx*)	*Zantac EFFERdose* (Glaxo Wellcome)
Injection: 0.5 and 25 mg (as HCl) per ml (*Rx*)	*Zantac* (Glaxo Wellcome)

Actions:

Pharmacology: Histamine H_2 antagonists are reversible competitive blockers of histamine at the H_2 receptors, particularly those in the gastric parietal cells. They also inhibit fasting and nocturnal secretions, and secretions stimulated by food, insulin, caffeine, pentagastrin and betazole. Cimetidine, ranitidine and famotidine have no effect on gastric emptying, and cimetidine and famotidine have no effect on lower esophageal sphincter pressure. Ranitidine, nizatidine and famotidine have little or no effect on fasting or postprandial serum gastrin.

Pharmacokinetics:

Pharmacokinetic Properties of Histamine H_2 Antagonists

H_2receptor antagonist	Bioavailability (%)	Time to peak plasma concentration (hrs)	Peak plasma concentration[1] (mcg/ml)	Half-life (hrs)	Protein binding (%)	Volume of distribution (L/kg)	Elimination (%)		
							Urine, unchanged		Metabolized
							Oral	IV	
Cimetidine	60-70	0.75-1.5	0.7-3.2 (300 mg dose) (3.5-7.5 IV)	≈ 2[2]	13-25	0.8-1.2	48	75	30-40
Famotidine	40-45	1-3	0.076-0.1 (40 mg dose)	2.5-3.5[3]	15-20	1.1-1.4	25-30	65-70	30-35
Nizatidine	>90	0.5-3	0.7-1.8/ 1.4-3.6 (150/300 mg dose)	1-2[3]	≈ 35	0.8-1.5	60	na[4]	< 18
Ranitidine	50-60 (90-100 IM)	1-3 (0.25 IM)	0.44-0.55 (0.58 IM)	2-3[3]	15	1.2-1.9	30-35	68-79	< 10

[1] Dose-dependent.
[2] Increased in renal and hepatic impairment and in the elderly.
[3] Increased in renal impairment.
[4] na = not applicable.

Indications:

Histamine H_2 Antagonists: Summary of Indications				
✓ – Labeled x Unlabeled	Cimetidine	Famotidine	Nizatidine	Ranitidine
Duodenal ulcer Treatment	✓	✓	✓	✓
Maintenance	✓	✓	✓	✓
GERD (including erosive esophagitis)	✓	✓	✓	✓
Gastric ulcer Treatment	✓	✓	✓	✓
Maintenance				✓
Pathological hypersecretory conditions	✓	✓		✓
Heartburn/acid indigestion/ sour stomach	✓[1,2]	✓[1,3]		
Erosive esophagitis, maintenance				✓
Prevent upper GI bleeding	✓	x		x
Peptic ulcer [4]	x	x	x	x
Prevent aspiration pneumonitis	x	x		x
Prophylaxis of stress ulcers	x	x		x
Prevent gastric NSAID damage				x
Hyperparathyroidism	x			
Secondary hyperparathyroidism in hemodialysis	x			
Tinea capitis	x			
Herpes virus infection	x			
Hirsute women	x			
Chronic idiopathic urticaria	x			
Anaphylaxis (dermatological)	x			
Acetaminophen overdose	x			
Dyspepsia	x			
Warts	x			
Colorectal cancer	x			

[1] *otc* use only.
[2] Relief of symptoms only.
[3] Relief and prevention of symptoms.
[4] As part of a multi-drug regimen to eradicate *Helicobacter pylori*.

Contraindications:

Hypersensitivity to individual agents or to other H_2-receptor antagonists.

Warnings:

Benzyl alcohol, contained in some of these products as a preservative, has been associated with a fatal "gasping syndrome" in premature infants.

Hypersensitivity: Rare cases of anaphylaxis have occurred as well as rare episodes of hypersensitivity (eg, bronchospasm, laryngeal edema, rash, eosinophilia).

Renal function impairment: Since these agents are excreted primarily via the kidneys, decreased clearance may occur; reduced dosage may be necessary.

Hepatic function impairment: Observe caution. Decreased clearance may occur; these agents are partly metabolized in the liver.

Elderly: Safety and efficacy appear similar to those of younger age; however, the elderly may have reduced renal function. Decreased **cimetidine** clearance may be more common.

Pregnancy: (Category B - cimetidine, famotidine, ranitidine. Category C - nizatidine). Cimetidine crosses the placenta.

Lactation: **Cimetidine** is excreted in breast milk with milk:plasma ratios of approximately 5:1 to 12:1. Potential daily infant ingestion is approximately 6 mg.

Ranitidine is excreted in breast milk with milk:plasma ratios of 1:1 to 6.7:1.

Nizatidine is excreted in breast milk in a concentration of 0.1% of the oral dose in proportion to plasma concentrations.

Famotidine is excreted in the breast milk of rats. It is not known whether it is excreted in human breast milk.

Children: Safety and efficacy are not established. **Cimetidine** is not recommended for children < 16 years old, unless anticipated benefits outweigh potential risks. In very limited experience, cimetidine 20 to 40 mg/kg/day has been used.

Precautions:

Gastric malignancy: Symptomatic response to these agents does not preclude gastric malignancy.

Reversible CNS effects (eg, mental confusion, agitation, psychosis, depression, anxiety, hallucinations, disorientation) have occurred with **cimetidine,** predominantly in severely ill patients. Advancing age (≥ 50 years) and preexisting liver or renal disease appear to be contributing factors.

Hepatocellular injury may occur with **nizatidine** as evidenced by elevated liver enzymes (AST, ALT or alkaline phosphatase).

Occasionally, reversible hepatitis, hepatocellular or hepatocanalicular or mixed, with or without jaundice have occurred with oral **ranitidine.**

Laboratory test monitoring for liver abnormalities is appropriate.

Antiandrogenic effect: **Cimetidine** has a weak antiandrogenic effect in animals. Gynecomastia in patients treated for ≥ 1 month may occur.

Immunocompromised patients: Decreased gastric acidity, including that produced by acid-suppressing agents such as H_2 antagonists, may increase the possibility of strongyloidiasis.

Drug Interactions:

Cimetidinereduces the hepatic metabolism of drugs metabolized via the cytochrome P-450 pathway, delaying elimination and increasing serum levels.

Cimetidine Drug Interactions (Decreased Hepatic Metabolism)		
Benzodiazepines[1]	Metronidazole	Sulfonylureas
Caffeine	Moricizine	Tacrine
Calcium channel blockers	Pentoxifylline	Theophyllines [2]
Carbamazepine	Phenytoin	Triamterene
Chloroquine	Propafenone	Tricyclic antidepressants
Labetalol	Propranolol	Valproic acid
Lidocaine	Quinidine	Warfarin
Metoprolol	Quinine	

[1] Does not include agents metabolized by glucuronidation (lorazepam, oxazepam, temazepam).
[2] Does not include dyphylline.

Ranitidine (which weakly binds to cytochrome P450 in vitro), **famotidine** and **nizatidine** do not inhibit the cytochrome P450-linked oxygenase enzyme system in the liver. Drug interactions with these agents mediated by inhibition of hepatic metabolism are not expected.

Drugs that may affect histamine H_2 antagonists include antacids, anticholinergics, metoclopramide and cigarette smoking. Drugs that may be affected by histamine H_2 antagonists include ferrous salts, indomethacin, ketoconazole, tetracyclines, carmustine, digoxin, flecainide, fluconazole, fluorouracil, narcotic analgesics, procainamide, succinylcholine, tocainide, salicylates, diazepam, sulfonylureas, theophyllines, warfarin and ethanol.

Drug/Lab test interactions: False-positive tests for urobilinogen may occur during **nizatidine** therapy. False-positive tests for urine protein with *Multistix* may occur during **ranitidine** therapy; testing with sulfosalicylic acid is recommended.

Drug/Food interactions: Food may increase bioavailability of **famotidine** and **nizatidine;** this is of no clinical consequence. **Cimetidine** and **ranitidine** are not affected.

Adverse Reactions:

Adverse reactions may include headache, somnolence/fatigue, dizziness, confusional states, hallucinations, insomnia, nausea, vomiting, abdominal discomfort, diarrhea, constipation, thrombocytopenia, alopecia, rash, gynecomastia, impotence, loss of libido and arthralgia.

Administration and Dosage:

CIMETIDINE:

Duodenal ulcer –

Short-term treatment of active duodenal ulcer: 800 mg at bedtime. Alternate regimens are 300 mg 4 times a day with meals and at bedtime, or 400 mg twice a day.

Maintenance therapy: 400 mg at bedtime.

Active benign gastric ulcer – For short-term treatment, 800 mg at bedtime or 300 mg 4 times a day with meals and at bedtime.

Erosive gastroesophageal reflux disease (GERD) –

Adults: 1600 mg daily in divided doses (800 mg twice daily or 400 mg 4 times a day) for 12 weeks. Use beyond 12 weeks has not been established.

Pathological hypersecretory conditions – 300 mg 4 times a day with meals and at bedtime. If necessary, give 300 mg doses more often. Do not exceed 2400 mg/day.

Prevention of upper GI bleeding – Continuous IV infusion of 50 mg/hour. Patients with creatinine clearance < 30 ml/min should receive half the recommended dose. Treatment beyond 7 days has not been studied.

Severely impaired renal function – Accumulation may occur. Use the lowest dose; 300 mg every 12 hours orally or IV has been recommended. Dosage frequency may be increased to every 8 hours or even further with caution.

Parenteral – The usual dose is 300 mg IM or IV every 6 to 8 hours. If it is necessary to increase dosage, do so by more frequent administration of a 300 mg dose, not to exceed 2400 mg/day.

IM: Administer undiluted.

IV: Dilute to a total volume of 20 ml; inject over ≥ 2 minutes.

Intermittent IV infusion: Dilute 300 mg in at least 50 ml of compatible IV solution; infuse over 15 to 20 minutes.

Continuous IV infusion: 37.5 mg/hour (900 mg/day).

FAMOTIDINE:

Duodenal ulcer –

Acute therapy: 40 mg/day at bedtime. 20 mg twice/day is also effective.

Maintenance therapy: 20 mg once a day at bedtime.

Benign gastric ulcer –

Acute therapy: 40 mg orally once a day at bedtime.

Pathological hypersecretory conditions – The adult starting dose is 20 mg every 6 hours.

GERD – 20 mg twice daily for up to 6 weeks. For esophagitis including erosions and ulcerations and accompanying symptoms due to GERD, 20 or 40 mg twice daily for up to 12 weeks.

Severe renal insufficiency –

Ccr < 10 ml/min: To avoid excess accumulation of the drug, the dose may be reduced to 20 mg at bedtime or the dosing interval may be prolonged to 36 to 48 hours, as indicated.

Parenteral –

IV: Give famotidine IV 20 mg every 12 hours.

NIZATIDINE:

Active duodenal ulcer – 300 mg once daily at bedtime. An alternative dosage regimen is 150 mg twice daily.

Maintenance of healed duodenal ulcer – 150 mg once daily at bedtime.

GERD – 150 mg twice daily.

Moderate to severe renal insufficiency –

Nizatidine Dosage in Renal Insufficiency		
	Dosage	
Creatinine clearance	Active duodenal ulcer	Maintenance therapy
20 to 50 ml/min	150 mg/day	150 mg every other day
< 20 ml/min	150 mg every other day	150 mg every 3 days

RANITIDINE:

Duodenal ulcer –

Short-term treatment of active duodenal ulcer: 150 mg orally twice daily. An alternate dosage of 300 mg once daily at bedtime can be used for patients in whom dosing convenience is important.

Maintenance therapy: 150 mg at bedtime.

Pathological hypersecretory conditions – 150 mg orally twice a day. More frequent doses may be necessary. Doses up to 6 g/day have been used.

Benign gastric ulcer (oral doseforms only) and GERD – 150 mg twice daily.

Erosive esophagitis – 150 mg 4 times daily.

Renal impairment – (Ccr < 50 ml/min): 150 mg orally every 24 hours or 50 mg parenterally every 18 to 24 hours. The frequency of dosing may be increased to every 12 hours or further with caution.

Parenteral –

IM: 50 mg (2 ml) every 6 to 8 hours. (No dilution necessary.)

IV injection: 50 mg (2 ml) every 6 to 8 hours. Dilute 50 mg to a total volume of 20 ml; inject over ≥ 5 min.

Intermittent IV infusion: 50 mg (2 ml) every 6 to 8 hours. Dilute 50 mg and infuse over 15 to 20 minutes; do not exceed 400 mg/day.

Continuous IV infusion: Add ranitidine injection to 5% Dextrose Injection or other compatible IV solution. Deliver at a rate of 6.25 mg/hr (eg, 150 mg [6 ml] ranitidine injection in 250 ml of 5% Dextrose Injection at 10.7 ml/hr).

MISOPROSTOL

Tablets: 100 and 200 mcg (*Rx*)	*Cytotec* (Searle)

Warning:

Misoprostol is contraindicated because of its abortifacient property in pregnant women. Advise patients of the abortifacient property and warn them not to give the drug to others. Do not use in women of childbearing potential unless the patient requires nonsteroidal anti-inflammatory drugs (NSAIDs) and is at high risk of complications from gastric ulcers associated with use of NSAIDs, or is at high risk of developing gastric ulceration. In such patients, misoprostol may be prescribed if the patient:

- Is capable of complying with effective contraceptive measures;
- Has received both oral and written warnings of the hazards of misoprostol, the risk of possible contraception failure and the danger to other women of childbearing potential should the drug be taken by mistake;
- Has had a negative *serum* pregnancy test within 2 weeks prior to beginning therapy;
- Will begin therapy only on second or third day of next normal menstrual period.

Actions:

Pharmacology: Misoprostol, a synthetic prostaglandin E_1 analog, has both antisecretory (inhibiting gastric acid secretion) and (in animals) mucosal protective properties. NSAIDs inhibit prostaglandin synthesis; a deficiency of prostaglandins within the gastric mucosa may lead to diminishing bicarbonate and mucous secretion and may contribute to the mucosal damage caused by these agents. Misoprostol can increase bicarbonate and mucus production.

Effects on gastric acid secretion – Misoprostol over the range of 50 to 200 mcg inhibits basal and nocturnal gastric acid secretion, and acid secretion in response to a variety of stimuli, including meals, histamine, pentagastrin and coffee. Activity is apparent 30 minutes after oral administration and persists for at least 3 hours. Only the 200 mcg dose had substantial effects on nocturnal secretion or on histamine and meal-stimulated secretion.

Uterine effects – Misoprostol produces uterine contractions that may endanger pregnancy.

Pharmacokinetics: Misoprostol is extensively absorbed, and undergoes rapid de-esterification to its free acid, which is responsible for its clinical activity and, unlike the parent compound, is detectable in plasma. In healthy volunteers, misoprostol is rapidly absorbed after oral administration with a time to reach peak concentration of misoprostol acid of 12 minutes and a terminal half-life of 20 to 40 minutes.

Mean plasma levels after single doses show a linear relationship with doses over the range of 200 to 400 mcg. No accumulation was noted in multiple-dose studies; plasma steady state was achieved within 2 days. After oral administration of radiolabeled misoprostol, ≈ 80% of detected radioactivity appears in urine.

Misoprostol does not affect the hepatic mixed function oxidase (cytochrome P-450) enzyme system in animals. The serum protein binding of misoprostol acid is < 90% and is concentration-independent in the therapeutic range.

Indications:

Prevention of NSAID- (including aspirin) induced gastric ulcers in patients at high risk of complications from a gastric ulcer, eg, the elderly and patients with concomitant debilitating disease, as well as patients at high risk of developing gastric ulceration, such as patients with a history of ulcer. Take misoprostol for the duration of NSAID therapy.

Unlabeled uses: In doses of at least 400 mcg/day, misoprostol appears effective in treating duodenal ulcers, and may be useful in treating duodenal ulcers unresponsive to histamine H_2 antagonists; however, it does not prevent duodenal ulcers in patients on NSAIDs.

In one study, misoprostol 200 mcg 4 times daily for 12 weeks (concurrently with cyclosporine and prednisone) reduced the incidence of acute graft rejection in renal transplant recipients by improving renal function.

Contraindications:

History of allergy to prostaglandins; pregnancy.

Warnings:

Duodenal ulcers: Misoprostol does not prevent duodenal ulcers in patients on NSAIDs. It had no effect, compared to placebo, on GI pain or discomfort associated with NSAIDs.

Renal function impairment: Pharmacokinetic studies in patients with varying degrees of renal impairment showed an approximate doubling of half-life, maximum concentration and area under the curve (AUC), but no clear correlation between degree of impairment and AUC was shown. No routine dosage adjustment is recommended, but dosage may need to be reduced if usual dose is not tolerated.

Fertility impairment: Results of animal studies suggest the possibility of a general adverse effect on fertility in males and females.

Elderly: In subjects > 64 years of age, the AUC for misoprostol acid is increased; however, no routine dosage adjustment is recommended. Reduce the dose if the usual dose is not tolerated.

Pregnancy: *Category X.* Misoprostol may cause miscarriage. Uterine contractions, uterine bleeding and expulsion of the products of conception occur. Miscarriages caused by misoprostol may be incomplete.

Lactation: It is unlikely that misoprostol is excreted in breast milk, since it is rapidly metabolized. However, it is not known if the active metabolite (misoprostol acid) is excreted in breast milk. Therefore, do not administer to nursing mothers because the potential excretion of misoprostol acid could cause significant diarrhea in nursing infants.

Children: Safety and efficacy in children < 18 years of age have not been established.

Precautions:

Women of childbearing potential: Advise women of childbearing potential that they must not be pregnant when misoprostol therapy is initiated, and that they must use an effective contraception method while taking misoprostol.

Diarrhea (13% to 40%) is dose-related and usually develops early in the course of therapy (after 13 days), usually is self-limiting (often resolving after 8 days), but sometimes requires discontinuation of misoprostol (2% of the patients). The incidence of diarrhea can be minimized by administering after meals and at bedtime, and by avoiding coadministration of misoprostol with magnesium-containing antacids.

Drug Interactions:

Antacids reduce the total availability of misoprostol acid but this does not appear clinically important.

Drug/Food interactions: Maximum plasma concentrations of misoprostol acid are diminished when taken with food.

Adverse Reactions:

Adverse reactions associated with misoprostol may include diarrhea, abdominal pain and nausea.

Administration and Dosage:

Adults: 200 mcg 4 times daily with food. If this dose cannot be tolerated, 100 mcg can be used. Take misoprostol for the duration of NSAID therapy as prescribed. Take with meals, the last dose of the day taken at bedtime.

OMEPRAZOLE

Capsules, sustained release: 10 and 20 mg (*Rx*) — *Prilosec* (Astra Merck)

Actions:

Pharmacology: Omeprazole belongs to a new class of antisecretory compounds, the substituted benzimidazoles, that suppress gastric acid secretion by specific inhibition of the H^+/K^+ ATPase enzyme system at the secretory surface of the gastric parietal cell. Because this enzyme system is the acid (proton) pump' within the gastric mucosa, omeprazole has been characterized as a gastric acid pump inhibitor; it blocks the final step of acid production.

Antisecretory activity – Onset after oral administration of omeprazole occurs within 1 hour, and is maximum within 2 hours. Inhibition of secretion is about 50% of maximum at 24 hours and the duration of inhibition lasts up to 72 hours.

Pharmacokinetics:

Absorption/Distribution – Omeprazole contains an enteric coated granule formulation (because omeprazole is acid-labile). Absorption is rapid, with peak plasma levels occurring within 0.5 to 3.5 hours. Absolute bioavailability is about 30% to 40% at doses of 20 to 40 mg, due to presystemic metabolism. Plasma half-life is 0.5 to 1 hour, and total body clearance is 500 to 600 ml/min. Protein binding is ≈ 95%.

Metabolism/Excretion – Little unchanged drug is excreted in urine. The majority of the dose (about 77%) is eliminated in urine as at least six metabolites.

Indications:

Active duodenal ulcer: Short-term treatment of active duodenal ulcer. Most patients heal within 4 weeks, although some may require an additional 4 weeks.

Gastroesophageal reflux disease (GERD):

Severe erosive esophagitis – Short-term treatment (4 to 8 weeks) of erosive esophagitis, diagnosed by endoscopy.

Poorly responsive symptomatic GERD – Short-term treatment (4 to 8 weeks) of symptomatic GERD (esophagitis) poorly responsive to customary medical treatment, usually including histamine H_2-receptor antagonists.

Eradication of H. pylori – In combination with clarithromycin for treatment of patients with H. pylori infection and active duodenal ulcer.

Maintenance – To maintain healing of erosive esophagitis.

Pathological hypersecretory conditions (eg, Zollinger-Ellison syndrome, multiple endocrine adenomas and systemic mastocytosis): Long-term treatment.

Gastric ulcer: Short-term treatment (4 to 8 weeks) of active benign gastric ulcer.

Contraindications:

Hypersensitivity to any component of the formulation.

Warnings:

Maintenance therapy: Omeprazole should not be used as maintenance therapy for treatment of patients with duodenal ulcer disease.

Duration of therapy (GERD): In the rare patient not responding to 8 weeks of treatment, an additional 4 weeks of treatment may help. If there is recurrence of severe or symptomatic GERD poorly responsive to customary medical treatment, an additional 4 to 8 week course of omeprazole may be considered.

Elderly: Bioavailability may be increased.

Pregnancy: Category C.

Lactation: It is not known whether omeprazole is excreted in breast milk.

Children: Safety and efficacy in children have not been established.

Precautions:

Gastric malignancy: Symptomatic response does not preclude gastric malignancy.

Drug Interactions:

Drugs that may interact with omeprazole include clarithromycin, diazepam, phenytoin and warfarin. There may be interactions with other drugs also metabolized via the cytochrome P–450 system. Omeprazole may interfere with absorption of drugs where gastric pH is a determinant of their bioavailability (eg, ketoconazole, ampicillin esters, iron salts).

Adverse Reactions:

Adverse reactions may include: Headache; diarrhea.

Administration and Dosage:

Active duodenal ulcer:

Adults – 20 mg daily for 4 to 8 weeks.

GERD:

Erosive esophagitis or poorly responsive GERD – Adults – 20 mg daily for 4 to 8 weeks.

Maintenance of healing erosive esophagitis – 20 mg daily.

Reduction of risk of duodenal ulcer recurrence:

Omeprazole and Clarithromycin: Combination Therapy	
Days 1 - 14	Days 15 - 28
Omeprazole 40 mg qd (in the morning) plus clarithromycin 500 mg tid	Omeprazole 20 mg qd

Gastric ulcer: The recommended adult oral dose is 40 mg once a day for 4 to 8 weeks.

Pathological hypersecretory conditions: Initial adult dose is 60 mg once a day. Doses up to 120 mg 3 times/day have been administered. Administer daily dosages > 80 mg in divided doses.

No dosage adjustment is necessary for patients with renal impairment, hepatic dysfunction or for the elderly.

Take before eating. Do not open, crush or chew the capsule; swallow whole.

LANSOPRAZOLE

Capsules, delayed release: 15 and 30 mg (*Rx*) *Prevacid* (TAP Pharm)

Actions:

Pharmacology: Lansoprazole belongs to a class of antisecretory compounds, the substituted benzimidazoles, that suppress gastric acid secretion by specific inhibition of the (H^+, K^+)-ATPase enzyme system at the secretory surface of the gastric parietal cell. Because this enzyme system is regarded as the acid (proton) pump within the parietal cell, lansoprazole is characterized as a gastric acid-pump inhibitor, in that it blocks the final step of acid production. The effect is dose-related and leads to inhibition of both basal and stimulated gastric acid secretion regardless of stimulus.

Pharmacokinetics:

Absorption/Distribution – Absorption of lansoprazole begins only after the granules leave the stomach. Absorption is rapid with mean peak plasma levels occurring after ≈ 1.7 hours and is relatively complete with absolute bioavailability over 80%. In healthy subjects, the mean plasma half-life was 1.5 hours. Lansoprazole is 97% bound to plasma proteins.

Metabolism – Lansoprazole is extensively metabolized in the liver. Two metabolites, which have little or no antisecretory activity, have been identified in measurable quantities in plasma. The plasma elimination half-life is < 2 hrs while the acid inhibitory effect lasts > 24 hrs.

Excretion – Following single-dose oral administration, virtually no unchanged lansoprazole was excreted in the urine. In one study, after a single oral dose, ≈ 33% was excreted in the urine and 66% was recovered in feces. This implies a significant biliary excretion of the metabolites.

Indications:

Duodenal ulcer: Short-term treatment (up to 4 weeks) for healing and symptomatic relief of active duodenal ulcer.

Erosive esophagitis: Short-term treatment (up to 8 weeks) for healing and symptomatic relief of all grades of erosive esophagitis.

Maintenance – Lansoprazole is indicated to maintain healing of erosive esophagitis. Controlled studies do not extend beyond 12 months.

Pathological hypersecretory conditions including Zollinger-Ellison syndrome: Long-term treatment of pathological hypersecretory conditions, including Zollinger-Ellison syndrome.

Contraindications:

Hypersensitivity to any component of the formulation.

Warnings:

Renal/Hepatic function impairment: In severe renal insufficiency, plasma protein binding decreased by 1% to 1.5% after use of 60 mg. Patients with renal insufficiency had a shortened elimination half-life and decreased total AUC (free and bound). In patients with various degrees of chronic hepatic disease, the mean plasma half-life of the drug was prolonged from 1.5 to 3.2 to 7.2 hours. An increase in mean AUC of up to 500% was observed at steady state in hepatically impaired patients compared with healthy subjects. Consider dose reduction in severe hepatic disease.

Elderly: The clearance of lansoprazole is decreased in the elderly, with elimination half-life increased ≈ 50% to 100%. The initial dosing regimen need not be altered, but subsequent doses > 30 mg/day should not be administered unless additional gastric acid suppression is necessary.

Pregnancy: Category B.

Lactation: It is not known whether lansoprazole is excreted in human breast milk.

Children: Safety and efficacy have not been established.

Precautions:

Gastric malignancy: Symptomatic response to therapy with lansoprazole does not preclude the presence of gastric malignancy.

Drug Interactions:

Drugs that may interact with lansoprazole include theophylline and sucralfate. Lansoprazole may interfere with the absorption of drugs where gastric pH is an important determinant of bioavailability (eg, ketoconazole, ampicillin, iron salts, digoxin).

Drug/Food interactions: Both C_{max} and AUC are diminished by about 50% if the drug is given 30 minutes after food as opposed to in the fasting condition. There is no significant food effect if the drug is given before meals.

Adverse Reactions:

In general, lansoprazole treatment has been well tolerated, and the only adverse reaction reported in ≥ 3% of patients was diarrhea.

Administration and Dosage:

Lansoprazole capsules can be opened, and the intact granules contained within can be sprinkled out on one tablespoon of applesauce and swallowed immediately. The granules should not be chewed or crushed. Take before eating.

Duodenal ulcer: 15 mg daily before eating for 4 weeks.

Erosive esophagitis: 30 mg daily before eating for up to 8 weeks. For patients who do not heal with lansoprazole for 8 weeks (5% to 10%) it may be helpful to give an additional 8 weeks of treatment. If there is a recurrence of erosive esophagitis, an additional 8 week course of lansoprazole may be considered.

Maintenance of healing of erosive esophagitis: 15 mg/day for adults.

Pathological hypersecretory conditions including Zollinger-Ellison syndrome: The recommended starting dose is 60 mg once a day. Adjust doses to individual patient needs and continue for as long as clinically indicated. Dosages up to 90 mg twice daily have been administered. Administer daily dosages of > 120 mg in divided doses. Some patients with Zollinger-Ellison syndrome have been treated continuously with lansoprazole for > 4 years.

Hepatic function impairment: Consider dosage adjustment in severe liver disease.

Elderly/Renal function impairment: No dosage adjustment is necessary.

METOCLOPRAMIDE

Tablets: 5 and 10 mg (*Rx*)	Various, *Reglan* (Robins), *Maxolon* (SK-Beecham)
Syrup: 5 mg/5 ml (*Rx*)	Various, *Reglan* (Robins)
Concentrated solution: 10 mg per ml (*Rx*)	*Metoclopramide Intensol* (Roxane)
Injection: 5 mg/ml (*Rx*)	Various, *Octamide PFS* (Adria), *Reglan* (Robins)

Actions:

Pharmacology: Metoclopramide stimulates motility of the upper GI tract without stimulating gastric, biliary or pancreatic secretions. Its mode of action is unclear, but it appears to sensitize tissues to the action of acetylcholine. The effect on motility does not depend on intact vagal innervation, but it can be abolished by anticholinergic drugs.

Pharmacokinetics:

Absorption/Distribution – Metoclopramide is rapidly and well absorbed. Onset of action is 1 to 3 minutes following an IV dose, 10 to 15 minutes following IM administration, and 30 to 60 minutes following an oral dose. Effects persist for 1 to 2 hours.

Relative to an IV dose of 20 mg, the absolute oral bioavailability of metoclopramide is 80% ± 15.5%. Peak plasma concentrations occur at about 1 to 2 hours after a single oral dose. Similar time to peak is observed after individual doses at steady state. The area under the drug concentration-time curve increases linearly with doses from 20 to 100 mg; peak concentrations also increase linearly with dose. The whole body volume of distribution is high (about 3.5 L/kg) which suggests extensive distribution of drug to the tissues.

Metabolism/Excretion – Approximately 85% of an orally administered dose appears in the urine within 72 hours. Of the 85% eliminated in the urine, about one-half is present as free or conjugated metoclopramide. The average elimination half-life in individuals with normal renal function is 5 to 6 hours. The drug is not extensively bound to plasma proteins (about 30%).

Indications:

Diabetic gastroparesis: Relief of symptoms associated with acute and recurrent diabetic gastroparesis (diabetic gastric stasis). Usual manifestations of delayed gastric emptying (ie, nausea, vomiting, heartburn, persistent fullness after meals, anorexia) respond within different time intervals. Significant relief of nausea occurs early and improves over 3 weeks. Relief of vomiting and anorexia may precede the relief of abdominal fullness by ≥ 1 week.

Oral:

Symptomatic gastroesophageal reflux – Short-term (4 to 12 weeks) therapy for adults with symptomatic documented gastroesophageal reflux who fail to respond to conventional therapy.

Parenteral: For prevention of nausea and vomiting associated with emetogenic cancer chemotherapy.

Prophylaxis of postoperative nausea and vomiting when nasogastric suction is undesirable.

Single doses may facilitate small bowel intubation when the tube does not pass the pylorus with conventional maneuvers.

Stimulates gastric emptying and intestinal transit of barium in cases where delayed emptying interferes with radiological examination of the stomach or small intestine.

Unlabeled uses: Used to improve lactation. Doses of 30 to 45 mg/day have increased milk secretion, possibly by elevating serum prolactin levels. (See Warnings.)

Studies have indicated some potential value of metoclopramide in the following conditions: Nausea and vomiting of a variety of etiologies (uncontrolled studies report 80% to 90% efficacy), including emesis during pregnancy and labor (see Warnings); gastric ulcer; anorexia nervosa (due to GI stimulation); to improve patient response to ergotamine, analgesics and sedatives in migraine, perhaps by enhancing absorption of the other medications; treatment of postoperative gastric bezoars (10 mg 3 or 4 times daily); diabetic cystoparesis (atonic bladder); esophageal variceal bleeding.

Contraindications:

When stimulation of GI motility might be dangerous (eg, in the presence of GI hemorrhage, mechanical obstruction or perforation); pheochromocytoma (the drug may cause a hypertensive crisis, probably due to release of catecholamines from the tumor; control such crises with phentolamine); sensitivity or intolerance to metoclopramide; epileptics or patients receiving drugs likely to cause extrapyramidal reactions (the frequency and severity of seizures or extrapyramidal reactions may be increased).

Warnings:

Depression has occurred in patients with and without prior history of depression. Give metoclopramide to patients with a prior history of depression only if the expected benefits outweigh the potential risks.

Extrapyramidal symptoms, manifested primarily as acute dystonic reactions, occur in ≈ 0.2% to 1% of patients treated with the usual adult dosages of 30 to 40 mg/day. These usually are seen during the first 24 to 48 hours of treatment, occur more frequently in children and young adults, and are even more frequent at the higher doses used in prophylaxis of vomiting due to cancer chemotherapy. If symptoms occur, they usually subside following 50 mg diphenhydramine IM. Benztropine 1 to 2 mg IM may also be used to reverse these reactions.

Parkinson-like symptoms have occurred, more commonly within the first 6 months after beginning treatment with metoclopramide, but occasionally after longer periods. These symptoms generally subside within 2 to 3 months following discontinuance of metoclopramide. Give metoclopramide cautiously, if at all, to patients with preexisting Parkinson's disease, since such patients may experience exacerbation of parkinsonian symptoms when taking metoclopramide.

Tardive dyskinesia, a syndrome consisting of potentially irreversible, involuntary, dyskinetic movements, may develop in patients treated with metoclopramide. Metoclopramide itself, however, may suppress (or partially suppress) the signs of tardive dyskinesia, thereby masking the underlying disease process. Therefore, the use of metoclopramide for the symptomatic control of tardive dyskinesia is not recommended.

Hypertension: In one study of hypertensive patients, IV metoclopramide released catecholamines. Use caution in hypertensive patients.

Anastomosis or closure of the gut: Giving a promotility drug such as metoclopramide could theoretically put increased pressure on suture lines following a gut anastomosis or closure. Consider the possibility when deciding whether to use metoclopramide or nasogastric suction in the prevention of postoperative nausea and vomiting.

Carcinogenesis: Elevated prolactin levels persist during chronic administration. Approximately one-third of human breast cancers are prolactin-dependent in vitro; use caution if metoclopramide is contemplated in a patient with previously detected breast cancer. Although galactorrhea, amenorrhea, gynecomastia and impotence have occurred with prolactin-elevating drugs, the clinical significance of elevated serum prolactin levels is unknown. An increase in mammary neoplasms has been found in rodents after chronic administration of prolactin-stimulating neuroleptic drugs; however, studies have not shown an association and evidence is not conclusive.

Pregnancy: Category B.

Lactation: Metoclopramide is excreted into breast milk and may concentrate at about twice the plasma level at 2 hours postdose. There appears to be no risk to the nursing infant with maternal doses ≤ 45 mg/day.

Children: Infants and children (ages 21 days to 3.3 years) with symptomatic gastroesophageal reflux have been treated with metoclopramide at a dosage of 0.5 mg/kg/day; symptoms improved, the duration of the disease was shortened, and surgery was avoided.

Methemoglobinemia has occurred in premature and full term neonates given metoclopramide orally, IV or IM, 1 to 4 mg/kg/day for 1 to ≥ 3 days; this did not occur at 0.5 mg/kg/day. Reverse methemoglobinemia by IV administration of methylene blue.

Precautions:

Hypoglycemia: Gastroparesis (gastric stasis) may be responsible for poor diabetic control. Exogenously administered insulins may act before food has left the stomach, leading to hypoglycemia.

Hazardous tasks: May cause drowsiness; observe caution while driving or performing other tasks requiring alertness, coordination or physical dexterity.

Drug Interactions:

Drugs that may affect metoclopramide include levodopa, anticholinergics and narcotic analgesics. Drugs that may be affected by metoclopramide include alcohol, cimetidine, cyclosporine, digoxin, levodopa, MAO inhibitors and succinylcholine.

Adverse Reactions:

Adverse reactions occurring in ≥ 3% of patients include restlessness; drowsiness; fatigue; lassitude; akathisia; dizziness; anxiety; dystonia; insomnia; headache; myoclonus; confusion; convulsive seizures; hallucinations; nausea; bowel disturbances, primarily diarrhea.

Administration and Dosage:

Diabetic gastroparesis: 10 mg 30 minutes before each meal and at bedtime for 2 to 8 weeks.

Determine initial route of administration by the severity of symptoms. With only the earliest manifestations of diabetic gastric stasis, initiate oral administration. If symptoms are severe, begin with parenteral therapy. Administer 10 mg IV over 1 to 2 minutes. Parenteral administration up to 10 days may be required before symptoms subside, then oral administration may be instituted. Reinstitute therapy at the earliest manifestation.

Symptomatic gastroesophageal reflux: 10 to 15 mg orally up to 4 times daily 30 minutes before each meal and at bedtime. If symptoms occur only intermittently or at specific times of the day, single doses up to 20 mg prior to the provoking situation may be preferred rather than continuous treatment. Occasionally, patients who are more sensitive to the therapeutic or adverse effects of metoclopramide (eg, elderly) will require only 5 mg per dose. Guide therapy directed at esophageal lesions by endoscopy. Therapy > 12 weeks has not been evaluated and cannot be recommended.

Prevention of postoperative nausea and vomiting: Inject IM near the end of surgery. The usual adult dose is 10 mg; however, doses of 20 mg may be used.

Prevention of chemotherapy-induced emesis: Infuse slowly IV over not less than 15 minutes, 30 minutes before beginning cancer chemotherapy; repeat every 2 hours for 2 doses, then every 3 hours for 3 doses.

The initial 2 doses should be 2 mg/kg if highly emetogenic drugs such as cisplatin or dacarbazine are used alone or in combination. For less emetogenic regimens, 1 mg/kg/dose may be adequate.

If extrapyramidal symptoms occur, administer 50 mg diphenhydramine IM.

IV admixture: When diluted in a parenteral solution, administer IV slowly over a period of not less than 15 minutes.

Direct IV injection: Inject undiluted metoclopramide slowly IV allowing 1 to 2 minutes for 10 mg, since a transient but intense feeling of anxiety and restlessness, followed by drowsiness, may occur with rapid administration.

Facilitation of small bowel intubation – If the tube has not passed the pylorus with conventional maneuvers in 10 minutes, administer a single undiluted dose slowly IV over 1 to 2 minutes.

Recommended single dose –

Adults: 10 mg (2 ml).

Children (6 to 14 years): 2.5 to 5 mg (0.5 to 1 ml).

Children (< 6 years): 0.1 mg/kg.

Radiological examinations – In patients where delayed gastric emptying interferes with radiological examination of the stomach or small intestine, a single dose may be administered slowly IV over 1 to 2 minutes.

Rectal administration: For outpatient treatment when oral dosing is not possible, suppositories containing 25 mg metoclopramide have been extemporaneously compounded (5 pulverized oral tablets in polyethylene glycol). Administer 1 suppository 30 to 60 minutes before each meal and at bedtime.

Renal/Hepatic function impairment: Since metoclopramide is excreted principally through the kidneys, in those patients whose creatinine clearance is < 40 ml/min, initiate therapy at approximately one-half the recommended dosage. Depending on clinical efficacy and safety considerations, the dosage may be increased or decreased as appropriate.

Metoclopramide undergoes minimal hepatic metabolism, except for simple conjugation. Its safe use has been described in patients with advanced liver disease whose renal function was normal.

Admixture compatibilities/incompatibilities:

Physically and chemically compatible up to 48 hours – Cimetidine; mannitol; potassium acetate; potassium chloride; potassium phosphate.

Physically compatible up to 48 hours – Ascorbic acid; benztropine; cytarabine; dexamethasone sodium phosphate; diphenhydramine; doxorubicin; heparin sodium; hydrocortisone sodium phosphate; lidocaine; magnesium sulfate; multi-vitamin infusion (must be refrigerated) vitamin B complex with ascorbic acid.

Incompatible – Cephalothin; chloramphenicol; sodium bicarbonate.

CISAPRIDE

Tablets: 10 and 20 mg (*Rx*)	*Propulsid* (Janssen)
Suspension: 1 mg/ml (*Rx*)	

Actions:

Pharmacology: Cisapride is an oral GI prokinetic agent. The mechanism of action appears to be primarily enhancement of release of acetylcholine at the myenteric plexus. In vitro cisapride is a serotonin-4 (5-HT_4) receptor agonist. This action may result in increased GI motility and cardiac rate.

Esophagus – Single doses of cisapride increased the lower esophageal sphincter pressure (LESP) and lower esophageal peristalsis compared to placebo or metoclopramide.

Stomach – Cisapride significantly accelerated gastric emptying of both liquids and solids.

Pharmacokinetics: Cisapride is rapidly absorbed after oral administration; peak plasma concentrations are reached 1 to 1.5 hours after dosing. Onset of action is ≈ 30 to 60 minutes after oral use. Absolute bioavailability is 35% to 40%. Cisapride is ≈ 98% bound to plasma proteins, mainly to albumin. Volume of distribution is ≈ 180 L, indicating extensive tissue distribution.

The plasma clearance is about 100 ml/min. The mean terminal half-life ranges from 6 to 12 hours. The drug is extensively metabolized; unchanged drug accounts for < 10% of urinary and fecal recovery following oral administration. Norcisapride, formed by N-dealkylation, is the principal metabolite in plasma, feces and urine.

Indications:

Heartburn: Symptomatic treatment of patients with nocturnal heartburn due to gastroesophageal reflux disease.

Contraindications:

Patients in whom an increase in GI motility could be harmful; hypersensitivity or intolerance to the drug; concomitant administration of ketoconazole, itraconazole, miconazole IV or troleandomycin.

Warnings:

Cardiac effects: Rare cases of serious cardiac arrhythmias, including ventricular arrhythmias and torsades de pointes associated with QT prolongation, have been observed in patients taking cisapride.

Concomitant use with ketoconazole is contraindicated because it has resulted in markedly elevated cisapride plasma concentrations and prolonged QT interval, and has rarely been associated with ventricular arrhythmias and torsades de pointes. Itraconazole, miconazole IV and troleandomycin are also expected to markedly raise cisapride plasma concentrations. Therefore, concomitant use with cisapride is also contraindicated.

Elderly: Steady-state plasma levels are generally higher in older than in younger patients, due to a moderate prolongation of the elimination half-life.

Pregnancy: Category C.

Lactation: Cisapride is excreted in breast milk at concentrations ≈ 1/20 of those observed in plasma.

Children: Safety and efficacy in children have not been established.

Precautions:

QT prolongation: Weigh potential benefits against risks prior to administration in patients with conditions associated with QT prolongation, such as congenital prolonged QT syndrome, uncorrected electrolyte disturbances or in patients who are taking other medications known to prolong QT interval.

Drug Interactions:

The acceleration of gastric emptying by cisapride could affect the rate of absorption of other drugs.

Drugs that may interact include anticholinergics, azole antifungals and macrolides (contraindicated), H_2 antagonists and anticoagulants.

Adverse Reactions:

Adverse reactions associated with cisapride may include: Diarrhea; abdominal pain; nausea; constipation; flatulence; rhinitis; sinusitis; pain; headache.

Administration and Dosage:

Adults: Initiate therapy with 10 mg 4 times daily at least 15 minutes before meals and at bedtime. In some patients the dosage will need to be increased to 20 mg, given as above, to obtain a satisfactory result.

LAXATIVES

BISACODYL	
Tablets, enteric coated: 5 mg (*otc*)	Various, *Dulcagen* (Goldline), *Dulcolax* (CIBA Cons.), *Fleet Laxative* (Fleet)
Suppositories: 10 mg (*otc*)	Various, *Bisacodyl Uniserts* (Upsher-Smith), *Bisco-Lax* (Raway), *Dulcagen* (Goldline), *Dulcolax* (CIBA Cons.), *Fleet Laxative* (Fleet)
BISACODYL TANNEX	
Powder: 1.5 mg bisacodyl and 2.5 g tannic acid per packet (*Rx*)	*Clysodrast* (Rhone-Poulenc Rorer)
CALCIUM SALTS OF SENNOSIDES A & B	
Tablets: 20 mg (*otc*)	*Ex-Lax Gentle Nature* (Sandoz)
CASCARA SAGRADA	
Tablets: 325 mg (*otc*)	Various
Liquid: (*otc*)	Various
CASTOR OIL	
Liquid: (*otc*)	Various, *Purge* (Fleming)
Emulsion: 67% and 95% castor oil with emulsifying agents (*otc*)	*Emulsoil* (Paddock), *Fleet Flavored Castor Oil* (Fleet)
Oil: 36.4% (*otc*)	*Neoloid* (Kenwood/Bradley)
CO_2 RELEASING SUPPOSITORIES	
Suppositories: Sodium bicarbonate and potassium bitartrate in a water soluble polyethylene glycol base (*otc*)	*Ceo-Two* (Beutlich)
DOCUSATE CALCIUM (DIOCTYL CALCIUM SULFOSUCCINATE)	
Capsules: 50 and 240 mg (*otc*)	Various, *Surfak Liquigels* (Upjohn)
DOCUSATE POTASSIUM (DIOCTYL POTASSIUM SULFOSUCCINATE)	
Tablets: 100 mg (*otc*)	*Dialose* (J & J-Merck), *Diocto-K* (Rugby) *Kasof* (J & J-Merck)
DOCUSATE SODIUM (DIOCTYL SODIUM SULFOSUCCINATE; DSS)	
Tablets: 100 mg (*otc*)	*Dialose* (J & J-Merck), *Regutol* (Schering-Plough)
Capsules: 50 and 100 mg (*otc*)	Various, *Colace* (Mead Johnson), *Disonate* (Lannett), *Modane Soft* (Adria), *Regulax SS* (Republic)
Capsules: 240 and 250 mg (*otc*)	Various, *Dioeze* (Century), *Disonate* (Lannett), *Regulax SS* (Republic)
Capsules, soft gel: 100 mg (*otc*)	*Correctol Extra Gentle* (Schering-Plough)
Syrup: 50 and 60 mg per 15 ml (*otc*)	Various, *Colace* (Mead Johnson), *Silace* (Silax)
GLYCERIN	
Suppositories: Glycerin and sodium stearate (*otc*)	Various, *Sani-Supp* (G & W Labs)
Liquid: 4 ml per applicator (*otc*)	*Fleet Babylax* (Fleet)
MINERAL OIL	
Liquid: Heavy mineral oil (*otc*)	Various
Jelly: Refined mineral oil (*otc*)	*Neo-Cultol* (Fisons)
Emulsion: Mineral oil with an emulsifier (*otc*)	*Agoral Plain* (Warner-Lambert), *Kondremul Plain* (Fisons), *Milkinol* (Schwarz Pharma Kremers Urban)
PHENOLPHTHALEIN	
Tablets: 60 and 130 mg phenolphthalein (*otc*)	*Alophen Pills* (Warner-Lambert), *Modane* (Adria)
Tablets: 90, 97.2 and 135 mg yellow phenolphthalein (*otc*)	*Ex-Lax Unflavored* (Sandoz Consumer), *Lax Pills* (G & W), *Espotabs* (Combe), *Feen-a-mint* (Schering-Plough), *Ex-Lax Maximum Relief* (Sandoz)
Tablets: 60 mg white phenolphthalein (*otc*)	*Prulet* (Mission)
Tablets, chewable: 65, 90 and 97.2 mg yellow phenolphthalein (*otc*)	*Feen-a-mint Chocolated* (Schering-Plough), *Ex-Lax Chocolated* (Sandoz Consumer), *Evac-U-Gen* (Walker), *Feen-a-mint* (Schering-Plough)
Tablets, chewable: 120 mg phenolphthalein (*otc*)	*Medilax* (Mission)
Wafers: 64.8 and 80 mg phenolphthalein (*otc*)	*Phenolax* (Upjohn) *Evac-U-Lax Tablets* (Hauck)
Gum: 97.2 mg yellow phenolphthalein (*otc*)	*Feen-a-mint* (Schering-Plough)

POLYCARBOPHIL	
Tablets: 500 mg (as calcium). Sodium free (*otc*)	*FiberCon* (Lederle)
Tablets, chewable: 500 mg (as calcium) (*otc*)	*Equalactin* (Numark), *Mitrolan* (Robins)
Tablets: 625 mg (*otc*)	*Fiber-Lax* (Rugby), *FiberNorm* (G & W), *Konsyl Fiber* (Konsyl)
Tablets, chewable: 1250 mg calcium carbophil (=1 g polycarbophil) (*otc*)	*Fiberall* (*Ciba Consumer*)
PSYLLIUM	
Powder: Psyllium (*otc*)	Various, *Fiberall Natural Flavor* (Ciba Consumer), *Fiberall Orange Flavor* (Ciba Consumer), *Hydrocil Instant* (Solvay Pharm.), *Konsyl*, *Konsyl-D* (Konsyl Pharm.), *Maalox Daily Fiber Therapy* (R-P Rorer), *Metamucil*, *Metamucil, Sugar Free* (Procter & Gamble), *Mylanta Natural Fiber Supplement* (J & J Merck), *Restore*, *Restore Sugar Free* (InAgra), *Serutan* (Menley & James), *Syllact* (Wallace)
Wafers: Psyllium (*otc*)	*Fiberall* (Ciba Consumer), *Metamucil* (Procter & Gamble)
Effervescent Powder: Psyllium (*otc*)	*Alramucil* (Alra), *Metamucil* (Procter & Gamble)
Granules: Psyllium (*otc*)	*Perdiem Fiber* (Rhone-Poulenc Rorer)
SALINE LAXATIVES	
Granules: Magnesium sulfate (*otc*)	*Epsom Salt* (Various)
Liquid: Magnesium hydroxide (*otc*)	Various, *Phillips' Milk of Magnesia*, *Phillips' Milk of Magnesia, Concentrated* (Glenbrook)
Solution: Magnesium citrate (*otc*)	*Citrate of Magnesia* (Dixon-Shane)
Solution: Sodium phosphates (*otc*)	Various, *Fleet Phospho-soda* (Fleet)
SENNA	
Tablets: 187, 217 and 374 mg senna concentrate (*otc*)	*Senexon* (Rugby), *Senolax* (Schein), *Senokot* (Purdue Frederick), *Senna-Gen* (Goldline), *Senokotxtra* (Purdue Fredrick)
Tablets: 600 mg senna equivalent (*otc*)	*Black-Draught* (Chattem)
Granules: 326 mg standardized senna concentrate per tsp (*otc*)	*Gentlax* (Blair), *Senokot* (Purdue Frederick)
Granules: 1.65 g senna equivalent per ½ tsp (*otc*)	*Black-Draught* (Chattem)
Liquid: 33.3 mg/ml senna concentrate (*otc*)	*Dr. Caldwell Senna Laxative* (Gebauer), *Fletcher's Castoria* (Mentholatum)
Syrup: 218 mg/5 ml standardized senna extract (*otc*)	*Senokot* (Purdue Frederick)
Syrup: Extract of senna fruit (*otc*)	*Dosalax* (Richwood)
Suppositories: 652 mg standardized (*otc*)	*Senokot* (Purdue Frederick)
MISCELLANEOUS BULK-PRODUCING LAXATIVES	
Powder: 2 mg methylcellulose per heaping tbsp (*otc*)	*Citrucel*, *Citrucel Sugar Free* (SK-Beecham)
Powder: Powdered cellulose (*otc*)	*Unifiber* (Dow B. Hickam)
Tablets: 750 mg adiastatic barley malt extract (*otc*)	*Maltsupex* (Wallace)
Powder: 8 g adiastatic barley malt extract/tbsp (*otc*)	*Maltsupex* (Wallace)
Liquid: 16 g adiastatic barley malt extract/tbsp (*otc*)	*Maltsupex* (Wallace)

Actions:

Pharmacology:

Pharmacologic Actions of Laxatives					
	Laxatives	Onset of action (hrs)	Site of action	Mechanism of action	Comments
Saline	Magnesium sulfate Magnesium hydroxide Magnesium citrate Sodium phosphate	0.5-3	Small & large intestine	Attract/retain water in intestinal lumen increasing intraluminal pressure; cholecystokinin release	May alter fluid and electrolyte balance. Sulfate salts are considered the most potent.
	Sod. phosphate/ biphosphate enema	0.03-0.25	Colon		
Irritant/Stimulant	Cascara Senna Phenolphthalein Bisacodyl Tablets Casanthranol	6-10	Colon	Direct action on intestinal mucosa; stimulate myenteric plexus; alters water and electrolyte secretion	Bile must be present for phenolphthalein to produce its effects. May prefer castor oil when more complete evacuation is required.
	Bisacodyl suppository	0.25-1			
	Castor oil	2-6	Small intestine		Castor oil is converted to ricinoleic acid (active com-ponent) in the gut.
Bulk-Producing	Methylcellulose Psyllium Polycarbophil	12-24 (up to 72)	Small & large intestine	Holds water in stool; mechanical distention; malt soup extract reduces fecal pH	Safest and most physiological.
Lubricant	Mineral oil	6-8	Colon	Retards colonic absorption of fecal water; softens stool	May decrease absorption of fat soluble vitamins.
Surfactants	Docusate	24-72	Small & large intestine	Detergent activity; facilitates admixture of fat & water to soften stool	Beneficial when feces are hard or dry, or in anorectal conditions where passage of a firm stool is painful.
Miscellaneous	Glycerin suppository	0.25-0.5	Colon	Local irritation; hyperosmotic action	Sodium stearate in preparation causes the local irritation.
	Lactulose	24-48	Colon	Delivers osmotically active molecules to colon	Also indicated in portal-systemic encephalopathy.

Indications:

Short-term treatment of constipation; certain stimulant, lubricant and saline laxatives are used to evacuate the colon for rectal and bowel examinations. Lubricant laxatives or fecal softeners are useful prophylactically in patients who should not strain during defecation (ie, following anorectal surgery, myocardial infarction). Psyllium is also useful in patients with irritable bowel syndrome, diverticular disease, spastic colon and hemorrhoids. Polycarbophil is indicated for constipation or diarrhea associated with conditions such as irritable bowel syndrome and diverticulosis; it is also for acute non-specific diarrhea. Mineral oil enema is indicated for relief of fecal impaction.

Unlabeled uses: Psyllium appears to be useful in the reduction of cholesterol levels as an adjunct to a dietary program.

Contraindications:

Hypersensitivity to any ingredient; nausea, vomiting or other symptoms of appendicitis; acute surgical abdomen; fecal impaction (except mineral oil enema); intestinal obstruction; undiagnosed abdominal pain.

Do not use bisacodyl tannex in patients with ulcerative lesions of the colon or in children < 10 years old.

Do not give **docusate sodium** if mineral oil is being given.

Warnings:

Fluid and electrolyte balance: Excessive laxative use may lead to significant fluid and electrolyte imbalance.

Preparations containing sodium should not be used by individuals on a sodium restricted diet or in the presence of edema, congestive heart failure, hypertension, megacolon or imperforate anus.

Megacolon, imperforate anus or CHF: Do not use sodium phosphate and sodium biphosphate in these patients; hypernatremic dehydration may occur.

Abuse/Dependency: Chronic use of laxatives, particularly stimulants, may lead to laxative dependency, which in turn may result in fluid and electrolyte imbalances, steatorrhea, osteomalacia, vitamin and mineral deficiencies and a poorly functioning colon. Also known as laxative abuse syndrome (LAS), it is difficult to diagnose.

Cathartic colon, a poorly functioning colon, results from the chronic abuse of stimulant cathartics.

Melanosis coli is a darkened pigmentation of the colonic mucosa resulting from chronic use of anthraquinone derivatives.

Bisacodyl tannex: Use with caution when multiple enemas are administered. Tannic acid is hepatotoxic if absorbed in sufficient quantity.

Lipid pneumonitis may result from oral ingestion and aspiration of mineral oil, especially when patient reclines. The young, elderly, debilitated and dysphagic are at greatest risk.

Renal function impairment: Up to 20% of the magnesium in magnesium salts may be absorbed. Do not use products containing phosphate, sodium, magnesium or potassium salts in the presence of renal dysfunction.

Pregnancy: Category C. (Docusate sodium, cascara sagrada, mineral oil, senna) Do not use castor oil during pregnancy; its irritant effect may induce premature labor. Mineral oil may decrease absorption of fat-soluble vitamins. Improper use of saline cathartics can lead to dangerous electrolyte imbalance. If needed, limit use to bulk forming or surfactant laxatives.

Lactation: Cascara sagrada is excreted in breast milk. There may be an increased incidence of diarrhea in the nursing infant.

Children: Physical manipulation of a glycerin suppository in infants often initiates defecation; hence, adverse effects are minimal. Do not administer enemas to children < 2 years of age. Do not use bisacodyl tannex in children < 10 years of age.

Precautions:

Rectal bleeding or failure to respond to therapy may indicate a serious condition which may require further medical attention.

Phenolphthalein may cause a skin hypersensitivity characterized by a fixed drug eruption.

Discoloration of acid urine to yellow-brown may occur with cascara sagrada or senna. Pink-red, red-violet or red-brown discoloration of alkaline urine may occur with phenolphthalein, cascara sagrada or senna.

Impaction or obstruction may be caused by bulk-forming agents if temporarily arrested in their passage through the alimentary canal (eg, patients with esophageal strictures).

Drug Interactions:

Drugs that may interact with laxatives include mineral oil, milk or antacids, lipid soluble vitamins (A, D, E and K) and tetracycline.

Adverse Reactions:

Excessive bowel activity (griping, diarrhea, nausea, vomiting); perianal irritation; weakness; dizziness; fainting; palpitations; sweating; bloating; flatulence; abdominal cramps.

Esophageal, gastric, small intestinal and rectal obstruction due to the accumulation of mucilaginous components of bulk laxatives have occurred.

Large doses of mineral oil may cause anal seepage, resulting in itching (pruritis ani), irritation, hemorrhoids and perianal discomfort.

Bisacodyl suppositories may cause proctitis and inflammation. Not recommended for long-term use.

Administration and Dosage:

BISACODYL: Swallow whole; do not chew. Do not take within 1 hour of antacids or milk.

Tablets – *Adults*- 10 to 15 mg in a single dose once daily. Up to 30 mg has been used for preparation of lower GI tract for special procedures.

Children (6 to < 12 years)- 5 to 10 mg once daily.

Suppositories – *Adults*- 10 mg once daily.

Children (6 to < 12 years)- 5 mg once daily.

BISACODYL TANNEX:

Cleansing enema – 2.5 g (1 packet) in 1 L warm water.

Barium enema – 2.5 or 5 g in 1 L barium suspension.

Total dosage for one colonic examination should not exceed 7.5 g. Do not give > 10 g within a 72–hour period.

Do not administer to children < 10 years of age.

CALCIUM SALTS OF SENNOSIDES A & B:

Adults – 1 to 2 tablets wtih water at bedtime.

Children (≥ 6 years) – 1 tablet/day.

CASCARA SAGRADA:

Tablets – 1 tablet at bedtime.

Liquid – 5 ml.

CASTOR OIL:

Liquid – *Adults*- Daily dose range, 15 to 60 ml.

Children (2 to 12 years)- 5 to 15 ml.

Infants- 2.5 to 7.5 ml.

Emulsion – *Adults*- 67%, 15 to 60 ml; 95%, 45 ml (should be mixed with ½ to 1 glass liquid).

Children (2 to 12 years)- 67%, 15 ml; 95%, 5 to 10 ml (should be mixed with ½ to 1 glass liquid).

DOCUSATE CALCIUM (Dioctyl Calcium Sulfosuccinate):

Adults – 240 mg daily until bowel movements are normal.

Children (≥ 6 years) – 50 to 150 mg daily.

DOCUSATE POTASSIUM (Dioctyl Potassium Sulfosuccinate):

Adults – 100 to 300 mg daily until bowel movements are normal.

Children (≥ 6 years) – 100 mg at bedtime.

DOCUSATE SODIUM (Dioctyl Sodium Sulfosuccinate; DSS):

Adults and older children – 50 to 500 mg.

Children (6 to 12) – 40 to 120 mg.

Children (3 to 6) – 20 to 60 mg.

Children (< 3) – 10 to 40 mg.

GLYCERIN:

Suppositories – Insert one suppository high in the rectum and retain 15 minutes; it need not melt to produce laxative action.

Rectal liquid – With gentle, steady pressure, insert stem with tip pointing twoards navel. Squeeze unit until nearly all the liquid is expelled, then remove. A small amount of liquid will remain in unit.

MINERAL OIL:

Dose –

Adults: 5 to 45 ml.

Children: 5 to 20 ml. Although usual directions are to give at bedtime, caution is advised because of lipid pneumonitis.

PHENOLPHTHALEIN: Yellow phenolphthalein is 2 to 3 times more potent than white phenolphthalein.

Dose – 60 to 194 mg, preferably at bedtime.

POLYCARBOPHIL:

Adults – 1 g 1 to 4 times daily or as needed. Do not exceed 6 g in 24 hours.

Children – 500 mg 1 to 3 times daily or as needed. Do not exceed 3 g/day.

(3 to < 6 years): 500 mg 1 to 2 times daily or as needed. Do not exceed 1.5 g/day.

For severe diarrhea, repeat the dose every 30 min; do not exceed maximum daily dose.

SALINE LAXATIVES:

Magnesium sulfate –

Adults: 10 to 15 g in glass of water.

Children: 5 to 10 g in glass of water.

Magnesium hydroxide –

Adults: Recommended dosage varies from product to product, ranging from 10 to 60 ml per day. See individual package labeling for specific dosing information.

Children (≥ 2 years): 5 to 30 ml, depending on age (must be at least 2 years old).

Magnesium citrate –

Adults: 1 glassful (approx. 240 ml) as needed.

Children: ½ the adult dose as needed; repeat if necessary.

Sodium phosphates –

Adults: 20 to 30 ml mixed with ½ glass cool water.

Children: 5 to 15 ml.

SENNA CONCENTRATE: The following dosages are for senna concentrate *only*. For other forms of senna, consult labeling. Dosages are different.

Tablets (187 and 217 mg) – Adults- 2 tablets, up to 8/day.

Children- 1 tablet, up to 4/day.

Tablets (374 mg) – Adults- 1 tablet at bedtime, up to 4/day

Granules – Adults- 1 tsp, up to 4/day.

Children-½ tsp, up 2 tsp/day.

Suppositories – Adults- 1 at bedtime; repeat in 2 hours if necessary.

Children-½ suppository at bedtime.

Liquid – Adults- 15 to 30 ml with or after meals or at bedtime.

Children *(6 to 15 years)*- 10 to 15 ml at bedtime.

Children *(2 to 5 years)*- 5 to 10 ml at bedtime.

Syrup – Adults- 10 to 15 ml at bedtime (up to 30 ml/day).

Children *(5 to 15 years)*- 5 to 10 ml at bedtime (up to 20 ml/day).

Children *(1 to 5 years)*- 2.5 to 5 ml at bedtime (up to 10 ml/day).

Children *(1 month to 1 year)*- 1.25 to 2.5 ml at bedtime (up to 5 ml/day).

MISCELLANEOUS BULK-PRODUCING LAXATIVES:

Citrucel –

Adults and children ≥ 12 years: 1 heaping tbsp (19 g) in 8 oz cold water, 1 to 3 times daily.

Children (6 to < 12 years): ½ the adult dose in 4 oz cold water, 1 to 3 times daily.

Unifiber is classified as a dietary fiber supplement. It is not FDA approved as a bulk-producing laxative. Dose is 1 to 2 tbsp in liquid once or twice daily.

Maltsupex –

Tablets: Adults, 12 to 64 g/day. Initially, 4 tabs 4 times daily (meals and bedtime).

Powder: 16 g = 1 heaping tablespoon

Adults, up to 32 g twice daily for 3 or 4 days, then 16 to 32 g at bedtime. Children 6 to 12 years, up to 16 g twice daily for 3 or 4 days; 2 to 6 years, 8 g twice daily for 3 or 4 days. Infants, > 1 month (bottlefed), 8 to 16 g daily in formula for 3 or 4 days, then 4 to 8 g daily in formula; > 1 month (breastfed), 4 g in 2 to 4 oz water or fruit juice twice daily for 3 or 4 days.

Liquid: Adults, 2 tbsp twice daily for 3 or 4 days, then 1 to 2 tbsp at bedtime. Children 6 to 12 years, 1 to 2 tbsp once or twice daily for 3 or 4 days; 2 to 6 years, ½ tbsp once or twice daily for 3 or 4 days. Infants, > 1 month (bottlefed), ½ to 2 tbsp daily in formula for 3 or 4 days, then 1 to 2 tsp daily in formula; > 1 month (breastfed), 1 to 2 tsp in 2 to 4 oz water or fruit juice once or twice daily for 3 or 4 days.

POLYETHYLENE GLYCOL-ELECTROLYTE SOLUTION (PEG-ES)

POLYETHYLENE GLYCOL-ELECTROLYTE SOLUTION (PEG-ES)	
Powder for solution: 60 g PEG 3350, 1.46 g NaCl, 0.745 g KCl, 1.68 g sodium bicarb and 5.68 g sodium sulfate per L. (*Rx*)	*Col-Lav* (Copley)
Powder for Oral Solution: 146 mg NaCl, 168 mg sodium bicarb, 568 mg sodium sulfate anhydrous, 74.5 mg KCl, 6 g PEG 3350/100 ml. (*Rx*)	*Colovage* (Dynapharm)
Powder for Oral Solution: 1 gal: 227.1 g PEG 3350, 21.5 g sodium sulfate, 6.36 g sodium bicarb, 5.53 g NaCl, 2.82 g KCl (*Rx*)	*CoLyte* (Schwarz Pharma)
4 L: 240 g PEG 3350, 22.72 g sodium sulfate, 6.72 g sodium bicarb, 5.84 g NaCl, 2.98 g KCl. (*Rx*)	
Powder for solution: 59 g PEG 3350, 5.685 g sodium sulfate, 1.685 sodium bicarb, 1.465 g sodium chloride and 0.743 g potassium chloride per L. (*Rx*)	*Go-Evac* (Copley)
Powder for Oral Solution: 236 g PEG 3350, 22.74 g sodium sulfate, 6.74 g sodium bicarb, 5.86 g NaCl, 2.97 g KCl. (*Rx*)	*GoLYTELY* (Braintree Labs)
Powder for Oral Solution: 420 g PEG 3350, 5.72 g sodium bicarb, 11.2 g NaCl, 1.48 g KCl. (*Rx*)	*NuLytely* (Braintree)
Oral Solution: 146 mg NaCl, 168 mg sodium bicarb, 1.29 g sodium sulfate decahydrate, 75 mg KCl, 6 g PEG 3350, 30 mg polysorbate-80/100 ml. (*Rx*)	*OCL* (Abbott)

Actions:

Pharmacology: Oral solution induces diarrhea (onset 30 to 60 min) which rapidly cleanses the bowel, usually within 4 hours. Polyethylene glycol 3350 (PEG 3350), a nonabsorbable solution, acts as an osmotic agent.

Indications:

For bowel cleansing prior to GI examination.

Unlabeled uses: PEG electrolyte solutions are useful in the management of acute iron overdose in children.

Contraindications:

GI obstruction; gastric retention; bowel perforation; toxic colitis, megacolon or ileus.

Warnings:

Pregnancy: Category C.

Children: Safety and efficacy for use in children have not been established.

Several studies in infants and children ranging in age from 3 weeks to 18 years showed that the use of PEG-electrolyte solutions are safe and effective in bowel evacuation.

Precautions:

Barium enema: Patient prep may be less satisfactory with this solution; it may interfere with barium coating of colonic mucosa using double-contrast technique.

Regurgitation/Aspiration: Observe unconscious or semiconscious patients with impaired gag reflex and those who are otherwise prone to regurgitation or aspiration during use, especially if given via a nasogastric tube. If GI obstruction or perforation is suspected, rule out these contraindications before administration.

Severe bloating: If a patient experiences severe bloating, distention or abdominal pain, slow or temporarily discontinue administration until symptoms abate.

Severe ulcerative colitis: Use with caution.

Drug Interactions:

Oral medication given within 1 hour of start of therapy may be flushed from the GI tract and not absorbed.

Adverse Reactions:

Nausea, abdominal fullness, bloating (≤ 50%); abdominal cramps, vomiting, anal irritation (less frequent).

Administration and Dosage:

The patient should fast approximately 3 to 4 hours prior to ingestion of the solution; solid foods should never be given < 2 hours before solution is administered.

One method is to schedule patients for midmorning exam, allowing 3 hours for drinking and 1 hour to complete bowel evacuation. Another method is to give the solution the evening before the exam, particularly if the patient is to have a barium enema. No foods except clear liquids are permitted after solution administration.

Adult dosage is 4 L orally of solution prior to GI exam. May be given via a nasogastric tube to patients unwilling or unable to drink the preparation. Drink 240 ml every 10 minutes until 4 L are consumed or until the rectal effluent is clear. Rapid drinking of each portion is preferred to drinking small amounts continuously. Nasogastric tube administration is at the rate of 20 to 30 ml/minutes (1.2 to 1.8 L/hour). The first bowel movement should occur in ≈ 1 hour.

LACTULOSE

Syrup: 10 g lactulose per 15 ml (*Rx*)	Various, *Cephulac*, *Chronulac* (HMR), *Cholac*, *Constilac* (Alra), *Duphalac* (Solvay Pharm.), *Evalose* (Copley), *Heptalac* (Copley)

Actions:

Pharmacology: Lactulose, a synthetic disaccharide analog of lactose containing galactose and fructose, decreases blood ammonia concentrations and reduces the degree of portal-systemic encephalopathy.

The human GI tissue does not have an enzyme capable of hydrolysis of this disaccharide; as a result, oral doses pass to the colon virtually unchanged. After reaching the colon, lactulose is metabolized by bacteria resulting in the formation of low molecular weight acids and carbon dioxide. These products produce an increased osmotic pressure and slightly acidify the colonic contents, resulting in an increase in stool water content and stool softening. Since the colonic contents are more acidic than the blood, ammonia can migrate from the blood into the colon. The acid colonic contents convert NH_3 to the ammonium ion $[NH_4]^+$, trapping it and preventing its absorption. The laxative action of the lactulose metabolites then expels the trapped ammonium ion from the colon.

Pharmacokinetics: Lactulose is poorly absorbed. When given orally, only small amounts reach the blood. Urinary excretion is ≤ 3% and is essentially complete within 24 hours. Lactulose does not exert its effect until it reaches the colon.

Indications:

Chronulac, Constilac, Duphalac: Treatment of constipation.

Cephulac, Cholac, Enulose: Prevention and treatment of portal-systemic encephalopathy, including the stages of hepatic pre-coma and coma.

Contraindications:

Patients who require a low galactose diet.

Warnings:

Electrocautery procedures: A theoretical hazard may exist for patients being treated with lactulose who may undergo electrocautery procedures during proctoscopy or colonoscopy. Accumulation of H_2 gas in significant concentration in the presence of an electrical spark may result in an explosion.

Pregnancy: Category B.

Lactation: It is not known whether lactulose is excreted in breast milk.

Children: Safety and efficacy for use in children have not been established. Infants receiving lactulose may develop hyponatremia and dehydration.

Precautions:

Monitoring: In the overall management of portal-systemic encephalopathy, there is serious underlying liver disease with complications such as electrolyte disturbance which may require other specific therapy. Elderly, debilitated patients who receive lactulose for > 6 months should have serum electrolytes (potassium, chloride) and carbon dioxide measured periodically.

Diabetics: Lactulose syrup contains galactose and lactose. Use with caution in these individuals.

Concomitant laxative use: Do not use other laxatives, especially during the initial phase of therapy for portal-systemic encephalopathy; the resulting loose stools may falsely suggest adequate lactulose dosage.

Drug Interactions:

Drugs that may affect lactulose include neomycin and other anti-infectives, and antacids.

Adverse Reactions:

Adverse reactions may include nausea and vomiting and gaseous distention with flatulence, belching and abdominal discomfort such as cramping. Excessive dosage can lead to diarrhea.

Administration and Dosage:

Chronulac, Constilac, Duphalac:

Treatment of constipation – 15 to 30 ml (10 to 20 g lactulose) daily, increased to 60 ml/day, if necessary.

Cephulac, Cholac, Enulose: Prevent and treat portal-systemic encephalopathy:

Oral –

Adults: 30 to 45 ml, 3 or 4 times daily. Adjust dosage every day or two to produce 2 or 3 soft stools daily. Hourly doses of 30 to 45 ml may be used to induce rapid laxation in the initial phase of therapy.

Children: Recommended initial daily oral dose in infants is 2.5 to 10 ml in divided doses. For older children and adolescents, the total daily dose is 40 to 90 ml. If the initial dose causes diarrhea, reduce immediately. If diarrhea persists, discontinue use.

Rectal – Administer to adults during impending coma or coma stage of portal-systemic encephalopathy when the danger of aspiration exists or when endoscopic or intubation procedures interfere with oral administration.

May be more palatable when mixed with fruit juice, water or milk.

DIFENOXIN HCl WITH ATROPINE SULFATE

Tablets: 1 mg difenoxin (as HCl) and 0.025 mg atropine sulfate (*c-iv*)	*Motofen* (Carnrick)

Actions:

Pharmacology: Difenoxin is an antidiarrheal agent chemically related to meperidine. Atropine sulfate is present to discourage deliberate overdosage.

Difenoxin manifests its antidiarrheal effect by slowing intestinal motility. The mechanism of action is by a local effect on the gastrointestinal wall.

Difenoxin is the principal active metabolite of diphenoxylate and is effective at one-fifth the dosage of diphenoxylate.

Pharmacokinetics: Difenoxin is rapidly and extensively absorbed orally. Mean peak plasma levels occur within 40 to 60 minutes. Plasma levels decline to less than 10% of their peak values within 24 hours and to less than 1% of their peak values within 72 hours. This decline parallels the appearance of difenoxin and its metabolites in the urine. Difenoxin is metabolized to an inactive hydroxylated metabolite. Both the drug and its metabolites are excreted, mainly as conjugates, in urine and feces.

Indications:

Adjunctive therapy in management of acute nonspecific diarrhea and acute exacerbations of chronic functional diarrhea.

Contraindications:

Diarrhea associated with organisms that penetrate the intestinal mucosa (eg, toxigenic *E coli, Salmonella* sp, *Shigella;*) and pseudomembranous colitis associated with broad-spectrum antibiotics. Antiperistaltic agents may prolong or worsen diarrhea.

Children under 2 years of age because of the decreased margin of safety of drugs in this class in younger age groups.

Hypersensitivity to difenoxin, atropine or any of the inactive ingredients; jaundice.

Warnings:

Difenoxin HCl with atropine sulfate is not innocuous; strictly adhere to dosage recommendations. Overdosage may result in severe respiratory depression and coma, possibly leading to permanent brain damage or death.

Fluid and electrolyte balance: The use of this drug does not preclude the administration of appropriate fluid and electrolyte therapy. Dehydration, particularly in children, may further influence the variability of response and may predispose to delayed difenoxin intoxication. Drug-induced inhibition of peristalsis may result in fluid retention in the colon, and this may further aggravate dehydration and electrolyte imbalance.

Ulcerative colitis: Agents which inhibit intestinal motility or delay intestinal transit time have induced toxic megacolon. Consequently, carefully observe patients with acute ulcerative colitis.

Liver and kidney disease: Use with extreme caution in patients with advanced hepatorenal disease and in all patients with abnormal liver function tests since hepatic coma may be precipitated.

Atropine: A subtherapeutic dose of atropine has been added to difenoxin to discourage deliberate overdosage. A recommended dose is not likely to cause prominent anticholinergic side effects, but avoid in patients in whom anticholinergic drugs are contraindicated. In children, signs of atropinism may occur even with recommended doses, particularly in patients with Down's Syndrome.

Pregnancy: Category C.

Lactation: Decide whether to discontinue nursing or to discontinue the drug, taking into account the importance of the drug to the mother.

Children: Contraindicated in children under 2 years of age. Safety and efficacy in children below the age of 12 have not been established.

Precautions:

Drug abuse and dependence: Addiction to (dependence on) difenoxin is theoretically possible at high dosage. Therefore, do not exceed recommended dosage.

Drug Interactions:

Drugs that may interact include MAO inhibitors, barbiturates, tranquilizers, narcotics and alcohol.

Adverse Reactions:

Adverse reactions may include nausea, dry mouth, dizziness, lightheadedness and drowsiness.

Administration and Dosage:

Adults: Recommended starting dose: 2 tablets, then 1 tablet after each loose stool; 1 tablet every 3 to 4 hours as needed. The total dosage during any 24 hour treatment period should not exceed 8 tablets. For diarrhea in which clinical improvement is not observed in 48 hours, continued administration is not recommended. For acute diarrhea and acute exacerbations of functional diarrhea, treatment beyond 48 hours is usually not necessary.

DIPHENOXYLATE HCl WITH ATROPINE SULFATE

Tablets: 2.5 mg diphenoxylate HCl and 0.025 mg atropine sulfate (*c-v*)	Various, *Logen* (Goldline), *Lomotil* (Searle), *Lonox* (Geneva)
Liquid: 2.5 mg diphenoxylate HCl and 0.025 mg atropine sulfate per 5 ml (*c-v*)	Various, *Lomotil* (Searle)

Actions:

Pharmacology: Diphenoxylate, a constipating meperidine congener, lacks analgesic activity. High doses cause opioid activity.

Pharmacokinetics: Bioavailability of tablet vs liquid is ≈ 90%. Diphenoxylate is rapidly, extensively metabolized to diphenoxylic acid (difenoxine), the active major metabolite. Elimination half-life is ≈ 12 to 14 hrs. An average of 14% of drug and metabolites are excreted over 4 days in urine, 49% in feces. Urinary excretion of unmetabolized drug is < 1%; difenoxine plus its glucuronide conjugate constitutes ≈ 6%.

Indications:

Adjunctive therapy in the management of diarrhea.

Contraindications:

Children < 2 years old due to greater variability of response; hypersensitivity to diphenoxylate or atropine; obstructive jaundice; diarrhea associated with pseudomembranous enterocolitis or enterotoxin-producing bacteria.

Warnings:

Diarrhea: Diphenoxylate may prolong or aggravate diarrhea associated with organisms that penetrate intestinal mucosa (ie, toxigenic *Escherichia coli*, *Salmonella*, *Shigella*) or in pseudomembranous enterocolitis associated with broad-spectrum antibiotics. Do not use diphenoxylate in these conditions. In some patients with acute ulcerative colitis, diphenoxylate may induce toxic megacolon.

Fluid/electrolyte balance: Dehydration, particularly in younger children, may influence variability of response and may predispose to delayed diphenoxylate intoxication. Inhibition of peristalsis may result in fluid retention in the intestine, which may further aggravate dehydration and electrolyte imbalance.

Hepatic function impairment: Use with extreme caution in patients with advanced hepatorenal disease or abnormal liver function; hepatic coma may be precipitated.

Pregnancy: Category C.

Lactation: Diphenoxylic acid may be excreted in breast milk and atropine is excreted in breast milk.

Children: Use with caution; signs of atropinism may occur with recommended doses, particularly in Down's syndrome patients. Use with caution in young children due to variable response. Not recommended in children < 2 years old.

Precautions:

Drug abuse and dependence: In recommended doses, diphenoxylate has not produced addiction and is devoid of morphine-like subjective effects. At high doses, it exhibits codeine-like subjective effects; therefore, addiction to diphenoxylate is possible. A subtherapeutic dose of atropine may discourage deliberate abuse.

Drug Interactions:

Drugs that may interact include MAO inhibitors, barbiturates, tranquilizers and alcohol.

Adverse Reactions:

Adverse reactions may include dry skin and mucous membranes, flushing, hyperthermia, tachycardia, urinary retention (especially in children), pruritus, gum swelling, angioneurotic edema, urticaria, anaphylaxis, dizziness, drowsiness, sedation, headache, malaise, lethargy, restlessness, euphoria, depression, numbness of extremities, confusion, anorexia, nausea, vomiting, abdominal discomfort, toxic megacolon and pancreatitis.

Administration and Dosage:

Adults: Individualize dosage. Initial dose is 5 mg 4 times a day.

Children: In children 2 to 12 years of age, use liquid form only. The recommended initial dosage is 0.3 to 0.4 mg/kg daily, in 4 divided doses.

Diphenoxylate w/Atropine Pediatric Dosage

Age (years)	Approximate weight kg	lb	Dosage (ml) (4 times daily)
2	11-14	24-31	1.5-3
3	12-16	26-35	2-3
4	14-20	31-44	2-4
5	16-23	35-51	2.5-4.5
6-8	17-32	38-71	2.5-5
9-12	23-55	51-121	3.5-5

Reduce dosage as soon as initial control of symptoms is achieved. Maintenance dosage may be as low as ¼ of the initial daily dosage. Do not exceed recommended dosage. Clinical improvement of acute diarrhea is usually observed within 48 hours. If clinical improvement of chronic diarrhea is not seen within 10 days after a maximum daily dose of 20 mg, symptoms are unlikely to be controlled by further use.

LOPERAMIDE HCl

Tablets: 2 mg (*otc*)	*Imodium A-D Caplets* (McNeil-CPC), *Kaopectate II Caplets* (Upjohn), *Maalox Anti-Diarrheal Caplets* (R-P Rorer)
Capsules: 2 mg (*Rx*)	Various, *Imodium* (Janssen)
Liquid: 1 mg/5 ml (*otc*)	Various, *Imodium A-D* (McNeil-CPC)
Liquid: 1 mg/ml (*otc*)	*Pepto Diarrhea Control* (Procter & Gamble)

Actions:

Pharmacology: Loperamide slows intestinal motility and affects water and electrolyte movement through the bowel. It inhibits peristalsis by a direct effect on the circular and longitudinal muscles of the intestinal wall. It reduces daily fecal volume, increases viscosity and bulk density and diminishes the loss of fluid and electrolytes.

Pharmacokinetics:

Absorption/Distribution – Loperamide is 40% absorbed after oral administration and does not penetrate well into the brain. Peak plasma levels occur approximately 5 hours after capsule administration, 2.5 hours after liquid administration and are similar for both formulations.

Metabolism/Excretion – The apparent elimination half-life is 10.8 hrs (range, 9.1 to 14.4 hrs). Of a 4 mg oral dose, 25% is excreted unchanged in the feces, and 1.3% is excreted in the urine as free drug and glucuronic acid conjugate within 3 days.

Indications:

Rx: Control and symptomatic relief of acute nonspecific diarrhea and of chronic diarrhea associated with inflammatory bowel disease.

For reducing the volume of discharge from ileostomies.

OTC: Control of symptoms of diarrhea, including Traveler's Diarrhea.

Contraindications:

Hypersensitivity to the drug and in patients who must avoid constipation.

OTC use: Bloody diarrhea; body temperature > 101°F.

Warnings:

Diarrhea: Do not use loperamide in acute diarrhea associated with organisms that penetrate the intestinal mucosa (enteroinvasive *Escherichia coli*, *Salmonella* and *Shigella*) or in pseudomembranous colitis associated with broad-spectrum antibiotics.

Acute ulcerative colitis: In some patients with acute ulcerative colitis, agents which inhibit intestinal motility or delay intestinal transit time may induce toxic megacolon.

Fluid/electrolyte depletion may occur in patients who have diarrhea. Loperamide use does not preclude administration of appropriate fluid and electrolyte therapy.

Pregnancy: Category B.

Lactation: It is not known whether loperamide is excreted in breast milk.

Children: Not recommended for use in children < 2 years old. Use special caution in young children because of the greater variability of response in this age group. Dehydration may further influence variability of response. Dosage has not been established for children in treatment of chronic diarrhea.

Precautions:

Acute diarrhea: If clinical improvement is not observed in 48 hours, discontinue use.

Hepatic dysfunction: Monitor patients with hepatic dysfunction closely for signs of CNS toxicity because of the apparent large first-pass biotransformation.

Adverse Reactions:

Adverse reactions may include abdominal pain, distention or discomfort, constipation, dry mouth, nausea, vomiting, tiredness, drowsiness or dizziness, hypersensitivity reactions (including skin rash).

Administration and Dosage:

Rx:

Acute diarrhea –

Adults: 4 mg followed by 2 mg after each unformed stool. Do not exceed 16 mg/day. Clinical improvement is usually observed within 48 hours.

Children:

Loperamide Pediatric Dosage (First Day Schedule)			
Age (years)	Weight (kg)	Doseform	Amount
2-5	13-20	liquid	1 mg tid
6-8	20-30	liquid or capsule	2 mg bid
8-12	> 30	liquid or capsule	2 mg tid

Subsequent doses: Administer 1 mg/10 kg only after a loose stool. Total daily dosage should not exceed recommended dosages for the first day.

Chronic diarrhea –

Adults: 4 mg followed by 2 mg after each unformed stool until diarrhea is controlled. When optimal daily dosage (average, 4 to 8 mg) has been established, administer as a single dose or in divided doses.

If clinical improvement is not observed after treatment with 16 mg/day for at least 10 days, symptoms are unlikely to be controlled by further use.

Children – Dose has not been established.

OTC:

Acute diarrhea, including Traveler's Diarrhea –

Adults: 4 mg after first loose bowel movement followed by 2 mg after each subsequent loose bowel movement but no more than 8 mg/day for no more than 2 days.

Children: 9 to 11 years old (60 to 95 lbs), 2 mg after first loose bowel movement followed by 1 mg after each subsequent loose bowel movement but no more than 6 mg/day for no more than 2 days; *6 to 8 years old (48 to 59 lbs)*, 1 mg after first loose bowel movement followed by 1 mg after each subsequent loose bowel movement but no more than 4mg/day for no more than 2 days; < *6 years old (up to 47 lbs)*, consult physician (not for use in children < 6).

BISMUTH SUBSALICYLATE (BSS)

Tablets, chewable: 262 mg (*otc*)	Various, *Pepto-Bismol* (Procter & Gamble)
Caplets: 262 mg (*otc*)	*Pepto-Bismol* (Procter & Gamble)
Liquid: 130 mg/15 ml (*otc*)	Various, *Pepto-Bismol* (Procter & Gamble)
262 mg/15 ml (*otc*)	
524 mg/15 ml (*otc*)	

Actions:

Pharmacology: Bismuth subsalicylate (BSS) appears to have antisecretory and antimicrobial effects in vitro and may have some anti-inflammatory effects. The salicylate moiety provides the antisecretory effect, while the bismuth moiety may exert direct antimicrobial effects against bacterial and viral enteropathogens.

Pharmacokinetics: BSS undergoes chemical dissociation in the GI tract. Two BSS tablets yield 204 mg salicylate. Following ingestion, salicylate is absorbed, with > 90% recovered in the urine; plasma levels are similar to levels achieved after a comparable dose of aspirin. Absorption of bismuth is negligible.

Indications:

For indigestion without causing constipation; nausea; control of diarrhea, including Traveler's Diarrhea, within 24 hours. Also relieves abdominal cramps.

Unlabeled uses: Bismuth subsalicylate has also been used in the prevention of Traveler's Diarrhea (enterotoxigenic *Escherichia coli*).

BSS has also been used for chronic infantile diarrhea and for symptoms of Norwalk virus-induced gastroenteritis.

Precautions:

Impaction may occur in infants and debilitated patients.

Radiologic examinations: May interfere with radiologic examinations of GI tract. Bismuth is radiopaque.

Drug Interactions:

Drugs that may be affected by bismuth include aspirin and tetracyclines.

Administration and Dosage:

Adults: 2 tablets or 30 ml.

Children: 9 to 12 years – 1 tablet or 15 ml.
6 to 9 years – ⅔ tablet or 10 ml.
3 to 6 years – ⅓ tablet or 5 ml.
< 3 years – Consult physician.

Repeat dosage every 30 min to 1 hour, as needed, up to 8 doses in 24 hrs.

MESALAMINE (5-aminosalicylic acid, 5–ASA)

Tablets, delayed release: 400 mg (*Rx*)	*Asacol* (Procter & Gamble)
Capsules, controlled release: 250 mg (*Rx*)	*Pentasa* (Hoechst-Marion Roussel)
Suppositories: 500 mg (*Rx*)	*Rowasa* (Solvay)
Rectal Suspension: 4 g per 60 ml (*Rx*)	*Rowasa* (Solvay)

Actions:

Pharmacology: Sulfasalazine is split by bacterial action in the colon into sulfapyridine and mesalamine (5–ASA). It is thought that the mesalamine component is therapeutically active in ulcerative colitis.

The mechanism of action of mesalamine (and sulfasalazine) is unknown, but appears to be topical rather than systemic, and it is possible that mesalamine diminishes inflammation by blocking cyclooxygenase and inhibiting prostaglandin production in the colon.

Pharmacokinetics:

Absorption/Distribution –

Rectal: Mesalamine administered rectally as a suspension enema is poorly absorbed from the colon and is excreted principally in the feces during subsequent bowel movements. At steady state, approximately 10% to 30% of the daily 4 g dose can be recovered in cumulative 24 hour urine collections.

Oral:

Tablets – Mesalamine tablets are coated with an acrylic-based resin that delays release of mesalamine until it reaches the terminal ileum and beyond. Approximately 28% is absorbed after oral ingestion, leaving the remainder available for topical action and excretion in the feces. Mesalamine from oral mesalamine tablets appears to be more extensively absorbed than that released from sulfasalazine.

Capsules – Mesalamine capsules are designed to release therapeutic quantities of the drug throughout the GI tract; 20% to 30% of mesalamine is absorbed. Plasma mesalamine concentration peaked at approximately 1 mcg/ml 3 hours after administration of a 1 g dose and declined in a biphasic manner. Mean terminal half-life was 42 minutes after IV administration.

Metabolism/Excretion –

Rectal: Whatever the metabolic site, most absorbed mesalamine is excreted in urine as the N-acetyl–5–ASA metabolite. While the elimination half-life of mesalamine is short (0.5 to 1.5 hr), the acetylated metabolite exhibits a half-life of 5 to 10 hours.

Oral:

Tablets – Following oral administration, the absorbed mesalamine is rapidly acetylated in the gut mucosal wall and by the liver. It is excreted mainly by the kidneys as N-acetyl-5-ASA. The half-lives of elimination for mesalamine and the metabolite are usually about 12 hours, but are variable ranging from 2 to 15 hours.

Capsules – Elimination of free mesalamine and salicylates in feces increased proportionately with the dose. N-acetyl-5–ASA was the primary compound excreted in the urine (19% to 30%).

Indications:

Chronic inflammatory bowel disease:

Oral – Remission and treatment of mildly to moderately active ulcerative colitis.

Rectal – Treatment of active mild to moderate distal ulcerative colitis, proctosigmoiditis or proctitis.

Contraindications:

Hypersensitivity to mesalamine, salicylates or any component of the formulation.

Warnings:

Intolerance/Colitis exacerbation: Mesalamine has been implicated in the production of an acute intolerance syndrome or exacerbation of colitis characterized by cramping, acute abdominal pain and bloody diarrhea, and occasionally fever, headache, malaise, pruritus, conjunctivitis and rash. Symptoms usually abate when mesalamine is discontinued.

Pancolitis: While using mesalamine some patients have developed pancolitis.

Hypersensitivity: Most patients who were hypersensitive to sulfasalazine were able to take mesalamine enemas without evidence of any allergic reaction. Nevertheless, exercise caution when mesalamine is initially used in patients known to be allergic to sulfasalazine.

Renal function impairment: Renal impairment, including minimal change nephropathy, and acute and chronic interstitial nephritis, has occurred.

Pregnancy: *Category* B. Mesalamine is known to cross the placental barrier.

Lactation: Low concentrations of mesalamine and higher concentrations of N-acetyl-5-ASA have been detected in breast milk.

Children: Safety and efficacy for use in children have not been established.

Precautions:

Pericarditis has occurred rarely with mesalamine-containing products including sulfasalazine.

Adverse Reactions:

Adverse reactions may include: Abdominal pain/cramps/discomfort; colitis exacerbation; constipation; diarrhea; dyspepesia; eructation; flatulence/gas; nausea; vomiting; asthenia; chills; dizziness; fever; headache; malaise/fatigue/weakness; sweating; pharyngitis; rhinitis; pruritus; rash/spots; arthralgia; back pain; hypertonia; myalgia; chest pain; dysmenorrhea; edema; flu syndrome; pain.

Administration and Dosage:

Oral:

Tablets – 800 mg 3 times daily for a total dose of 2.4 g/day for 6 weeks.

Capsules – 1 g 4 times daily for a total dose of 4 g for up to 8 weeks.

Suppository: One suppository (500 mg) 2 times daily. Retain the suppository in the rectum for 1 to 3 hours or more if possible to achieve maximum benefit. While the effect may be seen within 3 to 21 days, the usual course of therapy is 3 to 6 weeks depending on symptoms and sigmoidoscopic findings.

Suspension: The usual dosage of mesalamine suspension enema in 60 ml units is one rectal instillation (4 g) once a day, preferably at bedtime, and retained for ≈ 8 hours. While the effect may be seen within 3 to 21 days, the usual course of therapy is 3 to 6 weeks depending on symptoms and sigmoidoscopic findings.

OLSALAZINE SODIUM

Capsules: 250 mg (*Rx*)	*Dipentum* (Pharmacia)

Actions:

Pharmacology: Olsalazine sodium is a sodium salt of a salicylate compound that is effectively bioconverted to 5–aminosalicylic acid (mesalamine; 5–ASA), which has anti-inflammatory activity in ulcerative colitis. Approximately 98% to 99% of an oral dose will reach the colon where each molecule is rapidly converted into two molecules of 5-ASA by colonic bacteria. The liberated 5-ASA is absorbed slowly, resulting in very high local concentrations in the colon.

Mechanism of action of mesalamine is unknown, but appears topical rather than systemic. It may diminishes colonic inflammation by blocking cyclooxygenase and inhibiting colon prostaglandin production in bowel mucosa.

Pharmacokinetics: After oral administration approximately 2.4% of a single 1 g oral dose is absorbed. Maximum serum concentrations appear after approximately 1 hour, and are low even after a 1 g single dose. Olsalazine has a very short serum half-life of ≈ 0.9 hours and is > 99% bound to plasma proteins. Urinary recovery is < 1%. Total oral olsalazine recovery ranges from 90% to 97%.

Serum concentrations of 5-ASA are detected after 4 to 8 hours. Of the total urinary 5-ASA, > 90% is in the form of N-acetyl-5-ASA (Ac-5-ASA).

Indications:

Maintenance of remission of ulcerative colitis in patients intolerant of sulfasalazine.

Contraindications:

Hypersensitivity to salicylates.

Warnings:

Pregnancy: Category C.

Lactation: It is not known whether this drug is excreted in breast milk.

Children: Safety and efficacy in children have not been established.

Precautions:

Diarrhea: About 17%, resulting in drug withdrawal in 6%; appears dose-related, but may be difficult to distinguish from underlying disease symptoms.

Exacerbation of the symptoms of colitis thought to have been caused by mesalamine or sulfasalazine has been noted.

Renal abnormalities were not reported in clinical trials with olsalazine; however, the possibility of renal tubular damage due to absorbed mesalamine or its n-acetylated metabolite must be kept in mind, particularly for patients with pre-existing renal disease.

Adverse Reactions:

Adverse reactions may include: Headache; diarrhea; pain/cramps; nausea; dyspepsia; arthralgia.

Administration and Dosage:

1 g per day in 2 divided doses.

HELICOBACTER PYLORI AGENTS

Helicobacter pylori is found in ≈ 100% of chronic active antral gastritis cases, 90% to 95% of duodenal ulcer patients and 50% to 80% of gastric ulcer patients. The treatment of documented *H. pylori* infection in patients with confirmed peptic ulcer on first presentation or recurrence has been recommended by the National Institutes for Health in a 1994 Consensus Conference. Once *H. pylori* eradication has been achieved, reinfection rates are < 0.5% per year, and ulcer recurrence rates are dramatically reduced

Numerous clinical trials have been done to determine the optimal regimen for *H. pylori* eradication, but there remains no gold standard of therapy to date. When selecting a regimen, take into account efficacy, tolerability, compliance and cost. *H. pylori* is easily suppressed but, to ensure successful eradication, requires the use of two antimicrobial agents with either a bismuth compound, an antisecretory agent or both. These combinations have been shown to enhance *H. pylori* cure, shorten the duration of treatment and decrease treatment failure due to antimicrobial resistance.

The following is a brief description of the individual agents used in *H. pylori* eradication regimens and their role in eradication. Consult the individual drug monographs for complete prescribing information.

Amoxicillin: 500 mg 4 times daily.

This agent works by inhibiting the synthesis of bacterial cell walls. *H. pylori* is very sensitive to amoxicillin both in vitro and in vivo. Bacterial resistance to amoxicillin has not been reported

Tetracycline: 500 mg 4 times daily.

This agent works by inhibiting bacterial protein synthesis. *H. pylori* is very sensitive to tetracycline. Bacterial resistance to tetracycline has not been reported.

Metronidazole: 250 mg 4 times daily.

The exact mechanism of this agent is not well understood. It demonstrates selective toxicity to anaerobic or microaerophilic microorganisms and for anoxic or hypoxic cells. Resistance is very high in areas of the world where it is used frequently for other indications. Resistance develops less often when metronidazole is given with bismuth or a second antimicrobial agent.

Clarithromycin: 500 mg 2 or 3 times daily.

Clarithromycin is a macrolide antibiotic that inhibits bacterial protein synthesis. It is more acid stable than erythromycin, better absorbed and more effective against *H. pylori*. Resistance can develop when clarithromycin is used alone.

Bismuth: 525 mg 4 times daily.

Bismuth compounds are topical compounds that disrupt the integrity of bacterial cell walls. Bismuth compounds are thought to lyse *H. pylori* near the gastric surface; prevent the adhesion of *H. pylori* to the gastric epithelium; inhibit its urease, phospholipase and proteolytic activity; and decrease resistance development when used with antimicrobial agents such as metronidazole.

Antisecretory agents (H_2 antagonists, Proton pump inhibitors): Provide rapid symptom relief and accelerated ulcer healing when used with antimicrobial agents for *H. pylori* eradication. Proton pump inhibitors may have a direct effect on inhibiting the growth of *H. pylori* and also appear to have a synergistic effect when combined with antimicrobial agents.

Eradication of H. pylori:

Single antimicrobial agents: Monotherapy is not recommended because of the potential for the development of antimicrobial resistance.

Dual therapy:

Proton pump inhibitors plus amoxicillin – Eradication rates range from 30% to 80%. Therefore, dual therapy with these two agents is not recommended.

Proton pump inhibitors plus clarithromycin – Overall eradication appears to be ≈ 71%. Currently, the American College of Gastroenterology recommends adding a second antimicrobial agent to this regimen to enhance successful eradication.

Double antimicrobial therapy plus an antisecretory drug:

Regimens Used in the Eradication of *H. pylori*[1]

Regimen	Dosing	Duration	Eradication
Metronidazole	500 mg twice daily with meals	1 week	87% to 91%
Omeprazole	20 mg twice daily with meals		
Clarithromycin	500 mg twice daily with meals		
Amoxicillin	1 g twice daily with meals	1 to 2 weeks	77% to 83%
Omeprazole	20 mg twice daily before meals		
Clarithromycin	500 mg twice daily with meals		
Metronidazole	500 mg twice daily with meals	1 to 2 weeks	77% to 83%
Omeprazole	20 mg twice daily before meals		
Amoxicillin	1 g twice daily with meals		

[1] Extending therapy to 10 to 14 days in the above regimens may provide additional benefit. H_2 blockers may be used with two antibiotics, but a longer treatment course (10 to 14 days), higher antibiotic doses and 3 times daily administration are required.

Triple-therapy regimens: These regimens have proven to be very effective in eradicating *H. pylori*. The primary disadvantage of these regimens is compliance because of the variety and number of medications used. Likewise, adverse effects are more common in patients taking these regimens compared with alternatives.

Regimens Used in the Eradication of *H. pylori*[1]

Regimen	Dosing	Duration	Eradication
Bismuth subsalicylate	525 mg 4 times daily with meals and at bedtime	2 weeks 1 week	88% to 90% 86% to 90%
Metronidazole	250 mg 4 times daily with meals and at bedtime		
Tetracycline	500 mg 4 times daily		
Bismuth subsalicylate	525 mg 4 times daily with meals and at bedtime	1 week	94% to 98%
Metronidazole	250 mg 4 times daily with meals and at bedtime		
Tetracycline	500 mg 4 times daily		
Omeprazole	20 mg 2 times daily before meals		
Bismuth subsalicylate	525 mg 4 times daily with meals and at bedtime	2 weeks 1 week	80% to 86% 75% to 81%
Metronidazole	250 mg 4 times daily with meals and at bedtime		
Amoxicillin	500 mg 4 times daily with meals and at bedtime		

[1] One week of 4 times daily therapy may be sufficient in the absence of antibiotic resistance. Adding a proton pump inhibitor facilitates shorter treatment periods. Until more data is available, the use of H_2 antagonists or proton pump inhibitors with the above regimens is appropriate to enhance ulcer healing and provide symptomatic relief.

Quadruple therapy regimens (two antibiotics, bismuth, antisecretory agent): Like triple therapy regimens these have proven to be effective in *H. pylori* eradication. The primary disadvantage of these regimens is compliance. In addition, because of the variety and number of medications used, adverse effects are more common in patients taking these regimens compared with alternatives.

FDA Approved Regimens for the Eradication of *H. pylori*			
Regimen	Dosing	Eradication	Comments
Omeprazole	40 mg once daily followed by a 2-week course of 20 mg once daily	64% to 74%	The American College of Gastroenterology recommends that either tetracycline or amoxicillin be added to this regimen.
Clarithromycin	500 mg 3 times daily for 2 weeks		
Ranitidine bismuth citrate	400 mg twice daily for 4 weeks	82%	The American College of Gastroenterology recommends that either tetracycline or amoxicillin be added to this regimen.
Clarithromycin	500 mg 3 times daily for 2 weeks		
Metronidazole	250 mg 4 times daily at meals and bedtime	82%	*Helidac* therapy combines bismuth subsalicylate, metronidazole and tetracycline in a consumer-tested, patient-friendly kit.
Tetracycline HCl	500 mg 4 times daily at meals and bedtime		
Bismuth subsalicylate	525 mg 4 times daily at meals and bedtime		

Practice Guidelines from the American College of Gastroenterology: In the 1996 Consensus Statement on Medical Treatment of Peptic Ulcer Disease, the American College of Gastroenterology does not recommend single-antibiotic combinations of either clarithromycin or amoxicillin with proton pump inhibitors because efficacy is < 70% (cure), and a high-dose, 2–week treatment period is required. The Consensus Statement recommends a two-antibiotic combination of clarithromycin, metronidazole or amoxicillin in regimens that do not employ a bismuth compound. In addition, the American College of Gastroenterology suggests adding either tetracycline or amoxicillin to the recently approved ranitidine-bismuth citrate-clarithromycin combination to enhance successful *H. pylori* eradication. Combining a proton pump inhibitor, either omeprazole or lansoprazole, with two antibiotics is thought to enhance effectiveness and allow for a shorter duration of treatment.

There are a number of factors that limit the effectiveness of regimens designed to eradicate *H. pylori*. The first, antibiotic resistance, is seen with metronidazole and clarithromycin but has not been reported with bismuth, amoxicillin or tetracycline.

Second, mild adverse effects (eg, diarrhea, metallic taste, black stools) do occur in ≈ 30% to 50% of patients. Therefore, shorter treatment periods in this group of patients may be better tolerated.

Finally, patient compliance is often a problem because of cumbersome regimens and adverse effects.

Maintenance therapy with antisecretory agents: Currently, it is advisable to continue maintenance until *H. pylori* cure has been confirmed in patients with a history of complications, frequent or troublesome recurrences or refractory ulcers.

Confirming successful eradication is important in patients with a history of complicated or refractory ulcers but is controversial in those with uncomplicated ulcers who remain asymptomatic after therapy.

Refractory ulcers in patients receiving antibiotic therapy for H. pylori eradication is often due to failure to successfully eradicate *H. pylori* infection. Resistance patterns, as well as noncompliance, and concurrent NSAID use may play a role in refractory cases.

Chapter 8

ANTI-INFECTIVES

PENICILLINS

AMOXICILLIN	
Tablets, chewable: 125 and 250 mg (as trihydrate) (*Rx*)	Various, *Amoxil* (SK-Beecham)
Capsules: 250 and 500 mg (as trihydrate (*Rx*)	Various, *Amoxil* (SK-Beecham), *Wymox* (Wyeth-Ayerst)
Powder for Oral Suspension: 50 mg/ml, 125 and 250 mg/5 ml (as trihydrate) when reconstituted (*Rx*)	Various, *Amoxil* (SK-Beecham), *Wymox* (Wyeth-Ayerst)
AMOXICILLIN AND POTASSIUM CLAVULANATE	
Tablets: 250, 500 or 875 mg amoxicillin and 125 mg clavulanic acid (*Rx*)	*Augmentin* (SK-Beecham)
Tablets, chewable: 125 mg amoxicillin and 31.25 mg clavulanic acid, 250 mg amoxicillin and 62.5 mg clavulanic acid, 200 mg amoxicillin (as trihydrate) and 28.5 mg clavulanic acid, 400 mg amoxicillin (as trihydrate) and 57 mg clavulanic acid (*Rx*)	
Powder for Oral Suspension: 125 mg amoxicillin and 21.25 mg clavulanic acid/5 ml, 200 mg amoxicillin and 28.5 mg clavulanic acid per 5 ml, 250 mg amoxicillin and 62.5 mg clavulanic acid/5 ml, 400 mg amoxicillin and 57 mg clavulanic acid per 5 ml (*Rx*)	
AMPICILLIN, ORAL	
Capsules: 250 and 500 mg (as trihydrate or anhydrous (*Rx*)	Various, *Totacillin* (SK-Beecham), *Omnipen* (Wyeth-Ayerst), *Marcillin* (Marnel)
Powder for Oral Suspension: 100 mg/ml, 125, 250, 500 mg/5 ml (as trihydrate) when reconstituted (*Rx*)	Various, *Omnipen* (Wyeth-Ayerst), *Totacillin* (SK-Beecham), *Polycillin Pediatric Drops* (Apothecon)
Powder for Suspension: 250 mg/100 ml (as trihydrate) when reconstituted (*Rx*)	*Marcillin* (Marnel)
AMPICILLIN WITH PROBENECID	
Powder for Oral Suspension: 3.5 g ampicillin (as trihydrate) & 1 g probenecid per bottle (*Rx*)	*Polycillin-PRB* (Apothecon), *Probampacin* (Various)
AMPICILLIN SODIUM, PARENTERAL	
Powder for Injection: 125, 250, 500 mg and 1, 2, 10 g (*Rx*)	Various, *Omnipen-N* (Wyeth-Ayerst), *Totacillin-N* (SK-Beecham)
AMPICILLIN SODIUM AND SULBACTAM SODIUM	
Powder for Injection: 1.5 g (1 g ampicillin sodium/0.5 g sulbactam sodium), 3 g (2 g ampicillin sodium/1 g sulbactam sodium) (*Rx*)	*Unasyn* (Roerig)
BACAMPICILLIN HCl	
Tablets: 400 mg (chemically equivalent to 280 mg ampicillin) (*Rx*)	*Spectrobid* (Roerig)
Powder for Oral Suspension: 125 mg/5 ml reconstituted suspension (chemically equivalent to 87.5 mg ampicillin) (*Rx*)	
CARBENICILLIN INDANYL SODIUM	
Tablets, film coated: 382 mg carbenicillin (118 mg indanyl sodium ester) (*Rx*)	*Geocillin* (Roerig)
CLOXACILLIN SODIUM	
Capsules: 250 and 500 mg (*Rx*)	Various, *Cloxapen* (SK-Beecham), *Tegopen* (Apothecon)
Powder for Oral Suspension: 125 mg/5 ml when reconstituted (*Rx*)	Various, *Tegopen* (Apothecon)
DICLOXACILLIN SODIUM	
Capsules: 125, 250, 500 mg (*Rx*)	Various, *Dycill* (SK-Beecham), *Pathocil* (Wyeth-Ayerst), *Dynapen* (Apothecon)
Powder for Oral Suspension: 62.5 mg/5 ml reconstituted (*Rx*)	*Dynapen* (Apothecon), *Pathocil* (Wyeth-Ayerst)
METHICILLIN SODIUM	
Powder for Injection: 1, 4, 6, 10 g (*Rx*)	*Staphcillin* (Apothecon)
MEZLOCILLIN SODIUM	
Powder for Injection: 1, 2, 3, 4, 20 g (*Rx*)	*Mezlin* (Miles)

NAFCILLIN SODIUM	
Tablets: 500 mg (*Rx*)	*Unipen* (Wyeth-Ayerst)
Capsules: 250 mg (*Rx*)	
Powder for Injection: 500 mg, 1, 2, 10 g (*Rx*)	Various, *Nallpen* (SK-Beecham), *Unipen* (Wyeth-Ayerst)
OXACILLIN SODIUM	
Capsules: 250 and 500 mg (*Rx*)	Various, *Bactocill* (SK-Beecham), *Prostaphlin* (Apothecon)
Powder for Oral Solution: 250 mg/5 ml when reconstituted (*Rx*)	*Prostaphlin* (Apothecon)
Powder for Injection: 250 and 500 mg, 1, 2, 4 and 10 g (*Rx*)	*Oxacillin Sodium* (Apothecon), *Bactocill* (SK-Beecham), *Prostaphlin* (Apothecon)
PENICILLIN G (AQUEOUS), PARENTERAL	
Injection, premixed, frozen: 1, 2 and 3 million units (*Rx*)	*Penicillin G Potassium* (Baxter)
Powder for Injection: 1, 5, 10 and 20 million units per vial (*Rx*)	*Pfizerpen* (Roerig), *Penicillin G Potassium* (Apothecon), *Penicillin G Sodium* (Apothecon)
PENICILLIN G BENZATHINE, PARENTERAL	
Injection: 300,000 units/ml; 600,000 units; 1,200,000; 2,400,000 units/dose (*Rx*)	*Bicillin L-A* (Wyeth-Ayerst), *Permapen* (Roerig)
PENICILLIN G PROCAINE, AQUEOUS (APPG)	
Injection: 300,000; 500,000; 600,000 units per ml, 1,200,000; 2,400,000 units per dose (*Rx*)	*Pfizerpen-AS* (Roerig), *Wycillin* (Wyeth-Ayerst), *Crysticillin 300* A.S. (Apothecon), *Crysticillin 600* A.S. (Apothecon)
PENICILLIN G BENZATHINE AND PROCAINE COMBINED	
Injection: 300,000 units/ml; 600,000; 1,200,000; 2,400,000 units/dose; 900,000 units penicillin G benzathine and 300,000 units penicillin G procaine/dose (*Rx*)	*Bicillin C-R* (Wyeth-Ayerst), *Bicillin C-R 900/300* (Wyeth-Ayerst)
PENICILLIN V (PHENOXYMETHYL PENICILLIN)	
Tablets: 125, 250, 500 mg (*Rx*)	Various, *Beepen-VK* (SK-Beecham), *V-Cillin K* (Lilly)
Powder for Oral Solution: 125 or 250 mg/5 ml when reconstituted (*Rx*)	Various, *Beepen-VK* (SK-Beecham), *Pen•Vee K* (Wyeth-Ayerst)
PIPERACILLIN SODIUM	
Powder for injection: 2, 3, 4, 40 g (*Rx*)	*Pipracil* (Lederle)
PIPERACILLIN SODIUM AND TAZOBACTAM SODIUM	
Powder for Injection: 2 g piperacillin/ 0.25 g tazobactam, 3 g piperacillin/ 0.375 g tazobactam, 4 g piperacillin/ 0.5 g tazobactam (*Rx*)	*Zosyn* (Wyeth-Ayerst)
TICARCILLIN DISODIUM	
Powder for Injection: 1, 3, 6, 20, 30 g (*Rx*)	*Ticar* (SK-Beecham)
TICARCILLIN AND CLAVULANATE POTASSIUM	
Powder for Injection: 3 g ticarcillin and 0.1 g clavulanic acid (*Rx*)	*Timentin* (SK-Beecham)
Solution: 3 g ticarcillin and 0.1 g clavulanic acid (*Rx*)	

Actions:

Pharmacology: Penicillins inhibit the biosynthesis of cell wall mucopeptide. They are bactericidal against sensitive organisms when adequate concentrations are reached, and they are most effective during the stage of active multiplication. Inadequate concentrations may produce only bacteriostatic effects.

Penicillins					
	Routes of administration	Penicillinase-resistant	Acid stable	% Protein bound	May be taken with meals
Natural Penicillins					
Penicillin G	IM-IV	no	†[1]	60	†[1]
Penicillin V	Oral	no	yes	80	yes
Penicillinase-Resistant					
Cloxacillin	Oral	yes	yes	95	no
Dicloxacillin	Oral	yes	yes	98	no
Methicillin	IM-IV	yes	†[1]	40	†[1]
Nafcillin	IM-IV-Oral	yes	yes	87 to 90	no
Oxacillin	IM-IV-Oral	yes	yes	94	no
Aminopenicillins					
Amoxicillin	Oral	no	yes	20	yes
Amoxicillin/ potassium clavulanate	Oral	yes	yes	20/30	yes
Ampicillin	IM-IV-Oral	no	yes	20	no
Ampicillin/ sulbactam	IM-IV	yes	†[1]	28/38	†[1]
Bacampi-cillin	Oral	no	yes	20	yes[2]
Extended Spectrum					
Carbeni-cillin	Oral	no	yes	50	no
Mezlocillin	IM-IV	no	†[1]	16 to 42	†[1]
Piperacillin	IM-IV	no	†[1]	16	†[1]
Ticarcillin	IM-IV	no	†[1]	45	†[1]
Ticarcillin/ potassium clavulanate	IV	yes	†[1]	45/9	†[1]

[1] Available only for IM or IV use.
[2] Tablets only; not the suspension.

Pharmacokinetics:

Absorption – Peak serum levels occur approximately 1 hour after oral use. Parenteral penicillin G (sodium and potassium) gives rapid and high but transient blood levels; derivatives provide prolonged penicillin blood levels with IM use.

Distribution – Penicillins are bound to plasma proteins, primarily albumin, in varying degrees. They diffuse readily into most body tissues and fluids.

Excretion – Penicillins are excreted largely unchanged in the urine by glomerular filtration and active tubular secretion. Nonrenal elimination includes hepatic inactivation and excretion in bile; this is only a minor route for all penicillins except nafcillin and oxacillin. Excretion by renal tubular secretion can be delayed by coadministration of probenecid. Elimination half-life of most penicillins is short ($\le$ 1.5 hr). Impaired renal function prolongs the serum half-life of penicillins eliminated primarily by renal excretion.

Microbiology:

β-lactamase inhibitors (clavulanic acid and sulbactam) have weak antimicrobial activity, but irreversibly inactivate bacterial β-lactamase enzymes. Used with β-lactam antibiotics, they protect antibiotics from inactivation by β-lactamase-producing organisms.

Organisms Generally Susceptible to Penicillins

	Organisms	Natural penicillins		Penicillinase-resistant					Aminopenicillins					Extended spectrum				
	✓ = generally susceptible	Penicillin G	Penicillin V	Cloxacillin	Dicloxacillin	Methicillin	Nafcillin	Oxacillin	Amoxicillin	Ampicillin	Bacampicillin	Amoxicillin/potassium clavulanate	Ampicillin/sulbactam	Carbenicillin	Mezlocillin	Piperacillin	Ticarcillin	Ticarcillin/potassium clavulanate
Gram-positive	Staphylococci	✓[1]	✓[1]	✓	✓	✓	✓	✓	✓[1]	✓[1]	✓[1]	✓	✓	✓[1]		✓[1]	✓[1]	✓
	Staphylococcus aureus	✓[1]	✓[1]	✓	✓	✓	✓	✓				✓	✓	✓[1]	✓[1]	✓[1]	✓[1]	✓
	Streptococci	✓	✓			✓				✓			✓					
	Streptococcus pneumoniae	✓	✓	✓	✓	✓	✓	✓	✓	✓	✓	✓	✓	✓	✓	✓	✓	✓
	Beta-hemolytic streptococci	✓	✓				✓		✓	✓	✓	✓	✓	✓	✓	✓	✓	✓
	Streptococcus faecalis	✓	✓						✓	✓	✓	✓	✓	✓	✓	✓	✓	✓
	Streptococcus viridans	✓	✓				✓		✓	✓		✓	✓			✓		✓
	Corynebacterium diphtheriae	✓	✓															
	Bacillus anthracis	✓	✓							✓			✓					
	Listeria monocytogenes	✓	✓							✓			✓					
Gram-negative	Escherichia coli	✓							✓	✓	✓	✓	✓	✓	✓	✓	✓	✓
	Hemophilus influenzae								✓	✓	✓	✓	✓	✓	✓	✓[2]	✓	✓
	Klebsiella sp											✓	✓		✓	✓		✓
	Neisseria gonorrhoeae	✓[1]	✓						✓	✓	✓	✓	✓	✓	✓	✓	✓	✓
	Neisseria meningitidis	✓								✓		✓	✓			✓	✓	✓
	Proteus mirabilis	✓							✓	✓	✓	✓	✓	✓	✓	✓	✓	✓
	Salmonella sp	✓								✓			✓	✓	✓	✓	✓	✓
	Shigella sp	✓								✓			✓		✓	✓		
	Morganella morganii												✓	✓	✓	✓	✓	✓
	Proteus vulgaris												✓	✓	✓	✓	✓	✓
	Providencia sp																	
	Providencia rettgeri												✓	✓	✓	✓	✓	✓
	Providencia stuartii												✓		✓			✓
	Enterobacter sp	✓										✓	✓	✓	✓	✓	✓	✓
	Citrobacter sp													✓	✓	✓	✓	✓
	Pseudomonas aeruginosa													✓	✓	✓	✓	✓
	Serratia sp													✓	✓	✓	✓	✓
	Acinetobacter sp												✓		✓	✓		✓
	Streptobacillus moniliformis	✓	✓															
	Moraxella (Branhamella) catarrhalis											✓	✓			✓		✓

Organisms Generally Susceptible to Penicillins																		
	Organisms	Natural penicillins		Penicillinase-resistant					Aminopenicillins					Extended spectrum				
	✓ = generally susceptible	Penicillin G	Penicillin V	Cloxacillin	Dicloxacillin	Methicillin	Nafcillin	Oxacillin	Amoxicillin	Ampicillin	Bacampicillin	Amoxicillin/potassium clavulanate	Ampicillin/sulbactam	Carbenicillin	Mezlocillin	Piperacillin	Ticarcillin	Ticarcillin/potassium clavulanate
Anaerobic	Clostridium sp	✓	✓						✓	✓		✓	✓	✓	✓	✓	✓	✓
	Peptococcus sp	✓	✓						✓	✓		✓	✓	✓	✓	✓	✓	✓
	Peptostreptococcus sp	✓	✓						✓			✓	✓	✓	✓	✓	✓	✓
	Bacteroides sp	✓[3]											✓	✓	✓	✓	✓	✓
	Fusobacterium sp	✓											✓	✓	✓	✓	✓	✓
	Eubacterium sp	✓													✓	✓	✓	✓
	Treponema pallidum	✓	✓															
	Actinomyces bovis	✓	✓													✓		
	Veillonella sp														✓	✓		✓

[1] Non-penicillinase-producing.
[2] Non-beta-lactamase-producing.
[3] B fragilis is resistant.

Indications:

Oral: Penicillins are generally indicated in the treatment of mild to moderately severe infections due to penicillin-sensitive microorganisms.

Penicillinase-resistant penicillins: The percentage of staphylococcal isolates resistant to penicillin G outside the hospital is increasing, approximating the high percentage found in the hospital. Therefore, use a penicillinase-resistant penicillin as initial therapy for any suspected staphylococcal infection until culture and sensitivity results are known.

When treatment is initiated before definitive culture and sensitivity results are known, consider that these agents are only effective in the treatment of infections caused by pneumococci, group A beta-hemolytic streptococci and penicillin G-resistant and penicillin G–sensitive staphylococci.

Parenteral: In patients with severe infection, or when there is nausea, vomiting, gastric dilatation, cardiospasm or intestinal hypermotility.

Contraindications:

History of hypersensitivity to penicillins, cephalosporins or imipenem.

Do not treat severe pneumonia, empyema, bacteremia, pericarditis, meningitis and purulent or septic arthritis with an oral penicillin during the acute stage.

Warnings:

Bleeding abnormalities: **Ticarcillin, mezlocillin or piperacillin** may induce hemorrhagic manifestations associated with abnormalities of coagulation tests.

Cystic fibrosis patients have a higher incidence of side effects (eg, fever, rash) when treated with extended spectrum penicillins (eg, piperacillin, carbenicillin).

Hypersensitivity: Serious and occasionally fatal immediate hypersensitivity reactions have occurred. The incidence of anaphylactic shock is between 0.015% and 0.04%. Anaphylactic shock resulting in death has occurred in approximately 0.002% of the patients treated. These reactions are likely to be immediate and severe in penicillin-sensitive individuals with a history of atopic conditions.

Hypersensitivity myocarditis is not dose-dependent and may occur at any time during treatment.

An urticarial rash, not representing a true penicillin allergy, occasionally occurs with **ampicillin** (9%). Typically, the rash appears 7 to 10 days after the start of oral ampicillin therapy and remains for a few days to a week after drug discontinuance. In most cases, the rash is maculopapular, pruritic and generalized.

Desensitization: Patients with a positive skin test to one of the penicillin determinants can be desensitized, which is a relatively safe procedure. This is recommended in instances when penicillin must be given where no proven alternatives exist.

Cross-allergenicity with cephalosporins: Individuals with a history of penicillin hypersensitivity have experienced severe reactions when treated with a cephalosporin. The incidence of cross-allergenicity between penicillins and cephalosporins is estimated to range from 5% to 16%; however, it is possible the incidence is much lower, possibly 3% to 7%.

Renal function impairment: Since carbenicillin is primarily excreted by the kidney, patients with severe renal impairment (creatinine clearance, < 10 ml/min) will not achieve the therapeutic urine levels of carbenecillin.

In patients with creatinine clearance 10 to 20 ml/min, it may be necessary to adjust dosage to prevent accumulation of the drug.

Pregnancy: Category B. Penicillins cross the placenta.

Lactation: Penicillins are excreted in breast milk in low concentrations; use may cause diarrhea, candidiasis or allergic response in the nursing infant.

Children: Safety and efficacy of carbenicillin, piperacillin and the β-lactamase inhibitor/penicillin combinations have not been established in infants and children < 12 years old. Use caution in administering to newborns and evaluate organ system function frequently.

Precautions:

Monitoring: Obtain blood cultures, white blood cell and differential cell counts prior to initiation of therapy and at least weekly during therapy with penicillinase-resistant penicillins. Measure AST and ALT during therapy to monitor for liver function abnormalities.

Perform periodic urinalysis, BUN and creatinine determinations during therapy with penicillinase-resistant penicillins, and consider dosage alterations if these values become elevated.

Streptococcal infections: Therapy must be sufficient to eliminate the organism (a minimum of 10 days); otherwise, sequelae (eg, endocarditis, rheumatic fever) may occur.

Sexually transmitted diseases: When treating gonococcal infections in which primary and secondary syphilis are suspected, perform proper diagnostic procedures, including darkfield examinations and monthly serological tests for at least 4 months.

Resistance: The number of strains of staphylococci resistant to penicillinase-resistant penicillins has been increasing; widespread use of penicillinase-resistant penicillins may result in an increasing number of resistant staphylococcal strains.

Pseudomembranous colitis has occurred with the use of broad spectrum antibiotics due to overgrowth of clostridia; therefore, it is important to consider its diagnosis in patients who develop diarrhea in association with antibiotic use.

Procaine sensitivity: If sensitivity to the procaine in **penicillin G procaine** is suspected, inject 0.1 ml of a 1% to 2% procaine solution intradermally. Development of erythema, wheal, flare or eruption indicates procaine sensitivity; treat by the usual methods.

Parenteral administration: Inadvertent intravascular administration, including direct intra-arterial injection or injection immediately adjacent to arteries, has resulted in severe neurovascular damage, including transverse myelitis with permanent paralysis, gangrene requiring amputation of digits and more proximal portions of extremities, and necrosis and sloughing at and surrounding the injection site.

Electrolyte imbalance: Patients given continuous IV therapy with **potassium penicillin G** in high dosage (> 10 million units daily) may suffer severe or even fatal potassium poisoning particularly if renal insufficiency is present. High dosage of **sodium salts of penicillins** may result in or aggravate CHF due to high sodium intake. Individuals with liver disease or those receiving cytotoxic therapy or diuretics rarely demonstrated a decrease in serum potassium concentrations with high doses of **piperacillin. Sodium penicillin G** contains 2 mEq sodium per million units, **potassium penicillin G** contains 1.7 mEq potassium and 0.3 mEq sodium per million units. The sodium content of other IV penicillin derivatives is listed below:

Sodium Content of IV Penicillins

Penicillin	Maximum daily dose (g)	Sodium content (mEq/g)[1]	Sodium (mEq/day)[1,2]
Ampicillin sodium	12	2.9	34.8
Methicillin sodium	12	3	36
Mezlocillin sodium	24	1.85	44.4
Nafcillin sodium	9	2.9	26
Oxacillin sodium	12	2.5	30
Piperacillin sodium	24	1.85	44.4
Ticarcillin disodium	24	4.7 to 5	112.8 to 120

[1] 1 mEq sodium equals 23 mg.
[2] Based on maximum daily dose.

Hypokalemia has occurred in a few patients receiving **mezlocillin, ticarcillin** and **piperacillin.**

Drug Interactions:

Drugs that may affect penicillins include allopurinol, chloramphenicol, erythromycin, tetracycline, aminoglycosides (parenteral), beta blockers. Drugs that may be affected by penicillins include aminoglycosides (parenteral), anticoagulants, beta blockers, oral contraceptives, heparin, chloramphenicol, erythromycin.

Drug/Lab test interactions: False-positive **urine glucose** reactions may occur with penicillin therapy if Clinitest, Benedict's Solution or Fehling's Solution are used. It is recommended that enzymatic glucose oxidase tests (such as *Clinistix* or *Tes-Tape*) be used. Positive *Coombs' tests* have occurred. High urine concentrations of some penicillins may produce false-positive protein reactions (pseudoproteinuria) with the following methods: Sulfosalicylic acid and boiling test, acetic acid test, biuret reaction and nitric acid test. The bromphenol blue (*Multi-Stix*) reagent strip test has been reported to be reliable.

Drug/Food interactions: Absorption of most penicillins is affected by food; these medications are best taken on an empty stomach, 1 hour before or 2 hours after meals. Penicillin V may be given with meals; however, blood levels may be slightly higher when taken on an empty stomach. Amoxicillin, amoxicillin/potassium clavulanate and bacampicillin tablets may be given without regard to meals; absorption of bacampicillin suspension is affected by food.

Adverse Reactions:

Hypersensitivity: Adverse reactions (estimated incidence, 1% to 10%) are more likely to occur in individuals with previously demonstrated hypersensitivity. In penicillin-sensitive individuals with a history of allergy, asthma or hay fever, the reactions may be immediate and severe.

Allergic symptoms include urticaria, angioneurotic edema, laryngospasm, bronchospasm, hypotension, vascular collapse; death; maculopapular to exfoliative dermatitis; vesicular eruptions; erythema multiforme; reactions resembling serum sickness (chills, fever, edema, arthralgia, arthritis, malaise); laryngeal edema; skin rashes; prostration.

GI: Glossitis; stomatitis; gastritis; sore mouth or tongue; dry mouth; furry tongue; black "hairy" tongue; abnormal taste sensation; nausea; vomiting; abdominal pain or cramp; epigastric distress; diarrhea or bloody diarrhea; rectal bleeding; flatulence; enterocolitis; pseudomembranous colitis.

Hematologic/Lymphatic: Anemia; hemolytic anemia; thrombocytopenia; thrombocytopenic purpura; eosinophilia; leukopenia; granulocytopenia; neutropenia; bone marrow depression; agranulocytosis; a reduction of hemoglobin or hematocrit; prolongation of bleeding and prothrombin time; decrease in WBC and lymphocyte counts; increase in lymphocytes, monocytes, basophils and platelets.

CNS: Penicillins have caused neurotoxicity (manifested as lethargy, neuromuscular irritability, hallucinations, convulsions and seizures) when given in large IV doses especially in patients with renal failure.

Local: Pain (accompanied by induration) at the site of injection; ecchymosis; deep vein thrombosis; hematomas..

Miscellaneous: Vaginitis and anorexia.

Lab test abnormalities: Elevations of AST, ALT, bilirubin and LDH have been noted in patients receiving semisynthetic penicillins (particularly **oxacillin** and **cloxacillin**); such reactions are more common in infants. Elevations of serum alkaline phosphatase and hypernatremia, and reduction in serum potassium, albumin, total proteins and uric acid may occur.

Administration and Dosage:

Therapy may be initiated prior to obtaining results of bacteriologic studies when there is reason to believe the causative organisms may be susceptible. Once results are known, adjust therapy.

Continue treatment of all infections for a minimum of 48 to 72 hours beyond the time that the patient becomes asymptomatic or evidence of bacterial eradication has been obtained, unless single dose therapy is employed.

AMOXICILLIN: The children's dose is intended for individuals whose weight will not cause the calculated dosage to be greater than that recommended for adults; the children's dose should not exceed the maximum adult dose.

Amoxicillin Uses and Dosages	
Organisms/Infections	Dosage
Infections of the ear, nose and throat due to streptococci, pneumococci, nonpenicillinase-producing staphylococci and *H influenzae* *Infections of the GU tract due to E coli, P mirabilis and S faecalis* *Infections of the skin and soft tissues* due to streptococci, susceptible staphylocci and *E coli*	*Adults and children (> 20 kg)* - 250 to 500 mg every 8 hours. *Children* - 20 to 40 mg/kg/day in divided doses every 8 hours.
Infections of the lower respiratory tract due to streptococci, pneumococci, nonpenicillinase-producing staphylococci and *H influenzae*	*Adults and children (> 20 kg)* - 500 mg q 8 h. *Children* - 40 mg/kg/day in divided doses q 8 h.
Prevention of bacterial endocarditis: For dental, oral or upper respiratory tract procedures in patients at risk	
Standard regimen:	3 g 1 hour before procedure, then 1.5 g 6 hours after initial dose
Alternate regimen:	1 to 2 g (50 mg/kg for children) ampicillin plus 1.5 mg/kg gentamicin (2 mg/kg for children) not to exceed 80 mg, both IM or IV one-half hour prior to procedure, followed by 1.5 g amoxicillin (25 mg/kg for children) 6 hours after initial dose or, repeat parenteral dose 8 hours after initial dose.
For GU or GI procedures	
Standard regimen:	2 g ampicillin (50 mg/kg for children) plus 1.5 mg/kg gentamicin (2 mg/kg for children) not to exceed 80 mg, both IM or IV one-half hour prior to procedure, followed by 1.5 g amoxicillin (25 mg/kg for children)

Amoxicillin Uses and Dosages	
Organisms/Infections	Dosage
Alternate low-risk patient regimen	3 g 1 hour before procedure, then 1.5 g 6 hours after initial dose
Unlabeled use: *Chlamydia trachomatis* in pregnancy	As an alternative to erythromycin; 500 mg 3 times a day for 7 days.

AMOXICILLIN AND POTASSIUM CLAVULANATE: May be administered without regard to meals

Since both the 250 mg and 500 mg tablets contain the same amount of clavulanic acid (125 mg as potassium salt), two 250 mg tablets are not equivalent to one 500 mg tablet.

The 875 mg tablet also contains 125 mg potassium clavulanate. In addition, the 250 mg tablet and 250 mg chewable tablet do NOT contain the same amount of potassium clavulanate and should not be substituted for each other, as they are not interchangeable.

Usual dose – Children's dose is based on amoxicillin content.

Adults: One 250 mg tablet every 8 hours.

Suspension – Adults who have difficulty swallowing may be given the 125 mg/5 ml or 250 mg/5 ml suspension in place of the 500 mg tablet or give 200 mg/5 ml or 400 mg/5 ml suspension in place of the 875 mg tablet.

Children:

≥ 40 kg – Dose according to adult recommendations.

< 3 months old – 30 mg/kg/day divided every 12 hours, based on the amoxicillin component. Use of the 125 mg/5 ml oral suspension is recommended.

≥ 3 months old – Children's dose is based on amoxicillin content. Refer to the following table. Because of the different amoxicillin to clavulanic acid ratios in the 250 mg tablets (250/125) vs the 250 mg chewable tablets (250/62.5), do not use the 250 mg tablet until the child weighs ≥ 40 kg.

Amoxicillin/Potassium Clavulanate Dosing in Children ≥ 3 Months of Age		
	Dosing regimen	
Infections	200 mg/5 ml or 400 mg/5 ml (q12hr)[1,2]	125 mg/5 ml or 250 mg/5 ml (q8hr)[2]
Otitis media,[3] sinusitus, lower respiratory tract infections, severe infections	45 mg/kg/day	40 mg/kg/day
Less severe infections	25 mg/kg/day	20 mg/kg/day

[1] The every-12–hour regimen is associated with significantly less diarrhea; however, the 200 and 400 mg formulations (suspension and chewable tablets) contain aspartame and should not be used by phenylketonurics.
[2] Each strength of the suspension is available as a chewable tablet for use by older children.
[3] Recommended duration is 10 days.

Severe infections and respiratory tract infections –

Adults: One 500 mg tablet every 8 hours.

Children (< 40 kg): 40 mg/kg/day, in divided doses every 8 hours.

Otitis media, sinusitis and lower respiratory infections –

Children (< 40 kg): 40 mg/kg/day, in divided doses every 8 hours.

Chancroid (Hemophilus ducreyi infection) – One 500 mg tablet 3 times daily for 7 days as an alternative to erythromycin or ceftriaxone (not evaluated in the US).

Disseminated gonococcal infection – Following appropriate parenteral therapy with ceftriaxone, ceftizoxime or cefotaxime, reliable patients with uncomplicated disease may be discharged from the hospital 24 to 48 hours after all symptoms resolve and may complete the therapy (for a total of 1 week of antibiotic therapy) with an oral regimen of one 500 mg tablet 3 times a day.

AMPICILLIN:

Ampicillin Uses and Dosages	
Organisms/infections	Dosage
Labeled uses: *Respiratory tract and soft tissue infections:*	Parenteral: Patients ≥ 40 kg - 250 to 500 mg every 6 hours; < 40 kg - 25 to 50 mg/kg/day in divided doses at 6 to 8 hour intervals. Oral: Patients ≥ 20 kg - 250 mg every 6 hours; < 20 kg - 50 mg/kg/day in divided doses at 6 to 8 hour intervals.
Bacterial meningitis: H influenzae, S pneumoniae or N meningitidis	8 to 14 g/day (100 to 200 mg/kg/day for children) in divided doses every 3 to 4 hours. Initial treatment is usually by IV drip, followed by frequent (every 3 to 4 hour) IM injections.
Septicemia:	Parenteral: 150 to 200 mg/kg/day. Give IV at least 3 days; continue IM every 3 to 4 hrs.
Rape victims (prophylaxis of infection): Alternative regimen for pregnant women or when tetracycline is contraindicated.	3.5 g orally with 1 g probenecid.
Prevention of bacterial endocarditis: For dental, oral or upper respiratory tract procedures in patients at high risk: Alternate regimen.	1 to 2 g (50 mg/kg for children) plus gentamicin 1.5 mg/kg (2 mg/kg for children) not > 80 mg, both IM or IV 30 min pior to procedure, then 1.5 g amoxicillin (25 mg/kg for children) 6 hours after initial dose or repeat parenteral dose 8 hours after initial dose.
For GU or GI procedures: Standard regimen.	2 g (50 mg/kg for children) IM or IV plus gentamicin 1.5 mg/kg (not > 80 mg) IM or IV (2 mg/kg for children) 30 min prior to procedure, then 1.5 g amoxicillin (25 mg/kg for children) 6 hours after initial dose; or repeat parenteral dose 8 hours after initial dose.
Unlabeled use: Prophylaxis in cesarean section in certain high risk patients	Single IV dose, administered immediately after cord clamping.

Renal impairment – Increase dosing interval to 12 hours in severe renal impairment (creatinine clearance ≤ 10 ml/min).

Adults – 1 to 12 g daily in divided doses every 4 to 6 hours.

Children – 50 to 200 mg/kg/day in divided doses every 4 to 6 hours.

Infants (over 7 days and > 2000 g): 100 mg/kg/day in divided doses every 6 hours (meningitis 200 mg/kg/day).

Over 7 days and < 2000 g: 75 mg/kg/day in divided doses every 8 hours (meningitis 150 mg/kg/day).

Under 7 days and > 2000 g: 75 mg/kg/day in divided doses every 8 hours (meningitis 150 mg/kg/day).

Under 7 days and < 2000 g: 50 mg/kg/day in divided doses every 12 hours (meningitis 100 mg/kg/day).

AMPICILLIN AND PROBENECID: Administer 3.5 g ampicillin and 1 g probenecid as a single dose.

AMPICILLIN SODIUM AND SULBACTAM SODIUM: May be administered by either the IV or the IM routes. The recommended adult dosage is 1.5 g (1 g ampicillin plus 0.5 g sulbactam) to 3 g (2 g ampicillin plus 1 g sulbactam) every 6 hours. Do not exceed 4 g/day sulbactam.

Renal function impairment – The elimination kinetics of ampicillin and sulbactam are similarly affected; hence, the ratio of one to the other will remain constant whatever the renal function. In patients with renal impairment, give as follows:

Ampicillin/Sulbactam Dosage Guide For Patients With Renal Impairment		
Ccr (ml/min/1.72 m^2)	Half-life (hours)	Recommended dosage
≥ 30	1	1.5-3 g q 6-8 h
15-29	5	1.5-3 q 12 h
5-14	9	1.5-3 g q 24 h

Children – Safety and efficacy in children < 12 years old have not been established.

BACAMPICILLIN HCl: Tablets may be given without regard to meals; administer suspension to fasting patients.

Upper respiratory tract infections (including otitis media) due to streptococci, pneumococci, nonpenicillinase-producing staphylococci and H influenzae; urinary tract infections due to *E coli*, *P mirabilis* and *S faecalis*; skin and skin structure infections due to streptococci and susceptible staphylococci:

Adults (≥ 25 kg): 400 mg every 12 hours.

Children: 25 mg/kg/day in equally divided doses at 12 hour intervals.

Severe infections or those caused by less susceptible organisms –

Adults (≥ 25 kg): 800 mg every 12 hours.

Children: 50 mg/kg/day in equally divided doses at 12 hour intervals.

Lower respiratory tract infections due to streptococci, pneumococci, nonpenicillinase-producing staphylococci and *H influenzae:*

Adults (≥ 25 kg): 800 mg every 12 hours.

Children: 50 mg/kg/day in equally divided doses at 12 hour intervals.

Gonorrhea – The usual adult dosage (males and females) is 1.6 g bacampicillin plus 1 g probenecid as a single oral dose. No pediatric dosage has been established.

CARBENICILLIN INDANYL SODIUM:

Urinary tract infections –

E coli, Proteus species and Enterobacter: 382 to 764 mg 4 times daily.

Pseudomonas and enterococci: 764 mg 4 times daily.

Prostatitis due to E coli, P mirabilis, Enterobacter and enterococcus (S faecalis) – 764 mg 4 times daily.

CLOXACILLIN SODIUM:

Mild to moderate upper respiratory and localized skin and soft tissue infections –

Adults and children (> 20 kg): 250 mg every 6 hours.

Children (< 20 kg): 50 mg/kg/day in equally divided doses every 6 hours.

Severe infections (lower respiratory tract or disseminated infections) –

Adults and children (> 20 kg): ≥ 500 mg every 6 hours.

Children (< 20 kg): ≥ 100 mg /kg/day in equal doses every 6 hours.

Another suggested dosage for infants and children is 50 to 100 mg/kg/day, up to a maximum of 4 g/day, divided every 6 hours.

DICLOXACILLIN SODIUM:

For mild to moderate upper respiratory and localized skin and soft tissue infections –

Adults and children (> 40 kg): 125 mg every 6 hours.

Children (< 40 kg): 12.5 mg/kg/day in equal doses every 6 hours.

For more severe infections, such as lower respiratory tract or disseminated infections –

Adults and children (> 40 kg): 250 mg every 6 hours.

Children (< 40 kg): 25 mg/kg/day in equally divided doses every 6 hours.

Another suggested dosage for children is 12 to 25 mg/kg/day divided every 6 hours. Use in the newborn is not recommended.

METHICILLIN SODIUM:

Adults – 4 to 12 g/day in divided doses every 4 to 6 hours; in severe renal impairment (creatinine clearance ≤ 10 ml/min) do not exceed 2 g every 12 hours.

Children – 100 to 300 mg/kg/day in divided doses every 4 to 6 hours.

Infants –

Over 7 days and > 2000 g: 100 mg/kg/day in divided doses every 6 hours; for meningitis – 200 mg/kg/day.

Over 7 days and < 2000 g: 75 mg/kg/day in divided doses every 8 hours; for meningitis – 150 mg/kg/day.

Under 7 days and > 2000 g: 75 mg/kg/day in divided doses every 8 hours; for meningitis – 150 mg/kg/day.

Under 7 days and < 2000 g: 50 mg/kg/day in divided doses every 12 hours; for meningitis - 100 mg/kg/day.

MEZLOCILLIN SODIUM: Administer IV for serious infections. IM doses should not exceed 2 g/injection.

Adults – The recommended adult dosage for serious infections is 200 to 300 mg/kg/day given in 4 to 6 divided doses. The usual dose is 3 g given every 4 hours (18 g/day) or 4 g given every 6 hours (16 g/day).

Infants and children – Limited data are available on the safety and effectiveness in the treatment of infants and children with serious infection.

Mezlocillin Dosage Guidelines for Neonates

Body weight (g)	Age	
	≤ 7 Days	> 7 Days
≤ 2000	75 mg/kg every 12 hours (150 mg/kg/day)	75 mg/kg every 8 hours (225 mg/kg/day)
> 2000	75 mg/kg every 12 hours (150 mg/kg/day)	75 mg/kg every 6 hours (300 mg/kg/day)

For infants > 1 month of age and children < 12 years, administer 50 mg/kg every 4 hours (300 mg/kg/day); infuse IV over 30 minutes or administer by IM injection.

Renal function impairment – After an IV dose of 3 g, the serum half-life is approximately 1 hour in patients with creatinine clearances > 60 ml/min, 1.3 hours in those with clearances of 30 to 59 ml/min, 1.6 hours in those with clearances of 10 to 29 ml/min, and approximately 3.6 hours in patients with clearances of < 10 ml/min.

Mezlocillin Uses and Dosages

Organisms/Infections	Dosage
Urinary infection: Uncomplicated with normal renal function (creatinine clearance ≥ 30 ml/min).	100 to 125 mg/kg/day (6 to 8 g/day); 1.5 to 2 g every 6 hours IV or IM.
Uncomplicated with renal impairment	1.5 g every 8 hours
Complicated with normal renal function	150 to 200 mg/kg/day (12 g/day); 3 g every 6 hours IV.
Complicated with renal impairment - Creatinine clearance	
10 to 30 ml/min	1.5 g every 6 hours.
<10 ml/min	1.5 g every 8 hours.
Lower respiratory tract infection, intra-abdominal infection, gynecological infection, skin and skin structure infections, septicema:	225 to 300 mg/kg/day (16 to 18 g/day); 4 g every 6 hours or 3 g every 4 hours IV.
Serious systemic infection with renal impairment - Creatinine clearance	
10 to 30 ml/min	3 g every 8 hours.
< 10 ml/min	2 g every 8 hours.
Serious systemic infection undergoing hemodialysis for renal failure	3 g every 2 hours
peritoneal dialysis	
Life-threatening infections:	Up to 350 mg/kg/day; 4 g every 4 hours (24 g/day maximum).
In patients with renal impairment - Creatinine clearance	
10 to 30 ml/min	3 g every 6 hours.
<10 ml/min	2 g every 6 hours.

Mezlocillin Uses and Dosages	
Organisms/Infections	Dosage
Acute, uncomplicated gonococcal urethritis:	1 to 2 g IV or IM; plus 1 g probenecid at time of dosing or up to ½ hour before.
Prophylaxis: To prevent postoperative infection in contaminated or potentially contaminated surgery Cesarean section patients -	 4 g IV, ½ to 1½ hr prior to start of surgery; 4 g IV, 6 and 12 hours later. First dose: 4 g IV when umbilical cord is clamped; Second dose: 4 g IV, 4 hours after first dose; Third dose: 4 g IV, 8 hrs after first dose.

NAFCILLIN SODIUM:

Parenteral – IV: 3 to 6 g per 24 hours. Use this route for short-term therapy (24 to 48 hours) because of occasional occurrence of thrombophlebitis, particularly in the elderly.

IM: *Adults* – 500 mg every 4 to 6 hours.

Infants and children – 25 mg/kg twice daily.

Neonates – 10 mg/kg twice daily. Other suggested doses include: Weight < 2000 g - 50 mg/kg/day divided every 12 hours (age <7 days) or 75 mg/kg/day divided every 8 hours (age > 7 days).

Weight > 2000 g - 50 mg/kg/day divided every 8 hours (age < 7 days) or 75 mg/kg/day divided every 6 hours (age > 7 days).

Oral – Serum levels of nafcillin after oral administration are low and unpredictable.

Adults: 250 to 500 mg every 4 to 6 hours for mild to moderate infections. In severe infections – 1 g every 4 to 6 hours.

Children:

Staph infections – 50 mg/kg/day in 4 divided doses. For neonates, 10 mg/kg 3 to 4 times daily. If inadequate, change to parenteral nafcillin sodium.

Scarlet fever and pneumonia – 25 mg/kg/day in 4 divided doses.

Streptococcal pharyngitis – 250 mg, 3 times daily for 10 days. (Penicillin V is the drug of choice for streptococcal infections.)

OXACILLIN SODIUM:

Oral –

Mild to moderate infections of skin, soft tissue, or upper respiratory tract:

Adults and children (> 20 kg) – 500 mg every 4 to 6 hrs for at least 5 days.

Children (< 20 kg) – 50 mg/kg/day in divided doses every 6 hrs for at least 5 days.

In serious or life-threatening infections, such as staphylococcal septicemia or other deep-seated severe infection –

Adults: 1 g every 4 to 6 hours.

Children: ≥ 100 mg/kg/day in equally divided doses every 4 to 6 hours.

Parenteral –

Mild to moderate upper respiratory or localized skin or soft tissue infections:

Adults and children (≥ 40 kg) – 250 to 500 mg every 4 to 6 hours.

Children (< 40 kg) – 50 mg/kg/day in equally divided doses every 6 hours.

Absorption and excretion data indicate that 25 mg/kg/day in prematures and neonates provided adequate therapeutic levels.

Severe infections (lower respiratory tract or disseminated infections):

Adults and children (≥ 40 kg) – ≥ 1 g every 4 to 6 hours.

Children (< 40 kg) – ≥ 100 mg/kg/day in equally divided doses every 4 to 6 hrs.

Very severe infections may require very high doses and prolonged therapy. Maximum daily dose for adults is 12 g/day and for children 100 to 300 mg/kg/day.

Other suggested doses for children and neonates include:

Children – 50 to 100 mg/kg/day divided every 6 hours.

Neonates – Weight < 2000 g – 50 mg/kg/day divided every 12 hours (age < 7 days) or 100 mg/kg/day divided every 8 hours (age > 7 days).

Weight > 2000 g: 75 mg/kg/day divided every 8 hours (age < 7 days) or 150 mg/kg/day divided every 6 hours (age > 7 days).

PENICILLIN G (AQUEOUS), PARENTERAL:

Children – 100,000 to 250,000 units /kg/day in divided doses every 4 hours.

Infants –

(over 7 days and > 2000 g): 100,000 units/kg/day in divided doses every 6 hours (meningitis - 200,000 units).

Over 7 days and < 2000 g: 75,000 units/kg/day in divided doses every 8 hours (meningitis - 150,000 units).

Under 7 days and > 2000 g: 50,000 units/kg/day in divided doses every 8 hours (meningitis - 150,000 units).

Under 7 days and < 2000 g: 50,000 units/kg/day in divided doses every 12 hours (meningitis - 100,000 units).

Parenteral Penicillin G Use and Dosages	
Organisms/Infections	Dosage
Labeled uses:	
Meningococcal meningitis	1 to 2 million units IM every 2 hours; or 20 to 30 million units/day continuous IV drip for 14 days or until afebrile for 7 days; or 200,000 to 300,000 units/kg/day every 2 to 4 hours divided doses for a total of 24 doses.
Actinomycosis: For cervicofacial cases	1 to 6 million units/day
For thoracic and abdominal disease	12 to 20 million units/day IV for 6 weeks. May be followed by oral penicillin V, 500 mg 4 times daily for 2 to 3 months
Clostridial infections	20 million units/day as adjunct to antitoxin
Fusospirochetal infections: Severe infections of oropharynx, lower respiratory tract and genital area	5 to 10 million units/day
Rat-bite fever (Spirillum minus, Streptobacillus moniliformis), Haverhill fever	12 to 20 million units/day for 3 to 4 weeks
Listeria infections (Listeria monocytogenes):	
Meningitis (adults)	15 to 20 million units/day for 2 weeks
Endocarditis (adults)	15 to 20 million units/day for 4 weeks
Pasteurella infections (Pasteurella multocida): Bacteremia and meningitis	4 to 6 million units/day for 2 weeks
Erysipeloid (Erysipelothrix rhusiopathiae): Endocarditis	12 to 20 million units/day for 4 to 6 weeks
Gram-negative bacillary bacteremia (Escherichia coli, Enterobacter aerogenes, Alcaligenes faecalis, Salmonella, Shigella, Proteus mirabilis)	≥ 20 million units/day
Diphtheria: Adjunct to antitoxin to prevent carrier state	2 to 3 million units/day in divided doses for 10 to 12 days
Anthrax: (*B anthracis* is often resistant)	Minimum 5 million units/day; 12 to 20 million units/day have been used
Pneumococcal infections (S pneumoniae):	
Empyema	5 to 24 million units/day in divided doses every 4 to 6 hours
Meningitis	20 to 24 million units/day for 14 days
Suppurative arthritis, osteomyelitis, mastoiditis, endocarditis, peritonitis, pericarditis	12 to 20 million units/day for ≥ 2 to 4 weeks
Syphilis:	

Parenteral Penicillin G Use and Dosages	
Organisms/Infections	Dosage
Neurosyphilis	12 to 24 million units/day IV (2 to 4 million units every 4 hours) for 10 to 14 days. Many recommend benzathine penicillin G 2.4 million units IM weekly for 3 weeks following the completion of this regimen.
Congenital syphilis: Symptomatic or asymptomatic infants	*Newborns:*50,000 units/kg/day IV every 8 to 12 hours for 10 to 14 days. If > 1 day of therapy is missed, restart the entire course. *Infants (after newborn period):* 50,000 units/kg every 4 to 6 hours for 10 to 14 days.
Unlabeled uses: *Lyme disease (Borrelia burgdorferi):* Erythema chronicum migrans	Use oral penicillin V
Neurologic complications (eg, meningitis, encephalitis)	200,000 to 300,000 units/kg/day (up to 20 million units) IV for 10 to 14 days
Carditis	200,000 to 300,000 units/kg/day (up to 20 million units) IV for 10 days with cardiac monitoring and a temporary pacemaker for complete heart block
Arthritis	200,000 to 300,000 units/kg/day (up to 20 million units) IV for 10 to 20 days

PENICILLIN G BENZATHINE, PARENTERAL: Administer by deep IM injection in the upper outer quadrant of the buttock. In infants and small children, the midlateral aspect of the thigh may be preferable. Do not inject benzathine penicillin into the gluteal region of children < 2 years of age. When doses are repeated, rotate the injection site.

Adults – 1.2 million units in one dose.

Children (> 27 kg) – 900,000 to 1.2 million units in one dose.

Children and infants (< 27 kg) – 300,000 to 600,000 units in one dose.

Neonates – 50,000 units/kg in one dose.

Parenteral Penicillin G Benzathine Uses and Dosages	
Organisms/Infections	Dosage
Streptococcal (group A): Prevention of recurrent rheumatic fever.	1.2 million units every 4 weeks
Syphilis: *Early syphilis* - Primary, secondary or latent syphilis of < 1 year's duration	2.4 million units IM in single dose
Syphilis of > 1 year's duration, gummas and cardiovascular syphilis - Latent, cardiovascular or late benign syphilis.	2.4 million units once weekly for three weeks
Neurosyphilis	Aqueous penicillin G, 12 to 24 million units/day IV (2 to 4 million units every 4 hours) for 10 to 14 days. Many recommend benzanthine penicillin G, 2.4 million IM units weekly for 3 doses following completion of this regimen. or Aqueous procaine penicillin G, 2.4 million units/day IM *plus* probenecid 500 mg orally 4 times daily, both for 10 to 14 days. Many recommend benzathine penicillin G, 2.4 million units IM weekly for 3 doses following completion of this regimen.
Syphilis in pregnancy	Dosage schedule appropriate for stage of syphilis recommended for nonpregnant patients.

Parenteral Penicillin G Benzathine Uses and Dosages	
Organisms/Infections	Dosage
Congenital syphilis - Older children with definite acquired syphilis and a normal neurologic examination.	50,000 units/kg IM, up to the adult dose of 2.4 million units.
Yaws, bejel and pinta	1.2 million units in a single dose
Erysipeloid (Erysipelothrix rhusiopathiae): Uncomplicated infection.	1.2 million units in a single dose

PENICILLIN G PROCAINE, AQUEOUS (APPG): Administer by deep IM injection into the upper, outer quadrant of the buttock. In infants and small children, the midlateral aspect of the thigh may be preferable. When doses are repeated, rotate the injection site.

Adults and children – 600,000 to 1.2 million units/day IM in one or two doses (up to a maximum of 4.8 million units/day) for 10 days to 2 weeks.

Newborns – 50,000 units/kg IM once daily. Avoid use in these patients since sterile abscesses and procaine toxicity are of much greater concern than in older children.

Penicillin G Procaine Uses and Dosages	
Organisms/Infections	Dosage
Pneumococcal infections: Moderately severe uncomplicated pneumonia and middle ear and paranasal sinus infections	600,000 to 1.2 million units/day
Streptococcal infections (group A): Moderately severe to severe tonsillitis, erysipelas, scarlet fever, upper respiratory tract (ie, otitis media) and skin and skin structure infections	600,000 to 1.2 million units/day for a minimum of 10 days
Bacterial endocarditis - Only in extremely sensitive infections (*S viridans, S bovis*)	1.2 million units 4 times daily for 2 to 4 weeks plus streptomycin 500 mg twice daily for the first 2 weeks
Staphylococcal infections: Moderately severe to severe infections of the skin and skin structure	600,000 to 1.2 million units/day
Diphtheria: Adjunctive therapy with antitoxin	300,000 to 600,000 units/day
Carrier state	300,000 units/day for 10 days
Anthrax: Cutaneous	600,000 to 1.2 million units/day
Vincent's gingivitis and pharyngitis (fusospirochetosis):	600,000 to 1.2 million units/day. Obtain necessary dental care in infections involving gum tissue.
Erysipeloid:	600,000 to 1.2 million units/day
Rat-bite fever (Streptobacillus moniliformis and Spirillum minus):	600,000 to 1.2 million units/day
Gonorrheal infections (uncomplicated):	4.8 million units divided into at least two doses at one visit; 1 g oral probenecid is given 30 minutes before the injections. Obtain follow-up cultures form the original site(s) of infection 7 to 14 days after therapy. In women, it is also desirable to obtain culture test-of-cure from both the endocervical and anal canals. Note: Treat gonorrheal endocarditis intensively with aqueous penicillin G
Syphilis: Primary, secondary and latent with a negative spinal fluid (adults and children > 12 years of age):	600,000 units daily for 8 days; total 4.8 million units

Penicillin G Procaine Uses and Dosages	
Organisms/Infections	Dosage
Neurosyphilis[1] (as an alternative to the recommended regimen of penicillin G aqueous)	2 to 4 million units/day plus probenecid 500 mg orally 4 times daily, both for 10 to 14 days; many recommend benzathine penicillin G 2.4 million units weekly for 3 doses following the completion of this regimen.
Congenital syphilis:[1] Symptomatic and asymptomatic infants	50,000 units/kg/day (administered once IM) for 10 to 14 days
Yaws, Bejel and Pinta:	Treat same as syphilis in corresponding stage of disease

PENICILLIN G BENZATHINE AND PROCAINE COMBINED: Administer by deep IM injection in the upper outer quadrant of the buttock. In infants and small children, the midlateral aspect of the thigh may be preferable. when doses are repeated, rotate the injection site.

Streptococcal infections – Treatment with the recommended dosage is usually given in a single session using multiple IM sites when indicated. An alternative dosage schedule may be used, giving half the total dose on day 1 and half on day 3. This will also ensure adequate serum levels over a 10 day period; however use only when the patient's cooperation can be assured.

Adults and children (> 60 lbs; 27 kg): 2.4 million units.

Children (30 to 60 lbs; 14 to 27 kg): 900,000 to 1.2 million units.

Infants and children (< 30 lbs; 14 kg): 600,000 units.

Pneumococcal infections (except pneumococcal meningitis) –

Children: 600,000 units.

Adults: 1.2 million units. Repeat every 2 or 3 days until the patient has been afebrile for 48 hours.

PENICILLIN V (PHENOXYMETHYL PENICILLIN): 250 mg = 400,000 units.

Adults – 125 to 500 mg 4 times a day; in renal impairment (creatinine clearance, ≤ 10 ml/min) - Do not exceed 250 mg every 6 hours.

Children – 25 to 50 mg/kg/day in divided doses every 6 to 8 hours.

Penicillin V Uses and Dosages	
Organisms/Infections	Dosage
Labeled uses:	
Streptococcal infections: Infections of the upper respiratory tract, including scarlet fever and mild erysipelas	125 to 250 mg every 6 to 8 hours for 10 days for mild to modeately severe infections
Pharyngitis in children	250 mg 2 times daily for 10 days
Otitis media and sinusitis	250 to 500 mg every 6 hours for 2 weeks
Prevention of bacterial endocarditis[1] in patients with rheumatic, congential or other acquired valvular heart disease undergoing dental procedures or upper respiratory tract surgical procedures	Amoxicillin is the recommended agent; however, the choice of penicillin V is rational and acceptable
Pneumococcal infections: Mild to moderately severe respiratory tract infections including otitis media	250 to 500 mg every 6 hours until afebrile at least 2 days
Staphylococcal infections: Mild infections of skin and soft tissue	250 to 500 mg every 6 to 8 hours
Fusospirochetosis (Vincent's infection) of the oropharynx: Mild to moderately severe infections	250 to 500 mg every 6 to 8 hours
Unlabeled uses:	
Prophylactic treatment of children with sickle cell anemia (to reduce the incidence of *S pneumoniae* septicemia	125 mg 2 times daily
Anaerobic infections: Mild to moderate infections	250 mg 4 times daily
Lyme disease (Borrelia burgdorferi):	

Penicillin V Uses and Dosages	
Organisms/Infections	Dosage
Erythema chronicum migrans:	
Pregnant or lactating women, tetracycline treatment failures	250 to 500 mg 4 times a day for 10 to 20 days
Children < 2 years of age	50 mg/kg/day (up to 2 g/day) in 4 divided doses for 10 to 20 days
Neurologic complications (eg, meningitis, encephalitis), carditis, arthritis	Use penicillin G IV

[1] American Heart Association Statement. JAMA 1990;264:2919–2922.

PIPERACILLIN SODIUM: Administer IM or IV. For serious infections, give 3 to 4 g every 4 to 6 hours as a 20 to 30 minute IV infusion. Maximum daily dose is 24 g/day, although higher doses have been used. Limit IM injections to 2 g/site.

Hemodialysis – Maximum dose is 6 g/day (2 g every 8 hours). Hemodialysis removes 30% to 50% of piperacillin in 4 hours; administer an additional 1 g after dialysis.

Renal failure and hepatic insufficiency – Measure serum levels to provide additional guidance for adjusting dosage; however, this may not be practical.

Infants and children < 12 years of age – Dosages have not been established; however, the following doses have been suggested:

Neonates: 100 mg/kg/dose every 12 hours.

Children: Cystic fibrosis, 350 to 500 mg/kg/day divided every 4 to 6 hours.

Other conditions, 200 to 300 mg/kg/day, up to a maximum of 24 g/day divided every 4 to 6 hours.

Piperacillin Uses and Dosages	
Organisms/Infections	Dosage
Serious infections (septicemia, nosocomial pneumonia, intra-abdominal infections, aerobic and anaerobic gynecologic infections and skin and soft tissue infections):	12 to 18 g/day IV (200 to 300 mg/kg/day) in divided doses every 4 to 6 hours.
Renal impairment-	
Creatinine clearance 20 to 40 ml/min	12 g/day; 4 g every 8 hours.
< 20 ml/min	8 g/day; 4 g every 6 to 12 hours.
Urinary tract infections: Complicated (normal renal function)	8 to 16 g/day IV (125 to 200 mg/kg/day) in divided doses every 6 to 8 hours.
Renal impairment	
Creatinine clearance 20 to 40 ml/min	9 g/day; 3 g every 8 hours.
<20 ml/min	6 g/day; 3 g every 12 hours.
Uncomplicated UTI and most community-acquired pneumonia (normal renal function)	6 to 8 g/day IM or IV (100 to 125 mg/kg/d) in divided doses every 6 to 12 hours.
Uncomplicated UTI with renal impairment-Creatinine clearance < 20 ml/min	6 g/day; 3 g every 12 hours.
Uncomplicated gonorrhea infections:	2 g IM in a single dose with 1 g probenecid ½ hour prior to injection.
Prophylaxis: Intra-abdominal surgery	2 g IV just prior to surgery; 2 g during surgery; 2 g every 6 hours post-op for no more than 24 hours.
Vaginal hysterectomy	2 g IV just prior to surgery; 2 g 6 hrs after initial dose; 2 g 12 hrs after first dose.
Cesarean section	2 g IV after cord is clamped; 2 g 4 hours after initial dose; 2 g 8 hours after first dose.
Abdominal hysterectomy	2 g IV just prior to surgery; 2 g on return to recovery room; 2 g after 6 hours.

PIPERACILLIN SODIUM AND TAZOBACTAM SODIUM: Administer by IV infusion over 30 minutes. The usual total daily dose for adults is 12 g/1.5 g, given as 3.375 g every 6 hours.

Nosocomial pneumonia – Start with 3.375 g every 4 hours plus an aminoglycoside. Continue the aminoglycoside in patients from whom *P. aeruginosa* is isolated. If it is not isolated, the aminoglycoside may be discontinued at the discretion of the treating physician as guided by the severity of the infection and the patient's clinical and bacteriological progress.

Renal function impairment – In patients with renal insufficiency (Ccr < 40 ml/min), adjust the IV dose to the degree of actual renal function impairment. Measurement of serum levels of piperacillin and tazobactam will provide additional guidance for adjusting dosage.

Piperacillin Sodium and Tazobactam Sodium Dosage Recommendations	
Creatinine Clearance (ml/min)	Recommended Dosage Regimen
> 40	12 g/1.5 g/day in divided doses of 3.375 g every 6 hours
20 - 40	8 g/1 g/day in divided doses of 2.25 g every 6 hours
< 20	6 g/0.75 g/day in divided doses of 2.25 g every 8 hours

Hemodialysis – The maximum dose is 2.25 g every 8 hours. In addition, because hemodialysis removes 30% to 40% of a dose in 4 hours, give one additional dose of 0.75 g following each dialysis period.

TICARCILLIN DISODIUM: Use IV therapy in higher doses in serious urinary tract and systemic infections. Intramuscular injections should not exceed 2 g/injection.

Ticarcillin Uses and Dosages	
Organism/Infections	Dosage
Bacterial septicemia, respiratory tract infections, skin and soft tissue infections, intra-abdominal infections and infections of the female pelvis and genital tract	*Adults:* 200 to 300 mg/kg/day by IV infusion in divided doses every 3, 4 or 6 hours (3 g every 3, 4 or 6 hours), depending on weight of patient and severity of infection. *Children (< 40 kg):* 200 to 300 mg/kg/day by IV infusion in divided doses every 4 or 6 hours.[1]
Urinary tract infections: Complicated infections.	150 to 200 mg/kg/day IV infusion in divided doses every 4 or 6 hours. Usual dose for average adult (70 kg) is 3 g 4 times daily.
Uncomplicated infections.	*Adults:* 1 g IM or direct IV every 6 hours. *Children (< 40 kg):* 50 to 100 mg/kg/day IM or direct IV in divided doses every 6 or 8 hours.
Neonates: Severe infections (sepsis) due to susceptible strains of *Pseudomonas* species, *Proteus* species and *E coli*.	Give IM or by 10 to 20 minute IV infusions.
< 2 kg -	*< 7 days* - 75 mg/kg/12 hr (150 mg/kg/day). *> 7 days* - 75 mg/kg/8 hr (225 mg/kg/day).
> 2 kg -	*< 7 days* - 75 mg/kg/8 hr (225 mg/kg/day). *> 7 days* - 100 mg/kg/8 hr (300 mg/kg/day).
Dosage in renal insufficiency:[2]	Initial loading dose of 3 g IV followed by IV doses based on creatinine clearance and type of dialysis.
Creatinine clearance (ml/min) -	
> 60	3 g every 4 hours.
30 to 60	2 g every 4 hours.
10 to 30	2 g every 8 hours.
< 10	2 g every 12 hours or 1 g IM every 6 hours.
< 10 with hepatic dysfunction	2 g every 24 hours or 1 g IM every 12 hours.
Patients on peritoneal dialysis	3 g every 12 hours.

Ticarcillin Uses and Dosages	
Organism/Infections	Dosage
Patients on hemodialysis	2 g every 12 hours supplemented with 3 g after each dialysis.

[1] Daily dose for children should not exceed adult dosage.
[2] Half-life in patients with renal failure is approximately 13 hours.

TICARCILLIN AND CLAVULANATE POTASSIUM: Administer by IV infusion over 30 minutes.

Ticarcillin/Clavulanate Potassium Uses and Dosages	
Infection	Dosage
Systemic and urinary tract infections:	
Adults (≥ 60 kg)	3.1 g[1] every 4 to 6 hours
(≤ 60 kg)[2]	200 to 300 mg/kg/day (based on ticarcillin content) in divided doses every 4 to 6 hrs
Gynecologic infections:	
Adults (≥ 60 kg)	
moderate infections	200 mg/kg/day in divided doses every 6 hours
severe infections	300 mg/kg/day in divided doses every 4 hours

[1] 3 g ticarcillin plus 100 mg clavulanic acid.
[2] Dosage in children < 12 years of age is not established.

Dosage of Ticarcillin/Clavulanate Potassium in Renal Insufficiency[1]	
Initial loading dose is 3.1 g[2]. Follow with doses based on creatinine clearance and type of dialysis.	
Creatinine clearance (ml/min)	*Dosage*
> 60	3.1 g[2] every 4 hours
30 to 60	2 g every 4 hours
10 to 30	2 g every 8 hours
<10	2 g every 12 hours
< 10 with hepatic dysfunction	2 g every 24 hours
Patients on peritoneal dialysis	3.1 g[2] every 12 hours
Patients on hemodialysis	2 g every 12 hours supplemented with 3.1 g[2] after each dialysis

[1] Half-life of ticarcillin in patients with renal failure is ≈ 13 hours.
[2] 3 g ticarcillin plus 100 mg clavulanic acid.

CEPHALOSPORINS AND RELATED ANTIBIOTICS

CEFACLOR	
Tablets, extended release: 375 mg or 500 mg (*Rx*)	*Ceclor CD* (Lilly)
Capsules: 250 or 500 mg (*Rx*)	Various, *Ceclor Pulvules* (Lilly)
Suspension: 125, 187, 250 or 375 mg/5 ml (*Rx*)	Various, *Ceclor* (Lilly)
CEFADROXIL	
Capsules: 500 mg (*Rx*)	Various, *Duricef* (Mead Johnson)
Tablets: 1 g (*Rx*)	Various, *Duricef* (Mead Johnson)
Oral Suspension: 125, 250 or 500 mg/5 ml (*Rx*)	Various, *Ultracef* (Mead Johnson)
CEFAMANDOLE NAFATE	
Powder for injection: 1, 2 and 10 g (*Rx*)	*Mandol* (Lilly)
CEFAZOLIN SODIUM	
Powder for injection: 250 or 500 mg, 1, 5, 10 or 20 g (*Rx*)	Various, *Ancef* (SK-Beecham), *Zolicef* (Apothecon)
Injection: 500 mg or 1 g in 5% Dextrose in Water (*Rx*)	*Ancef* (SK-Beecham)
CEFEPIME HCl	
Powder for injection: 500 mg, 1 and 2 g (*Rx*)	*Maxipime* (Bristol-Myers Squibb)
CEFIXIME	
Tablets: 200 or 400 mg (*Rx*)	*Suprax* (Lederle)
Powder for oral suspension: 100 mg/5 ml (*Rx*)	*Suprax* (Lederle)
CEFMETAZOLE SODIUM	
Powder for injection: 1 or 2 g (*Rx*)	*Zefazone* (Upjohn)
CEFONICID SODIUM	
Powder for injection: 500 mg, 1 or 10 g (*Rx*)	*Monocid* (SmithKline Beecham)
CEFOPERAZONE SODIUM	
Powder for injection: 1 or 2 g (*Rx*)	*Cefobid* (Roerig)
Injection: 1 or 2 g (*Rx*)	*Cefobid* (Roerig)
CEFOTAXIME SODIUM	
Powder for injection: 1, 2 or 10 g (*Rx*)	*Claforan* (Hoechst-Marion Roussel)
Injection: 1 or 2 g (*Rx*)	*Claforan* (Hoechst-Marion Roussel)
CEFOTETAN DISODIUM	
Powder for injection: 1, 2 or 10 g (*Rx*)	*Cefotan* (Stuart)
CEFOXITIN SODIUM	
Powder for injection: 1, 2 or 10 g (*Rx*)	*Mefoxin* (Merck)
Injection: 1 or 2 g in 5% Dextrose in Water (*Rx*)	*Mefoxin* (Merck)
CEFPODOXIME PROXETIL	
Tablets: 100 or 200 mg (*Rx*)	*Vantin* (Upjohn)
Granules for suspension: 50 or 100 mg/5 ml (*Rx*)	*Vantin* (Upjohn)
CEFPROZIL	
Tablets: 250 or 500 mg (*Rx*)	*Cefzil* (Bristol Labs)
Powder for suspension: 125 or 250 mg/5 ml (*Rx*)	*Cefzil* (Bristol Labs)
CEFTAZIDIME	
Powder for injection: 349 or 500 mg, 1, 2 or 6 g (*Rx*)	*Fortaz* (Glaxo Wellcome)
Injection: 1 or 2 g (*Rx*)	*Fortaz* (Glaxo Wellcome)
CEFTIBUTEN	
Capsules: 400 mg (*Rx*)	*Cedax* (Schering)
Oral suspension: 90 or 180 mg/5 ml (*Rx*)	
CEFTIZOXIME SODIUM	
Powder for injection: 500 mg, 1, 2 or 10 g (*Rx*)	*Cefizox* (Fujisawa)
Injection: 1 or 2 g in 5% Dextrose in Water (*Rx*)	*Cefizox* (Fujisawa)
CEFTRIAXONE SODIUM	
Powder for injection: 250 or 500 mg, 1, 2 or 10 g (*Rx*)	*Rocephin* (Roche)
Injection: 1 or 2 g (*Rx*)	*Rocephin* (Roche)

Product	Manufacturer
CEFUROXIME	
Tablets: 125, 250 or 500 mg (*Rx*)	*Ceftin* (Glaxo Wellcome)
Suspension: 125 mg/5 ml (when reconstituted) (*Rx*)	*Ceftin* (Glaxo Wellcome)
Powder for injection: 750 mg, 1.5 or 7.5 g per vial (*Rx*)	Various, *Zinacef* (Glaxo Wellcome), *Kefurox* (Lilly)
Injection: 750 mg or 1.5 g (*Rx*)	*Zinacef* (Glaxo Wellcome)
CEPHALEXIN	
Capsules: 250 and 500 mg (*Rx*)	Various, *Keflex* (Dista)
Tablets: 250 and 500 mg and 1 g (*Rx*)	Various
Oral suspension: 100 or 200 mg (*Rx*)	Various, *Keflex* (Dista)
Powder for oral suspension: 125 or 250 mg/5 ml (when reconstituted) (*Rx*)	*Biocef* (Inter. Ethical Labs)
CEPHALEXIN HCl MONOHYDRATE	
Tablets: 500 mg (*Rx*)	*Keftab* (Dista)
CEPHALOTHIN SODIUM	
Injection: 1 or 2 g in 5% Dextrose (*Rx*)	*Cephalothin Sodium* (Baxter)
Powder for injection: 1 or 2 g (*Rx*)	Various, *Keflin, Neutral* (Lilly)
CEPHAPIRIN SODIUM	
Powder for injection: 500 mg, 1, 2, 4 or 20 g (*Rx*)	Various, *Cefadyl* (Apothecon)
CEPHRADINE	
Capsules: 250 or 500 mg (*Rx*)	Various, *Velosef* (Apothecon)
Oral suspension: 125 or 250 mg/5 ml (when reconstituted) (*Rx*)	Various, *Velosef* (Apothecon)
Powder for injection: 250 or 500 mg, 1 or 2 g (*Rx*)	*Velosef* (Apothecon)
LORACARBEF	
Pulvules (capsules): 200 and 400 mg (*Rx*)	*Lorabid* (Lilly)
Powder for suspension: 100 and 200 mg/5 ml (*Rx*)	*Lorabid* (Lilly)
Oral suspension: 100 and 200 mg/5 ml (*Rx*)	*Lorabid* (Lilly)

Actions:

Pharmacology: Structurally and pharmacologically related to penicillins. Cefoxitin and cefotetan (cephamycins) and loracarbef (a carbacephem) are included due to their similarity.

Cephalosporins inhibit mucopeptide synthesis in the bacterial cell wall, making it defective and osmotically unstable. The drugs are usually bactericidal, depending on organism susceptibility, dose, tissue concentrations and the rate at which organisms are multiplying. They are more effective against rapidly growing organisms forming cell walls.

Pharmacokinetics:

Pharmacokinetic Parameters of Cephalosporins

	Drug	Routes	Half-Life: Normal renal function (minutes)	Half-Life: ESRD [1] (hours)	Half-Life: Hemo-dialysis (hours)	Protein bound (%)	Recovered unchanged in urine (%)	Peak serum level 1 g IV dose (mcg/ml)	Sodium (mEq/g)
First	Cephalexin	Oral	50-80	19-22	4-6	10	> 90	–	-
	Cefadroxil	Oral	78-96	20-25	3-4	20	> 90	-	-
	Cephradine	Oral/IM-IV	48-80	8-15	-	8-17	> 90	86	6 [2]
	Cephalothin	IM-IV	30-50	3-15	3	70	68-70	30	2.8
	Cephapirin	IM-IV	24-36	1.8-4	1.8	54	68-70	73	2.4
	Cefazolin	IM-IV	90-120	3-7	9-14	80-86	80-96	185-189	2-2.1
Second	Cefaclor	Oral	35-54	2-3	1.6-2.1	25	60-85	-	-
	Cefamandole	IM-IV	30-60	8-11	7	70	65-85	139	3.3
	Cefoxitin	IM-IV	40-60	20	4	73	85-99	64-110	2.3
	Cefuroxime	Oral/IM-IV	80	16-22 [3]	3.5	33-50	66-100	100 [4]	2.4 [3]
	Cefonicid	IM-IV	270	11	-	98	95-99	221.3	3.7
	Cefmetazole	IV	72	-	-	65	85	-	2
	Cefotetan	IM-IV	180-276	13-35	5	88-90	51-81	158	3.5
	Cefprozil	Oral	78	5.2-5.9	de-creased	36	60	-	-
	Cefpodoxime [5]	Oral	120-180	9.8	-	21-29	29-33	-	-
	Loracarbef	Oral	60	32	4	25	> 90	-	-
Third	Cefixime	Oral	180-240	11.5	-	65	50	-	-
	Cefpodoxime[5]	Oral	120-180	9.8	-	21-29	29-33	-	-
	Cefoperazone	IM-IV	102-156	1.3-2.9	2	82-93	20-30	73-153	1.5
	Cefotaxime	IM-IV	60	3-11	2.5	30-40	20-36	42-102	2.2
	Ceftizoxime	IM-IV	84-114	25-30	6	30	80	60-87	2.6
	Ceftriaxone	IM-IV	348-522	15.7	14.7	85-95	33-67	151	3.6
	Ceftazidime	IM-IV	114-120	14-30	-	< 10-17	80-90	69-90	2.3
	Ceftibuten	Oral	144	13.4-22.3	2-4	65	56	-	-
	Cefepime	IM-IV	102-138	17-21	11-16	20	85	79	-

[1] ESRD = End stage renal disease (Ccr < 10 ml/min/1.73 m^2).
[2] Also available in sodium free form.
[3] Injection only.
[4] Following 1.5 g IV dose.
[5] Extended spectrum agent.

Cephalexin, cephradine, cefaclor, cefixime, cefprozil, cefadroxil, ceftibuten and loracarbef are well absorbed from the GI tract. Cephalosporins are widely distributed to most tissues and fluids. First and second generation agents do not readily enter cerebrospinal fluid (CSF), except cefuroxime, even when meninges are inflamed. Third generation compounds (little data for cefixime) readily diffuse into the CSF of patients with inflamed meninges. However, CSF levels of cefoperazone are relatively low. Most cephalosporins and metabolites are primarily excreted renally.

Microbiology:

Organisms Generally Susceptible to Cephalosporins

Organisms		First Generation						Second Generation				
✓= generally susceptible ‡ = demonstrated in vitro activity		Cephalexin	Cefadroxil	Cephradine	Cephalothin	Cephapirin	Cefazolin	Cefaclor	Cefamandole	Cefoxitin	Cefuroxime	Cefonicid
Gram-positive	*Staphylococci*[1]	✓[2]	✓	✓	✓	✓	✓	✓[2]	✓	✓	✓	✓[2]
	Streptococci, betahemolytic	✓	✓	✓	✓	✓	✓	✓	✓	✓	✓	✓
	Streptococcus pneumoniae	✓	✓	✓	✓	✓	✓	✓	✓	✓	✓	✓
	Streptococcus pyogenes											
Gram-negative	*Acinetobacter* sp											
	Citrobacter sp										✓[2]	‡
	Enterobacter sp						✓[2]		✓		✓[2]	‡
	Escherichia coli	✓	✓	✓	✓	✓	✓	✓	✓	✓	✓	✓
	Haemophilus influenzae	✓		✓	✓	✓	✓	✓[3]	✓[3]	✓[3]	✓[3]	✓[3]
	Haemophilus parainfluenzae										‡	
	Hafnia alvei											
	Klebsiella sp	✓	✓	✓	✓	✓	✓	✓	✓	✓	✓	✓
	Moraxella (Branhamella) catarrhalis	‡						✓			‡	
	Morganella (Proteus) morganii								✓	✓	✓[2]	✓
	Neisseria gonorrhoeae							‡		✓	✓	‡
	Neisseria meningitidis										✓	
	Proteus mirabilis	✓	✓	✓	✓	✓	✓	✓	✓	✓	✓	✓
	Proteus vulgaris								✓[2]	✓		✓
	Providencia sp									✓	✓	
	Providencia rettgeri								✓	✓	✓	✓
	Pseudomonas aeruginosa											
	Salmonella sp				✓						✓	
	Salmonella typhi											
	Serratia sp											
	Shigella sp				✓						✓	
Anaerobes	*Bacteroides* sp							✓	✓	✓	✓	
	Bacteroides fragilis									✓		
	Clostridium sp								✓	✓	✓	‡
	Clostridium difficile											
	Eubacterium sp											
	Fusobacterium sp								✓		✓	‡
	Peptococcus sp							‡	✓	✓	✓	‡
	Peptostreptococcus sp							‡	✓	✓	✓	‡

[1] Coagulase-positive, coagulase-negative and penicillinase-producing.
[2] Some strains are resistant.
[3] Including some β-lactamase-producing strains.

Organisms Generally Susceptible to Cephalosporins

Second Generation (Cont.)					Third Generation								Organisms	
Cefmetazole	Cefotetan	Cefprozil	Cefpodoxime[4]	Loracarbef	Cefixime	Cefoperazone	Cefotaxime	Ceftizoxime	Ceftriaxone	Ceftazidime	Ceftibuten	Cefepime	✓= generally susceptible ‡= demonstrated in vitro activity	
✓	✓	✓	✓[2]	✓		✓	✓[3]	✓	✓	✓		✓[5]	*Staphylococci*[1]	Gram-positive
✓	✓	✓	✓	✓	✓	✓	✓	✓	✓	✓		‡	*Streptococci*, betahemolytic	
✓	✓	✓	✓	✓	✓	✓	✓	✓	✓	✓	✓[6]	✓	*Streptococcus pneumoniae*	
											✓	✓[7]	*Streptococcus pyogenes*	
						✓[2]	✓	✓	✓	‡		‡	*Acinetobacter* sp	Gram-negative
‡	‡	‡	‡	‡	‡	✓	✓	‡	‡	✓		‡	*Citrobacter* sp	
‡	✓					✓	✓	✓	✓	✓		✓	*Enterobacter* sp	
✓	✓	‡	✓	✓	✓	✓	✓	✓	✓	✓		✓	*Escherichia coli*	
✓[3]	✓[3]	✓[3]	✓[3]	✓[3]	✓[3]	✓[3]	✓[3]	✓[3]	✓[3]	✓[3]	✓[3]	‡[3]	*Haemophilus influenzae*	
			‡	‡	‡[3]		✓		✓	‡			*Haemophilus parainfluenzae*	
												‡	*Hafnia alvei*	
✓	✓	‡	✓	‡	‡	✓	✓	✓	✓	✓		✓	*Klebsiella* sp	
‡		✓	✓	✓[3]	✓[3]			‡		✓	✓[3]	‡[3]	*Moraxella (Branhamella) catarrhalis*	
✓	✓					✓	✓	✓	✓	‡		‡	*Morganella (Proteus) morganii*	
‡	✓	‡	✓[2]	‡[1]	‡	✓[3]	✓	✓	✓	‡			*Neisseria gonorrhoeae*	
	‡					‡	✓	‡	✓	✓			*Neisseria meningitidis*	
✓	✓	‡	✓	‡	✓	✓	✓	✓	✓	✓		✓	*Proteus mirabilis*	
✓	✓		‡		‡	✓	✓	✓	✓	✓		‡	*Proteus vulgaris*	
✓	✓				‡		‡	‡	‡	‡		‡	*Providencia* sp	
‡	✓		‡		‡	✓	✓	✓	‡	‡		‡	*Providencia rettgeri*	
						✓	✓[2]	✓[2]	✓[2]	✓		✓	*Pseudomonas aeruginosa*	
‡	‡	‡		‡	‡	‡	‡	‡	‡	‡			*Salmonella* sp	
	‡						‡	‡	‡				*Salmonella typhi*	
	‡				‡	✓	✓	✓	✓	✓		‡	*Serratia* sp	
‡	‡	‡		‡	‡	‡	‡	‡	‡	‡			*Shigella* sp	
✓	✓[2]	‡				✓	✓	‡	✓				*Bacteroides* sp	Anaerobes
✓	✓					✓	✓	✓	‡				*Bacteroides fragilis*	
✓	✓	‡		‡		✓	✓	‡	‡	‡			*Clostridium* sp	
		‡				‡							*Clostridium difficile*	
						‡			‡				*Eubacterium* sp	
✓	✓	‡		‡		‡	✓	‡	‡				*Fusobacterium* sp	
‡	✓			‡		✓	✓	✓	‡	‡			*Peptococcus* sp	
‡	✓	‡	‡	‡		✓	✓	✓	‡	‡			*Peptostreptococcus* sp	

[1] Coagulase-positive, coagulase-negative and penicillinase-producing.
[2] Some strains are resistant.
[3] Including some β-lactamase-producing strains.
[4] Extended spectrum agent.
[5] Methicillin-susceptible strains only.
[6] Penicillin-susceptible strains only.
[7] Lancefield's Group A streptococci.

Indications:

For approved indications, refer to the Administration and Dosage section.

Contraindications:

Hypersensitivity to cephalosporins or related antibiotics.

Warnings:

Cefepime has a broad spectrum of activity against gram-positive and gram-negative bacteria but has a low affinity for chromosomally-encoded beta-lactamases.

Hypersensitivity: Reactions range from mild to life-threatening. Before therapy is instituted, inquire about previous hypersensitivity reactions to cephalosporins and penicillins.

Cross-allergenicity with penicillin: Administer cautiously to penicillin-sensitive patients. There is evidence of partial cross-allergenicity; cephalosporins cannot be assumed to be an absolutely safe alternative to penicillin in the penicillin-allergic patient. The estimated incidence of cross-sensitivity is 5% to 16%; however, it is possibly as low as 3% to 7%.

Serum sickness-like reactions: (erythema multiforme or skin rashes accompanied by polyarthritis, arthralgia and, frequently, fever) have been reported; these reactions usually occurred following a second course of therapy. Signs and symptoms occur after a few days of therapy and resolve a few days after drug discontinuation with no serious sequelae.

Seizures: Several cephalosporins have been implicated in triggering seizures, particularly in patients with renal impairment when the dosage was not reduced.

Coagulation abnormalities: **Cefamandole** and **cefoperazone** can interfere with hemostasis through three different mechanisms: Hypoprothrombinemia with or without bleeding; platelet dysfunction; very rarely, immune-mediated thrombocytopenia. Alterations in prothrombin times (PT) occur rarely in patients treated with **ceftriaxone.**

Predisposing factors to cephalosporin bleeding abnormalities include hepatic and renal dysfunction, thrombocytopenia and the concomitant use of "high dose" heparin (> 20,000 units/day), oral anticoagulants or other drugs that affect hemostasis (eg, aspirin). Elderly, malnourished or debilitated patients are more likely to experience bleeding abnormalities than other patients.

Pseudomembranous colitis occurs with the use of cephalosporins (and other broad spectrum antibiotics); therefore, consider its diagnosis in patients who develop diarrhea with antibiotic use.

Renal function impairment: Cephalosporins may be nephrotoxic; use with caution in the presence of markedly impaired renal function (creatinine clearance [Ccr] rate of < 50 ml/min/1.73 m^2).

Hepatic function impairment: Cefoperazone is extensively excreted in bile. Serum half-life increases twofold to fourfold in patients with hepatic disease or biliary obstruction.

Pregnancy: Category B; (*Category* C - Moxalactam). These agents cross the placenta; peak umbilical cord concentrations for the various agents range from 3 to 29 mcg/ml following doses of 0.5 to 2 g.

Lactation: Most of these agents are excreted in breast milk in small quantities. Levels range from 0.16 to 4 mcg/ml, or a breast milk:maternal serum ratio of 0.01 to 0.5 following 0.5 to 2 g doses.

Children: When using cephalosporins in infants, consider the relative benefit to risk. In neonates, accumulation of cephalosporin antibiotics (with resulting prolongation of drug half-life) has occurred.

Safety and efficacy in children < 1 month (**cefaclor, cefamandole, cefazolin** and **parenteral cephradine**), < 3 months (**cefuroxime**), < 6 months (**cefixime, cefpodoxime**), < 9 months (**oral cephradine**) and < 1 year (**ceforanide**) have not been established.

Safety and efficacy of **cefoperazone** and **cefotetan** in children not established.

Precautions:

Parenteral use: Inject IM preparations deep into musculature; properly dilute IV preparations and administer over an appropriate time interval.

Gonorrhea: In the treatment of gonorrhea, all patients should have a serologic test for syphilis. Patients with incubating syphilis (seronegative without clinical signs of syphilis) are likely to be cured by the regimens used for gonorrhea.

Drug Interactions:

Agents that may interact with cephalosporins include ethanol, aminoglycosides, anticoagulants, polypeptide antibiotics and probenecid.

Drug/Lab test interactions: A false-positive reaction for **urine glucose** may occur with Benedict's solution, Fehling's solution or with *Clinitest* tablets, but not with enzyme-based tests such as *Clinistix* and *Tes-Tape*. There may be a false-positive test for *proteinuria* with acid and denaturization-precipitation tests.

Cephradine may cause false-positive reactions in urinary protein tests that use sulfosalicylic acid.

Cefuroxime may cause a false-negative reaction in the ferricyanide test for *blood glucose*.

A false-positive direct *Coombs' test* has occurred in some patients receiving cephalosporins.

Cephalosporins may falsely elevate *urinary 17-ketosteroid* values.

High concentrations of **cephalothin** or **cefoxitin** (> 100 mcg/ml) may interfere with measurement of *creatinine levels* by the Jaffe reaction and produce false results. **Cefotetan** may also affect these measurements.

Drug/Food interactions: Food increases absorption of cefpodoxime, oral cefuroxime.

Adverse Reactions:

Most common: GI disturbances (nausea, vomiting, diarrhea); hypersensitivity phenomena (most common); hypotension; fever; dyspnea; candidal overgrowth consisting of oral candidiasis, vaginitis, genital moniliasis, vaginal discharge and genito-anal pruritus; nervousness; insomnia; confusion; hypertonia; dizziness; somnolence.

Hematologic: Eosinophilia; transient neutropenia; leukocytosis; leukopenia; thrombocythemia; thrombocytopenia; agranulocytosis; granulocytopenia; hemolytic anemia; bone marrow depression; pancytopenia; decreased platelet function; anemia; aplastic anemia; hemorrhage.

Hepatic: Elevated AST, ALT, GGTP, total bilirubin, alkaline phosphatase, LDH; hepatitis.

Renal: Transitory elevations in BUN with and without elevated serum creatinine (frequency increases in patients > 50 years old and in children < 3).

CNS: Headache; dizziness; lethargy; fatigue; paresthesia; confusion; diaphoresis; flushing.

Local: IM administration commonly results in pain, induration, temperature elevation and tenderness.

Administration and Dosage:

Duration of therapy: Continue administration for a minimum of 48 to 72 hours after fever abates or after evidence of bacterial eradication has been obtained.

Perioperative prophylaxis: Discontinue prophylactic use within 24 hours after the surgical procedure. In surgery where infection may be particularly devastating, may continue prophylactic use for 3 to 5 days following surgery completion.

CEFACLOR:

Adults – Usual dosage is 250 mg every 8 hours. In severe infections or those caused by less susceptible organisms, dosage may be doubled.

Tablets, extended release: Administer with food to enhance absorption. Do not cut, crush or chew.

Acute bacterial exacerbations of chronic bronchitis – 500 mg/12 hours for 7 days.
Secondary bacterial infection of acute bronchitis – 500 mg/12 hours for 7 days.
Pharyngitis or tonsillitis – 375 mg/12 hours for 10 days.

Uncomplicated skin and skin structure infections – 375 mg/12 hours for 7 to 10 days.

Children – Give 20 mg/kg/day in divided doses, every 8 hours. In more serious infections, otitis media and infections caused by less susceptible organisms, administer 40 mg/kg/day, with a maximum dosage of 1 g/day.

Twice daily treatment option: For otitis media and pharyngitis, the total daily dosage may be divided and administered every 12 hours.

CEFADROXIL: Can be given without regard to meals.

Urinary tract infections – For uncomplicated lower urinary tract infection (eg, cystitis), the usual dosage is 1 or 2 g/day in single or 2 divided doses. For all other urinary tract infections, the usual dosage is 2 g/day in 2 divided doses.

Skin and skin structure infections – 1 g/day in single or 2 divided doses.

Pharyngitis and tonsillitis –

Group A β-hemolytic streptococci: 1 g/day in single or 2 divided doses for 10 days.

Children –

Urinary tract infections, skin and skin structure infections: 30 mg/kg/day in divided doses every 12 hours.

Pharyngitis, tonsillitis: 30 mg/kg/day in single or 2 divided doses. For β-hemolytic streptococcal infections, continue treatment for at least 10 days.

Renal impairment – Adjust dosage according to creatinine clearance rates to prevent drug accumulation.

Initial adult dose: 1 g: the maintenance dose (based on creatinine clearance rate, ml/min/1.73 m^2) is 500 mg at the intervals below:

Cefadroxil Dosage in Renal Impairment

Creatinine clearance (ml/min)	Dosage interval (hours)
0-10	36
10-25	24
25-50	12
> 50	No adjustment

CEFAMANDOLE NAFTATE:

Adults – Usual dosage range is 500 mg to 1 g every 4 to 8 hours; 500 mg every 6 hours is adequate in uncomplicated skin and skin structure infections. In uncomplicated urinary tract infections, 500 mg every 8 hours; in more serious urinary tract infections, the dose may be increased to 1 g every 8 hours. In severe infections, administer 1 g at 4 to 6 hour intervals. In life-threatening infections or infections due to less susceptible organisms, up to 2 g every 4 hours may be needed.

Infants and children – 50 to 100 mg/kg/day in equally divided doses every 4 to 8 hours is effective for most infections susceptible to cefamandole. This may be incresed to 150 mg/kg/day (not to exceed the maximum adult dose) for severe infections.

Perioperative prophylaxis –

Adults: 1 or 2 g IM or IV, ½ to 1 hour prior to the surgical incision, followed by 1 or 2 g every 6 hours for 24 to 48 hours.

Children (3 months of age and older): 50 to 100 mg/kg/day in equally divided doses by the routes and schedule designated above.

Renal function impairment – Reduce dosages and monitor the serum levels. After an initial dose of 1 to 2 g (depending on the severity of infection), follow maintenance dosage in table.

Maintenance Cefamandole Dosage Guide for Patients with Renal Impairment			
Renal function	Creatinine clearance (ml/min/1.73 m ^{2})	Life-threatening infections (Maximum dosage)	Less severe infections
Normal impairment	> 80	2 g q 4 h	1-2 g q 6 h
Mild impairment	50-80	1.5 g q 4 h or 2 g q 6 h	0.75-1.5 g q 6 h
Moderate impairment	25-50	1.5 g q 6 h or 2 g q 8 h	0.75-1.5 g q 8 h
Severe impairment	10-25	1 g q 6 h or 1.25 g q 8 h	0.5-1 g q 8 h
Marked impairment	2-10	0.67 g q 8 h or 1 g q 12 h	0.5-0.75 g q 12 h
None	< 2	0.5 g q 8 h or 0.75 g q 12 h	0.25-0.5 g q 12 h

CEFAZOLIN SODIUM: Total daily dosages are the same for IM and IV administration.

Mild infections caused by susceptible gram-positive cocci – 250 to 500 mg every 8 hours.

Moderate to severe infections – 500 mg to 1 g every 6 to 8 hours.

Pneumococcal pneumonia – 500 mg every 12 hours.

Severe, life-threatening infections (eg, endocarditis, septicemia) – 1 to 1.5 g every 6 hours. Rarely, 12 g per day have been used.

Acute uncomplicated urinary tract infections – 1 g every 12 hours.

Perioperative prophylaxis –

Preoperative: 1 g IV or IM, ½ to 1 hour prior to surgery.

Intraoperative (≥ 2 hrs): 0.5 to 1 g IV or IM during surgery at appropriate intervals.

Postoperative: 0.5 to 1 g IV or IM every 6 to 8 hours for 24 hours after surgery.

Renal function impairment – All reduced dosage recommendations apply after an initial loading dose appropriate to the severity of the infection.

Cefazolin Dosage in Renal Impairment				
Serum Creatinine (mg %)	Ccr (ml/min)	Dose		Dosage Interval (hrs)
		≤1.5	≥ 55	
1.6-3	35-54	250 to 500	500 to 1000	≥ 8
3.1-4.5	11-34	125 to 250	250 to 500	12
≥ 4.6	≤ 10	125 to 250	250 to 500	18-24

Children –

Mild to moderately severe infections: A total daily dosage of 25 to 50 mg/kg (approximately 10 to 20 mg/lb) in 3 or 4 equal doses.

Severe infections: Total daily dosage may be increased to 100 mg/kg (45 mg/lb).

CEFEPIME:

Recommended Dosage Schedule for Cefepime			
Site and type of infection	Dose	Frequency	Duration (days)
Mild to moderate uncomplicated or complicated urinary tract infections, including pyelonephritis, due to *E. coli*, *K. pneumoniae* or *P. mirabilis*.[1]	0.5 to 1 g IV/IM [2]	q12h	7 to 10
Severe uncomplicated or complicated urinary tract infections, including pyelonephritis, due to *E. coli* or *K. pneumoniae*.	2 g IV	q12h	10
Moderate to severe pneumonia due to *S. pneumoniae*, *Pseudomonas aeruginosa*, *Klebsiella pneumoniae* or *Enterobacter* sp.	1 to 2 g IV	q12h	10
Moderate to severe uncomplicated skin and skin structure infections due to *S. aureus* or *S. pyogenes*.	2 g IV	q12h	10

[1] Including cases associated with concurrent bacteremia.
[2] IM route of administration is indicated only for mild to moderate, uncomplicated or complicated UTIs due to *E. coli* when the IM route is a more appropriate route of drug administration.

Renal function impairment – In patients with impaired renal function (creatinine clearance < 60 ml/min), adjust the dose of cefepime to compensate for the slower rate of renal elimination. The recommended initial dose should be the same as in patients with normal renal function.

In patients undergoing hemodialysis, ≈ 68% of the total amount of cefepime present in the body at the start of dialysis will be removed during a 3-hour dialysis period. A repeat dose, equivalent to the initial dose, should be given at the completion of each dialysis session.

In elderly patients with renal insufficiency, adjust dosage and administration.

In patients undergoing continuous ambulatory peritonial dialysis, administer cefepime at normal recommended doses at a dosage interval of every 48 hours.

<table>
<tr><th colspan="4">Recommended Cefepime Maintenance Schedule in Patients with Renal Impairment</th></tr>
<tr><th>Creatinine clearance (ml/min)</th><th colspan="3">Recommended maintenance schedule</th></tr>
<tr><td>> 60</td><td>500 mg q 12h [1]</td><td>1 g q 12h</td><td>2 g q 12h</td></tr>
<tr><td>30 to 60</td><td rowspan="2">500 mg q 24h</td><td>1 g q 24h</td><td>2 g q 24h</td></tr>
<tr><td>11 to 29</td><td>500 mg q 24h</td><td>1 g q 24h</td></tr>
<tr><td>≤ 10</td><td>250 mg q 24h</td><td>250 mg q 24h</td><td>500 mg q 24h</td></tr>
</table>

[1] Normal recommended dosing schedule.

IV administration – Administer over ≈ 30 minutes. Dilute with 50 to 100 ml of a compatible IV fluid. Cefepime is compatible at concentrations of 1 to 40 mg/ml with 0.9% Sodium Chloride Injection, 5% and 10% Dextrose Injection, M/6 Sodium Lactate Injection, 5% Dextrose and 0.9% Sodium Chloride Injection, Lactated Ringers and 5% Dextrose Injection, *Normosol-R* or *Normosol-M* in 5% Dextrose injection.

CEFIXIME:

Adults – 400 mg/day as a single 400 mg tablet (recommended for gonococcal infections) or as 200 mg every 12 hours.

Children – 8 mg/kg/day suspension as a single daily dose or as 4 mg/kg every 12 hours. Treat children > 50 kg or > 12 years of age with the recommended adult dose.

Treat otitis media with the suspension.

For S *pyogenes* infections, administer cefixime for at least 10 days.

Renal function impairment –

Cefixime Dosing in Renal Impairment	
Creatinine clearance (ml/min)	Dosage
> 60	Standard
21-60 or renal hemodialysis	75% of standard
≤ 20 or continuous ambulatory peritoneal dialysis	50% of standard

CEFMETAZOLE SODIUM:

Adults –

General guidelines: 2 g IV every 6 to 12 hours for 5 to 14 days.

Prophylaxis –

Cefmetazole Dosing Regimen for Prophylaxis	
Surgery	Dosing Regimen
Vaginal hysterectomy	2 g single dose 30 to 90 min before surgery or 1 g doses 30 to 90 min before surgery and repeated 8 and 16 hours later.
Abdominal hysterectomy	1 g doses 30 to 90 min before surgery and repeated 8 and 16 hours later.
Cesarean section	2 g single dose after clamping cord or 1 g doses after clamping cord; repeated at 8 and 16 hours.
Colorectal surgery	2 g single dose 30 to 90 minutes before surgery or 2 g doses 30 to 90 minutes before surgery and repeated 8 to 16 hours later.
Cholecystectomy (high risk)	1 g doses 30 to 90 minutes before surgery and repeated 8 and 16 hours later.

Renal function impairment –

Cefmetazole Dosage Guidelines in Renal Function Impairment			
Renal function	Creatinine clearance (ml/min/1.73 m^2)	Dose (g)	Frequency (hrs)
Mild impairment	50-90	1 to 2	q 12
Moderate impairment	30-49	1 to 2	q 16
Severe impairment	10-29	1 to 2	q 24
Essentially no function	< 10	1 to 2	q 48 [1]

[1] Administered after hemodialysis.

CEFONICID SODIUM:

Adults – Usual dose is 1 g/24 hours, IV or by deep IM injection. Doses > 1 g/day are rarely necessary; however, up to 2 g/day have been well tolerated.

General Cefonicid Dosage Guidelines (IM or IV)		
Type of infection	Daily dosage (g)	Frequency
Uncomplicated urinary tract	0.5	once every 24 hrs
Mild to moderate	1	once every 24 hrs
Severe or life-threatening	2[1]	once every 24 hrs
Surgical prophylaxis	1	1 hr preoperatively

[1] When administering 2 g IM doses once daily, divide dose in half and give each half in a different large muscle mass.

Preoperative prophylaxis – Administer 1 g 1 hour prior to appropriate surgical procedures, to provide protection from most infections due to susceptible organisms for approximately 24 hours after administration.

Renal function impairment requires modification of dosage. Following an initial loading dosage of 7.5 mg/kg, IM or IV, follow maintenance schedule below. It is not necessary to administer additional dosage following dialysis.

Cefonicid Dosage in Adults with Reduced Renal Function		
Creatinine Clearance (ml/min/1.73 [2])	Mild to moderate infections	Severe infections
60-79	10 mg/kg q 24 hr	25 mg/kg q 24 hr
40-59	8 mg/kg q 24 hr	20 mg/kg q 24 hr
20-39	4 mg/kg q 24 hr	15 mg/kg q 24 hr
10-19	4 mg/kg q 48 hr	15 mg/kg q 48 hr
5-9	4 mg/kg q 3 to 5 days	15 mg/kg q 3 to 5 days
< 5	3 mg/kg q 3 to 5 days	4 mg/kg q 3 to 5 days

CEFOPERAZONE SODIUM: Administer IM or IV.

Usual adult dose is 2 to 4 g/day administered in equally divided doses every 12 hours.

In severe infections or infections caused by less sensitive organisms, the total daily dose or frequency may be increased. Patients have been successfully treated with a total daily dosage of 6 to 12 g divided into 2, 3 or 4 administrations ranging from 1.5 to 4 g/dose. A total daily dose of 16 g by constant infusion has been given without complications.

Hepatic disease or biliary obstruction – In general, total daily dosage above 4 g should not be necessary.

Renal function impairment –

Hemodialysis: The half-life is reduced slightly during hemodialysis. Thus, schedule dosing to follow a dialysis period.

CEFOTAXIME SODIUM:

Adults – Administer IV or IM. Maximum daily dosage should not exceed 12 g.

Cefotaxime Dosage Guidelines for Adults		
Type of infection	Daily dosage (g)	Frequency and route
Gonorrhea	1	1 g IM (single dose)
Uncomplicated infections	2	1 g every 12 hours IM or IV
Moderate to severe	3 to 6	1 to 2 g every 8 hours IM or IV
Infections commonly needing higher dosage (eg, septicemia)	6 to 8	2 g every 6 to 8 hours IV
Life-threatening infections	up to 12	2 g every 4 hours IV

Perioperative prophylaxis: 1 g IV or IM, 30 to 90 minutes prior to surgery.

Cesarean section: Administer the first 1 g dose IV as soon as the umbilical cord is clamped. Administer the second and third doses as 1 g IV or IM at 6 and 12 hour intervals after the first dose.

Children –

Cefotaxime Dosage Guidelines in Pediatrics			
Age	Weight (kg)	Dosage schedule	Route
0 to 1 week	—	50 mg/kg every 12 hours	IV
1 to 4 weeks	—	50 mg/kg every 8 hours	IV
1 month to 12 years	< 50 [1]	50 to 180 mg/kg/day in 4 to 6 divided doses [2]	IV or IM

[1] For children ≥ 50 kg, use adult dosage.
[2] Use higher doses for more severe or serious infections including meningitis.

Renal function impairment – In patients with estimated creatinine clearances of less than 20 ml/min/1.73 m^2, reduce dosage by one-half.

CDC recommended treatment schedules for gonorrhea –

Disseminated gonococcal infection: Give 500 mg cefotaxime IV 4 times per day for at least 7 days.

Gonococcal ophthalmia in adults: For penicillinase-producing *Neisseria gonorrhoeae* (PPNG), give 500 mg, IV, 4 times per day.

CEFOTETAN DISODIUM:

Adults – The usual dosage is 1 or 2 g IV or IM every 12 hours for 5 to 10 days. Determine proper dosage and route of administration by the condition of the patient, severity of the infection and susceptibility of the causitive organism.

General Cefotetan Dosage Guidelines		
Type of infection	Daily dose	Frequency and route
Urinary tract	1 to 4 g	500 mg every 12 hours IV or IM 1 or 2 g every 24 hours IV or IM 1 or 2 g every 12 hours IV or IM
Other sites	2 to 4 g	1 or 2 g every 12 hours IV or IM
Severe	4 g	2 g every 12 hours IV
Life-threatening	6 g [1]	3 g every 12 hours IV

[1] Maximum daily dose should not exceed 6 g.

Prophylaxis – To prevent postoperative infection in clean contaminated or potentially contaminated surgery in adults, give a single 1 or 2 g IV dose 30 to 60 minutes prior to surgery. In patients undergoing cesarean section, give the dose as soon as the umbilical cord is clamped.

Renal function impairment – Reduce the dosage schedule using the following guidelines:

Cefotetan Dosage in Renal Impairment		
Ccr (ml/min)	Dose	Frequency
> 30	Usual recommended dose[1]	Every 12 hours
10-30	Usual recommended dose[1]	Every 24 hours
< 10	Usual recommended dose[1]	Every 48 hours

[1] Dose determined by the type and severity of infection and susceptibility of the causitive organism.

Alternatively, the dosing interval may remain constant at 12 hour intervals, but reduce dose by one-half for patients with a creatinine clearance of 10 to 30 ml/min, and by one-quarter for patients with a creatinine clearance of less than 10 ml/min.

Dialysis – Cefotetan is dialyzable; for patients undergoing intermittent hemodialysis, give one-quarter of the usual recommended dose every 24 hours on days between dialysis and one-half of the usual recommended dose on the day of dialysis.

CEFOXITIN SODIUM:

Adult dosage range is 1 to 2 g every 6 to 8 hours.

Cefoxitin Dosage Guidelines		
Type of infection	Daily dosage	Frequency and route
Uncomplicated (pneumonia, urinary tract, cutaneous) [1]	3 to 4 g	1 g every 6 to 8 hours IV or IM
Moderately severe or severe	6 to 8 g	1 g every 4 hours or 2 g every 6 to 8 hours IV
Infections commonly requiring higher dosage (eg, gas, gangrene)	12 g	2 g every 4 hours or 3 g every 6 hours IV

[1] Including patients in whom bacteremia is absent or unlikely.

Uncomplicated gonorrhea – 2 g IM with 1 g oral probenecid given concurrently or up to 30 minutes before cefoxitin.

Prophylactic use, surgery – Administer 2 g IV or IM 30 to 60 minutes prior to surgery followed by 2 g every 6 hours after the first dose for no more than 24 hours (continued for 72 hours after prosthetic arthroplasty).

Prophylactic use, cesarean section – Administer 2 g IV as soon as the umbilical cord is clamped. If a three dose regimen is used, give the second and third 2 g dose IV, 4 and 8 hours after the first dose.

Prophylactic use, transurethral prostatectomy – Administer 1 g prior to surgery; 1 g every 8 hours for up to 5 days.

Renal function impairment –

Adults:

Maintenance Cefoxitin Dosage in Renal Impairment			
Renal function	Ccr (ml/min/1.73 m^2)	Dose (g)	Frequency (hrs)
Mild impairment	30-50	1-2	8-12
Moderate impairment	10-29	1-2	12-24
Severe impairment	5-9	0.5-1	12-24
Essentially no function	< 5	0.5-1	24-48

Hemodialysis – Administer a loading dose of 1 to 2 g after each hemodialysis. Give the maintenance dose as indicated in the table above.

Infants and children ≥ 3 months: 80 to 160 mg/kg/day divided every 4 to 6 hours. Use higher dosages for more severe or serious infections. Do not exceed 12 g/day.

Prophylactic use (≥ 3 months) – 30 to 40 mg/kg/dose every 6 hours

Renal function impairment – Modify consistent with recommendation for adults.

CDC recommended treatment schedules for acute pelvic inflammatory disease (PID) – For hospitalized patients, give 100 mg doxycycline, IV, twice/day plus 2 g cefoxitin, IV, 4 times/day. Continue drugs IV for at least 4 days and at least 48 hours after patient improves. Continue 100 mg oral doxycyline, twice/day after discharge to complete 10 to 14 days of therapy. For outpatients, give 2 g cefoxitin IM with 1 g oral probenecid, then 100 mg oral doxycycline, twice/day for 10 to 14 days.

CEFPODOXIME PROXETIL: Administer with food to enhance absorption.

Dosage/Duration of Cefpodoxime			
Type of infection	Total daily dose	Dose frequency	Duration
Adults ≥ 13 years of age:			
Acute community-acquired pneumonia	400 mg	200 mg every 12 hrs	14 days
Acute bacterial exacerbations of chronic bronchitis	400 mg	200 mg every 12 hrs	10 days
Uncomplicated gonorrhea (men and women) and rectal gonococcal infections (women)	200 mg	single dose	
Skin and skin structure	800 mg	400 mg every 12 hrs	7 to 14 days
Pharyngitis/Tonsillitis	200 mg	100 mg every 12 hrs	5 to 10 days
Uncomplicated urinary tract infection	200 mg	100 mg every 12 hrs	7 days
Children (age 6 months through 12 years):			
Acute otitis media	10 mg/kg/day divided every 12 hr (max 400 mg/day)	5 mg/kg/dose (max 200 mg/dose)	10 days

Dosage/Duration of Cefpodoxime			
Type of infection	Total daily dose	Dose frequency	Duration
Pharyngitis/Tonsillitis	10 mg/kg/day divided every 12 hr (max 200 mg/day)	5 mg/kg/dose (max 100 mg/dose)	5 to 10 days

Renal dysfunction – For patients with severe renal impairment (creatinine clearance [Ccr] < 30 ml/min), increase the dosing intervals to every 24 hours. In patients maintained on hemodialysis, use a frequency of 3 times/week after hemodialysis.

CEFPROZIL:

Dosage and Duration of Cefprozil		
Population/Infection	Dosage (mg)	Duration (days)
Adults (≥ 13 years of age)		
Upper respiratory tract		
Pharyngitis/Tonsillitis	500 q 24 h	10[1]
Lower respiratory tract		
Secondary bacterial infection of acute bronchitis and acute bacterial exacerbation of chronic bronchitis	500 q 12 h	10
Skin and skin structure		
Uncomplicated skin and skin structure infections	250 q 12 h or 500 q 24 h or 500 q 12 h	10
Infants and children (6 months to 12 years)		
Otitis media	15 mg/kg q 12 h	10
Children (2 to 12 years)		
Pharyngitis/Tonsillitis	7.5 mg/kg q 12 h	10[1]

[1] In treatment of infections due to *Streptococcus pyogenes*, administer for at least 10 days.

Renal function impairment – Cefprozil may be administered to patients with impaired renal function. Use the following dosage schedule.

Cefprozil Dosage in Renal Impairment		
Creatinine clearance (ml/min)	Dosage (mg)	Dosing interval
30 to 120	standard	standard
0 to 30 [1]	50% of standard	standard

[1] Cefprozil is in part removed by hemodialysis; therefore, administer after the completion of hemodialysis.

CEFTAZIDIME:

Ceftazidime Dosage Guidelines		
Patient/infection site	Dose	Frequency
Adults Usual recommended dose	1 g IV or IM	q 8-12 h
Uncomplicated urinary tract infections	250 mg IV or IM	q 12 h
Complicated urinary tract infections	500 mg IV or IM	q 8-12 h
Uncomplicated pneumonia; mild skin and skin structure infections	500 mg to 1 g IV or IM	q 8 h
Bone and joint infections	2 g IV	q 12 h
Serious gynecological and intra-abdominal infections	2 g IV	q 8 h
Meningitis		
Very severe life-threatening infections, especially in immunocompromised patients		

Ceftazidime Dosage Guidelines		
Patient/infection site	Dose	Frequency
Pseudomonal lung infections in cystic fibrosis patients w/normal renal function [1]	30 to 50 mg/kg IV up to 6 g/day	q 8 h
Neonates (0 to 4 weeks)	30 mg/kg IV	q 12 h
Infants and children (1 month to 12 years)	30 to 50 mg/kg IV up to 6 g/day [2]	q 8 h

[1] Although clinical improvement has been shown, bacteriological cures cannot be expected in patients with chronic respiratory disease and cystic fibrosis.
[2] Reserve the higher dose for immunocompromised children or children with cystic fibrosis or meningitis.

Renal function impairment – Ceftazidime is excreted by the kidneys, almost exclusively by glomerular filtration. In patients with impaired renal function (GFR < 50 ml/min), reduce dosage to compensate for slower excretion. In patients with suspected renal insufficiency, give an initial loading dose of 1 g. Estimate GFR to determine the appropriate maintenance dose.

Ceftazidime Dosage in Renal Impairment		
Creatinine clearance (ml/min)	Recommended unit dose of ceftazidime	Frequency of dosing
31-50	1 g	q 12 h
16-30	1 g	q 24 h
6-15	500 mg	q 24 h
≤ 5	500 mg	q 48 h

In patients with severe infections who normally receive 6 g ceftazidime daily were it not for renal insufficiency, the unit dose given in the table above may be increased by 50% or the dosing frequency increased appropriately.

Dialysis – Give a 1 g loading dose, followed by 1 g after each hemodialysis period.

Ceftazidime can also be used in patients undergoing intraperitoneal dialysis (IPD) and continuous ambulatory peritoneal dialysis (CAPD). Give a loading dose of 1 g, followed by 500 mg every 24 hours. In addition to IV use, ceftazidime can be incorporated in the dialysis fluid at a concentration of 250 mg per 2 L of dialysis fluid.

CEFTIBUTEN: Ceftibuten suspension must be administered at least 2 hours before or 1 hour after a meal.

Ceftibutin Dosage and Duration			
Type of infection	Daily maximum dose	Dose and frequency	Duration
Adults ≥ 12 years of age			
Acute bacterial exacerbations of chronic bronchitis due to *H influenzae*, *M catarrhalis* or *Streptococcus pneumoniae*	400 mg	400 mg qd	10 days
Pharyngitis and tonsillitis due to *S pyogenes*			
Acute bacterial otitis media due to *H influenzae*, *M catarrhalis* or *S pyogenes*			
Children			
Pharyngitis and tonsillitis due to *S pyogenes*	400 mg	9 mg/kg qd	10 days
Acute bacterial otitis media due to *H influenzae*, *M catarrhalis* or *S pyogenes*			

Ceftibuten Oral Suspension Pediatric Dosage Chart [1]			
Weight			
kg	lb	90 mg/5 ml	180 mg/5 ml
10	22	5 ml (1 tsp) qd	2.5 ml (½ tsp) qd
20	44	10 ml (2 tsp) qd	5 ml (1 tsp) qd
40	88	20 ml (4 tsp) qd	10 ml (2 tsp) qd

[1] Children > 45 kg should receive the maximum daily dose of 400 mg.

Renal function impairment – Ceftibuten may be given at normal doses in impaired renal function with creatinine clearance of ≥ 50 ml/min. Dosing recommendations for patients with varying degrees of renal insufficiency are presented in the following table.

Ceftibuten Dosage in Renal Impairment	
Creatinine clearance (ml/min)	Recommended dosing schedules
> 50	9 mg/kg or 400 mg q 24 h (normal dosing schedule)
30 - 49	4.5 mg/kg or 200 mg q 24 h
5 - 29	2.25 mg/kg or 100 mg q 24 h

Hemodialysis patients – In patients undergoing hemodialysis two or three times weekly, a single 400 mg dose of ceftibuten capsules or a single dose of 9 mg/kg (maximum of 400 mg) oral suspension may be given at the end of each hemodialysis session.

CEFTIZOXIME SODIUM:

Adults – Usual dosage is 1 or 2 g every 8 to 12 hours.

Ceftizoxime Dosage Guidelines in Adults		
Type of infection	Daily dose (g)	Frequency and route
Uncomplicated urinary tract	1	500 mg every 12 hours IM or IV
PID [1]	6	2 g every 8 hours IV
Other sites	2-3	1 g every 8 to 12 hours IV or IM
Severe or refractory	3-6	1 g every 8 hours IM or IV 2 g every 8 to 12 hours IM [1] or IV
Life-threatening [2]	9-12	3 to 4 g every 8 hours IV

[1] Dosages up to 2 g every 4 hours have been given.
[2] Divide 2 g IM doses and give in different large muscle masses.

Urinary tract infections – Higher dosage is recommended.

Gonorrhea, uncomplicated – A single 1 g IM injection is the usual dose.

Life-threatening infections – The IV route may be preferable for patients with bacterial septicemia, localized parenchymal abscesses (such as intra-abdominal abscess), peritonitis or other severe or life-threatening infections.

In those patients with normal renal function, the IV dosage is 2 to 12 g daily. In conditions such as bacterial septicemia, 6 to 12 g/day IV may be given initially for several days, and the dosage gradually reduced according to clinical response and laboratory findings.

Pediatric –

Children (≥ 6 months): 50 mg/kg every 6 to 8 hours. Dosage may be increased to 200 mg/kg/day. Do not exceed the maximum adult dose for serious infection.

Renal function impairment requires modification of dosage. Following an initial loading dose of 500 mg to 1 g IM or IV, use the maintenance dosing schedule in the following table.

Hemodialysis – No additional supplemental dosing is required following hemodialysis; give the dose (according to the table below) at the end of dialysis.

Ceftizoxime Dosage in Adults with Renal Impairment			
Renal function	Creatinine clearance (ml/min)	Less severe infections	Life-threatening infections
Mild impairment	50-79	500 mg q 8 h	750 mg to 1.5 g q 8 h
Moderate to severe impairment	5-49	250 to 500 mg q 12 h	500 mg to 1 g q 12 h
Dialysis patients	0-4	500 mg q 48 h or 250 mg q 24 h	500 mg to 1 g q 48 h or 500 mg q 24 h

CEFTRIAXONE SODIUM: Administer IV or IM.

Adults – Usual daily dosage is 1 to 2 g once a day (or in equally divided doses twice a day) depending on type and severity of infection. Do not exceed a total daily dose of 4 g.

Uncomplicated gonococcal infections: Give a single IM dose of 250 mg.

Surgical prophylaxis: Give a single 1 g dose ½ to 2 hours before surgery.

Children – To treat serious infections other than meningitis, administer 50 to 75 mg/kg/day (not to exceed 2 g) in divided doses every 12 hours.

Meningitis: 100 mg/kg/day (not to exceed 4 g). Thereafter, a total daily dose of 100 mg/kg/day (not to exceed 4 g/day) is recommended. May give daily dose once per day or in equally divided doses every 12 hours. Usual duration is 7 to 14 days.

Skin and skin structure infections: Give 50 to 75 mg/kg once daily (or in equally divided doses twice daily), not to exceed 2 g.

CDC recommended treatment schedules for chancroid, gonorrhea and acute pelvic inflammatory disease (PID) –

Chancroid (Haemophilus ducreyi infection): 250 mg IM as a single dose.

Gonococcal infections:

Uncomplicated – 125 mg IM once plus doxycycline.

Conjunctivitis – 1 g IM single dose.

Disseminated – 1 g IM or IV every 24 hours.

Meningitis/Endocarditis – 1 to 2 g IV every 12 hours for 10 to 14 days (meningitis) or for at least 4 weeks (endocarditis).

Children (< 45 kg) – With bacteremia or arthritis, use 50 mg/kg (maximum, 1 g) IM or IV in a single dose for 7 days. For meningitis, increase duration to 10 to 14 days and maximum dose to 2 g.

Infants – 25 to 50 mg/kg/day IV or IM in a single daily dose, not to exceed 125 mg. For disseminated infection, continue for 7 days, with a duration of 7 to 14 days with documented meningitis.

Acute PID (ambulatory): 250 mg IM plus doxycycline.

CEFUROXIME:

Oral – Tablets and suspension are NOT bioequivalent and NOT substitutable on a mg/mg basis.

Tablets: The tablets may be given without regard to meals.

Suspension: Must be administered with food.

Dosage for Cefuroxime Axetil Tablets		
Population/Infection	Dosage	Duration (days)
Adults (≥ 13 years)		
Pharyngitis/tonsillitis	250 mg bid	10
Acute bacterial exacerbations of chronic bronchitis and secondary bacterial infections of acute bronchitis	250 or 500 mg bid	10
Uncomplicated skin and skin structure infections	250 or 500 mg bid	10
Uncomplicated urinary tract infections	125 or 250 mg bid	7 to 10
Uncomplicated gonorrhea	1000 mg once	single dose
Children who can swallow tablets whole		
Pharyngitis/tonsillitis	125 mg bid	10
Acute otitis media	250 mg bid	10

Dosage for Cefuroxime Axetil Suspension			
Population/Infection	Dosage	Daily maximum dose	Duration (days)
Infants and children (3 months to 12 years)			
Pharyngitis/tonsillitis	20 mg/kg/day divided bid	500 mg	10
Acute otitis media	30 mg/kg/day divided bid	1000 mg	10
Impetigo	30 mg/kg/day divided bid	1000 mg	10

Renal failure: Because cefuroxime is renally eliminated, its half-life will be prolonged in patients with renal failure.

Parenteral –

Dosage:

Adults – 750 mg to 1.5 g IM or IV every 8 hours, usually for 5 to 10 days.

Cefuroxime Dosage Guidelines		
Type of Infection	Daily dosage (g)	Frequency
Uncomplicated urinary tract, skin and skin structure, disseminated gonococcal, uncomplicated pneumonia	2.25	750 mg every 8 hours
Severe or complicated	4.5	1.5 g every 8 hours
Bone and joint	4.5	1.5 g every 8 hours
Life-threatening or due to less susceptible organisms	6	1.5 g every 6 hours
Bacterial meningitis	9	≤ 3 g every 8 hours
Uncomplicated gonococcal	1.5 g IM [1]	single dose

[1] Administered at 2 different sites together with 1 g oral probenecid.

Preoperative prophylaxis: For clean-contaminated or potentially contaminated surgical procedures, administer 1.5 g IV prior to surgery (≈ ½ to 1 hour before). Thereafter, give 750 mg IV or IM every 8 hours when the procedure is prolonged.

For preventative use during open heart surgery, give 1.5 g IV at the induction of anesthesia and every 12 hours thereafter for a total of 6 g.

Renal function impairment: Reduce dosage.

Parenteral Cefuroxime Dosage in Renal Impairment (Adults)	
Creatinine clearance (ml/min)	Dose and frequency
> 20	750 mg to 1.5 g every 8 hours
10-20	750 mg every 12 hours
< 10	750 mg every 24 hours [1]

[1] Because cefuroxime is dialyzable, give patients on hemodialysis a further dose at the end of the dialysis.

Infants and children (> 3 months) – 50 to 100 mg/kg/day in equally divided doses every 6 to 8 hours. Use 100 mg/kg/day (not to exceed maximum adult dose) for more severe or serious infections.

Bone and joint infections: 150 mg/kg/day (not to exceed maximum adult dose) in equally divided doses every 8 hours.

Bacterial meningitis: Initially, 200 to 240 mg/kg/day IV in divided doses every 6 to 8 hours.

In renal insufficiency, modify dosage frequency per adult guidelines.

CEPHALEXIN:

Adults – 1 to 4 g/day in divided doses.

Usual dose: 250 mg every 6 hours.

Streptococcal pharyngitis, skin and skin structure infections, uncomplicated cystitis in patients > 15 years: 500 mg every 12 hours.

May need larger doses for more severe infections or less susceptible organisms.

If dose is > 4 g/day, use parenteral drugs.

Children –

Monohydrate: 25 to 50 mg/kg/day in divided doses. For streptococcal pharyngitis in patients > 1 year and skin and skin structure infections, divided total daily dose and give every 12 hours. In severe infections, double dose.

Otitis media – 75 to 100 mg/kg/day in 4 divided doses.

β-hemolytic streptococcal infections – Continue treatment for at least 10 days.

HCl monohydrate: Safety and efficacy not established for use in children.

CEPHALOTHIN SODIUM:

Adults – 500 mg to 1 g every 4 to 6 hours.

Uncomplicated pneumonia, furunculosis with cellulitis, most urinary tract infections: 500 mg every 6 hours.

Severe infections: Increase the dose to 1 g or administer 500 mg every 4 hours.

Life-threatening infections: Up to 2 g every 4 hours.

Normal renal function (bacteremia, septicemia or other severe life-threatening infections) – The IV dosage is 4 to 12 g daily. In conditions such as septicemia, 6 to 8 g per day may be administered IV for several days at the beginning of therapy; reduce the dosage gradually.

Infants and children – The dosage is proportionately less according to age, weight and severity of infection. Daily administration of 100 mg/kg (80 to 160 mg/kg or 40 to 80 mg/lb) in divided doses is effective for most infections susceptible to cephalothin.

Perioperative prophylaxis –

Preoperative: 1 to 2 g administered IV ½ to 1 hour prior to initial incision.

Intraoperative: 1 to 2 g during surgery, administered according to the duration of the surgery.

Postoperative: 1 to 2 g every 6 hours; discontinue within 24 hours after surgery.

Children: 20 to 30 mg/kg given at the times designated above.

Renal function impairment – Give an IV loading dose of 1 to 2 g. Determine the continued dosage schedule by degree of renal impairment, severity of infection and susceptibility of the causative organism. Base maximum doses on the following recommendations:

Cephalothin Dosage in Renal Impairment

Renal function	Creatinine clearance (ml/min)	Maximum adult dosage (maintenance)
Mild impairment	50-80	2 g every 6 hours
Moderate impairment	25-50	1.5 g every 6 hours
Severe impairment	10-25	1 g every 6 hours
Marked impairment	2-10	0.5 g every 6 hours
Essentially no function	< 2	0.5 g every 8 hours

CEPHAPIRIN SODIUM:

Adults – 500 mg to 1 g every 4 to 6 hours IM or IV. The lower dose is adequate for certain infections, such as skin and skin structure and most urinary tract infections; the higher dose is recommended for more serious infections.

Serious or life-threatening infections – Up to 12 g daily. Use the IV route when high doses are indicated.

Renal function impairment: Patients with reduced renal function (moderately severe oliguria or serum creatinine > 5 mg/100 ml) may be treated adequately with a lower dose, 7.5 to 15 mg/kg every 12 hours. Patients who are to be dialyzed should receive the same dose just prior to dialysis and every 12 hours thereafter.

Perioperative prophylaxis: 1 to 2 g IM or IV administered ½ to 1 hour prior to the start of surgery; 1 to 2 g during surgery (administration modified depending on duration of operation); 1 to 2 g IV or IM every 6 hours for 24 hours postoperatively.

Children – Recommended total daily dose is 40 to 80 mg/kg (20 to 40 mg/lb) administered in 4 equally divided doses.

Infants – Cephapirin has not been extensively studied in infants; therefore, in the treatment of children < 3 months of age, consider the relative benefit to risk.

CEPHRADINE:

Oral – May be given without regard to meals.

Adults:

Skin, skin structures and repiratory tract infections (other than lobar pneumonia) – Usual dose is 250 mg every 6 hours or 500 mg every 12 hours.

Lobar pneumonia – 500 mg every 6 hours or 1 g every 12 hours.

Uncomplicated urinary tract infections – The usual dose is 500 mg every 12 hours. In more serious infections and prostatitis, 500 mg every 6 hours or 1 g every 12 hours. Severe or chronic infections may require larger doses (up to 1 g every 6 hours).

Children: No adequate information is available on the efficacy of twice a day regimens in children less than 9 months of age. For children over 9 months, the usual dose is 25 to 50 mg/kg/day, in equally divided doses every 6 or 12 hours. For otitis media due to *H influenzae*, 75 to 100 mg/kg/day in equally divided doses every 6 or 12 hours is recommended; do not exceed 4 g/day.

All patients regardless of age and weight: Larger doses (up to 1 g 4 times/day) may be given for severe or chronic infections.

Parenteral – Parenteral therapy may be followed by oral. To minimize pain and induration, inject IM deep into a large muscle mass.

Adults: Daily dose is 2 to 4 g in equally divided doses 4 times/day, IM or IV. In bone infections, the usual dosage is 1 g IV, 4 times/day. A dose of 500 mg, 4 times/day is adequate in uncomplicated pneumonia, skin and skin structure infections and most urinary tract infections. In severe infections, dose may be increased by giving every 4 hours or by increasing dose up to a maximum of 8 g/day.

Perioperative prophylaxis – Recommended doses are 1 g IV or IM administered 30 to 90 minutes prior to the start of surgery, followed by 1 g every 4 to 6 hours after the first dose for 1 or 2 doses, or for up to 24 hours postoperatively.

Cesarean section – Give 1 g IV as soon as the umbilical cord is clamped. Give the second and third doses as 1 g IM or IV at 6 to 12 hours after the first dose.

Infants and children – 50 to 100 mg/kg/day in 4 equally divided doses; determine by age, weight and infection severity.

Renal impairment dosage –

Patients not on dialysis:

Cephradine Dosage in Renal Impairment		
Ccr (ml/min)	Dose (mg)	Time interval (hours)
> 20	500	6
5 to 20	250	6
< 5	250	12

Patients on chronic, intermittent dialysis: 250 mg initially; repeat at 12 hours and after 36 to 48 hours.

LORACARBEF: Administer at least 1 hour before or 2 hours after a meal.

Dosage/Duration of Loracarbef

Population/Infection	Dosage (mg)	Duration (days)
Adults ≥ 13 years of age		
Lower respiratory tract		
Secondary bacterial infection of acute bronchitis	200 - 400 q 12 h	7
Acute bacterial exacerbation of chronic bronchitis	400 q 12 h	7
Pneumonia	400 q 12 h	14
Upper respiratory tract		
Pharyngitis/Tonsillitis	200 q 12 h	10[1]
Sinusitis	400 q 12 h	10
Skin and skin structure		
Uncomplicated	200 q 12 h	7
Urinary tract		
Uncomplicated cystitis	200 q 24 h	7
Uncomplicated pyelonephritis	400 q 12 h	14
Infants and children (6 months to 12 years)		
Upper respiratory tract		
Acute otitis media [2]	30 mg/kg/day in divided doses q 12 h	10
Pharyngitis/Tonsillitis	15 mg/kg/day in divided doses q 12 h	10[1]
Skin and skin structure		
Impetigo	15 mg/kg/day in divided doses q 12 h	7

[1] In treatment of infections due to *S pyogenes*, administer for at least 10 days.
[2] Use suspension; It is more rapidly absorbed than capsules, resulting in higher peak plasma concentrations when given at the same dose.

Renal function impairment – Use usual dose and schedule in patients with creatinine clearance (Ccr) levels ≥ 50 ml/min. Patients with Ccr between 10 and 49 ml/min may be given half the recommended dose at the usual dosage interval. Patients with Ccr levels < 10 ml/min may receive recommended dose given every 3 to 5 days; patients on hemodialysis should receive another dose following dialysis.

MEROPENEM

Powder for injection: 500 mg or 1 g (*Rx*)	*Merrem IV* (Zeneca)

Actions:

Pharmacology: Meropenem is a broad-spectrum carbapenem antibiotic. The bactericidal activity of meropenem results from the inhibition of cell-wall synthesis. Meropenem readily penetrates the cell wall of most gram-positive and gram-negative bacteria to reach penicillin-binding-protein (PBP) targets.

Pharmacokinetics: Meropenem has dose-dependent kinetics.

In subjects with normal renal function, the elimination half-life of meropenem is ≈ 1 hour. Meropenem is excreted by the kidney with a half-life of 0.8 to 1.24 hours; 65% to 83% of the dose is recovered in the urine as meropenem and 20% to 28% as the inactive open β-lactam metabolite.

Plasma protein binding of meropenem is ≈ 2%. The volume of meropenem distribution is 15.7 to 26.68 L. Meropenem penetrates well into most body fluids and tissues, including cerebrospinal fluid, achieving concentrations matching or exceeding those required to inhibit most susceptible bacteria.

The pharmacokinetics of meropenem in pediatric patients ≥ 2 years of age are essentially similar to those in adults. In infants and children ages 2 months to 12 years, no age- or dose-dependent effects on pharmacokinetic parameters were observed. Mean half-life was 1.13 hours, mean volume of distribution at steady-state was 0.43 L/kg, mean residence time was 1.57 hours, clearance was 5.63 ml/min/kg and renal clearance was 2.53 ml/min/kg. The elimination half-life is slghtly prolonged (1.5 hours) in pediatric patients 3 months to 2 years of age.

Microbiology: Meropenem has significant stability to hydrolysis by β-lactamases of most categories, both penicillinases and cephalosporinases produced by gram-positive and gram-negative bacteria, with the exception of matallo-β-lactamases. Do not use to treat methicillin-resistant staphylococci. Cross resistance is sometimes observed with strains resistant to other carbapenems. In vitro tests show meropenem to act synergistically with aminoglycoside antibiotics against some isolates of *P. aeruginosa*.

Indications:

For the treatment of the following infections when caused by susceptible strains of the designated microorganisms:

Intra-abdominal infections: Complicated appendicitis and peritonitis caused by viridans group streptococci, *E. coli*, *K. pneumoniae*, *P. aeruginosa*, *B. fragilis*, *B. thetaiotaomicron* and *Peptostreptococcus* sp.

Bacterial meningitis (pediatric patients ≥ 3 months only): Bacterial meningitis caused by *S. pneumoniae*, *H. influenzae* (β-lactamase and non-β-lactamase-producing strains) and *N. meningitidis*.

Contraindications:

Hypersensitivity to any component of this product or to other drugs in the same class or in patients who have demonstrated anaphylactic reactions to β-lactams.

Warnings:

Pseudomembranous colitis has been reported with nearly all antibacterial agents, including meropenem and may range in severity from mild to life-threatening. Therefore, it is important to consider this diagnosis in patients who develop diarrhea subsequent to the administration of antibacterial agents.

Hypersensitivity: Serious and occasionally fatal hypersensitivity (anaphylactic) reactions have been reported in patients receiving therapy with β-lactams. These reactions are more likely to occur in individuals with a history of sensitivity to multiple allergens.

There have been reports of individuals with a history of penicillin hypersensitivity who have experienced severe hypersensitivity reactions when treated with other β-lactams.

Renal function impairment: Plasma clearance of meropenem correlates with creatinine clearance. In moderate renal dysfunction (Ccr 30 to 80 ml/min), mean half-life has been prolonged to 1.93 to 3.36 hours. In patients with greater dysfunction (Ccr 2 to 30 mg/min), mean half-life has been further prolonged to 3.82 to 5.73 hours. Patients undergoing hemodialysis (patients with end-stage renal disease) had mean predialysis half-lives of 7 to 10 hours. Hemodialysis shortened elimination half-life to 1.4 to 2.9 hours during the dialysis period.

Elderly: Elderly patients with renal insufficiency have shown a reduction in plasma clearance of meropenem that correlates with age-associated reduction in creatinine clearance. The mean terminal half-life is prolonged slightly to 1.27 hours.

Pregnancy: Category B.

Lactation: It is not known whether this drug is excreted in breast milk.

Children: The safety and efficacy of meropenem have not been established for children < 3 months of age (see Administration and Dosage).

Precautions:

Monitoring: Periodic assessment of organ system functions, including renal, hepatic and hematopoietic is advisable during prolonged therapy.

Seizures and other CNS adverse experiences have been reported during treatment with meropenem. These adverse experiences have occurred most commonly in patients with CNS disorders (eg, brain lesions or history of seizures) or with bacterial meningitis or compromised renal function.

Superinfection: As with other broad-spectrum antibiotics, prolonged use of meropenem may result in overgrowth of nonsusceptible organisms.

Drug Interactions:

Probenecid may interact with meropenem.

Adverse Reactions:

Adverse reactions occurring in ≥ 3% of patients include inflammation at the injection site, diarrhea, nausea and vomiting.

Adverse reactions occuring in ≥ 3% of pediatric patients include diarrhea, vomiting and rash (mostly diaper area moniliasis).

Administration and Dosage:

Adults: 1 g by IV administration every 8 hours. Give over ≈ 15 to 30 minutes or as an IV bolus injection (5 to 20 ml) over ≈ 3 to 5 minutes.

Renal function impairment: Reduce dosage in patients with creatinine clearance < 50 ml/min.

Recommended Meropenem IV Dosage Schedule for Adults with Impaired Renal Function

Creatinine clearance (ml/min)	Dose (dependent on type of infection)	Dosing interval
26 to 50	recommended dose (100 mg)	every 12 hours
10 to 25	one-half recommended dose	every 12 hours
< 10	one-half recommended dose	every 24 hours

When only serum creatinine is available the Cockcroft and Gault equation may be used to estimate creatinine clearance.

$$\text{Males: } \frac{\text{Weight (kg)} \times (140 - \text{age})}{72 \times \text{serum creatinine (mg/dl)}} = \text{Ccr}$$

Females: 0.85 × above value

Use in pediatric patients: For pediatric patients from ≥ 3 months of age, the meropenem dose is 20 or 40 mg/kg every 8 hours (maximum dose is 2 g every 8 hours), depending on the type of infection (intra-abdominal or meningitis). Administer pediatric patients weighing > 50 kg 1 g every 8 hours for intra-abdominal infections and 2 g every 8 hours for meningitis. Give over ≈ 15 to 30 minutes or as an IV bolus injection (5 to 20 ml) over ≈ 3 to 5 minutes.

Recommended Meropenem IV dosage Schedule for Pediatrics with Normal Renal Function		
Type of infection	Dose (mg/kg)	Dosing interval
Intra-abdominal	20	every 8 hours
Meningitis	40	every 8 hours

IMIPENEM-CILASTATIN

Powder for Injection: 250 mg, 500 mg and 750 mg imipenem equivalent and cilastatin equivalent. (*Rx*) — *Primaxin I.V.* (Merck), *Primaxin I.M.* (Merck)

Actions:

Pharmacology: This product is a formulation of imipenem, a thienamycin antibiotic, and cilastatin sodium, the inhibitor of the renal dipeptidase, dehydropeptidase-1, which is responsible for the extensive metabolism of imipenem when it is administered alone. Cilastatin prevents the metabolism of imipenem, increasing urinary recovery and decreasing possible renal toxicity. The bactericidal activity of imipenem results from the inhibition of cell wall synthesis, related to binding to penicillin binding proteins (PBP) 2 and 1B.

Pharmacokinetics:

Absorption/Distribution –

IV: IV infusion over 20 minutes results in peak plasma levels of imipenem antimicrobial activity that range from 14 to 83 mcg/ml, depending on the dose. Plasma levels declined to ≤ 1 mcg/ml in 4 to 6 hours. Peak plasma levels of cilastatin following a 20 minute IV infusion range from 15 to 88 mcg/ml, depending on the dose. The plasma half-life of each component is ≈ 1 hour.

IM: Following IM administration of 500 or 750 mg doses, peak plasma levels of imipenem antimicrobial activity occur within 2 hours and average 10 and 12 mcg/ml, respectively. When compared to IV administration, imipenem is ≈ 75% bioavailable following IM administration while cilastatin is ≈ 95% bioavailable. The prolonged absorption of imipenem following IM use results in an effective plasma half-life of ≈ 2 to 3 hours and plasma levels which remain above 2 mcg/ml for at least 6 or 8 hours following a 500 or 750 mg dose, respectively.

Imipenem urine levels remain above 10 mcg/ml for the 12 hour dosing interval following IM administration of 500 or 750 mg doses. Total urinary excretion of imipenem and cilastatin averages 50% and 75%, respectively, following either dose.

Metabolism/Excretion – Cilastatin prevents renal metabolism of imipenem. The protein binding of imipenem and cilastatin is ≈ 20% and 40%, respectively. Approximately 70% of imipenem and cilastatin is recovered in urine within 10 hours of administration.

Microbiology: It has a high degree of stability in the presence of β-lactamases, including penicillinases and cephalosporinases produced by gram-negative and gram-positive bacteria.

Indications:

IV:

Lower respiratory tract infections – *S aureus* (penicillinase-producing), *E coli*, *Klebsiella* sp, *Enterobacter* sp, *H influenzae*, *H parainfluenzae*, *Acinetobacter* sp, *S marcescens*.

Urinary tract infections (complicated and uncomplicated) – *Enterococcus faecalis*, *S aureus* (penicillinase-producing), group D streptococci (enterococci), *E coli*, *Klebsiella* sp, *Enterobacter* sp, *P vulgaris*, *P rettgeri*, *M morganii*, *P aeruginosa*.

Intra-abdominal infections – *E. faecalis*, *S aureus* (penicillinase-producing), *Staphylococcus epidermidis*,*E coli*, *Klebsiella* sp, *Enterobacter* sp, *Proteus* sp (indole-positive and indole-negative), *M morganii*, *P aeruginosa*, *Citrobacter* sp, *Clostridium* sp, gram-positive anaerobes including *Peptococcus* sp, *Peptostreptococcus* sp, *Eubacterium* sp, *Propionibacterium* sp, *Bifidobacterium* sp, *Bacteroides* sp including *B fragilis*, *Fusobacterium* sp.

Gynecologic infections – *E. faecalis*; *S aureus* (penicillinase-producing), *S epidermidis*, *Streptococcus agalactiae* (group B streptococcus), *E coli*, *Klebsiella* sp, *Proteus* sp (indole-positive and indole-negative), *Enterobacter* sp, gram-positive anaerobes including *Peptococcus* sp, *Peptostreptococcus* sp, *Propionibacterium* sp, *Bifidobacterium* sp, *Bacteroides* sp, *B fragilis*, *Gardnerella vaginalis*.

Bacterial septicemia – *E. faecalis*, *S aureus* (penicillinase-producing), group D streptococci (enterococci), *E coli*, *Klebsiella* sp, *P aeruginosa*, *Serratia* sp, *Enterobacter* sp, *Bacteroides* sp, *B fragilis*.

Bone and joint infections – *E. faecalis*, *S aureus* (penicillinase-producing), *S epidermidis*, group D streptococci (enterococci), *Enterobacter* sp, *P aeruginosa*.

Skin and skin structure infections – *E. faecalis*, *S aureus* (penicillinase-producing), *S epidermidis*, group D streptococci (enterococci), *E coli*, *Klebsiella* sp, *Enterobacter* sp, *P vulgaris*, *P rettgeri*, *M morganii*, *P aeruginosa*, *Serratia* sp, *Citrobacter* sp, *Acinetobacter* sp, gram-positive anaerobes including *Peptococcus* sp and *Peptostreptococcus* sp, *Bacteroides* sp including *B fragilis*, *Fusobacterium* sp.

Endocarditis – *S aureus* (penicillinase-producing).

Polymicrobic infections, including those in which *S pneumoniae* (pneumonia, septicemia), group A β–hemolytic streptococcus (skin and skin structure) or nonpenicillinase-producing *S aureus* is one of the causative organisms.

IM: Not intended for severe or life-threatening infections, including bacterial sepsis or endocarditis, or in instances of major physiological impairments (eg, shock).

Contraindications:

Hypersensitivity to any component of this product.

IM: Hypersensitivity to local anesthetics of the amide type and in patients with severe shock or heart block due to the use of lidocaine HCl diluent.

Warnings:

Resistance: As with other β-lactam antibiotics, some strains of *Pseudomonas aeruginosa* may develop resistance fairly rapidly during treatment with imipenem-cilastatin.

Pseudomembranous colitis has occurred with virtually all antibiotics.

Hypersensitivity: Serious and occasionally fatal hypersensitivity reactions have occurred in patients receiving therapy with β-lactams. They are more apt to occur in persons with a history of sensitivity to multiple allergens. Patients with a history of penicillin hypersensitivity have experienced severe reactions when treated with another β-lactam.

Renal function impairment: Do not give imipenem-cilastatin IV to patients with creatinine clearance (Ccr) of ≤ 5 ml/min/1.73 m^2, unless hemodialysis is instituted within 48 hours. For patients on hemodialysis, imipenem-cilastatin IV is recommended only when the benefit outweighs the potential risk of seizures.

Pregnancy: Category C.

Lactation: It is not known whether this drug is excreted in breast milk.

Children: Safety and efficacy for use in children < 12 are not established.

Precautions:

Monitoring: Periodically assess organ system function during prolonged therapy.

CNS adverse experiences have occurred with the IV formulation, especially when recommended dosages were exceeded. They are most common in patients with CNS disorders who also have compromised renal function and are rare when no underlying CNS disorder exists. Continue anticonvulsants in patients with a known seizure disorder.

Drug Interactions:

Drugs that may interact with imipenem-cilistatin include ganciclovir and probenecid.

Adverse Reactions:

Adverse reactions occurring in ≥ 3% of patients include: Phlebitis/thrombophlebitis.

Administration and Dosage:

Dosage recommendations represent the quantity of imipenem to be administered. An equivalent amount of cilastatin is also present in the solution.

Renal function impairment:

Imipenem-Cilastatin IV Dosage in Renal Impairment			
Ccr (ml/min/1.73 m^2)	Renal function impairment	Fully susceptible organisms including gram-positive and gram-negative aerobes and anaerobes	Moderately susceptible organisms, primarily some strains of *P aeruginosa*
31-70	Mild	500 mg q 8 h	500 mg q 6 h
21-30	Moderate	500 mg q 12 h	500 mg q 8 h
6-20	Severe to marked	250 mg q 12 h	500 mg q 12 h
0-5[1]	None, but on hemodialysis		

[1] Do not administer imipenem-cilastatin unless hemodialysis is instituted within 48 hours.

IV: Give a 125, 250 or 500 mg dose by IV infusion over 20 to 30 min. Infuse a 750 or 1 g dose over 40 to 60 min. In patients who develop nausea, slow the infusion rate.

Due to high antimicrobial activity, do not exceed 50 mg/kg/day or 4 g/day, whichever is lower.

Imipenem-Cilastatin IV Dosing Schedule for Adults with Normal Renal Function		
Type or severity of infection	Fully susceptible organisms including gram-positive and gram-negative aerobes and anaerobes	Moderately susceptible organisms, primarily some strains of *P aeruginosa*
Mild	250 mg q 6 h	500 mg q 6 h
Moderate	500 mg q 8 h - 500 mg q 6 h	500 mg q 6 h - 1 g q 8 h
Severe, life-threatening	500 mg q 6 h	1 g q 8 h - 1 g q 6 h
Uncomplicated UTI	250 mg q 6 h	250 mg q 6 h
Complicated UTI	500 mg q 6 h	500 mg q 6 h

IM: Total daily IM dosages > 1500 mg/day are not recommended.

Administer by deep IM injection into a large muscle mass (such as the gluteal muscles or lateral part of the thigh) with a 21 gauge 2" needle.

Imipenem-Cilastatin IM Dosage Guidelines		
Type/Location of infection	Severity	Dosage regimen
Lower respiratory tract Skin and skin structure Gynecologic	Mild/Moderate	500 or 750 mg q 12 h depending on the severity of infection
Intra-abdominal	Mild/Moderate	750 mg q 12 h

Children – 25 mg/kg/dose every sixth hour to children aged 3 months to 3 years with a maximal daily dose of 2 g. In children ≥ 3 years, the recommended dose is 15 mg/kg/dose every sixth hour.

Hemodialysis – Imipenem-cilastatin is cleared by hemodialysis. The patient should receive imipenem-cilastatin after hemodialysis and at 12 hour intervals timed from the end of that dialysis session.

AZTREONAM

Powder for Injection: 500 mg, 1 g and 2g (*Rx*) *Azactam* (Squibb)

Actions:

Pharmacology: Aztreonam, a synthetic bactericidal antibiotic, is the first of a class identified as monobactams. The monobactams have a monocyclic β-lactam nucleus. Aztreonam's bactericidal action results from the inhibition of bacterial cell wall synthesis due to a high affinity of aztreonam for penicillin binding protein 3 (PBP3).

Pharmacokinetics:

Absorption/Distribution – Following single IM injections of 500 mg and 1 g, maximum serum concentrations occur at about 1 hour.

The serum half-life averaged 1.7 hours in subjects with normal renal function. In healthy subjects, the serum clearance was 91 ml/min and renal clearance was 56 ml/min; the apparent mean volume of distribution at steady state averaged 12.6 L.

Metabolism/Excretion – In healthy subjects, aztreonam is excreted in the urine about equally by active tubular secretion and glomerular filtration. Approximately 60% to 70% of an IV or IM dose was recovered in the urine by 8 hours; recovery was complete by 12 hours.

Administration IV or IM of a single 500 mg or 1 g dose every 8 hours for 7 days to healthy subjects produced no apparent accumulation; serum protein binding averaged 56% and was independent of dose.

Indications:

Urinary tract infections (complicated and uncomplicated), including pyelonephritis and cystitis (initial and recurrent) caused by *E coli, K pneumoniae, P mirabilis, P aeruginosa, E cloacae, K oxytoca, Citrobacter* sp and *S marcescens.*

Lower respiratory tract infections, including pneumonia and bronchitis caused by *E coli, K pneumoniae, P aeruginosa, H influenzae, P mirabilis, Enterobacter* sp and *S marcescens.*

Septicemia caused by *E coli, K pneumoniae, P aeruginosa, P mirabilis, S marcescens* and *Enterobacter* sp.

Skin and skin structure infections, including those associated with postoperative wounds, ulcers and burns caused by *E coli, P mirabilis, S marcescens, Enterobacter* sp, *P aeruginosa, K pneumoniae* and *Citrobacter* sp.

Intra-abdominal infections, including peritonitis caused by *E coli, Klebsiella* sp including *K pneumoniae, Enterobacter* sp including *E cloacae, P aeruginosa, Citrobacter* sp including *C freundii* and *Serratia* sp including *S marcescens.*

Gynecologic infections, including endometritis and pelvic cellulitis caused by *E coli, K pneumoniae, Enterobacter* sp including *E cloacae* and *P mirabilis.*

Surgery: For adjunctive therapy to surgery to manage infections caused by susceptible organisms.

Concurrent initial therapy with other antimicrobials and aztreonam is recommended before the causative organism(s) is known in seriously ill patients who are also at risk of having an infection due to gram-positive aerobic pathogens. If anaerobic organisms are also suspected, initiate therapy concurrently with aztreonam.

Unlabeled uses: 1 g IM may be beneficial for acute uncomplicated gonorrhea in patients with penicillin-resistant gonococci, as an alternative to spectinomycin.

Contraindications:

Hypersensitivity to aztreonam or any other component in the formulation.

Warnings:

Pseudomembranous colitis has been reported with nearly all antibacterial agents, including aztreonam, and may range in severity from mild to life-threatening.

Epidermal necrolysis: Rarely reported in association with aztreonam in patients undergoing bone marrow transplant with multiple risk factors.

Hypersensitivity: Make careful inquiry for a history of hypersensitivity reactions. Monitor patients who have had immediate hypersensitivity reactions to penicillins or cephalosporins. If an allergic reaction occurs, discontinue the drug and institute supportive treatment.

Renal/Hepatic function impairment: Appropriate monitoring is recommended.

In patients with impaired renal function, the serum half-life is prolonged.

Pregnancy: Category B. Aztreonam crosses the placenta and enters fetal circulation.

Lactation: Aztreonam is excreted in breast milk in concentrations that are < 1% of maternal serum. Consider temporary discontinuation of nursing.

Children: Safety and efficacy for use in infants and children have not been established. However, aztreonam has been used in children.

Drug Interactions:

Drugs that may interact include other β-lactamase-inducing antibiotics and aminoglycosides.

Adverse Reactions:

There have been no adverse reactions reported in ≥ 3% of patients.

Administration and Dosage:

Give IM or IV.

Aztreonam Dosage Guide (Adults)

Type of infection	Dose[1]	Frequency (hours)
Urinary tract infection	500 mg or 1 g	8 or 12
Moderately severe systemic infections	1 or 2 g	8 or 12
Severe systemic or life-threatening infections	2 g	6 or 8

[1] Maximum recommended dose is 8 g/day.

IV route is recommended for patients requiring single doses > 1 g or those with bacterial septicemia, localized parenchymal abscess (eg, intra-abdominal abscess), peritonitis or other severe systemic or life-threatening infections. For infections due to *P aeruginosa*, a dosage of 2 g every 6 or 8 hours is recommended, at least upon initiation of therapy.

Duration of therapy depends on the severity of infection. Generally, continue aztreonam for at least 48 hours after the patient becomes asymptomatic or evidence of bacterial eradication has been obtained. Persistent infections may require treatment for several weeks.

Children: 30 mg/kg every 6 to 8 hours has been used in children for various infections; 50 mg/kg every 4 to 6 hours has been used for *P aeruginosa* infections.

Renal function impairment: Reduce dosage by 50% in patients with estimated creatinine clearances (Ccr) between 10 and 30 ml/min/1.73 m^2 after an initial loading dose of 1 or 2 g.

In patients with severe renal failure, give 500 mg, 1 or 2 g initially. The maintenance dose should be 25% of the usual initial dose given at the usual fixed interval of 6, 8 or 12 hours. For serious or life-threatening infections, in addition to the maintenance doses, give 12.5% of the initial dose after each hemodialysis session.

Elderly: Obtain estimates of Ccr and make appropriate dosage modifications.

IV: Bolus injection may be used to initiate therapy. Slowly inject directly into a vein, or into the tubing of a suitable administration set, over 3 to 5 minutes.

IM: Inject deeply in large muscle mass.

CHLORAMPHENICOL

Capsules: 250 mg (*Rx*)	Various, *Chloromycetin Kapseals* (Parke-Davis)
Powder for Injection: 100 mg/ml (as sodium succinate) when reconstituted (*Rx*)	Various, *Chloromycetin Sodium Succinate* (Parke-Davis)

Warning:

Serious and fatal blood dyscrasias occur after both short-term and prolonged therapy with chloramphenicol. Aplastic anemia, which later terminated in leukemia, has been reported. Chloramphenicol must not be used when less potentially dangerous agents are effective. *It must not be used to treat trivial infections, infections other than indicated or as prophylaxis for bacterial infections.*

Actions:

Pharmacology: Chloramphenicol binds to 50 S ribosomal subunits of bacteria and interferes with or inhibits protein synthesis.

Pharmacokinetics:

Absorption – Chloramphenicol base is absorbed rapidly from the intestinal tract and is 75% to 90% bioavailable. The inactive prodrug, chloramphenicol palmitate, is rapidly hydrolyzed to active chloramphenicol base. Bioavailability is ≈ 80% for the palmitate ester. The bioavailability of the IV succinate is ≈ 70%. Approximately 30% is eliminated in the urine as unhydrolyzed ester.

Distribution – The therapeutic range for total serum chloramphenicol concentration is: Peak, 10 to 20 mcg/ml; trough, 5 to 10 mcg/ml. The drug is ≈ 60% bound to plasma proteins. Chloramphenicol enters the cerebrospinal fluid (CSF), even in the absence of meningeal inflammation.

Metabolism/Excretion – Total urinary excretion of chloramphenicol ranges from 68% to 99% over 3 days. Most chloramphenicol detected in the blood is in the active free form. The elimination half-life of chloramphenicol is ≈ 4 hours.

Indications:

Serious infections for which less potentially dangerous drugs are ineffective or contraindicated caused by susceptible strains of *Salmonella* species; *H influenzae*, specifically, meningeal infections; rickettsiae; lymphogranuloma-psittacosis group; various gram-negative bacteria causing bacteremia, meningitis or other serious gram-negative infections; infections involving anaerobic organisms, when *Bacteroides fragilis* is suspected; other susceptible organisms which have been demonstrated to be resistant to all other appropriate antimicrobial agents.

If presumptive therapy is initiated, perform in vitro sensitivity tests concurrently, so that the drug may be discontinued if less potentially dangerous agents are indicated.

Acute infections caused by *S typhi*. Chloramphenicol is a drug of choice.

Cystic fibrosis regimens.

Contraindications:

History of hypersensitivity to, or toxicity from, chloramphenicol.

Chloramphenicol must not be used to treat trivial infections, infections other than indicated, or as prophylaxis for bacterial infections.

Warnings:

Blood dyscrasias: An irreversible type of marrow depression leading to aplastic anemia with a high rate of mortality is characterized by appearance of bone marrow aplasia or hypoplasia weeks or months after therapy. Peripherally, pancytopenia is most often observed, but only one or two of the three major cell types may be depressed.

A dose-related reversible type of bone marrow depression may occur and is associated with sustained serum levels at peak ≥ 25 mcg/ml, trough ≥ 10 mcg/ml.

Renal/Hepatic function impairment: Excessive blood levels may result in patients with impaired liver or kidney function, including that due to immature metabolic processes in the infant.

Pregnancy: Chloramphenicol readily crosses the placental barrier; cautious use is particularly important during pregnancy at term or during labor because of potential toxic effects on the fetus.

Lactation: Chloramphenicol appears in breast milk with a milk:plasma ratio of 0.5. Use with caution, if at all, during lactation.

Children: Use with caution and in reduced dosages in premature and full-term infants to avoid gray syndrome toxicity. Monitor drug serum levels carefully during therapy of the newborn.

Precautions:

Hematology: Evaluate baseline and periodic blood studies approximately every 2 days during therapy. Discontinue the drug upon appearance of reticulocytopenia, leukopenia, thrombocytopenia, anemia or any other findings attributable to chloramphenicol. Avoid concurrent therapy with other drugs that may cause bone marrow depression.

Avoid repeated courses if at all possible. Do not continue treatment longer than required to produce a cure.

Acute intermittent porphyria or glucose-6-phosphate dehydrogenase deficiency: Use with caution in patients with these conditions.

Drug Interactions:

Drugs that may affect chloramphenicol include barbiturates, rifampin and hydantoins. Drugs that may be affected by chloramphenicol include barbiturates, anticoagulants, cyclophosphamide, hydantoins, iron salts, penicillins, sulfonylureas and vitamin B_{12}.

Adverse Reactions:

Adverse reactions may include: Nausea; vomiting; glossitis; stomatitis; diarrhea; headache; mild depression; mental confusion; fever; macular/vesicular rashes; angioedema; urticaria; anaphylaxis; optic and peripheral neuritis.

Toxic reactions including fatalities (approximately 40%) have occurred in the premature infant and newborn; the signs and symptoms associated with these reactions have been referred to as the "gray syndrome."

Administration and Dosage:

Therapeutic concentrations generally should be maintained as follows: Peak 10 to 20 mcg/ml; trough 5 to 10 mcg/ml.

Monitoring serum levels is important because of the variability of chloramphenicol's pharmacokinetics. Monitor serum concentrations weekly; monitor more often in patients with hepatic dysfunction, in therapy > 2 weeks or with potentially interacting drugs.

Adults: 50 mg/kg/day in divided doses every 6 hours for typhoid fever and rickettsial infections. Exceptional infections (ie, meningitis, brain abscess) due to moderately resistant organisms may require dosage up to 100 mg/kg/day to achieve blood levels inhibiting the pathogen; decrease high doses as soon as possible.

Renal/hepatic function impairment – An initial loading dose of 1 g followed by 500 mg every 6 hours has been recommended in impaired hepatic function.

Children: 50 to 75 mg/kg/day in divided doses every 6 hours has been recommended for most indications. For meningitis, 50 to 100 mg/kg/day in divided doses every 6 hours has been recommended.

Newborns 25 mg/kg/day in 4 doses every 6 hours usually produces and maintains adequate concentrations in blood and tissues. Give increased dosage demanded by severe infections only to maintain the blood concentration within an effective range. After the first 2 weeks of life, full-term infants ordinarily may receive up to 50 mg/kg/day in 4 doses every 6 hours.

Neonates (< 2 kg) – 25 mg/kg once daily.

Neonates from birth to 7 days (> 2 kg) – 25 mg/kg once daily.

Neonates over 7 days (> 2 kg) – 50 mg/kg/day in divided doses every 12 hours.

These dosage recommendations are extremely important because blood concentration in all premature and full-term infants < 2 weeks of age differs from that of other infants due to variations in the maturity of the metabolic functions of the liver and kidneys.

Infants and children with immature metabolic processes: 25 mg/kg/day usually produces therapeutic concentrations. In this group particularly, carefully monitor the concentration of drug in the blood.

IV administration: Chloramphenicol sodium succinate is intended for IV use only; it is ineffective when given IM. Administer IV as a 10% solution injected over at least 1 minute. Substitute oral dosage as soon as feasible.

FLUOROQUINOLONES

CIPROFLOXACIN	
Tablets: 250, 500 or 750 mg (*Rx*)	*Cipro* (Bayer)
Injection: 200 or 400 mg (*Rx*)	*Cipro IV* (Bayer)
NORFLOXACIN	
Tablets: 400 mg (*Rx*)	*Noroxin* (Roberts)
OFLOXACIN	
Tablets: 200, 300 or 400 mg (*Rx*)	*Floxin* (Ortho)
Injection: 200 or 400 mg (*Rx*)	*Floxin* (Ortho)
ENOXACIN	
Tablets: 200 or 400 mg (*Rx*)	*Penetrex* (Rhone-Poulenc Rorer)
LOMEFLOXACIN HCl	
Tablets: 400 mg (*Rx*)	*Maxaquin* (Searle)
SPARFLOXACIN	
Tablets: 200 mg (*Rx*)	*Zagam* (Rhone-Poulenc Rorer)
LEVOFLOXACIN	
Tablets: 250 or 500 mg (*Rx*)	*Levaquin* (McNeil Pharmaceutical)
Injection: 500 mg (*Rx*)	*Levaquin* (McNeil Pharmaceutical)
Injection (premix): 250 or 500 mg (*Rx*)	*Levaquin* (McNeil Pharmaceutical)

Actions:

Pharmacology: The fluoroquinolones are synthetic, broad-spectrum antibacterial agents related to the other quinolones, nalidixic acid and cinoxacin. These agents are bactericidal; they interfere with the enzyme DNA gyrase needed for the synthesis of bacterial DNA.

Pharmacokinetics:

Pharmacokinetics of Fluoroquinolones

Fluoroquinolone	Bioavailability (%)	Max urine concentration (mcg/ml) (dose)	Mean peak plasma concentration (mcg/ml) (dose)	Area under curve (AUC) (mcg • hr/ml) (dose)	Protein binding (%)	t½ (hr)	Urine recovery unchanged (%)
Ciprofloxacin Oral	70-80	160-700 (500 mg)	1.2 (250 mg) 2.4 (500 mg) 4.3 (750 mg) 5.4 (1000 mg)	4.8 (250 mg) 11.6 (500 mg) 20.2 (750 mg) 30.8 (1000 mg)	20-40	4	40-50
IV		> 200 (200 mg) > 400 (400 mg)	4.3 (400 mg)	4.8 (200 mg) 11.6 (400 mg)	20-40	5-6	50-70
Enoxacin	90	nd	0.83 (200 mg) 2 (400 mg)	16 (400 mg)	40	3-6	> 40
Lomefloxacin	95-98	> 300 (400 mg)	4.2 (400 mg)	5.6 (100 mg) 10.9 (200 mg) 26.1 (400 mg)	10	8	65
Norfloxacin	30-40	200-500 (400 mg)	0.8 (200 mg) 1.5 (400 mg)	5.4 (400 mg)	10-15	3-4.5	26-32
Ofloxacin Oral	≈ 98	220 (200 mg)	1.5 (200 mg) 2.4 (300 mg) 2.9 (400 mg)	14.1 (200 mg) 21.2 (300 mg) 31.4 (400 mg)	32	5-7	70-80
IV		nd[1]	2.7 (200 mg) 4 (400 mg)	43.5 (400 mg)	32	5-10	nd[1]

[1] nd = no data.

Microbiology:

Table I: Organisms Generally Susceptible to Fluoroquinolones In Vitro

	Organism	Ciprofloxacin	Enoxacin	Lomefloxacin	Norfloxacin	Ofloxacin
Gram-negative	Acinetobacter sp	✓			✓	✓
	Aeromonas sp	✓	✓[1]	✓[1]	✓[1]	✓
	Alcaligenes sp				✓	
	Brucella melitensis	✓				
	Campylobacter sp	✓			✓	✓[1]
	Citrobacter sp	✓	✓[1]	✓[1]	✓[1]	✓[1]
	Edwardsiella tarda	✓			✓	
	Enterobacter sp	✓	✓[1]	✓	✓[1]	✓[1]
	Escherichia coli	✓	✓	✓	✓	✓
	Flavobacterium sp				✓	
	Hafnia alvei			✓	✓	
	Haemophilus ducreyi	✓	✓			
	Haemophilus influenzae	✓		✓	✓	✓
	Haemophilus parainfluenzae	✓		✓	✓	✓
	Klebsiella pneumoniae	✓	✓[1]	✓	✓[1]	✓[1]
	Klebsiella sp	✓	✓	✓	✓	✓
	Legionella sp	✓		✓	✓	✓
	Listeria monocytogenes	✓				
	Moraxella (Branhamella) catarrhalis	✓		✓	✓	✓
	Morganella morganii	✓	✓	✓	✓	✓
	Neisseria gonorrhoeae	✓	✓		✓	✓
	Neisseria meningitidis	✓			✓	✓
	Pasteurella multocida	✓				
	Plesiomonas shigelloides					✓
	Proteus mirabilis	✓	✓	✓	✓	✓
	Proteus vulgaris	✓	✓	✓	✓	✓
	Providencia alcalifaciens		✓	✓	✓	
	Providencia rettgeri	✓		✓	✓	✓
	Providencia stuartii	✓	✓		✓	✓
	Pseudomonas aeruginosa	✓	✓	✓	✓	✓
	Pseudomonas fluorescens					✓
	Salmonella sp	✓			✓	✓
	Serratia sp	✓	✓[1]	✓	✓[1]	✓[1]
	Shigella sp	✓			✓	✓
	Vibrio sp	✓			✓[1]	✓[1]
	Xanthomonas (Pseudomonas) maltophilia					✓
	Yersinia enterocolitica	✓			✓	✓

Table I: Organisms Generally Susceptible to Fluoroquinolones In Vitro						
	Organism	Ciprofloxacin	Enoxacin	Lomefloxacin	Norfloxacin	Ofloxacin
Gram-positive	Staphylococcus aureus	✓[2]		✓[2]	✓[2]	✓[2]
	coagulase-negative sp	✓				
	epidermidis	✓	✓	✓[2]	✓	✓[2]
	hemolyticus	✓			✓	
	saprophyticus	✓	✓	✓	✓	✓
	Streptococci group D				✓	
	agalactiae				✓	✓
	faecalis	✓			✓	✓
	pneumoniae	✓				✓
	pyogenes	✓				✓
	Bacillus cereus				✓	

[1] May be species-dependent.
[2] Including methicillin-susceptible and methicillin-resistant strains.

Indications:

For specific approved indications, refer to the Administration and Dosage section.

Unlabeled uses:

Ciprofloxacin appears effective in patients with cystic fibrosis who have pulmonary exacerbations associated with susceptible microorganisms. It may also be useful in the treatment of malignant external otitis (750 mg twice daily) and for tuberculosis in combination with rifampin and other antituberculosis agents. It has been used as part of a multi-drug regimen for the treatment of *Mycobacterium avium* complex infection, a common infection in AIDS patients.

Fluoroquinolones may also be useful in the following conditions (some agents are specifically indicated for these conditions; refer to drug monographs): Bronchitis; pneumonia (including Legionella and Mycoplasma); prostatitis; osteomyelitis (selected types); prophylaxis in urological surgery; traveler's diarrhea; gonorrheal cervicitis or urethritis; pelvic inflammatory disease; sinusitis; otitis media; septic arthritis; bacterial meningitis; bacteremia (pseudomonal or staphylococcal); endocarditis. Further study is needed.

Contraindications:

Hypersensitivity to fluoroquinolones or the quinolone group of antibacterial agents (cinoxacin and nalidixic acid).

Warnings:

Photosensitivity: Moderate to severe phototoxic reactions have occurred in patients exposed to direct or indirect sunlight or to artificial ultraviolet light (eg, sunlamps) during or following treatment with **lomefloxacin.**

Avoid direct exposure to direct or indirect sunlight (even when using sunscreens or sunblocks) while taking lomefloxacin and other fluoroquinolones for several days following therapy. Discontinue therapy at first signs or symptoms of phototoxicity.

Convulsions, increased intracranial pressure and toxic psychosis have occurred. CNS stimulation may also occur, which may lead to tremor, restlessness, lightheadedness, confusion and hallucinations.

Syphilis: **Ofloxacin** and **enoxacin** are not effective for syphilis. High doses of antimicrobial agents for short periods of time to treat gonorrhea may mask or delay symptoms of incubating syphilis.

Chronic bronchitis due to S pneumoniae: **Lomefloxacin** is not indicated for the empiric treatment of acute bacterial exacerbation of chronic bronchitis when it is probable that *S pneumoniae* is a causative pathogen since it exhibits in vitro resistance to lomefloxacin.

Hypersensitivity reactions, serious and occasionally fatal, have occurred in patients receiving quinolone therapy, some following the first dose. Refer to Management of Acute Hypersensitivity Reactions.

Pseudomembranous colitis has been reported with nearly all antibacterial agents, including fluoroquinolones, and may range from mild to life-threatening in severity.

Renal function impairment: Alteration in dosage regimen is necessary. See Administration and Dosage.

Elderly: Norfloxacin is eliminated more slowly because of decreased renal function; absorption appears unaffected. The apparent half-life of **ofloxacin** is 6 to 8 hours, compared to ≈ 5 hours in younger adults; absorption is unaffected. **Lomefloxacin** plasma clearance was reduced by ≈ 25% and the AUC was increased by ≈ 33% in the elderly, which may be due to decreased renal function in this population. **Enoxacin** plasma concentrations are 50% higher in the elderly than in young adults.

Pregnancy: Category C.

Lactation: **Norfloxacin** was not detected in breast milk. **Ciprofloxacin** is excreted in breast milk; however, the amount ingested by the infant appears to be low. **Ofloxacin** as a single 200 mg dose resulted in breast milk concentrations in nursing females that were similar to those found in plasma. It is not known whether **lomefloxacin** or **enoxacin** are excreted in breast milk.

Children: Do not use in children. Safety and efficacy of **lomefloxacin**, **enoxacin** and **ofloxacin** in children < 18 years of age have not been established.

Precautions:

Monitoring: Periodic assessment of organ system functions, including renal, hepatic and hematopoietic is advisable during prolonged therapy.

Ophthalmologic abnormalities, including cataracts and multiple punctate lenticular opacities, have occurred during therapy with some quinolones.

Crystalluria: Needle-shaped crystals were found in the urine of some volunteers who received either placebo or 800 or 1600 mg norfloxacin. While crystalluria is not expected to occur under usual conditions with 400 mg twice daily, do not exceed the daily recommended dosage. Crystalluria related to ciprofloxacin has occurred only rarely in man because human urine is usually acidic. The patient should drink sufficient fluids to ensure proper hydration and adequate urinary output.

Drug Interactions:

Drugs that may affect fluoroquinolones include antacids, didanosine, iron salts, sucralfate, zinc salts, antineoplastic agents, azlocillin, bismuth subsalicylate, cimetidine, nitrofurantoin and probenecid.

Drugs that may be affected by fluoroquinolones include caffeine, cyclosporine, digoxin, hydantoins, anticoagulants, cyclosporine and theophylline.

Drug/Food interactions: Food may decrease the absorption of **norfloxacin**. Food delays the absorption of **ciprofloxacin**, resulting in peak concentrations that are closer to 2 hours after dosing rather than 1 hour; however, overall absorption is not substantially affected. Dairy products such as milk and yogurt reduce the absorption of ciprofloxacin; avoid concurrent use. The bioavailability of ciprofloxacin may also be decreased by enteral feedings. Food delays the rate of absorption of **lomefloxacin** and decreases the extent of absorption (AUC) by 12%.

Adverse Reactions:

Fluoroquinolone AdverseReactions (%)					
Adverse reactions	Ciprofloxacin[1]	Enoxacin	Lomefloxacin	Norfloxacin	Ofloxacin[1]
Nausea	5.2	2-9	3.7	2.8	3-10
Abdominal pain/ discomfort	1.7	≤ 2	< 1	0.3-1	1-3
Diarrhea	2.3	1-2	1.4	✓[2]	1-4
Vomiting	2	6-9	< 1	✓[2]	1-3
Dry/painful mouth	< 1	< 1	< 1	✓[2]	1-3
Flatulence	✓[2]	< 1	< 1	0.3-1	1-3
Headache	1.2	≤ 2	3.2	2.7	1-9
Dizziness	< 1	≤ 3	2.3	1.8	1-5
Fatigue/Lethargy/Malaise	< 1	< 1	< 1	0.3-1	1-3
Somnolence/Drowsiness	< 1	< 1	< 1	0.3-1	1-3
Insomnia	< 1	1	< 1	0.3-1	3-7
Rash	1.1	≤ 1	< 1	0.3-1	1-3
Pruritus		1	<1	✓[2]	1-3
Visual disturbances	< 1	< 1	< 1	✓[2]	1-3
Vaginitis	< 1	< 1	< 1		1-3

[1] Includes data for oral and IV formulations.
[2] ✓ = Adverse reaction observed, incidence not reported.
[3] See Warnings or Precautions.

Administration and Dosage:

Ciprofloxacin:

Ciprofloxacin Dosage Guidelines				
Location of infection	Type or severity	Unit dose	Frequency	Daily dose
Urinary tract	mild/moderate	250 mg (200 mg IV)	12 h	500 mg (400 mg IV)
	severe/complicated	500 mg (400 mg IV)	q 12 h	1000 mg (800 mg IV)
Lower respiratory tract Bone and joint Skin & skin structure	mild/moderate	500 mg (400 mg IV)	q 12 h	1000 mg (800 mg IV)
	severe/complicated	750 mg	q 12 h	1500 mg
Infectious diarrhea	mild/moderate/severe	500 mg	q 12 h	1000 mg
Typhoid fever	mild/moderate	500 mg	q 12 h	1000 mg
Urethral/Cervical gonococcal infections	uncomplicated	250 mg	single dose	

The duration of treatment depends upon the severity of infection. Generally, continue ciprofloxacin for at least 2 days after the signs and symptoms of infection have disappeared. The usual duration is 7 to 14 days; however, for severe and complicated infections, more prolonged therapy may be required. Bone and joint infections may require treatment for 4 to 6 weeks or longer. Infectious diarrhea may be treated for 5 to 7 days. Typhoid fever should be treated for 10 days.

Renal function impairment –

Ciprofloxacin Dosage in Impaired Renal Function	
Creatinine clearance (ml/min)	Dose
> 50 (oral); ≥ 30 (IV)	See usual dosage
30 - 50	250 - 500 mg q 12 h
5 - 29	250 - 500 mg q 18 h (oral); 200 - 400 mg q 18-24 h (IV)
Hemodialysis or peritoneal dialysis	250 - 500 mg q 24 h (after dialysis)

In patients with severe infections and severe renal impairment, 750 mg may be administered orally at the intervals noted in the table.

CDC recommended treatment schedules for chancroid and gonorrhea –

Chancroid (H ducreyi infection): 500 mg orally 2 times a day for 3 days (alternative regimen).

Gonococcal infections:

Disseminated – 500 mg orally 2 times a day to complete a full week of therapy after treatment with initial regimen (ceftriaxone 1 g IM or IV every 24 hours) for 24 to 48 hours after improvement begins.

Uncomplicated – 500 mg orally single dose plus doxycycline

IV: Administer by IV infusion over 60 minutes. Slow infusion of a dilute solution into a large vein will minimize patient discomfort and reduce the risk of venous irritation.

Norfloxacin: Take 1 hour before or 2 hours after meals with glass of water. Patients should be well hydrated.

Recommended Norfloxacin Dosage

Infection	Description	Dose	Frequency	Duration	Daily dose
Urinary tract infections (UTI)	Uncomplicated (cystitis) due to *E coli, K pneumoniae* or *P mirabilis*.	400 mg	q 12 h	3 days	800 mg
	Uncomplicated due to other organisms	400 mg	q 12 h	7 - 10 days	800 mg
	Complicated	400 mg	q 12 h	10 - 21 days	800 mg
Sexualy transmitted diseases	Uncomplicated gonorrhea	800 mg	single dose	1 day	800 mg

Renal Function impairment – In patients with a Ccr rate ≤ 30 ml/min/1.73 m^2, administer 400 mg once daily for the duration given above.

Elderly – Dose based on normal or impaired renal function.

CDC recommended treatment schedules for gonorrhea –

Gonococcal infections, uncomplicated: 800 mg as a single dose (alternative regimen to ciprofloxacin or ofloxacin).

Ofloxacin: Usual daily dose is 200 to 400 mg every 12 hours as described in the following table:

Ofloxacin Dosage Guidelines (Oral and IV)

Infection	Description	Unit dose	Frequency	Duration	Daily dose
Lower respiratory tract	Exacerbation of chronic bronchitis	400 mg	q 12 h	10 days	800 mg
	Pneumonia	400 mg	q 12 h	10 days	800 mg
Sexually transmitted diseases	Acute, uncomplicated gonorrhea	400 mg	single dose	1 day	400 mg
	Cervicitis/urethritis due to C *trachomatis*	300 mg	q 12 h	7 days	600 mg
	Cervicitis/urethritis due to C *trachomatis and N gonorrhoeae*	300 mg	q 12 h	7 days	600 mg
Skin and skin structure	Mild to moderate	400 mg	q 12 h	10 days	800 mg
Urinary tract	Cystitis due to *E coli* or *K pneumoniae*	200 mg	q 12 h	3 dyas	400 mg
	Cystitis due to other organisms	200 mg	q 12 h	7 days	400 mg
	Complicated UTIs	200 mg	q 12 h	10 days	400 mg
Prostatitis		300 mg	q 12 h	6 weeks[1]	600 mg

[1] Because there are no safety data presently available to support the use of the IV formulation for > 10 days, switch to oral therapy or other appropriate therapy after 10 days.

Renal function impairment – Adjust dosage in patients with a Ccr value of ≤ 50 ml/min. After a normal initial dose, adjust the dosing interval as follows: Ccr 10 - 50 ml/min, use a 24 hour interval and do not adjust the dosage; Ccr < 10 ml/min, use a 24 hour interval and one-half the recommended dosage.

CDC recommended treatment schedules for chlamydia, epididymitis, pelvic inflammatory disease (PID) and gonorrhea –

Chlamydia: 300 mg orally 2 times a day for 7 days (alternative regimen).

Epididymitis: 300 mg orally 2 times a day for 10 days (alternative regimen).

PID, outpatient: 400 mg orally 2 times a day for 14 days plus clindamycin or metronidazole.

Gonococcal infections, uncomplicated: 400 mg orally in a single dose plus doxycycline.

IV – Administer by IV infusion only. Do not give IM, intrathecally, intraperitoneally or SC. Avoid rapid or bolus IV infusion; administer slowly over a period of not less than 60 min.

Enoxacin: Take at least 1 hour before or 2 hours after a meal.

Enoxacin Dosage Guidelines					
Infection	Description	Dose	Frequency	Duration	Daily dose
Urinary tract infections	Uncomplicated (cystitis)	200 mg	q 12 h	7 days	400 mg
	Complicated	400 mg	q 12 h	14 days	800 mg
Sexually transmitted diseases	Uncomplicated gonorrhea	400 mg	single dose	1 day	400 mg

Renal function impariment – Adjust dosage in patients with a creatinine clearance (Ccr) $\leq$ 30 ml/min/1.73 m^2. After a normal initial dose, use a 12 hour interval and one-half the recommended dose.

Elderly – Dosage adjustment is not necessary with normal renal function.

CDC recommended treatment schedules for gonorrhea –

Gonococcal infections, uncomplicated: 400 mg as a single dose (alternative regimen to ciprofloxacin or ofloxacin).

Lomefloxacin HCl: Lomefloxacin may be taken without regard to meals.

Recommended Daily Dose of Lomefloxacin					
Body system	Infection	Dose	Frequency	Duration	Daily dose
Lower respiratory tract	Acute bacterial exacerbation of chronic bronchitis	400 mg	once daily	10 days	400 mg
Urinary tract	Cystitis	400 mg	once daily	10 days	400 mg
	Complicated urinary tract infections	400 mg	once daily	14 days	400 mg

Elderly – No dosage adjustment needed for elderly patients with normal renal function (Ccr $\geq$ 40 ml/min/1.73 m^2).

Renal function impairment – Lomefloxacin is primarily eliminated by renal excretion. Modification of dosage is recommended in patients with renal dysfunction. In patients with a Ccr > 10 but < 40 ml/min/1.73 m^2, the recommended dosage is an initial loading dose of 400 mg followed by daily maintenance doses of 200 mg once daily for the duration of the treatment.

Dialysis patients – Hemodialysis removes only a negligable amount of lomefloxacin (3% in 4 hours). Hemodialysis patients should receive an initial loading dose of 400 mg followed by maintenance dose of 200 mg once daily for duration of treatment.

Prophylaxis – A single 400 mg dose 2 to 6 hrs prior to surgery when oral preoperative prophylaxis for transurethral surgical procedures is considered appropriate.

CDC recommended treatment schedules for gonorrhea –

Gonococcal infections, uncomplicated: 400 mg as a single dose (alternative regimen to ciprofloxacin or ofloxacin).

Sparfloxacin: Sparfloxacin can be taken with or without food.

Community-acquired pneumonia; acute bacterial exacerbations of chronic bronchitis – The recommended daily dose of sparfloxacin in patients with normal renal function is two 200 mg tablets taken on the first day as a loading dose. Thereafter, take one 200 mg tablet every 24 hours for a total of 10 days of therapy (11 tablets).

Renal function impairment – The recommended daily dose of sparfloxacin in patients with renal impairment (creatinine clearance < 50 ml/min) is two 200 mg tablets taken on the first day as a loading dose. Thereafter, take one 200 mg tablet every 48 hours for a total of 9 days of therapy (6 tablets).

Levofloxacin:

Tablets – The usual dose is 500 mg orally every 24 hours as described in the following dosing chart. These recommendations apply to patients with normal renal function. Administer oral doses at least 2 hours before or 2 hours after antacids containing magnesium or aluminum, as well as sucralfate, metal cations such as iron and multivitamin preparations with zinc.

Levofloxacin Dosing				
Infection*	Unit dose	Frequency	Duration	Daily dose
Acute exacerbation of chronic bronchitis	500 mg	every 24 hours	7 days	500 mg
Community acquired pneumonia	500 mg	every 24 hours	7-14 days	500 mg
Acute maxillary sinusitis	500 mg	every 24 hours	10-14 days	500 mg
Uncomplicated SSSI	500 mg	every 24 hours	7-10 days	500 mg
Complicated UTI	250 mg	every 24 hours	10 days	250 mg
Acute pyelonephritis	250 mg	every 24 hours	10 days	250 mg

* Due to the designated pathogens (see Indications).

Levofloxacin Dosing with Renal Function Impairment		
Renal status	Initial dose	Subsequent dose
Acute bacterial exacerbation of chronic bronchitis/Community acquired pneumonia/Acute maxillary sinusitis/Uncomplicated SSSI		
Ccr[1] from 50 to 80 ml/min	No dosage adjustment required	
Ccr[1] from 20 to 49 ml/min	500 mg	250 mg every 24 hours
Ccr[1] from 10 to 19 ml/min	500 mg	250 mg every 48 hours
Hemodialysis	500 mg	250 mg every 48 hours
CAPD[2]	500 mg	250 mg every 48 hours
Complicated UTI/Acute pyelonephritis		
Ccr[1] ≥ 20 ml/min	No dosage adjustment required	
Ccr[1] from 10 to 19 ml/min	250 mg	250 mg every 48 hours

[1] Ccr = creatinine clearance.
[2] CAPD = chronic ambulatory peritoneal dialysis.

TETRACYCLINES

TETRACYCLINE HCl	
Oral suspension: 125 mg/5 ml (*Rx*)	Various, *Achromycin V* (Lederle)
Capsules: 100, 250 or 500 mg (*Rx*)	Various, *Achromycin V* (Lederle)
Tablets: 250 or 500 mg (*Rx*)	*Sumycin 250 or 500* (Apothecon)
DEMECLOCYCLINE HCl	
Capsules: 50 or 100 mg (*Rx*)	*Declomycin* (Lederle)
Tablets: 150 or 300 mg (*Rx*)	*Declomycin* (Lederle)
DOXYCYCLINE	
Capsules: 50 or 100 mg (*Rx*)	Various, *Monodox* (Oclassen), *Vibramycin* (Pfizer)
Tablets: 50 or 100 mg (as hyclate) (*Rx*)	Various, *Vibra-Tabs* (Pfizer), *Bio-Tab* (Inter. Ethical Labs)
Capsules, coated pellets: 100 mg (as hyclate) (*Rx*)	*Doryx* (Parke-Davis)
Capsules: 50 or 100 mg (as monohydrate) (*Rx*)	*Monodox* (Oclassen)
Powder for oral suspension: 25 mg/5 ml (as monohydrate when reconstituted) (*Rx*)	*Vibramycin* (Pfizer)
Syrup: 50 mg/5 ml (as calcium) (*Rx*)	*Vibramycin* (Pfizer)
Powder for injection: 100 or 200 mg (as hyclate) (*Rx*)	Various, *Vibramycin IV* (Pfizer)
MINOCYCLINE	
Capsules: 50 or 100 mg (*Rx*)	Various, *Dynacin* (Medicis Dermatologics)
Capsules, pellet filled: 50 or 100 mg (*Rx*)	*Minocin* (Lederle)
Oral suspension: 50 mg/5 ml (*Rx*)	*Minocin* (Lederle)
Powder for injection: 100 mg (*Rx*)	*Minocin IV* (Lederle)
OXYTETRACYCLINE	
Capsules: 250 mg (*Rx*)	Various, *Terramycin* (Pfizer)
Injection: 50 or 125 mg/ml (*Rx*)	*Terramycin IM* (Roerig)

Actions:

Pharmacology: The tetracyclines are bacteriostatic. They exert their antimicrobial effect by inhibition of protein synthesis.

Pharmacokinetics:

Tetracycline Pharmacokinetic Variables and Dosage Regimens

Tetracyclines	Serum Protein Binding (%)	Normal Serum Half-Life (hrs)	% Excreted Unchanged in Urine	Usual Oral Adult Maintenance Dosage	Lipid Solubility
Tetracycline	65	16 to 12	60	250 mg q 6 h or 500 mg q 6 to 12 h	Intermediate
Demeclocycline	65 to 91	12 to 16	39	150 mg q 6 h or 300 mg q 12 h	Intermediate
Doxycycline	80 to 95	15 to 25	30 to 42	150 mg q 12 h or 100 mg q 24 h	High
Minocycline	70 to 80	11 to 18	16 to 12	100 mg q 12 h	High
Oxytetracycline	20 to 40	16 to 12	70	250 to 500 mg q 6 h	Low

Indications:

Infections caused by the following microorganisms: Rickettsiae (Rocky Mountain spotted fever, typhus fever and the typhus group, Q fever, rickettsialpox and tick fevers); Mycoplasma pneumoniae (PPLO, Eaton agent); agents of psittacosis and ornithosis; agents of lymphogranuloma venereum and granuloma inguinale; the spirochetal agent of relapsing fever (*Borrelia recurrentis*).

Infections caused by the following gram-negative microorganisms: *Haemophilus ducreyi* (chancroid); *Yersinia pestis* and *Francisella tularensis* (formerly *Pasteurella pestis* and *P tularensis*); *Bartonella bacilliformis*; *Bacteroides* sp; *Campylobacter fetus* (formerly *Vibrio fetus*); *V cholerae* (formerly *V comma*); *Brucella* sp (in conjunction with streptomycin).

Infections caused by the following microorganisms, when bacteriologic testing indicates appropriate susceptibility to the drug:

Gram-negative – *Escherichia coli*; *Enterobacter aerogenes* (formerly *Aerobacter aerogenes)*; *Shigella* sp; *Acinetobacter calcoaceticus* (formerly *Mima* and *Herellea* sp); *H influenzae* (respiratory infections); *Klebsiella* sp (respiratory and urinary infections).

Gram-positive – *Streptococcus* sp including *S pneumoniae*. Up to 44% of strains of *S pyogenes* and 74% of *S faecalis* are resistant to tetracyclines.

Staphylococcus aureus, skin and soft tissue infections. Tetracyclines are not the drugs of choice in the treatment of any type of staphylococcal infection.

Treatment of trachoma, although the infectious agent is not always eliminated, as judged by immunofluorescence.

When penicillin is contraindicated,: tetracyclines are alternatives for treatment of infections due to: *Neisseria gonorrhoeae*; *Treponema pallidum* and *T pertenue* (syphilis and yaws); *Listeria monocytogenes*; *Clostridium* sp; *Bacillus anthracis*; *Fusobacterium fusiforme* (Vincent's infection); *Actinomyces* sp; *N meningitidis* (IV only).

Acute intestinal amebiasis: Tetracyclines may be a useful adjunct to amebicides.

Oral tetracyclines:

Adults – Treatment of uncomplicated urethral, endocervical or rectal infections caused by *Chlamydia trachomatis*.

Severe acne (where it may be useful as adjunctive therapy).

Inclusion conjunctivitis (which may be treated with oral tetracyclines or with a combination of oral and topical agents).

Doxycycline, oral – Treatment of uncomplicated gonococcal infections in adults (except for anorectal infections in men); gonococcal arthritis-dermatitis syndrome; acute epididymo-orchitis caused by *N gonorrhoeae* and *C trachomatis*; nongonococcal urethritis caused by *C trachomatis* and *Ureaplasma urealyticum*.

Minocycline, oral – Treatment of asymptomatic carriers of *N meningitidis* to eliminate meningococci from the nasopharynx. *Not* indicated for the treatment of meningococcal infection.

Oral minocycline has been successful in *Mycobacterium marinum* infections.

Minocycline is also indicated for the treatment of uncomplicated urethral, endocervical or rectal infections in adults caused by *U urealyticum*; uncomplicated gonococcal urethritis in men due to *N gonorrhoeae*.

Unlabeled uses: **Demeclocycline** has been used successfully in the treatment of chronic hyponatremia associated with the syndrome of inappropriate antidiuretic hormone (SIADH) secretion.

Doxycycline has been used to prevent "Traveler's Diarrhea" commonly caused by enterotoxigenic *E coli*.

Minocycline has been used as an alternative to sulfonamides in nocardiosis.

Tetracycline and **doxycycline** instilled through a chest tube are employed as a pleural sclerosing agent in malignant pleural effusions. Tetracycline plus gentamicin is recommended for *V vulnificus* infections caused by wound infection after trauma or by ingestion of contaminated seafood.

Tetracycline suspension has been used as a mouthwash in the treatment of nonspecific mouth ulcerations, aphthous ulcers and canker sores. Dosages have ranged from 5 to 10 ml of 125 mg/ml 3 times/day for 5 to 7 days.

Lyme disease (the etiologic agent is a spirochete, *Borrelia burgdorferi*): Oral **tetracycline** 250 mg daily for 10 days is the drug of choice for stage I disease in adults; **doxycycline** has also been recommended for early disease. Both agents have been recommended for stage II disease, and they are being evaluated for treatment of stage III disease. However, the efficacy of tetracycline at the recommended dose for early Lyme disease has been questioned.

Contraindications:

Hypersensitivity to any of the tetracyclines.

Warnings:

Photosensitivity: Photosensitivity manifested by an exaggerated sunburn reaction has been observed in some individuals taking tetracyclines. Advise patients who are apt to be exposed to direct sunlight or ultraviolet light that this reaction can occur with tetracycline drugs, and discontinue treatment at the first evidence of skin erythema.

Phototoxic reactions are most frequent with demeclocycline, and occur less frequently with the other tetracyclines; minocycline is least likely to cause phototoxic reactions.

Parenteral therapy: Reserve for situations in which oral therapy is not indicated. Institute oral therapy as soon as possible. If given IV over prolonged periods, thrombophlebitis may result. IM use produces lower blood levels than recommended oral dosages.

Nephrogenic diabetes insipidus: Administration of **demeclocycline** has resulted in appearance of the diabetes insipidus syndrome (polyuria, polydipsia and weakness) in some patients on long-term therapy.

Hazardous tasks: Lightheadedness, dizziness or vertigo may occur with **minocycline.** Patients should observe caution while driving or performing other tasks requiring alertness.

Renal function impairment: If renal impairment exists, even usual doses may lead to excessive systemic accumulation of the tetracyclines (with the exception of doxycycline and minocycline) and possible liver toxicity. Use lower than usual doses.

Hepatic function impairment: Doses > 2 g/day IV can be extremely dangerous. In the presence of renal dysfunction, and particularly in pregnancy, IV tetracycline > 2 g/day has been associated with death secondary to liver failure.

Pregnancy: Category D (doxycycline). Do not use during pregnancy. They readily cross the placenta; concentrations of oxytetracycline in cord blood are ≈ 50% of those of the mother. Tetracyclines are found in fetal tissues and can have toxic effects on the developing fetus (retardation of skeletal development).

Lactation: Tetracyclines are excreted in breast milk. A dosage of 2 g/day for 3 days has achieved a milk:plasma ratio of 0.6 to 0.8.

Children: Tetracyclines should not generally be used in children under 8 years of age, unless other drugs are not likely to be effective, or are contraindicated.

Teeth – The use of tetracyclines during the period of tooth development (from the last half of pregnancy through the eighth year of life) may cause permanent discoloration (yellow-gray-brown) of deciduous and permanent teeth. Doxycycline and oxytetracycline may be less likely to affect teeth.

Bone – Tetracycline forms a stable calcium complex in any bone-forming tissue. Decreased fibula growth rate occurred in premature infants given 25 mg/kg oral tetracycline every 6 hrs.

Precautions:

Pseudotumor cerebri (benign intracranial hypertension) in adults has been associated with tetracycline use.

Outdated products: Under no circumstances should outdated tetracyclines be administered; the degradation products of tetracyclines are highly nephrotoxic and have, on occasion, produced a Fanconi-like syndrome.

Drug Interactions:

Drugs that may affect tetracyclines include antacids containing aluminum, calcium, zinc, magnesium, bismuth salts, divalent and trivalent cations, barbiturates, carbamazepine, hydantoins, cimetidine, oral iron salts, methoxyflurane and sodium bicarbonate.

Drugs that may be affected by tetracyclines include oral anticoagulants, digoxin, insulin, lithium, methoxyflurane, oral contraceptives and penicillins.

Drug/Food interactions: Food and some dairy products interfere with absorption of tetracyclines. Administer oral tetracycline 1 hour before or 2 hours after meals. Doxycycline has a low affinity for calcium binding. Gastrointestinal absorption of minocycline and doxycycline is not significantly affected by food or dairy products.

Adverse Reactions:

GI:

Oral and parenteral – Anorexia; nausea; vomiting; diarrhea; epigastric distress; bulky loose stools; stomatitis; sore throat; glossitis; hoarseness.

Oral – Esophageal ulcers, most commonly in patients with an esophageal obstructive element or hiatal hernia.

Dermatologic: Maculopapular and erythematous rashes.

Hepatic: Fatty liver; increases in liver enzymes.

CNS: Lightheadedness, dizziness or vertigo has been reported with **minocycline**.

Hypersensitivity: Urticaria; angioneurotic edema; anaphylaxis; anaphylactoid purpura; pericarditis; exacerbated systemic lupus erythematosus; polyarthralgia; serum sickness-like reactions, (eg, fever, rash, arthralgia).

Hematologic: Hemolytic anemia; thrombocytopenia; thrombocytopenic purpura; neutropenia; eosinophilia.

Miscellaneous: Pseudotumor cerebri (adults); bulging fontanels (infants). Nephrogenic diabetes insipidus has been reported with **demeclocycline**.

Administration and Dosage:

Avoid rapid IV administration. Thrombophlebitis may result from prolonged IV therapy.

Continue therapy at least 24 to 48 hours after symptoms and fever subside. Treat all infections due to group A β-hemolytic streptococci for at least 10 days.

TETRACYCLINE HCl:

Adults –

Usual dose: 1 to 2 g/day in 2 or 4 equal doses.

Children (over 8 years of age) – Daily dose is 10 to 20 mg/lb (25 to 50 mg/kg in 4 equal doses.

Brucellosis – 500 mg 4 times/day for 3 weeks, accompanied by 1 g streptomycin IM twice/day the first week, and once daily the second week.

Syphilis – 30 to 40 g in equally divided doses over 10 to 15 days. Perform close follow-up and laboratory tests.

Gonorrhea – 1.5 g initially, then 500 mg every 6 hours, to a total of 9 g.

Gonorrhea in patients sensitive to penicillin – Initially, 1.5 g; follow with 500 mg every 6 hours for 4 days to a total of 9 g.

Uncomplicated urethral, endocervical or rectal infections caused by Chlamydia trachomatis – 500 mg 4 times/day for at least 7 days.

Severe acne (long-term therapy) – Initially, 1 g/day in divided doses. For maintenance, give 125 to 500 mg/day.

CDC-recommended treatment schedules for sexually transmitted diseases –

Chlamydia trachomatis-Uncomplicated urethral, endocervical or rectal infections in adults: 500 mg 4 times/day for 7 days.

Gonococcal infections-Uncomplicated urethral, endocervical or rectal infections in adults: 3 g amoxicillin, 3.5 g oral ampicillin, 4.8 million units IM aqueous procaine penicillin G or 250 mg IM ceftriaxone. Each (except ceftriaxone) should be accompanied by 1 g oral probenecid. Follow with 500 mg tetracycline, 4 times/day for 7 days.

In adults allergic to penicillins, cephalosporins or probenecid – 500 mg 4 times/day for 7 days.

Penicillinase-producing Neisseria gonorrheae (PPNG): 2 g IM spectinomycin or 250 mg IM ceftriaxone. Follow with 500 mg tetracycline, 4 times/day for 7 days.

Children – 40 mg/kg/day in 4 divided doses for 5 days.

In PPNG-endemic and -hyperendemic areas: 250 mg IM ceftriaxone plus 100 mg oral doxycycline twice daily for 7 days or 500 mg oral tetracycline 4 times a day for 7 days. If tetracyclines are contraindicated or not tolerated, follow the single-dose regimen with erythromycin.

Disseminated gonococcal infections in patients allergic to penicillins or cephalosporins: 500 mg 4 times/day for at least 7 days.

Lymphogranuloma venereum-Genital, inguinal or anorectal: 500 mg 4 times/day for at least 2 weeks.

Nongonococcal urethritis: 500 mg 4 times/day for 7 days.

Acute pelvic inflammatory disease-Ambulatory treatment: 2 g IM cefoxitin, 3 g amoxicillin, 3.5 g oral ampicillin, 4.8 million units IM aqueous procaine penicillin G at 2 sites or 250 mg IM ceftriaxone. Each (except for ceftriaxone) should be accompanied by 1 g oral probenecid. Follow with 500 mg tetracycline 4 times/day. (However, doxycycline is preferred.)

Children over 7 years of age – 150 mg/kg/day IV cefuroxime or 100 mg/kg/day IV ceftriaxone followed by 30 mg/kg/day IV tetracycline in 3 doses, continued for at least 4 days. Thereafter, continue tetracycline orally to complete at least 14 days of therapy.

Syphilis (penicillin-allergic patients):

Early – 500 mg 4 times/day for 15 days.

More than 1 year's duration – 500 mg 4 times/day for 30 days.

Sexually transmitted epididymo-orchitis: 3 g oral amoxicillin, 3.5 g oral ampicillin, 4.8 million units IM aqueous procaine penicillin G at 2 sites (each with 1 g oral probenecid), 2 g IM spectinomycin or 250 mg ceftriaxone followed by 500 mg tetracycline, 4 times/day for 10 days.

Urethral syndrome in women: 500 mg 4 times/day for 7 days.

Rape victims-Prophylaxis: 500 mg 4 times/day for 7 days.

DEMECLOCYCLINE HCl:

Adults –

Daily dose: 4 divided doses of 150 mg each or 2 divided doses of 300 mg each.

Children (over 8 years of age) –

Usual daily dose: 3 to 6 mg/lb (6 to 12 mg/kg), depending upon the severity of the disease, divided into 3 or 4 doses.

Gonorrhea patients sensitive to penicillin – Initially, 600 mg; follow with 300 mg every 12 hours for 4 days to a total of 3 g.

DOXYCYCLINE:

Oral –

Adults:

Usual dose – 200 mg on the first day of treatment (100 mg every 12 hours); follow with a maintenance dose of 100 mg/day. The maintenance dose may be administered as a single dose or as 50 mg every 12 hours.

More severe infections (particularly chronic urinary tract infections) – 100 mg every 12 hours.

Children (over 8 years of age):

100 lbs or less (< 45 kg) – 2 mg/lb (4.4 mg/kg) divided into 2 doses on the first day of treatment; follow with 1 mg/lb (2.2 mg/kg) given as a single daily dose or divided into 2 doses on subsequent days.

More severe infections – Up to 2 mg/lb (4.4 mg/kg) may be used. For children over 100 lbs (45 kg), use the usual adult dose.

Acute gonococcal infection: 200 mg immediately, then 100 mg at bedtime on the first day. Follow by 100 mg 2 times/day for 3 days.

Single visit dose – Immediately give 300 mg; follow with 300 mg in 1 hour, which may be administered with food, milk or carbonated beverage.

Primary and secondary syphilis: 300 mg/day in divided doses for at least 10 days.

Uncomplicated urethral, endocervical or rectal infections in adults caused by Chlamydia trachomatis: 100 mg twice daily for at least 7 days.

Unlabeled use: Doxycycline has been used to prevent "Traveler's Diarrhea" commonly caused by enterotoxigenic *Escherichia coli*. In limited trials, this prophylactic (100 mg/day) therapy appears to be superior to placebo.

Endometritis, salpingitis, parametritis or peritonitis: Give 100 mg doxycycline IV, twice daily and 2 g cefoxitin IV, 4 times/day. Continue IV administration for at least 4 days and for at least 48 hours after patient improves. Then continue oral doxycycline (100 mg), twice daily to complete 10 to 14 days total therapy.

Parenteral – Do not inject IM or SC. The duration of IV infusion may vary with the dose (100 to 200 mg per day), but is usually 1 to 4 hours. A recommended minimum infusion time for 100 mg of a 0.5 mg/ml solution is 1 hour.

Adults: The usual dosage is 200 mg IV on the first day of treatment, administered in 1 or 2 hour infusions. Subsequent daily dosage is 100 to 200 mg, depending upon the severity of infection, with 200 mg administered in 1 or 2 infusions.

Primary and secondary syphilis – 300 mg daily for at least 10 days.

Children (> 8 years): ≤ 100 lbs (45 kg), give 2 mg/lb (4.4 mg/kg) on the first day of treatment, in 1 or 2 infusions. Subsequent daily dosage is 1 to 2 mg/lb (2.2 to 4.4 mg/kg) given as 1 or 2 infusions, depending on the severity of the infection. For children > 100 lbs (45 kg), use the usual adult dose.

Children (< 8 years): Safety of IV use has not been established.

CDC-recommended treatment schedules for sexually transmitted diseases –

Chlamydia trachomatis-Uncomplicated urethral, endocervical or rectal infections in adults: 100 mg 2 times/day for 7 days.

Gonococcal infections:

Uncomplicated urethral, endocervical or rectal infections in adults – 3 g oral amoxicillin, 3.5 g oral ampicillin, 4.8 million units IM aqueous procaine penicillin G or 250 mg IM ceftriaxone. Each (except for ceftriaxone) should be accompanied by 1 g oral probenecid. Follow with 100 mg doxycycline, twice daily for 7 days.

In adults allergic to penicillins, cephalosporins or probenecid: 100 mg, twice daily for 7 days.

In PPNG-endemic and -hyperendemic areas: 250 mg IM ceftriaxone plus 100 mg oral doxycycline twice daily for 7 days. If tetracyclines are contraindicated or not tolerated, follow the single-dose regimen with erythromycin.

Penicillinase-producing Neisseria gonorrhea: 2 g IM spectinomycin or 250 mg IM ceftriaxone. Follow with 100 mg doxycycline, twice daily for 7 days.

Disseminated gonococcal infections in patients allergic to penicillins or cephalosporins: 100 mg, twice daily for at least 7 days.

Lymphogranuloma venereum:

Genital, inguinal or anorectal – 100 mg, twice daily for at least 2 weeks.

Nongonococcal urethritis: 100 mg, twice daily for 7 days.

Acute pelvic inflammatory disease:

Ambulatory treatment – 250 mg single IM dose of ceftriaxone plus 100 mg oral doxycycline twice daily for 10 to 14 days. Other effective third generation cephalosporins may be substituted in the appropriate doses for ceftriaxone.

Inpatient treatment – 100 mg IV doxycycline twice daily, plus 2 g IV cefoxitin 4 times a day. Continue drugs IV for at least 4 days and at least 48 hours after patient improves. Then continue doxycycline 100 mg orally twice daily to complete 10 to 14 days of total therapy.

Sexually transmitted epididymo-orchitis: 3 g oral amoxicillin, 3.5 g oral ampicillin, 4.8 million units IM aqueous procaine penicillin G at 2 sites (each with 1 g oral probenecid), 2 g IM spectinomycin or 250 mg IM ceftriaxone followed by 100 mg doxycycline, twice daily for 7 days.

Rape victims prophylaxis: 100 mg twice daily for 7 days.

MINOCYCLINE:

Oral –

Usual dosage:

Adults – 200 mg initially, followed by 100 mg every 12 hours. If more frequent doses are preferred, give 100 or 200 mg initially; follow with 50 mg 4 times/day.

Children (over 8 years of age) – Initially, 4 mg/kg; follow with 2 mg/kg every 12 hours.

Syphilis: Administer usual dose over a period of 10 to 15 days. Close follow-up, including laboratory tests, is recommended.

Uncomplicated urethral, endocervical or rectal infections in adults caused by Chlamydia trachomatis: 100 mg, 2 times/day for at least 7 days.

Uncomplicated gonococcal urethritis in men: 100 mg, 2 times/day for 5 days.

Mycobacterium marinum infections: Although optimal doses are not established, 100 mg twice daily for 6 to 8 weeks has been successful in a limited number of cases.

Parenteral –

Adults: 200 mg followed by 100 mg every 12 hours; do not exceed 400 mg in 24 hours.

Children (over 8 years of age): Usual pediatric dose is 4 mg/kg, followed by 2 mg/kg every 12 hours.

OXYTETRACYCLINE:

Oral – See Tetracycline HCl.

Parenteral –

Adults: The usual daily dose is 250 mg administered once every 24 hours or 300 mg given in divided doses at 8 to 12 hour intervals.

Children (over 8 years of age): 15 to 25 mg/kg, up to a maximum of 250 mg per single daily injection. Dosage may be divided and given at 8 to 12 hour intervals.

MACROLIDES

AZITHROMYCIN	
Capsules: 250 mg (*Rx*)	*Zithromax* (Pfizer)
CLARITHROMYCIN	
Tablets: 250 or 500 mg (*Rx*)	*Biaxin* (Abbott)
Granules for oral suspension: 125 or 250 mg/5 ml (*Rx*)	*Biaxin* (Abbott)
DIRITHROMYCIN	
Tablets, enteric coated: 250 mg (*Rx*)	*Dynabac* (Bock)
ERYTHROMYCIN	
IV	
Powder for injection: 500 mg or 1 g erythromycin lactobionate (*Rx*)	Various
Injection: 1 g erythromycin gluceptate (*Rx*)	Various
ORAL	
ERYTHROMYCIN ETHYLSUCCINATE	
Tablets, chewable: 200 mg (*Rx*)	*EryPed* (Abbott)
Tablets: 400 mg (*Rx*)	*E.E.S. 400* (Various)
Suspension: 200 or 400 mg/5 ml (*Rx*)	Various, *EryPed Drops* (Abbott)
Drops, suspension: 100 mg/2.5 ml (*Rx*)	*EryPed Drops* (Abbott)
Powder for oral suspension: 200 mg/5 ml when reconstituted (*Rx*)	*E.E.S. Granules* (Abbott)
Granules for oral suspension: 400 mg/5 ml when reconstituted (*Rx*)	*EryPed* (Abbott)
ERYTHROMYCIN STEARATE	
Tablets, film coated: 250 or 500 mg (*Rx*)	Various, *Eramycin* (Wesley)
TROLEANDOMYCIN	
Capsules: 250 mg (*Rx*)	*Tao* (Roerig)

Actions:

Pharmacology: Macrolide antibiotics reversibly bind to the P site of the 50S ribosomal subunit of susceptible organisms and inhibit RNA-dependent protein synthesis by stimulating the dissociation of peptidyl t-RNA from ribosomes. They may be bacteriostatic or bactericidal, depending on such factors as drug concentration.

Despite differing structures, macrolides have similar antibacterial spectrum, mechanisms of action and resistance, but relatively different pharmacokinetics (see table).

Pharmacokinetics:

Various Pharmacokinetic Parameters of Macrolides

Macrolide	Protein binding (%)	Metabolism	Elimination	Bioavailability (%)	Effect of food	C_{max}* (mcg/ml)	T_{max}* (hr)	Half-life (hr)
Azithromycin	50 (0.02 mg/L) 7 (1 mg/L)		4.5% excreted unchanged in urine; primarily excreted unchanged in bile	≈ 40	Food decreases absorption, C_{max} and AUC by ≈ 50%; take on empty stomach	0.4	2-3	68[1]
Clarithromycin		Metabolized to active metabolite (14-OH clarithromycin)	Primarily renal; rate approximates normal GFR	≈ 50	Food delays onset of absorption and formation of metabolite; does not affect extent of bioavailability. Take without regard to meals	1-3	1.7	3-7
Dirithromycin	15-30 [2]	Non-enzymatic conversion to erythromycylamine	81%-97% fecal/hepatic [2]	≈ 10	Take with food or within an hour of having eaten	0.3 - 0.4[2]	3.9 - 4.1[2]	2-36

Various Pharmacokinetic Parameters of Macrolides								
Macrolide	Protein binding (%)	Metabolism	Elimination	Bioavailability (%)	Effect of food	C_{max}* (mcg/ml)	T_{max}* (hr)	Half-life (hr)
Erythromycin	70-74	Hepatic; demethylation	< 5% (oral) and 12% to 15% (IV) excreted unchanged in urine; significant quantity excreted in bile		Base or stearate: Take on an empty stomach. Estolate, ethylsuccinate, delayed release base: Take without regard to meals			1.4
Troleandomycin			20% excreted in urine; significant quantity excreted in bile		Take on an empty stomach	2	2	

* C_{max} = Maximum concentration; T_{max} = Time to reach maximum concentration.
[1] Average terminal half-life.
[2] Value listed for erythromycylamine, the active moiety.

Microbiology:

Organisms Generally Susceptible to Macrolides In Vitro						
	Organisms (✓ = generally susceptible)	Azithromycin	Clarithromycin	Dirithromycin	Erythromycin	Troleandomycin[1]
Gram-positive aerobes	*Staphylococcus aureus*	✓	✓	✓	✓	
	Streptococcus pyogenes	✓	✓	✓	✓	✓
	Streptococcus pneumoniae	✓	✓	✓	✓	✓
	Streptococcus agalactiae	✓	✓	✓	✓	
	Streptococcus sp	✓	✓	✓		
	Streptococcus viridans	✓	✓	✓	✓	
	Listeria monocytogenes		✓	✓	✓	
	Corynebacterium diphtheriae				✓	
	Corynebacterium minutissimum				✓	
Gram-negative aerobes	*Haemophilus influenzae*	✓	✓		†[2]	
	Haemophilus ducreyi	✓				
	Moraxella catarrhalis	✓	✓	✓	✓	
	Bordetella pertussis	✓	✓	✓	✓	
	Legionella pneumophila	✓	✓	✓	✓	
	Campylobacter jejuni	✓	✓			
	Neisseria gonorrhoeae		✓		✓	
	Pasteurella multocida		✓			
Anaerobes	*Bacteroides bivius*	✓				
	Bacteroides melaninogenicus		✓			
	Clostridium perfringens	✓	✓			
	Propionibacterium acnes		✓	✓		
	Peptococcus niger		✓			
	Peptostreptococcus sp	✓				

Organisms Generally Susceptible to Macrolides In Vitro						
	Organisms (✔ = generally susceptible)	Azithro-mycin	Clarithro-mycin	Dirithro-mycin	Erythro-mycin	Trolean-domycin[1]
Other	*Borrelia burgdorferi*	✔				
	Chlamydia trachomatis	✔	✔		✔	
	Mycobacterium kansasii		✔			
	Mycoplasma pneumoniae	✔	✔	✔	✔	
	Treponema pallidum	✔			✔	
	Ureaplasma urealyticum	✔			✔	
	Entamoeba histolytica				✔	

[1] Data is limited for troleandomycin.
[2] Many strains resistant to erythromycin alone; may be susceptible to erythromycin plus a sulfonamide.

The in vitro spectrum of erythromycin covers primarily gram-positive microorganisms and gram-negative cocci.

Azithromycin is less active than erythromycin against most *Staphylococcus* and *Streptococcus* sp, but it is more potent against other organisms, including many gram-negative bacteria considered resistant to erythromycin. Azithromycin may expand the therapeutic range traditionally assigned to macrolides.

Clarithromycin exhibits the same spectrum of in vitro activity as erythromycin, but appears to have significantly increased potency against those organisms.

Troleandomycin, an acetylated ester of oleandomycin, is less active than erythromycin and offers no advantage. It can also cause hepatotoxicity.

Indications:

For specific approved indications, refer to the Administration and Dosage sections.

Contraindications:

Hypersensitivity to any of the macrolide antibiotics; patients receiving terfenadine or astemizole who have preexisting cardiac abnormalities or electrolyte disturbances.

Erythromycin estolate: Preexisting liver disease.

Warnings:

Pseudomembranous colitis has occurred with nearly all antibacterial agents and may range in severity from mild to life-threatening. Consider this diagnosis in patients who present with diarrhea subsequent to the administration of antibacterial agents.

Azithromycin:

Pneumonia – Azithromycin is only safe and effective in the treatment of community-acquired pneumonia of mild severity due to *S pneumoniae* and *H influenzae* in patients appropriate for outpatient oral therapy. Do not use in patients with pneumonia who are judged to be inappropriate for outpatient oral therapy because of moderate to severe illness or risk factors.

Gonorrhea or syphilis – Azithromycin at the recommended dose should not be relied upon to treat gonorrhea or syphilis.

Cardiac effects – Ventricular arrhythmias in individuals with prolonged QT intervals has occurred with macrolide products.

Hypersensitivity – Rare serious allergic reactions, including angioedema and anaphylaxis have been reported in patients on azithromycin.

Dirithromycin:

Terfenadine drug interaction – Serious cardiac dysrhythmias, some resulting in death, have occurred in patients receiving terfenadine concomitantly with other macrolide antibiotics. Until further use data are available, it is prudent to monitor the terfenadine levels when dirithromycin and terfenadine are coadministered.

Bacteremias – Dirithromycin should not be used in patients with known, suspected or potential bacteremias as serum levels are inadequate to provide antibacterial coverage of the blood stream.

Respiratory infections – Dirithromycin is NOT indicated for the empiric treatment of acute bacterial exacerbations of chronic or secondary bacterial infection of acute bronchitis.

Skin/Skin structure infections – Dirithromycin is NOT indicated for the empiric treatment of uncomplicated skin and skin structure infections.

Erythromycin:

Hepatotoxicity – Erythromycin administration has been associated with the infrequent occurrence of cholestatic hepatitis. This effect is most common with erythromycin estolate; however, it has also occurred with other erythromycin salts.

Although initial symptoms have developed after a few days of treatment, they generally have followed 1 or 2 weeks of continuous therapy. Symptoms reappear promptly, usually within 48 hours after the drug is readministered to sensitive patients. The syndrome seems to result from a form of sensitization, occurs chiefly in adults, and is reversible when medication is discontinued.

Troleandomycin:

Hepatic effects – Troleandomycin has been associated with an allergic cholestatic hepatitis. Some patients receiving troleandomycin for > 2 weeks or in repeated courses have developed jaundice accompanied by right upper quadrant pain, fever, nausea, vomiting, eosinophilia and leukocytosis. These have reversed on drug discontinuance. Readministration reproduces hepatotoxicity, often within 24 to 48 hours.

Renal/Hepatic function impairment:

Clarithromycin – In the presence of severe renal impairment (creatinine < 30 ml/min) with or without coexisting hepatic impairment, decrease dosage or prolonged dosing intervals may be appropriate.

Azithromycin and troleandomycin – Exercise caution when administering to patients with impaired renal or hepatic function.

Erythromycin – Erythromycin is principally excreted by the liver. Exercise caution in administering to patients with impaired hepatic function.

Dirithromycin – No dosage adjustment should be necessary in patients with impaired renal function, including dialysis patients. In patients with mild hepatic impairment, mean peak serum concentration, AUC and volume of distribution increased somewhat with multiple-dose administration; however, based on the magnitude of these changes, no dosage adjustment should be necessary in patients with mildly impaired hepatic function.

Elderly:

Clarithromycin – Studies show age-related decreases in renal function. Consider dosage adjustment in elderly patients with severe renal impairment.

Azithromycin – Dosage adjustment does not appear to be necessary for older patients with normal renal and hepatic function.

Dirithromycin – No dosage adjustment should be necessary in elderly patients.

Pregnancy: Category B (azithromycin, erythromycin); *Category* C (clarithromycin, dirithromycin).

Troleandomycin – Safety for use during pregnancy has not been established.

Lactation:

Clarithromycin, dirithromycin and azithromycin – It is not known whether these agents are excreted in breast milk.

Erythromycin – Erythromycin is excreted in breast milk, and may concentrate (observed milk:plasma ratio of 0.5 to 3). Erythromycin is considered compatible with breastfeeding by the American Academy of Pediatrics.

Children:

Dirithromycin – Safety and efficacy in children < 12 years of age have not been established.

Clarithromycin – Safety and efficacy in children < 6 months of age have not been established.

Azithromycin – Safety and efficacy in children < 6 months of age (acute otitis media) or < 2 years of age (pharyngitis/tonsilitis) have not been established.

Precautions:

Azithromycin: Photosensitization (photoallergy or phototoxicity) may occur.

Drug Interactions:

Clarithromycin: Drugs that may be affected by clarithromycin include anticoagulants, astemizole, carbamazepine, cisapride, cyclosporine, digoxin, ergot alkaloids, tacrolimus, terfenadine, theophylline, triazolam, zidovudine, alfentanil and hexobarbital. Also consider all drug interactions with erythromycin.

Azithromycin: Drugs that may interact with azithromycin include antacids, tacrolimus, theophyllines and warfarin. Drugs that may affect clarithromycin include fluconazole. Also consider all drug interactions with erythromycin.

Dirithromycin: Drugs that may be affected by dirithromycin include terfenedine and theophylline. Drugs that may affect dirithromycin include antacids and H_2 antagonists. Also consider all drug interactions with erythromycin.

Erythromycin: Drugs that may be affected by erythromycin include alfentanil, anticoagulants, antihistamines, astemizole, terfenadine, bromocriptine, carbamazepine, cyclosporine, digoxin, disopyramide, ergot alkaloids, lincosamides, methylprednisolone, penicillins, theophyllines and triazolam.

Troleandomycin: Drugs that may be affected by troleandomycin include carbamazepine, oral contraceptives, ergot alkaloids, methylprednisolone, theophyllines and triazolam.

Drug/Food interactions:

Clarithromycin – Following tablet administration, food delays both the onset of clarithromycin absorption and the formulation of 14 OH clarithromycin, but does not affect bioavailability. Following the suspension, food decreases mean peak clarithromycin levels and extent of absorption.

Azithromycin – Food decreases the absorption of azithromycin capsules, reducing the maximum concentration by 52% and bioavailability by 43%. When azithromycin suspension was administered with food, the rate of absorption (C_{MAX}) was increased by 56% while the extent of absorption (AUC) was unchanged. Take 1 hour before or 2 hours after a meal. Do not take with food.

Dirithromycin – Dirithromycin should be administered with food or within an hour of having eaten. After administration of two 250 mg tablets 1 or 4 hours before food and immediately after a standard breakfast indicated an increase in absorption of erythromycylamine when dirithromycin was administered after food, while a significant decrease in C_{max} (33%) and AUC (31%) occurred when administered 1 hour before food.

Erythromycin – Antimicrobial effectiveness of erythromycin stearate and certain formulations of erythromycin base may be reduced. Take at least 2 hours before or after a meal. Erythromycin estolate and ethylsuccinate and the base in a delayed release form may be administered without regard to meals.

Adverse Reactions:

Clarithromycin: Adverse reactions occurring in ≥ 3% of patients include diarrhea, nausea, abdominal pain, rash and abnormal taste.

Azithromycin: Adverse reactions occurring in ≥ 3% of patients include diarrhea/loose stools, vomiting, nausea and abdominal pain.

Dirithromycin:

Dirithromycin Adverse Reactions (%): Dirithromycin vs Erythromycin

Adverse reaction	Dirithromycin	Erythromycin
Abdominal pain	9.7	7.5
Headache	8.6	8.2
Nausea	8.3	7.5
Diarrhea	7.7	7.3
Platelet count increased	3.8	4.8
Vomiting	3	2.8

Erythromycin:

Local – Venous irritation and phlebitis have occurred with parenteral administration, but the risk of such reactions may be reduced if the infusion is given slowly, in dilute solution, by continuous IV infusion or intermittent infusion over 20 to 60 minutes.

GI – The most frequent dose-related side effects following oral use include abdominal cramping and discomfort, anorexia, nausea, vomiting and diarrhea. Pseudomembranous colitis associated with erythromycin therapy has occurred (see Warnings). Several cases of nausea and vomiting following IV erythromycin lactobionate have occurred.

Hepatic – Hepatotoxicity is most commonly associated with erythromycin estolate.

Administration and Dosage:

AZITHROMYCIN: Administer at least 1 hour before or 2 hours after a meal. Do not give with food.

Adults –

Mild to moderate acute bacterial exacerbations of chronic obstructive pulmonary disease, pneumonia, pharyngitis/tonsillitis (as second-line therapy), and uncomplicated skin and skin structure infections (≥ 16 years of age): 500 mg as a single dose on the first day followed by 250 mg once daily on days 2 through 5 for a total dose of 1.5 g.

Nongonococcal urethritis and cervicitis due to C *trachomatis:* Give a single 1 g dose.

CDC recommended treatment schedules for chancroid and chlamydia: 1 g as a single dose.

Children –

Acute otitis media: The recommended dose for oral suspension is 10 mg/kg as a single dose on the first day (not to exceed 500 mg/day, followed by 5 mg/kg on days 2 through 5 (not to exceed 250 mg/day). See the following table.

Pediatric Dosage Guidelines for Otitis Media (≥ 6 months of age)						
Dosing calculated on 10 mg/kg on day 1 dose, followed by 5 mg/kg on days 2 to 5						
Weight		Amount of 100 mg/5 ml Suspension		Amount of 200 mg/5 ml Suspension		Total ml per treatment course
kg	lbs	Day 1	Days 2 to 5	Day 1	Days 2 to 5	
10	22	5 ml	2.5 ml			15 ml
20	44			5 ml	2.5 ml	15 ml
30	66			7.5 ml	3.75 ml	22.5 ml
40	88			10 ml	5 ml	30 ml

Pharyngitis/tonsillitis: The recommended dose for children with pharyngitis/tonsillitis is 12 mg/kg qd for 5 days (not to exceed 500 mg/day). See the following.

Pediatric Dosage Guidelines for Pharyngitis/Tonsillitis (≥ 2 years of age)			
Dosing calculated on 12 mg/kg once daily days 1 through 5			
Weight		Amount of 200 mg/5 ml suspension	
kg	lbs	Days 1 to 5	Total ml per treatment course
8	18	2.5 ml	12.5 ml
17	37	5 ml	25 ml
25	55	7.5 ml	37.5 ml
33	73	10 ml	50 ml
40	88	12.5	62.5 ml

CLARITHROMYCIN: Clarithromycin may be given with or without meals.

Helicobacter pylori – Clarithromycin in combination with omeprazole is indicated for the treatment of patients with an active duodenal ulcer associated with *H. pylori* infection. The eradication of *H. pylori* has been demonstrated to reduce the risk of duodenal ulcer recurrence.

Clarithromycin Dosage Regimen for Active Duodenal Ulcer Associated with *H. pylori Infection* (28-Day Therapy)	
Days 1 - 14	Days 15 - 28
500 mg tablet three times daily plus omeprazole 2 × 20 mg every morning	Omeprazole 20 mg every morning

Adults –

Clarithromycin Dosage Guidelines		
Infection	Dosage (every 12 hr)	Normal duration (days)
Pharyngitis/Tonsillitis	250 mg	10
Acute maxillary sinusitis	500 mg	14
Lower respiratory tract	250-500 mg	7 to 14
Acute exacerbation of chronic bronchitis due to:		
S pneumoniae	250 mg	7 to 14
M catarrhalis	250 mg	7 to 14
H influenzae	500 mg	7 to 14
Pneumonia due to:		
S pneumoniae	250 mg	7 to 14
M pneumoniae	250 mg	7 to 14
Uncomplicated skin and skin structure	250 mg	7 to 14

Children – Usual recommended daily dosage is 15 mg/kg/day divided every 12 hours for 10 days.

Pediatric Dosage Guidelines (based on body weight)				
Dosing calculated on 7.5 mg/kg q 12 h				
Weight		Dose	125 mg/5 ml	250 mg/5 ml
kg	lb	(q 12 h)	(q 12 h)	(q 12 h)
9	20	62.5 mg	2.5 ml	1.25 ml
17	37	125 mg	5 ml	2.5 ml
25	55	187.5 mg	7.5 ml	3.75 ml
33	73	250 mg	10 ml	5 ml

Mycobacterial infections – Recommended as the primary agent for the treatment of disseminated *Mycobacterium avium* complex (MAC). Use in combination with other antimycobacterial drugs that have shown an in vitro activity against MAC. Continue therapy for life if clinical and mycobacterial improvments are observed.

Dosage:

Adults – 500 mg twice daily.

Children – 7.5 mg/kg twice daily up to 500 mg twice daily. Refer to the Pediatric Dosing table.

Renal/Hepatic function impairment – In the presence of severe renal impairment with or without coexisting hepatic impairment, halved doses or prolongation of dosing intervals may be needed.

DIRITHROMYCIN: Administer with food or within 1 hour of having eaten. Do not cut, crush or chew the tablets.

Recommended Dosage Schedule for Dirithromycin (≥ 12 years of age)			
Infection (Mild to Moderate Severity)	Dose	Frequency	Duration (days)
Acute bacterial exacerbations of chronic bronchitis due to *Moraxella catarrhalis* or *Streptococcus pneumoniae*. Not for empiric therapy (see Warnings).	500 mg	once a day	7
Secondary bacterial infection of acute bronchitis due to *M catarrhalis* or *S pneumoniae*. Not for empiric therapy (see Warnings).	500 mg	once a day	7

Recommended Dosage Schedule for Dirithromycin (≥ 12 years of age)			
Infection (Mild to Moderate Severity)	Dose	Frequency	Duration (days)
Community-acquired pneumonia due to *Legionella pneumophila*, *Mycoplasma pneumoniae* or *S pneumoniae*	500 mg	once a day	14
Pharyngitis/Tonsillitis due to *Streptococcus pyogenes*	500 mg	once a day	10
Uncomplicated skin and skin structure infections due to *Staphylococcus aureus* (methicillin-susceptible). Not for empiric therapy (see Warnings).	500 mg	once a day	7

ERYTHROMYCIN, IV:

Erythromycin IV is indicated when oral use is impossible, or when severity of the infection requires immediate high serum levels. Replace IV therapy with oral as soon as possible.

Continuous infusion is preferable, but intermittent infusion in 20 to 60 minute periods at intervals of ≤ 6 hours is also effective. Due to irritative properties of erythromycin, IV push is unacceptable.

Severe infections – 15 to 20 mg/kg/day. Up to 4 g/day in very severe infections.

ERYTHROMYCIN, ORAL: Dosages and product strengths are expressed as erythromycin base equivalents. Because of differences in absorption and biotransformation, varying quantities of each salt form are required to produce the same free erythromycin serum levels.

Optimal serum levels of erythromycin are reached when erythromycin base or stearate is taken in the fasting state or immediately before meals. Erythromycin ethylsuccinate, estolate and enteric coated erythromycin may be administered without regard to meals.

Usual dosage –

Adults: 250 mg (or 400 mg ethylsuccinate) every 6 hours, or 500 mg every 12 hours, or 333 mg every 8 hours. May increase up to ≥ 4 g/day, according to severity of infection. If twice-a-day dosage is desired, the recommended dose is 500 mg every 12 hours. Twice-a-day dosing is not recommended when doses > 1 g daily are administered.

Children: 30 to 50 mg/kg/day in divided doses.

Erythromycin Uses and Dosages	
Indication (Organism)	Dosage (Stated as erythromycin base)
Labeled uses: Upper respiratory tract infections of mild to moderate severity	
Streptococcus pyogenes (Group A beta-hemolytic streptococcus)	250 to 500 mg 4 times a day or 20 to 50 mg/kg/day in divided doses for 10 days.
S pneumoniae	250 to 500 mg every 6 hours.
Haemophilus influenzae (used concomitantly with a sulfonamide)	Erythromycin ethylsuccinate: 50 mg/kg/day. Sulfisoxazole: 150 mg/kg/day. Combination given for 10 days.
Lower respiratory tract infections of mild to moderate severity	
S pyogenes	250 to 500 mg 4 times a day or 20 to 50 mg/kg/day in divided doses for 10 days.
S pneumoniae	250 to 500 mg every 6 hours.
Respiratory tract infections *Mycoplasma pneumoniae* (Eaton agent, PPLO)	500 mg every 6 hours for 5 to 10 days. Treat severe infections for up to 3 weeks.
Skin and skin structure infections of mild to moderate severity	
S pyogenes	250 to 500 mg 4 times a day or 20 to 50 mg/kg/day in divided doses for 10 days.

Erythromycin Uses and Dosages	
Indication (Organism)	Dosage (Stated as erythromycin base)
Staphylococcus aureus (resistant organisms may emerge)	250 mg every 6 hours or 500 mg every 12 hours, maximum 4 g/day.
Pertussis (whooping cough) *Bordetella pertussis:*Effective in eliminating the organism from the nasopharynx of infected patients. May be helpful in prophylaxis of pertussis in exposed individuals.	40 to 50 mg/kg/day in divided doses for 5 to 14 days, or 500 mg 4 times a day for 10 days.
Diphtheria *Corynebacterium diphtheriae:* Adjunct to anti- toxin to prevent establishment of carriers and to eradicate organism in carriers.	500 mg every 6 hours for 10 days.
Erythrasma C *minutissimum*	250 mg 3 times daily for 21 days.
Intestinal amebiasis *Entamoeba histolytica:* Oral erythromycin only.	*Adults:* 250 mg 4 times daily for 10 to 14 days. *Children:*30 to 50 mg/kg/day in divided doses for 10 to 14 days.
Pelvic inflammatory disease (PID), acute *Neisseria gonorrhoeae:*Erythromycin lactobionate IV followed by oral erythromycin [1]	500 mg IV every 6 hours for 3 days, then 250 mg orally every 6 hours for 7 days. An alternative regimen for ambulatory management of PID is 500 mg orally 4 times a day for 10 to 14 days.
Conjunctivitis of the newborn, pneumonia of infancy, urogenital infections during pregnancy caused by *Chlamydia trachomatis*.	50 mg/kg/day in 4 divided doses for 14 days (conjunctivitis) or 21 days (pneumonia); 500 mg 4 times daily for 7 days or 250 mg 4 times daily for 14 days (urogenital infections).
Urethral, endocervical or rectal infections, uncomplicated C *trachomatis*[1]	500 mg 4 times daily for 7 days or 250 mg 4 times daily for 14 days.
Nongonococcal urethritis *Ureaplasma urealyticum*[1]	500 mg 4 times daily for at least 7 days.
Primary syphilis *Treponema pneumophila:* (Oral only) [1]	20 g in divided doses over 10 days.
Legionnaire's disease *Legionella pneumophila:* No controlled clinical efficacy studies have been conducted, but data suggest effectiveness.	1 to 4 g daily in divided doses or 500 mg to 1 g 4 times daily for 21 days.
Rheumatic fever S *pyogenes* (group A beta-hemolytic streptococci): Prevention of initial or recurrent attacks. [1]	250 mg 2 times daily.
Bacterial endocarditis *Alpha-hemolytic streptococcus* (Viridans)	*Adults:* 1 g 2 hours prior to procedure, then 500 mg 6 hours after initial dose. *Children:* 20 mg/kg 2 hours prior to procedure, then 10 mg/kg 6 hours after initial dose.
Listeria monocytogenes	*Adults:* 250 mg every 6 hours or 500 mg every 12 hours, maximum 4 g/day.
Unlabeled uses: *Campylobacter jejuni:* Has been successful with severe or prolonged diarrhea associated with *Campylobacter enteritis* or enterocolitis.	500 mg 4 times a day for 7 days.
Lymphogranuloma venereum: Genital, inguinal or anorectal. *Hemophilus ducreyi (chancroid):* Treat until ulcers or lymph nodes are healed.	500 mg 4 times a day for 21 days. 500 mg 4 times a day for 7 days.

Erythromycin Uses and Dosages	
Indication (Organism)	Dosage (Stated as erythromycin base)
Neisseria gonorrhoeae:	
Uncomplicated urethral, endocervical or rectal infections and in penicillinase-producing *N gonorrhoeae* (PPNG).	500 mg 4 times a day for 7 days or spectinomycin 2 g IM followed by erythromycin regimen.
In pregnancy	500 mg 4 times a day for 7 days.
Treponema pallidum:	
Early syphilis (primary, secondary or latent syphilis of < 1 year duration).	500 mg 4 times a day for 14 days.
Prior to elective colorectal surgery, to reduce wound complications.	Combination of erythromycin base and neomycin is a popular preoperative preparation.
Clostridium tetani:	
Tetanus.[1]	500 mg every 6 hours for 10 days.

[1] Use as an alternative drug in penicillin or tetracycline hypersensitivity or when penicillin or tetracycline are contraindicated or not tolerated.

ERYTHROMYCIN ETHYLSUCCINATE: Expressed in base equivalents, 400 mg erythromycin ethylsuccinate produces the same free erythromycin serum levels as 250 mg or erythromycin base, stearate or estolate.

TROLEANDOMYCIN: Continue therapy for 10 days when used for streptococcal infection.

Adults – 250 to 500 mg, 4 times a day.

Children – 125 to 250 mg (6.6 to 11 mg/kg) every 6 hours.

SPECTINOMYCIN

Powder for Injection: 400 mg per ml when reconstituted (*Rx*) *Trobicin* (Upjohn)

Actions:

Pharmacology: Spectinomycin inhibits protein synthesis in bacterial cell.

Pharmacokinetics: Rapidly absorbed after IM injection. The majority of drug is excreted in urine in biologically active form.

Indications:

Acute gonorrheal urethritis and proctitis in the male and acute gonorrheal cervicitis and proctitis in the female due to susceptible strains of N gonorrhoeae.

Contraindications:

Hypersensitivity to spectinomycin.

Warnings:

Syphilis: Not effective in the treatment of syphilis. All patients with gonorrhea should have a serologic test for syphilis at time of diagnosis and a follow-up test after 3 months.

Pharyngeal infections: Not effective in pharyngeal infections due to *N gonorrhoeae*.

Pregnancy: Safety for use during pregnancy has not been established.

Children: Safety for use has not been established.

Precautions:

Monitoring: Monitor clinical effectiveness to detect resistance by *N gonorrhoeae*.

Benzyl alcohol: The diluent provided with this product contains benzyl alcohol which has been associated with a fatal gasping syndrome in infants.

Hypersensitivity: A few cases of anaphylaxis or anaphylactoid reactions have been reported. Have epinephrine immediately available.

Adverse Reactions:

Adverse reactions may include: Urticaria; dizziness; nausea; chills; fever; decrease in hemoglobin, hematocrit and creatinine clearance; elevation of alkaline phosphatase, BUN and ALT.

Administration and Dosage:

For IM use only. Shake vials vigorously immediately after adding diluent and before withdrawing dose. Inject 5 ml (2 g) IM deep into upper outer quadrant of gluteus. Also recommended for patients being treated after failure of previous antibiotic therapy. In geographic areas where antibiotic resistance is prevalent, initial treatment with 4 g (10 ml) IM is preferred, and may be divided between 2 gluteal injection sites.

CDC recommended treatment schedules for gonorrhea:

Uncomplicated urethral, endocervical or rectal gonococcal infections, alternative regimen – For patients who cannot take ceftriaxone, the preferred alternative is spectinomycin 2 g IM as a single dose followed by doxycycline.

Children ≥ 45 kg (100 lbs) should receive adult regimens. *Children < 45 kg* with uncomplicated vulvovaginitis, cervicitis, urethritis, pharyngitis or proctitis and who cannot tolerate ceftriaxone may receive 40 mg/kg IM once.

Gonococcal infections in pregnancy – Treat pregnant women allergic to β-lactams with 2 g IM followed by erythromycin.

Disseminated gonococcal infection – Treat patients allergic to β-lactams with 2 g IM every 12 hours.

VANCOMYCIN

Pulvules: 125 mg, 250 mg (*Rx*)	*Vancocin* (Lilly)
Powder for Oral Solution: 1 g, 10 g (*Rx*)	*Vancocin* (Lilly)
Powder for Injection: 500 mg, 1 g, 5 g, 10 g (*Rx*)	Various, *Vancocin* (Lilly), *Lyphocin* (Lyphomed)

Actions:

Pharmacology: Vancomycin is a tricyclic glycopeptide antibiotic which inhibits cell-wall biosynthesis. It also alters bacterial-cell-membrane permeability and RNA synthesis.

Pharmacokinetics:

Absorption/Distribution – Systemic absorption of oral vancomycin is generally poor.

Metabolism/Excretion – In the first 24 hours, about 75% of a dose is excreted in urine by glomerular filtration. Elimination half-life is 4 to 6 hours in adults. About 60% of an intraperitoneal dose administered during peritoneal dialysis is absorbed systemically in 6 hours.

Indications:

Parenteral: Serious or severe infections not treatable with other antimicrobials, including the penicillins and cephalosporins.

Severe staphylococcal infections (including methicillin-resistant staphylococci) in patients who cannot receive or who have failed to respond to penicillins and cephalosporins, or who have infections with resistant staphylococci. Infections may include endocarditis, bone infections, lower respiratory tract infections, septicemia and skin and skin structure infections.

Endocarditis –

Staphylococcal: Vancomycin is effective alone.

Streptococcal: Vancomycin is effective alone or in combination with an aminoglycoside for endocarditis caused by Streptococcus viridans or *S bovis*. It is only effective in combination with an aminoglycoside for endocarditis caused by enterococci (eg, *S faecalis*).

Diphtheroid: Vancomycin is effective for diphtheroid endocarditis, and has been used successfully with rifampin, an aminoglycoside or both in early onset prosthetic valve endocarditis caused by *S epidermidis* or diphtheroids.

Prophylactic: IV vancomycin has been suggested for prophylaxis against bacterial endocarditis in penicillin-allergic patients who have congenital heart disease or rheumatic or other acquired or valvular heart disease when these patients undergo dental procedures or surgical procedures of the upper respiratory tract.

Pseudomembranous colitis/staphylococcal enterocolitis caused by C difficile – The parenteral form may be administered orally; parenteral use alone is unproven.

Oral: Staphylococcal enterocolitis and antibiotic-associated pseudomembranous colitis produced by C *difficile*. The parenteral product may also be given orally for these infections. Oral vancomycin is *not* effective for other types of infection.

Contraindications:

Hypersensitivity to vancomycin.

Warnings:

Ototoxicity has occurred in patients receiving vancomycin. It may be transient or permanent. It has occurred mostly in patients who have been given excessive doses, who have an underlying hearing loss, or who are receiving concomitant therapy with another ototoxic agent.

Hypotension: Rapid bolus administration may be associated with exaggerated hypotension, including shock, and, rarely, cardiac arrest. To avoid hypotension, administer in a dilute solution over ≥ 60 minutes. Stopping the infusion usually results in prompt cessation of these reactions. Frequently monitor blood pressure and heart rate.

Pseudomembranous colitis: In rare instances, pseudomembranous colitis has occurred due to C *difficile* developing in patients who received IV vancomycin.

Reversible neutropenia has occurred in patients receiving vancomycin.

Tissue irritation: Vancomycin is irritating to tissue and must be given by a secure IV route of administration. Pain, tenderness and necrosis occur with IM injection or inadvertent extravasation.

Renal function impairment: Because of its nephrotoxicity, use carefully in renal insufficiency.

Pregnancy: Category C.

Lactation: Vancomycin is excreted in breast milk.

Children: In premature and full-term neonates it may be appropriate to confirm desired vancomycin serum concentrations.

Precautions:

Monitoring: Perform serial tests of auditory function and monitor serum levels. When monitoring serum levels, draw a serum sample 1.5 to 2.5 hours after the completion of a 1 hour infusion. Peak levels are generally expected to be in the 30 to 40 ng/ml range.

Systemic absorption: Clinically significant serum concentrations may occur in some patients who have taken multiple oral doses for active C difficile-induced pseudomembranous colitis or who have inflammatory disorders of the intestinal mucosa; the risk is greater with the presence of renal impairment.

Red Man (or Redneck) syndrome is usually stimulated by a too rapid IV infusion (dose given over a few minutes), but it has been reported rarely when given as recommended and following oral or intraperitoneal administration. The onset may occur anytime within a few minutes of starting an IV infusion, to a short time after infusion completion. The rash generally resolves several hours after termination of administration.

Drug Interactions:

Drugs that may interact with vancomycin include aminoglycosides, anesthetics, neurotoxic/nephrotoxic agents and nondepolarizing muscle relaxants.

Adverse Reactions:

Adverse reactions may include: Vertigo; dizziness; anaphylaxis; drug fever; nausea; chills; eosinophilia; rashes; hypotension; wheezing; dyspnea; urticaria; inflammation at injection site; Redneck or Red Man syndrome.

Administration and Dosage:

Complete full course of therapy; do not discontinue therapy without notifying physician.

Oral:

Adults – 500 mg to 2 g/day given in 3 or 4 divided doses for 7 to 10 days.

Alternatively, dosages of 125 mg 3 or 4 times daily for C *difficile* colitis may be as effective as the 500 mg dose regimen.

Children – 40 mg/kg/day in 3 or 4 divided doses for 7 to 10 days. Do not exceed 2 g/day.

Neonates – 10 mg/kg/day in divided doses.

Parenteral: Administer each dose over at least 60 minutes. Intermittent infusion is the preferred administration method.

Adults – 500 mg IV every 6 hours or 1 g every 12 hours.

Children – 10 mg/kg per dose given every 6 hours.

Infants and neonates – Initial dose of 15 mg/kg, followed by 10 mg/kg every 12 hours for neonates in the first week of life and every 8 hours thereafter up to the age of 1 month.

Prevention of bacterial endocarditis: Dental, oral or upper respiratory tract procedures (alternate regimen, penicillin-allergic patients considered high risk) – 1 g IV over 1 hour (children, 20 mg/kg), starting 1 hour before procedure; no repeat dose is necessary.

GU/GI *procedures (penicillin allergic patients)* – 1 g IV over 1 hour (children, 20 mg/kg) plus 1.5 mg/kg (children, 2 mg/kg) gentamicin IV or IM (not to exceed 80 mg) 1 hour before procedure; may repeat once 8 hours after initial dose.

Renal function impairment: Adjust dosage; check serum levels regularly. In premature infants and the elderly, dosage reduction may be necessary due to decreasing renal function.

Vancomycin Dosage in Impaired Renal Function	
Ccr (ml/min)	Dose (mg/24 hr)
100	1545
90	1390
80	1235
70	1080
60	925
50	770
40	620
30	465
20	310
10	155

The table is not valid for functionally anephric patients on dialysis. For such patients, give a loading dose of 15 mg/kg to achieve therapeutic serum levels promptly and a maintenance dose of 1.9 mg/kg/24 hr. In patients with marked renal impairment, it may be more convenient to give maintenance doses of 250 to 1000 mg once every several days rather than administering the drug on a daily basis. In anuria a dose of 1000 mg every 7 to 10 days has been recommended.

LINCOSAMIDES

LINCOMYCIN	
Capsules: 500 mg (*Rx*)	*Lincocin* (Upjohn)
Capsules, pediatric: 250 mg (*Rx*)	*Lincocin* (Upjohn)
Injection: 300 mg/ml (*Rx*)	*Lincocin* (Upjohn), *Lincorex* (Hyrex)
CLINDAMYCIN	
Capsules: 75, 150 and 300 mg (*Rx*)	Various, *Cleocin* (Upjohn)
Granules for Oral Solution: 75 mg/5 ml (*Rx*)	*Cleocin Pediatric* (Upjohn)
Injection: 150 mg/ml (*Rx*)	Various. *Cleocin Phosphate* (Upjohn)

Warning:

These agents can cause severe and possibly fatal colitis, characterized by severe persistent diarrhea, severe abdominal cramps and possibly, the passage of blood and mucus.

Reserve for serious infections where less toxic antimicrobial agents are inappropriate. Do not use in patients with nonbacterial infections (ie, most upper respiratory tract infections).

Actions:

Pharmacology: Lincomycin and clindamycin, known collectively as lincosamides, bind exclusively to the 50 S subunit of bacterial ribosomes and suppress protein synthesis. Cross-resistance has been demonstrated between these two agents. Clindamycin is preferred because it is better absorbed and more potent.

Pharmacokinetics: Administration with food markedly impairs lincomycin (but not clindamycin) oral absorption.

Dialysis –

Select Pharmacokinetic Parameters of Lincosamides

Lincosamides	Bioavailability (%)	Mean peak serum level[1] (mcg/ml)	Time to peak serum level (hours)	Protein binding (%)	Half-Life (hours): Normal	Half-Life (hours): Anephric	Half-Life (hours): Liver disease	Elimination (%): Hepatic	Elimination (%): Unchanged in urine (range)	Elimination (%): Feces
Clindamycin[2]										
Oral	23-38	4	1-2							
IM		4.9	1-3	≈ 90	2.4-3	3.5-5	7-14	85	10-15	3.6
IV		14.7	0[3]							
Lincomycin										
Oral	30	2.6	2-4						4 (1-31)	
IM		9.5	0.5	70-72	4.4-6.4	10	11.8	50-70	17.3 (2-25)	40
IV		19	0						13.8 (5-30)	

[1] Clindamycin 300 mg; lincomycin, oral 500 mg, IM/IV 600 mg.
[2] Clindamycin palmitate and phosphate are rapidly hydrolyzed to the base.
[3] By end of infusion, peak levels are reached.

Microbiology:

Organisms Generally Susceptible to Lincosamides			
✓ = generally susceptible		Lincosamides	
Microorganism		Lincomycin	Clindamycin
Gram-positive	Staphylococcus aureus	✓	✓
	S epidermidis[1]	✓	✓
	Streptococcus pneumoniae	✓	✓
	S pyogenes	✓	✓
	β-hemolytic streptococci	✓	
	S viridans	✓	✓
	Pneumococci		✓
	Corynebacterium diphtheriae	✓	✓
	Nocardia asteroides	✓	✓
Anaerobes	Bacteroides sp	✓	✓[2]
	Fusobacterium		✓
	Propionibacterium (same as C acnes)	✓	✓
	Eubacterium	✓	✓
	Actinomyces sp	✓	✓
	Peptococcus	✓	✓
	Peptostreptococcus	✓	✓
	Microaerophilic streptococci		✓
	Clostridium perfringens	✓	✓
	C tetani	✓	✓
	Veillonella		✓

[1] Penicillinase and nonpenicillinase.
[2] Including B fragilis and B melaninogenicus.

Indications:

For the treatment of serious infections due to susceptible strains of streptococci, pneumococci and staphylococci. Reserve use for penicillin-allergic patients or when penicillin is inappropriate.

For approved indications, refer to the Administration and Dosage section.

Unlabeled uses:

Clindamycin – Clindamycin may be beneficial as an alternative to sulfonamides in combination with pyrimethamine in the acute treatment of CNS toxoplasmosis in AIDS patients.

Clindamycin with primaquine may be beneficial in *Pneumocystitis carinii* pneumonia.

Clindamycin is effective in the treatment of *Chlamydia trachomatis* infections in women.

Clindamycin is effective in bacterial vaginosis due to *Gardnerella vaginalis* and may be an alternative to metronidazole.

Contraindications:

Hypersensitivity to lincosamides; treatment of minor bacterial or viral infections.

Warnings:

Meningitis: Clindamycin does not diffuse adequately into CSF; do not use for meningitis.

Hypersensitivity: Use with caution in patients with a history of asthma or significant allergies. Refer to Management of Acute Hypersensitivity Reactions.

Renal function impairment: Cautiously give **clindamycin** to patients with severe renal or hepatic disease accompanied by severe metabolic aberrations. Use of **lincomycin** in preexisting liver disease is not recommended unless special clinical circumstances so indicate.

Elderly: Older patients with associated severe illness may not tolerate diarrhea well.

Pregnancy: Category B.

Lactation: Clindamycin and lincomycin appear in breast milk. The American Academy of Pediatrics considers clindamycin to be compatible with breastfeeding.

Children: **Lincomycin** is not indicated for use in the newborn. When **clindamycin** is administered to newborns and infants, monitor organ system functions.

Precautions:

Monitoring: In prolonged therapy, perform liver/kidney function tests, blood counts.

IV infusion: Do NOT inject IV undiluted as a bolus; infuse over at least 10 to 60 minutes as directed in Administration and Dosage.

Drug Interactions:

Drugs that may interact with lincosamides include erythromycin, kaolin-pectin and neuromuscular blockers (non-depolarizing).

Drug/Food interactions: Food impairs the absorption of lincomycin; do not take anything by mouth (except water) for 1 to 2 hours before and after lincomycin. Clindamycin absorption is not affected by food.

Adverse Reactions:

Nausea; vomiting; diarrhea (clindamycin 3.4% to 30%); pseudomembranous colitis (clindamycin 0.01% to 10%; 3 to 4 times more frequent with oral administration); neutropenia (sometimes transient); leukopenia; agranulocytosis; thrombocytopenic purpura; skin rashes, urticaria, erythema multiforme; anaphylaxis; jaundice; liver function test abnormalities (serum transaminase elevations).

Administration and Dosage:

LINCOMYCIN:

Oral – Take at least 1 to 2 hours before or after eating to ensure optimum absorption.

Adults: Serious infections – 500 mg every 8 hours.

More severe nfections – ≥ 500 mg every 6 hours.

Children > 1 month of age: Serious infections – 30 mg/kg/day (15 mg/lb/day) divided into 3 or 4 equal doses.

More severe infections – 60 mg/kg/day (30 mg/lb/day) divided into 3 or 4 equal doses.

IM –

Adults: Serious infections – 600 mg every 24 hours.

More severe infections – 600 mg every 12 hours or more often.

Children > 1 month of age: Serious infections – 10 mg/kg (5 mg/lb) every 24 hours.

More severe infections – 10 mg/kg (5 mg/lb) every 12 hours or more often.

IV – Dilute to 1 g/100 ml (minimum) and infuse over 1 hour. Severe cardiopulmonary reactions have occurred when given at greater than the recommended concentration and rate.

Adults: Serious infections – 600 mg to 1 g every 8 to 12 hours.

Severe to life-threatening situations – Doses of 8 g/day have been given.

Maximum recommended dose – 8 g/day.

Children > 1 month of age: Infuse 10 to 20 mg/kg/day (5 to 10 mg/lb/day), depending on severity of infection, in divided doses as described above for adults.

Subconjunctival injection – 75 mg/0.25 ml injected subconjunctivally results in ocular fluid levels of antibiotic (lasting for at least 5 hours) with MICs sufficient for most susceptible pathogens.

Renal function impairment – When required, an appropriate dose is 25% to 30% of that recommended for patients with normal renal function.

CLINDAMYCIN:

Oral – Take with a full glass of water or with food to avoid esophageal irritation. Clindamycin absorption is not affected by food.

Adults: Serious infections – 150 to 300 mg every 6 hours.

More severe infections – 300 to 450 mg every 6 hours.

Children:

Clindamycin HCl – Serious infections: 8 to 16 mg/kg/day divided into 3 or 4 equal doses.

More severe infections: 16 to 20 mg/kg/day divided into 3 or 4 equal doses.

Clindamycin palmitate HCl – Serious infections: 8 to 12 mg/kg/day divided into 3 or 4 equal doses.

Severe infections: 13 to 25 mg/kg/day divided into 3 or 4 equal doses. In children weighing ≤ 10 kg, administer 37.5 mg 3 times daily as the minimum dose.

Parenteral –

Adults: Serious infections due to aerobic gram-positive cocci and the more sensitive anaerobes: 600 to 1200 mg/day in 2 to 4 equal doses.

More severe infections, particularly those due to *B fragilis*, *Peptococcus* sp or *Clostridium* sp other than *C perfringens:* 1.2 to 2.7 g/day in 2 to 4 equal doses.

In life-threatening situations due to aerobes or anaerobes, doses of 4.8 g/day have been given IV to adults. Single IM injections > 600 mg are not recommended.

Children (> 1 month of age): 20 to 40 mg/kg/day in 3 or 4 equal doses, depending on the severity of infection.

Alternatively, children may be dosed based on body surface area:

Serious infections – 350 mg/m^2/day; *more serious infections* – 450 mg/m^2/day.

Neonates (< 1 month of age): 15 to 20 mg/kg/day in 3 to 4 equal doses.

CDC recommendation for acute pelvic inflammatory disease – 900 mg IV every 8 hours plus gentamicin loading dose 2 mg/kg IV or IM, followed by 1.5 mg/kg every 8 hours.

After discharge from hospital, continue with oral doxycycline 100 mg 2 times a day for 10 to 14 days total. Alternatively, continue with oral clindamycin 450 mg 5 times daily for 10 to 14 days.

AMINOGLYCOSIDES, PARENTERAL

STREPTOMYCIN SULFATE	
Injection: 400 mg/ml (*Rx*)	*Streptomycin Sulfate* (Pfizer)
KANAMYCIN SULFATE	
Injection: 500 mg or 1 g (*Rx*)	Various, *Kantrex* (Apothecon)
Pediatric Injection: 75 mg (*Rx*)	Various, *Kantrex* (Apothecon)
GENTAMICIN	
Injection: 2, 10 or 40 mg/ml (*Rx*)	Various, *Garamycin* (Schering)
TOBRAMYCIN SULFATE	
Injection: 10 or 40 mg/ml (*Rx*)	Various, *Nebcin* (Lilly)
Pediatric Injection: 10 mg/ml (*Rx*)	Various, *Nebcin* (Lilly)
Powder for Injection: 30 mg/ml (after reconstitution) (*Rx*)	*Nebcin* (Lilly)
AMIKACIN SULFATE	
Injection: 250 mg/ml (*Rx*)	Various, *Amikin* (Apothecon)
Pediatric Injection: 50 mg/ml (*Rx*)	Various, *Amikin* (Apothecon)
NETILMICIN SULFATE	
Injection: 100 mg/ml (*Rx*)	*Netromycin* (Schering)

Actions:

Pharmacology: The aminoglycosides are bactericidal antibiotics used primarily in the treatment of gram-negative infections.

Pharmacokinetics:

Absorption – Absorption from IM injection is rapid, with peak blood levels achieved within 1 hour.

Excretion is by glomerular filtration, largely as unchanged drug; thus, high urine levels are attained. Aminoglycosides are removed by hemodialysis (4 to 6 hours removes approximately 50%) and peritoneal dialysis (range, removal of 23% in 8 hours to only 4% in 22 hours).

Serum levels: Because of the narrow range between therapeutic and toxic serum levels, careful attention to dosage calculations is essential, especially in patients with renal impairment, geriatric and female patients, those requiring high peak serum levels, patients on prolonged (> 10 days) therapy, patients with unstable renal function or those undergoing dialysis, those with abnormal extracellular fluid volume, or with prior exposure to ototoxic or nephrotoxic drugs. Age markedly affects peak concentration in children; it is generally lower in young children and infants. Monitor drug serum levels. Peak levels indicate therapeutic levels. Trough serum level determinations (just before next dose) best indicate drug accumulation. Obtain serum levels within 48 hours of start of therapy and every 3 to 4 days assuming stable renal function; also, levels are indicated when dose is changed or in changing renal function. Generally, to measure peak levels, draw a serum sample about 30 minutes after IV infusion or 1 hour after an IM dose. For trough levels, obtain serum samples at 8 hours or just prior to the next dose.

Various Pharmacokinetic Parameters of the Aminoglycosides

Aminoglycoside	Half-life (hrs)		Therapeutic serum levels (peak) (mcg/ml)	Toxic serum levels (mcg/ml)		Dose (mg/kg/day) (normal Ccr)
	Normal	ESRD		Peak[1]	Trough[2]	
Amikacin	2-3	24-60	16-32	> 35	> 10	15
Gentamicin	2	24-60	4-8	> 12	> 2	3-5
Kanamycin	2-3	24-60	15-40	> 35	> 10	15
Netilmicin	2-2.7	40	6-10	> 16	> 4	3-6.5
Streptomycin	2.5	100	20-30	> 50	—	15
Tobramycin	2-2.5	24-60	4-8	> 12	> 2	3-5

[1] Measured 1 hour after IM administration.
[2] Measured immediately prior to next dose.

Microbiology:

Organisms Generally Susceptible to Aminoglycosides

	Organisms	Amikacin	Gentamicin	Kanamycin	Netimicin	Streptomycin	Tobramycin
Gram-positive	Mycobacterium tuberculosis	✓[1]				✓[2]	
	Staphylococci	✓[3]	✓[3]		✓[3]		✓
	S aureus	✓	✓	✓[3]	✓[3]		✓
	S epidermidis	✓		✓	✓		
	Streptococci					✓[2]	
	S faecalis		✓[2]		✓[2]	✓[2]	✓[2]
Gram-negative	Acinetobacter sp	✓		✓	✓		
	Brucella sp					✓	
	Citrobacter sp	✓	✓	✓	✓	✓	✓
	Enterobacter sp	✓	✓	✓	✓	✓	✓
	Escherichia coli	✓	✓	✓	✓	✓	✓
	Hemophilus influenzae	✓		✓		✓[2]	
	Hemophilus ducreyi					✓	
	Klebsiella sp	✓	✓	✓	✓	✓[2]	✓
	Morganella morganii						✓
	Neisseria sp	✓		✓	✓	✓	
	Proteus sp	✓[4]	✓[4]	✓[4]	✓	✓	✓[4]
	Providencia sp	✓	✓	✓	✓	✓	✓
	Pseudomonas sp	✓			✓		
	P aeruginosa	✓	✓[2]		✓	✓	✓
	Salmonella sp	✓	✓	✓	✓	✓	✓
	Serratia sp	✓	✓	✓	✓	✓	✓
	Shigella sp	✓	✓	✓	✓	✓	✓
	Yersinia (Pasteurella) pestis	✓	✓	✓	✓	✓	✓

[1] ✓ = generally susceptible
[2] Usually used concomitantly with other anti-infectives.
[3] Penicillinase-producing and nonpenicillinase-producing.
[4] Indole-positive and indole-negative.

Indications:

Reserve these drugs for treatment of infections caused by organisms not sensitive to less toxic agents. Safety for treatment periods > 14 days has not been established.

For approved indications, refer to the Administration and Dosage section.

Unlabeled uses: In cystic fibrosis patients, inhaled aminoglycosides may be beneficial in certain populations (eg, younger patients). Clinical outcome is not improved but deterioration of pulmonary function tests may be slowed or prevented.

Streptomycin, amikacin or kanamycin may be used as part of a multi-drug regimen for *Mycobacterium avium* complex, a common infection in AIDS patients.

Gentamicin – An alternative regimen for pelvic inflammatory disease is gentamicin plus clindamycin. Continue for at least 4 days and at least 48 hours after patient improves; then continue clindamycin 450 mg orally 4 times daily for 10 to 14 days total therapy.

Amikacin sulfate – Intrathecal/intraventricular administration has been suggested at 8 mg/24 hours.

Contraindications:

Previous reactions to these agents. With the exception of the use of streptomycin in tuberculosis, these agents are generally not indicated in long-term therapy because of the ototoxic and nephrotoxic hazards of extended administration.

Warnings:

Toxicity: Aminoglycosides are associated with significant nephrotoxicity or ototoxicity. These agents are excreted primarily by glomerular filtration; thus, the serum half-life will be prolonged and significant accumulation will occur in patients with impaired renal function. Toxicity may develop even with conventional doses, particularly in prerenal azotemia or impaired renal function.

Ototoxicity – Neurotoxicity, manifested as both auditory (cochlear) and vestibular ototoxicity, can occur with any of these agents. Auditory changes are irreversible, usually bilateral and may be partial or total. Risk of hearing loss increases with degree of exposure to either high peak or high trough serum concentrations and continues to progress after drug withdrawal. Risk is greater with renal impairment and with preexisting hearing loss. High frequency deafness usually occurs first and can be detected by audiometric testing. Relative ototoxicity is: Streptomycin = Kanamycin > Amikacin = Gentamicin = Tobramycin > Netilmicin.

Renal toxicity may be characterized by decreased creatinine clearance, cells or casts in the urine, decreased urine specific gravity, oliguria, proteinuria or evidence of nitrogen retention. Renal damage is usually reversible. The relative nephrotoxicity of these agents is estimated to be: Kanamycin = Amikacin = Gentamicin = Netilmicin > Tobramycin > Streptomycin.

Monitoring – Closely observe all patients treated with aminoglycosides. Monitoring renal and eighth cranial nerve function at onset of therapy is essential for patients with known or suspected renal impairment and also in those whose renal function is initially normal, but who develop signs of renal dysfunction.

Burn patients: In patients with extensive burns, altered pharmacokinetics may result in reduced serum concentrations of aminoglycosides.

Hypomagnesemia may occur in more than ⅓ of patients whose oral diet is restricted or who are eating poorly.

Neuromuscular blockade: Neurotoxicity can occur. Aminoglycosides may aggravate muscle weakness because of a potential curare-like effect on the neuromuscular junction.

Neuromuscular blockade resulting in respiratory paralysis has occurred with these agents, especially if given with or soon after anesthesia or muscle relaxants.

Nephrotoxicity may occur. Risk factors include the elderly, patients with a history of renal impairment who are treated for longer periods or with higher doses than those recommended, a recent course of aminoglycosides (within 6 weeks), concurrent use of other nephrotoxic agents, frequent dosing, potassium depletion and decreased intravascular volume. Adverse renal effects can occur in patients with initially normal renal function. Of patients receiving an aminoglycoside for several days or more, approximately 8% to 26% will develop mild renal impairment which is generally reversible.

Hydration – These drugs reach high concentrations in the renal system; keep patients well hydrated to minimize chemical irritation of tubules.

Dosing interval: Preliminary evidence indicates that aminoglycosides may be administered on a once-daily basis without compromising efficacy and without increasing the potential for nephrotoxicity and ototoxicity. It is possible that the incidence of nephrotoxicity may even be decreased.

Elderly patients may have reduced renal function that is not evident in the results of routine screening tests, such as BUN or serum creatinine. A Ccr determination may be more useful.

Pregnancy: *Category D* (amikacin, gentamicin, kanamycin, netilmicin, tobramycin).

Lactation: Small amounts of **streptomycin, kanamycin** and **netilmicin** are excreted in breast milk.

Children: Use with caution in premature infants and neonates because of their renal immaturity and the resulting prolongation of serum half-life of these drugs.

Precautions:

Intrathecal gentamicin: Use of excessive (40 to 160 mg) doses of intrathecal gentamicin has produced neuromuscular disturbances (eg, ataxia, paresis, incontinence).

Cross-allergenicity among the aminoglycosides has been demonstrated.

Monitoring: Monitor peak and trough serum concentrations periodically to assure adequate levels and to avoid potentially toxic levels. Also monitor serum calcium, magnesium and sodium (see Adverse Reactions).

Eighth cranial nerve function testing – Serial audiometric tests are suggested, particularly when renal function is impaired or prolonged aminoglycoside therapy is required; also repeat such tests periodically after treatment if there is evidence of a hearing deficit or vestibular abnormality before or during therapy, or when consecutive or concomitant use of other potentially ototoxic drugs is unavoidable.

Syphilis: In the treatment of sexually transmitted disease, if concomitant syphilis is suspected, perform a darkfield examination before treatment is started. Perform monthly serologic tests for at least 4 months.

Topical use: Aminoglycosides are quickly and almost totally absorbed when applied topically in association with surgical procedures, except to the urinary bladder.

Drug Interactions:

Drugs that may affect aminoglycosides include cephalosporins, enflurane, methoxyflurane, vancomycin, indomethacin IV, loop diuretics and penicillins.

Drugs that may be affected by aminoglycosides include depolarizing and nondepolarizing neuromuscular blockers and polypeptide antibiotics.

Adverse Reactions:

Aminoglycoside Adverse Reactions (%)

	Adverse Reaction	Amikacin	Gentamicin	Kanamycin	Netimicin	Streptomycin	Tobramycin
Central/Peripheral nervous system	Headache	rare	✓[1]	rare	< 0.1		✓
	Confusion		✓				✓
	Fever		✓		0.1	✓	✓
	Lethargy		✓				✓
	Disorientation				< 0.1		✓
	Neuromuscular blockade[2]	✓		✓	✓	✓	
	Paresthesia	rare		rare	< 0.1		
GI	Vomiting	rare	✓	rare	< 0.1	✓	✓
	Nausea	rare	✓	rare		✓	✓
	Diarrhea			rare	< 0.1		✓
Hematologic	Anemia	rare	✓		< 0.1		✓
	Eosinophilia	rare	✓		0.4	✓	✓
	Leukopenia		✓		< 0.1	✓	✓
	Thrombocytopenia		✓		< 0.1	✓	✓
Hypersensitivity	Rash	rare	✓	rare	≤ 0.5	✓	✓
	Urticaria		✓			✓	✓
	Itching		✓		≤ 0.5		✓

Aminoglycoside Adverse Reactions (%)							
	Adverse Reaction	Amikacin	Gentamicin	Kanamycin	Netimicin	Streptomycin	Tobramycin
Special senses	Dizziness		✓		✓		✓
	Tinnitus		✓		✓		✓
	Vertigo		✓		✓	✓	✓
	Hearing loss/deafness	✓	✓	✓[3]		✓	✓
Renal[1]	Oliguria	✓	✓	✓	✓		✓
	Proteinuria	✓	✓	✓	✓		✓
	Rising serum creatinine[2]	✓	✓	✓	✓		✓
	Casts	✓	✓		✓		
	Rising BUN[2]		✓	✓	✓		✓
	Red and white cells in urine	✓		✓	✓		
	Azotemia	✓				✓	
Lab test abnormalities	Increased AST/ALT		✓		1.5		✓
	Increased bilirubin		✓		1.5		✓
Other	Apnea	✓	✓	✓	✓	✓	✓
	Pain/Irritation at injection site		✓	✓	≈ 0.4		✓
	Hypotension	rare	✓		< 0.1		

[1] ✓ = Reported; no incidence given
[2] See Warnings
[3] Partially reversible to irreversible bilateral hearing loss.

Administration and Dosage:

Synergism: In vitro studies indicate that aminoglycosides combined with penicillins or cephalosporins act synergistically against some strains of gram-negative organisms and enterococci (*Streptococcus faecalis*). Aminoglycosides may exhibit a synergistic effect when combined with carbenicillin or ticarcillin for *Pseudomonas* infections.

STREPTOMYCIN SULFATE: Administer IM only.

Tuberculosis – The standard regimen for the treatment of drug-susceptible TB has been 2 months of INH, rifampin and pyrazinamide followed by 4 months of INH and rifampin. When streptomycin is added to this regimen because of suspected or proven drug resistence, the recommended dosing for streptomycin is as follows:

Streptomycin Dosing for TB			
	Daily	Twice weekly	Thrice weekly
Children	20 - 40 mg/kg max 1 g	25 - 30 mg/kg max 1.5 g	25 - 30 mg/kg max 1.5 g
Adults	15 mg/kg max 1 g	25 - 30 mg/kg max 1.5 g	25 - 30 mg/kg max 1.5 g

Streptomycin is usually administered daily as a single IM injection. Give a total dose of < 120 g over the course of therapy unless there are no other therapeutic options. In patients > 60 years of age, use a reduced dosage. The total period of drug treatment of TB is a minimum of 1 year.

Tularemia – 1 to 2 g/day in divided doses for 7 to 14 days, or until is afebrile 5 to 7 days.

Plague – 2 g daily in two divided doses for a minimum of 10 days.

Bacterial endocarditis –

Streptococcal: In penicillin-sensitive alpha and non-hemolytic streptococci, use streptomycin for 2 weeks with penicillin: 1 g twice daily for 1 week, 0.5 g twice daily for the second week. If patient is > 60 years of age, give 0.5 g twice daily for the entire 2–week period.

Enterococcal: 1 g twice daily for 2 weeks and 0.5 g twice daily for 4 weeks in combination with penicillin.

Adults – 1 to 2 g in divided doses every 6 to 12 hours for moderate to severe infections. Doses should generally not exceed 2 g per day.

Children – 20 to 40 mg/kg/day in divided doses every 6 to 12 hours.

KANAMYCIN SULFATE: Do not exceed total 1.5 g/day by any route.

IM – For adults or children, 7.5 mg/kg every 12 hrs (15 mg/kg/day). If continuously high blood levels are desired, give daily dose of 15 mg/kg in equally divided doses every 6 or 8 hours. Usual treatment duration is 7 to 10 days. Doses of 7.5 mg/kg give mean peak levels of 22 mcg/ml. At 8 hours after a 7.5 mg/kg dose, mean serum levels are 3.2 mcg/ml.

IV –

Adults: Do not exceed 15 mg/kg/day. Give slowly over 30 to 60 minutes. Divide daily doses into 2 to 3 equal doses.

Children: Use sufficient diluent to infuse drug over 30 to 60 minutes.

Renal failure – Calculate the dosage interval with the following formula: Serum creatinine (mg/dl) × 9 = dosage interval (in hours).

Intraperitoneal (following exploration for peritonitis or after peritoneal contamination caused by fecal spill during surgery) – 500 mg in 20 ml sterile distilled water instilled through a polyethylene catheter into wound.

Aerosol treatment – 250 mg 2 to 4 times a day.

Other routes – Concentrations of 0.25% have been used as irrigating solutions in abscess cavities, pleural space, peritoneal and ventricular cavities.

GENTAMICIN:

Dosage – May be given IM or IV. For patients with serious infections and normal renal function, give 3 mg/kg/day in 3 equal doses every 8 hours. For patients with life-threatening infections, administer up to 5 mg/kg/day in 3 or 4 equal doses. Reduce dosage to 3 mg/kg/day as soon as clinically indicated.

Obese patients: Base dosage on an estimate of lean body mass.

Children: 6 to 7.5 mg/kg/day (2 to 2.5 mg/kg every 8 hours).

Infants and neonates: 7.5 mg/kg/day (2.5 mg/kg every 8 hours).

Premature or full term neonates (≤ 1 week of age): 5 mg/kg/day (2.5 mg every 12 hours). A regimen of either 2.5 mg/kg every 18 hours or 3 mg/kg every 24 hours may also provide satisfactory peak and trough levels in preterm infants < 32 weeks gestational age.

Prevention of bacterial endocarditis –

In dental, oral or upper respiratory tract procedures (alternate regimen): 1 to 2 g (50 mg/kg for children) ampicillin plus 1.5 mg/kg (2 mg/kg for children) gentamicin not to exceed 80 mg, both IM or IV one-half hour prior to procedure, followed by 1.5 g (25 mg/kg for children) amoxicillin 6 hours after initial dose or repeat parenteral dose 8 hours after initial dose.

GU or GI procedures (standard regimen): 2 g (50 mg/kg for children) ampicillin plus 1.5 mg/kg (2 mg/kg for children) gentamicin not to exceed 80 mg, both IM or IV one-half hour prior to procedure followed by 1.5 mg (25 mg/kg for children) amoxicillin.

Renal function impairment –

Rule of eights: Approximate the interval between doses (in hours) by multiplying the serum creatinine level (mg/dl) by 8. For example, a patient weighing 60 kg with a serum creatinine level of 2 mg/dl could be given 60 mg (1 mg/kg) every 16 hours (2 × 8).

IV – A 1 to 2 mg/kg loading dose may be used, followed by a maintenance dose.

Intrathecal – In general, the recommended dose for infants and children ≥ 3 months of age is 1 to 2 mg once a day. For adults, administer 4 to 8 mg once a day.

TOBRAMYCIN SULFATE:

Dosage – Use the patient's ideal body weight for dosage calculation.

Adults with serious infections – Administer 3 mg/kg/day in 3 equal doses every 8 hours.

Life-threatening infections: Administer up to 5 mg/kg/day in 3 or 4 equal doses. Reduce dosage to 3 mg/kg/day as soon as clinically indicated.

Children – Administer 6 to 7.5 mg/kg/day in 3 or 4 equally divided doses (2 to 2.5 mg/kg every 8 hours or 1.5 to 1.9 mg/kg every 6 hours).

Premature or full term infants (≤ 1 year of age) – Administer up to 4 mg/kg/day in 2 equal doses every 12 hours. Preliminary data suggest that 2.5 mg/kg every 18 hours or 3 mg/kg every 24 hours may achieve safe and effective peak and trough serum concentrations in newborn infants weighing < 1 kg at birth.

Renal function impairment – Following a loading dose of 1 mg/kg, adjust subsequent dosage, either with reduced doses administered at 8–hour intervals or with normal doses given at prolonged levels.

An alternative guide for determining reduced dosage at 8–hour intervals (for patients whose steady-state serum creatinine values are known) is to divide the normally recommended dose by the patient's serum creatinine.

Hemodialysis removes approximately 50% of a dose in 6 hours. In patients maintained by regular dialysis, the usual dose of 1.5 to 2 mg/kg given after every dialysis usually maintains therapeutic, nontoxic serum levels. In patients receiving intermittent peritoneal dialysis, patients dialyzed twice weekly should receive a 1.5 to 2 mg/kg loading dose followed by 1 mg/kg every 3 days. Where dialysis occurs every 7 days, a 1.5 mg/kg loading dose is given after the first dialysis and 0.75 mg/kg after each subsequent dialysis.

IV administration – The IV dose is the same as the IM dose. Infuse the diluted solution over a period of 20 to 60 minutes. Infusion periods of < 20 minutes are not recommended because peak serum levels may exceed < 20 mcg/ml.

AMIKACIN SULFATE:

Adults and children – Use the patient's ideal body weight for dosage calculation. Administer IM or IV. Administer 15 mg/kg/day divided into 2 or 3 equal doses at equally divided intervals. Treatment of heavier patients should not exceed 1.5 g/day. In uncomplicated UTIs, use 250 mg twice daily.

Neonates: A loading dose of 10 mg/kg is recommended, followed by 7.5 mg/kg every 12 hours. Lower dosages may be safer during the first 2 weeks of life.

Renal function impairment – Adjust doses in patients with impaired renal function by administering normal doses at prolonged intervals or by administering reduced doses at a fixed interval.

Normal dosage at prolonged intervals: If the Ccr is not available and the patient's condition is stable, calculate a dosage interval (in hours) for the normal dose by multiplying the patient's serum creatinine by 9.

Reduced dosage at fixed time intervals: Measure serum concentration to assure accurate administration and to avoid concentrations > 35 mcg/ml. Initiate therapy by administering a normal dose, 7.5 mg/kg, as a loading dose.

To determine maintenance doses administered every 12 hours, reduce the loading dose in proportion to the reduction in the patient's Ccr:

$$\text{Maintenance dose every 12 hours} = \frac{\text{observed Ccr (ml/min)}}{\text{normal Ccr (ml/min)}} \times \text{calculated loading dose (mg)}$$

Dialysis: Approximately half the normal mg/kg dose can be given after hemodialysis; in peritoneal dialysis, a parenteral dose of 7.5 mg/kg is given, and then amikacin is instilled in peritoneal dialysate at a concentration desired in serum.

NETILMICIN SULFATE:

Dosage – Administer IM or IV. The recommended dosage for both methods is identical.

Obtain the patient's pretreatment body weight for calculation of correct dosage. Base the dosage in obese patients on an estimate of the lean body mass.

Patients with normal renal function –

Adults: Complicated UTIs: 1.5 to 2 mg/kg every 12 hours (3 to 4 mg/kg/day).

Serious systemic infections – 1.3 to 2.2 mg/kg every 8 hours or 2 to 3.25 mg/kg every 12 hours (4 to 6.5 mg/kg/day).

Infants and children (6 weeks through 12 years of age): Administer 1.8 to 2.7 mg/kg every 8 hours or 2.7 to 4 mg/kg every 12 hours (5.5 to 8 mg/kg/day).

Neonates (< 6 weeks of age): Administer 2 to 3.25 mg/kg every 12 hours (4 to 6.5 mg/kg/day).

Renal function impairment – If netilmicin serum concentrations are not available and renal function is stable, serum creatinine and Ccr values are the most reliable, readily available indicators of the degree of renal impairment to guide dosage adjustment. The BUN level is much less reliable for this purpose. Periodically reassess renal function during therapy.

Hemodialysis – In adults with renal failure who are undergoing hemodialysis, the amount of netilmicin removed from the blood may vary, depending upon the dialysis equipment and methods used. In adults, a dose of 2 mg/kg at the end of each dialysis period is recommended until the results of tests measuring serum levels become available.

AMINOGLYCOSIDES, ORAL

KANAMYCIN SULFATE	
Capsules: 500 mg (*Rx*)	*Kantrex* (Apothecon)
NEOMYCIN SULFATE	
Tablets: 500 mg (*Rx*)	Various, *Neo-Tabs* (Pharma-Tek)
Oral Solution: 125 mg per 5 ml (*Rx*)	*Mycifradin* (Upjohn), *Neo-Fradin* (Pharma-Tek)
PAROMOMYCIN SULFATE	
Capsules: 250 mg (*Rx*)	*Humatin* (Parke-Davis)

For complete information on the aminoglycosides, refer to the Aminoglycosides, Parenteral monograph.

Actions:

Pharmacokinetics: Oral aminoglycosides are poorly absorbed; therefore use only for suppression of GI bacterial flora.

Indications:

Suppression of intestinal bacteria.

Hepatic coma.

Neomycin sulfate: Many studies have documented lipid-lowering efficacy of neomycin. Alone, it reduced LDL cholesterol levels by 24%. Combined with niacin, it reduced LDL cholesterol levels to below the 90th percentile in 92% of patients.

Contraindications:

Presence of intestinal obstruction; hypersensitivity to aminoglycosides.

Warnings:

Increased absorption: Although negligible amounts are absorbed through intact mucosa, consider the possibility of increased absorption from ulcerated or denuded areas.

Nephrotoxicity/Ototoxicity: Because of reported cases of deafness and potential nephrotoxic effects, closely observe patients. Refer to the Warning Box in the Aminoglycosides, Parenteral monograph concerning aminoglycoside toxicity.

Pregnancy:

Neomycin – Category D.

Lactation: It is not known whether neomycin is excreted in breast milk. Other aminoglycosides are excreted in breast milk.

Children: The safety and efficacy of oral neomycin in patients < 18 years of age have not been established. If treatment is necessary, use with caution; do not exceed a treatment period of 3 weeks because of absorption from the GI tract.

Precautions:

Muscular disorders: Use with caution in patients with muscular disorders such as myasthenia gravis or parkinsonism.

GI effects:

Neomycin – Orally administered neomycin increases fecal bile acid excretion and reduces intestinal lactase activity.

Paromomycin – Use with caution in individuals with ulcerative lesions of the bowel to avoid renal toxicity through inadvertent absorption.

Drug Interactions:

Drugs that may be affected by aminoglycosides include anticoagulants, digoxin, methotrexate, neuromuscular blockers (depolarizing and nondepolarizing).

Adverse Reactions:

Nausea, vomiting, diarrhea (most common); "malabsorption syndrome" characterized by increased fecal fat, decreased serum carotene and fall in xylose absorption. *Clostridium difficile*—associated colitis (following neomycin therapy); nephrotoxicity and ototoxicity (following prolonged and high dosage therapy in hepatic coma).

Administration and Dosage:

KANAMYCIN SULFATE:

Suppression of intestinal bacteria – As an adjunct to mechanical cleansing of the large bowel in short-term therapy — 1 g for every hour for 4 hours, followed by 1 g every 6 hours for 36 to 72 hours.

Hepatic coma – 8 to 12 g/day in divided doses.

NEOMYCIN SULFATE:

Preoperative prophylaxis for elective colorectal surgery –

Recommended Bowel Preparation Regimen (Proposed Surgery Time 8 am)[1]			
Therapy	Day 3 before surgery	Day 2 before surgery	Day 1 before surgery
Diet	Minimum residue or clear liquid	Minimum residue or clear liquid	Clear liquid
Bisacodyl, 1 oral cap	6 pm (-62 hrs)		
Magnesium sulfate, 30 ml of a 50% solution orally		10 am (-46 hrs). Repeat at 2 pm (-42 hrs) and 6 pm (-38 hrs)	10 am (-22 hrs). Repeat at 2 pm (-18 hrs).
Enema		7 pm (-37 hrs) & 8 pm (-36 hrs). Repeat hourly until no solid feces return with last enema	None
Supplemental IV fluids			As needed
Neomycin and erythromycin tablets, 1 g each, orally			1 pm (-19 hrs). Repeat at 2 pm (-18 hrs) and 11 pm (-9 hrs)

[1] On day of surgery, patient should evacuate rectum at 6:30 am (-1½ hrs) for 8 am procedure.

Heptaic coma (as adjunct) –

Adults: 4 to 12 g/day in divided doses.

Children: 50 to 100 mg/kg/day in divided doses. Continue treatment over a period of 5 to 6 days; during this time, return protein to the diet incrementally. Chronic hepatic insufficiency may require up to 4 g/day over an indefinite period.

PAROMOMYCIN SULFATE:

Intestinal amebiasis –

Adults and children: Usual dose is 25 to 35 mg/kg/day, in 3 doses with meals for 5 to 10 days.

Management of hepatic coma –

Adults: Usual dose: 4 g/day in divided doses at regular intervals for 5 to 6 days.

Paromomycin sulfate has been recommended for other parasitic infections — *Dientamoeba fragilis* (25 to 30 mg/kg/day in 3 doses for 7 days); *Diphyllobothrium latum, Taenia saginata, T solium, Dipylidium caninum* (*adults:* 1 g every 15 min for 4 doses; *pediatric:* 11 mg/kg every 15 min for 4 doses); *Hymenolepis nana* (45 mg/kg/day for 5 to 7 days).

METRONIDAZOLE

Tablets: 250 mg, 500 mg (*Rx*)	Various, *Flagyl* (Searle)
Capsules: 375 mg (*Rx*)	*Flagyl 375* (Searle)
Powder for Injection. lyophilized: 500 mg (as HCl) (*Rx*)	*Flagyl I.V.* (Schiapparelli Searle)
Injection, ready-to-use: 500 mg per 100 ml (*Rx*)	Various, *Metronidazole* (Abbott), *Flagyl I.V. RTU* (Schiapparelli Searle)

Metronidazole is also available for topical and intravaginal use and is also used orally as an amebicide.

Warning:
Metronidazole is carcinogenic in rodents. Avoid unnecessary use.

Actions:

Pharmacology: Metronidazole, a nitroimidazole, is active against various anaerobic bacteria and protozoa.

Pharmacokinetics:

Absorption – Metronidazole is well absorbed after oral administration. Peak serum levels occur at about 1 to 2 hours. Food delays peak serum levels up to 2 hours.

Distribution – Metronidazole has a large apparent volume of distribution. It diffuses well into all tissues.

Excretion – The major route of elimination of metronidazole and its metabolites is via the urine (60% to 80% of the dose), fecal excretion accounts for 6% to 15% of the dose. Renal clearance is approximately 10 ml/min/1.73 m^2. Metronidazole has an average elimination half-life in healthy subjects of 8 hours. Patients with Ccr < 10 ml/min (not receiving dialysis) will accumulate both metabolites. Metronidazole and its two major metabolites are removed by hemodialysis. Metronidazole is also removed by peritoneal dialysis.

Indications:

Anaerobic infections: Teatment of serious infections caused by susceptible anaerobic bacteria. Effective in B fragilis infections resistant to clindamycin, chloramphenicol and penicillin.

Intra-abdominal infections (peritonitis, intra-abdominal abscess and liver abscess) caused by *Bacteroides* sp (*B fragilis, B distasonis, B ovatus, B thetaiotaomicron, B vulgatus*), *Clostridium* sp, *Eubacterium* sp, *Peptostreptococcus* sp and *Peptococcus* sp.

Skin and skin structure infections, caused by *Bacteroides* sp including the *B fragilis* group, *Clostridium* sp, *Peptococcus* sp, *Peptostreptococcus* sp and *Fusobacterium* sp.

Gynecologic infections (endometritis, endomyometritis, tubo-ovarian abscess and postsurgical vaginal cuff infection), caused by *Bacteroides* sp including the *B fragilis* group, *Clostridium* sp, *Peptococcus* sp and *Peptostreptococcus* sp.

Bacterial septicemia caused by *Bacteroides* sp including the *B fragilis* group and *Clostridium* sp.

Bone and joint infections caused by *Bacteroides* sp including the *B fragilis* group, as adjunctive therapy.

CNS infections (meningitis and brain abscess), caused by *Bacteroides* sp including the *B fragilis* group.

Lower respiratory tract infections (pneumonia, empyema and lung abscess) caused by *Bacteroides* sp including the *B fragilis* group.

Endocarditis caused by *Bacteroides* sp including the *B fragilis* group.

Prophylaxis: Preoperative, intraoperative and postoperative IV metronidazole may reduce the incidence of postoperative infection in patients undergoing elective colorectal surgery which is classified as contaminated or potentially contaminated.

Metronidazole is also indicated for amebiasis and trichomoniasis, intravaginally for bacterial vaginosis and topically for acne rosacea.

Unlabeled uses: Metronidazole has shown efficacy, alone and in combination, as prophylaxis in reducing infection rates in gynecologic and abdominal surgery.

Hepatic encephalopathy – Metronidazole has compared favorably to neomycin.

Crohn's disease – Metronidazole has been successful, with particular improvement of perianal manifestations.

Antibiotic-associated pseudomembranous colitis – Metronidazole is as effective as vancomycin.

Helicobacter pylori – A combination of metronidazole and bismuth for 4 weeks appears to be effective in the eradication of *H pylori* for up to 12 months. The addition of tetracycline may increase the length of remission.

The CDC has recommended the use of oral metronidazole for bacterial vaginosis (500 mg twice daily for 7 days). Single-dose therapy for bacterial vaginosis (2 g) also appears to be as effective as multiple-dose therapy.

Contraindications:

Hypersensitivity to metronidazole or other nitroimidazole derivatives; pregnancy (first trimester in patients with trichomoniasis).

Warnings:

Neurologic effects: Seizures (associated with high cumulative doses) and peripheral neuropathy (characterized by numbness or paresthesia of an extremity) have occurred. In some cases, neuropathy is not reversible.

Hepatic function impairment: Patients with severe hepatic disease metabolize metronidazole slowly. Accumulation of the drug and its metabolites may occur.

Elderly: Since the pharmacokinetics of metronidazole may be altered in the elderly, monitoring of serum levels may be necessary to adjust the dosage accordingly.

Pregnancy: Category B. Restrict metronidazole for trichomoniasis in the second and third trimesters to those in whom local palliative treatment has been inadequate to control symptoms.

Lactation: Safety for use in nursing mothers has not been established. A nursing mother should express and discard any breast milk produced while on the drug and resume nursing 24 to 48 hours after the drug is discontinued.

Children: Safety and efficacy in children have not been established, except for the treatment of amebiasis. Newborns demonstrate a diminished capacity to eliminate metronidazole; half-life may be as high as 22 hours.

Precautions:

Crohn's disease patients are known to have an increased incidence of GI and certain extraintestinal cancers.

Candidiasis, may present more prominent symptoms during therapy and requires treatment with a candicidal agent.

Hematologic effects: Metronidazole is a nitroimidazole; use with care in patients with evidence or history of blood dyscrasia. Perform total and differential leukocyte counts before and after therapy.

Amebic liver abscess: Metronidazole does not obviate the need for aspiration of pus.

Drug Interactions:

Drugs that may affect metronidazole include barbiturates and cimetidine. Drugs that may be affected by metronidazole include anticoagulants, disulfiram, ethanol, hydantoins and lithium.

Drug/Lab test interactions: The drug may interfere with chemical analyses for AST, ALT, LDH, triglycerides and hexokinase glucose.

Adverse Reactions:

Adverse reactions may include: Dysuria; cystitis; polyuria; incontinence; proliferation of *Candida* in the vagina; dyspareunia; darkened urine; seizures and peripheral neuropathy; dizziness; vertigo; incoordination; ataxia; confusion; irritability; depression; weakness; insomnia; headache; syncope; nausea; diarrhea; epigastric distress; constipation; proctitis; glossitis; stomatitis; unpleasant metallic taste; urticaria; erythematous rash; flushing; nasal congestion.

Administration and Dosage:

May cause GI upset; take with food. Avoid alcoholic beverages.

Anaerobic bacterial infections: In the treatment of most serious anaerobic infections, metronidazole is usually administered IV initially.

Loading dose – 15 mg/kg infused over 1 hour (≈ 1 g for a 70 kg adult).

Maintenance dose – 7.5 mg/kg infused over 1 hour every 6 hours (≈ 500 mg for a 70 kg adult). Administer the first maintenance dose 6 hours following the initiation of loading dose. Do not exceed a maximum of 4 g in 24 hours.

The usual duration of therapy is 7 to 10 days; however, infections of the bone and joints, lower respiratory tract and endocardium may require longer treatment.

Administer by slow IV, continuous or intermittent drip infusion only. Do not give by direct IV bolus injection because of the low pH (0.5 to 2) of the reconstituted product. The drug must be further diluted and neutralized for infusion.

Oral – Following IV therapy, use oral metronidazole when conditions warrant. The usual adult oral dosage is 7.5 mg/kg every 6 hours. Do not exceed a maximum of 4 g in 24 hours.

Prophylaxis: To prevent postoperative infection in contaminated or potentially contaminated colorectal surgery, the recommended adult dosage is 15 mg/kg infused over 30 to 60 minutes and completed ≈ 1 hour before surgery, followed by 7.5 mg/kg infused over 30 to 60 minutes at 6 and 12 hours after the initial dose.

It has also been suggested that a dose of 1500 mg infused at the beginning of surgery achieves significantly higher concentrations against B fragilis than the 500 mg infusion and may be beneficial in ensuring adequate metronidazole levels.

Hepatic disease patients metabolize metronidazole slowly; accumulation of metronidazole and its metabolites occurs. Therefore, reduce doses below those usually recommended

Renal disease: Do not specifically reduce the dose in anuric patients because accumulated metabolites may be rapidly removed by dialysis.

NYSTATIN, ORAL

Tablets: 500,000 units (*Rx*)	Various, *Nilstat* (Lederle), *Mycostatin* (Apothecon)

Actions:

Pharmacology: A polyene antibiotic with antifungal activity. Nystatin probably acts by binding to sterols in the cell membrane of the fungus, with a resultant change in membrane permeability allowing leakage of intracellular components.

Pharmacokinetics: Sparingly absorbed after oral use.

Indications:

Treatment of intestinal candidiasis.

Contraindications:

Hypersensitivity to nystatin.

Adverse Reactions:

Nystatin is virtually nontoxic and nonsensitizing and is well tolerated by all age groups including debilitated infants, even on prolonged administration.

Administration and Dosage:

500,000 to 1,000,000 units 3 times daily. Continue treatment for at least 48 hours after clinical cure to prevent relapse.

MICONAZOLE

Injection: 10 mg per ml (*Rx*)	*Monistat i.v.* (Janssen)

Actions:

Pharmacology: Miconazole, an imidazole derivative, exerts a fungicidal effect by altering the permeability of the fungal cell membrane.

Pharmacokinetics:

Absorption/Distribution – CSF levels following IV administration are undetectable. Penetration of the drug into inflamed joints, the vitreous body of the eye and the peritoneal cavity is good. Greater than 90% is bound to serum protein.

Metabolism/Excretion – Miconazole is rapidly metabolized in the liver. About 14% to 22% of the administered dose is excreted in the urine, mainly as inactive metabolites. The terminal elimination half-life is 20 to 25 hours.

Indications:

Use only to treat severe systemic fungal disease: Coccidioidomycosis, candidiasis, cryptococcosis, pseudoallescheriosis (petriellidiosis, allescheriosis), paracoccidioidomycosis and for the treatment of chronic mucocutaneous candidiasis.

In the treatment of fungal meningitis or *Candida* urinary bladder infections, IV infusion alone is inadequate. It must be supplemented with intrathecal administration or bladder irrigation.

Contraindications:

Hypersensitivity to miconazole.

Warnings:

Cardiac effects: Cardiorespiratory arrest or anaphylaxis has occurred, possibly due to excessively rapid administration in some cases. Rapid injection of undiluted miconazole may produce transient tachycardia or arrhythmia.

Pregnancy: Category C.

Children: Safety for use in children < 1 year of age has not been extensively studied.

Precautions:

Give by IV infusion. Start treatment under stringent conditions of hospitalization. Subsequently, it may be given to suitable patients under ambulatory conditions with close clinical monitoring. Monitor hemoglobin, hematocrit, electrolytes and lipids.

Systemic fungal mycoses may be complications of chronic underlying conditions which, in themselves, may require appropriate measures.

Drug Interactions:

Drugs that may interact with miconazole include amphotericin B, astemizole, cisapride, oral anticoagulants, phenytoin and terfenadine.

Adverse Reactions:

Adverse reactions occurring in ≥ 3% of patients include phlebitis at infusion site, pruritus/rash (if severe, discontinuation may be necessary), nausea, vomiting, fever and chills.

Administration and Dosage:

Adults: The following daily doses are recommended:

Recommended Miconazole Daily Doses		
Organism	Total daily dosage range[1] (mg)	Duration of therapy (weeks)
Coccidioidomycosis	1800 to 3600	3 to > 20
Cryptococcosis	1200 to 2400	3 to > 12
Pseudoallescheriosis	1600 to 3000	5 to > 20
Candidiasis	1600 to 1800	1 to > 20
Paracoccidioidomycosis	1200 to 1200	2 to > 16

[1] May be divided over 3 infusions.

Repeated courses may be necessitated by relapse or reinfection.

Children:

< 1 year old – 15 to 30 mg/kg/day.

1 to 12 years old – 20 to 40 mg/kg/day. Do not exceed 15 mg/kg/dose.

IV: For doses ≤ 2400 mg/day, infuse at a rate of approximately 2 hours/amp. For doses > 2400 mg/day, adjust infusion rate and diluent according to patient tolerability.

Intrathecal: Administer undiluted solution by various intrathecal routes (20 mg per dose) as an adjunct to IV treatment in fungal meningitis. Succeeding intrathecal injections may be alternated between lumbar, cervical and cisternal punctures every 3 to 7 days.

Bladder instillation: 200 mg diluted solution for *Candida* of the urinary bladder.

KETOCONAZOLE

Tablets: 200 mg (*Rx*)	*Nizoral* (Janssen)

Warning:

Ketoconazole has been associated with hepatic toxicity, including some fatalities. Closely monitor patients and inform them of the risk.

Actions:

Pharmacology: Ketoconazole, an imidazole broad-spectrum antifungal agent, impairs the synthesis of ergosterol, the main sterol of fungal cell membranes, allowing increased permeability and leakage of cellular components.

Pharmacokinetics:

Absorption/Distribution – Bioavailability depends on an acidic pH for dissolution and absorption. In vitro, plasma protein binding is about 95% to 99%, mainly to albumin.

Metabolism/Excretion – The drug undergoes extensive hepatic metabolism to inactive metabolites. Plasma elimination is biphasic; half-life is 2 hours during the first 10 hours, 8 hours thereafter. The major excretory route is enterohepatic. From 85% to 90% is excreted in bile and feces, 10% to 15% in urine.

Indications:

Treatment of the following systemic fungal infections: Candidiasis, chronic mucocutaneous candidiasis, oral thrush, candiduria, blastomycosis, coccidioidomycosis, histoplasmosis, chromomycosis and paracoccidioidomycosis.

Treatment of severe recalcitrant cutaneous dermatophyte infections not responding to topical therapy or oral griseofulvin or in patients unable to take griseofulvin.

Unlabeled uses: Ketoconazole has been used successfully in the treatment of onychomycosis (caused by *Trichophyton* and *Candida* sp); pityriasis versicolor (Tinea versicolor); tinea pedis, corporis and cruris; tinea capitis; and vaginal candidiasis.

High-dose ketoconazole has shown some success in treating CNS fungal infections.

Ketoconazole has been used in the treatment of advanced prostate cancer.

Ketoconazole has been used to effectively treat Cushing's syndrome due to its ability to inhibit adrenal steroidogenesis.

Contraindications:

Hypersensitivity to ketoconazole. Do not use for the treatment of fungal meningitis because it penetrates poorly into the CSF.

Warnings:

Hepatotoxicity, primarily of the hepatocellular type, has been associated with ketoconazole including rare fatalities. Measure liver function before starting treatment and frequently during treatment. Monitor patients receiving ketoconazole concurrently with other potentially hepatotoxic drugs, particularly those patients requiring prolonged therapy or those with a history of liver disease. Transient minor elevations in liver enzymes have occurred.

Hypersensitivity: Anaphylaxis occurs rarely after the first dose. Hypersensitivity reactions, including urticaria, have been reported.

Pregnancy: *Category* C.

Lactation: Ketoconazole is probably excreted in breast milk; mothers who are under treatment should not nurse.

Children: Safety for use in children < 2 years of age has not been established.

Precautions:

Hormone levels: Testosterone levels are impaired with doses of 800 mg/day and abolished by 1600 mg/day. It also decreases ACTH-induced corticosteroid serum levels at similar high doses.

Gastric acidity: Ketoconazole requires acidity for dissolution and absorption. In achlorhydria, dissolve each tablet in 4 ml aqueous solution of 0.2 N HCl. Use a glass or plastic straw to avoid contact with teeth. Follow with a glass of water.

Drug Interactions:

Drugs that may affect ketoconazole include antacids, histamine H_2 antagonists, isoniazid and rifampin. Drugs that may be affected by ketoconazole include cisapride, oral anticoagulants, antihistamines (astemizole, terfenadine), corticosteroids, cyclosporine and theophylline.

Adverse Reactions:

Adverse reactions occurring in ≥ 3% of patients include nausea and vomiting.

Administration and Dosage:

If antacids, anticholinergics or H_2 blockers are needed, give at least 2 hours after administration. Take with food to alleviate GI disturbance.

Adults: Initially, 200 mg once daily. In very serious infections, or if clinical response is insufficient, increase dose to 400 mg once daily.

Children:

(*> 2 years*) – 3.3 to 6.6 mg/kg/day as a single daily dose.
(*< 2 years*) – Daily dosage has not been established.

Minimum treatment for candidiasis is 1 or 2 weeks and for the other indicated systemic mycoses, 6 months. Chronic mucocutaneous candidiasis usually requires maintenance therapy.

Minimum treatment of recalcitrant dermatophyte infections is 4 weeks in cases involving glabrous skin. Palmar and plantar infections may respond more slowly.

AMPHOTERICIN B

Injection: 50 mg (as deoxycholate) (*Rx*)	*Amphotericin B* (Pharmatek), *Fungizone Intravenous* (Bristol-Myers)
Suspension for Injection: Amphotericin B liposomal complex 100 mg/20 ml (*Rx*)	*Abelcet* (Liposome)
Powder for Injection, lyophilized: 50 mg (as cholesteryl)	*Amphotec* (Sequus Pharmaceuticals)

Warning:

Use primarily for treatment of patients with progressive and potentially fatal fungal infections. Do not use to treat the common clinically inapparent forms of fungal disease which show only positive skin or serologic tests.

Actions:

Pharmacology: Amphotericin B is fungistatic or fungicidal, depending on the concentration obtained in body fluids and on the susceptibility of the fungus. It probably acts by binding to sterols in the fungal cell membrane with a resultant change in membrane permeability, allowing leakage of a variety of small molecules.

Pharmacokinetics:

Absorption/Distribution – Amphotericin B is highly protein bound (> 90%) and is poorly dialyzable.

Metabolism/Excretion – Amphotericin B has a relatively short initial serum half-life of 24 hours, followed by a second elimination phase with a half-life of about 15 days. The drug is very slowly excreted by the kidneys with 2% to 5% as the biologically active form.

Indications:

Amphotericin B: Administer amphotericin B for injection primarily to those patients with progressive, potentially life-threatening fungal infections.

May be helpful in the treatment of American mucocutaneous leishmaniasis, but it is not the drug of choice in primary therapy.

Liposomal amphotericin B is indicated for the treatment of aspergillosis in patients refractory to or intolerant of conventional amphotericin B therapy.

Amphotericin B cholesteryl: For the treatment of invasive aspergillosis in patients where renal impairment or unacceptable toxicity precludes the use of amphotericin B deoxycholate in effective doses and in patients with invasive aspergillosis where prior amphotericin B deoxycholate therapy has failed.

Unlabeled uses: Prophylactic use to prevent fungal infection in patients with bone marrow transplantation.

Contraindications:

Hypersensitivity to amphotericin B, unless the condition requiring treatment is life-threatening and amenable only to amphotericin B therapy.

Warnings:

Fatal fungal diseases: Amphotericin B is frequently the only effective treatment for potentially fatal fungal diseases. Balance its possible lifesaving effect against its dangerous side effects.

Nephrotoxicity: Renal damage, the most important toxic effect, is a limiting factor for the use of amphotericin B. Renal dysfunction usually improves upon interruption of therapy, dose reduction or increased dosing interval; however, some permanent impairment often occurs, especially in patients receiving large doses (> 5 g). Decreased glomerular filtration rate and renal blood flow, increased serum creatinine and renal tubular dysfunction are prominent. In some patients, hydration and sodium repletion prior to amphotericin B administration may reduce the risk of developing nephrotoxicity.

Nephrocalcinosis is also commonly observed and usually improves upon interruption of therapy; however, some permanent impairment often occurs, especially in those patients receiving large amounts (> 5 g) of amphotericin B deoxycholate. Supplemental alkali medication may decrease renal tubular acidosis complications.

Acute reactions: Acute infusion-related reactions can be managed by pretreatment with antihistamines and corticosteroids or by reducing the rate of infusion and by prompt administration of antihistamines and corticosteroids.

Pregnancy: Category B.

Lactation: It is not known whether amphotericin B is excreted in breast milk; however, consider discontinuing nursing.

Children: Safety and efficacy in children have not been established. Limit administration to the least amount compatible with an effective therapeutic regimen.

Precautions:

Monitoring: Perform BUN and serum creatinine or endogenous creatinine clearance tests at least weekly during therapy. If BUN exceeds 40 mg/dl or if serum creatinine exceeds 3 mg/dl, discontinue the drug or reduce dosage until renal function improves. Weekly hemograms, serum potassium and magnesium determinations are also advisable. Discontinue therapy if liver function test results are abnormal.

Prolonged therapy is usually necessary. Unpleasant reactions are common and some are potentially dangerous. Use only in hospitalized patients or in those under close medical observation. Reserve use for those patients in whom a diagnosis of the progressive, potentially fatal forms of susceptible mycotic infections has been firmly established, preferably by positive culture or histologic study.

Therapy interruption: Whenever medication is interrupted for > 7 days, resume therapy with the lowest dosage level; increase gradually.

Pulmonary reactions characterized by acute dyspnea, hypoxemia and interstitial infiltrates have been observed in neutropenic patients receiving amphotericin B and leukocyte transfusions. Separate the infusion as far as possible from the time of a leukocyte transfusion.

Laboratory tests:

Serum electrolyte abnormalities – Hypomagnesemia, hyperkalemia, hypocalcemia, hypercalcemia, hypokalemia.

Liver function test abnormalities – Increased AST, ALT, GGT, bilirubin, alkaline phosphatase and LDH.

Renal function impairment – Increased BUN and serum creatinine.

Other test abnormalities – Acidosis, hypermylasemia, hypoglycemia, hyperglycemia, hyperuricemia, hypophosphatemia.

Drug Interactions:

Drugs that may interact with amphotericin B include antineoplastic agents, corticosteroids, zidovudine, other nephrotoxic agents, digitalis glycosides, flucytocine and neuromuscular blocking agents.

Adverse Reactions:

Adverse reactions may include: Fever (sometimes with shaking chills); headache; anorexia; malaise; generalized pain, including muscle and joint pains; hypokalemia; azotemia; hyposthenuria; nephrocalcinosis; renal tubular acidosis; nausea; vomiting; dyspepsia; diarrhea; cramping; epigastric pain; normochromic, normocytic anemia; venous pain at the injection site with phlebitis and thombophlebitis; weight loss.

Administration and Dosage:

Conventional amphotericin B:

Test dose – An initial test dose of 1 mg in 20 ml of dextrose injection 5% administered IV over 20 to 30 minutes may be preferred.

Administer by slow IV infusion over 6 hours at a concentration of 0.1 mg/ml.

Therapy is usually instituted with a daily dose of 0.25 mg/kg and gradually increased as tolerance permits. Do not exceed a total daily dose of 1.5 mg/kg. Total daily dosage may range up to 1 mg/kg; alternate day dosages range up to 1.5 mg/kg. Several months of therapy are usually necessary; a shorter period of therapy may be inadequate and lead to relapse.

Severe and rapidly progressive fungal infection – Therapy may be initiated with a daily dose of 0.3 mg/kg IV over 2 to 6 hours.

Impaired cardio-renal function or a severe reaction to the test dose – Therapy should be initiated with smaller daily doses (eg, 5 to 10 mg). Depending on the patient's cardiorenal status, doses may gradually be increased by 5 to 10 mg/day to a final daily dosage of 0.5 to 0.7 mg/kg. Do not exceed a total daily dose of 1.5 mg/kg.

Sporotrichosis – Usual dose per injection is 20 mg. Therapy has ranged up to 9 months.

Aspergillosis has been treated for ≤ 11 months with a total dose of ≤ 3.6 g per day.

Rhinocerebral phycomycosis – A cumulative dose of at least 3 g per day amphotericin B is recommended.

Liposomal amphotericin B: The recommended daily dosage for adults and children is 5 mg/kg given as a single infusion. Administer IV at a rate of 2.5 mg/kg/hr. If the infusion time exceeds 2 hours, mix the contents by shaking the infusion bag every 2 hours.

Amphotericin B cholesteryl: For adults and children, therapy may begin at a daily dose of 3 to 4 mg/kg as required. The dose may be increased to 6 mg/kg/day if there is not improvement or if there is evidence of progression of the fungal infection.

Administer diluted in 5% Dextrose for Injection by IV infusion at a rate of 1 mg/kg/hr. A test dose immediately preceding the first dose is advisable when commencing all new courses of treatment. Infuse a small amount of drug (eg, 10 ml of the final preparation containing between 1.6 to 8.3 mg) over 15 to 30 minutes, and observe the patient carefully for the next 30 minutes.

The infusion time may be shortened to a minimum of 2 hours for patients who show no evidence of intolerance or infusion-related reactions. If the patient experiences acute reactions or cannot tolerate the infusion volume, the infusion time may be extended.

GRISEOFULVIN

GRISEOFULVIN MICROSIZE	
Tablets: 250 and 500 mg (*Rx*)	*Fulvicin U/F* (Schering), *Grifulvin V* (Ortho Derm), *Grisactin 500* (Wyeth-Ayerst)
Capsules: 250 mg (*Rx*)	*Grisactin 250* (Wyeth-Ayerst)
Oral Suspension: 125 mg/5 ml (*Rx*)	*Grifulvin V* (Ortho Derm)
GRISEOFULVIN ULTRAMICROSIZE	
Tablets: 125, 165, 250 and 330 mg (*Rx*)	Various, *Fulvicin P/G* (Schering), *Grisactin Ultra* (Wyeth-Ayerst), *Gris-PEG* (Allergan Herbert)

Actions:

Pharmacology: Griseofulvin, an antibiotic derived from a species of *Penicillium*, is deposited in the keratin precursor cells, which are gradually exfoliated and replaced by noninfected tissue; it has a greater affinity for diseased tissue.

Pharmacokinetics: The peak serum level found in fasting adults given 0.5 g griseofulvin microsize occurs at about 4 hours and ranges between 0.5 to 2 mcg/ml. Some individuals are consistently "poor absorbers" and tend to attain lower blood levels at all times. The serum level may be increased by giving the drug with a meal with a high fat content.

Indications:

Treatment of ringworm infections of the skin, hair and nails, namely: Tinea corporis, tinea pedis, tinea cruris, tinea barbae, tinea capitis, tinea unguium (onychomycosis) when caused by one or more of the following genera of fungi: *Trichophyton rubrum; T tonsurans; T mentagrophytes; T interdigitalis; T verrucosum; T megnini; T gallinae; T crateriform; T sulphureum; T schoenleini; Microsporum audouini; M canis; M gypseum; Epidermophyton floccosum.*

Note: Prior to therapy, identify the types of fungi responsible for the infection. Use of this drug is not justified in minor or trivial infections which will respond to topical agents alone.

Griseofulvin is NOT effective in bacterial infections; candidiasis (moniliasis); histoplasmosis; actinomycosis; sporotrichosis; chromoblastomycosis; coccidioidomycosis; North American blastomycosis; cryptococcosis (torulosis); tinea versicolor; nocardiosis.

Contraindications:

Hypersensitivity to griseofulvin; porphyria; hepatocellular failure.

Warnings:

Hypersensitivity reactions (eg, skin rashes, urticaria, angioneurotic edema) may occur and necessitate withdrawal of therapy. Institute appropriate counter measures.

Pregnancy: Category C.

Precautions:

Prolonged therapy: Closely observe patients on prolonged therapy. Periodically monitor renal, hepatic and hematopoietic function.

Penicillin cross-sensitivity is possible since griseofulvin is derived from species of *Penicillium.*

Lupus erythematosus, lupus-like syndromes or exacerbation of lupus erythematosus have occurred in patients receiving griseofulvin.

Photosensitivity may occur. Photosensitivity reactions may aggravate lupus erythematosus.

Drug Interactions:

Drugs that may interact with griseofulvin include anticoagulants, oral contraceptives, cyclosporine, salicylates and barbiturates.

Adverse Reactions:

Adverse reactions may include: Hypersensitivity reactions such as skin rashes and urticaria; oral thrush; nausea; vomiting; epigastric distress; diarrhea; headache; fatigue; dizziness; insomnia; mental confusion; impairment of performance of routine activities.

Administration and Dosage:

Duration of therapy: Representative treatment periods are: Tinea capitis, 4 to 6 weeks; tinea corporis, 2 to 4 weeks; tinea pedis, 4 to 8 weeks; tinea unguium (depending on rate of growth) – fingernails, at least 4 months, toenails, at least 6 months.

Adults:

Tinea corporis, tinea cruris, tinea capitis – A single or divided daily dose of 500 mg microsize (330 to 375 mg ultramicrosize) will give a satisfactory response in most patients.

Tinea pedis, tinea unguium – 0.75 to 1 g microsize (660 to 750 mg ultramicrosize) per day in divided doses.

Children: Approximately 11 mg microsize/kg/day (5 mg/lb/day) or 7.3 mg ultramicrosize/kg/day (3.3 mg/lb/day) is an effective dose for most children.

Griseofulvin Dosage for Children Based on Weight			
Weight		Daily dose (mg)	
lb	kg	microsize	ultramicrosize
30 to 50	13.6 to 23	125 to 250	82.5 to 165
> 50	> 23	250 to 500	165 to 330

Clinical experience indicates that a single daily dose is effective in children with tinea capitis.

Children (≤ 2 years of age) – Dosage not established.

FLUCONAZOLE

Tablets: 50, 100, 150 and 200 mg (*Rx*) **Powder for oral suspension:** 10 and 40 mg/ml when reconstituted (*Rx*) **Injection:** 2 mg/ml (*Rx*)	*Diflucan* (Roerig)

Actions:

Pharmacology: Fluconazole, a synthetic broad spectrum bis-triazole antifungal agent, is a highly selective inhibitor of fungal cytochrome P-450 and sterol C-14 alpha-demethylation.

Pharmacokinetics:

Absorption/Distribution – The pharmacokinetic properties of fluconazole are similar following administration by the IV or oral routes. In healthy volunteers, the bioavailability of oral fluconazole is > 90% compared with IV administration.

Peak plasma concentrations (C_{max}) in fasted healthy volunteers occur between 1 and 2 hours with a terminal plasma elimination half-life of ≈ 30 hrs (range, 20 to 50) after oral administration.

Steady-state concentrations are reached within 5 to 10 days following oral doses of 50 to 400 mg given once daily. The apparent volume of distribution approximates that of total body water. Plasma protein binding is low (11% to 12%).

Metabolism/Excretion – Fluconazole is cleared primarily by renal excretion, with ≈ 80% of the dose appearing in the urine unchanged, ≈ 11% as metabolites. The dose may need to be reduced in patients with impaired renal function. A 3 hour hemodialysis session decreases plasma concentrations by ≈ 50%.

Indications:

Candidiasis:

Treatment – Oropharyngeal and esophageal candidiasis.

Candidal urinary tract infections, peritonitis and systemic candidal infections including candidemia, disseminated candidiasis and pneumonia.

Vaginal candidiasis (vaginal yeast infections due to *Candida*).

Prophylaxis – To decrease the incidence of candidiasis in patients undergoing bone marrow transplantation who receive cytotoxic chemotherapy or radiation therapy.

Cryptococcal meningitis: Treatment of cryptococcal meningitis.

Contraindications:

Hypersensitivity to fluconazole or to any excipients in the product. There is no information regarding cross hypersensitivity between fluconazole and other azole antifungal agents; use with caution in patients with hypersensitivity to other azoles.

Warnings:

Hepatic injury: Fluconazole has been associated with rare cases of serious hepatic toxicity. Instances of fatal hepatic reactions occurred primarily in patients with serious underlying medical conditions (predominantly AIDS or malignancy) and often while taking multiple concomitant medications.

Anaphylaxis: In rare cases, anaphylaxis has occurred.

Dermatologic changes: Patients have rarely developed exfoliative skin disorders during treatment with fluconazole.

Pregnancy: *Category* C.

Lactation: The use of fluconazole in nursing mothers is not recommended.

Children: Efficacy has not been established in children. A small number of patients from age 3 to 13 years have been treated safely with fluconazole using doses of 3 to 6 mg/kg daily. Safety and efficacy of the single-dose regimen for vaginal candidiasis in patients < 18 years of age have not been established.

Precautions:

Single-dose use: Weigh the convenience and efficacy of the single dose regimen for treatment of vaginal yeast infections against the acceptability of a higher incidence of adverse reactions with fluconazole (26%) vs intravaginal agents (16%).

Drug Interactions:

Drugs that may affect fluconazole include cimetidine, hydrochlorothiazide and rifampin. Drugs that may be affected by fluconazole include nonsedating antihistamines, cisapride, oral contraceptives, cyclosporine, phenytoin, theophylline, sulfonylureas, warfarin and zidovudine.

Adverse Reactions:

Adverse reactions occurring in ≥ 3% of patients include: Headache; nausea; abdominal pain; diarrhea.

Administration and Dosage:

Single dose:

Vaginal candidiasis – 150 mg as a single oral dose.

Multiple dose: The daily dose of fluconazole is the same for oral and IV administration. In general, a loading dose of twice the daily dose is recommended on the first day of therapy to result in plasma levels close to steady state by the second day of therapy.

Patients with AIDS and cryptococcal meningitis or recurrent oropharyngeal candidiasis usually require maintenance therapy to prevent relapse.

Adults –

Oropharyngeal candidiasis: 200 mg on the first day, followed by 100 mg once daily. Continue treatment for at least 2 weeks to decrease the likelihood of relapse.

Esophageal candidiasis: 200 mg on the first day, followed by 100 mg once daily. Doses up to 400 mg/day may be used, based on the patient's response. Treat patients with esophageal candidiasis for a minimum of 3 weeks and for at least 2 weeks following resolution of symptoms.

Candidiasis, other: For candidal UTIs and peritonitis, 50 to 200 mg/day has been used. For systemic candidal infections (including candidemia, disseminated candidiasis and pneumonia), optimal dosage and duration have not been determined, although doses up to 400 mg/day have been used.

Prevention of candidiasis in bone marrow transplant: 400 mg once daily. In patients who are anticipated to have severe granulocytopenia (< 500 neutrophils/mm^3), start fluconazole prophylaxis several days before the anticipated onset of neutropenia, and continue for 7 days after the neutrophil count rises above 1000 cells/mm^3.

Cryptococcal meningitis: 400 mg on the first day, followed by 200 mg once daily. A dosage of 400 mg once daily may be used, based on the patient's response to therapy. The duration of treatment for initial therapy of cryptococcal meningitis is 10 to 12 weeks after the cerebrospinal fluid becomes culture negative. The dosage of fluconazole for suppression of relapse of cryptococcal meningitis in patients with AIDS is 200 mg once daily.

Children –

Fluconazole Dosage in Children	
Pediatric Patients	Adults
3 mg/kg	100 mg
6 mg/kg	200 mg
12 mg/kg[1]	400 mg

[1] Some older children may have clearances similar to that of adults. Absolute doses exceeding 600 mg/day are not recommended.

Based on the prolonged half-life seen in premature newborns (gestational age 26 to 29 weeks), these children, in the first 2 weeks of life, should receive the same dosage (mg/kg) as older children, but administered every 72 hours. After the first 2 weeks, dose these children once daily.

Oropharyngeal candidiasis: The recommended dosage is 6 mg/kg on the first day, followed by 3 mg/kg once daily. Administer treatment for at least 2 weeks.

Esophageal candidiasis: The recommended dosage is 6 mg/kg on the first day followed by 3 mg/kg once daily. Doses up to 12 mg/kg/day may be used based on medical judgment of the patient's response to therapy. Treat patients with esophageal candidiasis for a minimum of 3 weeks and for at least 2 weeks following the resolution of symptoms.

Systemic Candida infections: For the treatment of candidemia and disseminated Candida infections, daily doses of 6 to 12 mg/kg/day have been used.

Cryptococcal meningitis: The recommended dosage is 12 mg/kg on the first day, followed by 6 mg/kg once daily. A dosage of 12 mg/kg once daily may be used. The recommended duration of treatment for initial therapy of cryptococcal meningitis is 10 to 12 weeks after the CSF becomes culture negative. For suppression of relapse of cryptococcal meningitis in children with AIDS, the recommended dose is 6 mg/kg once daily.

Renal function impairment: There is no need to adjust single dose therapy for vaginal candidiasis in patients with impaired renal function. In patients with impaired renal function who will receive multiple doses, give an initial loading dose of 50 to 400 mg. After the loading dose, base the daily dose on the following table:

Fluconazole Dose in Impaired Renal Function

Creatinine clearance (ml/min)	Percent of recommended dose
> 50	100%
11-50	50%
Patients receiving regular hemodialysis	One recommended dose after each dialysis

Injection: Fluconazole injection has been used safely for up to 14 days of IV therapy. Administer the IV infusion of fluconazole at a maximum rate of ≈ 200 mg/hr, given as a continuous infusion. Fluconazole injections are intended only for IV administration.

ITRACONAZOLE

Capsules: 100 mg (*Rx*) *Sporanox* (Janssen)

Warning:

Coadministration of terfenadine or cisapride with itraconazole is contraindicated. Serious cardiovascular adverse events, including death, ventricular tachycardia and torsade de pointes have occurred.

Another oral azole antifungal, ketoconazole, inhibits the metabolism of astemizole, resulting in elevated plasma concentrations of astemizole and its active metabolite desmethylastemizole, which may prolong QT intervals.

Actions:

Pharmacology: Itraconazole is a synthetic triazole antifungal agent. In vitro, itraconazole inhibits the cytochrome P-450-dependent synthesis of ergosterol, which is a vital component of fungal cell membranes.

Pharmacokinetics: Itraconazole may undergo saturation metabolism with multiple dosing. Doubling the dose results in ≈ 3-fold increase in the itraconazole plasma concentrations. Itraconazole is extensively metabolized by the liver.

The plasma protein binding of itraconazole is 99.8% and that of hydroxyitraconazole is 99.5%. Itraconazole is not removed by hemodialysis.

Indications:

Antifungal: Treatment of the following fungal infections in immunocompromised and nonimmunocompromised patients:

Blastomycosis (pulmonary and extrapulmonary).

Histoplasmosis (including chronic cavitary pulmonary disease and disseminated, nonmeningeal histoplasmosis).

Aspergillosis (pulmonary and extrapulmonary) in patients who are intolerant of or refractory to amphotericin B therapy.

Onychomycosis due to dermatophytes (tinea unguium) of the toenail with or without fingernail involvement.

Unlabeled uses: Itraconazole appears to be beneficial in the treatment of the following conditions.

Itraconazole Unlabeled Uses		
Superficial mycoses	Systemic mycoses	Miscellaneous
Dermatophytoses	Candidiasis	Subcutaneous mycoses
Tinea capitis	Cryptococcal infections	Sporotrichosis
Tinea corporis	Meningitis	Chromomycosis
Tinea cruris	Disseminated	Leishmaniasis, cutaneous
Tinea pedis	Dimorphic infections	Fungal keratitis
Tinea manuum	Paracoccidioidomycosis	Alternariosis
Pityriasis versicolor	Coccidioidomycosis	Zygomycosis
Sebopsoriasis		
Candidiasis		
Vaginal		
Chronic mucocutaneous		

Contraindications:

Coadministration of terfenadine or astemizole; hypersensitivity to the drug or its excipients (there is no information regarding cross hypersensitivity between itraconazole and other azole antifungal agents; use caution in prescribing to patients with hypersensitivity to other azoles).

Warnings:

Hepatitis: If clinical signs and symptoms consistent with liver disease develop that may be attributable to itraconazole, discontinue the drug.

HIV-infected patients: The response rate of histoplasmosis in HIV-infected patients appears to be similar to non-HIV-infected patients. The clinical course of histoplasmosis in HIV-infected patients is more severe and usually requires maintenance therapy to prevent relapse. Because hypochlorhydria has occurred in HIV-infected individuals, the absorption of itraconazole in these patients may be decreased.

Pregnancy: Category C.

Lactation: Do not administer to a nursing woman.

Children: Safety and efficacy have not been established. A small number of patients from age 3 to 16 years have been treated with 100 mg/day for systemic fungal infections and no serious adverse effects have been reported.

Precautions:

Monitoring: Monitor hepatic enzyme test values in patients with preexisting hepatic function abnormalities. Monitor hepatic enzyme test values periodically in all patients receiving continuous treatment for > 1 month or at any time a patient develops signs or symptoms suggestive of liver dysfunction.

Decreased gastric acidity: Under fasted conditions, itraconazole absorption was decreased in the presence of decreased gastric acidity. The absorption of itraconazole may be decreased with the concomitant administration of antacids or gastric acid secretion suppressors.

Drug Interactions:

Both itraconazole and its major metabolite, hydroxyitraconazole, are inhibitors of the cytochrome P450 3A4 enzyme system. Coadministration of itraconazole and drugs primarily metabolized by the cytochrome P450 3A4 enzyme system may result in increased plasma concentrations of the drugs that could increase or prolong both therapeutic and adverse effects.

Drugs that may affect itraconazole include H_2 antagonists, phenytoin and rifampin. Drugs that may be affected by itraconazole include astemizole, terfenadine, calcium blockers, cyclosporine plus HMG-CoA reductase inhibitors, digoxin, oral midazolam, triazolam, quinidine, sulfonylureas, tacrolimus, warfarin, phenytoin and cisapride.

Drug/Food interactions: Absorption of itraconazole under fasted conditions in individuals with relative or absolute achlorhydria, such as patients with AIDS or volunteers taking gastric acid secretion suppressors (eg, H_2 antagonists), was increased when itraconazole was administered with a cola beverage.

Adverse Reactions:

Adverse reactions occurring in ≥ 3% of patients include: Nausea; vomiting; elevated liver enzymes; GI disorders; diarrhea; edema; hypertension; rash; headache.

Administration and Dosage:

Take with a full meal to ensure maximal absorption.

Blastomycosis/Histoplasmosis: The recommended dose is 200 mg once daily. If there is no obvious improvement or there is evidence of progressive fungal disease, increase the dose in 100 mg increments to a maximum of 400 mg daily. Give doses > 200 mg/day in two divided doses.

Aspergillosis: Recommended daily dose is 200 to 400 mg.

Life-threatening situations: It is recommended that a loading dose of 200 mg 3 times a day (600 mg/day) be given for the first 3 days.

Continue treatment for a minimum of 3 months and until clinical parameters and laboratory tests indicate that the active fungal infection has subsided.

Onychomycosis: Recommended dose is 200 mg once daily for 12 consecutive weeks.

TERBINAFINE HCl

Tablet: 250 mg (*Rx*)	*Lamisil* (Sandoz)

Actions:

Pharmacology: Terbinafine is a synthetic allylamine derivative, which exerts its antifungal effect by inhibiting squalene epoxidase, a key enzyme in sterol biosynthesis in fungi. This action results in a deficiency in ergosterol and a corresponding accumulation of squalene within the fungal cell and causes fungal cell death.

Pharmacokinetics: Terbinafine is well absorbed (> 70%). First-pass metabolism is ≈ 40%. Peak plasma concentrations of 1 mcg/ml appear ≤ 2 hours after a single 250 mg dose, the AUC is ≈ 4.56 mcg•hr/ml. An increase in the AUC of terbinafene of < 20% is observed when terbinafine is taken with food.

In plasma, terbinafine is > 99% bound to plasma proteins. At steady-state, in comparison with a single dose, the peak concentration of terbinafine is 25% higher and plasma AUC increases by a factor of 2.5; the increase in plasma AUC is consistent with an effective half-life of ≈ 36 hours.

Prior to excretion, terbinafine is extensively metabolized. No metabolites have been identified that have antifungal activity similar to terbinafine. Approximately 70% of the administered dose is eliminated in the urine.

Microbiology: Terbinafine is active against most strains of the following organisms both in vitro and in clinical infections: *Trichophyton mentagrophytes; Trichophyton rubrum.* Terbinafine exceeds in vitro MICs against most strains of the following organisms which can infect the nail; however, safety and efficacy of terbinafine in treating nail infections due to these organisma have not been established: *Microsporum gypseum and nanum; Trichophyton verrucosum; Epidermophyton floccosum; Candida albicans; Scopulariopsis brevicaulis.*

Indications:

Onychomycosis: Treatment of onychomycosis of the toenail or fingernail due to dermatopytes.

Contraindications:

Hypersensitivity to terbinafine or any component of the product; pre-existing liver disease or renal impairment (creatinine clearance ≤ 50 ml/min).

Warnings:

Ophthalmic: Changes in the ocular lens and retina have been reported following the use of terbinafine.

Neutropenia: Isolated cases of severe neutropenia have been reported but were reversible with discontinuation of treatment with or without supportive therapy. If the neutrophil count is ≤ 1000 cells/mm^3, discontinue treatment and start supportive management.

Dermatologic: There have been isolated reports of serious skin reactions (eg, Stevens-Johnson syndrome and toxic epidermal necrolysis).

Renal/Hepatic function impairment: In patients with renal impairment (creatinine clearance ≤ 50 ml/min) or hepatic cirrhosis, the clearance of terbinafine is decreased by ≈ 50%.

Pregnancy: Category B.

Lactation: After oral administration, terbinafine is present in the breast milk of nursing mothers. Treatment with terbinafine tablets is not recommended in nursing mothers.

Children: Safety and efficacy in children have not been established.

Precautions:

Monitoring:

Immunodeficiency – Monitor CBC in patients receiving treatment for > 6 weeks.

Hepatic – Monitor hepatic function (hepatic enzyme) test in patients administered terbinafine for > 6 weeks.

Symptomatic hepatobiliary dysfunction: If hepatobiliary dysfunction or cholestatic hepatitis develops, discontinue treatment.

Drug Interactions:

Drugs that may interact with terbinafine include cimetidine, rifampin, terfenadine, caffeine and cyclosporine.

Adverse Reactions:

Adverse reactions occurring in ≥ 3% of patients include diarrhea, dyspepsia, rash, liver enzyme abnormalities and headache.

Lab test abnormalities: Decreases in absolute lymphocyte counts.

Administration and Dosage:

Onychomycosis:

Fingernail – 250 mg/day for 6 weeks.

Toenail – 250 mg/day for 12 weeks.

The optimal clinical effect is seen some months after mycological cure and cessation of treatment. This is related to the period required for outgrowth of healthy nail.

SULFONAMIDES

SULFADIAZINE	
Tablets: 500 mg (*Rx*)	Various, *Sulfadiazine* (Stanley)
SULFISOXAZOLE	
Tablets: 500 mg (*Rx*)	Various, *Gantrisin* (Roche)
SULFAMETHOXAZOLE	
Tablets: 500 mg (*Rx*)	Various, *Gantanol* (Roche), *Urobak* (Shionogi)
Oral Suspension: 500 mg per 5 ml (*Rx*)	*Gantanol* (Roche)
SULFAMETHIZOLE	
Tablets: 500 mg (*Rx*)	*Thiosulfil Forte* (Wyeth-Ayerst)
SULFASALAZINE	
Tablets: 500 mg (*Rx*)	Various, *Azulfidine* (Pharmacia)
Tablets, enteric coated: 500 mg (*Rx*)	Various, *Azulfidine EN-tabs* (Pharmacia)

Actions:

Pharmacology: Sulfonamides exert their bacteriostatic action by competitive antagonism of para-aminobenzoic acid (PABA), an essential component in folic acid synthesis.

Pharmacokinetics:

Absorption/Distribution – The oral sulfonamides are readily absorbed from the GI tract. Approximately 70% to 100% of an oral dose is absorbed. Sulfonamides are bound to plasma proteins in varying degrees.

Metabolism – Metabolism occurs in the liver by conjugation, acetylation and other metabolic pathways to inactive metabolites.

Excretion – Renal excretion is mainly by glomerular filtration; tubular reabsorption occurs in varying degrees.

Microbiology: Sulfonamides have a broad antibacterial spectrum which includes both gram-positive and gram-negative organisms.

Indications:

Sulfonamide Indications

✓ – Labeled Indications	Multiple Sulfas	Sulfadiazine	Sulfamethizole	Sulfamethoxazole	Sulfasalazine	Sulfisoxazole
Chancroid	✓	✓		✓		✓
Colitis, ulcerative					✓	
Inclusion conjunctivitis	✓	✓		✓		✓
Malaria[1]	✓	✓		✓		✓
Meningitis, *H influenzae*[2]	✓	✓				✓
Meningitis, meningococcal[3]	✓	✓		✓		✓
Nocardiosis	✓	✓		✓		✓
Otitis media, acute[4]	✓	✓		✓		✓
Rheumatic fever		✓				
Toxoplasmosis[5]	✓	✓		✓		✓
Trachoma	✓	✓		✓		✓
Urinary tract infections[6] (pyelonephritis, cystitis)	✓	✓	✓	✓		✓

[1] As adjunctive therapy due to chloroquine-resistant strains of *P falciparum*.
[2] As adjunctive therapy with parenteral streptomycin.
[3] When the organism is susceptible and for prophylaxis when sulfonamide-sensitive group A strains prevail.
[4] Due to *H influenzae* when used with penicillin or erythromycin.
[5] As adjunctive therapy with pyrimethamine.
[6] In the absence of obstructive uropathy or foreign bodies, when caused by *E coli*, *Klebsiella-Enterobacter*, *S aureus*, *P mirabilis* and *P vulgaris*.

Unlabeled uses: Sulfasalazine may be beneficial in the following: Ankylosing spondylitis; collagenous colitis; Crohn's disease; rheumatoid arthritis. Sulfisoxazole may be useful for recurrent otitis media.

Contraindications:

Hypersensitivity to sulfonamides or chemically related drugs (eg, sulfonylureas, thiazide and loop diuretics, carbonic anhydrase inhibitors, sunscreens with PABA, local anesthetics); pregnancy at term; lactation; infants < 2 months old (except in congenital toxoplasmosis as adjunct with pyrimethamine); porphyria; salicylate hypersensitivity; intestinal/urinary obstruction (**sulfasalazine**).

Warnings:

Group A beta-hemolytic streptococcal infections: Do not use for treatment of these infections.

Severe reactions including deaths due to sulfonamides have been associated with hypersensitivity reactions, agranulocytosis, aplastic anemia, other blood dyscrasias and renal and hepatic damage. Irreversible neuromuscular and CNS changes and fibrosing alveolitis may occur.

Porphyria: In patients with porphyria, these drugs have precipitated an acute attack.

Photosensitivity: Photosensitization (photoallergy or phototoxicity) may occur.

Renal/Hepatic function impairment: Use with caution. The frequency of renal complications is considerably lower in patients receiving the more soluble sulfonamides (sulfisoxazole and sulfamethizole).

Fertility impairment: Oligospermia and infertility have been described in men treated with **sulfasalazine**.

Pregnancy: Category B; Category D near term. Significant levels may persist in the neonate if these drugs are given near term; jaundice, hemolytic anemia and kernicterus may occur. Do not use at term.

Lactation: According to the American Academy of Pediatrics, breast feeding and sulfonamide use are compatible. However, do not nurse premature infants or those with hyperbilirubinemia or G–6–PD deficiency.

Children: Do not use in infants < 2 months old (except for congenital toxoplasmosis as adjunctive therapy with pyrimethamine). **Sulfacytine** is not recommended for children < 14 years.

Precautions:

Allergy or asthma: Give with caution to patients with severe allergy or bronchial asthma.

Hemolytic anemia, frequently dose-related, may occur in G-6-PD deficient individuals.

Drug Interactions:

Drugs that may interact with sulfonamides include anticoagulants, oral, cyclosporine, hydantoins, methotrexate and sulfonylureas.

Drugs that may interact with sulfisoxazole include barbiturate anesthetics.

Drugs that may interact with sulfasalazine include folic acid.

Drug/Lab test interactions: Sulfonamides may produce false-positive **urinary glucose tests** when performed by Benedict's method. Sulfisoxazole may interfere with the **Urobilistix test** and may produce false-positive results with sulfosalicylic acid tests for urinary protein.

Adverse Reactions:

Agranulocytosis; aplastic anemia; thrombocytopenia; leukopenia; hemolytic anemia; purpura; hypoprothrombinemia; cyanosis; methemoglobinemia; megaloblastic (macrocytic) anemia; Stevens-Johnson type erythema multiforme; generalized skin eruptions; epidermal necrolysis; urticaria; serum sickness; pruritus; exfoliative dermatitis; anaphylactoid reactions; periorbital edema; nausea; emesis; abdominal pains; diarrhea; bloody diarrhea; anorexia; pancreatitis; stomatitis; hepatitis; pseudomembranous enterocolitis; glossitis; headache; peripheral neuropathy; mental depression; convulsions; ataxia; hallucinations; tinnitus; vertigo; insomnia; hearing loss; drowsiness; apathy; crystalluria; hematuria; proteinuria; elevated creatinine; drug fever; chills; pyrexia; alopecia; arthralgia; myalgia.

Administration and Dosage:

CDC recommended treatment schedules for sexually transmitted diseases:

Lymphogranuloma venereum – As an alternative regimen to doxycycline, sulfisoxazole 500 mg 4 times a day for 21 days or equivalent sulfonamide course.

Treatment of uncomplicated urethral, endocervical or rectal Chlamydia trachomatic infections – As an alternative regimen to doxycycline or tetracycline (or if erythromycin is not tolerated), sulfisoxazole 500 mg 4 times a day for 10 days or equivalent sulfonamide course.

SULFADIAZINE:

Adults – *Loading dose* - 2 to 4 g. *Maintenance dose* - 4 to 8 g/day in 4 to 6 divided doses.

Children (> 2 months) – *Loading dose* - 75 mg/kg (or 2 g/m^2). *Maintenance dose* - 120 to 150 mg/kg/day (4 g/m^2/day) in 4 to 6 divided doses. *Maximum dose* - 6 g/day.

Infants (< 2 months) – Contraindicated, except as adjunctive therapy with pyrimehtamine in the treatment of congenital toxoplasmosis. *Loading dose* - 75 to 100 mg/kg. *Maintenance dose* - 100 to 150 mg/kg/day in 4 divided doses.

Other recommended doses for toxoplasmosis (for 3 to 4 weeks) include – *Infants (< 2 months)* - 25 mg/kg/dose 4 times daily. *Children (> 2 months)* - 25 to 50 mg/kg/dose 4 times daily.

Prevention of recurrent attacks of rheumatic fever (not for initial treatment of streptococcal infections): Patients > 30 kg (> 66 lbs) - 1 g/day; < 30 kg (< 66 lbs) - 0.5 g/day.

SULFISOXAZOLE:

Loading dose – 2 to 4 g. *Maintenance dose* - 4 to 8 g/day in 4 to 6 divided doses. Although recommended, a loading dose is unnecessary because sulfisoxazole is rapidly absorbed and appears in high concentrations in the urine.

Children and infants (> 2 months) – *Initial dose* - 75 mg/kg. *Maintenance dose* - 120 to 150 mg/kg/day (4 g/m^2/day) in 4 to 6 divided doses (max, 6 g/day).

SULFAMETHOXAZOLE:

Adults – *Mild to moderate infections* - 2 g initially; maintenance dose is 1 g morning and evening therafter. *Severe infections* - 2 g initially, then 1 g 3 times daily.

Children and infants (> 2 months) – Initially, 50 to 60 mg/kg; maintenance dose is 25 to 30 mg/kg morning and evening. Do not exceed 75 mg/kg/day.

Another recommended dose is 50 to 60 mg/kg/day divided every 12 hours, not to exceed 3 g/24 hours.

SULFAMETHIZOLE:

Adults – 0.5 to 1 g 3 or 4 times daily.

Children and infants (> 2 months) – 30 to 45 mg/kg/day in 4 divided doses.

MULTIPLE SULFONAMIDES (Trisulfapyrimidines):

Adults – 2 to 4 g initially, then 2 to 4 g daily in 3 to 6 dividded doses. *Children or infants (> 2 months)* - 75 mg/kg initially, then 120 to 150 mg/kg/day (4 g/m^2/day) in 4 to 6 divided doses. Do not exceed 6 g daily.

Recommended doses for toxoplasmosis (with pyrimethamine) for 3 to 4 wks:

Infants: 100 mg/kg/day divided 4 times; *children* - 25 to 50 mg/kg 4 times/day.

SULFASALAZINE: Intervals between nighttime doses should not exceed 8 hours. Administer after meals. Doses of ≥ 4 g/day tend to increase adverse reactions.

Initial therapy – *Adults* - 3 to 4 g/day in evenly divided doses; however, initial doses of 1 to 2 g/day may lessen adverse GI effects. Doses of ≥ 4 g/day increase the risk of toxicity. *Children (≥ 2 years old)* - 40 to 60 mg/kg/24 hours in 4 to 6 divided doses.

Maintenance therapy – *Adults* - 2 g/day (500 mg 4 times daily). *Children* - 20 to 30 mg/kg/day, in 4 divided doses, maximum 2 g/day.

ANTITUBERCULOUS DRUGS

Antituberculous drugs are categorized as primary and retreatment agents, indicating their approximate place and usefulness in treatment of tuberculosis. The foundation of treatment should include the primary agents, most of which are bactericidal (ie, destructive to mycobacteria) and are necessary for sterilization of the tuberculous lesions.

The retreatment agents are generally less effective or more toxic than the primary group. A number of these agents are bacteriostatic (ie, inhibit the growth or multiplication of mycobacteria). They are indicated for use in combination with the primary drugs for partial or complete drug-resistant organisms or to treat extrapulmonary tuberculosis.

Antituberculosis Drugs

Drugs	Activity	Route	Pediatric Daily Dose (mg/kg)	Adult Daily Dose (mg/kg/day)	Usual Adult Daily Dose	Max. Daily Dose (Children & Adults)	Toxicity
Primary Agents							
Isoniazid[1]	Bactericidal	oral	10-20 (20-40 twice weekly)	5-10 once daily (15 mg/kg twice weekly)	300 mg	300 mg (900 mg twice wkly)	Hepatic Neurologic
Rifampin	Bactericidal	oral	10-20 (10-20 twice weekly)	10 once daily (10 mg/kg twice weekly)	600 mg	600 mg	Hepatic Hematologic
Ethambutol[2]	Bacteriostatic	oral	15-25 (50 twice weekly)	15-25 once daily (50 twice weekly)	800-1600 mg	2.5 g	Optic neuritis
Pyrazinamide[2]	Bactericidal	oral	15-30 (50-70 twice weekly)	15-30 once daily (50-70 twice weekly)	1-2 g	2 g	Hepatic Hyperuricemia
Streptomycin[2]	Bactericidal	IM	20-40 (25-30 twice weekly)	7-15 once daily (25-30 twice weekly)	0.75-1 g	1 g (750 mg > 60 yrs)	Eighth nerve Renal
Retreatment Agents							
P–aminosalicylic acid	Bacteriostatic	oral	150-200	200, 4 equal doses 6–hourly	12-16 g	12 g	GI intolerance
Ethionamide	Bacteriostatic	oral	15-20	7-15, 4 equal doses 6–hourly	0.75-1 g	1 g	GI intolerance Hepatic
Cycloserine	Bacteriostatic	oral	10-20	10-15, 4 equal doses 6–hourly	0.75-1 g	1 g	Psychoses Seizures
Capreomycin	Bactericidal	IM	15	15 once daily	1 g	1 g	Eighth nerve Renal
Kanamycin	Bactericidal	IM	7.5-15	15 once daily	0.5-1 g	1 g	Eighth nerve Renal

[1] Always include in retreatment regimen if susceptibility remains.
[2] May use as primary or retreatment.

ISONIAZID (Isonicotinic acid hydrazide; INH)

Tablets: 50, 100 and 300 mg (*Rx*)	Various, *Laniazid* C.T. (Lannett)
Syrup: 50 mg per 5 ml (*Rx*)	Various, *Laniazid* (Lannett)
Injection: 100 mg per ml (*Rx*)	Various, *Nydrazid* (Apothecon)

Warning:

Severe and sometimes fatal hepatitis associated with isoniazid therapy may occur or develop even after many months of treatment. The risk of developing hepatitis is age-related. Risk of hepatitis increases with daily alcohol consumption.

Carefully monitor and interview patients at monthly intervals. Serum transaminase concentration becomes elevated in about 10% to 20% of patients, usually during the first few months of therapy but can occur at any time. Enzyme levels generally return to normal despite continuance of the drug, but in some cases, progressive liver dysfunction occurs. If signs suggestive of hepatic damage are detected, discontinue isoniazid promptly since continued use of the drug in such cases may cause a more severe form of liver damage.

Reinstitute isoniazid after symptoms and laboratory abnormalities have become normal. Restart the drug in very small doses; gradually increase doses and withdraw immediately if there is any indication of recurrent liver involvement.

Defer preventive treatment in persons with acute hepatic diseases.

Actions:

Pharmacology: Isoniazid (INH) acts against actively growing tubercle bacilli. It is bactericidal and interferes with lipid and nucleic acid biosynthesis in growing organisms.

Pyridoxine (vitamin B_6) deficiency is sometimes observed in adults taking high doses of INH, and is probably due to the drug's competition with pyridoxal phosphate for the enzyme apotryptophanase.

Pharmacokinetics:

Absorption – INH is rapidly and completely absorbed orally and parenterally and produces peak blood levels within 1 to 2 hours.

Metabolism – The half-life of INH is widely variable and dependent on acetylator status. Isoniazid is primarily acetylated by the liver; this process is genetically controlled. Fast acetylators metabolize the drug about 5 to 6 times faster than slow acetylators. Several minor metabolites have been identified, one or more of which may be "reactive" (monoacetylhydrazine is suspected), and responsible for liver damage. The rate of acetylation does not significantly alter the effectiveness of INH. However, slow acetylation may lead to higher blood levels of the drug, and thus to an increase in toxic reactions. Rapid acetylators may be more likely to develop hepatitis, since hepatotoxicity is caused by the acetylated metabolite of INH; however, this remains controversial.

Excretion – Approximately 50% to 70% of a dose of isoniazid is excreted as unchanged drug and metabolites by the kidneys in 24 hours. Elimination is largely independent of renal function.

Indications:

Used for all forms of tuberculosis in which organisms are susceptible.

Also recommended as preventive therapy (chemoprophylaxis) for specific situations.

IM administration is intended for use whenever oral is not possible.

Unlabeled uses: Isoniazid may improve severe tremor in patients with MS.

Contraindications:

Patients with previous isoniazid-associated hepatic injury or other severe adverse reactions.

Warnings:

Hypersensitivity: Stop all drugs and evaluate at the first sign of a hypersensitivity reaction.

Renal/Hepatic function impairment: Monitor patients with active chronic liver disease or severe renal dysfunction.

Carcinogenesis: Isoniazid induces pulmonary tumors in a number of strains of mice.

Pregnancy: Prescribe during pregnancy only when therapeutically necessary.

Lactation: Since isoniazid appears in breast milk, observe breastfed infants of isoniazid-treated mothers for any evidence of adverse effects.

Precautions:

Periodic ophthalmologic examinations during isoniazid therapy are recommended even when visual symptoms do not occur.

Pyridoxine administration is recommended in individuals likely to develop peripheral neuropathies secondary to INH therapy. Prophylactic doses of 6 to 50 mg of pyridoxine daily have been recommended.

Drug Interactions:

Drugs that may interact with isoniazid include alcohol, aluminum salts, oral anticoagulants, benzodiazepines, carbamazepine, cycloserine, disulfiram, enflurane, halothane, hydantoins, ketoconazole, meperidine and rifampin.

Drug/Food interactions: Rate and extent of INH absorption is decreased by food.

Adverse Reactions:

Toxic effects are usually encountered with higher doses of isoniazid; the most frequent are those affecting the nervous system and the liver.

Adverse reactions include pyridoxine deficiency; hyperglycemia; gynecomastia; peripheral neuropathy; convulsions; optic neuritis and atrophy; memory impairment; toxic psychosis; nausea; vomiting; epigastric distress; elevated AST, ALT; bilirubinemia; jaundice; anorexia; fatigue; malaise; weakness; agranulocytosis; hemolytic, sideroblastic or aplastic anemia; thrombocytopenia; eosinophilia; fever; skin eruptions; lymphadenopathy; vasculitis.

Administration and Dosage:

Treatment of tuberculosis: Use in conjunction with other effective antituberculosis agents.

Adults – 5 mg/kg/day (up to 300 mg total) in a single dose.

Infants and children – 10 to 20 mg/kg/day (300 mg total) in a single dose, depending on the severity of infection.

Preventive treatment:

Adults – 300 mg/day in a single dose.

Infants and children – 10 mg/kg/day (up to 300 mg total) in a single dose.

RIFAMPIN

Capsules: 150 and 300 mg (*Rx*)	*Rifadin* (Hoechst-Marion Roussel), *Rimactane* (Ciba)
Powder for Injection: 600 mg (*Rx*)	*Rifadin* (Hoechst-Marion Roussel)

Actions:

Pharmacology: Rifampin inhibits DNA-dependent RNA polymerase activity in susceptible cells. Specifically, it interacts with bacterial RNA polymerase, but does not inhibit the mammalian enzyme. Cross-resistance has only been shown with other rifamycins.

Pharmacokinetics:

Oral –

Absorption/Distribution: Rifampin is almost completely absorbed and achieves mean peak plasma levels within 1 to 4 hours. It is 80% protein bound but very lipid soluble; it penetrates and concentrates in many body tissues.

Metabolism: Rifampin is metabolized in the liver by deacetylation; the metabolite is still active against *Mycobacterium tuberculosis*. About 40% is excreted in bile and undergoes enterohepatic circulation; however, the deacetylated metabolite is poorly absorbed. The half-life is ≈ 3 hours after a 600 mg oral dose, up to 5.1 after a 900 mg oral dose. With repeated administration, the half-life decreases and averages ≈ 2 to 3 hours.

Excretion: 6% to 30% of rifampin is excreted in the urine; 30% to 60% in the deacetylated form, approximately 50% unchanged.

Indications:

Tuberculosis:

Oral – Treatment of all forms of tuberculosis in conjunction with at least one other antituberculous drug.

IV – Initial treatment and retreatment of tuberculosis when the drug cannot be taken by mouth.

Neisseria meningitidis carriers: Treatment of asymptomatic carriers of *N meningitidis* to eliminate meningococci from the nasopharynx. Not indicated for treatment of meningococcal infection.

Unlabeled uses: Rifampin has a broad antibacterial spectrum. Some uses showing promise with a reasonable amount of human data include: Infections caused by *Staphylococcus aureus* and *S epidermidis* (eg, endocarditis, osteomyelitis, prostatitis), usually in combination with other effective drugs; gram-negative bacteremia in infancy; Legionella (*Legionella pneumophilia*) when not responsive to erythromycin; leprosy (in combination with dapsone); prophylaxis of meningitis due to *Haemophilus influenzae*.

Contraindications:

Hypersensitivity to any rifamycin.

Warnings:

Hepatotoxicity: There have been fatalities associated with jaundice in patients with liver disease or patients receiving rifampin concomitantly with other hepatotoxic agents. Carefully monitor liver function, especially AST and ALT, prior to therapy and then every 2 to 4 weeks during therapy.

Hyperbilirubinemia, resulting from competition between rifampin and bilirubin for excretory pathways of the liver at the cell level, can occur in the early days of treatment.

Porphyria: Isolated reports have associated porphyria exacerbation with rifampin administration.

Meningococci resistance: The possibility of rapid emergence of resistant meningococci restricts use to short-term treatment of asymptomatic carrier state. Not for treatment of meningococcal disease.

Hypersensitivity reactions have occurred during intermittent therapy or when treatment was resumed following accidental or intentional interruption and were reversible with rifampin discontinuation and appropriate therapy.

Hepatic function impairment: Dosage adjustment is necessary.

Pregnancy: Category C.

Lactation: Rifampin is excreted in breast milk with a milk/plasma ratio of 0.2 to 0.6.

Precautions:

Monitoring: Obtain a complete blood count prior to instituting therapy and periodically throughout the course of therapy.

Intermittent therapy may be used if the patient cannot or will not self-administer drugs on a daily basis.

Urine, feces, saliva, sputum, sweat and tears may be colored red-orange. Soft contact lenses may be permanently stained. Advise patients of these possibilities. Rifampin may impart a yellow color to cerebrospinal fluid.

IV: For IV infusion only. Must not be administered by IM or SC route.

Thrombocytopenia has occurred, primarily with high dose intermittent therapy, but has also been noted after resumption of interrupted treatment. Cerebral hemorrhage and fatalities have occurred when rifampin administration has continued or resumed after appearance of purpura.

Drug Interactions:

Rifampin is known to induce the hepatic microsomal enzymes that metabolize various drugs such as acetaminophen, oral anticoagulants, barbiturates, benzodiazepines, beta-blockers, chloramphenicol, clofibrate, oral contraceptives, corticosteroids, cyclosporine, digitoxin, disopyramide, estrogens, hydantoins, methadone, mexiletine, quinidine, sulfones, sulfonylureas, theophyllines, tocainide and verapamil, digoxin, enalapril and ketoconazole. The therapeutic effects of these drugs may be decreased.

Drug/Lab test interactions: Therapeutic levels of rifampin inhibit standard assays for serum **folate** and **vitamin B_{12}**.

Transient abnormalities in liver function tests (eg, elevation in serum bilirubin, abnormal bromsulphalein [BSP] excretion, alkaline phosphatase and serum transaminases), and reduced biliary excretion of contrast media used for visualization of the gallbladder have also been observed.

Drug/Food interactions: Food interferes with the absorption of rifampin, possibly resulting in decreased peak plasma concentrations. Take on an empty stomach.

Adverse Reactions:

Adverse reactions may include: "flu-like" syndrome, hematopoietic reactions, cutaneous, GI and hepatic reactions, shortness of breath, shock, renl failure; asymptomatic elevations of liver enzymes (≤ 14 %); rash (1% to 5%).

Administration and Dosage:

Oral: Administer once daily, either 1 hour before or 2 hours after meals.

Data is not available to determine dosage for children < 5 years of age.

Oral and IV:

Tuberculosis: Adults – 600 mg once daily.

Children – 10 to 20 mg/kg, not to exceed 600 mg/day.

In patients who cannot be relied upon for compliance, intermittent therapy with 600 mg/day 2 or 3 times per week under close supervision may be prescribed and substituted for the daily regimen after 1 to 2 months of an initial daily phase of therapy.

The 6 month regimen ordinarily consists of an initial 2 month phase of rifampin, isoniazid and pyrazinamide and, if clinically indicated, streptomycin or ethambutol, followed by 4 months of rifampin and isoniazid.

The 9 month regimen ordinarily consists of rifampin and isoniazid, usually supplemented during the initial phase by pyrazinamide, streptomycin or ethambutol.

Either of the above regimens is recommended as standard therapy.

Meningococcal carriers: Once daily for 4 consecutive days in the following doses:

Adults – 600 mg.

Children – 10 to 20 mg/kg, not to exceed 600 mg/day.

The following dosage has also been recommended –

Adults: 600 mg every 12 hours for 2 days; *children (≥ 1 month of age)* – 10 mg/kg every 12 hours for 2 days; *children (< 1 month of age)* – 5 mg/kg every 12 hours for 2 days.

RIFABUTIN

Capsules: 150 mg (*Rx*)	*Mycobutin* (Adria)

Actions:

Pharmacology: Rifabutin, an antimycobacterial agent, is a semisynthetic ansamycin antibiotic derived from rifamycin S. Rifabutin inhibits DNA-dependent RNA polymerase in susceptible strains of *Escherichia coli* and *Bacillus subtilis* but not in mammalian cells. In resistant strains of *E coli*, rifabutin, like rifampin, did not inhibit this enzyme. It is not known whether rifabutin inhibits DNA-dependent RNA polymerase in *Mycobacterium avium* or in M. *intracellulare* which comprise M. *avium* complex (MAC).

Pharmacokinetics: Following a single oral dose of 300 mg to healthy adult volunteers, rifabutin was readily absorbed from the GI tract with mean peak plasma levels (C_{max}) of 375 ng/ml attained in 3.3 hours. Plasma concentrations post-C_{max} declined in an apparent biphasic manner. Kinetic dose-proportionality has been established over the 300 to 600 mg dose range in healthy adult volunteers and in early symptomatic HIV-positive patients over a 300 to 900 mg dose range. Rifabutin was slowly eliminated from plasma in healthy adult volunteers, presumably because of distribution-limited elimination, with a mean terminal half-life of 45 hours. Although the systemic levels of rifabutin following multiple dosing decreased by 38%, its terminal half-life remained unchanged. Estimates of apparent steady-state distribution volume (9.3 L/kg) in HIV-positive patients, following IV dosing, exceed total body water by ≈ 15-fold. About 85% of the drug is bound in a concentration-independent manner to plasma proteins over a concentration range of 0.05 to 1 mcg/ml.

Mean systemic clearance in healthy adult volunteers following a single oral dose was 0.69 L/hr/kg; renal and biliary clearance of unchanged drug each contribute ≈ 5%. About 30% of the dose is excreted in the feces; 53% of the oral dose is excreted in the urine, primarily as metabolites. Of the five metabolites that have been identified, 25-O-desacetyl and 31-hydroxy are the most predominant, and show a plasma metabolite:parent AUC ratio of 0.1 and 0.07, respectively. The 25-O-desacetyl metabolite has an activity equal to the parent drug and contributes ≤ 10% to the total antimicrobial activity.

Absolute bioavailability assessed in HIV-positive patients averaged 20%. At least 53% of the orally administered dose is absorbed from the GI tract. High-fat meals slow the rate without influencing the extent of absorption. The overall pharmacokinetics are modified only slightly by alterations in hepatic function or age. Compared to healthy volunteers, steady-state kinetics are more variable in elderly patients (> 70 years of age) and in symptomatic HIV-positive patients. Somewhat reduced drug distribution and faster drug elimination in compromised renal function may result in decreased drug concentrations.

Indications:

Prevention of disseminated MAC disease in patients with advanced HIV infection.

Contraindications:

Hypersensitivity to this drug or to any other rifamycins.

Warnings:

Active tuberculosis: Rifabutin prophylaxis must not be administered to patients with active tuberculosis. Patients are likely to have a nonreactive purified protein derivative (PPD) despite active disease. Chest X-ray, sputum culture, blood culture, urine culture or biopsy of a suspicious lymph node may be useful in the diagnosis of tuberculosis of tuberculosis in the HIV-positive patient.

Immediately evaluate patients who develop complaints consistent with active tuberculosis while on rifabutin prophylaxis, so that those with active disease may be given an effective combination regimen of antituberculosis medications.

There is no evidence that rifabutin is effective prophylaxis against M *tuberculosis*. Patients requiring prophylaxis against both M *tuberculosis* and M *avium* complex may be given isoniazid and rifabutin concurrently.

Pregnancy: Category B.

Lactation: It is not known whether rifabutin is excreted in breast milk. Because of the potential for serious adverse reactions in nursing infants, decide whether to discontinue nursing or discontinue the drug, taking into account the importance of the drug to the mother.

Children: Safety and efficacy in children have not been established. Limited safety data are available from treatment use in 22 HIV-positive children with MAC who received rifabutin in combination with at least two other antimycobacterials for periods from 1 to 183 weeks. Mean doses (mg/kg) for these children were: 18.5 for infants 1 year of age; 8.6 for children 2 to 10 years of age; and 4 for adolescents 14 to 16 years of age. There is no evidence that doses > 5 mg/kg/day are useful.

Precautions:

Monitoring: Because rifabutin may be associated with neutropenia, and more rarely thrombocytopenia, consider obtaining hematologic studies periodically in patients receiving prophylaxis.

Drug Interactions:

Drugs that may interact with rifabutin include zidovudine and didanosine.

Drug/Food interactions: High-fat meals slow the rate of absorption without influencing the extent. Rifabutin doses may be mixed with foods such as applesauce.

Adverse Reactions:

Rifabutin is generally well tolerated. Discontinuation of therapy due to an adverse event was required in 16% of patients receiving rifabutin vs 8% with placebo.

Adverse reactions occurring in ≥ 3% of patients include: Abdominal pain, headache, diarrhea, dyspepsia, eructation, nausea, vomiting, rash, taste perversion, discolored urine, increased AST and ALT, anemia, leukopenia, neutropenia and thrombocytopenia.

Administration and Dosage:

Usual dose: 300 mg once daily. For those patients with propensity to nausea, vomiting or other GI upset, administration of rifabutin at doses of 150 mg twice daily taken with food may be useful.

ETHAMBUTOL HCl

Tablets: 100 and 400 mg (*Rx*)	*Myambutol* (Lederle)

Actions:

Pharmacology: Ethambutol diffuses into actively growing mycobacterium cells such as tubercle bacilli. It inhibits the synthesis of one or more metabolites, thus causing impairment of cell metabolism, arrest of multiplication, and cell death. No cross-resistance with other agents has been demonstrated.

Pharmacokinetics:

Absorption/Distribution – Ethambutol absorption is not influenced by food. Following a single oral dose of 15 to 25 mg/kg, ethambutol attains a peak of 2 to 5 mcg/ml in serum 2 to 4 hours after administration. Serum levels are similar after prolonged dosing. The serum level is undetectable 24 hours after the last dose except in some patients with abnormal renal function. Cerebrospinal fluid concentrations may attain 10% to 50% of simultaneous serum concentrations in the presence of meningeal inflammation.

Metabolism – During the 24 hours following oral administration, about 20% of ethambutol is metabolized by the liver.

Excretion – Unchanged drug is excreted (≈ 50%) in the urine, 8% to 15% as metabolites and 20% to 25% unchanged in the feces. Marked accumulation may occur with renal insufficiency.

Indications:

Pulmonary tuberculosis: Use in conjunction with at least one other antituberculous drug.

In patients who have received previous therapy, mycobacterial resistance to other drugs used in initial therapy is frequent. In retreatment patients, combine ethambutol with at least one of the second-line drugs not previously administered to the patient, and to which bacterial susceptibility has been indicated.

Contraindications:

Hypersensitivity to ethambutol; known optic neuritis, unless clinical judgment determines that it may be used.

Warnings:

Renal function impairment: Patients with decreased renal function require reduced dosage (as determined by serum levels) since this drug is excreted by the kidneys.

Pregnancy: Category B.

Children: Not recommended for use in children < 13 years of age.

Precautions:

Monitoring: Perform periodic assessment of renal, hepatic and hematopoietic systems during long-term therapy.

Visual effects: This drug may have adverse effects on vision. The effects are generally reversible when the drug is discontinued promptly. In rare cases, recovery may be delayed for up to 1 year or more, and the effect may possibly be irreversible. Patients have then received the drug again without recurrence of loss of visual acuity. Acuity changes may be unilateral or bilateral; therefore, each eye must be tested separately and both eyes tested together. Perform testing before beginning therapy and periodically during drug administration (monthly when a patient is receiving > 15 mg/kg/day).

Advise patients to report promptly any change in visual acuity. Changes in color perception are probably the first signs of toxicity. If evaluation confirms visual change and fails to reveal other causes, discontinue drug and reevaluate patient at frequent intervals.

Patients developing visual abnormality during treatment may show subjective visual symptoms before, or simultaneously with, the demonstration of decreases in visual acuity; periodically question all patients receiving ethambutol about blurred vision and other subjective eye symptoms.

Drug Interactions:

Aluminum salts may delay and reduce the absorption of ethambutol. Separate their administration by several hours.

Adverse Reactions:

Adverse reactons may include: Anaphylactoid reactions, dermatitis, pruritus, decreases in visual acuity, anorexia, nausea, vomiting, GI upset, abdominal pain, fever, malaise, headache, dizziness, mental confusion, disorientation, possible hallucinations, peripheral neuritis, elevated serum uric acid levels, precipitation of acute gout, transient impairment of liver function, toxic epidermal necrolysis, thrombocytopenia, joint pain.

Administration and Dosage:

Do not use ethambutol alone. Administer once every 24 hours only. Absorption is not significantly altered by administration with food. Continue therapy until bacteriological conversion has become permanent and maximal clinical improvement has occurred.

Initial treatment: In patients who have not received previous antituberculous therapy, administer 15 mg/kg (7 mg/lb) as a single oral dose once every 24 hours. Isoniazid has been administered concurrently in a single, daily oral dose.

Retreatment: In patients who have received previous antituberculous therapy, administer 25 mg/kg (11 mg/lb) as a single oral dose once every 24 hours. Concurrently administer at least one other antituberculous drug to which the organisms have been demonstrated to be susceptible by in vitro tests. Suitable drugs usually include those not previously used in the treatment of the patient. After 60 days of administration, decrease the dose to 15 mg/kg and administer as a single oral dose once every 24 hours.

PYRAZINAMIDE

Tablets: 500 mg (*Rx*)	*Pyrazinamide* (Lederle)

Actions:

Pharmacology: Pyrazinamide, the pyrazine analog of nicotinamide, may be bacteriostatic or bactericidal against *Mycobacterium tuberculosis* depending on the concentration of the drug attained at the site of infection. The mechanism of action is unknown.

Pharmacokinetics:

Absorption/Distribution – Pyrazinamide is well absorbed from the GI tract and attains peak plasma concentrations within 2 hours. Plasma concentrations generally range from 30 to 50 mcg/ml with doses of 20 to 25 mg/kg. It is widely distributed in body tissues and fluids including the liver, lungs and cerebrospinal fluid.

Metabolism/Excretion – The half-life is 9 to 10 hours; it may be prolonged in patients with impaired renal or hepatic function. Pyrazinamide is hydrolyzed in the liver to its major active metabolite, pyrazinoic acid. Pyrazinoic acid is hydroxylated to the main excretory product, 5-hydroxypyrazinoic acid.

Approximately 70% of an oral dose is excreted in urine, mainly by glomerular filtration, within 24 hours.

Indications:

Initial treatment of active tuberculosis in adults and children when combined with other antituberculous agents.

Contraindications:

Severe hepatic damage; hypersensitivity; acute gout.

Warnings:

Combination therapy: Use only in conjunction with other effective antituberculous agents.

Hyperuricemia: Pyrazinamide inhibits renal excretion of urates, frequently resulting in hyperuricemia which is usually asymptomatic. Patients started on pyrazinamide should have baseline serum uric acid determinations. Discontinue the drug and do not resume if signs of hyperuricemia accompanied by acute gouty arthritis appear.

Renal function impairment: It does not appear that patients with impaired renal function require a reduction in dose. It may be prudent to select doses at the low end of the dosing range, however.

Hepatic function impairment: Patients started on pyrazinamide should have baseline liver function determinations. Closely follow those patients with preexisting liver disease or those at increased risk for drug-related hepatitis. Discontinue pyrazinamide and do not resume if signs of hepatocellular damage appear.

Elderly: In general, dose selection for an elderly patient should be cautious, usually starting at the low end of the dosing range, reflecting the greater frequency of decreased hepatic or renal function, and of concomitant disease or other drug therapy.

Pregnancy: Category C.

Lactation: Pyrazinamide has been found in small amounts in breast milk. Therefore, it is advised that pyrazinamide be used with caution in nursing mothers, taking into account the risk-benefit of this therapy.

Children: Pyrazinamide regimens employed in adults are probably equally effective in children. Pyrazinamide appears to be well tolerated in children.

Precautions:

Monitoring: Determine baseline liver function studies and uric acid levels prior to therapy. Perform appropriate laboratory testing at periodic intervals and if any clinical signs or symptoms occur during therapy.

HIV infection: In patients with concomitant HIV infection, be aware of current recommendations of CDC. It is possible these patients may require a longer course of treatment.

Diabetes mellitus: Use with caution in patients with a history of diabetes mellitus, as management may be more difficult.

Primary resistance of M tuberculosis to pyrazinamide is uncommon. In cases with known or suspected drug resistance, perform in vitro susceptibility tests with recent cultures of *M tuberculosis* against pyrazinamide and the usual primary drugs.

Drug Interactions:

Drug/Lab test interactions: Pyrazinamide has been reported to interfere with Acetest and *Ketostix* urine tests to produce a pink-brown color.

Adverse Reactions:

Adverse reactions may include: Fever; porphyria; dysuria; gout; hepatic reaction; nausea; vomiting; anorexia; thrombocytopenia and sideroblastic anemia with erythroid hyperplasia, vacuolation of erythrocytes, increased serum iron concentration and adverse effects on blood clotting mechanisms; mild arthralgia and myalgia; hypersensitivity reactions including rashes, urticaria, pruritus; fever; acne; photosensitivity; porphyria; dysuria; interstitial nephritis.

Administration and Dosage:

Administer pyrazinamide with other effective antituberculous drugs. It is administered for the initial 2 months of a 6 month or longer treatment regimen for drug susceptible patients. Treat patients who are known or suspected to have drug-resistant disease with regimens individualized to their situation. Pyrazinamide frequently will be an important component of such therapy.

HIV infection: Patients with concomitant HIV infection may require longer courses of therapy. Be alert to any revised recommendations from CDC for this group of patients.

Usual dose: 15 to 30 mg/kg once daily. Older regimens employed 3 to 4 divided doses daily, but the most current recommendations are once a day. Do not exceed 3 g/day. The CDC recommendations do not exceed 2 g/day when given as a daily regimen.

Alternative dosing: Alternatively, a twice weekly dosing regimen (50 to 70 mg/kg twice weekly based on lean body weight) has been developed to promote patient compliance on an outpatient basis. In studies evaluating the twice weekly regimen, doses of pyrazinamide in excess of 3 g twice weekly have been administered. This exceeds the recommended maximum 3 g/daily dose. However, an increased incidence of adverse reactions has not been reported.

AMINOSALICYLATE SODIUM (Para-Aminosalicylate Sodium)

Tablets: 0.5 g (*Rx*)	*Sodium PAS* (Lannett)

Aminosalicylate sodium is the sodium salt of para-aminosalicylic acid (PAS). It contains 73% aminosalicylic acid equivalent and 10.9% sodium (54.5 mg sodium/500 mg tab).

Actions:

Pharmacology: Aminosalicylate sodium is bacteriostatic against *Mycobacterium tuberculosis*. It inhibits the onset of bacterial resistance to streptomycin and isoniazid.

Pharmacokinetics:

Absorption/Distribution – PAS is readily absorbed from GI tract; the sodium salt is absorbed more rapidly than free acid. It is widely distributed, concentrates in pleural and caseous tissue, but achieves low cerebrospinal fluid concentration.

Metabolism – The half-life of PAS is about 1 hour. It is metabolized in the liver; > 50% is acetylated.

Excretion – Over 80% is excreted through the kidneys as metabolites and free acid. Excretion is retarded in the presence of renal dysfunction.

Indications:

Treatment of tuberculosis in combination with other antituberculous drugs when due to susceptible strains of tubercle bacilli.

Unlabeled uses: PAS has been shown to have serum lipid-lowering activity.

Contraindications:

Severe hypersensitivity to aminosalicylate sodium and its congeners.

Warnings:

Hypersensitivity: Stop all medication if symptoms of hypersensitivity develop. After the symptoms have abated, restart medications one at a time, in very small but gradually increasing doses, to determine if the symptoms were drug-induced and, if so, which medication was responsible. Oral hyposensitization can only occasionally be accomplished.

Renal/Hepatic function impairment: Use with caution.

Precautions:

Gastric ulcer: Use cautiously in patients with gastric ulcer.

Crystalluria may be prevented by maintaining the urine at a neutral or alkaline pH.

Tablet deterioration: Aminosalicylate sodium deteriorates rapidly in contact with water, heat and sunlight. A brownish or purplish color of powder or tablets, especially of a solution made with them, is indicative of such deterioration. If deterioration is evident, discard the drug.

Use with caution in patients with known or impending CHF and in other situations in which excess sodium is potentially harmful.

Drug Interactions:

Digoxin and oral vitamin B_{12} may interact with PAS.

Adverse Reactions:

Adverse reactions may include: Nausea; vomiting; diarrhea; abdominal pain; fever; various skin eruptions; infectious mononucleosis-like syndrome; leukopenia; agranulocytosis; thrombocytopenia; hemolyutic anemia; jaundice; hepatitis; encephalopathy; Loffler's syndrome; vasculitis; goiter with or without myxedema.

Administration and Dosage:

Administer aminosalicylate sodium with other antituberculous drugs.

Adults: 14 to 16 g/day in 2 to 3 divided doses.

Children: 275 to 420 mg/kg/day in 3 to 4 divided doses daily.

ETHIONAMIDE

Tablets: 250 mg (*Rx*)	*Trecator-SC* (Wyeth-Ayerst)

Actions:

Pharmacology: Bacteriostatic against Mycobacterium tuberculosis.

Pharmacokinetics: Oral administration of ethionamide yields peak plasma concentrations in 3 hours. It is widely and rapidly distributed, including into the cerebrospinal fluid. The drug is metabolized in the liver and < 1% is excreted in the urine unchanged.

Indications:

Recommended for any form of active tuberculosis when treatment with first-line drugs (isoniazid, rifampin) has failed. Use only with other effective antituberculous agents.

Contraindications:

Severe hypersensitivity to ethionamide; severe hepatic damage.

Warnings:

Pregnancy: Category C.

Children: Optimum dosage for children has not been established.

Precautions:

Monitoring: Make determinations of serum transaminase (AST, ALT) prior to and every 2 to 4 weeks during therapy.

Pretreatment examinations should include in vitro susceptibility tests of recent cultures of M *tuberculosis* from the patient as measured against ethionamide and the usual first-line antituberculous drugs.

Diabetes mellitus: Management of the diabetes may be more difficult and hepatitis occurs more frequently.

Adverse Reactions:

Adverse reactions may include: Depression, drowsiness and asthenia, convulsions, peripheral neuritis and neuropathy, olfactory disturbances, blurred vision, diplopia, optic neuritis, dizziness, headache, restlessness, tremors, psychosis, anorexia, nausea and vomiting, diarrhea, metallic taste, hepatitis, jaundice, stomatitis, postural hypotension, skin rash, acne, alopecia, thrombocytopenia, pellagra-like syndrome, gynecomastia, impotence, menorrhagia, increased difficulty managing diabetes mellitus.

Administration and Dosage:

Administer with at least 1 other effective antituberculous drug.

Average adult dose: 0.5 to 1 g/day in divided doses.

Children: A dose of 15 to 20 mg/kg/day (maximum 1 g) has been recommended.

Concomitant administration of pyridoxine is recommended.

CYCLOSERINE

Capsules: 250 mg (*Rx*)	*Seromycin Pulvules* (Dura)

Actions:

Pharmacology: Inhibits cell wall synthesis in susceptible strains of gram-positive and gram-negative bacteria and in *Mycobacterium tuberculosis*.

Pharmacokinetics:

Absorption/Distribution – When given orally, cycloserine is rapidly absorbed, reaching peak plasma concentrations in 3 to 8 hours. It is widely distributed throughout body fluids and tissues; cerebrospinal fluid levels are similar to plasma.

Metabolism/Excretion – Approximately 35% of the drug is metabolized; 50% of a parenteral dose is excreted unchanged in the urine in the first 12 hours. About 65% of the drug is recoverable in 72 hours. Renal insufficiency will lead to toxic accumulation; it may be removed by dialysis.

Indications:

Treatment of active pulmonary and extrapulmonary tuberculosis (including renal disease) when organisms are susceptible, after failure of adequate treatment with the primary medications. Use in conjunction with other effective chemotherapy.

May be effective in the treatment of acute urinary tract infections caused by susceptible strains of gram-positive and gram-negative bacteria, especially *Enterobacter* sp and *Escherichia coli*. It is usually less effective than other antimicrobial agents in the treatment of urinary tract infections caused by bacteria other than mycobacteria. Consider using only when the more conventional therapy has failed and when the organism has demonstrated sensitivity.

Contraindications:

Hypersensitivity to cycloserine; epilepsy; depression, severe anxiety or psychosis; severe renal insufficiency; excessive concurrent use of alcohol.

Warnings:

CNS toxicity: Discontinue or reduce dosage if patient develops allergic dermatitis or symptoms of CNS toxicity, such as convulsions, psychosis, somnolence, depression, confusion, hyperreflexia, headache, tremor, vertigo, paresis or dysarthria. The risk of convulsions is increased in chronic alcoholics.

Toxicity is closely related to excessive blood levels (> 30 mcg/ml), which are due to high dosage or inadequate renal clearance. The therapeutic index in tuberculosis is small.

Renal function impairment: Patients will accumulate cycloserine and may develop toxicity if the dosage regimen is not modified. Patients with severe impairment should not receive the drug.

Pregnancy: Category C.

Lactation: Because of the potential for serious adverse reactions in nursing infants, decide whether to discontinue nursing or to discontinue the drug.

Children: Safety and dosage not established for pediatric use.

Precautions:

Monitoring: Monitor patients by hematologic, renal excretion, blood level and liver function studies.

Obtain cultures and determine susceptibility before treatment.

Determine blood levels weekly for patients having reduced renal function, for individuals receiving > 500 mg/day, and for those with symptoms of toxicity. Adjust dosage to maintain blood level < 30 mcg/ml.

Anticonvulsant drugs or sedatives may be effective in controlling symptoms of CNS toxicity, such as convulsions, anxiety and tremor. Closely observe patients receiving > 500 mg/day for such symptoms. Pyridoxine may prevent CNS toxicity, but its efficacy has not been proven.

Anemia: Administration has been associated in a few cases with vitamin B_{12} or folic acid deficiency, megaloblastic anemia and sideroblastic anemia. If evidence of anemia develops, institute appropriate studies and therapy.

Drug Interactions:

Drugs that may interact with cycloserine include alcohol and isoniazid.

Adverse Reactions:

Adverse reactions may include: Convulsions; drowsiness and somnolence; headache; tremor; dysarthria; vertigo; confusion and disorientation with loss of memory; psychoses, possibly with suicidal tendencies, character changes, hyperirritability, aggression; paresis; hyperreflexia; paresthesias; major and minor (localized) clonic seizures; coma; sudden development of congestive heart failure; skin rash; elevated transaminase.

Administration and Dosage:

Administer 500 mg to 1 g daily in divided doses monitored by blood levels. The usual initial dosage is 250 mg twice daily at 12 hour intervals for the first 2 weeks. Do not exceed 1 g/day.

Pyridoxine 200 to 300 mg/day may prevent the neurotoxic effects.

Children: A recommended dose of 10 to 20 mg/kg/day (maximum 0.75 to 1 g).

STREPTOMYCIN SULFATE

For a complete listing of streptomycin sulfate products, refer to individual monograph in Aminoglycosides, Parenteral section.

Indications:

Recommended in the treatment of all forms of Mycobacterium tuberculosis when the infecting organisms are susceptible. Use only in combination with other antituberculous drugs.

For nontuberculous infection indications, see individual monograph in Aminoglycosides, Parenteral section.

Administration and Dosage:

Administer by the IM route only.

Combined therapy for adults: 1g streptomycin and an appropriate dosage of additional antitubercular drugs (usually isoniazid, ethambutol or rifampin). Elderly patients should have a smaller daily dose of streptomycin in accordance with age, renal function and eighth nerve function.

Discontinue the streptomycin or reduce dosage to 1 g 2 to 3 times weekly. Therapy with streptomycin may be terminated when toxic symptoms appear, impending toxicity is feared, organisms have become resistant, or full therapeutic effect has been obtained. The total period of treatment for tuberculosis is a minimum of 1 year; however, indications for terminating streptomycin therapy may occur at any time.

Children: A recommended dose of 20 to 40 mg/kg/day (maximum 0.75 to 1g).

As with other aminoglycosides, reduce dosage in patients with impaired renal function.

CAPREOMYCIN

Powder for Injection: 1 g (as sulfate) per 10 ml vial (*Rx*) *Capastat Sulfate* (Dura)

Warning:

The use of capreomycin in patients with renal insufficiency or preexisting auditory impairment must be undertaken with great caution, and weigh the risk of additional eighth nerve impairment or renal injury against benefits to be derived from therapy.

Since other parenteral antituberculous agents (eg, streptomycin) also have similar and sometimes irreversible toxic effects, particularly on eighth cranial nerve and renal function, simultaneous administration of these agents with capreomycin is not recommended. Use concurrent nonantituberculous drugs (eg, aminoglycoside antibiotics) having ototoxic or nephrotoxic potential only with great caution.

Actions:

Pharmacology: A polypeptide antibiotic isolated from *Streptomyces capreolus*.

Pharmacokinetics:

Distribution – Capreomycin sulfate is not absorbed in significant quantities from the GI tract and must be administered IM. Peak serum concentrations following IM administration of 1g are achieved in 1 to 2 hours. Low serum concentrations are present at 24 hours. Doses of 1 g daily for ≥ 30 days produce no significant accumulation in subjects with normal renal function.

Excretion – Capreomycin is excreted essentially unaltered; 52% is excreted in the urine within 12 hours. Urine concentrations average 1680 mcg/ml during the 6 hours following a 1 g dose.

Indications:

Intended for use concomitantly with other antituberculous agents in pulmonary infections caused by capreomycin-susceptible strains of *M. tuberculosis*, when the primary agents (eg, isoniazid, rifampin) have been ineffective or cannot be used because of toxicity or the presence of resistant tubercle bacilli.

Contraindications:

Hypersensitivity to capreomycin.

Warnings:

Hypersensitivity: Has occurred when capreomycin and other antituberculous drugs were given concomitantly.

Pregnancy: Category C.

Lactation: It is not known whether this drug is excreted in breast milk.

Children: Safety for use in infants and children has not been established.

Precautions:

Ototoxicity: Perform audiometric measurements and assessment of vestibular function prior to initiation of therapy and at regular intervals during treatment.

Nephrotoxicity: Perform regular tests of renal function throughout treatment, and reduce dose in patients with renal impairment. Renal injury with tubular necrosis, elevation of BUN or serum creatinine and abnormal sediment has been noted. Monitor renal function both before therapy is started and on a weekly basis during treatment. The appearance of casts, red cells and white cells in the urine has been noted in a high percentage.

Elevation of the BUN > 30 mg/dl or any other evidence of decreasing renal function with or without a rise in BUN level should indicate careful evaluation of the patient; reduce the dosage or withdraw the drug.

Hypokalemia may occur during therapy; therefore, determine serum potassium levels frequently.

Drug Interactions:
Drugs that may interact with capreomycin include aminoglycosides and nondepolarizing neuromuscular blocking agents.

Adverse Reactions:
Adverse reactions may include: Ototoxicity, tinnitus, vertigo, pain and induration and excessive bleeding at the injection sites, sterile abscesses, leukocytosis, leukopenia, eosinophilia, abnormal results in liver function tests, urticaria and maculopapular skin rashes.

Administration and Dosage:
Give by deep IM injection into a large muscle mass; superficial injections may be associated with increased pain and sterile abscesses. Always administer in combination with at least one other antituberculous agent to which the patient's strain of tubercle bacilli is susceptible.

Usual dose: 1 g daily (not to exceed 20 mg/kg/day) given IM for 60 to 120 days, followed by 1 g IM 2 or 3 times weekly.

Note: Maintain therapy for tuberculosis for 12 to 24 months. If facilities for administering injectable medication are not available, a change to oral therapy is indicated upon the patient's release from the hospital.

Children: A dose of 15mg/kg/day (maximum 1 g) has been recommended.

Renal function impairment: Reduce the dosage based on creatinine clearance (Ccr) using the guidelines in the table. These dosages are designed to achieve a mean steady-state capreomycin level of 10 mg/L.

Capreomycin Dosage in Renal Function Impairment

Ccr (ml/min)	Capreomycin clearance (L/kg/h × 10^{-2})	Half-life (hours)	Dose[1] (mg/kg) for the following dosing intervals		
			24 hr	48 hr	72 hr
0	0.54	55.5	1.29	2.58	3.87
10	1.01	29.4	2.43	4.87	7.31
20	1.49	20.0	3.58	7.16	10.7
30	1.97	15.1	4.72	9.45	14.2
40	2.45	12.2	5.87	11.7	
50	2.92	10.2	7.01	14	
60	3.40	8.8	8.16		
80	4.35	6.8	10.4		
100	5.31	5.6	12.7		
110	5.78	5.2	13.9		

[1] Initial maintenance dose estimates are given for optional dosing intervals; longer dosing intervals are expected to provide greater peak and lower trough serum capreomycin levels than shorter dosing intervals.

Preparation of solution: Dissolve in 2 ml of 0.9% Sodium Chloride Injection or Sterile Water for Injection. Allow 2 to 3 minutes for complete dissolution. For administration of a 1 g dose, give the entire contents of the vial. For dosages < 1 g, the following dilution table may be used.

Preparation of Capreomycin Solution

Concentration[1] (Approx.)	Diluent added to 1 g vial	Volume of solution
350 mg/ml	2.15 ml	2.85 ml
300 mg/ml	2.63 ml	3.33 ml
250 mg/ml	3.3 ml	4 ml
200 mg/ml	4.3 ml	5 ml

[1] Stated in terms of mg of capreomycin activity.

FAMCICLOVIR

Tablets: 125, 250 and 500 mg (*Rx*) *Famvir* (SmithKline Beecham)

Actions:

Pharmacology: Famciclovir undergoes rapid biotransformation to the active antiviral compound penciclovir, which has inhibitory activity against herpes simplex virus types 1 (HSV-1) and 2 (HSV-2) and varicella-zoster virus (VZV). In HSV-1-, HSV-2- and VZV-infected cells, viral thymidine kinase phosphorylates penciclovir to a monophosphate form which, in turn, is converted to penciclovir triphosphate by cellular kinases. In vitro, penciclovir triphosphate inhibits HSV-2 polymerase competitively with deoxyguanosine triphosphate. Consequently, herpes viral DNA synthesis and, therefore, replication are selectively inhibited.

Pharmacokinetics:

Absorption – The absolute bioavailability of famciclovir is 77%. The area under the plasma concentration-time curve (AUC) was 8.6 mcg•hr/ml. The maximum concentration (C_{max}) was 3.3 mcg/ml and the time to C_{max} (T_{max}) was 0.9 hours.

After a 1–hour intravenous infusion of penciclovir at doses of 5 to 20 mg/kg, the volume of distribution (Vd_b) of penciclovir was 83.1 and 125 L, respectively. Penciclovir is < 20% bound to plasma proteins over the concentration range of 0.1 to 20 mcg/ml. The blood/plasma ratio of penciclovir is ≈ 1.

Metabolism – Famciclovir given orally is deacetylated and oxidized to form penciclovir. Inactive metabolites include 6-deoxy penciclovir, monoacetylated penciclovir and 6-deoxy monoacetylated penciclovir (each < 0.5% of the dose). Cytochrome P–450 does not play an important role in famciclovir metabolism.

Excretion – Following a single 500 mg oral dose of radio-labeled famciclovir, 73% and 27% of administered radioactivity were recovered in urine and feces over 72 hours, respectively. Penciclovir accounted for 82% and 6-deoxy penciclovir accounted for 7% of the radioactivity excreted in the urine. Approximately 60% of the administered radiolabeled dose was collected in urine in the first 6 hours.

Renal clearance of penciclovir following the oral administration of a single 500 mg dose of famciclovir was 27.7 L/hr.

The plasma elimination half-life of penciclovir was 2 hours after IV penciclovir and 2.3 hours after 500 mg oral famciclovir. The half-life in 7 herpes zoster patients was 3 hrs.

Indications:

Acute herpes zoster: Management of acute herpes zoster (shingles).

Genital herpes: Treatment of recurrent episodes of genital herpes.

Contraindications:

Hypersensitivity to famciclovir.

Warnings:

Renal function impairment: Apparent plasma clearance, renal clearance and the plasma-elimination rate constant of penciclovir decreased linearly with reductions in renal function. After a single 500 mg oral famciclovir dose to healthy volunteers and to volunteers with varying degrees of renal insufficiency, the following results were obtained.

Pharmacokinetics of Famciclovir in Patients with Renal Function Impairment				
Parameter (mean)	CL_{CR}[1] ≥ 60 (ml/min; n = 15)	CL_{CR} 40-59 (ml/min; n = 5)	CL_{CR} 20-39 (ml/min; n = 4)	CL_{CR} < 20 (ml/min; n = 3)
CL_{CR} (ml/min	88.1	49.3	26.5	12.7
CL_R (L/hr)	30.1	13[2]	4.2	1.6
CL/F[3] (L/hr)	66.9	27.3	12.8	5.8
Half-life (hr)	2.3	3.4	6.2	13.4

[1] CL_{CR} is measured creatinine clearance.
[2] n = 4
[3] CL/F consists of bioavailability factor and famciclovir to penciclovir conversion factor.

Dosage adjustment is recommended in renal insufficiency (see Administration & Dosage).

Hepatic function impairment: Well compensated chronic liver disease (chronic hepatitis, chronic ethanol abuse or primary biliary cirrhosis) had no effect on extent of availability (AUC) of penciclovir following a single dose of 500 mg famiciclovir. However, there was a 44% decrease in penciclovir mean maximum plasma level and the time to maximum plasma concentration was increased by 0.75 hrs in patients with hepatic insufficiency compared with normal volunteers. No dosage adjustment is recommended in well compensated hepatic impairment. Penciclovir pharmacokinetics have not been evaluated in severe uncompensated hepatic impairment.

Elderly: Mean penciclovir AUC was 40% larger and penciclovir renal clearance was 22% lower after the oral administration of famciclovir in elderly volunteers (ages 65 to 79 years) compared with younger volunteers.

Pregnancy: Category B.

Lactation: It is not known whether it is excreted in human breast milk. Because of the potential for tumorigenicity shown for famciclovir in rats, discontinue nursing or the drug, taking into account the importance of the drug to the mother.

Children: Safety and efficacy in children < 18 years of age have not been established.

Drug Interactions:

The conversion of 6-deoxy penciclovir to penciclovir is catalyzed by aldehyde oxidase. Interactions with other drugs metabolized by this enzyme could occur.

Drugs that may affect famciclovir include cimetidine, probenecid and theophylline.

Famciclovir may affect digoxin.

Drug/Food interactions: When famciclovir was administered with food, penciclovir C_{max} decreased ≈ 50%. Because the systemic availability of penciclovir (AUC) was not altered, it appears that famciclovir may be taken without regard to meals.

Adverse Reactions:

Adverse reactions occurring in ≥ 3% of patients include dizziness, diarrhea, abdominal pain, dyspepsia, constipation, vomiting, fatigue, fever, pruritus.

The most frequent adverse events were headache and nausea.

Administration and Dosage:

Herpes Zoster: The recommended dosage is 500 mg every 8 hours for 7 days. Therapy should be initiated promptly as soon as herpes zoster is diagnosed.

Genital herpes (recurrent episodes): The recommended dosage is 125 mg twice daily for 5 days. Initiate therapy at the first sign or symptom if medical management of a genital herpes recurrence is indicated.

Famciclovir Dosage in Renal Function Impairment

Creatinine clearance (ml/min)	Dose regimen
Herpes zoster	
≥ 60	500 mg every 8 hours
40 to 59	500 mg every 12 hours
20 to 39	500 mg every 24 hours
< 20	250 mg every 48 hours
Recurrent genital herpes	
≥40	125 mg every 12 hours
20 to 39	125 mg every 24 hours
< 20	125 mg every 48 hours

Hemodialysis patients: The recommended dose of famciclovir is 250 mg (herpes zoster) or 125 mg (genital herpes) administered following each dialysis treatment.

STAVUDINE (d4T)

Capsules: 15, 20, 30, 40 mg (*Rx*) *Zerit* (Bristol-Myers Squibb)

Warning:

Stavudine is indicated for the treatment of adults with advanced HIV infection who are intolerant of approved therapies with proven clinical benefit or who have experienced significant clinical or immunologic deterioration while receiving these therapies or for whom such therapies are contraindicated. At present, there are no results from controlled trials evaluating the effect of stavudine therapy on the clinical progression of HIV infection, such as the incidence of opportunistic infections or survival. Because therapy with zidovudine prolongs survival in patients with advanced HIV disease, consider zidovudine initial therapy for the treatment of HIV infection.

The major clinical toxicity of stavudine is peripheral neuropathy. This occurred in 15% to 21% of patients in the controlled trials.

Actions:

Pharmacology: Stavudine, a synthetic thymidine nucleoside analog active against HIV, inhibits the replication of HIV in human cells in vitro. Stavudine is phosphorylated by cellular kinases to stavudine triphosphate which exerts antiviral activity. Stavudine triphosphate has an intracellular half-life of 3.5 hours in CEM and peripheral blood mononuclear cells. Stavudine triphosphate inhibits HIV replication in that it inhibits HIV reverse transcriptase by competing with the natural substrate deoxythymidine triphosphate; it inhibits viral DNA synthesis by causing DNA chain termination because stavudine lacks the 3'-hydroxyl group, necessary for DNA elongation. Stavudine triphosphate also inhibits cellular DNA polymerase beta and gamma, and markedly reduces mitochondrial DNA synthesis.

Pharmacokinetics:

Adults –

Absorption: Following oral administration to 25 HIV-infected patients, stavudine was rapidly absorbed with a mean absolute bioavailability of 86.4%. Peak plasma concentrations (C_{max}) increased in a dose-related manner for doses ranging from 0.03 to 4 mg/kg and occurred ≤ 1 hour after dosing. Area under the plasma concentration-time curve (AUC) increased in proportion to dose after both single and multiple doses. When 70 mg stavudine was administered to 16 asymptomatic HIV-infected patients under fasting conditions, 1 hour before a standardized high-fat meal (773 Kcal, 53% fat) or immediately after the meal, systemic exposure (AUC) was similar. Mean C_{max} of stavudine was reduced from 1.44 mcg/ml in the fasting state to 0.75 mcg/ml after the meal, and the median time to reach C_{max} was prolonged from 0.6 to 1.5 hours.

Distribution: Following 1 hour IV infusions of 0.0625 to 1 mg/kg, mean volume of distribution (Vd) was 58 L, suggesting that stavudine distributes into extravascular spaces. Mean apparent Vd following single oral doses ranging from 0.03 to 4 mg/kg was 66 L. Binding to serum proteins was negligible. Stavudine distributes equally between red blood cells and plasma.

Metabolism: After incubation of [^{14}C]-stavudine for 6 hours with human liver slices, 87% of radioactivity was accounted for by parent drug, 2% was metabolized to thymine and 7% was associated with unidentified polar compounds.

Excretion: Plasma clearance and terminal elimination half-life were independent of dose over an IV dosing range of 0.0625 to 1 mg/kg and an oral dosing range of 0.03 to 4 mg/kg. After single oral doses, the mean terminal elimination half-life was 1.44 hours. Following single-dose oral administration, mean apparent oral clearance was independent of dose, having a value of 559 ml/min. Renal elimination accounted for ≈ 40% of the overall clearance regardless of the route of administration; there is active tubular secretion in addition to glomerular filtration. Mean cumulative urinary excretion of unchanged drug over 6 to 24 hours after administration of an oral dose was 39% of the dose.

Children –

Absorption: Stavudine was rapidly absorbed following oral administration to HIV-infected children with a mean absolute bioavailability of 78.5% for capsules and 69.2% for solution, respectively. First-dose and multiple-dose pharmacokinetic profiles were similar, indicating no accumulation.

Distribution: Following IV infusions of 0.125 to 2 mg/kg, mean Vd was 13.2 L, suggesting that stavudine distributes into extravascular spaces. After 12 weeks of treatment, the stavudine concentration in CSF samples from 7 patients ranged from 0.01 to 0.12 mcg/ml at times ranging from 2 to 3 hours post-dose. CSF concentrations corresponded to 16% to 97% of the level in simultaneous plasma samples.

Elimination: Plasma concentrations declined with a mean terminal elimination half-life of 1.09 hours following the end of a 1-hour infusion. After a single oral dose, mean terminal half-life was 0.91 hours. Mean total body clearance after IV infusion was 181.13 ml/min. Mean apparent oral clearance after administration of solution (n = 10; age < 6 years) and capsule (n = 8; age > 6 years) formulations was 16.45 and 11.01 ml/min/kg, respectively.

Renal insufficiency – The apparent oral clearance of stavudine decreased as creatinine clearance (Ccr) decreased. The terminal elimination half-life was prolonged up to 8 hours. C_{max} and T_{max} were not significantly affected by reduced renal function. Based on these preliminary observations, it is recommended that stavudine dosage be modified in patients with reduced Ccr (see Administration and Dosage).

Indications:

HIV infection: Treatment of adults with advanced HIV infection who are intolerant of approved therapies with proven clinical benefit or who have experienced significant clinical or immunologic deterioration while receiving these therapies or for whom such therapies are contraindicated.

Contraindications:

Hypersensitivity to stavudine or to any components of the formulation.

Warnings:

Progression of HIV: At present, there are no results from controlled trials evaluating the effect of stavudine therapy on the clinical progression of HIV infection, such as the incidence of opportunistic infections or survival.

Initial therapy for HIV: Because therapy with zidovudine prolongs survival in patients with advanced HIV disease, consider zidovudine initial therapy for treating HIV.

Peripheral neuropathy: The major clinical toxicity of stavudine is peripheral neuropathy. Monitor patients for development of neuropathy, usually characterized by numbness, tingling or pain in feet or hands. Stavudine-related peripheral neuropathy may resolve if therapy is withdrawn promptly. Symptoms may worsen temporarily following therapy discontinuation. If symptoms resolve completely, resumption of treatment may be considered at a reduced dose. Patients with a history of peripheral neuropathy are at increased risk for developing neuropathy; careful monitoring is essential.

Pancreatitis was reported in 1% of patients enrolled in controlled clinical trials and was associated with 14 deaths, five of which were attributed to drug toxicity.

Pregnancy: Category C.

Lactation: It is not known whether stavudine is excreted in breast milk. Because of the potential for adverse reactions from stavudine in nursing infants, instruct mothers to discontinue nursing if they are receiving stavudine.

Children: Safety and efficacy of stavudine for treatment of HIV in children have not been established. Limited data are available from 37 children aged 5 months to 15 years who received stavudine in doses ranging from 0.125 to 4 mg/kg/day for a median duration of 37 weeks. Serious adverse events that have been observed include AST and ALT elevations and one case of neuropathy.

Precautions:

Laboratory tests: Mild to moderate increases in AST and ALT occurred commonly in clinical trials, and tended to resolve following interruption of therapy.

Drug Interactions:

Drug/Food interactions: C_{max} of stavudine was decreased by ≈ 45% when administered with food; however, systemic availability (AUC) was unchanged.

Adverse Reactions:

In Phase I trials, peripheral neuropathy occurred in 29%, 19%, 53%, 70%, 67% and 64% of patients at doses of 0.5, 1, 2, 4, 8 and 12 mg/kg/day, respectively. Modest hepatic transaminase elevations were common in controlled trials.

Adverse reactions occurring in ≥ 3% of patients include headache, chills/fever, asthenia, abdominal pain, back pain, pain, malaise, weight loss, allergic reaction, flu syndrome, lymphadenopathy, neoplasma, death, chest pain, vasodilation, diarrhea, nausea/vomiting, anorexia, dyspepsia, constipation, ulcerative stomatitis, myalgia, arthralgia, other peripheral neurologic symptoms, insomnia, anxiety, neuropathy, depression, nervousness, dizziness, confusion, migraine, dyspnea, pneumonia, rash, sweating, pruritus, maculopapular rash, skin benign neoplasm, urticaria, conjunctivitis, abnormal vision, dysuria.

Administration and Dosage:

Adults: The interval between oral doses should be 12 hours. Stavudine may be taken without regard to meals. Recommended starting dose based on body weight:

Patients ≥ 60 kg – 40 mg twice daily.

Patients < 60 kg – 30 mg twice daily.

Dosage adjustment: Monitor patients for the development of peripheral neuropathy. If these symptoms develop, interrupt stavudine therapy. Symptoms may resolve if therapy is withdrawn promptly. In some cases symptoms may worsen temporarily following discontinuation of therapy. If symptoms resolve completely, resumption of treatment may be considered using the following dosage schedule:

Patients ≥ 60 kg – 20 mg twice daily.

Patients < 60 kg – 15 mg twice daily.

Manage clinically significant elevations of hepatic transaminases in the same way.

Renal function impairment – Stavudine may be administered to adult patients with impaired renal function. The following schedule is recommended:

Stavudine Dosage in Renal Function Impairment

Creatinine clearance (ml/min)	Recommended stavudine dose by patient weight	
	≥ 60 kg	< 60 kg
> 50	40 mg every 12 hours	30 mg every 12 hours
26 - 50	20 mg every 12 hours	15 mg every 12 hours
10 - 25	20 mg every 24 hours	15 mg every 24 hours

There are insufficient data to recommend a dose for patients with Ccr < 10 ml/min or for patients undergoing dialysis.

VALACYCLOVIR HCl

Caplets: 500 mg (*Rx*)	*Valtrex* (Glaxo Wellcome)

Actions:

Pharmacology: Valacyclovir is the hydrochloride salt of L-valyl ester of the antiviral drug acyclovir. Valacyclovir is rapidly converted to acyclovir, which has in vitro and in vivo inhibitory activity against herpes simplex virus types I (HSV-1) and II (HSV-2) and varicella-zoster virus (VZV). In cell culture, acyclovir has the highest antiviral activity against HSV-1, followed by (in decreasing order of potency) HSV-2 and VZV.

The inhibitory activity of acyclovir is highly selective due to its affinity for the enzyme thymidine kinase (TK). This viral enzyme converts acyclovir into acyclovir monophosphate, a nucleotide analog. The monophosphate is further converted into diphosphate by cellular guanylate kinase and into triphosphate by a number of cellular enzymes. In vitro, acyclovir triphosphate stops replication of herpes viral DNA in three ways: 1) Competitive inhibition of viral DNA polymerase, 2) incorporation and termination of the growing viral DNA chain and 3) inactivation of the viral DNA polymerase.

Pharmacokinetics:

Absorption/Distribution – After oral administration, valacyclovir is rapidly absorbed from the GI tract and is rapidly and nearly completely converted to acyclovir and L-valine by first-pass intestinal or hepatic metabolism.

The absolute bioavailability of acyclovir after administration of valacyclovir is 54.5%. Acyclovir bioavailability from the administration of valacyclovir is not altered by administration with food (30 minutes after an 873 Kcal breakfast, which included 51 g of fat).

The binding of valacyclovir to human plasma proteins ranged from 13.5% to 17.9%.

Metabolism – Acyclovir is converted to a small extent to inactive metabolites by aldehyde oxidase and by alcohol and aldehyde dehydrogenase. Neither valacyclovir nor acyclovir metabolism is associated with liver microsomal enzymes. Plasma concentrations of unconverted valacyclovir are low and transient, generally becoming non-quantifiable by 3 hours after administration. Peak plasma valacyclovir concentrations are generally < 0.5 mcg/ml at all doses. After single-dose administration of 1 g, average plasma valacyclovir concentrations were 0.5, 0.4 and 0.8 mcg/ml in patients with hepatic dysfunction, renal insufficiency, and in healthy volunteers who received concomitant cimetidine and probenecid, respectively.

Excretion – The pharmacokinetic disposition of acyclovir from valacyclovir is consistent with previous experience from IV and oral acyclovir. Following the oral administration of a single 1 g valacyclovir dose to four healthy subjects, 45.6% and 47.12% was recovered in urine and feces over 96 hours, respectively. Acyclovir accounted for 88.6% excreted in the urine. Renal clearance of acyclovir following the administration of a single 1 g valacyclovir dose to 12 healthy volunteers was ≈ 255 ml/min, which represents 41.9% of total acyclovir apparent plasma clearance.

The plasma elimination half-life of acyclovir typically averaged 2.5 to 3.3 hours in volunteers with normal renal function.

End-stage renal disease (ESRD): Following administration of valacyclovir to volunteers with ESRD, the average acyclovir half-life is ≈ 14 hours. During hemodialysis, the acyclovir half-life is ≈ 4 hours. Apparent plasma clearance of acyclovir in dialysis patients and healthy volunteers was 86.3 ml/min/1.73 m^2 and 679.16 ml/min/1.73 m^2, respectively.

HIV disease: In nine patients with advanced HIV disease (CD4 cell counts < 50 cells/mm^3) who received valacyclovir at a dosage of 1 g 4 times daily for 30 days, the pharmacokinetics of valacyclovir and acyclovir were not different from that observed in healthy volunteers.

Indications:

Herpes zoster: Treatment of herpes zoster (shingles) in immunocompetent adults.

Recurrent genital herpes: Episodic treatment of recurrent genital herpes in immunocompetent adults.

Contraindications:

Hypersensitivity or intolerance to valacyclovir, acyclovir or any component of the formulation.

Warnings:

Thrombotic thrombocytopenic purpura/hemolytic uremic syndrome (TTP/HUS), in some cases resulting in death, has been reported in patients with advanced HIV disease and in bone marrow and renal transplant recipients. Valacyclovir is not indicated for the treatment of immunocompromised patients. TTP/HUS has not been seen in immunocompetent patients receiving valacyclovir in clinical trials.

Renal function impairment: Exercise caution when giving valacyclovir to patients with renal impairment or those receiving potentially nephrotoxic agents as this may increase the risk of renal dysfunction or the risk of reversible CNS symptoms such as those that occur infrequently in patients treated with IV acyclovir.

Hepatic function impairment: Administration of valacyclovir to patients with moderate (biopsy-proven cirrhosis) or severe (with and without ascites and biopsy-proven cirrhosis) liver disease indicated that the rate but not the extent of conversion of valacyclovir to acyclovir was reduced, and the acyclovir half-life was not affected. Dosage modification is not recommended for patients with cirrhosis.

Elderly: The pharmacokinetics of acyclovir following single- and multiple-dose oral administration of valacyclovir in geriatric volunteers varied with renal function. Dosage reduction may be required in geriatric patients, depending on the underlying renal status of the patient.

Pregnancy: Category B.

Lactation: There is no experience with valacyclovir. However, acyclovir concentrations have been documented in breast milk in two women following oral administration of acyclovir and ranged from 0.6 to 4.1 times corresponding plasma levels. These concentrations would potentially expose the nursing infant to a dose of acyclovir as high as 0.3 mg/kg/day. Give consideration to temporary discontinuation of nursing, as the safety of valacyclovir has not been established in infants.

Children: Safety and efficacy have not been established.

Drug Interactions:

Drugs that may affect valacyclovir include cimetidine/probenecid.

Adverse Reactions:

Adverse reactions occurring in ≥ 3% of patients include nausea, headache, vomiting, diarrhea, constipation, asthenia, dizziness, abdominal pain and anorexia.

Administration and Dosage:

Valacyclovir may be given without regard to meals.

Herpes zoster: The recommended dosage is 1 g 3 times daily for 7 days. Initiate therapy at the earliest sign or symptom of herpes zoster; it is most effective when started within 48 hours of the onset of zoster rash. No data are available on efficacy of treatment started > 72 hours after rash onset.

Recurrent genital herpes: The recommended dosage is 500 mg twice daily for 5 days. If medical management of a genital herpes recurrence is indicated, advise patients to initiate therapy at the first sign or symptom of an episode. There are no data on the efficacy of treatment started > 24 hours after the onset of signs or symptoms.

Acute or chronic renal impairment:

Valacyclovir Dosage Adjustments for Renal Impairment

Creatinine clearance (ml/min)	Herpes zoster		Genital herpes	
	Dose	Frequency	Dose	Frequency
≥ 50	1 g	every 8 hours	500 mg	every 12 hours
30 to 49	1 g	every 12 hours	500 mg	every 12 hours
10 to 29	1 g	every 24 hours	500 mg	every 24 hours
< 10	500 mg	every 24 hours	500 mg	every 24 hours

Hemodialysis: During hemodialysis, the half-life of acyclovir after administration of valacyclovir is ≈ 4 hours. About 33% of acyclovir in the body is removed by dialysis during a 4 hour hemodialysis session. Patients requiring hemodialysis should receive the recommended dose of valacyclovir after hemodialysis.

Peritoneal dialysis: Supplemental doses of valacyclovir should not be required following chronic ambulatory peritoneal dialysis (CAPD) or continuous arteriovenous hemofiltration/hemodialysis (CAVHD).

RITONAVIR

Capsules: 100 mg (*Rx*) — *Norvir* (Abbott)
Oral Solution: 80 mg/ml (*Rx*)

Warning:

Coadministration of ritonavir with certain nonsedating antihistamines, sedative hypnotics or antiarrhythmics may result in potentially serious or life-threatening adverse events due to possible effects of ritonavir on the hepatic metabolism of certain drugs.

Actions:

Pharmacology: Ritonavir is an inhibitor of HIV protease with activity against HIV. Ritonavir is a petidomimetic inhibitor of both the HIV-1 and HIV-2 proteases. Inhibition of HIV protease renders the enzyme incapable of processing the *gag-pol* polyprotein precursor which leads to production of non-infectious immature HIV particles. Cross-resistance between ritonavir and reverse transcriptase inhibitors is unlikely because of the different enzyme targets involved.

Pharmacokinetics: After a 600 mg dose of oral solution, peak concentrations of ritonavir were achieved ≈ 2 hours and 4 hours after dosing under fasting and nonfasting conditions, respectively. When the oral solution was given under non-fasting conditions, peak ritonavir concentrations decreased 23% and the extent of absorption decreased 7% relative to fasting conditions. Dilution of the oral solution, within 1 hour of administration, with 240 ml of chocolate milk, *Advera* or *Ensure* did not significantly affect the extent and rate of ritonavir absorption. After a single 600 mg dose under non-fasting conditions, in two separate studies, the capsule and oral solution formulations yielded mean areas under the plasma concentration-time curve (AUCs) of 129.5 and 129 mcg•hr/ml, respectively. Relative to fasting conditions, the extent of absorption of ritonavir from the capsule formulation was 15% higher when administered with a meal.

Nearly all of the plasma radioactivity after a single oral 600 mg dose of ^{14}C-ritonavir oral solution was attributed to unchanged ritonavir. Five ritonavir metabolites have been identified in urine and feces. The isopropylthiazole oxidation metabolite (M-2) is the major metabolite and has antiviral activity similar to that of the parent drug; however, the concentrations of this metabolite in plasma are low. Studies utilizing human liver microsomes demonstrate that cytochrome P450 3A (CYP3A) is a major isoform involved in ritonavir metabolism, although CYP2D6 also contributes to the formation of M-2.

Ritonavir Pharmacokinetic Characteristics

Parameter	Values (mean)	Parameter	Values (mean)
C_{max} SS [1]	11.2 mcg/ml	CL/F[2]	4.6 L/h
C_{trough} SS[1]	3.7 mcg/ml	CL_R	< 0.1 L/h
V_{β}/F[2]	0.41 L/kg	RBC/Plasma ratio	0.14
CL/F[2]	8.8 L/h	Percent bound[3]	98% to 99%

[1] SS = Steady state; ritonavir doses of 600 mg q 12 h.
[2] Single ritonavir 600 mg dose.
[3] Primarily bound to human serum albumin and alpha-1 acid glycoprotein over the ritonavir concentration range of 0.01 to 30 μg/ml.

Indications:

HIV infection: Combination with nucleoside analogs or as monotherapy for the treatment of HIV infection when therapy is warranted.

Contraindications:

Hypersensitivity to the drug or any of its ingredients.

Ritonavir is expected to produce large increases in the plasma concentrations of amiodarone, astemizole, bepridil, bupropion, cisapride, clozapine, encainide, flecainide, meperidine, piroxicam, propafenone, propoxyphene, quinidine, rifabutin and terfenadine. These agents have recognized risks of arrhythmias, hematologic abnormalities, seizures or other potentially serious adverse effects. Do not administer these drugs concomitantly with ritonavir.

Coadministration is likely to produce large increases in these highly metabolized sedatives and hypnotics: Alprazolam, clorazepate, diazepam, estazolam, flurazepam, midazolam, triazolam and zolpidem. Due to the potential for extreme sedation and respiratory depression from these agents, do not administer with ritonavir.

Warnings:

Hepatic function impairment: Ritonavir is principally metabolized by the liver. Exercise caution when administering this drug to patients with impaired hepatic function.

Pregnancy: Category B.

Lactation: It is not known whether this drug is excreted in breast milk. The CDC advises HIV-infected women not to breastfeed to avoid postnatal transmission of HIV to a child who may not be infected.

Children: Safety and efficacy in children < 12 years of age have not been established.

Precautions:

Lab test abnormalities: Ritonavir has been associated with alterations in triglycerides, AST, ALT, GGT, CPK and uric acid. Perform appropriate laboratory testing prior to initiating ritonavir therapy and at periodic intervals or if any clinical signs and symptoms occur during therapy.

Percentage of Patients with Marked Chemistry and Hematology Laboratory Value Abnormalities with Ritonavir Therapy

		Naive patients			Advanced patients	
Variable	Limit	Ritonavir + AZT	Ritonavir	AZT	Ritonavir	Placebo
Chemistry values	high					
Uric acid	(> 12 mg/dl)	—	—	—	3.6	0.2
AST	(> 180 IU/L)	2.9	6.5	1.7	3.8	4.3
ALT	(> 215 IU/L)	3.9	3.6	2.6	6.1	2.6
GGT	(> 300 IU/L)	2	2.8	0.9	14.7	6.7
Triglycerides	(> 1500 mg/dl)	1	2.8	—	10.1	0.2
Triglycerides fasting	(> 1500 mg/dl)	2.1	1.4	—	7.9	0.4
CPK	(> 1000 IU/L)	7	7.5	7.1	8.6	4.5
Hematology values	low					
Hematocrit	(< 30%)	2	—	—	11.7	16
RBC	(< 3 x 10^{12}/L)	1	—	1.7	14.9	19.7
WBC	(< 2.5 x 10^9/L)	—	—	3.5	25.1	51.4
Neutrophils	(≤ 0.5 x 10^9/L)	—	—	—	4	6.9

— Indicates no events reported.

Drug Interactions:

Drugs that may affect ritonavir include clarithromycin, didanosine, fluconazole, fluoxetine and rifampin.

Drugs that may be affected by ritonavir include clarithromycin, didanosine, desipramine, disulfiram, metronidazole, ethinyl estradiol, narcotic analgesics, rifabutin, saquinavir, sulfamethoxazole, theophylline, trimethoprim and zidovudine.

Agents Whose AUCs May be Increased by Ritonavir		
Alpha blockers	Antimalarials	Erythromycin
Antiarrhythmatics	Antineoplastics	Immunosuppressants
Antidepressants	Beta blockers	Methylphenidiate
Antiemetics	Calcium blockers	Pentoxifylline
Antifungals	Cimetidine	Phenothiazines
Antihyperlipidemics	Corticosteroids	Warfarin

Agents Whose AUCs May be Decreased by Ritonavir	
Atovaquone	Diphenoxylate
Clofibrate	Metoclopramide
Daunorubicin	Sedatives/Hypnotics

Drug/Food interactions: When the oral solution was given under non-fasting conditions, peak ritonavir concentrations decreased 23% and extent of absorption decreased 7% relative to fasting conditions. Extent of absorption of ritonavir from the capsule was 15% higher when given with a meal relative to fasting conditions. If possible, take ritonavir with meals.

Adverse Reactions:

The most frequent clinical adverse events, other than asthenia, among patients receiving ritonavir were GI and neurological disturbances including nausea, diarrhea, vomiting, anorexia, abdominal pain, taste perversion and circumoral and peripheral paresthesias.

Administration and Dosage:

The recommended dosage is 600 mg twice daily. If possible, take with food. Some patients experience nausea upon initiation of 600 mg twice daily dosing; dose escalation may provide some relief: 300 mg twice daily for 1 day, 400 mg twice daily for 2 days, 500 mg twice daily for 1 day and then 600 mg twice daily thereafter. In addition, patients initiating combination regimens with ritonavir and nucleosides may improve GI tolerance by initiating ritonavir alone and subsequently adding nucleosides before completing 2 weeks of ritonavir monotherapy.

INDINAVIR SULFATE

Capsules: 200 and 400 mg (*Rx*)	*Crixivan* (Merck)

Warning:

Indinavir is indicated for the treatment of HIV infection in adults when antiretroviral therapy is warranted. This indication is based on analyses of surrogate endpoints in studies of up to 24 weeks in duration. At present, there are no results from controlled clinical trials evaluating the effect of therapy with indinavir on clinical progression of HIV infection, such as survival or the incidence of opportunistic infections.

Actions:

Pharmacology: Indinavir is an inhibitor of the HIV protease. HIV protease is an enzyme required for the proteolytic cleavage of the viral polyprotein precursors into the individual functional proteins found in infectious HIV. Indinavir binds to the protease active site and inhibits the activity of the enzyme. This inhibition prevents cleavage of the viral polyproteins resulting in the formation of immature noninfectious viral particles. The relationship between in vitro susceptibility of HIV to indinavir and inhibition of HIV replication in humans has not been established.

Drug resistance – Isolates of HIV with reduced susceptibility to the drug have been recovered from some patients treated with indinavir.

Cross-resistance between indinavir and HIV reverse transcriptase inhibitors is unlikely because the enzyme targets involved are different. Cross-resistance was noted between indinavir and the protease inhibitor ritonavir. Varying degrees of cross-resistance have been observed between indinavir and other HIV-protease inhibitors.

Pharmacokinetics:

Absorption – Indinavir was rapidly absorbed in the fasted state with a time to peak plasma concentration (T_{max}) of 0.8 hours. A greater than dose-proportional increase in indinavir plasma concentrations was observed over the 200 to 1000 mg dose range. At a dosing regimen of 800 mg every 8 hours, steady-state AUC was 30,691 nM•hour, C_{max} was 12,617 nM and plasma concentration 8 hours post-dose (trough) was 251 nM.

Distribution – Indinavir was ≈ 60% bound to human plasma proteins over a concentration range of 81 to 16,300 nM.

Metabolism – Following a 400 mg dose of ^{14}C-indinavir, 83% and 19% of the total radioactivity was recovered in feces and urine, respectively; radioactivity due to parent drug in feces and urine was 19.1% and 9.4%, respectively. Seven metabolites have been identified, one glucuronide conjugate and six oxidative metabolites. In vitro studies indicate that cytochrome P450 3A4 (CYP3A4) is the major enzyme responsible for formation of the oxidative metabolites.

Excretion – Indinavir is excreted (< 20%) unchanged in the urine. Mean urinary excretion of unchanged drug was 10.4% and 12% following a single 700 and 1000 mg dose, respectively. Indinavir was rapidly eliminated with a half-life of 1.8 hours. Significant accumulation was not observed after multiple dosing at 800 mg every 8 hours.

Indications:

HIV infection: Treatment of HIV infection in adults when antiretroviral therapy is warranted.

Contraindications:

Hypersensitivity to any component of the product.

Warnings:

Concomitant agents: Do not administer indinavir concurrently with terfenadine, astemizole, cisapride, triazolam and midazolam because competition for CYP3A4 by indinavir could result in inhibition of the metabolism of these drugs and create the potential for serious or life-threatening events.

Renal function impairment: Nephrolithiasis, including flank pain with or without hematuria (including microscopic hematuria), has been reported in ≈ 4% of patients. In general, these events were not associated with renal dysfunction and resolved with hydration and temporary interruption of therapy (eg, 1 to 3 days). Following the acute episode, 9.2% of patients discontinued therapy.

To ensure adequate hydration, it is recommended that the patient drink at least 1.5 liters (≈ 48 ounces) of liquids during the course of 24 hours.

Hepatic function impairment: Patients with mild to moderate hepatic insufficiency and clinical evidence of cirrhosis had evidence of decreased metabolism of indinavir resulting in ≈ 60% higher mean AUC following a single 400 mg dose. The half-life increased to 2.8 hours.

Pregnancy: Category C.

Lactation: Although it is not known whether indinavir is excreted in breast milk, there exists the potential for adverse effects from indinavir in nursing infants. Instruct mothers to discontinue nursing if they are receiving indinavir. This is consistent with the recommendation by the CDC that HIV-infected mothers not breastfeed their infants to avoid risking postnatal transmission of HIV.

Children: Safety and efficacy have not been established.

Precautions:

Hyperbilirubinemia: Asymptomatic hyperbilirubinemia (total bilirubin ≥ 2.5 mg/dl), reported predominantly as elevated indirect bilirubin, has occurred in ≈ 10% of patients. In < 1%, this was associated with elevations in ALT or AST.

Drug Interactions:

Drugs that may affect indinavir include clarithromycin, didanosine, fluconazole, ketoconazole, quinidine, rifampin, rifabutin and zidovudine.

Drugs that may be affected by indinavir include astemizole, cisapride, midazolam, terfenadine, triazolam, clarithromycin, isoniazid, lamivudine, oral contraceptives, rifabutin, stavudine, TMP-SMZ and zidovudine.

Drug/Food interactions: Administration of indinavir with a meal high in calories, fat and protein (784 kcal, 48.6 g fat, 31.3 g protein) resulted in a 77% reduction in AUC and an 84% reduction in C_{max}. Administration with lighter meals resulted in little or no change in AUC, C_{max} or trough concentration. A single 400 mg dose of indinavir with 8 oz of grapefruit juice resulted in a decrease in indinavir AUC (26%).

Adverse Reactions:

Adverse reactions occurring in ≥ 3% of patients include: Abdominal pain; asthenia/fatigue; nausea; diarrhea; vomiting; headache; insomnia.

Indinavir vs Zidovudine: Selected Lab Test Abnormalities (%)

Lab test abnormalities	Indinavir (n = 196)	Indinavir + zidovudine (n = 196)	Zidovudine (n = 195)
Hematology			
Decreased hemoglobin < 8 g/dl	0.5	1.1	0.5
Decreased platelet count <50 THS/mm ^{3}	0.5	0.5	0
Decreased neutrophil < 0.75 THS/mm ^{3}	1.1	1.6	3.8
Blood chemistry			
Increased ALT > 500% ULN [1]	3.1	3.2	2.1
Increased AST > 500% ULN	2.1	2.1	1.1
Total serum bilirubin > 2.5 mg/dl	7.8	7.4	0.5
Increased serum amylase > 200% ULN	1	2.1	0.5

[1] Upper limit of the normal range.

Administration and Dosage:

The recommended dosage is 800 mg (two 400 mg capsules) orally every 8 hours. The dosage is the same whether indinavir is used alone or in combination with other antiretroviral agents. The antiretroviral activity of indinavir may be increased when used in combination with approved reverse transcriptase inhibitors.

Administer at intervals of 8 hours. For optimal absorption, administer without food but with water 1 hour before or 2 hours after a meal or administer with other liquids such as skim milk, juice, coffee or tea, or with a light meal (eg, dry toast with jelly, juice and coffee with skim milk and sugar; or corn flakes, skim milk and sugar).

If indinavir and didanosine are administered concomitantly, they should be administered at least 1 hour apart on an empty stomach.

In addition to adequate hydration, medical management in patients who experience nephrolithiasis may include temporary interruption of therapy (eg, 1 to 3 days) during the acute episode of nephrolithiasis or therapy discontinuation.

Cirrhosis: Reduce the dosage of indinavir to 600 mg every 8 hours in patients with mild-to-moderate hepatic insufficiency due to cirrhosis.

ZIDOVUDINE (Azidothymidine; AZT; Compound S)

Capsules: 100 mg (*Rx*) — *Retrovir* (Glaxo Wellcome)
Syrup: 50 mg/5 ml (*Rx*)
Injection: 10 mg/ml (*Rx*)

Warning:

Zidovudine may be associated with hematologic toxicity including granulocytopenia and severe anemia particularly in patients with advanced human immunodeficiency (HIV) disease. Prolonged use of zidovudine has been associated with symptomatic myopathy similar to that produced by HIV.

Rare occurrences of lactic acidosis in the absence of hypoxemia, and severe hepatomegaly with steatosis have occurred with antiretroviral nucleoside analogs, including zidovudine and zalcitabine, and are potentially fatal.

Actions:

Pharmacology: Zidovudine is a thymidine analog and an inhibitor of the in vitro replication of some retroviruses, including HIV. Cellular thymidine kinase converts zidovudine into zidovudine monophosphate and finally to the triphosphate derivative by other cellular enzymes. Zidovudine triphosphate interferes with the HIV viral RNA-dependent DNA polymerase (reverse transcriptase) and inhibits viral replication. It also inhibits cellular α-DNA polymerase, but at concentrations 100-fold higher than those required to inhibit reverse transcriptase. In vitro, zidovudine triphosphate is incorporated into growing chains of DNA by viral reverse transcriptase, and the DNA chain is terminated.

Pharmacokinetics:

Absorption/Distribution – Overall, the pharmacokinetics in pediatric patients > 3 months of age are similar to that in adults. Zidovudine is rapidly absorbed from the GI tract with peak serum concentrations occurring within 0.5 to 1.5 hours. As a result of first-pass metabolism, the average oral capsule bioavailability is 65% (range, 52% to 75%). The rate of absorption of the syrup is greater than that of the capsules. Dose-dependent kinetics were observed over the range of 2 mg/kg every 8 hours to 10 mg/kg every 4 hours. Zidovudine plasma protein binding is 34% to 38%. Mean steady-state predose and 1.5 hours post-dose concentrations were 0.16 mcg/ml (range, 0 to 0.84 mcg/ml) and 0.62 mcg/ml (range, 0.05 to 1.46 mcg/ml), respectively, following chronic oral use of 250 mg every 4 hours (n=21; 3 to 5.4 mg/kg).

Metabolism/Excretion – Zidovudine is rapidly metabolized in the liver to an inactive metabolite which has an apparent elimination half-life of 1 hr (range, 0.61 to 1.73). The mean zidovudine half-life was ≈ 1 hr (range, 0.78 to 1.93). Urinary recovery of zidovudine and its metabolite was 14% and 74% of an oral dose, respectively, and the total urinary recovery averaged 90% (range, 63% to 95%).

Following IV dosing (1 to 5 mg/kg) total body clearance averaged 1900 ml/min/70 kg and the apparent volume of distribution was 1.6 L/kg. Renal clearance is ≈ 400 ml/min/70 kg, indicating glomerular filtration and active tubular secretion by the kidneys. The zidovudine CSF/plasma concentration ratios measured at 2 to 4 hours following IV dosing of 2.5 and 5 mg/kg were 0.2 and 0.64, respectively.

Indications:

Oral:

Monotherapy –

Adults: Initial treatment of HIV-infected adults with CD4 cell count ≤ 500/mm^3. Monotherapy with zidovudine was found to be clinically superior to didanosine or zalcitabine monotherapy for the initial management of HIV-infected patients who have not received previous antiretroviral treatment. However, for some patients with advanced disease on prolonged zidovudine therapy, modifying the antiviral regimen may be more effective in delaying disease progression than remaining on zidovudine monotherapy.

Children: For HIV-infected children > 3 months of age who have HIV-related symptoms or who are asymptomatic with abnormal laboratory values indicating significant HIV-related immunosuppression.

Maternal-Fetal HIV transmission: Prevention of maternal-fetal HIV transmission as part of a regimen that includes oral zidovudine beginning between 14 and 34 weeks of gestation, IV zidovudine during labor, and zidovudine syrup to the newborn after birth. However, transmission to infants may still occur in some cases despite the use of this regimen.

Combination therapy with zalcitabine – Treatment of selected patients with advanced HIV disease (CD4 cell count ≤ 300 cells/mm^3). In patients without prior exposure to zidovudine, this indication is based on greater increases in CD4 cell counts that were maintained longer for patients treated with combination therapy vs monotherapy with zidovudine.

IV: For the management of certain adult patients with symptomatic HIV infection (AIDS and advanced ARC) who have a history of cytologically confirmed *Pneumocystis carinii* pneumonia (PCP) or an absolute CD4 lymphocyte count of < 200/mm^3 in the peripheral blood before therapy is begun.

Contraindications:

Life-threatening allergic reactions to any of the components of the product.

Warnings:

Hematologic effects: Use with extreme caution in patients who have bone marrow compromise evidenced by granulocyte count < 1000/mm^3 or hemoglobin < 9.5 g/dl. Anemia and granulocytopenia are the most significant adverse events observed. Reversible pancytopenia has been reported.

Myopathy and myositis with pathological changes, similar to that produced by HIV disease, have been associated with prolonged use of zidovudine.

Lactic acidosis/severe hepatomegaly with steatosis: Rare occurrences of lactic acidosis in the absence of hypoxemia, and severe hepatomegaly with steatosis have been reported with the use of antiretroviral nucleoside analogs, including zidovudine and zalcitabine, and are potentially fatal.

Combination therapy: No benefit from combination therapy with zalcitabine has been observed in a study of patients with extensive prior exposure to zidovudine (median 18 months) and CD4 cell counts < 150 cells/mm^3; combination therapy is therefore not recommended for these patients.

Hypersensitivity: Sensitization reactions, including anaphylaxis in one patient, have occurred with zidovudine therapy. Patients experiencing a rash should undergo medical evaluation.

Renal/Hepatic function impairment: Zidovudine is eliminated from the body primarily by renal excretion following metabolism in the liver (glucuronidation). In patients with severely impaired renal function, dosage reduction is recommended. Although very little data are available, patients with severely impaired hepatic function may be at greater risk of toxicity.

Carcinogenesis/Mutagenesis: In cultured human lymphocytes, zidovudine caused dose-related structural chromosomal abnormalities at concentrations ≥ 3 mcg/ml.

Pregnancy: Category C.

Lactation: It is not known whether zidovudine is excreted in breast milk or whether zidovudine reduces the potential for transmission of HIV in breast milk. The US Public Health Centers for Disease Control and Prevention advises HIV-infected women not to breastfeed to avoid postnatal transmission of HIV to a child who may not yet be infected.

Children: A positive test for HIV-antibody in children < 15 months of age may represent passively acquired maternal antibodies, rather than an active antibody response to infection in the infant. Thus, the presence of HIV-antibody in a child < 15 months of age must be interpreted with caution, especially in the asymptomatic infant. Pursue confirmatory tests such as serum P_{24} antigen or viral culture in such children.

Drug Interactions:

Drugs that may affect zidovudine include acetaminophen, bone marrow, suppressive/cytotoxic agents (eg, adriamycin, dapsone), fluconazole, ganciclovir, interferon alfa, interferon beta-1b, nucleoside analogs, probenecid, rifamycins, trimethoprim and phenytoin.

Drugs that may be affected by zidovudine include acyclovir and phenytoin.

Drug/Food interactions: Administration of capsules with food decreased peak plasma concentrations by > 50%; however, bioavailability as determined by AUC may not be affected.

Adverse Reactions:

The most frequent adverse events and abnormal laboratory values reported in the placebo controlled clinical trial of oral zidovudine were granulocytopenia and anemia. Several serious adverse reactions have been reported in clinical practice. Myopathy and myositis with pathological changes, similar to these produced by HIV disease, have been associated with prolonged use. Reports of hepatomegaly with steatosis, hepatitis, pancreatitis, lactic acidosis, sensitization reactions (including anaphylaxis in one patient), hyperbilirubinemia, vasculitis and seizures have been rare. A single case of macular edema has been reported.

Adverse reactions occurring in ≥ 3% of patients include: Asthenia; diaphoresis; fever; headache; malaise; dizziness; insomnia; paresthesia; somnolence; anorexia; diarrhea; dyspepsia; GI pain; nausea; vomiting; dyspnea; myalgia; rash; taste perversion.

Administration and Dosage:

Oral:

Monotherapy –

Adults:

Symptomatic HIV infection (including AIDS) – 100 mg (one 100 mg capsule or 2 teaspoonfuls [10 ml] syrup) every 4 hours (600 mg daily dose). The effectiveness of this dose compared to higher dosing regimens in improving neurologic dysfunction associated with HIV disease is unknown. A small study found a greater effect of higher doses on improvement of neurological symptoms in patients with preexisting neurological disease.

Asymptomatic HIV infection – 100 mg every 4 hours while awake (500 mg/day).

Children (3 months to 12 years): The recommended starting dose is 180 mg/m^2 every 6 hours (720 mg/m^2/day), not to exceed 200 mg every 6 hours.

Maternal-Fetal HIV transmission:

Maternal dosing (> 14 weeks of pregnancy) – 100 mg orally 5 times per day until the start of labor. During labor and delivery, administer IV zidovudine at 2 mg/kg over 1 hour followed by a continuous IV infusion of 1 mg/kg/hr until clamping of the umbilical cord.

Infant dosing – 2 mg/kg orally every 6 hours starting within 12 hours after birth and continuing through 6 weeks of age. Infants unable to receive oral dosing may be given zidovudine IV at 1.5 mg/kg, infused over 30 minutes, every 6 hours.

Combination therapy with zalcitabine – Zidovudine 200 mg orally with zalcitabine 0.75 mg every 8 hours.

Monitor hematologic indices every 2 weeks to detect serious anemia or granulocytopenia. In patients with hematologic toxicity, reduction in hemoglobin may occur as early as 2 to 4 weeks, and granulocytopenia usually occurs after 6 to 8 weeks. Hematologic toxicities appear to be related to pretreatment bone marrow reserve and to dose and duration of therapy.

Dose adjustment – Significant anemia (hemoglobin of < 7.5 g/dl or reduction of > 25% of baseline) or significant granulocytopenia (granulocyte count of < 750/mm^3 or reduction of > 50% from baseline) may require a dose interruption until evidence of marrow recovery is observed. For less severe anemia or granulocytopenia, dose reduction may be adequate. In patients who develop significant anemia, dose modification does not necessarily eliminate the need for transfusion. If marrow recovery occurs following dose modification, gradual increases in dose may be appropriate depending on hematologic indices and patient tolerance.

Renal function impairment: In end-stage renal disease patients maintained on hemodialysis or peritoneal dialysis, recommended dosing is 100 mg every 6 to 8 hours.

IV: 1 to 2 mg/kg infused over 1 hour at a constant rate; administer every 4 hours around the clock (6 times daily). Avoid rapid infusion or bolus injection. Do not give IM. Patients should receive the IV infusion only until oral therapy can be administered. The IV dosing regimen equivalent to the oral administration of 100 mg every 4 hours is ≈ 1 mg/kg IV every 4 hours.

LAMIVUDINE (3TC)

Tablets: 150 mg (*Rx*)	*Epivir* (Glaxo Wellcome)
Oral Solution: 10 mg/ml (*Rx*)	

Warning:

Lamivudine is indicated for use in combination with zidovudine (AZT) for the treatment of HIV infection when antiretroviral therapy is warranted based on clinical or immunological evidence of disease progression. This indication is based on analyses of surrogate endpoints. At present, there are no results from controlled clinical trials evaluating the effect of therapy with lamivudine plus zidovudine on the clinical progression of HIV infection, such as the incidence of opportunistic infections or survival.

Patients receiving lamivudine plus AZT may continue to develop opportunistic infections and other complications of HIV infection, and should remain under close observation by physicians experienced in treating HIV-associated diseases.

Actions:

Pharmacology: Lamivudine is a synthetic nucleoside analog with activity against HIV. In vitro, lamivudine is phosphorylated to its active 5'-triphosphate metabolite (L-TP), which has an intracellular half-life of 10.5 to 15.5 hours. The principal mode of action of L-TP is inhibition of HIV reverse transcription via viral DNA chain termination. L-TP also inhibits the RNA- and DNA-dependent DNA polymerase activities of reverse transcriptase.

Pharmacokinetics:

Absorption/Distribution – Absolute bioavailability in 12 adult HIV-infected patients was 86% for the tablet and 87% for the oral solution. After oral administration of 2 mg/kg twice a day to nine adults with HIV, C_{max} was 1.5 mcg/ml. The area under the plasma concentration vs time curve (AUC) and C_{max} increased in proportion to oral dose over the range from 0.25 to 10 mg/kg.

The apparent volume of distribution after IV administration to 20 patients was 1.3 L/kg, suggesting that lamivudine distributes into extravascular spaces. Volume of distribution was independent of dose and did not correlate with body weight. Binding of lamivudine to human plasma proteins is < 36%. In vitro, over the concentration range of 0.1 to 100 pg/ml, the amount of lamivudine associated with erythrocytes ranged from 53% to 57% and was independent of concentration.

Children: Lamivudine pharmacokinetics after monotherapy were assessed after 1, 2, 4, 8, 12 and 20 mg/kg/day. In the nine infants and children receiving 8 mg/kg/day, absolute bioavailability was 66% (86% observed in adolescents and adults). The mechanism for this diminished absolute bioavailability in infants and children is unknown. Systemic clearance decreased with increasing age in pediatric patients.

After oral administration of 8 mg/kg/day to 11 pediatric patients ranging from 4 months to 14 years of age, C_{max} was 1.1 mcg/ml and half-life was 2 hours (in adults with similar blood sampling, the half-life was 3.7 hours). Total exposure to lamivudine, as reflected by mean AUC values, was comparable between pediatric patients receiving an 8 mg/kg/day dose and adults receiving a 4 mg/kg/day dose.

Metabolism – Metabolism of lamivudine is a minor route of elimination. The only known metabolite of lamivudine is the trans-sulfoxide metabolite. Within 12 hours after a single oral dose of lamivudine in six HIV-infected adults, 5.2% of the dose was excreted as the trans-sulfoxide metabolite in the urine. Serum concentrations of this metabolite have not been determined.

Excretion – The majority is eliminated unchanged in urine. In 20 patients given a single IV dose, renal clearance was 0.22 L/hr•kg, representing 71% of total clearance. In most single dose studies, the observed mean elimination half-life ranged from 5 to 7 hours. Total clearance was 0.37 L/hr•kg. Oral clearance and elimination half-life were independent of dose and body weight from 0.25 to 10 mg/kg.

Renal function impairment:

Lamivudine Pharmacokinetics in Renal Function Impairment (Single 300 mg Oral Dose)

Parameter	Creatinine clearance criterion		
	> 60 ml/min (n = 6)	10 to 30 ml/min (n = 4)	< 10 ml/min (n = 6)
Creatinine clearance (ml/min)	111	28	6
C_{max} (mcg/ml)	2.6	3.6	5.8
AUC (mcg·h/ml)	11	48	157
Cl/F (ml/min)	464	114	36

Exposure (AUC), C_{max} and half-life increased with diminishing renal function (as expressed by Ccr). Apparent total oral clearance (Cl/F) of lamivudine decreased as Ccr decreased. T_{max} was not significantly affected by renal function. Based on these observations, it is recommended that the dosage of lamivudine be modified in patients with renal impairment. The effects of renal impairment on lamivudine pharmacokinetics in pediatric patients are not known.

Indications:

HIV infection: Lamivudine in combination with zidovudine is indicated for the treatment of HIV infection when therapy is warranted based on clinical or immunological evidence of disease progression. At present, there are no results from controlled trials evaluating the effect of lamivudine plus zidovudine on clinical progression of HIV infection, such as the incidence of opportunistic infections or survival.

Contraindications:

Hypersensitivity to any of the components of the products.

Warnings:

Pregnancy: Category C.

Antiretroviral pregnancy registry – To monitor maternal-fetal outcomes of pregnant women exposed to lamivudine, an Antiretroviral Pregnancy Registry has been established. Physicians are encouraged to register patients by calling (800) 722-9292, ext 58465.

Lactation: Although it is not known if lamivudine is excreted in breast milk, there is the potential for adverse effects from lamivudine in nursing infants. Instruct mothers to discontinue nursing if they are receiving lamivudine.

Children: There are no data on the use of lamivudine in combination with zidovudine in pediatric patients.

Pancreatitis – In children with a history of pancreatitis or other significant risk factors for development of pancreatitis, use the combination of lamivudine and zidovudine with extreme caution and only if there is no satisfactory alternative therapy. Stop treatment with lamivudine immediately if clinical signs, symptoms or laboratory abnormalities suggestive of pancreatitis occur.

Drug Interactions:

Drugs that may interact with lamivudine include zidovudine and trimethoprim- sulfamethoxazole.

Drug/Food interactions: An investigational 25 mg dosage form of lamivudine was given orally to 12 asymptomatic HIV-infected patients on two occasions, once in the fasted state and once with food (1099 kcal; 75 g fat, 34 g protein, 72 g carbohydrate). Lamivudine may be administered with or without food.

Adverse Reactions:

Adverse reactions occurring in ≥ 3% of patients include: Headache; malaise and fatigue; fever or chills; skin rashes; nausea; diarrhea; nausea and vomiting; anorexia or decreased appetite; abdominal pain; abdominal cramps; dyspepsia; neuropathy; insomnia and other sleep disorders; dizziness; depressive disorders; nasal signs and symptoms; cough; musculoskeletal pain; myalgia; arthralgia; neutropenia; amylase; elevated ALT.

Children: Limited information on the incidence of adverse events in children receiving monotherapy is available from one open-label uncontrolled study. Of 97 patients, 14% developed pancreatitis while receiving monotherapy.

Paresthesias and peripheral neuropathies were reported in 13 patients (13%) and resulted in treatment discontinuation in 3 patients.

Selected Laboratory Abnormalities in Pediatric Patients (%; n = 97)		
Test (abnormal level)	Patients with normal baselines	Patients with abnormal baselines
Neutropenia (ANC < 750/mm^3)	22	45
Anemia (Hgb < 8 g/dl)	2	24
Thrombocytopenia (platelets < 40,000/mm^3)	0	25
ALT (> 5 x ULN)	4	29
AST (> 5 x ULN)	0	19
Amylase (> 2 ULN)	3	23

Administration and Dosage:

Adults and adolescents (12 to 16 years of age): The recommended dose is 150 mg twice daily in combination with zidovudine. Consult the complete prescribing information for zidovudine for information on its dosage and administration.

For adults with low body weights (< 50 kg; < 110 lbs), the recommended dose is 2 mg/kg twice daily in combination with zidovudine. No data are available to support a dosage recommendation for adolescents with low body weight (< 50 kg).

Children (3 months to 12 years of age): The recommended dose is 4 mg/kg twice daily (up to a maximum of 150 mg twice a day) administered with zidovudine.

Renal function impairment: It is recommended that doses of lamivudine be adjusted in accordance with renal function in patients > 16 years of age.

Adjustment of Lamivudine Dosage in Patients with Renal Function Impairment	
Creatinine clearance (ml/min)	Recommended lamivudine dosage
≥50	150 mg twice daily
30 - 49	150 mg once daily
15 - 29	150 mg first dose, then 100 mg once daily
5 - 14	150 mg first dose, then 50 mg once daily
< 5	50 mg first dose, then 25 mg once daily

Insufficient data are available to recommend a dosage in dialysis.

SAQUINAVIR MESYLATE

Capsules: 200 mg (*Rx*)	*Invirase* (Roche)

Warning:

The indication for saquinavir for the treatment of HIV infection is based on changes in surrogate markers. At present, there are no results from controlled clinical trials evaluating the effect of regimens containing saquinavir on patient survival or the clinical progression of HIV infection, such as the occurrence of opportunistic infections or malignancies.

Actions:

Pharmacology: Saquinavir is an inhibitor of HIV protease which cleaves viral polyprotein precursors to generate functional proteins in HIV-infected cells. The cleavage of viral polyprotein precursors is essential for maturation of infectious virus. Saquinavir is a synthetic peptide-like substrate analog that inhibits the activity of HIV protease and prevents the cleavage of viral polyproteins.

Pharmacokinetics:

Absorption – Following multiple dosing (600 mg 3 times daily) in HIV-infected patients, the steady-state AUC was 2.5 times higher than that observed after a single dose. HIV-infected patients administered saquinavir 600 mg 3 times daily, after a meal or substantial snack, had AUC C_{max} values which were about twice those observed in healthy volunteers receiving the same treatment regimen.

Distribution – The mean steady-state volume of distribution following IV administration of a 12 mg dose was 700 L, suggesting saquinavir partitions into tissues. Saquinavir was ≈ 98% bound to plasma proteins over a concentration range of 15 to 700 ng/ml. In two patients receiving saquinavir 600 mg 3 times daily, CSF concentrations were negligible.

Metabolism/Excretion – In vitro, the metabolism of saquinavir is cytochrome P450 mediated with specific isoenzyme, CYP3A4, responsible for > 90% of the hepatic metabolism. In vitro, saquinavir is rapidly metabolized to a range of mono- and di-hydroxylated inactive compounds; 88% and 1% of the orally administered dose was recovered in feces and urine, respectively, within 48 hours of dosing; 81% and 3% of an IV dose was recovered in feces and urine, respectively, within 48 hours of dosing. In mass balance studies, 13% of circulating radioactivity in plasma was attributed to unchanged drug after oral administration and the remainder attributed to saquinavir metabolites. Following IV administration, 66% of ciculating radioactivity was attributed to unchanged drug and the remainder attributed to saquinavir metabolites, suggesting that saquinavir undergoes extensive first-pass metabolism.

Systemic clearance of saquinavir was rapid, 1.14 L/hr/kg after IV doses of 6, 36 and 72 mg. The mean residence time of saquinavir was 7 hours.

Indications:

HIV infection: In combination with nucleoside analogs for the treatment of advanced HIV infection in selected patients. This indication is based on changes in surrogate markers in patients who initiated saquinavir concomitantly with either AZT (in previously untreated patients) or ddC (in patients previously treated with prolonged zidovudine therapy). At present, no results are available from trials evaluating the activity of saquinavir in combination with nucleoside analogs other than AZT of ddC. There are no results available from clinical trials confirming the clinical benefit of combination therapy with saquinavir on HIV disease progression or survival.

Contraindications:

Clinically significant hypersensitivity to saquinavir or to any of the components in the capsule.

Photosensitization (photoallergy or phototoxicity) may occur; therefore, caution patients to take protective measures against exposure to ultraviolet or sunlight (ie, sunscreens, protective clothing) until tolerance is determined.

Warnings:

Hepatic function impairment: Exercise caution when administering saquinavir to patients with hepatic insufficiency because patients with baseline liver function tests > 5 times the normal upper limit were not included in clinical studies.

Pregnancy: Category B.

Lactation: It is not known whether saquinavir is excreted in breast milk. Because of the potential for serious adverse reactions in nursing infants from saquinavir, decide whether to discontinue nursing or discontinue the drug, taking into account the importance of saquinavir to the mother.

Children: Safety and efficacy in HIV-infected children or adolescents < 16 years of age have not been established.

Precautions:

Monitoring: Perform clinical chemistry tests prior to initiating saquinavir therapy and at appropriate intervals thereafter

Toxicity: If a serious or severe toxicity occurs during treatment with saquinavir, interrupt therapy until the etiology of the event is identified or the toxicity resolves. At the time, resumption of treatment with full dose saquinavir may be considered.

Drug Interactions:

Drugs that may interact with saquinavir include ketoconazole and rifamycins.

Other drugs that induce CYP3A4 (eg, phenobarbital, phenytoin, dexamethasone, carbamazepine) may reduce saquinavir plasma concentrations.

Coadministration of terfenadine or astemizole with drugs that are known to be potent inhibitors of the cytochrome P450–3A pathway (eg, ketoconazole, itraconazole) may lead to elevated plasma concentrations of terfenadine or astemizole, which may in turn prolong QT intervals leading to rare cases of serious cardiovascular adverse events. Other compounds that are substrates of CYP3A4 (eg, calcium channel blockers, clindamycin, dapsone, quinidine, triazolam) may have elevated plasma concentrations when coadministered with saquinavir; therefore, monitor patients for toxicities associated with such drugs.

Drug/Food interactions: Absolute bioavailability averaged 4% in eight healthy volunteers who received a single 600 mg dose following a high fat breakfast. The low bioavailability may be due to a combination of incomplete absorption and extensive first-pass metabolism. The mean 24 hour AUC after a single 600 mg oral dose in healthy volunteers was increased from 24 (under fasting conditions) to 161 ng•hr/ml when saquinavir was given following a high fat breakfast. Saquinavir 24 hour AUC and C_{max} following the administration of a higher calorie meal (943 kcal, 54 g fat) were on average two times higher than after a lower calorie, lower fat meal. The effect of food persists for up to 2 hours.

Adverse Reactions:

Adverse reactions occurring in ≥ 3% of patients include: Diarrhea, abdominal discomfort; nausea; buccal mucosa ulceration; paresthesia; peripheral neuropathy; asthenia; rash; lab test abnormalities of creatine phosphokinase, glucose (low), AST, ALT and neutrophils (low).

Administration and Dosage:

The recommended dose for saquinavir in combination with a nucleoside analog is three 200 mg capsules 3 times daily taken within 2 hours after a full meal. The recommended doses of ddC of AZT as part of combination therapy are: ddC 0.75 mg 3 times daily, or AZT 200 mg 3 times daily as appropriate.

Dose adjustment for combination therapy with saquinavir: For toxicities that may be associated with saquinavir, interrupt the drug. Saquinavir at doses < 600 mg 3 times daily are not recommended since lower doses have not shown antiviral activity. For recipients of combination therapy with saquinavir and nucleoside analogs, dose adjustment of the nucleoside analog should be based on the known toxicity profile of the individual drug.

NEVIRAPINE

Tablets: 200 mg (*Rx*)	*Viramune* (Roxane)

Warning:

The duration of benefit from antiretroviral therapy may be limited. Consider alteration of antiretroviral therapies if disease progression occurs while patients are receiving nevirapine.

Resistant HIV virus emerges rapidly and uniformly when nevirapine is administered as monotherapy. Therefore, always administer nevirapine in combination with at least one additional antiretroviral agent.

Nevirapine has been associated with severe rash, which in some cases, has been life-threatening. When severe rash occurs, discontinue nevirapine.

Actions:

Pharmacology: Nevirapine is a non-nucleoside reverse transcriptase inhibitor (NNRTI) with activity against human immunodeficiency virus type 1 (HIV-1).

Nevirapine binds directly to reverse transcriptase (RT) and blocks the RNA-dependent and DNA-dependent DNA polymerase activities by causing a disruption of the enzyme's catalytic site. The activity of nevirapine does not compete with template or nucleoside triphosphates. HIV-2 RT and eukaryotic DNA polymerases are not inhibited by nevirapine.

Pharmacokinetics:

Absorption – Nevirapine is readily absorbed (> 90%) after oral administration. Peak plasma nevirapine concentrations of 2 mcg/ml (7.5 µM) were attained within 4 hours following a single 200 mg dose. Following multiple doses, nevirapine peak concentrations appear to increase linearly in the dose range of 200 to 400 mg/day. Steady-state trough nevirapine concentrations of 4.5 mcg/ml were attained at 400 mg/day.

Distribution – Nevirapine is highly lipophilic and is essentially nonionized at physiologic pH. Following IV administration to healthy adults, the volume of distribution of nevirapine was 1.21 L/kg, suggesting that nevirapine is widely distributed in humans.

Metabolism/Excretion – Nevirapine is extensively biotransformed via cytochrome P450 (oxidative) metabolism to several hydroxylated metabolites.

Nevirapine has been shown to be an inducer of hepatic cytochrome P450 metabolic enzymes. The pharmacokinetics of autoinduction are characterized by an ≈ 1.5- to 2-fold increase in the apparent oral clearance of nevirapine as treatment continues from a single dose to 2 to 4 weeks of dosing with 200 to 400 mg/day. Autoinduction also results in a corresponding decrease in the terminal phase half-life of nevirapine in plasma from ≈ 45 hours (single dose) to ≈ 25 to 30 hours following multiple dosing with 200 to 400 mg/day.

Indications:

HIV-1 infection: In combination with nucleoside analogs for the treatment of HIV-1 infected adults who have experienced clinical and immunologic deterioration.

Contraindications:

Hypersensitivity to any of the components contained in the product.

Warnings:

Skin reactions: Severe and life-threatening skin reactions have occurred in patients treated with nevirapine including Stevens-Johnson syndrome (SJS). Discontinue nevirapine in patients developing a severe rash accompanied by constitutional symptoms such as fever, blistering, oral lesions, conjunctivitis, swelling muscle or joint aches or general malaise.

The majority of rashes associated with nevirapine occur within the first 6 weeks of initiation of therapy. Instruct patients not to increase the 200 mg/day dosage if any rash occurs during the 2–week lead-in dosing period until the rash resolves.

Rashes are usually mild to moderate, maculopapular, erythematous cutaneous eruptions with or without pruritus, located on the trunk, face and extremities.

Renal/Hepatic function impairment: Use with caution in these patient populations.

Hepatotoxicity – Abnormal liver function tests have been reported with nevirapine, some in the first few weeks of therapy, including cases of hepatitis. Interrupt administration in patients experiencing moderate or severe liver function test abnormalities until liver function tests return to baseline values. Discontinue treatment permanently if liver function abnormalities recur on readministration.

Pregnancy: Category C.

Lactation: Nevirapine readily crosses the placenta and is found in breast milk. Instruct patients receiving nevirapine to discontinue nursing.

Children: Safety and efficacy have not been established. Nevirapine is metabolized more rapidly in pediatric patients than in adults.

Precautions:

Monitoring: Perform clinical chemistry tests, which include liver function tests, prior to initiating nevirapine therapy and at appropriate intervals during therapy.

Drug Interactions:

Drugs that may affect nevirapine include rifampin and rifabutin.

Nevirapine may affect protease inhibitors and oral contraceptives.

Adverse Reactions:

The most frequent adverse events related to nevirapine therapy are rash, fever, nausea, headache and abnormal liver function tests. Others include: Diarrhea, abdominal pain, ulcerative stomatitis, peripheral neuropathy, paresthesia, myalgia and hepatits.

Lab test abnormalities: Decreased H_2, platelets and neutrophils. Increase ALT, AST, GGT and total bilirubin.

Administration and Dosage:

Initial therapy: 200 mg tablet daily for 14 days.

Maintenance: 200 mg tablet twice daily in combination with nucleoside analog antiretroviral agents. For concomitantly administered nucleoside therapy, the manufacturer's recommended dosage and monitoring should be followed.

Missed doses: Patients who interrupt nevirapine dosing for more than 7 days should restart the recommended dosing, using one 200 mg tablet daily for the first 14 days (lead-in), followed by one 200 mg twice daily.

RIBAVIRIN

Lyophilized powder for aerosol reconstitution: 6 g ribavirin/100 ml vial. Contains 20 mg/ml when reconstituted with 300 ml sterile water (*Rx*)	*Virazole* (ICN)

Warning:

In patients requiring mechanical ventilator assistance, pay strict attention to procedures that have been shown to minimize the accumulation of drug precipitate that can result in mechanical ventilator dysfunction and associated increased pulmonary pressures.

Deterioration of respiratory function has been associated with ribavirin use in infants, and in adults with chronic obstructive lung disease or asthma. Carefully monitor respiratory function during treatment. If ribavirin aerosol treatment produces sudden deterioration of respiratory function, stop treatment and reinstitute only with extreme caution and continuous monitoring.

Actions:

Pharmacology:

Antiviral effects – Ribavirin has antiviral inhibitory activity in vitro against respiratory syncytial virus (RSV), influenza virus and herpes simplex virus. The mechanism of action is unknown.

Immunologic effects – Neutralizing antibody responses to RSV were decreased in ribavirin-treated infants compared to placebo treated infants; clinical significance of this observation is unknown.

Pharmacokinetics:

Absorption – Ribavirin administered by aerosol is absorbed systemically. Four pediatric patients inhaling ribavirin aerosol by face mask for 2.5 hours each day for 3 days had plasma concentrations ranging from 0.44 to 1.55 μM (mean, 0.76 μM). The plasma half-life was 9.5 hours. Three pediatric patients inhaling ribavirin aerosol by face mask or mist tent for 20 hours/day for 5 days had plasma concentrations ranging from 1.5 to 14.3 μM (mean, 6.8 μM).

Distribution – Bioavailability of the aerosol is unknown and may depend on mode of delivery. After aerosol use, peak plasma concentrations are less than the concentration that reduced RSV plaque formation in tissue culture by 85% to 98%. Respiratory tract secretions are likely to contain ribavirin in concentrations many times higher than those required to reduce plaque formation. However, RSV is an intracellular virus and serum concentrations may better reflect intracellular concentrations in the respiratory tract than respiratory secretion concentrations.

Accumulation of drug or metabolites in red blood cells occurs, with plateauing in red cells in ≈ 4 days. Accumulation gradually declines with an apparent half-life of 40 days. Accumulation following inhalation is not well defined.

Indications:

Lower respiratory tract infection: Treatment of carefully selected hospitalized infants and young children with severe lower respiratory tract infections due to RSV.

Unlabeled uses: Aerosol ribavirin has shown some success against influenza A and B.

Oral ribavirin (600 mg to 1800 mg/day for 10 to 14 days) has been variously effective against other viral diseases including acute and chronic hepatitis, herpes genitalis, measles and Lassa fever.

Contraindications:

Hypersensitivity to the drug or its components.

Females who are, or who may become pregnant during exposure to the drug. Ribavirin may cause fetal harm and RSV infection is self-limited in this population. Although there are no pertinent human data, ribavirin has been found to be teratogenic (malformation of skull, palate, eye, jaw, limbs, skeleton and GI tract) or embryolethal in nearly all species in which it has been tested in dosages of 1 to 10 mg/kg.

Warnings:

Assisted ventilation: Some subjects requiring assisted ventilation have experienced serious difficulties because of inadequate ventilation and gas exchange. Drug precipitation within the ventilatory apparatus, including the endotracheal tube, has resulted in increased positive and expiratory pressure and increased positive inspiratory pressure. Accumulation of fluid in tubing ("rain out") has also been noted.

Respiratory function: Carefully monitor respiratory function during treatment. If ribavirin aerosol treatment produces sudden deterioration of respiratory function, stop treatment and reinstitute only with extreme caution, continuous monitoring and consideration of concomitant administration of bronchodilators.

Deaths: Deaths during or shortly after treatment with aerosolized ribavirin have been reported in 20 cases.

Anemia: Although anemia has not been reported with aerosol use, it occurs frequently with oral and IV ribavirin.

Carcinogenesis/Mutagenesis/Fertility impairment: Ribavirin induces cell transformation in an in vitro mammalian system. However, in vivo carcinogenicity studies are incomplete. Ribavirin causes testicular lesions (tubular atrophy) in adult rats at oral dose levels as low as 16 mg/kg/day, but fertility of ribavirn-treated animals is unknown.

Pregnancy: Category X.

Lactation: Use of ribavirin aerosol in nursing mothers is not indicated because RSV infection is self-limited in this population. Ribavirin is toxic to lactating animals and their offspring. It is not known whether the drug is excreted in breast milk.

Adverse Reactions:

Adverse reactions may include: Bacterial pneumonia; pneumothorax; apnea; ventilator dependence; cardiac arrest; hypotension; digitalis toxicity; rash; conjunctivitis; reticulocytosis; dyspnea; chest soreness; bigeminy; bradycardia; tachycardia; bronchospasm; pulmonary edema; hypoventilation; cyanosis; dyspnea; atelectasis; ventilator dependence

Health care workers: Headache (51%); conjunctivitis (32%); rhinitis, nausea, rash, dizziness, pharyngitis, lacrimation (10 to 20%).

Administration and Dosage:

For aerosol administration only.

Mechanically ventilated infants: The recommended dose and administration schedule for infants who require mechanical ventilation is the same as for those who do not. Either a pressure or volume cycle ventilator may be used in conjunction with the SPAG-2. In either case, suction endotracheal tubes every 1 to 2 hours and monitor pulmonary pressures frequently (every 2 to 4 hours). For both pressure and volume ventilators, heated wire connective tubing and bacteria filters in series in the expiratory limb of the system (which must be changed frequently, eg, every 4 hours) must be used to minimize the risk of ribavirin precipitation in the system and the subsequent risk of ventilator circuit for pressure cycled ventilators. They may also be utilized with volume cycled ventilators.

Before use, read thoroughly the Viratek Small Particle Aerosol Generator (SPAG) Model SPAG-2 Operator's Manual for operating instructions.

Treatment was effective when instituted within the first 3 days of RSV lower respiratory tract infection.

Treatment is carried out for 12 to 18 hours per day for at least 3, but no more than 7 days, and is part of a total treatment program. The aerosol is delivered to an infant oxygen hood from the SPAG-2 aerosol generator. Administration by face mask or oxygen tent may be necessary if a hood cannot be used. However, the volume of distribution and condensation area are larger in a tent, and efficacy of this method has been evaluated in only a few patients. Ribavirin aerosol is not to be administered with any other aerosol generating device or together with other aerosolized medications. Not for patients requiring simultaneous assisted ventilation.

Solubilize drug with sterile USP water for injection or inhalation in the 100 ml vial. Transfer to the clean, sterilized 500 ml wide-mouth Erlenmeyer flask (SPAG-2 Reservoir) and further dilute to a final volume of 300 ml with sterile USP water for injection or inhalation. The final concentration should be 20 mg/ml.

Reconstitute drug with a minimum of 75 ml of sterile water for injection or inhalation in the original 100 ml vial. Shake well. *Important:* This water should not have any antimicrobial agent or other substance added. Discard solutions placed in the SPAG-2 unit at least every 24 hours and when the liquid level is low before adding newly reconstituted solution. Using the recommended drug concentration of 20 mg/ml ribavirin as the starting solution in the SPAG unit's drug reservoir, the average aerosol concentration for a 12 hour period is 190 mcg/L of air.

AMANTADINE HCl

Capsules: 100 mg (*Rx*)	Various, *Symadine* (Solvay)
Syrup: 50 mg/5 ml (*Rx*)	*Symmetrel* (DuPont)

Actions:

Pharmacology: Amantadine's antiviral activity against influenza A virus is not completely understood. Its mode of action appears to be the prevention of the release of infectious viral nucleic acid into the host cell. It may also interfere with viral penetration into cells. The reaction appears to be virus specific (for influenza A) but not host specific.

Amantadine is 70% to 90% effective in preventing illnesses caused by circulating strains of type A influenza viruses.

Pharmacokinetics:

Absorption/Distribution – After administration of a single dose of 100 mg, maximum blood levels are reached in ≈ 4 hours, based on the mean time of the peak urinary excretion rate; the peak excretion rate is ≈ 5 mg/hr; the mean half-life of the excretion rate is ≈ 15 hours.

Clearance of amantadine is significantly reduced in adults with renal insufficiency. Elimination half-life increases two- to threefold when creatinine clearance is < 40 ml/min/1.73 m^2 and averages 8 days in patients on chronic maintenance hemodialysis.

Metabolism/Excretion – Amantadine is readily absorbed, is not metabolized, and is excreted in the urine. The renal clearance of amantadine is reduced and plasma levels are increased in otherwise healthy elderly patients age 65 years and older. The drug plasma levels in elderly patients receiving 100 mg daily have been reported to approximate those determined in younger adults taking 200 mg daily.

Indications:

Influenza A virus respiratory tract illness: Prevention or chemoprophylaxis of and treatment of respiratory tract illness caused by influenza A virus strains. Indicated especially for high risk patients because of underlying disease (eg, cardiovascular, pulmonary, metabolic, neuromuscular or immunodeficiency disease), close household or hospital ward contacts of index cases, immunocompromised patients and health care and community services personnel. Early immunization is the prophylaxis method of choice. When early immunization is contraindicated, not feasible or not available, amantadine can be used for chemoprophylaxis.

Amantadine prophylaxis recommendations:

1.) Short-term prophylaxis during the course of a presumed influenza A outbreak (eg, in institutions for persons at high risk), particularly when the vaccine may be relatively ineffective.

2.) Adjunct to late immunization of high risk individuals. It is not too late to immunize even when influenza A is known to be in the community. Since the development of a protective response following vaccination takes about 2 weeks, use amantadine in the interim.

3.) To reduce disruption of medical care and to reduce spread of virus to high risk persons when influenza A virus outbreaks occur. Prophylaxis is desirable for those physicians, nurses and other personnel who have extensive contact with high risk patients but who failed to receive the recommended annual influenza vaccination before the onset of influenza A activity.

4.) To supplement vaccination protection in those with impaired immune responses. Consider chemoprophylaxis for high risk patients who may have a poor response to influenza vaccine, eg, those with severe immunodeficiency.

5.) As chemoprophylaxis throughout the influenza season for those few high risk individuals for whom influenza vaccine is contraindicated because of anaphylactic hypersensitivity to egg protein or prior severe reactions associated with influenza vaccination.

Parkinson's disease and drug-induced extrapyramidal reactions: See amantadine in the Antiparkinson Agents section.

Contraindications:

Hypersensitivity to amantadine.

Warnings:

Seizures: Closely observe patients with a history of epilepsy or other seizures for increased seizure activity. Dosage reduction is recommended.

Use caution in patients with liver disease, history of recurrent eczematoid rash, or psychosis or severe psychoneurosis not controlled by chemotherapeutic agents.

CHF or peripheral edema requires careful observation and dosage titration; patients have developed CHF while receiving amantadine.

Renal function impairment: Reduce the dose in renal impairment.

Elderly: Reduce dose in individuals ≥ 65 years of age and older.

Pregnancy: Category C.

Lactation: Amantadine is excreted in breast milk.

Children: Safety and efficacy for use in neonates and infants < 1 year of age have not been established.

Precautions:

Discontinuing treatment: Do not discontinue abruptly; a few patients with Parkinson's disease experienced a parkinsonian crisis when this medication was stopped suddenly.

Drug Interactions:

Drugs that may interact with amantadine include anticholinergic drugs and hydrochlorothiazide plus triamterene.

Anticholinergic drugs: Reduce the dose of anticholinergic drugs or of amantadine if atropine-like effects appear when these drugs are used concurrently.

Hydrochlorothiazide plus triamterene: Decreased urinary excretion of amantadine with subsequent increased plasma concentrations occurred when hydrochlorothiazide plus triamterene was administered concurrently with amantadine.

Adverse Reactions:

Adverse reactions occurring in ≥ 3% of patients include: Nausea; dizziness; lightheadedness; insomnia; depression; anxiety; irritability; hallucinations; confusion; anorexia; dry mouth; constipation; ataxia; livedo reticularis; peripheral edema; orthostatic hypotension; headache.

Administration and Dosage:

Influenza A virus illness:

Prophylaxis – Start in anticipation of contact or as soon as possible after exposure. Use daily for ≥ 10 days following a known exposure. The infectious period extends from shortly before onset of symptoms to up to 1 week after. Because amantadine does not appear to suppress antibody response, it can be used in conjunction with inactivated influenza A virus vaccine until protective antibody responses develop; administer for 2 to 3 weeks after vaccine has been given. When inactivated influenza A virus vaccine is unavailable or contraindicated, administer amantadine for up to 90 days in case of possible repeated and unknown exposures.

Symptomatic management – Start as soon as possible after onset of symptoms and continue for 24 to 48 hours after symptoms disappear.

The following table may serve as a guideline for dosage:

Amantadine Dosage by Patient Age and Renal Function	
Renal function	Dosage[1]
No recognized renal disease	
1 to 9 yrs[2]	4.4 to 8.8 mg/kg/day once daily or divided twice daily, not to exceed 150 mg/day
10 to 64 yrs[3]	200 mg once daily or divided twice daily
≥ 65 yrs	100 mg once daily[4]
Renal function impairment Ccr: (ml/min/1.73m^2)	
30 to 50	200 mg 1st day; 100 mg daily thereafter
15 to 29	200 mg 1st day; then 100 mg on alternate days
<15	200 mg every 7 days
Hemodialysis patients	200 mg every 7 days

[1] For prophylaxis, take amantadine each day for the duration of influenza A activity in the community (generally 6 to 12 weeks). For therapy, institute amantadine as soon as possible after onset of symptoms and continue for 24 to 48 hours after symptoms disappear (generally 5 to 7 days).

[2] Use in children < 1 year old is not evaluated adequately. In one study, a dose of 6.6 mg/kg/day was well tolerated by children > 2 years old.

[3] Reduce dosage to 100 mg/day for persons with an active seizure disorder, because they may be at increased risk of seizure frequency when given 200 mg/day.

[4] Recommended to minimize risk of toxicity; renal function normally declines with age, and side effects are more frequent in the elderly.

FOSCARNET SODIUM (Phosphonoformic acid)

Injection: 24 mg/ml (*Rx*) — *Foscavir* (Astra)

Warning:

Renal impairment, the major toxicity, occurs to some degree in most patients. Continual assessment of a patient's risk and frequent monitoring of serum creatinine with dose adjustment for changes in renal function are imperative.

Foscarnet causes alterations in plasma minerals and electrolytes that have led to seizures. Monitor patients frequently for such changes and their potential sequelae.

Actions:

Pharmacology: Foscarnet exerts its antiviral activity by a selective inhibition at the pyrophosphate binding site on virus-specific DNA polymerases and reverse transcriptases at concentrations that do not affect cellular DNA polymerases. CMV strains resistant to ganciclovir may be sensitive to foscarnet.

Pharmacokinetics: Foscarnet is 14% to 17% bound to plasma protein at plasma drug concentrations of 1 to 1000 mcM.

Approximately 80% to 90% of IV foscarnet is excreted unchanged in the urine of patients with normal renal function. Both tubular secretion and glomerular filtration account for urinary elimination of foscarnet.

Plasma half-life increases with the severity of renal impairment. Half-lives of 2 to 8 hours occurred in patients having estimated or measured 24 hour Ccr of 44 to 90 ml/min. Careful monitoring of renal function and dose adjustment is imperative.

Variable penetration into cerebrospinal fluid (CSF) has been observed. Disease-related defects in the blood-brain barrier may be responsible for the variations seen.

Indications:

CMV retinitis: Treatment of CMV retinitis in patients with AIDS.

HSV infections: Treatment of acyclovir-resistant mucocutaneous HSV infections in immunocompromised patients.

Contraindications:

Hypersensitivity to foscarnet.

Warnings:

Mineral and electrolyte imbalances: Foscarnet has been associated with changes in serum electrolytes including hypocalcemia (15%), hypophosphatemia (8%) and hyperphosphatemia (6%), hypomagnesemia (15%) and hypokalemia (16%). Foscarnet is associated with a transient, dose-related decrease in ionized serum calcium, which may not be reflected in total serum calcium.

Neurotoxicity and seizures: Foscarnet was associated with seizures in AIDS patients.

Statistically significant risk factors associated with seizures were low baseline absolute neutrophil count (ANC), impaired baseline renal function and low total serum calcium. Several cases of seizures were associated with death.

Other CMV infections: Safety and efficacy have not been established for the treatment of other CMV infections (eg, pneumonitis, gastroenteritis); congenital or neonatal CMV disease; non-immunocompromised individuals.

Renal function impairment: The major toxicity of foscarnet is renal impairment, which occurs to some degree in most patients. Approximately 33% of 189 patients with AIDS and CMV retinitis who received IV foscarnet in clinical studies developed significant impairment of renal function, manifested by a rise in serum creatinine concentration to ≥ 2 mg/dl.

Elderly: Since these individuals frequently have reduced glomerular filtration, pay particular attention to assessing renal function before and during administration.

Pregnancy: Category C.

Lactation: It is not known whether foscarnet is excreted in breast milk.

Children: The safety and efficacy of foscarnet in children have not been studied.

Precautions:

Monitoring: The majority of patients will experience some decrease in renal function due to foscarnet administration. Therefore it is recommended that Ccr be determined at baseline, 2 to 3 times per week during induction therapy and at least once every 1 to 2 weeks during maintenance therapy, with foscarnet dose adjusted accordingly. More frequent monitoring may be required for some patients. It is also recommended that a 24 hour Ccr be determined at baseline and periodically thereafter to ensure correct dosing. Discontinue foscarnet if Ccr drops to < 0.4 ml/min/kg.

Due to foscarnet's propensity to chelate divalent metal ions and alter levels of serum electrolytes, closely monitor patients for such changes. It is recommended that a schedule similar to that recommended for serum creatinine be used to monitor serum calcium, magnesium, potassium and phosphorus.

Careful monitoring and appropriate management of creatinine are of particular importance in patients with conditions that may predispose them to seizures.

Diagnosis of CMV retinitis should be established by an ophthalmologist familiar with the retinal presentation of these conditions.

Toxicity/local irritation: The maximum single-dose administered was 120 mg/kg by IV infusion over 2 hours. It is likely that larger doses, or more rapid infusions, would result in increased toxicity. Infuse solutions containing foscarnet only into veins with adequate blood flow to permit rapid dilution and distribution, and avoid local irritation. Local irritation and ulcerations of penile epithelium have occurred in patients receiving foscarnet, possibly because of drug in urine. One case of vulvovaginal ulceration in a female has occurred. Adequate hydration with close attention to personal hygiene may minimize the occurrence of such events.

Anemia occurred in 33% of patients. Granulocytopenia occurred in 17% of patients.

Drug Interactions:

Drugs that may interact with foscarnet include nephrotoxic drugs (eg, aminoglycosides, amphotericin B, IV pentamidine), pentamidine and zidovudine.

Foscarnet decreases serum levels of ionized calcium. Exercise particular caution when other drugs known to influence serum calcium levels are used concurrently.

Adverse Reactions:

Adverse reactions occurring in ≥ 3% of patients include: Fever; nausea; anemia; diarrhea; abnormal renal function including acute renal failure, decreased Ccr and increased serum creatinine; vomiting; headache; seizure; death; marrow suppression; injection site pain or inflammation; paresthesia; dizziness; involuntary muscle contractions; hypoesthesia; neuropathy; sensory disturbances; influenza-like symptoms; bacterial/fungal infections; rectal hemorrhage; dry mouth; melena; flatulence; ulcerative stomatitis; pancreatitis; granulocytopenia; leukopenia; thrombocytopenia; platelet abnormalities; thrombosis; WBC abnormalities; lymphadenopathy; electrolyte abnormalities; neurotoxicity; renal impairment; decreased weight, increased alkaline phosphatase, LDH and BUN; acidosis; cachexia; thirst; depression; confusion; anxiety; aggressive reaction; hallucination; coughing; dyspnea; pneumonia; sinusitis; pharyngitis; rhinitis; respiratory disorders or insufficiency; pulmonary infiltration; stridor; pneumothorax; hemoptysis; bronchospasm; rash; increased sweating; pruritus; skin ulceration; seborrhea; erythematous rash; maculopapular rash; vision anbormalities; taste perversions; eye abnormalities; eye pain; conjunctivitis; hypertension; palpitations; ECG abnormalities.

Administration and Dosage:

HSV infections: Foscarnet is not a cure for HSV infections. While complete healing may occur, relapse occurs in most patients.

Caution: Do not administer by rapid or bolus IV injection. Toxicity may be increased as a result of excessive plasma levels. An infusion pump must be used.

Induction treatment: The recommended initial dose for patients with normal renal function is 60 mg/kg, adjusted for individual patients' renal function, given IV at a constant rate over a minimum of 1 hour every 8 hours for 2 to 3 weeks depending on clinical response.

Maintenance treatment: 90 to 120 mg/kg/day (individualized for renal function) given as an IV infusion over 2 hours. It is recommended that most patients be started on maintenance treatment with a dose of 90 mg/kg/day. Escalation to 120 mg/kg/day may be considered should early reinduction be required because of retinitis progression.

Patients who experience progression of retinitis while receiving maintenance therapy may be retreated with the induction and maintenance regimens given above.

Dose adjustment in renal impairment: To use this dosing guide, actual 24 hour Ccr (ml/min) must be divided by body weight (kg) or the estimated Ccr in ml/min/kg can be calculated from serum creatinine (mg/dl) using the modified Cockcroft and Gault equation.

$$\text{Males: } \frac{140 - \text{age}}{\text{serum creatinine}} \times 72 = \text{Ccr}$$

Females: 0.85 × above value

Foscarnet Dosing Guide Based on CCR for Induction			
	HSV: Equivalent to		CMV: Equivalent to
Ccr (ml/min/kg)	80 mg/kg/day	120 mg/kg/day	180 mg/kg/day
> 1.4	40 q 12 hr	40 q 8 hr	60 q 8 hr
> 1 to 1.4	30 q 12 hr	30 q 8 hr	45 q 8 hr
> 0.8 to 1	20 q 12 hr	35 q 12 hr	50 q 12 hr
> 0.6 to 0.8	35 q 24 hr	25 q 12 hr	40 q 12 hr
> 0.5 to 0.6	25 q 24 hr	40 q 24 hr	60 q 24 hr
≥ 0.4 to 0.5	20 q 24 hr	35 q 24 hr	50 q 24 hr
< 0.4	Not recommended	Not recommended	Not recommended

Foscarnet Dosing Guide Based on Ccr for Maintenance		
Ccr (ml/min/kg)	CMV: Equivalent to	
	90 mg/kg/day	120 mg/kg/day
> 1.4	90 q 24 hr	120 q 24 hr
> 1 to 2.4	70 q 24 hr	90 q 24 hr
> 0.8 to 1	50 q 24 hr	65 q 24 hr
> 0.6 to 0.8	80 q 48 hr	105 q 48 hr
> 0.5 to 0.6	60 q 48 hr	30 q 48 hr
≥ 0.4 to 0.5	50 q 48 hr	65 q 48 hr
< 0.4	Not recommended	Not recommended

DIDANOSINE (ddI; dideoxyinosine)

Tablets, buffered, chewable/dispersible: 25, 50, 100 and 150 mg (*Rx*) — *Videx* (Bristol-Myers Squibb)
Powder for Oral Solution, buffered: 100, 167, 250 and 375 mg (*Rx*)
Powder for Oral Solution, pediatric: 2 and 4 g (*Rx*)

Warning:

Pancreatitis, which has been fatal in some cases, is the major clinical toxicity associated with didanosine therapy. Consider pancreatitis whenever a patient receiving didanosine develops abdominal pain and nausea, vomiting or elevated biochemical markers. Under these circumstances, suspend use until the diagnosis of pancreatitis is excluded.

Patients receiving didanosine or any antiretroviral therapy may continue to develop opportunistic infections and other complications of HIV infection, and should remain under close clinical observation by physicians experienced in the treatment of patients with HIV-associated diseases.

Actions:

Pharmacology: Didanosine, 2',3'-dideoxyinosine or ddI, is a synthetic purine nucleoside analog of deoxyadenosine. It inhibits in vitro replication of HIV (ie, HTLV III or LAV) in human primary cell cultures and in established cell lines. After didanosine enters the cell, it is converted by cellular enzymes to the active antiviral metabolite, dideoxyadenosine triphosphate (ddATP). The intracellular half-life of ddATP varies from 8 to 24 hours.

A common feature of dideoxynucleosides is the lack of a free 3'-hydroxyl group. The 3'-hydroxyl is required for continued DNA chain extension. Because ddATP lacks a 3'-hydroxyl group, incorporation of ddATP into viral DNA leads to chain termination and, thus, inhibition of viral replication. ddATP further contributes to inhibition of viral replication through interference with the HIV-RNA dependent DNA polymerase by competing with the natural nucleoside triphosphate, dATP, for binding to the active site of the enzyme.

Pharmacokinetics:

Bioequivalence of dosage formulations – A 375 mg dose of the buffered powder for oral solution produced similar plasma concentrations to a 300 mg (2 x 150 mg tablets) dose of the tablets indicating that didanosine is 20% to 25% more bioavailable from the tablet than the solution. Mean peak plasma concentrations (C_{max}) for both formulations were 1.6 mcg/ml. Mean area under the plasma concentration vs time curve (AUC) values were 3 mcg•hr/ml (range, 1.6 to 5.1) for the buffered solution and 2.6•hr/ml (range, 1.1 to 3.9) for the chewable tablet.

Effect of food on oral absorption – Didanosine is rapidly degraded at acidic pH. Administer all didanosine formulations on an empty somach. The administration of didanosine tablets within 5 minutes of a meal results in a 50% decrease in mean C_{max} and AUC values.

Adults – The pharmacokinetics of didanosine were evaluated in 69 adult patients with AIDS or severe AIDS-Related Complex (ARC) after single and multiple IV and oral doses. Patients received a 60 minute IV infusion once or twice a day for 2 weeks, at total daily doses ranging from 0.8 to 33 mg/kg. Oral doses equivalent to twice the IV dose were administered for an additional 4 weeks. Plasma concentrations were obtained on the first day of dosing and at steady state after IV and oral dosing.

Absorption: At doses of ≤ 7 mg/kg, the average absolute bioavailability was 33% after a single dose and 37% after 4 weeks of dosing. Pharmacokinetic parameters at steady state were not significantly different from values obtained after the initial IV or oral dose.

Distribution: The steady-state volume of distribution after IV administration averaged 54 L (range, 22 to 103). In a study of five adults, the concentration in the CSF 1 hour after infusion averaged 21% of the simultaneous plasma concentration.

Elimination: After oral administration, average elimination half-life was 1.6 hours. Total body clearance averaged 800 ml/min. Renal clearance represented ≈ 50% of total body clearance (average, 400 ml/min) when didanosine was given either IV or orally. This indicates that active tubular secretion, in addition to glomerular filtration, is responsible for the renal elimination. Urinary recovery after a single dose was ≈ 55%, and 20% of the dose after IV and oral administration, respectively. There was no evidence of accumulation after either IV or oral dosing.

Children – The pharmacokinetics of didanosine have been evaluated in two pediatric studies. In one study, 16 children and 4 adolescents received a single IV dose ranging from 40 to 90 mg/m^2 and multiple, twice-daily oral doses of 80 to 180 mg/m^2 of didanosine. In another study, 48 pediatric patients received a single IV dose and then multiple, 3 times daily oral doses ranging from 20 to 180 mg/m^2.

Absorption: The absolute bioavailability varied between patients in one study and averaged 32% and 42%, after the first oral dose and at steady state, respectively. The other study also demonstrated significant variability in the oral absorption of didanosine with an average absolute bioavailability of 19%. In one study, the average steady-state AUC was 1.4, 1.6 and 2.3 mcg•hr/ml after the administration of oral doses of 80, 120 and 180 mg/m^2, respectively. The average corresponding steady-state C_{max} values were 0.8, 1.4 and 1.7 mcg/ml, respectively.

Distribution: In one study, the volume of distribution after IV administration averaged 35.6 L/m^2 (range, 18.4 to 60.7). In this study, the concentration of didanosine ranged from 0.04 to 0.12 mcg/ml in CSF samples collected from seven patients at times ranging from 1.5 to 3.5 hours after a single IV or oral dose. These CSF concentrations corresponded to 12% to 85% of the concentration in a simultaneous plasma sample.

Elimination: In one study, the elimination half-life following oral administration averaged 0.8 hours. Total body clearance following IV administration averaged 532 ml/min/m^2 (range, 294 to 920). Mean renal clearance ranged from 190 to 319 ml/min/m^2 after the first oral dose and from 231 to 265 ml/min/m^2 at steady state. Urinary recovery averaged 17% at steady state. There was no evidence of accumulation of didanosine after the administration of oral doses for an average of 26 days.

Metabolism: The metabolism of didanosine has not been evaluated in humans. Based on data from animal studies, it is presumed that the metabolism of didanosine in humans will occur by the same pathways responsible for elimination of endogenous purines.

The intracellular half-life of ddATP, the metabolite presumed to be responsible for the antiretroviral activity of didanosine, is 8 to 24 hours in vitro.

In vitro human plasma protein binding is < 5%.

Indications:

For the treatment of adult patients with advanced HIV infection who have received prolonged prior zidovudine therapy.

For the treatment of adult and pediatric patients (> 6 months of age) with advanced HIV infection who have demonstrated intolerance or significant clinical or immunologic deterioration during zidovudine therapy.

Because zidovudine prolongs survival and decreases the incidence of opportunistic infections in patients with advanced HIV disease, consider zidovudine as initial therapy for the treatment of advanced HIV infection, unless contraindicated.

Contraindications:

Hypersensitivity to any of the components of the formulations.

Warnings:

Peripheral neuropathy occurs in patients treated with didanosine; the frequency appears to be dose-related. Monitor patients for the development of a neuropathy that is usually characterized by distal numbness, tingling, or pain in the feet or hands.

Incidence of Neuropathy with Didanosine

Parameter	All phase I (n = 170)	≤ 12.5 mg/kg/day (n = 91)	Phase I > 12.5 mg/kg/day (n = 79)
Neuropathy	42%	34%	51%
Neuropathy requiring dose modification	22%	12%	34%

Neuropathy occurred more frequently in patients with a history of neuropathy or neurotoxic drug therapy. These patients may be at increased risk of neuropathy during didanosine therapy.

Pancreatitis must be considered whenever a patient receiving didanosine develops abdominal pain, nausea, vomiting or elevated biochemical markers. Incidence ranges from 2% to 9% (recommended dose) to 3.2% to 27% (high dose). Under these circumstances, suspend use of didanosine until the diagnosis of pancreatitis is excluded. When treatment with other drugs known to cause pancreatic toxicity is required (eg, IV pentamidine), consider suspension of didanosine.

Closely follow patients with a heightened risk of pancreatitis, such as those with a history of pancreatitis, alcohol consumption, elevated triglycerides or evidence of advanced HIV infection. Patients with renal impairment may be at greater risk for pancreatitis if treated without dose adjustment.

In pediatric studies, pancreatitis occurred in 3% of patients treated at entry doses < 300 mg/m²/day and in 13% treated at higher doses. In pediatric patients with symptoms similar to those described above, suspend didanosine until the diagnosis of pancreatitis is excluded.

Hepatic failure: In a controlled clinical trial comparing two doses of didanosine to zidovudine, the 1 year rates of grade 3 to 4 liver function test alteration was 21% for high-dose didanosine, 13% for didanosine at the recommended dose and 14% for zidovudine. Fatal liver failure of unknown etiology occurred during didanosine therapy in 1/170 patients in the Phase I studies and 14/7806 in the Expanded Access Program.

Retinal depigmentation: Four pediatric patients demonstrated retinal depigmentation at doses > 300 mg/m²/day. Two of the patients, treated at doses of 540 mg/m²/day, had progression of disease when treated with lower doses. One patient treated at lower doses has continued therapy without progression of disease. Children receiving didanosine should undergo dilated retinal examination every 6 months or if a change in vision occurs.

Myopathy: Evidence of a dose-limiting skeletal muscle toxicity has been observed in mice and rats (but not in dogs) following long-term (> 90 days) dosing with didanosine at doses that were ≈ 1.2 to 12 times the estimated human exposure. Human myopathy has been associated with administration of other nucleoside analogs.

Renal function impairment: Patients with renal impairment (serum creatinine > 1.5 mg/dl or creatinine clearance < 60 ml/min) may be at greater risk of toxicity from didanosine due to decreased drug clearance; consider a dose reduction. The magnesium hydroxide content of each tablet (15.7 mEq) may present an excessive magnesium load to patients with significant renal impairment, particularly after prolonged dosing.

Hepatic function impairment: Patients with hepatic impairment may be at greater risk for toxicity due to altered metabolism; a dose reduction may be necessary.

Pregnancy: *Category B.*

Lactation: It is not known whether didanosine is excreted in breast milk. Because of the potential for serious adverse reactions from didanosine in nursing infants, instruct mothers to discontinue nursing when taking didanosine.

Children: Neuropathy has occurred rarely in children treated with didanosine. However, because signs and symptoms of neuropathy are difficult to assess in children, alert physicians of this possibility.

Precautions:

Opportunistic infections: Patients receiving didanosine or any other antiretroviral therapy may continue to develop opportunistic infections and other complications of HIV infection should remain under close clinical observation by physicians experienced in the treatment of patients with associated HIV diseases.

Phenylketonuria: Didanosine tablets contain 22.5 mg phenylalanine (33.7 mg in the 150 mg tablet).

Sodium-restricted diets: Each buffered tablet contains 264.5 mg sodium. Each single-dose packet of buffered powder for oral solution contains 1380 mg sodium.

Hyperuricemia: Didanosine has been associated with asymptomatic hyperuricemia; consider suspending treatment if clinical measures aimed at reducing uric acid levels fail.

Diarrhea: Didanosine buffered powder for oral solution was associated with diarrhea in 34% of adult patients. No data are available to demonstrate whether other formulations are associated with lower rates of diarrhea. However, if diarrhea develops in a patient receiving buffered powder for oral solution, consider a trial of chewable/dispersible buffered tablets.

Drug Interactions:

Drugs that may interact with didanosine include fluoroquinolones and tetracyclines.

Administer drugs whose absorption can be affected by the level of acidity in the stomach (eg, ketoconazole, dapsone) at least 2 hours prior to dosing with didanosine.

Coadministration of didanosine with drugs that are known to cause peripheral neuropathy or pancreatitis may increase the risk of these toxicities. Closely observe patients who receive these drugs.

Drug/Food interactions: Ingestion of didanosine with food reduces the absorption of didanosine by as much as 50%. Therefore, administer on an empty stomach.

Adverse Reactions:

The major toxicities are pancreatitis and peripheral neuropathy (see Warnings).

Adverse reactions ocurring in ≥ 3% of adult patients include diarrhea, neuropathy (all grades), chills/fever, rash/pruritis, abdominal pain, asthenia, headache, pain, nausea/vomiting, infection, pancreatitis, pneumonia, sarcoma, myopathy, dry mouth; dyspnea, and laboratory abnormalities including leukopenia, amylase, granulocytopenia, thrombocytopenia, ALT, AST, hemoglobin.

Adverse reactions occurring in ≥ 3% of pediatric patients include chills/fever, anorexia, asthenia, pain, malaise, failure to thrive, weight loss, flu syndrome, change in appetite, alopecia, dehydration, increased appetite; diarrhea, nausea/vomiting, liver abnormalities, abdominal pain, stomatitis/ mouth sores, pancreatitis, constipation, oral thrush, melena, dry mouth, ecchymosis, hemorrhage, petechiae; arthritis, myalgia, muscle atrophy decreased strength, vasodilation, arrhythmia; headache, nervousness, insomnia, dizziness, poor coordination, lethargy; cough, rhinitis, dyspnea, asthma, rhinorrhea, epistaxis, pharyngitis, hypoventilation, sinusitis, rhonchi/rales, congestion; rash/pruritus, skin disorder, eczema, sweating, impetigo, excoriation, erythema; ear pain/otitis, photophobia, strabismus, visual impairment; urinary frequency.

Children: In pediatric studies, pancreatitis occurred in 3% of patients treated at entry doses < 300 mg/m^2/day and in 13% of patients treated at higher doses.

Administration and Dosage:

Dosage: Use a 12 hour dosing interval. Administer all formulations on an empty stomach.

Chewable/dispersible buffered tablets – Thoroughly chew tablets or manually crush or disperse 2 tablets in at least 1 ounce of water prior to consumption. To disperse tablets, add 2 tablets to at least 1 ounce of water. Stir until a uniform dispersion forms, and drink entire dispersion immediately.

Buffered powder for oral solution –

1.) Open packet carefully and pour contents into ≈ 4 ounces of water. Do not mix with fruit juice or other acid-containing liquid.
2.) Stir until the powder completely dissolves (≈ 2 to 3 minutes).
3.) Drink the entire solution immediately.

Adults: Take 2 tablets at each dose so that adequate buffering is provided to prevent gastric acid degradation of didanosine. The recommended starting dose in adults is dependent on weight as outlined in the table below:

Adult Didanosine Dosing		
Patient weight (kg)	Tablets	Buffered powder
≥ 60	200 mg bid	250 mg bid
< 60	125 mg bid	167 mg bid

Children: To prevent gastric acid degradation, children > 1 year of age should receive a 2 tablet dose; children < 1 year old should receive a 1 tablet dose. The recommended dose in children is dependent on body surface area as outlined in the table below. Doses equivalent to 100 to 300 mg/m^2/day of the pediatric powder are being further evaluated in controlled clinical trials. The optimal dose has not been established; some investigators recommend doses of up to 300 mg/m^2/day divided into 3 daily doses.

Pediatric Didanosine Dosing (based on 200 mg/m^2/day average recommended dose)[1]			
		Pediatric powder (m^2)	
Body surface area (m^2)	Tablets	Dose	Vol/10 mg/ml admixture
1.1-1.4	100 mg bid	125 mg bid	12.5 ml bid
0.8-1	75 mg bid	94 mg bid	9.5 ml bid
0.5-0.7	50 mg bid	62 mg bid	6 ml bid
< 0.4	25 mg bid	31 mg bid	3 ml bid

[1] Based on didanosine pediatric powder.

Dose adjustment: If clinical signs suggest pancreatitis, suspend dose and carefully evaluate the possibility of pancreatitis. Resume dosing only after pancreatitis has been ruled out.

Many patients who have presented with symptoms of neuropathy will tolerate a reduced dose after resolution of these symptoms following drug discontinuation.

There are insufficient data to recommend dose adjustment in patients with impaired renal or hepatic function. Consider a dose reduction in patients with renal insufficiency or hepatic impairment.

ACYCLOVIR (Acycloguanosine)

Tablets: 400, 800 mg (*Rx*) — *Zovirax* (Glaxo Wellcome)
Capsules: 200 mg (*Rx*)
Suspension: 200 mg/5 ml (*Rx*)
Powder for Injection: 500 and 1000 mg/vial (as sodium) (*Rx*)

Actions:

Pharmacology: A synthetic acyclic purine nucleoside analog, acyclovir has in vitro inhibitory activity against HSV–1 and HSV–2, varicella zoster, Epstein-Barr and cytomegalovirus. Acyclovir is preferentially taken up and selectively converted to the active triphosphate form by HSV-infected cells. Acyclovir triphosphate interferes with HSV DNA polymerase and inhibits viral DNA replication. In vitro, acyclovir triphosphate can be incorporated into growing chains of DNA by viral DNA polymerase and, to a much smaller extent, by cellular DNA polymerase. When incorporation occurs, the DNA chain is terminated.

Pharmacokinetics:

Absorption/Distribution – When acyclovir was administered to adults at 5 mg/kg (≈ 250 mg/m^2) by 1 hour infusions every 8 hours, mean steady-state peak and trough concentrations were 9.8 mcg/ml (5.5 to 13.8 mcg/ml) and 0.7 mcg/ml (0.2 to 1 mcg/ml), respectively. Similar concentrations are achieved in children > 1 year old when doses of 250 mg/m^2 are given every 8 hours. Oral acyclovir is slowly and incompletely absorbed from the GI tract. Peak concentrations are reached in 1.5 to 2 hours; absorption is unaffected by food. Bioavailability is between 15% and 30% and decreases with increasing doses. Concentrations achieved in CSF are ≈ 50% of plasma values. Plasma protein binding is 9% to 33%. Acyclovir is widely distributed in tissues and body fluids, including brain, kidney, lung, liver, muscle, spleen, uterus, vaginal mucosa, vaginal secretions, CSF and herpetic vesicular fluid.

Metabolism/Excretion – Renal excretion of unchanged drug by glomerular filtration and tubular secretion following IV use accounts for 62% to 91% of the dose. Mean renal excretion of unchanged drug following oral use is 14.4% (8.6% to 19.8%). The only major urinary metabolite may account for up to 14% of the dose in patients with normal renal function. An insignificant amount is recovered in feces and expired CO_2; there is no evidence of tissue retention.

Half-life and total body clearance depend on renal function:

Acyclovir Half-Life and Total Body Clearance Based on Renal Function		
Creatinine clearance (ml/min/1.73 m^2)	Half-life (hr)	Total body clearance (ml/min/1.73 m^2)
> 80	2.5	327
50-80	3	248
15-50	3.5	190
0 (Anuric)	19.5	29

The half-life and total body clearance of acyclovir in pediatric patients > 1 year of age is similar to those in adults with normal renal function.

Indications:

Parenteral: Treatment of initial and recurrent mucosal and cutaneous HSV-1 and HSV-2 and varicella-zoster (shingles) infections in immunocompromised patients.

Herpes simplex encephalitis in patients > 6 months of age.

Severe initial clinical episodes of genital herpes in patients who are not immunocompromised.

Oral: Treatment of initial episodes and management of recurrent episodes of genital herpes in certain patients. Severity of the disease depends upon the immune status of the patient, frequency and duration of episodes and degree of cutaneous or systemic involvement.

Acute treatment of herpes zoster (shingles) and chickenpox (varicella).

Unlabeled uses: Other potential uses of oral or parenteral acyclovir include: Cytomegalovirus and HSV infection following bone marrow or renal transplantation, disseminated primary eczema herpeticum, herpes simplex-associated erythema multiforme, herpes simplex labialis, herpes simplex ocular infections; herpes simplex proctitis, herpes simplex whitlow, herpes zoster encephalitis, infectious mononucleosis and varicella pneumonia.

Contraindications:

Hypersensitivity to acyclovir or any component of the formulation.

Warnings:

Pregnancy: Category C.

Lactation: Acyclovir concentrations in breast milk in women following oral administration have ranged from 0.6 to 4.1 times corresponding plasma levels. These concentrations would potentially expose the nursing infant to a dose of acyclovir up to 0.3 mg/kg/day.

Children: Safety and efficacy of oral acyclovir in children < 2 years of age have not been established.

Precautions:

Diagnosis: Proof of HSV infection rests on viral isolation and identification in tissue culture. Although the cutaneous vesicular lesions associated with HSV are often characteristic, other etiologic agents can cause similar lesions.

Genital herpes: Avoid sexual intercourse when visible lesions are present.

Herpes zoster infections: Adults ≥ 50 years of age tend to have more severe shingles, and acyclovir treatment showed more significant benefit for older patients. Treatment was more useful if started within the first 48 hours of rash onset.

Chickenpox: Although chickenpox in otherwise healthy children is usually a self-limited disease of mild to moderate severity, adolescents and adults tend to have more severe disease. Treatment was initiated within 24 hours of the typical chickenpox rash in the controlled studies, and there is no information regarding the effects of treatment begun later in the disease course. It is unknown whether the treatment of chickenpox in childhood has any effect on long-term immunity. However, there is no evidence to indicate that acyclovir treatment of chickenpox would have any effect on either decreasing or increasing the incidence or severity of subsequent recurrences of herpes zoster (shingles) later in life.

Do not exceed the recommended dosage, frequency or length of treatment. Base dosage adjustments on estimated creatinine clearance.

Renal effects: Precipitation of acyclovir crystals in renal tubules can occur if the maximum solubility of free acyclovir is exceeded or if the drug is administered by bolus injection. Serum creatinine and blood urea nitrogen (BUN) rise and creatinine clearance decreases.

Bolus administration of the drug leads to a 10% incidence of renal dysfunction, while infusion of 5 mg/kg (250 mg/m^2) over an hour was associated with a lower frequency (4.6%). Concomitant use of other nephrotoxic drugs, preexisting renal disease and dehydration make further renal impairment with acyclovir more likely. In most instances, alterations of renal function were transient and resolved spontaneously or with improvement of water and electrolyte balance, with drug dosage adjustments or with drug discontinuation. However, these changes may progress to acute renal failure.

Hydration: Accompany IV infusion by adequate hydration. Since maximum urine concentration occurs within the first 2 hours following infusion, establish sufficient urine flow during that period to prevent precipitation in renal tubules.

Encephalopathic changes: Patients (1%) receiving acyclovir IV have manifested encephalopathic changes characterized by either lethargy, obtundation, tremors, confusion, hallucinations, agitation, seizures or coma. Use with caution in those patients who have underlying neurologic abnormalities; those with serious renal, hepatic or electrolyte abnormalities or significant hypoxia; and those who have manifested prior neurologic reactions to cytotoxic drugs.

Resistance: Exposure of HSV isolates to acyclovir in vitro can lead to the emergence of less sensitive viruses. In severely immunocompromised patients, prolonged or repeated courses of acyclovir may result in resistant viruses which may not fully respond to continued acyclovir therapy.

Drug Interactions:

Drugs that may affect acyclovir include probenecid and zidovudine.

Adverse Reactions:

Adverse reactions (parenteral) occurring in ≥ 3% of patients include inflammation or phlebitis at injection site, transient elevations of serum creatinine or BUN and nausea or vomiting.

Adverse reactions (oral) occurring in ≥ 3% of patients include malaise, nausea and headache.

Administration and Dosage:

Parenteral: For IV infusion only. Avoid rapid or bolus IV, IM or SC injection. Administer over at least 1 hour to prevent renal tubular damage. Initiate therapy as soon as possible following onset of signs and symptoms.

IV Acyclovir Dosage/Management Guidelines

Indication	Dosage	
	Adults	Children (< 12 years)
Mucosal and cutaneous HSV infections in immunocompromised patients	5 mg/kg infused at a constant rate over 1 hour every 8 hours (15 mg/kg/day) for 7 days[1]	250 mg/m² infused at a constant rate over 1 hour every 8 hours (750 mg/m²/day) for 7 days[1]
Varicella-zoster infections (shingles) in immunocompromised patients[2]	10 mg/kg infused at a constant rate over 1 hour every 8 hours for 7 days[3]	500 mg/m² infused at a constant rate over at least 1 hour every 8 hours for 7 days[3]
Herpes simplex encephalitis	10 mg/kg infused at a constant rate over at least 1 hour every 8 hours for 10 days	500 mg/m² infused at a constant rate over at least 1 hour every 8 hours for 10 days[4]

[1] For severe initial clinical episodes of herpes genitalis, use the same dose for 5 days.
[2] Base dosage for obese patients on ideal body weight (10 mg/kg).
[3] Do not exceed 500 mg/m² every 8 hours.
[4] > 6 months of age.

Renal function impairment, acute or chronic – Adjust the dosing interval as indicated below:

Parenteral Acyclovir Dosage in Renal Function Impairment

Creatinine clearance (ml/min/1.73 m²)	Percent of recommended dose	Dosing interval (hours)
> 50	100%	8
25-50	100%	12
10-25	100%	24
0-10	50%	24

Hemodialysis – The mean plasma half-life of acyclovir during hemodialysis is ≈ 5 hours; a 60% decrease in plasma concentrations follows a 6 hour dialysis period. Therefore, administer a dose after each dialysis.

Oral:

Herpes simplex –

Initial genital herpes: 200 mg every 4 hours 5 times daily for 10 days. In patients with extremely severe episodes in which prostration, CNS involvement, urinary retention or inability to take oral medication requires hospitalization and more aggressive management, initiate therapy with IV acyclovir (see above).

Chronic suppressive therapy for recurrent disease: 400 mg 2 times daily for up to 12 months, followed by reevaluation. Reevaluate the frequency and severity of the patient's HSV after 1 year of therapy to assess the need for continuation of therapy; frequency and severity of episodes of untreated genital herpes may change over time. Reevaluation usually requires a trial off acyclovir to assess the need for reinstitution of suppressive therapy. Some patients, such as those with very frequent or severe episodes before treatment, may warrant uninterrupted suppression for > 1 year.

Alternative regimens have included doses ranging from 200 mg 3 times daily to 200 mg 5 times daily.

Intermittent therapy: 200 mg every 4 hours 5 times daily for 5 days. Initiate therapy at the earliest sign or symptom (prodrome) of recurrence.

Herpes zoster, acute treatment – 800 mg every 4 hours 5 times daily for 7 to 10 days.

Chickenpox – 20 mg/kg (not to exceed 800 mg) 4 times daily for 5 days. Initiate at earliest sign or symptom.

Renal impairment, acute or chronic –

Oral Acyclovir Dosage in Renal Function Impairment

Normal dosage regimen (5x daily)	Creatinine clearance (ml/min/1.73 m^2)	Adjusted dosage regimen	
		Dose (mg)	Dosing interval
200 mg every 4 hours	> 10 0-10	200 200	Every 4 hours, 5x daily Every 12 hours
400 mg every 12 hours	> 10 0-10	400 200	Every 12 hours Every 12 hours
800 mg every 4 hours	> 25 10-25 0-10	800 800 800	Every 4 hours, 5x daily Every 8 hours Every 12 hours

Hemodialysis – For patients that require hemodialysis, adjust dosing schedule so that a dose is administered after each dialysis. No supplemental dose is necessary after peritoneal dialysis.

GANCICLOVIR (DHPG)

Capsules: 250 mg (*Rx*) — *Cytovene* (Roche)
Powder for Injection, lyophilized: 500 mg/vial ganciclovir (*Rx*)

Warning:

The clinical toxicity of ganciclovir includes granulocytopenia and thrombocytopenia. In animal studies, ganciclovir was carcinogenic, teratogenic and caused aspermatogenesis.

Ganciclovir IV is indicated for use only in the treatment of cytomegalovirus (CMV) retinitis in immunocompromised patients and for the prevention of CMV disease in transplant patients at risk for CMV disease.

Ganciclovir capsules are indicated only for prevention of CMV disease in patients with advanced HIV infection at risk for CMV disease and for maintenance treatment of CMV retinitis in immunocompromised patients.

Because oral ganciclovir is associated with a risk of more rapid rate of CMV retinitis progression, use only in those patients for whom this risk is balanced by the benefit associated with avoiding daily IV infusions.

Actions:

Pharmacology: Ganciclovir, a synthetic guanine derivative active against CMV, is an acyclic nucleoside analog of 2'-deoxyguanosine that inhibits replication of herpes viruses both in vitro and in vivo. Sensitive human viruses include CMV, HSV-1 and -2, herpes virus type 6, Epstein-Barr virus, varicella-zoster virus and hepatitis B virus.

Pharmacokinetics:

Absorption – Absolute bioavailability of oral ganciclovir under fasting conditions was ≈ 5%; following food it was 6% to 9%. When given with a high-fat meal, steady-state AUC increased and there was a significant prolongation of time to peak serum concentrations.

At the end of a 1–hour IV infusion of 5 mg/kg, total AUC and C_{max} ranged between 22.1 and 26.8 mcg•hr/ml and 8.27 and 9 mcg/ml, respectively.

Distribution – The steady-state volume of distribution after IV administration was 0.74 L/kg. Cerebrospinal fluid concentrations obtained 0.25 and 5.67 hours post-dose in three patients who received 2.5 mg/kg ganciclovir IV every 8 or 12 hours ranged from 0.31 to 0.68 mcg/ml, representing 24% to 70% of the respective plasma concentrations. Binding to plasma proteins was 1% to 2% over ganciclovir concentrations of 0.5 and 51 mcg/ml.

Metabolism – Following oral administration of a single 1000 mg dose, 86% of the administered dose was recovered in the feces and 5% was recovered in the urine.

Excretion – When administered IV, ganciclovir exhibits linear pharmacokinetics over the range of 1.6 to 5 mg/kg and when administered orally, it exhibits linear kinetics up to a total daily dose of 4 g/day. Renal excretion of unchanged drug by glomerular filtration and active tubular secretion is the major route of elimination. In patients with normal renal function, 91.3% of IV ganciclovir was recovered unmetabolized in the urine. After oral administration, steady-state is achieved within 24 hours. Renal clearance following oral administration was 3.1 ml/min/kg. Half-life was 3.5 hours following IV administration and 4.8 following oral use.

Children: At an IV dose of 4 or 6 mg/kg in 27 neonates (aged 2 to 49 days), the pharmacokinetic parameters were, respectively, C_{max} of 5.5 and 7 mcg/ml, systemic clearance of 3.14 and 3.56 ml/min/kg and half-life of 2.4 hours for both.

Indications:

IV:

CMV *retinitis* – Treatment of CMV retinitis in immunocompromised patients, including patients with AIDS.

CMV *disease* – Prevention of CMV disease in transplant recipients at risk for CMV disease.

Oral:

CMV *retinitis* – Alternative to the IV formulation for maintenance treatment of CMV retinitis in immunocompromised patients, including patients with AIDS, in whom retinitis is stable floowing appropriate induction therapy and for whom the risk of more rapid progression is balanced by the benefit associated with avoiding daily IV infusions.

CMV *disease* – Prevention of CMV disease in individuals with advanced HIV infection at risk for developing CMV disease.

Unlabeled uses: Ganciclovir may also be beneficial in some immunocompromised patients in the treatment of other CMV infections.

Contraindications:

Hypersensitivity to ganciclovir or acyclovir.

Warnings:

CMV *disease:* Safety and efficacy have not been established for congenital or neonatal CMV disease nor for the treatment of established CMV disease other than retinitis nor for use in nonimmunocompromised individuals. The safety and efficacy of oral ganciclovir have not been established for treating any manifestation of CMV disease other than maintenance treatment of CMV retinitis.

Retinal detachment has been observed in subjects with CMV retinitis both before and after initiation of therapy with ganciclovir. Its relationship to therapy is unknown. Patients with CMV retinitis should have frequent ophthalmologic evaluations to monitor the status of their retinitis and to detect any other retinal pathology.

Hematologic: Do not administer if the absolute neutrophil count is < $500/mm^3$ or the platelet count is < $25,000/mm^3$. Granulocytopenia (neutropenia), anemia and thrombocytopenia have been observed in patients treated with ganciclovir. The frequency and severity of these events vary widely in different patient populations. Therefore, use with caution in patients with pre-existing cytopenias or with a history of cytopenic reactions to other drugs, chemicals or irradiation. Granulocytopenia usually occurs during the first or second week of treatment, but may occur at any time during treatment. Cell counts usually begin to recover within 3 to 7 days of discontinuing the drug. Colony-stimulating factors have increased neutrophil and WBC counts in patients receiving IV ganciclovir for CMV retinitis.

Renal function impairment: Because the major elimination pathway for ganciclovir is renal, dosage must be reduced according to creatinine clearance.

Hemodialysis reduces plasma concentrations of ganciclovir by about 50% after both IV and oral administration.

Use ganciclovir with caution because the half-life and plasma/serum concentrations of ganciclovir will be increased due to reduced renal clearance.

Carcinogenesis/Mutagenesis/Fertility impairment: Consider ganciclovir a potential carcinogen.

Because of the mutagenic and teratogenic potential of ganciclovir, advise women of childbearing potential to use effective contraception during treatment. Similarly, advise men to practice barrier contraception during and for at least 90 days following treatment with ganciclovir.

Although data in humans have not been obtained regarding this effect, it is considered probable that ganciclovir, at recommended doses, causes temporary or permanent inhibition of spermatogenesis.

Elderly: Pharmacokinetic profile in elderly patients is not established. Since elderly individuals frequently have a reduced glomerular filtration rate, pay particular attention to assessing renal function before and during ganciclovir therapy.

Pregnancy: Category C.

Lactation: It is not known whether ganciclovir is excreted in breast milk. The possibility of serious adverse reactions from ganciclovir in nursing infants is considered likely. Instruct mothers to discontinue nursing if they are receiving ganciclovir. The minimum interval before nursing can safely be resumed after the last dose of ganciclovir is unknown.

Children: Safety and efficacy in children have not been established. The use of ganciclovir in children warrants extreme caution to the probability of long-term carcinogenicity and reproductive toxicity. Administer to children only after careful evaluation and only if the potential benefits of treatment outweigh the risks. Oral ganciclovir has not been studied in children < 13 years of age.

There has been very limited clinical experience using ganciclovir for the treatment of CMV retinitis in patients < 12 years of age.

The spectrum of adverse reactions reported in 120 immunocompromised pediatric clinical trial participants with serious CMV infections receiving IV ganciclovir were similar to those reported in adults. Granulocytopenia (17%) and thrombocytopenia (10%) were most commonly reported.

Precautions:

Monitoring: Due to the frequency of neutropenia, anemia and thrombocytopenia in patients receiving ganciclovir, it is recommended that complete blood counts and platelet counts be performed frequently, especially in patients in whom ganciclovir or other nucleoside analogs have previously resulted in leukopenia, or in whom neutrophil counts are < 1000/mm^3 at the beginning of treatment. Patients should also have serum creatinine or creatinine clearance values followed carefully.

Large doses/rapid infusion: The maximum single dose administered was 6 mg/kg by IV infusion over 1 hour. Larger doses have resulted in increased toxicity. It is likely that more rapid infusions would also result in increased toxicity.

Phlebitis/Pain at injection site: Initially, reconstituted ganciclovir solutions have a high pH (pH 11). Despite further dilution in IV fluids, phlebitis or pain may occur at the site of IV infusion. Take care to infuse solutions containing ganciclovir only into veins with adequate blood flow to permit rapid dilution and distribution.

Hydration: Since ganciclovir is excreted by the kidneys and normal clearance depends on adequate renal function, administration of ganciclovir should be accompanied by adequate hydration.

Photosensitivity: Photosensitization (photoallergy or phototoxicity) may occur; therefore, caution patients to take protective measures against exposure to ultraviolet or sunlight (eg, sunscreens, protective clothing) until tolerance is determined.

Drug Interactions:

Drugs that may affect ganciclovir include imipenem-cilastatin, nephrotoxic drugs, probenecid, didanosine and zidovudine. Drugs that may be affected by ganciclovir include cytotoxic drugs and zidovudine.

Adverse Reactions:

Adverse reactions occurring in ≥ 3% of AIDS patients include: Fever; abdominal pain; infection; chills; sepsis; diarrhea; nausea; anorexia; vomiting; flatulence; leukopenia; anemia; thrombocytopenia; neuropathy; paresthesia; rash; sweating; pruritus; vitreous disorder; pneumonia; neutropenia; asthenia; headache; aphthous stomatitis; abnormal dreams; abnormal gait; abnormal thinking; agitation; amnesia; anxiety; ataxia; coma; confusion; depression; dizziness; dry mouth; euphoria; hypertonia; hypesthesia; insomnia; libido decreased; manic reaction; myoclonus; nervousness; psychosis; seizures; somnolence; tremor; trismus.

Fatal: Pancreatitis, sepsis and multiple organ failure.

Administration and Dosage:

IV: Do not administer by rapid or bolus IV injection. The toxicity may be increased as a result of excessive plasma levels. Do not exceed the recommended infusion rate. IM or SC injection of reconstituted ganciclovir may result in severe tissue irritation due to high pH.

CMV *retinitis treatment (normal renal function):*

Induction – Recommended initial dose is 5 mg/kg (given IV at a constant rate of 1 hr) every 12 hours for 14 to 21 days. Do not use oral ganciclovir for induction.

Maintenance –

IV: Following induction, the recommended maintenance dose is 5 mg/kg given as a constant rate IV infusion over 1 hour once per day 7 days per week, or 6 mg/kg once per day 5 days/week.

Oral: Following induction, the recommended maintenance dose of oral ganciclovir is 1000 mg 3 times daily with food. Alternatively, the dosing regimen of 500 mg 6 times daily every 3 hours with food, during waking hours, may be used.

For patients who experience progression of CMV retinitis while receiving maintenance treatment with either formulation of ganciclovir, reinduction treatment is recommended.

Prevention of CMV *disease in transplant recipients:* The recommended initial dose of IV ganciclovir for patients with normal renal function is 5 mg/kg (given IV at a constant rate over 1 hour) every 12 hours for 7 to 14 days, followed by 5 mg/kg once daily 7 days/week, or 6 mg/kg once daily 5 days/week.

The duration of treatment with IV ganciclovir in transplant recipients is dependent on the duration and degree of immunosuppression. In controlled clinical trials in bone marrow allograft recipients, treatment was continued until day 100 to 120 post-transplantation. CMV disease occurred in several patients who discontinued treatment with ganciclovir prematurely. In heart allograft recipients, the onset of newly diagnosed CMV disease occurred after treatment with ganciclovir was stopped at day 28 post-transplant, suggesting that continued dosing may be necessary to prevent late occurrence of CMV disease in this patient population.

Prevention of CMV *disease in patients with advanced HIV infection and normal renal function:* The recommended dose of ganciclovir capsules is 1000 mg 3 times daily with food.

Renal function impairment:

IV – Refer to the table for recommended doses and adjust the dosing interval as indicated.

IV Ganciclovir Dose in Renal Impairment				
Creatinine clearance (ml/min)	Ganciclovir induction dose (mg/kg)	Dosing interval (hours)	Ganciclovir maintenance dose (mg/kg)	Dosing interval (hours)
≥ 70	5	12	5	24
50 to 69	2.5	12	2.5	24
25 to 49	2.5	24	1.25	24
10 to 24	1.25	24	0.625	24
< 10	1.25	3 times/week following hemodialysis	0.625	3 times/week following hemodialysis

Hemodialysis: Dosing for patients undergoing hemodialysis should not exceed 1.25 mg/kg 3 times/week, following each hemodialysis session, Give shortly after completion of the hemodialysis session, since hemodialysis reduces plasma levels by ≈ 50%.

Oral: In renal impairment, modify the dose of oral ganciclovir as follows:

Oral Ganciclovir Dose in Renal Impairment	
Creatinine clearance (ml/min)	Ganciclovir doses
≥ 70	1000 mg TID or 500 mg q3h, 6x/day
50 to 69	1500 mg QD or 500 mg TID
25 to 49	1000 mg QD or 500 mg BID
10 to 24	500 mg QD
< 10	500 mg 3 times/week, following hemodialysis

Reduction of dose: Dose reductions are required for patients with renal impairment and for those with neutropenia or thrombocytopenia. Therefore, perform frequent white blood cell counts. Severe neutropenia (ANC < 500 mm^3) or severe thrombocytopenia (platelets < 25,000 mm^3) require a dose interruption until evidence of marrow recovery is observed (ANC > 750/ mm^3).

ZALCITABINE (Dideoxycytidine; ddC)

Tablets: 0.375 and 0.75 mg (*Rx*) — *Hivid* (Roche)

Warning:

The use of zalcitabine has been associated with significant clinical adverse reactions, some of which are potentially fatal. Zalcitabine can cause severe peripheral neuropathy; therefore use with extreme caution in patients with preexisting neuropathy. Zalcitabine may also rarely cause pancreatitis, and patients who develop any symptoms suggestive of pancreatitis while using zalcitabine should have therapy suspended immediately until this diagnosis is excluded.

Rare occurrences of lactic acidosis in the absence of hypoxemia and severe hepatomegaly with steatosis have been reported with the use of nucleoside analogs, including zidovudine and zalcitabine, and are potentially fatal. In addition, rare cases of hepatic failure and death considered possibly related to underlying hepatitis B and zalcitabine monotherapy have been reported (see Warnings).

Because of clinical uncertainty regarding the most appropriate use of nucleoside analogs, it is recommended that the decisions regarding the use of zalcitabine therapy be made in consultation with a physician experienced in the treatment of HIV-infected persons.

Actions:

Pharmacology: Zalcitabine, active against HIV, is a synthetic pyrimidine nucleoside analog of the naturally occurring nucleoside 2'-deoxycytidine in which the 3'-hydroxyl group is replaced by hydrogen. Within cells, zalcitabine is converted to the active metabolite, dideoxycytidine 5'-triphosphate (ddCTP), by cellular enzymes. ddCTP serves as an alternative substrate to deoxycytidine triphosphate (dCTP) for HIV-reverse transcriptase and inhibits the in vitro replication of HIV-1 by inhibition of viral DNA synthesis.

Pharmacokinetics:

Adults –

Absorption/Distribution: Following oral administration to HIV-infected patients, the mean absolute bioavailability of zalcitabine was > 80%. The absorption rate of a 1.5 mg oral dose was reduced when administered with food. This resulted in a 39% decrease in mean maximum plasma concentrations (Cmax) from 25.2 to 15.5 ng/ml, and a twofold increase in time to achieve Cmax from a mean of 0.8 hours under fasting conditions to 1.6 hours when the drug was given with food. The extent of absorption was decreased by 14% (from 72 to 62 ng•hr/ml).

The steady-state volume of distribution following IV administration of a 1.5 mg dose averaged 0.534 L/kg. Cerebrospinal fluid obtained from 9 patients at 2 to 3.5 hours following 0.06 or 0.09 mg/kg IV infusion showed measurable concentrations of zalcitabine. The CSF:plasma concentration ratio ranged from 9% to 37% (mean, 20%), demonstrating drug penetration through the blood-brain barrier.

Metabolism/Excretion: Zalcitabine is phosphorylated intracellularly to zalcitabine triphosphate, the active substrate for HIV-reverse transcriptase. Concentrations of zalcitabine triphosphate are too low for quantitation. Metabolism has not been fully evaluated. Zalcitabine does not appear to undergo a significant degree of metabolism by the liver. Renal excretion appears to be the primary route of elimination, and accounted for ≈ 70% of an orally administered dose within 24 hours after dosing. The mean elimination half-life is 2 hours. Total body clearance following an IV dose averages 285 ml/min. Less than 10% of a dose appears in the feces.

Children – Limited pharmacokinetic data have been reported for five HIV-positive children using doses of 0.03 and 0.04 mg/kg administered orally every 6 hours. The mean bioavailability of zalcitabine in this study was 54% and mean apparent systemic clearance was 150 ml/min/m^2.

Indications:

Monotherapy: Treatment of HIV infection in adults with advanced HIV disease who either are intolerant to zidovudine or who have disease progression while receiving zidovudine.

Combination therapy with zidovudine: For the treatment of selected patients with advanced HIV infection (CD4 cell count ≤ 300/mm^3).

Contraindications:

Hypersensitivity to zalcitabine or any components of the product.

Warnings:

Peripheral neuropathy: The major clinical toxicity is peripheral neuropathy (22% to 35%) of subjects. By comparison, neuropathy occurred in ≤ 14% of zidovudine-treated patients. Rates were similar among patients treated with zalcitabine monotherapy and in combination with zidovudine.

In some patients, symptoms of neuropathy may initially progress despite discontinuation of zalcitabine. With prompt discontinuation, the neuropathy is usually slowly reversible.

Use with extreme caution in patients with pre-existing peripheral neuropathy. Avoid zalcitabine in individuals with moderate or severe peripheral neuropathy, as evidenced by symptoms accompanied by objective findings.

Oral ulcers: Severe oral ulcers occurred in ≈ 3% of patients in two trials. Less severe oral ulcerations occurred at higher frequencies in other clinical trials.

Esophageal ulcers: Infrequent cases of esophageal ulcers have been attributed to zalcitabine therapy. Consider interruption of therapy in patients who develop esophageal ulcers that do not respond to specific treatment for opportunistic pathogens in order to assess a possible relationship to zalcitabine.

Cardiomyopathy/CHF have occurred with the use of nucleoside antiretroviral agents in AIDS patients; infrequent cases have occurred in patients receiving zalcitabine. Approach treatment with caution in patients with baseline cardiomyopathy or history of CHF.

Anaphylactoid reaction: There has been one report of an anaphylactoid reaction occurring in a patient receiving both zalcitabine and zidovudine. In addition, there have been several reports of urticaria without other signs of anaphylaxis.

Combination therapy: Because severe adverse effects may be attributable to either zalcitabine or zidovudine components of combination therapy, or to their combination, consult complete product information for zidovudine before initiating combination therapy or reinstituting zidovudine monotherapy after an adverse reaction.

No benefit from combination therapy has been observed from studies of zidovudine-exposed patients with CD4 cell counts < 150 cells/mm^3. Combination therapy is not recommended in these patients.

Mutagenesis: Human peripheral blood lymphocytes were exposed to zalcitabine, and at ≥ 1.5 mcg/ml, dose-related increases in chromosomal aberrations were seen. Oral doses of zalcitabine at 2500 and 4500 mg/kg were clastogenic in the mouse micronucleus assay.

Pregnancy: Category C.

Lactation: It is not known whether zalcitabine is excreted in breast milk. Decide whether to discontinue nursing or the drug, taking into account the importance of the drug to the mother. It is currently recommended in the US that HIV-infected women do not breastfeed infants regardless of the use of antiretroviral agents.

Children: Safety and efficacy of zalcitabine in combination with zidovudine or as monotherapy in HIV-infected children < 13 years of age has not been established.

Precautions:

Monitoring: Perform periodic complete blood counts and clinical chemistry tests. Monitor serum amylase levels in those individuals who have a history of elevated amylase, pancreatitis, ethanol abuse, who are on parenteral nutrition or who are otherwise at high risk of pancreatitis.

Drug Interactions:

Drugs that may affect zalcitabine include antacids, chloramphenicol, cisplatin, dapsone, didanosine, disulfiram, ethionamide, glutethimide, gold, hydralazine, iodoquinol, isoniazid, metronidazole, nitrofurantoin, phenytoin, ribavirin, vincristine, cimetidine, metoclopramide, pentamidine and probenecid.

Drug/Food interactions: The absorption rate of a 1.5 mg dose is reduced when administered with food resulting in a 39% decrease in mean C_{max} and a twofold increase in time to achieve C_{max}. The extent of absorption is decreased by 14%.

Adverse Reactions:

Adverse reactions occurring in ≥ 3% of patients include: Malaise/fatigue; abdominal pain; oral lesions/stomatitis; vomiting/nausea; peripheral neuropathy; elevated amylase; rash/pruritus/urticaria; diarrhea; oral ulcers; dysphagia; hypoglycemia; hyponatremia; bilirubin increased; loss of appetite; abnormal weight loss; abnormal hepatic function; hyperglycemia; myalgia; headache; nasal discharge; cough; pruritic disorder; fever.

Administration and Dosage:

Monotherapy: 0.75 mg every 8 hours (2.25 mg total daily dose).

Combination therapy with zidovudine: 0.75 mg given concomitantly with 200 mg zidovudine every 8 hours (2.25 mg zalcitabine total daily dose and 600 mg zidovudine total daily dose).

Renal function impairment: Dosage reduction is recommended: Ccr 10 to 40 ml/min, 0.75 mg every 12 hours; Ccr < 10 ml/min, 0.75 mg every 24 hours.

Dose adjustment:

Monotherapy and combination therapy – For toxicities likely to be associated with zalcitabine, interrupt or reduce dose. For severe toxicities or those persisting after dose reduction, interrupt zalcitabine therapy. For recipients of combination therapy with zalcitabine and zidovudine, base dose adjustments for either drug on the known toxicity profile of the individual drugs. For toxicities that are associated with either zidovudine or zalcitabine, interrupt or reduce dose of both drugs. For any interruption of zalcitabine (especially if zalcitabine is permanently discontinued), adjust zidovudine dosage schedule from 200 mg every 8 hours to 100 mg every 4 hours. For severe toxicities or toxicities in which the causative drug is unclear or which persist after dose interruption or reduction of one drug, interrupt or reduce dose of the other drug.

Peripheral neuropathy – Patients developing moderate discomfort with signs or symptoms of peripheral neuropathy should stop zalcitabine. Zalcitabine-associated peripheral neuropathy may continue to worsen despite interruption of therapy. Reintroduce at 50% dose (0.375 mg every 8 hours) only if all findings related to peripheral neuropathy have improved to mild symptoms. Permanently discontinue the drug when patients experience severe discomfort related to peripheral neuropathy or moderate discomfort progresses. If other moderate to severe clinical adverse reactions or lab abnormalities occur, interrupt zalcitabine (or both zalcitabine and zidovudine in combination therapy) until the reaction abates. Carefully reintroduce therapy at lower doses if appropriate. If adverse reactions recur, discontinue therapy.

Hematologic toxicities – In patients with poor bone marrow reserve, particularly those patients with advanced symptomatic HIV disease, frequent monitoring of hematologic indices is recommended to detect serious anemia or granulocytopenia. Significant toxicities, such as anemia (hemoglobin < 7.5 g/dl or reduction > 25% of baseline) or granulocytopenia (granulocyte count < 750/mm^3 or reduction of > 50% from baseline), may require a treatment interruption of zalcitabine and zidovudine until evidence of marrow recovery is observed. For less severe anemia or granulocytopenia, a reduction in the zidovudine daily dose may be adequate. In patients who experience hematologic toxicity, reduction in hemoglobin may occur as early as 2 to 4 weeks after initiation of therapy and granulocytopenia usually occurs after 6 to 8 weeks of therapy. In patients who develop significant anemia, dose modification does not necessarily eliminate the need for transfusion. If marrow recovery occurs following dose modification, gradual increases in dose may be appropriate depending on hematologic indices and patient intolerance.

RIMANTADINE HCl

Tablets: 100 mg (*Rx*)	*Flumadine* (Forest)
Syrup: 50 mg/5 ml (*Rx*)	

Actions:

Pharmacology: Rimantadine is a synthetic antiviral agent. The mechanism of action is not fully understood. It appears to exert its inhibitory effect early in the viral replicative cycle, possibly inhibiting the uncoating of the virus. Genetic studies suggest that a virus protein specified by the virion M_2 gene plays an important role in the susceptibility of influenza A virus to inhibition by rimantadine.

Rimantadine is safe and effective in preventing signs and symptoms of infection caused by various strains of influenza A virus. Since rimantadine does not completely prevent the host immune response to influenza A infection, individuals who take this drug may still develop immune responses to natural disease or vaccination and may be protected when later exposed to antigenically related viruses. Following vaccination during an influenza outbreak, consider rimantadine prophylaxis for the 2 to 4 week time period required to develop an antibody response. However, the safety and efficacy of prophylaxis have not been shown for > 6 weeks.

Consider rimantadine therapy for adults who develop an influenza-like illness during known or suspected influenza A infection in the community. When given within 48 hours after onset of signs and symptoms of infection caused by influenza A virus strains, rimantadine reduces the duration of fever and systematic symptoms.

Pharmacokinetics: There are no data establishing a correlation between plasma concentration and antiviral effect. The tablet and syrup formulations of rimantadine are equally absorbed after oral administration. The mean peak plasma concentration after a single 100 mg dose was 74 ng/ml. The time to peak concentration was 6 hours in healthy adults. The single dose elimination half-life in this population was 25.4 hours. The single-dose elimination half-life in a group of healthy 71- to 79-year-old subjects was 32 hours. Plasma protein binding is about 40%.

In a group (n = 10) of children 4 to 8 years old who were given a single dose (6.6 mg/kg) of syrup, plasma concentrations ranged from 446 to 988 ng/ml at 5 to 6 hours and from 170 to 424 ng/ml at 24 hours. In some children, the drug was detected in plasma 72 hours after the last dose. Following oral administration, rimantadine is extensively metabolized in the liver with < 25% of the dose excreted in the urine as unchanged drug. Three hydroxylated metabolites have been found in plasma. These metabolites, an additional conjugated metabolite and parent drug account for 74% of a single 200 mg dose excreted in urine over 72 hours.

Indications:

Adults: Prophylaxis/treatment of illness caused by various strains of influenza A virus.

Children: Prophylaxis against influenza A virus.

Contraindications:

Hypersensitivity to drugs of the adamantine class, including rimantadine and amantadine.

Warnings:

Renal/Hepatic function impairment: The safety and pharmacokinetics of rimantadine in renal and hepatic insufficiency have only been evaluated after single dose administration. In a single dose study of patients with anuric renal failure, the apparent clearance was ≈ 40% lower and the elimination half-life was 1.6-fold greater than that in healthy controls. In a study of 14 persons with chronic liver disease (mostly stabilized cirrhotics), no alterations in the pharmacokinetics were observed after a single dose of rimantadine. However, the apparent clearance of rimantadine following a single dose to 10 patients with severe liver dysfunction was 50% lower than that reported for healthy subjects. Because of the potential for accumulation of rimantadine and its metabolites in plasma, exercise caution when patients with renal or hepatic insufficiency are treated with rimantadine.

Pregnancy: Category C.

Lactation: Rimantadine should not be administered to nursing mothers because of the adverse affects noted in offspring of rats treated with rimantadine during the nursing period.

Children: Prophylaxis studies with rimantadine have not been performed in children < 1 year of age.

Precautions:

Seizures: An increased incidence of seizures has been reported in patients with a history of epilepsy who received the related drug amantadine. In clinical trials, the occurrence of seizure-like activity was observed in a small number of patients with a history of seizures who were not receiving anticonvulsant medication while taking rimantadine. If seizures develop, discontinue the drug.

Resistance: Consider transmission of rimantadine-resistant virus when treating patients whose contacts are at high risk for influenza A illness. Influenza A virus strains resistant to rimantadine can emerge during treatment and may be transmissible and cause typical influenza illness. Of patients with initially sensitive virus upon treatment with rimantadine, 10% to 30% shed rimantadine-resistant virus. Clinical response, although slower in those patients, was not significantly different from those who did not shed resistant virus.

Drug Interactions:

Drugs that may affect rimantadine include acetaminophen, aspirin and cimetidine.

Adverse Reactions:

The most frequently reported adverse events involved the GI and CNS. Rates increased significantly using higher than recommended doses. In most cases, symptoms resolved rapidly with discontinuation of treatment. Adverse reactions occurring in ≥ 3% of patients include insomnia.

Administration and Dosage:

Adults: Prophylaxis/treatment — The recommended dose of rimantadine is 100 mg twice a day. In patients with severe hepatic dysfunction, renal failure (Ccr ≤ 10 ml/min) and elderly nursing home patients, a dose reduction to 100 mg daily is recommended. For treatment, initiate therapy as soon as possible, preferably within 48 hours after onset of signs and symptoms of influenza A infection. Continue therapy for ≈ 7 days from the initial onset of symptoms.

Children: Prophylaxis — Administer once a day at a dose of 5 mg/kg, not exceeding 150 mg. For children ≥ 10 years of age, use the adult dose.

TRIMETHOPRIM AND SULFAMETHOXAZOLE (Co-Trimoxazole; TMP-SMZ)

Tablets: 80 mg trimethoprim and 400 mg sulfomethoxazole (*Rx*)	Various, *Bactrim* (Roche), *Septra* (Glaxo Wellcome)
Tablets, Double Strength: 160 mg trimethoprim and 800 mg sulfamethoxazole (*Rx*)	Various, *Bactrim DS* (Roche), *Septra DS* (Glaxo Wellcome)
Oral Suspension: 40 mg trimethoprim and 200 mg sulfamethoxazole per 5 ml (*Rx*)	Various, *Bactrim Pediatric* (Roche), *Septra* (Glaxo Wellcome)
Injection: 80 mg trimethoprim and 400 mg sulfamethoxazole per 5 ml (*Rx*)	Various, *Bactrim IV* (Roche), *Septra IV* (Glaxo Wellcome)

Actions:

Pharmacology: Sulfamethoxazole (SMZ) inhibits bacterial synthesis of dihydrofolic acid by competing with para-aminobenzoic acid. Trimethoprim (TMP) blocks the production of tetrahydrofolic acid by inhibiting the enzyme dihydrofolate reductase.

Pharmacokinetics:

Absorption/Distribution – TMP-SMZ is rapidly and completely absorbed following oral administration. Approximately 44% of TMP and 70% of SMZ are protein bound. Following oral administration, the half-lives of TMP (8 to 11 hours) and SMZ (10 to 12 hours) are similar. Following IV administration, the mean plasma half-life was 11.3 hours for TMP and 12.8 hours for SMZ.

Metabolism/Excretion – TMP is metabolized to a small extent; SMZ undergoes biotransformation to inactive compounds.

Urine concentrations are considerably higher than serum concentrations.

Indications:

Oral and parenteral:

Urinary tract infections (UTIs) due to susceptible strains of E coli, Klebsiella and Enterobacter species, M morganii, P mirabilis and P vulgaris –

Shigellosis enteritis caused by susceptible strains of *S flexneri* and *S sonnei* in children and adults.

Pneumocystis carinii pneumonia (PCP) – Treatment in children and adults.

Oral:

Pneumocystis carinii pneumonia – Prophylaxis in individuals who are immunosuppressed and considered to be at increased risk.

Acute otitis media in children due to susceptible strains of *H influenzae* or *S pneumoniae*. There are limited data on the safety of repeated use in children < 2 years of age. Not indicated for prophylactic use or prolonged administration.

Acute exacerbations of chronic bronchitis in adults due to susceptible strains of *H influenzae* and *S pneumoniae*.

Travelers' diarrhea in adults due to susceptible strains of enterotoxigenic *E coli*.

Unlabeled uses: Treatment of cholera and salmonella-type infections and nocardiosis.

TMP 40 mg and SMZ 200 mg daily at bedtime, a minimum of 3 times weekly or postcoitally has been used to prevent recurrent UTIs in females.

Low-dose TMP–SMZ has been studied in the prophylaxis of neutropenic patients with *P carinii* infections or leukemia patients to reduce the incidence of gram-negative rod bacteremia.

Prophylaxis with TMP-SMZ appears beneficial in reducing the incidence of bacterial infection (especially of the urinary tract and blood) following renal transplantation, and may provide protection against *P carinii* pneumonia.

Treatment of acute and chronic prostatitis – 160 mg TMP/800 mg SMZ twice daily has been used for chronic bacterial prostatitis for up to 12 weeks.

Contraindications:

Hypersensitivity to TMP or SMZ; megaloblastic anemia due to folate deficiency; pregnancy at term and lactation; infants < 2 months old.

The sulfonamides are chemically similar to some goitrogens, diuretics (acetazolamide and the thiazides) and oral hypoglycemic agents. Goiter production, diuresis and hypoglycemia occur rarely in patients receiving sulfonamides. Cross-sensitivity may exist with these agents.

Warnings:

Streptococcal pharyngitis: Do not use to treat streptococcal pharyngitis.

Hematologic effects: Sulfonamide-associated deaths, although rare, have occurred from hypersensitivity of the respiratory tract, Stevens-Johnson syndrome, toxic epidermal necrolysis, fulminant hepatic necrosis, agranulocytosis, aplastic anemia and other blood dyscrasias.

IV use at high doses or for extended periods of time may cause bone marrow depression manifested as thrombocytopenia, leukopenia or megaloblastic anemia.

Pneumocystis carinii pneumonitis in patients with Acquired Immunodeficiency Syndrome (AIDS): AIDS patients may not tolerate or respond to TMP–SMZ.

Renal/Hepatic function impairment: Use with caution. Maintain adequate fluid intake to prevent crystalluria and stone formation. Patients with severely impaired renal function exhibit an increase in the half-lives of both TMP and SMZ, requiring dosage regimen adjustment.

Elderly: There may be an increased risk of severe adverse reactions, particularly when complicating conditions exist.

Pregnancy: Category C.

Lactation: TMP–SMZ is not recommended in the nursing period because sulfonamides are excreted in breast milk and may cause kernicterus. Premature infants and infants with hyperbilirubinemia or G–6–PD deficiency are also at risk for adverse effects.

Children: Not recommended for infants < 2 months old. See Indications.

Precautions:

Special risk patients: Use with caution in patients with possible folate deficiency, severe allergy or bronchial asthma. In G-6-PD deficient individuals, hemolysis may occur; it is frequently dose-related.

Extravascular infiltration: If local irritation and inflammation due to extravascular infiltration of the infusion occurs, discontinue the infusion and restart at another site.

Benzyl alcohol, contained in some of these products as a preservative, has been associated with a fatal "gasping syndrome" in premature infants.

Drug Interactions:

Drugs that may be affected by TMP-SMZ include anticoagulants, cyclosporine, dapsone, diuretics, hydantoins, methotrexate, sulfonylureas and zidovudine. Drugs that may affect TMP-SMZ include dapsone.

Adverse Reactions:

Adverse reactions may include: GI disturbances; allergic skin reactions; agranulocytosis; aplastic, hemolytic or megaloblastic anemia; thrombocytopenia; leukopenia; neutropenia; hypoprothrombinemia; eosinophilia; methemoglobinemia; hyperkalemia; hyponatremia; erythema multiforme; Stevens-Johnson syndrome; generalized skin eruptions; rash; toxic epidermal necrolysis; urticaria; pruritus; exfoliative dermatitis; anaphylactoid reactions; photosensitization; allergic myocarditis; angioedema; drug fever; chills; systemic lupus erythematosus; generalized allergic reactions; glossitis; anorexia; stomatitis; pancreatitis; elevation of serum transaminase and bilirubin; headache; mental depression; convulsions; ataxia; hallucinations; tinnitus; vertigo; insomnia; apathy; fatigue; weakness; nervousness; peripheral neuritis; renal failure; interstitial nephritis; BUN and serum creatinine elevation; toxic nephrosis with oliguria and anuria; crystalluria; arthralgia; myalgia.

ATOVAQUONE

Suspension: 750 mg/5 ml (*Rx*)	*Mepron* (Burroughs Wellcome)

Actions:

Pharmacology: Atovaquone, an analog of ubiquinone, is an antiprotozoal with antipneumocystis activity.

Pharmacokinetics: Absorption is enhanced approximately twofold when given with food. Atovaquone is extensively bound to plasma proteins (> 99.9%). CSF concentratons are < 1% of plasma concentrations. Half-life ranged from 67 to 77.6 hours following the suspension. The long half-life is due to presumed enterohepatic cycling and eventual fecal elimination. There is indirect evidence that atovaquone may undergo limited metabolism; however, a specific metabolite has not been identified.

Indications:

Pneumocystitis carinii pneumonia (PCP): Acute oral treatment of mild to moderate PCP in patients who are intolerant to TMP-SMZ.

Contraindications:

Development or history of potentially life-threatening allergic reactions to any of the components of the formulation.

Warnings:

Severe PCP: Clinical experience has been limited to patients with mild to moderate PCP. Treatment of more severe episodes of PCP has not been systematically studied.

Elderly: Exercise caution when treating elderly patients reflecting the greater frequency of decreased hepatic, renal and cardiac function.

Pregnancy: Category C.

Lactation: It is not known whether atovaquone is excreted into breast milk.

Children: Safety and efficacy have not been established. Preliminary analysis suggests that the pharmacokinetics are age-dependent.

Precautions:

Absorption of orally administered atovaquone is limited but can be significantly increased when the drug is taken with food. Plasma concentrations correlate with the likelihood of successful treatment and survival. GI disorders may limit absorption of orally administered drugs. Patients with these disorders also may not achieve plasma concentrations of atovaquone associated with response to therapy in controlled trials.

Concurrent pulmonary conditions: Atovaquone is not effective therapy for concurrent pulmonary conditions such as bacterial, viral or fungal pneumonia or mycobacterial diseases. Clinical deterioration in patients may be due to infections with other pathogens, as well as progressive PCP.

Drug Interactions:

Use caution when administering atovaquone concurrently with other highly plasma protein bound drugs with narrow therapeutic indices as competition for binding sites may occur.

Drugs that may interact include rifamycins, TMP-SMZ and zidovudine.

Drug/Food interactions: Administering atovaquone with food enhances its absorption by apporximately twofold.

Adverse Reactions:

Adverse reactions occurring in ≥ 3% of patients include rash (including maculopapular), nausea, diarrhea, headache, vomiting, fever, cough, insomnia, asthenia, pruritus, monilia (oral), abdominal pain, constipation, dizziness, anemia, neutropenia, elevated ALT and AST, elevated alkaline phosphatase, elevated amylase, hyponatremia, pain, sweating, anxiety, anorexia, sinusitis, dyspepsia, rhinitis and taste perversion.

Administration and Dosage:

Adults: 750 mg administered with food 3 times a day for 21 days (total daily dose 2250 mg). Failure to administer atovaquone with food may result in lower atovaquone plasma concentrations and may limit response to therapy.

TRIMETREXATE GLUCURONATE

Powder for injection, lyophilized: 25 mg trimetrexate (*Rx*) *Neutrexin* (US Bioscience)

Warning:

Trimetrexate must be used with concurrent leucovorin (leucovorin protection) to avoid potentially serious or life-threatening toxicities.

Actions:

Pharmacology: Trimetrexate, a 2.4-diaminoquinazoline, non-classical folate antagonist, is a synthetic inhibitor of the enzyme dihydrofolate reductase (DHFR). The end result is disruption of DNA, RNA and protein synthesis, with consequent cell death.

Pharmacokinetics: Clearance was 38 ± 15 ml/min/m^2 and volume of distribution at steady state (Vd_{ss}) was 20 ± 8 L/m^2. The plasma concentration time profile declined in a biphasic manner over 24 hours with a terminal half-life of 11 ± 4 hours.

Renal clearance in cancer patients has varied from about 4 ± 2 to 10 ± 6 ml/min/m^2 and 10% and 30% is excreted unchanged in the urine. Considering the free fraction of trimetrexate, active tubular secretion may possibly contribute to the renal clearance.

Indications:

As an alternative therapy with concurrent leucovorin administration (leucovorin protection) for the treatment of moderate-to-severe *Pneumocystis carinii* pneumonia (PCP) in immunocompromised patients, including patients with acquired immunodeficiency syndrome (AIDS), who are intolerant of, or are refractory to TMP-SMZ therapy or for whom TMP/SMZ is contraindicated.

Unlabeled uses: Trimetrexate is being investigated for treatment of non-small cell lung, prostate and colorectal cancer.

Contraindications:

Clinically significant sensitivity to trimetrexate, leucovorin or methotrexate.

Warnings:

Concurrent leucovorin: Trimetrexate must be used with concurrent leucovorin to avoid potentially serious or life-threatening complications including bone marrow suppression, oral and GI mucosal ulceration, and renal and hepatic dysfunction. Leucovorin therapy must extend for 72 hours past the last dose of trimetrexate. Inform patients that failure to take the recommended dose and duration of leucovorin can lead to fatal toxicity. Closely monitor patients for the development of serious hematologic adverse reactions.

Pregnancy: Category D.

Lactation: It is not known if trimetrexate is excreted in breast milk.

Children: Safety and efficacy of trimetrexate for the treatment of histologically confirmed PCP has not been established for patients < 18 years of age.

Precautions:

Monitoring: Perform blood tests at least twice a week during therapy to assess the following parameters: Hematology (absolute neutrophil counts [ANC], platelets); renal function (serum creatinine, BUN); hepatic function (AST, ALT, alkaline phosphatase).

Special risk patients: Patients receiving trimetrexate may experience hematologic, hepatic, renal and GI toxicities. Use caution in treating patients with impaired hematologic, renal or hepatic function.

Pulmonary conditions: Trimetrexate has not been evaluated clinically for the treatment of concurrent pulmonary conditions such as bacterial, viral or fungal pneumonia or mycobacterial diseases.

Drug Interactions:

Since trimetrexate is metabolized by a P–450 enzyme system, drugs that induce or inhibit this drug metabolizing enzyme system may elicit important drug interactions that may alter trimetrexate plasma concentrations, which include erythromycin, rifampin, rifabutin, ketoconazole, fluconazole, cimetidine, nitrogen substituted imidazole drugs (eg, clotrimazole, ketoconazole, miconazole).

Adverse Reactions:

Adverse reactions occurring in ≥ 3% of patients include fever, rash/pruritus, nausea/vomiting, neutropenia, thrombocytopenia, anemia, increased AST and ALT, increased alkaline phosphatase, hyponatremia.

Administration and Dosage:

Trimetrexate must be given with concurrent leucovorin (leucovorin protection) to avoid potentially serious or life-threatening toxicities. Leucovorin must be given daily during trimetrexate treatment and for 72 hours past the last trimetrexate dose.

Trimetrexate is administered at a dose of 45 mg/m^2 once daily by IV infusion over 60 to 90 minutes. Leucovorin may be administered IV at a dose of 20 mg/m^2 over 5 to 10 minutes every 6 hours for a total daily dose of 80 mg/m^2, or orally as 4 doses of 20 mg/m^2 spaced equally throughout the day. Round up the oral dose to the next higher 25 mg increment. The recommended course of therapy is 21 days of trimetrexate and 24 days of leucovorin.

Dosage modifications:

Hematologic toxicity – Modify trimetrexate and leucovorin doses based on the worst hematologic toxicity according to the following table. If leucovorin is given orally, round up doses to the next higher 25 mg increment.

Dose Modifications for Hematologic Toxicity

Toxicity Grade	Neutrophils per mm^3	Platelets per mm^3	Trimetrexate	Leucovorin
1	> 1,000	> 75,000	45 mg/m^2 once daily	20 mg/m^2 every 6 hours
2	750-1,000	50,000-75,000	45 mg/m^2 once daily	40 mg/m^2 every 6 hours
3	500-749	25,000-49,999	22 mg/m^2 once daily	40 mg/m^2 every 6 hours
4	< 500	< 25,000	Day 1-9 discontinue Day 10-21 interrupt up to 96 hours[1]	40 mg/m^2 every 6 hours

[1] If Grade 4 hematologic toxicity occurs prior to day 10, discontinue trimetrexate. Administer leucovorin (40 mg/m^2 every 6 hours) for an additional 72 hours. If Grade 4 hematologic toxicity occurs at day 10 or later, trimetrexate may be held up to 96 hours to allow counts to recover. If counts recover to Grade 3 within 96 hours, administer trimetrexate at a dose of 22 mg/m^2 and maintain leucovorin at 40 mg/m^2 every 6 hours. When counts recover to Grade 2 toxicity, trimetrexate dose may be increased to 45 mg/m^2, but the leucovorin dose should be maintained at 40 mg/m^2 for the duration of treatment. If counts do not improve to ≤ Grade 3 toxicity within 96 hours, discontinue trimetrexate. Administer leucovorin at a dose of 40 mg/m^2 every 6 hours for 72 hours following the last dose of trimetrexate.

DAPSONE (DDS)

Tablets: 25 and 100 mg (*Rx*)	*Dapsone* (Jacobus)

Actions:

Pharmacology: Dapsone, a sulfone, is bactericidal as well as bacteriostatic against *Mycobacterium leprae*.

Pharmacokinetics:

Absorption/Distribution – Dapsone is rapidly and nearly completely absorbed from the GI tract; peak plasma concentrations are reached in 4 to 8 hours. Daily administration of 200 mg for at least 8 days is necessary to achieve a plateau level of 0.1 to 7 mcg/ml (average 2.3). Approximately 70% to 90% of dapsone is plasma protein bound. Enterohepatic circulation accounts for appreciable tissue levels of dapsone 3 weeks after therapy is discontinued.

Metabolism/Excretion – Dapsone is acetylated in the liver, and the degree of acetylation is genetically determined. The plasma half-life ranges from 10 to 50 hours (average 28 hours).

About 70% to 85% is excreted in urine as conjugates and unidentified water-soluble metabolites.

Indications:

Dermatitis herpetiformis.

Leprosy: All forms of leprosy (Hansen's disease) except for cases of proven dapsone resistance.

Unlabeled uses: Treatment of relapsing polychondritis; prophylaxis of malaria; inflammatory bowel disorders; Leishmaniasis; *Pneumocystis carinii* pneumonia; rheumatic/connective tissue disorders; brown recluse spider bites.

Contraindications:

Hypersensitivity to dapsone or its derivatives.

Warnings:

Hematologic effects: Deaths associated with dapsone administration have been reported from agranulocytosis, aplastic anemia and other blood dyscrasias. Sore throat, fever, pallor, purpura or jaundice may occur.

Severe anemia – Treat prior to initiation of therapy and monitor hemoglobin. Hemolysis and methemoglobin may be poorly tolerated by patients with severe cardiopulmonary disease.

Hypersensitivity: Cutaneous reactions (especially bullous), include exfoliative dermatitis, toxic erythema, erythema multiforme, toxic epidermal necrolysis, morbilliform and scarlatiniform reactions, urticaria and erythema nodosum.

Sulfone syndrome is an unusual and potentially fatal hypersensitivity reaction. It consists of fever, malaise, jaundice with hepatic necrosis, exfoliative dermatitis, lymphadenopathy, methemoglobinemia and hemolytic anemia.

Leprosy reactional states, including cutaneous, are not hypersensitivity reactions to dapsone and do not require discontinuation (see Precautions).

Pregnancy: Category C.

Lactation: Dapsone is excreted in breast milk in substantial amounts. Hemolytic reactions can occur in neonates. Discontinue nursing or discontinue the drug.

Precautions:

Monitoring: Perform blood counts weekly for the first month, monthly for 6 months and semi-annually thereafter. If a significant reduction in leukocytes, platelets or hematopoiesis occurs, discontinue dapsone.

Hemolysis and Heinz body formation may be exaggerated in individuals with glucose-6-phosphate dehydrogenase (G-6-PD) deficiency, methemoglobin reductase deficiency or hemoglobin M. This reaction is frequently dose-related. Give with caution to these patients or patients exposed to other agents or conditions such as infection or diabetic ketosis capable of producing hemolysis.

Hepatic effects: Toxic hepatitis and cholestatic jaundice have been reported early in therapy. Hyperbilirubinemia may occur more often in G-6-PD deficient patients. When feasible, baseline and subsequent monitoring of liver function is recommended.

Peripheral neuropathy is an unusual complication in nonleprosy patients. Motor loss is predominant. If muscle weakness appears, withdraw dapsone.

Phototosensitivity: Phototoxicity may occur.

Leprosy reactional states are abrupt changes in clinical activity occurring in leprosy with any effective treatment and are classified into two groups.

Type 1 (reversal reaction; downgrading) may occur in borderline or tuberculoid leprosy patients soon after chemotherapy is started, and is presumed to result from a reduction in the antigenic load. The patient has an enhanced delayed hypersensitivity response to residual infection leading to swelling ("reversal") of existing skin and nerve lesions.

Type 2 (erythema nodosum leprosum; ENL; lepromatous reaction) occurs mainly in lepromatous patients and small numbers of borderline patients. Treated patients (≈ 50%) show this reaction in the first year. In general, antileprosy treatment is continued.

Drug Interactions:

Drugs that may affect dapsone include activated charcoal, didanosine, folic acid antagonists, para-aminobenzoic acid, probenecid, rifampin and trimethoprim. Drugs that may be affected by dapsone include trimethoprim.

Adverse Reactions:

Adverse reactions may include: Dose-related hemolysis, hemolytic anemia, hypoalbuminemia without proteinuria, drug-induced lupus erythematosus, phototoxicity, peripheral neuropathy, headache, psychosis, insomnia, vertigo, paresthesia, nausea, vomiting, abdominal pain, anorexia, albuminuria, the nephrotic syndrome, renal papillary necrosis, blurred vision, tinnitus, fever, male infertility, tachycardia, an infectious mononucleosis-like syndrome, pancreatitis, pulmonary eosinophilia.

Administration and Dosage:

Dermatitis herpetiformis: Start with 50 mg daily in adults and correspondingly smaller doses in children. If full control is not achieved within the range of 50 to 300 mg daily, higher doses may be tried. Reduce dosage to a minimum maintenance level as soon as possible.

Maintenance dosage may be reduced or eliminated on a strict gluten free diet; the average time for dosage reduction is 8 months with a range of 4 months to 2½ years and for dosage elimination 29 months with a range of 6 months to 9 years.

Leprosy:

Recommended dosage – The schedule amounts to 50 to 100 mg daily in adults, with correspondingly smaller doses for children.

Bacteriologically negative tuberculoid and indeterminate disease – An adult dosage of 100 mg daily with 6 months of rifampin 600 mg/day is recommended. Under WHO, daily rifampin may be replaced by 600 mg rifampin monthly if supervised. After all signs of clinical activity are controlled (usually after an additional 6 months), continue dapsone therapy a minimum of 3 years for tuberculoid and indeterminate patients.

Lepromatous and borderline patients – Administer dapsone (100 mg/day) for 2 years with rifampin 600 mg daily. Under WHO daily rifampin may be replaced by 600 mg rifampin monthly, if supervised. One may elect the concurrent administration of a third anti-leprosy drug, usually either clofazimine 50–100 mg daily or ethionamide 250–500 mg daily. Dapsone 100 mg daily is continued 3–10 years until all signs of clinical activity are controlled with skin scrapings and biopsies negative for one year. Dapsone should then be continued for an additional 10 years for borderline patients and for life for lepromatous patients.

Children: The recommended dosage is 1 to 2 mg/kg/day for a minimum of 3 years; maximum is usual adult dosage of 100 mg/day.

CLOFAZIMINE

Capsules: 50 and 100 mg (*Rx*) — *Lamprene* (Geigy)

Actions:

Pharmacology: Clofazimine exerts a slow bactericidal effect on *Mycobacterium leprae* (Hansen's bacillus). The drug also exerts anti-inflammatory properties in controlling erythema nodosum leprosum reactions.

Pharmacokinetics:

Absorption/Distribution – Absorption rate ranges from 45% to 62% after oral administration.

Metabolism/Excretion – Clofazimine is retained in the human body for a long time. Half-life after repeated doses is estimated to be at least 70 days.

Indications:

Leprosy: Treatment of lepromatous leprosy, including dapsone-resistant lepromatous leprosy and lepromatous leprosy complicated by erythema nodosum leprosum.

Combination drug therapy has been recommended for initial treatment of multibacillary leprosy to prevent the development of drug resistance.

Warnings:

GI effects: Severe abdominal symptoms have necessitated exploratory laparotomies in patients receiving clofazimine. Autopsies have revealed crystalline deposits of clofazimine in the intestinal mucosa, liver, gallbladder, bile, spleen, adrenals, subcutaneous fat, mesenteric lymph nodes, muscles, bone and skin.

Use with caution in patients who have GI problems such as abdominal pain and diarrhea. Give dosages of > 100 mg daily for as short a period as possible and only under close medical supervision. If a patient complains of colicky or burning pain in the abdomen, nausea, vomiting or diarrhea, reduce the dose and, if necessary, increase the interval between doses or discontinue the drug.

Pregnancy: Category C.

Lactation: Clofazimine is excreted in breast milk. Do not administer to a nursing woman unless clearly indicated.

Children: Safety and efficacy in children have not been established.

Precautions:

Skin discoloration due to the drug may result in depression.

Drug Interactions:

Dapsone: If leprosy-associated inflammatory reactions develop in patients being treated with dapsone and clofazimine, it is still advisable to continue treatment with both drugs.

Adverse Reactions:

Adverse reactions occurring in ≥ 3% of patients include: Pigmentation (pink to brownish black); ichthyosis; dryness; rash; pruritus; abdominal/epigastric pain; diarrhea; nausea; vomiting; GI intolerance.

Administration and Dosage:

Take with meals.

Dapsone-resistant leprosy: 100 mg clofazimine/day in combination with one or more other antileprosy drugs for 3 years, then monotherapy with 100 mg clofazimine/day.

Dapsone-sensitive multibacillary leprosy: Combination therapy with two other antileprosy drugs is recommended. Give the triple-drug regimen for at least 2 years and continue, if possible, until negative skin smears are obtained. At this time, monotherapy with an appropriate antileprosy drug can be instituted.

Erythema nodosum leprosum: Treatment depends on severity of symptoms. In general, continue basic antileprosy treatment; if nerve injury or skin ulceration is threatened, give corticosteroids. Where prolonged corticosteroid therapy is necessary, clofazimine 100 to 200 mg/day for up to 3 months may be useful in eliminating or reducing corticosteroid requirements. Dosages > 200 mg daily are not recommended; taper dosage to 100 mg daily as soon as possible after the reactive episode is controlled.

ANTHELMINTICS

The following table lists the major parasitic infections, causative organisms and drugs of choice for treatment.

Major Parasite Infections

	Infection (common name)	Organism	Drug(s) of Choice
Intestinal Nematodes	Ascariasis[1] (Roundworm)	*Ascaris lumbricoides*	Mebendazole, Pyrantel pamoate or Diethylcarbamazine
	Uncinariasis (hookworm)	*Ancylostoma duodenale* *Necator americanus*	Mebendazole or Pyrantel pamoate[2]
	Strongyloidiasis (Threadworm)	*Strongyloides stercoralis*	Thiabendazole
	Trichuriasis (Whipworm)	*Trichuris trichiura*	Mebendazole
	Enterobiasis[3] (Pinworm)	*Enterobius vermicularis*	Mebendazole, Pyrantel pamoate or Albendazole
	Capillariasis	*Capillaria philippinensis*	Mebendazole or Thiabendazole
Tissue Nematodes	Trichinosis	*Trichinella spiralis*	Steroids for severe symptoms plus Thiabendazole, Albendazole, Flubendazole[6] or Mebendazole[2]
	Cutaneous larva migrans (creeping eruption)	*Ancylostoma braziliense* and others	Thiabendazole, Albendazole or Ivermectin[4]
	Onchocerciasis (River blindness)	*Onchocerca volvulus*	Suramin[5], Diethylcarbamazine or Ivermectin[4]
	Dracontiasis (guinea worm)	*Dracunculus medinensis*	Thiabendazole or Mebendazole
	Angiostrongyliasis (rat lungworm)	*Angiostrongylus cantonensis*	Thiabendazole or Mebendazole
	Loiasis	*Loa loa*	Diethylcarbamazine
Cestodes	Taeniasis (Beef tapeworm)	*Taenia saginata*	Praziquantel[2] or Niclosamide
	(Pork tapeworm)	*Taenia solium*	Praziquantel[2], Niclosamide or Albendazole
	Diphyllobothriasis (Fish tapeworm)	*Diphyllobothrium latum*	Praziquantel[2] or Niclosamide
	Dog tapeworm	*Dipylidium caninum*	Praziquantel[2]
	Hymenolepiasis (Dwarf tapeworm)	*Hymenolepis nana*	Praziquantel[2] or Niclosamide[6]
	Hydatid cysts	*Echinococcus granulosus*	Albendazole or Praziquantel
Trematodes	Schistosomiasis	*Schistosoma mansoni*	Praziquantel or Oxamniquine
		Schistosoma japonicum	Praziquantel
		Schistosoma haematobium	Praziquantel
		Schistosoma mekongi	Praziquantel
	Hermaphroditic Flukes Fasciolopsiasis (Intestinal fluke)	*Fasciolopsis buski*	Praziquantel
		Heterophyes heterophyes *Metagonimus yokogawai*	Praziquantel
	Clonorchiasis (Chinese liver fluke)	*Clonorchis sinensis*	Praziquantel
	Fascioliasis (Sheep liver fluke)	*Fasciola hepatica*	Praziquantel or Bithionol[4]
	Opisthorchiasis (Liver fluke)	*Opisthorchis viverrini*	Praziquantel
	Paragonimiasis (Lung fluke)	*Paragonimus westermani*	Praziquantel or Bithionol[4] (alternate)

[1] These are also indicated in Ascariasis: Piperazine citrate (if intestinal or biliary obstruction); thiabendazole.
[2] Unlabeled use.
[3] The following drugs are also indicated in Enterobiasis: Piperazine and thiabendazole.
[4] Available from the CDC.
[5] Available from the CDC, although generally not recommended.
[6] Not available in the US.

NITROFURANTOIN

NITROFURANTOIN	
Oral Suspension: 25 mg/5 ml (*Rx*)	*Furadantin* (Procter & Gamble Pharm)
NITROFURANTOIN MACROCRYSTALS	
Capsules: 25, 50 and 100 mg (*Rx*)	Various, *Macrodantin* (Procter & Gamble Pharm)
Capsules: 100 mg (as 25 mg macrocrystals, 75 mg monohydrate) (*Rx*)	*Macrobid* (Procter & Gamble Pharm)

Actions:

Pharmacology: Nitrofurantoin is a synthetic nitrofuran that is bacteriostatic in low concentrations (5 to 10 mcg/ml) and bactericidal in higher concentrations.

Pharmacokinetics:

Absorption/Distribution – Well absorbed from the GI tract after oral administration. The macrocrystalline form is absorbed more slowly due to slower dissolution and causes less GI distress. Therapeutic serum and tissue concentrations are not achieved after usual oral doses, except in the urinary tract. Protein binding is about 60%.

Metabolism/Excretion – The plasma half-life is about 20 minutes in healthy individuals and increases to 60 minutes in the anephric patient. In patients with impaired renal function, nitrofurantoin accumulates in the serum. About 30% to 50% of a dose is excreted unchanged in the urine. Acid urine enhances tubular reabsorption of nitrofurantoin, enhancing antibacterial activity in the renal tissues and lowering urinary concentrations.

Indications:

Urinary tract infections: Treatment of urinary tract infections due to susceptible strains of *E coli*, enterococci, *S aureus* (not for treatment of pyelonephritis or perinephric abscesses) and certain strains of *Klebsiella* and *Enterobacter species*.

Contraindications:

Renal function impairment (creatinine clearance < 60 ml/min), anuria or oliguria; hypersensitivity to nitrofurantoin.

Pregnant patients at term, during labor and delivery, or when the onset of labor is imminent, and in infants under 1 month of age.

Warnings:

Pulmonary reactions:

Acute – Manifested by sudden onset of dyspnea, chest pain, cough, fever and chills, pulmonary infiltration with consolidation or pleural effusion on x-ray; elevated sedimentation rate and eosinophilia are also present. Rechallenge is dangerous and will produce similar symptoms.

Subacute/chronic – Associated with prolonged therapy. These reactions are characterized by insidious development of dyspnea, nonproductive cough and malaise after 1 to 6 months or more of therapy.

Hemolysis: Hemolytic anemia of the primaquine sensitivity type has been induced by nitrofurantoin.

Renal impairment: In patients with impaired renal function, nitrofurantoin accumulates in the serum. Renal excretion is via glomerular filtration and tubular secretion.

Hepatic reactions including hepatitis, cholestatic jaundice, chronic active hepatitis, and hepatic necrosis, occur rarely. Fatalities have been reported.

Pregnancy: Category B. Contraindicated in pregnant patients at term and during labor and delivery.

Lactation: Nitrofurantoin is excreted into breast milk in very low concentrations.

Children: Contraindicated in infants < 1 month of age.

Precautions:

Peripheral neuropathy may occur and may become severe or irreversible. Fatalities have been reported.

Drug Interactions:

Drugs that may interact with nitrofurantoin include anticholinergics, magnesium salts and uricosurics.

Drug/Lab test interactions: A false-positive reaction for glucose in the urine may occur. This has been observed with Benedict's and Fehling's solutions but not with the glucose enzymatic test.

Adverse Reactions:

Adverse reactions may include: Anorexia; nausea; emesis; abdominal pain; diarrhea; parotitis; pancreatitis; maculopapular, erythematous or eczematous eruption; pruritus; urticaria; angioedema; anaphylaxis; drug fever; arthralgia; myalgia; chills; glucose-6–phosphate dehydrogenase deficiency anemia; granulocytopenia; agranulocytosis; leukopenia; thrombocytopenia; eosinophilia; megaloblasic anemia; hemolytic anemia; peripheral neuropathy; headache; dizziness; nystagmus; drowsiness; asthenia; vertigo; confusion; depression; increased AST; increased ALT; decreased hemoglobin; increased serum phosphorus.

Administration and Dosage:

Give with food or milk to improve drug absorption and, in some patients, tolerance.

Adults: 50 to 100 mg 4 times/day with meals and at bedtime. For long-term suppressive therapy, reduce dosage (50 to 100 mg at bedtime).

Children: 5 to 7 mg/kg/24 hrs given in 4 divided doses. For long-term suppressive therapy, doses as low as 1 mg/kg/24 hrs, given in single or in 2 divided doses, may be adequate.

The following table is based on an average weight in each range receiving 5 to 6 mg/kg per 24 hours, given in four divided doses. It can be used to calculate an average dose of oral suspension (5 mg/ml).

Nitrofurantoin Dosage in Children Based on Body Weight

Body weight		No. of teaspoonsful 4 times a day
lbs	kg	
15 to 26	7 to 11	½ (2.5 ml)
27 to 46	12 to 21	1 (5 ml)
47 to 68	22 to 30	1½ (7.5 ml)
69 to 91	31 to 41	2 (10 ml)

METHENAMINE

METHENAMINE HIPPURATE	
Tablets: 1 g (*Rx*)	*Hiprex* (Hoechst Marion Roussel), *Urex* (3M Pharmaceuticals)
METHENAMINE MANDELATE	
Tablets, enteric coated: 0.5 and 1 g (*Rx*)	Various
Suspension: 0.5 g/5 ml (*Rx*)	Various

Actions:

Pharmacology: In acid urine, methenamine is hydrolyzed to ammonia and formaldehyde, which is bactericidal.

Pharmacokinetics:

Absorption – Methenamine is readily absorbed following oral administration; 10% to 30% of the drug will be hydrolyzed by the gastric juices unless it is protected by an enteric coating.

Metabolism/Excretion – Methenamine is metabolized in the liver (≈ 10% to 25%) and has a half-life of 3 to 6 hours.

Excretion occurs via glomerular filtration and tubular secretion. The methenamine moiety is excreted in the urine (≈ 90%) within 24 hours.

Microbiology: The nonspecific antibacterial action of formaldehyde is effective against gram-positive and gram-negative organisms and fungi. *Escherichia coli*, enterococci and staphylococci are usually susceptible.

Methenamine is effective clinically against most common urinary tract pathogens since most bacteria are sensitive to free formaldehyde concentrations of 20 mcg/ml.

Indications:

Urinary tract infections: Prophylaxis or suppression/elimination of frequently recurring urinary tract infections when long-term therapy is considered necessary.

Contraindications:

Renal insufficiency; severe dehydration; severe hepatic insufficiency; use alone for acute infections with parenchymal involvement causing systemic symptoms; hypersensitivity to the drug; concurrent sulfonamides since an insoluble precipitate may form with formaldehyde in the urine.

Warnings:

Pregnancy: Category C.

Lactation: Methenamine passes into breast milk; levels are about equivalent to maternal serum and peak in 1 hour.

Precautions:

Large doses (8 g daily for 3 to 4 weeks) have caused bladder irritation, painful and frequent micturition, proteinuria and gross hematuria.

Acid urine pH should be maintained, especially when treating infections due to urea-splitting organisms such as *Proteus* and strains of *Pseudomonas*.

Serum transaminases have elevated mildly during treatment in a few instances and returned to normal while patients were still receiving methenamine hippurate.

Gout: Methenamine salts may cause precipitation of urate crystals in the urine.

Drug Interactions:

Drugs that may interact with methenamine include sulfonamides and urinary alkalinizers.

Drug/Lab test interactions: Methenamine may interfere with laboratory urine determinations of **17-hydroxycorticosteroids**, catecholamines and **vanillylmandelic acid** (false increases); and **5-hydroxyindoleacetic acid** (false decrease).

Methenamine taken during pregnancy can interfere with laboratory tests of **urine estriol** (resulting in unmeasurably low values) when an acid hydrolysis procedure is used. Use enzymatic hydrolysis in place of acid hydrolysis.

Adverse Reactions:

Adverse reactions may include: Nausea, vomiting, cramps, stomatitis, anorexia, bladder irritation, dysuria, proteinuria, hematuria, urinary frequency/urgency and crystalluria, urticaria, erythematous eruptions, rash, headache, dyspnea.

Administration and Dosage:

Methenamine hippurate:

Adults and children > 12 years of age – 1 g twice daily.

Children (6 to 12 years of age) – 0.5 to 1 g twice daily.

Methenamine mandelate:

Adults – 1 g 4 times daily, after meals and at bedtime.

Children (6 to 12 years of age) – 0.5 g, 4 times daily.

Children (< 6 years of age) – 0.25 g/30 lb (14 kg), 4 times daily.

Chapter 9

BIOLOGICALS

IMMUNE SERUMS

Actions:

Pharmacology: Standard immune globulins contain ≈ 16.5% gamma globulin. Immune globulin IV contains 5% immune globulins. These products are obtained, purified and standardized from human serum or plasma. They are obtained from pooled plasma either of donors from the general population or of hyperimmunized donors (for immune globulins for specific diseases).

Indications:

To provide passive immunization to one or more infectious diseases. Protection derived will be of rapid onset, but of short duration (1 to 3 months).

Contraindications:

Allergic response to gamma globulin or anti-immunoglobulin A (IgA) antibodies; allergic response to thimerosal; people with isolated immunoglobulin A (IgA) deficiency.

Immune globulin, intramuscular: Patients who have severe thrombocytopenia or any coagulation disorder that would contraindicate IM use.

Warnings:

Route of administration: Do not give these products IV (except immune globulin IV). IV injections can cause a precipitous fall in blood pressure and a picture similar to anaphylaxis. Give IM.

Hypersensitivity:

Anaphylactic reactions (rare) may occur following injection of human immune globulin preparations. Anaphylaxis is more likely if immune globulin is given IV.

Give with caution to patients with prior systemic allergic reactions following use of human immunoglobulin preparations.

Pregnancy: Category C.

Lactation: It is not known whether immune globulin is excreted in breast milk.

Precautions:

Skin testing should not be performed because intradermal injection of concentrated gamma globulin causes a localized area of inflammation which can be misinterpreted as a positive allergic reaction.

Drug Interactions:

Live virus vaccines my interact with immune globulins.

Adverse Reactions:

Adverse reactions may include: Tenderness; pain; muscle stiffness at injection site; urticaria; angioedema.

IMMUNE GLOBULIN INTRAVENOUS (IGIV)

Injection: 5% and 10% (*Rx*)	*Gamimune N* (Bayer)
Solution: ≈ 5% protein containing ≥ 90% gamma globulin, 5% immune globulin IV (human) (*Rx*)	*Gammagard S/D* (Baxter)
Solution for Injection (solvent/detergent treated): 5% and 10% immune globulin IV (human) (*Rx*)	*Venoglobulin-S* (Alpha Therapeutics)
Powder for Injection (freeze-dried, solvent/detergent treated): 50 mg/ml (*Rx*)	*Gammagard S/D* (Baxter)
Powder for Injection (freeze-dried) 50 mg/ml; 90% gammaglobulin (*Rx*)	*Polygam S/D* (American Red Cross)
Powder for Injection (lyophilized) 1 and 5 g immune globulin G (*Rx*)	*Gammar-IV* (Armour), *Sandoglobulin* (American Red Cross, Sandoz), *Venoglobulin-I* (Alpha Therapeutic), *Gammar-P I.V.* (Centeon)
Powder for Injection (freeze-dried) 50 mg/ml (*Rx*)	*Iveegam* (Immuno)

IGIV provides immediate antibody levels, whereas IM administration involves a 2 to 5 day delay before adequate serum levels are attained. Half-life is ≈ 3 weeks.

Administration and Dosage:

Administer IV only.

Sandoglobulin:

Immunodeficiency syndrome – 200 mg/kg once a month by IV infusion. If clinical response or the IgG level achieved is insufficient (minimum serum level, 300 mg/dl), increase to 300 mg/kg or repeat the infusion more frequently.

Idiopathic thrombocytopenic purpura – 400 mg/kg for 2 to 5 consecutive days.

Gammagard S/D:

Immunodeficiency syndrome – 200 to 400 mg/kg. Monthly doses of at least 100 mg/kg are recommended.

B-Cell CLL – 400 mg/kg every 3 to 4 weeks.

Idiopathic thrombocytopenic purpura – 1000 mg/kg. Give up to 3 doses on alternate days if required.

Gammar-P.I.V.:

Immunodeficiency syndrome – 200 to 400 mg/kg every 3 to 4 weeks. An initial loading dose of at least 200 mg/kg at more frequent intervals, 200 to 600 mg/kg at 3 week intervals once a therapeutic plasma level has been established can be used.

Venoglobulin-I:

Immunodeficiency syndrome – 200 mg/kg, administered monthly. If clinical response or the level of IgG achieved is insufficient, increase to 300 to 400 mg/kg monthly or repeat infusion more frequently than once a month.

Idiopathic thrombocytopenic purpura –

Induction: Up to 2000 mg/kg/day for 2 to 7 consecutive days.

Acute – Patients who respond to induction therapy by manifesting a platelet count of 30,000 to 50,000/mm^3 may be discontinued after 2 to 7 daily doses.

Maintenance – If platelet count falls to < 30,000/mm^3 or clinically significant bleeding occurs, give as a single 2000 mg/kg infusion every 2 weeks or less as needed to maintain platelet count > 30,000/mm^3 in children or 20,000/mm^3 in adults.

Gamimune N:

Immunodeficiency syndrome – 100 to 200 mg/kg administered once a month by IV infusion. If clinical response or the level of IgG achieved is insufficient, increase to 400 mg/kg or repeat the infusion more frequently than once a month.

Idiopathic thrombocytopenic purpura – 400 mg/kg for 5 consecutive days.

Iveegam:

Immunodeficiency syndrome – 200 mg/kg per month. If desired clinical results are not obtained, the dosage may be increased up to fourfold or intervals shortened. Doses up to 800 mg/kg per month have been tolerated.

Polygam S/D:

Immunodeficiency syndrome – 100 mg/kg/month. An initial dose of 200 to 400 mg/kg may be administered.

B-Cell CLL – 400 mg/kg every 3 to 4 weeks.

Idiopathic thrombocytopenic purpura – 1 g/kg. Give up to 3 separate doses on alternate days as required.

Venoglobulin-S:

Immunodeficiency syndrome – 200 mg/kg/month. If clinical response or the level of IgG achieved is insufficient, increase to 300 to 400 mg/kg or repeat the infusion more frequently than once a month.

Idiopathic thrombocytopenic purpura – 2000 mg/kg over a maximum of 5 days for induction therapy.

Maintenance therapy – 1000 mg/kg may be given as needed to maintain platelet counts of 30,000/mm^3 in children and 20,000/mm^3 in adults, or to prevent bleeding episodes in the interval between infusions.

IMMUNE GLOBULIN IM (IG; Gamma Globulin; ISG)

Injection (*Rx*) — *Gamastan* (Cutter Biological), *Gammar* (Armour)

Administration and Dosage:

For IM injection only.

Hepatitis A: A dose of 0.02 ml/kg (0.01 ml/lb) is recommended for household and institutional hepatitis A case contacts, and for persons who plan to travel for < 3 months in areas where hepatitis A is common; for prolonged travel (> 3 months), the dose is 0.06 ml/kg (repeat every 4 to 6 months).

Measles (Rubeola): To prevent or modify measles in a susceptible person exposed less than 6 days previously, give 0.25 ml/kg (0.11 ml/lb). If a susceptible child who is also immunocompromised is exposed to measles, give 0.5 ml/kg (15 ml maximum) immediately.

Immunoglobulin deficiency: The usual dosage consists of an initial dose of 1.3 ml/kg followed in 3 or 4 weeks by 0.66 ml/kg (at least 100 mg/kg) to be given every 3 to 4 weeks. Some patients may require more frequent injections.

Varicella: Give 0.6 to 1.2 ml/kg promptly, if zoster immune globulin is unavailable.

Rubella: Some studies suggest that the use of IG in exposed susceptible women can lessen the likelihood of infection and fetal damage; therefore, a dose of 0.55 ml/kg within 72 hours of exposure has been recommended and may benefit those women who do not consider a therapeutic abortion.

HEPATITIS B IMMUNE GLOBULIN (HBIG)

Injection (*Rx*) — *H-BIG* (Abbott), *Hep-B-Gammagee* (Merck), *HyperHep* (Cutter Biological)

Administration and Dosage:

Give injections IM, preferably in the gluteal or deltoid region.

Postexposure prophylaxis: The recommended dose is 0.06 ml/kg; the usual adult dose is 3 to 5 ml. Administer the appropriate dose as soon after exposure as possible (preferably within 7 days) and repeat 28 to 30 days after exposure.

Prophylaxis of infants born to HB_SAG-positive mothers: The recommended dose for at-risk newborns is 0.5 ml IM into the anterolateral thigh, as soon after birth as possible, preferably within 12 hours.

Prevention of carrier state: A similar or higher rate of prevention of the carrier state may be achieved in at-risk infants by administering HBIG 0.5 ml IM as soon after birth as possible, preferably no later than 24 hours and repeated at 3 months of age. At this time, an active vaccination program with hepatitis B vaccine is begun.

Individuals at increased risk: HBIG may be administered at the same time (but at a different site), or up to 1 month preceding hepatitis B vaccination without impairing the active immune response from hepatitis B vaccination.

Hepatitis B Virus Postexposure Recommendations

Exposure	Hepatitis B Immune Globulin		Vaccine	
	Dose (IM)	Recommended Timing	Dose (IM)	Recommended Timing
Perinatal	0.5 ml	Within 12 hrs of birth	0.5 ml	Within 12 hrs of birth;[1] repeat at 1 and 6 months
Percutaneous[2]	0.06 ml/kg	Single dose within 24 hours	1 ml[3]	Within 7 days; repeat at 1 and 6 months
Sexual	0.06 ml/kg	Single dose within 14 days of sexual contact[4]	1 ml[5]	Within 7 days; repeat at 1 and 6 months

[1] First dose can be given the same time as the HBIG dose, but at a different site.
[2] Needlestick, ocular or mucosal exposure.
[3] < 10 years old, give 0.5 ml.
[4] In heterosexuals, if vaccine is not given, give a second dose of HBIG and a course of the vaccine if the index patient remains HB_sAG-positive for 3 months after detection.
[5] Vaccine recommended for homosexual men and for regular sexual contacts of HBV carriers. Vaccine optional in initial treatment of heterosexual contacts of persons with acute HBV.

TETANUS IMMUNE GLOBULIN

Injection: (*Rx*) Hyper-Tet (Cutter Biological)

Administration and Dosage:

Administer IM. Do NOT inject IV.

Prophylaxis:

Adults – 250 units.

Children – In small children, the dose may be calculated by the body weight (4 units/kg). However, it may be advisable to administer the entire contents of the vial or syringe (250 units) regardless of the child's size, since theoretically the same amount of toxin will be produced in his body by the infecting tetanus organisms as in an adult.

Therapy: Several studies suggest the value of human tetanus antitoxin in the actual treatment of active tetanus using single doses of 3000 to 6000 units in combination with other accepted clinical procedures.

Guide to Tetanus Prophylaxis in Wound Management

History of Tetanus Immunization (Doses)	Clean, Minor Wounds		All Other Wounds	
	Tetanus Toxoid	Tetanus Immune Globulin	Tetanus Toxoid	Tetanus Immune Globulin
Uncertain	Yes	No	Yes	Yes
0 to 1	Yes	No	Yes	Yes
2	Yes	No	Yes	No[1]
3 or more	No[2]	No	No[3]	No

[1] Unless wound is more than 24 hours old.
[2] Unless more than 10 years since last dose.
[3] Unless more than 5 years since last dose.

AGENTS FOR ACTIVE IMMUNIZATION

In contrast to the immune serums and antitoxins, which contain exogenous antibodies to provide passive immunity, the Agents for Active Immunization include specific antigens which induce the endogenous production of antibodies. Agents which induce active immunity include vaccines and toxoids.

Vaccines contain whole (killed or attenuated live) microorganisms capable of inducing antibody formation, but which are not pathogenic. Toxoids are detoxified by-products derived from organisms which induce disease primarily through the elaboration of exotoxins. Although toxoids are not toxic, they are antigenic, and therefore, stimulate specific antibody production. Active immunization induced through inoculation with vaccines and toxoids provides prolonged immunity, whereas passive immunization with immune sera or antitoxins is of short duration.

The table below indicates the recommended immunization schedule for infants and children. This schedule has been approved by the Advisory Committee on Immunization Practices (ACIP), The American Academy of Pediatrics (AAP) and the American Academy of Family Physicians (AAFP).

Recommended Immunization Schedules[1]

Vaccine	Birth	2 months	4 months	6 months	12 months	15 months	18 months	4-6 years	11-12 years	14-16 years
Hepatitis B	HB-1									
		HB-2		HB-3						
Diphtheria, tetanus, pertussis		DTP	DTP	DTP	DTP or DTaP at 15 months			DTP or DTaP	Td	
H influenzae type b		Hib	Hib	Hib	Hib					
Poliovirus		OPV	OPV	OPV				OPV		
Measles, mumps, rubella					MMR			MMR[2]		

[1] Recommended childhood immunization schedule-United States, January 1995. MMWR 1995 Jan 6;43:959–60.
[2] The second dose of measles-mumps-rubella vaccine should be administered either at 4 to 6 years or at 11 to 12 years.

Hypersesitivity to vaccine components: Vaccine antigens produced in systems containing allergenic substances, (ie, embryonated chicken eggs) may cause hypersensitivity reactions including anaphylaxis. In contrast, influenza vaccine antigens (whole or split), although prepared in embryonated eggs, are highly purified and only rarely are associated with hypersensitivity reactions.

Live virus vaccines prepared by growing viruses in cell cultures are essentially devoid of allergenic substances.

Some vaccines contain preservatives (eg, thimerosal) or trace amounts of antibiotics (eg, neomycin) to which patients may be hypersensitive.

Altered immunocompetence: Virus replication after administration of live, attenuated virus vaccines may be enhanced in persons with immune deficiency diseases, and in those with suppressed capability for immune response (eg, leukemia, lymphoma, generalized malignancy or therapy with corticosteroids, alkylating agents, antimetabolites or radiation). Do not give live, attenuated virus vaccines to such patients.

HIV infection: Special immunization recommendations are appropriate for persons infected with HIV.

Live bacterial or viral vaccines: Persons infected with HIV and persons who have developed AIDS are theoretically at risk of disseminated infection following immunization with a live, albeit attenuated, bacterial or viral vaccine.

Inactivated vaccines or toxoids: In general, immunization with an inactivated vaccine or toxoid poses no additional risk to persons infected with HIV and persons who have developed AIDS. But these persons may be less likely to develop an adequate immune response to vaccination and may remain susceptible to the disease at issue.

Immunization of HIV-infected persons: No clinical data have substantiated the concern about antigenic stimulation causing deterioration of clinical status. CDC and WHO continue to recommend immunization of HIV-infected persons when the benefits of immunization outweigh the risks of infection.

Summary Recommendations for Routine Immunization of HIV-infected Persons in the US

Drug	Known asymptomatic	Symptomatic
DTP/Td	yes	yes
OPV	no	no
e-IPV[1]	yes	yes
MMR	yes	yes[2]
MMR	yes	yes
Hib[3]	yes	yes
Pneumococcal	yes	yes
Influenza	yes[2]	yes

[1] For adults ≥ 18 years of age, use only if indicated.
[2] Consider risk and benefit.
[3] Consider for HIV-infected adults also.

Severe febrile illnesses: Immunization of persons with severe febrile illnesses should generally be deferred until they have recovered.

Vaccination during pregnancy: On the grounds of a theoretical risk to the developing fetus, live, attenuated virus vaccines are not generally given to pregnant women or to those likely to become pregnant within 3 months after receiving vaccine(s). With some of these vaccines, particularly rubella, measles and mumps, pregnancy is a contraindication. When vaccine is to be given during pregnancy, waiting until the second or third trimester to minimize any concern over teratogenicity is a reasonable precaution.

Measles, mumps, rubella or oral polio vaccines may be safely administered to children of pregnant women.

There is no convincing evidence of risk to the fetus from immunization of pregnant women using inactivated virus vaccines, bacterial vaccines or toxoids. Tetanus and diphtheria toxoid (Td) should be given to inadequately immunized pregnant women because it affords protection against neonatal tetanus.

HAEMOPHILUS b CONJUGATE VACCINE

Injection: 10 mcg capsular oligosaccharide and ≈ 25 mcg diphtheria CRM_{197} protein per 0.5 ml dose (*Rx*)	*HibTITER* (Lederle/Praxis Biologicals)
Powder for Injection, lyophilized: 10 mcg purified capsular polysaccharide and 24 mcg tetanus toxoid per 0.5 ml (*Rx*)	*OmniHIB* (SK-Beecham), *ActHIB* (Connaught)
Powder for Injection: 15 mcg purified capsular polysaccharide and 250 mcg *Neisseria meningitidis* OMPC per dose when reconstituted (*Rx*)	*PedvaxHIB* (MSD)
Injection: 25 mcg purified capsular polysaccharide and 18 mcg conjugated diphtheria toxoid protein per 0.5 ml dose (*Rx*)	*ProHIBiT* (Connaught)

Haemophilus influenzae type b (Haemophilus b; Hib) is a leading cause of serious systemic bacterial disease in the US. Most cases of *H influenzae* meningitis among children are caused by capsular strains of type b. In addition to bacterial meningitis, Haemophilus b is responsible for other invasive diseases, including epiglottitis, sepsis, septic arthritis, osteomyelitis, pericarditis and pneumonia.

Approximately 17% of all cases of Hib occur in infants < 6 months of age, 47% by 1 year of age and the remaining 53% over the next 4 years. Peak incidence occurs between 6 to 11 months of age. Incidence rates of Hib disease are increased in high-risk groups, such as daycare attendees, household contacts of cases, Caucasians who lack the G2m (n or 23) immunoglobulin allotype, Native Americans, blacks, individuals of lower socioeconomic status and patients with asplenia, sickle cell disease and antibody deficiency syndromes.

Actions:

Pharmacology: An antibody concentration of ≥ 0.15 mcg/ml is correlated with protection; in 3 week post-vaccination serum, antibody levels ≥ 1 mcg/ml were correlated with long-term protection.

Indications:

For the routine immunization of children 2 months to 5 years of age (*HibTITER*), 2 to 71 months of age (*PedvaxHIB*) and 18 months to 5 years of age (*ProHIBiT*) against invasive diseases caused by *H influenzae* type b. The duration of protection and need for booster doses have not yet been determined.

Administration may be considered for children as young as 15 months of age (*ProHIBiT*) when it is expected that the child will not return at 18 months for Haemophilus b immunization. However, the percentage of children at 15 months of age responding with > 1 mcg/ml may not be as high as in children ≥ 18 months of age.

The Immunization Practices Advisory Committee (ACIP) recommends that all children receive one of the conjugate vaccines licensed for infant use beginning routinely at 2 months of age. The vaccine series may be initiated as early as age 6 weeks.

Children < 24 months of age who have had invasive Hib disease should still receive the vaccine, since many children of that age fail to develop adequate immunity following natural disease. The vaccine can be initiated (or continued) at the time of hospital discharge.

Chemoprophylaxis of household or daycare classroom contacts of children with Hib disease should be directed at both vaccinated and unvaccinated contacts because immune individuals may asymptomatically carry and transmit the organism.

Conjugate vaccines may be given simultaneously with diphtheria and tetanus toxoids and pertussis vaccine adsorbed (DPT); combined measles, mumps and rubella vaccine (MMR); oral poliovirus vaccine (OPV); or inactivated poliovirus vaccine (IPV).

Haemophilus b conjugate vaccines will not protect children against *H influenzae* other than type b or other microorganisms that cause meningitis or septic disease.

Contraindications:

Hypersensitivity to diphtheria toxoid or any component of the vaccine, including thimerosal.

Warnings:

Deficient antibodies: The expected immune response may not be attained in persons deficient in producing antibody, whether due to genetic defect or to immunosuppressive therapy.

Illness or infection: Any febrile illness or active infection is reason for delaying vaccine.

Haemophilus b disease may occur in the week after vaccination, prior to the onset of the protective effects of the vaccine.

Although some immune response to the diphtheria toxoid component of the conjugate vaccine may occur, it does not substitute for routine diphtheria immunization.

Hypersensitivity: Have epinephrine 1:1000 available for immediate use if an anaphylactoid reaction occurs. Refer to Management of Acute Hypersensitivity Reactions.

Pregnancy: *Category* C.These vaccines are NOT recommended for use in pregnant patients.

Children: *ProHIBiT* is not recommended for use in children < 15 months of age. *Hib TITER* and *PedvaxHIB* are not recommended in children < 2 months of age; however, the ACIP states that the vaccine series may be initiated as early as age 6 weeks.

Drug Interactions:

Drug/Lab test interactions: Sensitive tests (eg, Latex Agglutination Kits) may detect PRP derived from the vaccine in urine of some vaccinees for up to 7 days following vaccination with *PedvaxHIB*.

Adverse Reactions:

Adverse reactions may include fever, erythema and tenderness.

Administration and Dosage:

Administer IM doses in the outer aspect area of the vastus lateralis (mid-thigh) or deltoid. Do not inject IV.

Data are not available regarding the interchangeability of haemophilus b conjugate vaccines with regard to safety, immunogenicity or efficacy. Ideally, use the same conjugate vaccine throughout the entire vaccination series. However, situations will arise in which the vaccine provider does not know which vaccine was previously used. Under these circumstances, it is prudent for vaccine providers to ensure that, at a minimum, an infant 2 to 6 months of age receives a primary series of three doses of conjugate vaccine.

Vaccination Schedule for Haemophilus b Conjugate Vaccines

	HibTITER		*PedvaxHIB*		*ProHIBiT*	
Age at first dose (mos)	Primary series	Booster	Primary series	Booster	Primary series	Booster
2-6	3 doses, 2 months apart	15 mos.[1]	2 doses, 2 months apart	12 mos.[1]		
7-11	2 doses, 2 months apart	15 mos.[1]	2 doses, 2 months apart	15 mos.[1]		
12-14	1 dose	15 mos.[1]	1 dose	15 mos.[1]		
15-59	1 dose	—	1 dose	—	1 dose	—

[1] At least 2 months after previous dose.

INFLUENZA VIRUS VACCINE

Injection (split-virus, whole-virus or purified surface antigen): 15 mcg A/Texas/36/91 (H1N1), 15 mcg A/Johannesburg/33/94 (H3N2) and 15 mcg B/Harbin/7/94 (B/Beijing/184/93-like) hemagglutinin antigens per 0.5 ml (*Rx*)	*Fluogen* (Parke-Davis), *Flu-Shield* (Wyeth-Ayerst), *Fluzone* (Connaught), *Fluvirin* (Adams)

Actions:

Pharmacology: Inoculation of antigens prepared from inactivated influenza virus stimulates the production of specific antibodies. Protection is afforded only against those strains from which the vaccine is prepared or against closely related strains. Having received a vaccination for the previous flu season does not preclude the need to be revaccinated for the current season to provide optimal protection.

Indications:

Groups at increased risk of influenza-related complications:

1.) People ≥ 65 years of age.

2.) Residents of nursing homes and other chronic-care facilities housing persons of any age with chronic medical conditions.

3.) Adults and children with chronic disorders of the pulmonary or cardiovascular systems, including children with asthma.

4.) Adults and children who have required regular medical follow-up or hospitalization during the preceding year because of chronic metabolic diseases (including diabetes mellitus), renal dysfunction, hemoglobinopathies or immunosuppression (including immunosuppression caused by medications).

5.) Children and teenagers (6 months to 18 years of age) who are receiving long-term aspirin therapy and, therefore, may be at risk of developing Reye's syndrome after influenza.

Groups that can transmit influenza to high-risk persons: Persons who are clinically or subclinically infected and who attend or live with high-risk persons can transmit influenza virus to them. Therefore, the following groups should be vaccinated:

1.) Physicians, nurses and other personnel in both hospital and outpatient-care settings who have contact with high-risk persons in all age groups, including infants.

2.) Employees of nursing homes and chronic-care facilities who have contact with patients or residents.

3.) Providers of home care to high-risk persons (eg, visiting nurses, volunteer workers).

4.) Household members (including children) of high-risk persons.

General population: Any individual wishing to reduce the chance of acquiring an influenza infection.

Persons infected with human immunodeficiency virus (HIV): Because influenza may result in serious illness and complications, vaccination is a prudent precaution and will result in protective antibody levels in many recipients.

Foreign travelers: The risk of exposure to influenza varies, depending on season and destination. Consult information for their intended destination.

Contraindications:

The use of products prepared from the embryonic fluid of chicken eggs is contraindicated in persons with a history of allergy to eggs or egg products; hypersensitivity to any component of the vaccine.

Defer immunization in the presence of acute respiratory disease or other active infection or acute febrile illness.

Warnings:

Hypersensitivity: Refer to Management of Acute Hypersensitivity Reactions.

Immunosuppressed patients may experience a lower than expected antigenic response, although in one study, appropriate antibody responses occurred in patients with HIV who received trivalent influenza vaccine.

Pregnancy: Category C.

Children: Safety and efficacy of *Fluvirin* in children 6 months to 4 years of age have not been established; do not administer unless potential benefits clearly outweigh the risks. Do not administer *Fluvirin* to chidren < 6 months. Safety and efficacy of other available products in children < 6 months have not been established.

Precautions:

Concurrent vaccination: Pneumococcal vaccine and influenza vaccine can be given at the same time at different sites without increasing side effects..

High-risk children may receive influenza vaccine at the same time as measles-mumps-rubella, *Hemophilus b*, pneumococcal and oral polio vaccines, at different sites. Do not give influenza vaccine within 3 days of vaccination with pertussis vaccine.

Febrile reaction: Because of the possibility of a febrile reaction following immunization, weigh the value of immunizing patients with a history of febrile convulsions. Persons with acute febrile illnesses should not usually be vaccinated until their temporary symptoms have abated.

Sero-conversion: Vaccination may not result in sero-conversion in all individuals.

Guillain-Barre syndrome (GBS), characterized by ascending paralysis, is usually self-limited and reversible. Although most persons recover without residual weakness, approximately 5% of cases are fatal. Since 1978, vaccines have not been associated with an increased frequency of GBS.

Other neurologic disorders, including encephalopathies, have been temporally associated with influenza vaccination.

Drug Interactions:

Drugs that may be affected by influenza virus vaccine include phenytoin, theophylline and warfarin.

Adverse Reactions:

Adverse reactions may include soreness at injection site for up to 1 or 2 days, and fever, malaise, myalgia and other symptoms of toxicity (occur more often in children and those not exposed to the vaccine influenza virus antigen).

Administration and Dosage:

Do not inject IV. Give injections IM, preferably in the deltoid muscle for adults and older children; for infants and young children, the preferred site is the anterolateral aspect of the thigh.

Vaccination schedules: Organized vaccination campaigns where high-risk persons are routinely accessible, such as in chronic-care facilities or worksites, may be optimally undertaken in November. Vaccination is desirable in September or October (1) if warranted by regional experience of earlier than normal epidemic activity (eg, in Alaska); or (2) for other persons recommended for vaccination who receive medical check-ups or treatment during September or October and who may not be seen again until after November.

Influenza Vaccine Dosage Recommendations by Age Group

Age	Product type[1]	Dosage (ml)	Number of doses
> 12 years	whole-virus, split-virus or purified surface antigen	0.5	1
9-12 years	split-virus or purified surface antigen only	0.5	1
3-8 years	split-virus or purified surface antigen only	0.5	1 or 2[2]
6-35 months	split-virus or purified surface antigen only	0.25	1 or 2[2]

[1] Because of the lower potential for causing febrile reactions, use only split (subvirion) or purified surface antigen vaccine in children. Immunogenicity and side effects of split, whole and purified surface antigen virus vaccine are similar in adults when used as recommended.

[2] ≥ 4 weeks between doses; both doses are recommended for maximum protection. However, if the individual received at least 1 dose of the 1978-1979 or later influenza vaccine, 1 dose is sufficient.

HEPATITIS B VACCINE

Injection (adult formulation): 10 mcg/ml (*Rx*)	*Recombivax HB* (Merck)
Injection (pediatric formulation): 2.5 mcg/0.5 ml (*Rx*)	
Injection (adolescent/high-risk infant formulation): 5 mcg/0.5 ml (*Rx*)	
Injection (dialysis formulation): 40 mcg/ml (*Rx*)	
Injection (adult formulation): 20 mcg/ml (*Rx*)	*Engerix-B* (SK-Beecham)
Injection (pediatric formulation): 10 mcg/0.5 ml (*Rx*)	

Actions:

Pharmacology: The recombinant hepatitis vaccines are derived from HBsAg produced in yeast cells.

Antibody titers ≥ 10 mIU/ml against HBsAg are recognized as conferring protection against hepatitis B. Seroconversion is defined as antibody titers ≥ 1 mIU/ml. Duration of protective effect is unknown.

The vaccines, injected into the deltoid, induced protective antibody levels in 93% to 99% of healthy adults, adolescents, children and neonates who received the recommended regimen; in adults ≥ 40 years of age, the protective level is lower (88% to 89%).

Interchangeability with hepatitis B vaccines – It is possible to interchange the use of vaccines for completion of a series or for booster doses since studies indicate the antibody produced in response to each type of vaccine is comparable. However, the quantity of antigen or the dosage volume will vary.

Indications:

For immunization against infection caused by all known subtypes of hepatitis B virus. Since hepatitis D virus (caused by the delta virus) can only infect and cause illness in persons infected with hepatitis B, immunity to hepatitis B also protects against hepatitis D.

Vaccination is recommended in persons of all ages, especially in those at increased risk of infection with hepatitis B virus.

Healthcare personnel: Dentists; oral surgeons, physicians; surgeons; nurses; paramedical personnel and custodial staff who may be exposed via blood or patient specimens; dental hygienists and nurses; blood bank and plasma fractionation workers; laboratory personnel handling blood, its products and patient specimens; dental, medical and nursing students.

Selected patients and patient contacts: Patients and staff in hemodialysis units and hematology/oncology units; patients requiring frequent or large volume blood transfusions or clotting factor concentrates; residents and staff of institutions for the mentally handicapped; classroom contacts of deinstitutionalized mentally handicapped persons who have persistent hepatitis B antigenemia and who show aggressive behavior; household and other intimate contacts of persons with persistent hepatitis B antigenemia.

Adolescents: Because a vaccination strategy limited to high-risk individuals has failed to substantially lower the overall incidence of hepatitis B infection, both the Immunization Practices Advisory Committee (ACIP) and the Committee on Infectious Diseases of the American Academy of Pediatrics (AAP) have endorsed universal infant immunization as part of a comprehensive strategy for the control of hepatitis B infection.

Infants, including those born to HBsAg-positive mothers whether HBeAg-positive or -negative: CDC, ACIP and AAP recommend routine vaccination of all infants against hepatitis B.

Populations with high incidence of the disease: Alaskan Eskimos; Pacific islanders, Indochinese refugees; Haitian refugees; refugees from other HBV endemic areas; all infants of women born in areas where the infection is highly endemic.

Persons at increased risk due to their sexual practices: Persons who have heterosexual activity with multiple partners (eg, > 1 partner in a 6 month period), persons who repeatedly contract sexually transmitted diseases, homosexually active males and female prostitutes.

Others at increased risk: Certain military personnel; morticians and embalmers; prisoners; users of illicit injectable drugs; police and fire department personnel who render first aid or medical assistance; blood bank and plasma-fractionation workers; adoptees from countries of high HBV endemicity.

Contraindications:

Hypersensitivity to yeast or any component of the vaccines.

Warnings:

Hypersensitivity: Refer to Management of Acute Hypersensitivity Reactions.

Immunosuppressed patients may require larger vaccine doses and may not respond as well as healthy individuals.

Unrecognized hepatitis B infection may be present at the time the vaccine is given, and the vaccine may not prevent hepatitis B in such patients because of the long incubation period.

Limitations: No hepatitis B vaccine will protect against hepatitis A, C and E viruses or other viruses known to infect the liver.

Elderly: Immunogenicity of hepatitis B vaccine is somewhat reduced in persons > 40 years of age.

Pregnancy: Category C.

Lactation: Safety for use in the nursing mother has not been established.

Children: Hepatitis B vaccine is well tolerated and highly immunogenic in infants and children of all ages. Newborns also respond well.

Precautions:

Infection: Serious active infection is reason to delay use of hepatitis B vaccine, except when withholding the vaccine entails a greater risk.

Special risk patients: Give cautiously in severely compromised cardiopulmonary status or when a febrile or systemic reaction could be a significant risk.

Drug Interactions:

Other vaccines: ACIP states that, in general, simultaneous administration of certain live and inactivated pediatric vaccines has not resulted in impaired antibody responses or increased rates of adverse reactions.

Drugs that may interact include immunosuppressants, yellow fever vaccine, anticoagulants and interleukin-2.

Adverse Reactions:

Adverse reactions may include: Erythema; swelling; warmth; induration; pain; tenderness; pruritus; nausea; vomiting; abdominal pain/cramps; dyspepsia; diminished appetite; anorexia; diarrhea; headache; lightheadedness; vertigo; dizziness; insomnia; disturbed sleep; somnolence; irritability; agitation; migraine; arthralgia; myalgia; back/neck/shoulder pain; fatigue/weakness; fever; malaise; hypotension; tachycardia/palpitations; visual disturbances.

Administration and Dosage:

Route and site: For IM use. Never inject IV. The deltoid muscle is the preferred site in adults. Injections given in the buttocks frequently are given into fatty tissue instead of into muscle and have resulted in a lower seroconversion rate than expected. The anterolateral thigh is the recommended site in infants and young children. May be given SC to persons at risk of hemorrhage following IM injection (eg, hemophiliacs).

Immunization Regimen of Hepatitis B Vaccine Doses						
	Initial		1 month		6 months	
Age group	*Recombivax HB*	*Engerix-B*	*Recombivax HB*	*Engerix-B*	*Recombivax HB*	*Engerix-B*
Birth[1] to 10 years	2.5 mcg/0.25 ml or 2.5 mcg/0.5 ml	10 mcg/ 0.5 ml	2.5 mcg/0.25 ml or 2.5 mcg/0.5 ml	10 mcg/ 0.5 ml	2.5 mcg/0.25 ml or 2.5 mcg/0.5 ml	10 mcg/ 0.5 ml
11 to 19 years	5 mcg/0.5 ml	20 mcg/ml	5 mcg/0.5 ml	20 mcg/ml	5 mcg/0.5 ml	20 mcg/ml
≥ 20 years[2]	10 mcg/ml	20 mcg/ml	10 mcg/ml	20 mcg/ml	10 mcg/0.5 ml	20 mcg/ml
Dialysis/ immuno-compromised	40 mcg	40 mcg/ 2 ml[3]	40 mcg	40 mcg/ 2 ml[4]	40 mcg	40 mcg/ 2 ml[3]

[1] Infants born of HBsAg negative mothers. If the infant is born of an HBsAg-positive mother, give 0.5 ml of HBIG at birth and 5 mcg/0.5 ml of vaccine within 7 days of birth, with additional 10 mcg/0.5 ml vaccine doses 1 month and 6 months later or 1, 2 and 12 months later.
[2] *Engerix-B* dose for 11–19 years age group is the same.
[3] Two 1 ml doses given at different sites.
[4] Two 1 ml doses given at different sites, plus an additional dose at 2 months.

Post-exposure prophylaxis:

Alternate schedule –

Engerix-B: Designed for certain populations (eg, neonates born of hepatitis B infected mothers, others who have or might have been recently exposed to the virus, certain travelers to high-risk areas).

Alternate Dosing Schedule for *Engerix-B*				
Age Group	Initial	1 month	2 months	12 months
Birth-10 yrs	10 mcg/0.5 ml	10 mcg/0.5 ml	10 mcg/0.5 ml	10 mcg/0.5 ml[1]
Children > 10 yrs and adults	20 mcg/ml	20 mcg/ml	20 mcg/ml	20 mcg/ml[1]

[1] Recommended for infants born of infected mothers and for others for whom prolonged maintenance of protective titers is desired.

Recombivax HB: An alternate schedule has been recommended. Give doses at 0, 1 and 2 months to provide rapid induction of immunity. On this alternate schedule, give an additional dose 12 months after the first dose if prolonged protection is needed.

Post-exposure prophylaxis: See also the HBIG monograph. In response to known or presumed exposure to hepatitis B surface antigen, give previously unvaccinated persons post-exposure prophylaxis. This consists of 0.06 ml/kg HBIG as soon as possible or within 24 hours after exposure, if possible (within 14 days in the case of sexual contact). Give the appropriate volume of either hepatitis B vaccine based on age within 7 days of exposure, with additional vaccine doses either 1 and 6 months after the first dose or 1, 2 and 12 months later.

Revaccination (booster): The antibody response to properly administered vaccine is excellent, and protection lasts for at least 5 years. Booster doses are not routinely recommended, nor is routine serologic testing to assess antibody levels in vaccine recipients necessary during this period.

Engerix-B – Children ≤ 10 years of age – 10 mcg. *Adults and children ≥ 10 years of age* – 20 mcg.

Hemodialysis patients – The vaccine-induced protection is less complete and may persist only as long as antibody levels remain above 10 mIU/ml. Assess need by semi-annual antibody testing. Give 40 mcg (two 20 mcg doses) when antibody levels decline below 10 mIU/ml.

Vaccinated persons who experience percutaneous or needle exposure to HBsAg-positive blood – Serologic testing to assess immune status is recommended unless testing within the previous 12 months has indicated adequate antibody levels. If inadequate levels exist, treatment with HBIG or a booster dose of vaccine is indicated.

Nonresponders – Revaccination of persons who do not respond to the primary series produces adequate antibody in only one-third when the primary vaccination has been given in the deltoid. Therefore, revaccination of nonresponders to deltoid injection is not recommended.

Prophylaxis of perinatal hepatitis B:

Recommended Schedule for Prophylaxis of Perinatal Hepatitis B in Infants Born to Mothers Known to be HBsAg-Positive		
Age of infant	Vaccine dose	HBIG dose
Birth (within 12 hrs)	First	First
1 month	Second	
6 months[1]	Third	

[1] If the 4–dose schedule for *Engerix-B* is used, give the third dose at 2 months of age and the fourth dose at 12 to 18 month.

Recommended Schedule for Prophylaxis of Perinatal Hepatitis B in Infants Born of Mothers Not Screened or Known to be HBsAg-Negative		
Age of infant	Vaccine dose[1]	HBIG dose
Birth (within 12 hours)	First	See footnote[2]
1 to 2 months[3]	Second	
6 months[4]	Third	

[1] If mother was not screened, use appropriate dose for an infant of an HBsAg-positive mother. If the mother is later found to be HBsAg-positive, continue that dose. If the mother is later found to be HBsAg-negative, decrease *Recombivax HB* vaccine dose to appropriate level.
[2] If mother is later found to be HBsAg-positive, administer HBIG to infants as soon as possible, not later than 1 week after birth.
[3] Vaccinate infants of women who are HBsAg-negative beginning at birth or at 2 months of age.

Recombivax HB dialysis formulation is intended only for adult predialysis/dialysis patients.

Dosage – Recommended vaccination schedule is as follows: 1 ml initially, than 1 ml at 1 and 6 months.

Revaccination – A booster dose may be considered if the anti-HBs level is < 10 mIU/ml 1 to 2 months after the third dose.

HEPATITIS A VACCINE, INACTIVATED

Injection (pediatric formulation): 360 ELU./0.5 ml or 25 U/0.5 ml of viral antigen (*Rx*)
Injection (adult formulation): 1440 ELU./1 ml or 50 U/1 ml of viral antigen (*Rx*)

Havrix (SmithKline Beecham), *Vaqta* (Merck)

Indications:

Hepatitis A virus (HAV): For active immunization of persons ≥ 2 years of age against disease caused by HAV.

Primary immunization should be completed at least 2 weeks prior to expected exposure to HAV. Immunization with hepatitis A vaccine is indicated for those people desiring protection against hepatitis A who are, or will be, at increased risk of infection by HAV:

Travelers – Persons traveling to areas of higher endemicity for hepatitis A.

Populations with high incidence of the disease – Native peoples of Alaska and the Americas.

Persons at increased risk due to their employment – Certain institutional workers (eg, caretakers for the developmentally challenged); employees of child day-care centers; laboratory workers who handle live hepatitis A virus; handlers of primate animals that may be harboring HAV.

Others – Persons engaging in high-risk sexual activity (such as homosexually active males); users of illicit injectable drugs; residents of a community experiencing an outbreak of hepatitis A; military personnel; people living in, or relocating to areas of high endemicity.

Contraindications:

Hypersensitivity to any component of the vaccine.

Warnings:

Hepatitis: Hepatitis A vaccine will not prevent hepatitis caused by other agents such as hepatitis B, C or E virus or other pathogens known to infect the liver.

Hypersensitivity: Epinephrine should be available for use in case of anaphylaxis or anaphylactoid reaction.

Pregnancy: Category C.

Lactation: It is not known whether the vaccine is excreted in breast milk.

Children: Hepatitis A vaccine is well tolerated and highly immunogenic and effective in children ≥ 2 years of age.

Precautions:

Febrile illness: is reason to delay use of hepatitis A vaccine, except when withholding the vaccine entails a greater risk.

Bleeding disorders: Administer cautiously to people with thrombocytopenia or a bleeding disorder as bleeding may occur following IM use.

Immunosuppressed persons: or persons receiving immunosuppressive therapy may not obtain the expected immune response.

Injection site: Do not inject into a blood vessel.

Drug Interactions:

When concomitant administration of other vaccines or IG is required, they should be given with different syringes and at different injection sites.

Adverse Reactions:

Adverse reactions occurring in ≥ 3% of patients include: Injection site soreness/pain, tenderness, induration, redness, swelling, fatigue, fever, malaise, anorexia, nausea and headache.

Administration and Dosage:

Route and site: For IM use. Do not inject IV, ID or SC. In adults, give the injection in the deltoid region. It should not be administered in the gluteal region; such injections may result in suboptimal response.

Primary immunization regimen:

Adults – A single dose of 1440 EL.U.

Children (2 to 18 years of age) – Two doses, each containing 360 EL.U. given 1 month apart.

Booster dose – A booster dose is recommended anytime between 6 and 12 months after the initiation of the primary course in order to ensure the highest Antibody titers.

In those with an impaired immune system, adequate anti-HAV response may not be obtained after the primary immunization course. Such patients may therefore require administration of additional doses of vaccine.

VARICELLA VIRUS VACCINE

Powder for Injection: 1350 PFU of Oka/Merck varicella virus (live) (*Rx*) *Varivax* (Merck)

Actions:

Pharmacology: Varicella virus vaccine is a preparation of the Oka/Merck strain of live, attenuated varicella virus.

Indications:

Varicella: Vaccination against varicella in individuals ≥ 12 months of age.

Contraindications:

Hypersensitivity to any component of the vaccine, including gelatin; history of anaphylactoid reaction to neomycin; individuals with blood dyscrasia, leukemia, lymphomas of any type, or other malignant neoplasms affecting the bone marrow or lymphatic systems; concomitant immunosuppressive therapy; individuals with primary and acquired immunodeficiency states, including those who are immunosuppressed in association with AIDS or other clinical manifestations of infection with HIV, cellular immune deficiencies, and hypogammaglobulinemic and dysgammaglobulinemic states; family history of congenital or hereditary immunodeficiency, unless the immune competence of the potential vaccine recipient is demonstrated; active untreated tuberculosis; any febrile respiratory illness or other active febrile infection; pregnancy.

Warnings:

Booster doses: The duration of protection of varicella vaccine is unknown at present and the need for booster doses is not defined. Post-marketing surveillance studies are ongoing to evaluate the need and timing for booster vaccination.

Protection/Prevention: Vaccination with varicella vaccine may not result in protection of all healthy, susceptible children, adolescents and adults. It is not known whether varicella vaccine given immediately after exposure to natural varicella virus will prevent illness.

Acute lymphoblastic leukemia (ALL): Children and adolescents with ALL in remission can receive the vaccine under an investigational protocol.

Hypersensitivity: Have adequate treatment provisions, including epinephrine injection (1:1000), available for immediate use should an anaphylactoid reaction occur

Pregnancy: Category C.

Lactation: It is not known whether varicella vaccine virus is excreted in breast milk.

Children: Administration to infants < 1 year of age is not recommended.

Precautions:

Reye's syndrome: Vaccine recipients should avoid use of salicylates for 6 weeks after vaccination with varicella vaccine as Reye's syndrome has been reported following the use of salicylates during natural varicella infections.

Transmission: Individuals vaccinated with varicella vaccine may potentially be capable of transmitting the vaccine virus to close contacts. Therefore, vaccine recipients should avoid close association with susceptible high-risk individuals.

Immunodeficiency: The safety and efficacy of varicella vaccine have not been established in children and young adults who are known to be infected with HIV with and without evidence of immunosuppression. Vaccination should be deferred in patients with a family history of congenital or hereditary immunodeficiency until the patient's own immune system has been evaluated.

Drug Interactions:

Drugs that may interact with varicella vaccine include immune globulins, immunosuppressants and salicylates.

Concomitant vaccines: Results from clinical studies indicate that varicella vaccine can be administered concomitantly with MMR II.

Limited data from an experimental product containing varicella vaccine suggest that varicella vaccine can be administered concomitantly with DTaP and *PedvaxHIB* (haemophilus b conjugate vaccine) using separate sites and syringes.

Adverse Reactions:

Adverse reactions occurring in ≥ 3% of patients include: Fever, injection site complaints and varicella-like rash.

Administration and Dosage:

For SC administration; the outer aspect of the upper arm (deltoid) is the preferred site of injection. Do not inject IV. During clinical trials, some children received varicella vaccine IM resulting in seroconversion rates similar to those in children who received the vaccine by the SC route.

Children (1 to 12 years of age): A single 0.5 ml dose administered SC.

Adults and adolescents (≥ 13 years of age): A 0.5 ml dose administered SC at elected date and a second 0.5 ml dose 4 to 8 weeks later.

INTERFERON GAMMA-1B

Injection: 100 mcg (3 million U) (*Rx*)	*Actimmune* (Genentech)

Actions:

Pharmacology: Interferon gamma-1b, a biologic response modifier, is a single-chain polypeptide containing 140 amino acids. Interferon gamma has potent phagocyte-activating effects not seen with other interferon preparations, including generation of toxic oxygen metabolites within phagocytes, which are capable of mediating the killing of microorganisms such as *Staphylococcus aureus*, *Toxoplasma gondii*, *Leishmania donovani*, *Listeria monocytogenes* and Mycobacterium *avium* intracellulare.

Pharmacokinetics: After IM or SC injection, the apparent fraction of dose absorbed was > 89%. The mean elimination half-life after IV administration was 38 minutes. The mean elimination half-lives for IM and SC dosing were 2.9 and 5.9 hours, respectively after IM dosing and 7 hours after SC dosing.

Indications:

For reducing the frequency and severity of serious infections associated with chronic granulomatous disease.

Contraindications:

Hypersensitivity to interferon gamma, *E coli* derived products or any component of the product.

Warnings:

Seizure disorders/compromised CNS function: Exercise caution in patients with these conditions. CNS adverse reactions including decreased mental status, gait disturbance and dizziness have been observed, particularly in patients receiving doses > 250 mcg/m^2/day.

Cardiac disease: Use with caution in patients with pre-existing cardiac disease, including symptoms of ischemia, CHF or arrhythmia.

Myelosuppression: Exercise caution in patients with myelosuppression. Reversible neutropenia and elevation of hepatic enzymes can be dose-limiting at doses > 250 mcg/m^2/day.

Hypersensitivity: Acute serious hypersensitivity reactions have not been observed in patients receiving interferon gamma; however, if such an acute reaction develops, discontinue the drug immediately and institute appropriate medical therapy. Refer to Management of Acute Hypersensitivity Reactions.

Pregnancy: Category C.

Lactation: It is not known whether interferon gamma is excreted in breast milk.

Children: Safety and efficacy in children < 1 year of age has not been established.

Precautions:

Monitoring: In addition to tests normally required for monitoring patients with chronic granulomatous disease, the following laboratory tests are recommended for all patients prior to beginning therapy and at 3 month intervals during treatment: Hematologic tests including complete blood counts, differential and platelet counts; blood chemistries including renal and liver function tests; urinalysis.

Drug Interactions:

Exercise caution when administering interferon gamma in combination with other potentially myelosuppressive agents.

Adverse Reactions:

Adverse reactions may include fever, headache, rash, chills, injection site erythema or tenderness, fatigue, diarrhea, vomiting, nausea, abdominal pain, weight loss, myalgia, anorexia and depression.

Administration and Dosage:

Chronic granulomatous disease: 50 mcg/m^2 (1.5 million U/m^2) for patients whose body surface area is > 0.5 m^2 and 1.5 mcg/kg/dose for patients whose body surface area is ≤ 0.5 m^2. Administer SC 3 times weekly (eg, Monday, Wednesday, Friday). The optimum sites of injection are the right and left deltoid and anterior thigh.

Higher doses are not recommended. Safety and efficacy have not been established for interferon gamma given in doses greater or less than the recommended dose of 50 mcg/m^2. The minimum effective dose has not been established.

If severe reactions occur, modify the dosage (50% reduction) or discontinue therapy until the adverse reaction abates.

INTERFERON BETA

INTERFERON BETA-1a

Powder for Injection, lyophilized: 33 mcg (6.6 mIU) (*Rx*) *Avonex* (Biogen)

INTERFERON BETA-1b

Powder for Injection, lyophilized: 0.3 mg (9.6 mIU) (*Rx*) *Betaseron* (Berlex)

Actions:

Pharmacology: Interferon beta–1a and beta–1b have both antiviral and immunoregulatory activities. The mechanisms by which they exert their actions in multiple sclerosis (MS) are not clearly understood.

Pharmacokinetics:

Interferon beta-1a – Biological response marker levels increase within 12 hours of dosing and remain elevated for at least 4 days. Peak biological response marker levels are typically observed 48 hours after dosing.

Pharmacokinetic Parameters Following 60 mcg Administration of Interferon beta-1a				
Route	AUC (IU-hr/ml)	C_{max} (IU/ml)	T_{max} (range [hr])	Elimination half-life (hr)
IM	1352	45	9.8 (3-15)	10
SC	478	30	7.8 (3-18)	8.6

Interferon beta-1b – Peak serum concentrations occurred between 1 to 8 hours. Bioavailability, based on a total dose of 0.5 mg given as two SC injections at different sites, was approximately 50%.

Mean serum clearance values ranged from 9.4 to 28.9 ml/min/kg and were independent of dose. Mean terminal elimination half-life values ranged from 8 minutes to 4.3 hours and mean steady-state volume of distribution values ranged from 0.25 to 2.88 L/kg. IV dosing 3 times a week for 2 weeks resulted in no accumulation of interferon beta-1a or beta-1b in the serum of patients.

Indications:

Interferon beta-1a:

Multiple sclerosis (MS) – For the treatment of relapsing forms of MS to slow the accumulation of physical disability and decrease the frequency of clinical exacerbations.

Interferon beta-1b:

Multiple sclerosis (MS) – For use in ambulatory patients with relapsing-remitting MS to reduce the frequency of clinical exacerbations. Relapsing-remitting MS is characterized by recurrent attacks of neurologic dysfunction followed by complete or incomplete recovery.

Unlabeled uses: Interferon beta is being investigated in the treatment of AIDS, AIDS-related Kaposi's sarcoma, metastatic renal-cell carcinoma, malignant melanoma, cutaneous T-cell lymphoma, herpes of the lips or genitals and acute non-A/non-B hepatitis.

Contraindications:

Hypersensitivity to natural or recombinant interferon beta, albumin human or any other component of the formulation.

Warnings:

Chronic progressive MS: The safety and efficacy of interferon beta in chronic progressive MS have not been evaluated.

Suicide/Mental disorders: Inform patients to be treated with interferon beta that depression and suicidal ideation can be a side effect of the treatment and that they should report these symptoms immediately. Other mental disorders have been observed and can include anxiety, emotional lability, depersonalization and confusion.

Seizures: Exercise caution when administering interferon beta to patients with preexisiting seizure disorder. It is not known whether these events were related to the effects of MS alone, to interferon beta or to a combination of both.

Cardiac disease: Closely monitor patients with cardiac disease, such as angina, CHF or arrhythmia, for worsening of their clinical condition during initiation. Interferon beta does not have any known direct-acting cardiac toxicity; however, symptoms of flu syndrome seen with interferon beta therapy may prove stressful to patients with severe cardiac conditions.

Pregnancy: Category C.

Lactation: It is not known whether interferon beta is excreted in breast milk.

Children: Safety and efficacy in children < 18 years of age have not been established.

Precautions:

Monitoring: The following laboratory tests are recommended prior to initiating therapy and at periodic intervals thereafter: Hemoglobin; complete and differential white blood cell counts; platelet counts and blood chemistries including liver function tests.

Self-administration: Instruct patients in injection techniques to ensure the safe self-administration of interferon beta.

Flu-like symptoms complex was reported in 61% to 76% of the patients treated with interferon beta. A patient was defined as having a flu-like symptom complex if at least two of the following symptoms were concurrently reported: Fever, chills, myalgia, malaise, sweating or flu-like syndrome. Only myalgia, fever and chills were reported as severe in > 5% of the patients.

Photosensitivity: Photosensitization (photoallergy or phototoxicity) may occur.

Adverse Reactions:

Adverse reactions occurring in ≥ 3% of patients may include: Injection site reaction, headache, fever, flu-like symptoms, pain, asthenia, chills, infection, abdominal pain, chest pain, malaise, generalized edema, pelvic pain, injection site necrosis/inflammation, cyst/ovarian cyst, suicide attempt, hypersensitivity reaction, migraine, palpitation, hypertension, tachycardia, peripheral vascular disorder, hemmorhage, syncope, vasodilation, lymphocytes < 1500/mm^3, ANC < 3000/mm^3, lymphadenopathy, anemia, eosinophils ≥ 10%, HCT (%) ≤ 37, sinusitis, upper respiratory tract infection, dyspnea, laryngitis, myalgia, myasthenia, arthralgia, nausea, diarrhea, constipation, vomiting, dyspepsia, anorexia, GI disorder, ALT > 5 x baseline, glucose < 55 mg/dl, total bilirubin > 2.5 x baseline, urine protein > 1 +, AST > 5 x baseline, weight gain/loss, AST ≥ 3 x ULN, mental symptoms, hypertonia, sleep difficulty, dizziness, muscle spasm, somnolence, speech disorder, convulsion, sweating, urticaria, alopecia, nevus, herpes zoster, conjunctivitis, abnormal vision, otitis media, hearing decreased, dysmenorrhea, menstrual disorder, metorrhagia, cystitis, breast pain, menorrhagia, urinary urgency, vaginitis, fibrocystic breast.

Administration and Dosage:

Interferon beta-1a:

Relapsing/Remitting MS – 30 mcg IM once a week.

Interferon beta-1b:

Relapsing/Remitting MS – 0.25 mg (8 mIU) SC every other day. The effectiveness of lower doses is undocumented. Evidence of efficacy > 2 years is not known.

Administration: Withdraw 1 ml of reconstituted solution from the vial into a sterile syringe fitted with a 27-gauge needle and inject the solution subcutaneously. Sites for self-injection include arms, abdomen, hips and thighs.

Chapter 10
TOPICALS

TOPICAL OPHTHALMICS

General Considerations in Topical Ophthalmic Drug Therapy: Proper administration essential to optimal therapeutic response. In many instances, health professionals may be too casual when instructing patients on proper use of ophthalmics. The administration technique used often determines drug safety and efficacy.

- The normal eye retains ≈ 10 mcl of fluid (adjusted for blinking). The average dropper delivers 25 to 50 mcl/drop. The value of more than one drop is questionable.
- Minimize systemic absorption of ophthalmic drops by compressing lacrimal sac for 3 to 5 minutes after instillation. This retards passage of drops via nasolacrimal duct into areas of potential absorption such as nasal and pharyngeal mucosa.
- Because of rapid lacrimal drainage and limited eye capacity, if multiple drop therapy is indicated, the best interval between drops is 5 min. This ensures the first drop is not flushed away by the second or the second is not diluted by the first.
- Topical anesthesia will increase the bioavailability of ophthalmic agents by decreasing the blink reflex and the production and turnover of tears.
- Factors that may increase absorption from ophthalmic dosage forms include lax eyelids of some patients, usually the elderly, which creates a greater reservoir for retention of drops, and hyperemic or diseased eyes.
- Eyecup use is discouraged due to risk of contamination and spreading disease.
- Ophthalmic suspensions mix with tears less rapidly and remain in the cul-de-sac longer than solutions.
- Ophthalmic ointments maintain contact between the drug and ocular tissues by slowing the clearance rate to as little as 0.5% per minute. Ophthalmic ointments provide maximum contact between drug and external ocular tissues.
- Ophthalmic ointments may impede delivery of other ophthalmic drugs to the affected side by serving as a barrier to contact.
- Ointments may blur vision during the waking hours. Use with caution in conditions where visual clarity is critical (eg, operating motor equipment, reading).
- Monitor expiration dates closely. Do not use outdated medication.
- Solutions and ointments are frequently misused. Do not assume that patients know how to maximize safe and effective use of these agents. Combine appropriate patient education and counseling with prescribing and dispensing of ophthalmics.

Topical application is the most common route of administration for ophthalmic drugs. Advantages include convenience, simplicity, noninvasive nature and the ability of the patient to self-administer. Because of blood and aqueous losses of drug, topical medications do not typically penetrate in useful concentrations to posterior ocular structures and therefore are of no therapeutic benefit for diseases of retina, optic nerve and other posterior segment structures.

Medications:

Solutions and suspensions – Most topical ocular preparations are commercially available as solutions or suspensions that are applied directly to the eye from the bottle, which serves as the eye dropper. Avoid touching the dropper tip to the eye because this can lead to contamination of the medication and may also cause ocular injury. Resuspend suspensions (notably, many ocular steroids) by shaking to provide an accurate dosage of drug.

Recommended procedures for administration of solutions or suspensions:

- Wash hands thoroughly before administration.
- Tilt head backward or lie down and gaze upward.
- Gently grasp lower eyelid below eyelashes and pull the eyelid away from the eye to form a pouch.
- Place dropper directly over eye. Avoid contact of the dropper with the eye, finger or any surface.
- Look upward just before applying a drop.

- After instilling the drop, look downward for several seconds.
- Release the lid slowly.
- With eyes closed, apply gentle pressure with fingers to the inside corner of eye for 3 to 5 min. This retards drainage of solution from intended solution.
- Do not rub the eye. Minimize blinking.
- Do not rinse the dropper.
- Do not use eye drops that have changed color.
- If more than one type of ophthalmic drop is used, wait ≥ 5 minutes before administering the second agent.
- When the instillation of eye drops is difficult (eg, pediatric patients, adults with particularly strong blink reflex), the close-eye method may be used. This involves lying down, placing the prescribed number of drops on the eyelid in the inner corner of the eye, then opening eye so that drops will fall into the eye by gravity.

Ointments – The primary purpose for an ophthalmic ointment vehicle is to prolong drug contact time with the external ocular surface. This is particularly useful for treating children, who may "cry out" topically applied solutions, and for medicating ocular injuries, such as corneal abrasions, when the eye is to be patched. Administer solutions before ointments. Ointments preclude entry of subsequent drops.

Recommended procedures for administration of ointments:

- Wash hands thoroughly before administration.
- Holding the ointment tube in the hand for a few minutes will warm the ointment and facilitate flow.
- When opening the ointment tube for the first time, squeeze out and discard the first 0.25 inch of ointment as it may be too dry.
- Tilt head backward or lie down and gaze upward.
- Gently pull down the lower lid to form a pouch.
- Place 0.25 to 0.5 inch of ointment with a sweeping motion inside the lower lid by squeezing the tube gently.
- Close the eye for 1 to 2 minutes and roll the eyeball in all directions.
- Temporary blurring of vision may occur. Avoid activities requiring visual acuity until blurring clears.
- Remove excessive ointment around the eye or ointment tube tip with a tissue.
- If using more than one kind of ointment, wait about 10 minutes before applying the second drug.

AGENTS FOR GLAUCOMA

Glaucoma is a condition of the eye in which an elevation of the intraocular pressure (IOP) leads to progressive cupping and atrophy of the optic nerve head, deterioration of the visual fields and ultimately, to blindness. Primary open-angle glaucoma is the most common type of glaucoma. Angle-closure glaucoma and congenital glaucoma are treated primarily by surgical methods, although short-term drug therapy is used to decrease IOP prior to surgery.

Drugs used in the therapy of primary open-angle glaucoma include a variety of agents with different mechanisms of action. The therapeutic goal in treating glaucoma is reducing the elevated IOP, a major risk factor in the pathogenesis of glaucomatous visual field loss. The higher the level of IOP, the greater the likelihood of glaucomatous visual field loss and optic nerve damage. Reduction of IOP may be accomplished by: 1) Decreasing the rate of production of aqueous humor or 2) increasing the rate of outflow (drainage) of aqueous humor from the anterior chamber of the eye.

The five groups of agents used in therapy of primary open-angle glaucoma are listed in the table, which summarizes their mechanism of decreasing IOP, effects on pupil size and ciliary muscle and duration of action.

Agents for Glaucoma

Drug	Strength	Duration (hrs)	Decrease aqueous production	Increase aqueous outflow	Effect on pupil	Effect on ciliary muscle
Sympathomimetics						
Apraclonidine[1]	0.5 -1%	7-12	+++	NR	NR	NR
Epinephrine	0.1%-2%	12-24	+	++	mydriasis	NR
Dipivefrin	0.1%	12	+	++	mydriasis	NR
Brimonidine	0.2%	12	++	++	NR	NR
Beta Blockers						
Betaxolol	0.25%-0.5%	12	+++	NR	NR	NR
Carteolol	1%	12	+++	nd	NR	NR
Levobunolol	0.25%-0.5%	12-24	+++	NR	NR	NR
Metipranolol	0.3%	12-24	+++	+	NR	NR
Timolol	0.25%-0.5%	12-24	+++	+	NR	NR
Miotics, Direct-Acting						
Acetylcholine[2]	1%	10-20 min	NR	+++	miosis	accommodation
Carbachol[2]	0.75%-3%	6-8	NR	+++	miosis	accommodation
Pilocarpine[3]	0.25%-10%	4-8	NR	+++	miosis	accommodation
Miotics, Cholinesterase Inhibitors						
Physostigmine	0.25%-0.5%	12-36	NR	+++	miosis	accommodation
Demecarium	0.125%-0.25%	days/wks	NR	+++	miosis	accommodation
Echothiophate	0.03%-0.25%	days/wks	NR	+++	miosis	accommodation
Carbonic Anhydrase Inhibitors[3]						
Dichlorphenamide	50 mg	6-12	+++	NR	NR	NR
Acetazolamide	125-500 mg	8-12	+++	NR	NR	NR
Methazolamide	25-50 mg	10-18	+++	NR	NR	NR
Dorzolamide	2%	≈ 8	+++	NR	NR	NR
Prostaglandin analogue						
Latanoprost	0.0005%	24	NR	+++	NR	NR

+++ = significant activity ++ = moderate activity + = some activity
NR = no activity reported nd = No data available

[1] 1% used only to decrease IOP in surgery.
[2] Intraocular administration only for miosis during surgery; carbachol also available as a topical agent.
[3] Also available as a gel and an insert; the duration of these doseforms is longer (18 to 24 hours and 1 week, respectively) than the solution.
[4] Systemic agents; for detailed information, see group monograph in Cardiovascular section.
[5] Topical ophthalmic agent.

Prostaglandin analogues increase uveoscleral outflow through a new mechanism of action; selective prostanoid receptor agonism. Latanoprost, currently the only agent avalable in this class, can be used concurrently with other topical ophthalmic drug products to reduce IOP.

BRIMONIDINE TARTRATE

Solution: 0.2% (*Rx*)	*Alphagan* (Allergan)

Actions:

Pharmacology: Brimonidine tartrate is an alpha-2 adrenergic receptor agonist. It has a peak ocular hypotensive effect occurring at 2 hours post-dosing. Brimonidine has a dual mechanism of action by reducing aqueous humor production and increasing uveoscleral outflow.

Pharmacokinetics: After ocular administration of a 0.2% solution, plasma concentrations peaked within 1 to 4 hours and declined with a systemic half-life of ≈ 3 hours.

It is metabolized primarily by the liver. Urinary excretion is the major route of elimination of the drug and its metabolites. Approximately 87% of an orally administered radioactive dose was eliminated within 120 hours, with 74% found in the urine.

Indications:

Intraocular pressure (IOP): Lowering IOP in patients with open-angle glaucoma or ocular hypertension.

Contraindications:

Hypersensitivity to brimonidine tartrate or any component of this medication; patients receiving monoamine oxidase (MAO) inhibitor therapy.

Warnings:

Soft contact lenses: The preservative in brimonidine tartrate, benzalkonium chloride, may be absorbed by soft contact lenses. Instruct patients wearing soft contact lenses to wait at least 15 minutes after instilling brimonidine tartrate to insert soft contact lenses.

Renal/Hepatic function impairment: Use caution when treating patients with hepatic or renal impairment.

Pregnancy: Category B.

Lactation: It is not known whether brimonidine tartrate is excreted in breast milk.

Children: Safety and efficacy in pediatric patients have not been established.

Precautions:

Cardiovascular disease: Exercise caution in treating patients with severe cardiovascular disease.

Use with caution in patients with depression, cerebral or coronary insufficiency, Raynaud's phenomenon, orthostatic hypotension or thromboangiitis obliterans.

Loss of effect in some patients may occur. The IOP-lowering efficacy observed with brimonidine tartrate during the first month of therapy may not always reflect the long-term level of IOP reduction. Therefore, routinely monitor IOP.

Drug Interactions:

Drugs that may be affected by brimonidine tartrate include CNS depressants, beta-blockers, antihypertensives and cardiac glycosides.

Drugs that may affect brimonidine tartrate include tricyclic antidepressants.

Adverse Reactions:

Adverse events occurring in ≈ 10% to 30% of patients in descending order include: Oral dryness, ocular hyperemia, burning and stinging, headache, blurring, foreign body sensation, fatigue/drowsiness, conjunctival follicles, ocular allergic reactions and ocular pruritus.

Adverse events occurring in ≈ 3% to 9% in descending order include: Corneal staining/erosion, photophobia, eyelid erythema, ocular ache/pain, ocular dryness, tearing, upper respiratory symptoms, eyelid edema, conjunctival edema, dizziness, blepharitis, ocular irritation, GI symptoms, asthenia, conjunctival blanching, abnormal vision and muscular pain.

Administration and Dosage:
The recommended dose is one drop of brimonidine tartrate in the affected eye(s) 3 times daily, ≈ 8 hours apart.

EPINEPHRINE

EPINEPHRINE (as HCl)	
Solution: 0.1%, 1% and 2% (*Rx*)	**Epinephrine HCl (Ciba Vision),** *Glaucon* (Alcon)
Solution: 0.5%, 1% and 2% (as base) (*Rx*)	*Epifrin* (Allergan)
EPINEPHRINE (as Borate)	
Solution: 0.5%, 1% and 2% (*Rx*)	*Epinal* (Alcon)

Actions:
Pharmacology: Epinephrine, a direct-acting sympathomimetic agent, acts on α and β receptors. Topical application, therefore, causes conjunctival decongestion (vasoconstriction), transient mydriasis (pupillary dilation) and reduction in intraocular pressure (IOP). It is believed IOP reduction is primarily due to reduced aqueous production and increased aqueous outflow. The duration of decrease in IOP is 12 to 24 hours.

Indications:
Glaucoma: Management of open-angle (chronic simple) glaucoma; may be used in combination with miotics, beta blockers, hyperosmotic agents or carbonic anhydrase inhibitors.

Contraindications:
Hypersensitivity to epinephrine or any component of the formulation; narrow- or shallow-angle (angle Y closure) glaucoma; aphakia; patients with a narrow angle but no glaucoma; if the nature of the glaucoma is not clearly established. Do not use while wearing soft contact lenses; discoloration of lenses may occur.

Warnings:
For ophthalmic use only. Not for injection or intraocular use.

Gonioscopy: Since pupil dilation may precipitate an acute attack of narrow-angle glaucoma, evaluate anterior chamber angle by gonioscopy prior to beginning therapy.

Anesthesia: Discontinue use prior to general anesthesia with anesthetics which sensitize the myocardium to sympathomimetics (eg, cyclopropane, halothane).

Aphakic patients: Maculopathy with associated decrease in visual acuity may occur in the aphakic eye; if this occurs, promptly discontinue use.

Elderly: Use with caution.

Pregnancy: Category C.

Lactation: It is not known whether this drug is excreted in breast milk.

Children: Safety and efficacy for use in children have not been established.

Precautions:
Instillation discomfort: Epinephrine is relatively uncomfortable upon instillation. Discomfort lessens as concentration of epinephrine decreases.

Special risk patients: Use with caution in the presence or history of: Hypertension; diabetes; hyperthyroidism; heart disease; cerebral arteriosclerosis; bronchial asthma.

Potentially hazardous tasks: Epinephrine may cause temporarily blurred or unstable vision after instillation; observe caution while driving, operating machinery or performing other tasks requiring physical dexterity.

Drug Interactions:

Consider interactions that occur with systemic use of epinephrine, including beta blockers and chymotrypsin.

Adverse Reactions:

Adverse reactions may include transient stinging and burning; eye pain/ache; browache; headache; allergic lid reaction; conjunctival hyperemia; conjunctival or corneal pigmentation; ocular irritation (hypersensitivity); localized adrenochrome deposits in conjunctiva and cornea (prolonged use); reversible cystoid macular edema may result from use in aphakic patients; palpitations; tachycardia; extrasystoles; cardiac arrhythmia; hypertension; faintness.

Administration and Dosage:

Instill 1 drop into affected eye(s) once or twice daily. Determine frequency of instillation by tonometry.

More frequent instillation than 1 drop twice daily does not usually elicit any further improvement in therapeutic response.

When used in conjunction with miotics, instill the miotic first.

DIPIVEFRIN HCl (Dipivalyl epinephrine)

Solution: 0.1% (*Rx*)	Various, *Propine* (Allergan), *AKPro* (Akorn)

Actions:

Pharmacology: Dipivefrin is a prodrug of epinephrine. Dipivefrin, converted to epinephrine in the eye by enzymatic hydrolysis, appears to act by decreasing aqueous production and enhancing outflow facility. It has the same therapeutic effects as epinephrine with fewer local and systemic side effects.

Pharmacokinetics: The onset of action with 1 drop occurs about 30 minutes after treatment, with maximum effect seen at about 1 hour.

Indications:

Glaucoma: Initial therapy or as an adjunct with other antiglaucoma agents for the control of IOP in chronic open-angle glaucoma.

Contraindications:

Hypersensitivity to dipivefrin or any formulation component; narrow angle glaucoma.

Warnings:

Pregnancy: Category B.

Lactation: It is not known whether this drug is excreted in breast milk.

Children: Safety and efficacy for use in children have not been established.

Precautions:

Aphakic patients: Macular edema occurs in up to 30% of aphakic patients treated with epinephrine. Discontinuation generally results in reversal of the maculopathy.

Adverse Reactions:

Adverse reactions may include tachycardia; arrhythmias; hypertension; burning and stinging; conjunctival injection.

Administration and Dosage:

Initial glaucoma therapy: Instill 1 drop into the eye(s) every 12 hours.

APRACLONIDINE HYDROCHLORIDE

Solution: 0.5% and 0.01% (*Rx*)	*Iopidine* (Alcon)

Actions:

Pharmacology: Apraclonidine HCl is a relatively selective α-adrenergic agonist. When instilled into the eyes, apraclonidine reduces intraocular pressure (IOP) and has minimal effect on cardiovascular parameters.

Pharmacokinetics: Topical use of apraclonidine 0.5% leads to systemic absorption. The onset of action is usually within 1 hour and the maximum IOP reduction occurs 3 to 5 hours after application of a single dose.

Indications:

1%: To control or prevent postsurgical elevations in IOP that occur in patients after argon laser trabeculoplasty or iridotomy.

0.5%: Short-term adjunctive therapy in patients on maximally tolerated medical therapy who require additional IOP reduction.

Contraindications:

Hypersensitivity to any component of this medication or to **clonidine**; concurrent monamine oxidase inhibitor therapy.

Warnings:

Concomitant therapy: The addition of apraclonidine 0.5% to patients already using two aqueous suppressing drugs (eg, beta-blocker plus carbonic anhydrase inhibitor) as part of their maximally tolerated medical therapy may not provide additional benefit.

Tachyphylaxis: The IOP lowering efficacy of apraclonidine 0.5% diminishes over time in some patients. The benefit for most patients is < 1 month.

Hypersensitivity: Apraclonidine can lead to an allergic-like reaction characterized wholly or in part by the symptoms of hyperemia, pruritus, discomfort, tearing, foreign body sensation and edema of the lids and conjunctiva. If ocular allergic-like symptoms occur, discontinue therapy.

Renal/Hepatic function impairment: Although the topical use of apraclonidine has not been studied in renal failure patients, structurally related clonidine undergoes a significant increase in half-life in patients with severe renal impairment. Close monitoring of cardiovascular parameters in patients with impaired renal function is advised if they are candidates for topical apraclonidine therapy. Close monitoring of cardiovascular parameters in patients with impaired liver function is also advised as the systemic dosage form of clonidine is partly metabolized in the liver.

Pregnancy: Category C.

Lactation: Consider discontinuing nursing for the day on which apraclonidine is used.

Children: Safety and efficacy for use in children have not been established.

Precautions:

Monitoring: Glaucoma patients on maximally tolerated medical therapy who are treated with apraclonidine 0.5% to delay surgery should have their visual fields monitored periodically. Discontinue treatment if IOP rises significantly.

IOP reduction: Since apraclonidine is a potent depressor of IOP, closely monitor patients who develop exaggerated reductions in IOP.

Cardiovascular disease: Acute administration of two drops of apraclonidine has had minimal effect on heart rate or blood pressure; however, observe caution in treating patients with severe cardiovascular disease, including hypertension.

Use apraclonidine 0.5% with caution in patients with coronary insufficiency, recent myocardial infarction, cerebrovascular disease, chronic renal failure, Raynaud's disease or thromboangiitis obliterans.

Depression: Caution and monitor depressed patients since apraclonidine has been infrequently associated with depression.

Drug Interactions:

Drugs that may interact include cardiovascular agents and MAOIs.

Adverse Reactions:

Adverse reactions from 1% solution may include: Upper lid elevation; conjunctival blanching; mydriasis; burning; discomfort; foreign body sensation; dryness; itching; hypotony; blurred or dimmed vision; allergic response; conjunctival microhemorrhage; dry mouth; bradycardia; vasovagal attack; palpitations; orthostatic episode; headache; taste abnormalities; nasal burning or head cold sensation; shortness of breath.

Adverse reactions from 0.5% solution may include: Hyperemia; pruritus; discomfort; tearing; taste perversion; use can lead to an allergic-type reaction.

Administration and Dosage:

0.5%: Instill one to two drops in the afected eye(s) 3 times daily. Since apraclonidine 0.5% will be used with other ocular glaucoma therapies, use an approximate 5 minute interval between instillation of each medication to prevent washout of the previous dose. Not for injection into the eye.

1%: Instill 1 drop in scheduled operative eye 1 hour before initiating anterior segment laser surgery. Instill second drop into same eye immediately upon completion of surgery.

BETA-ADRENERGIC BLOCKING AGENTS

BETAXOLOL HCL	
Solution: 5.6 mg (equiv. to 5 mg base) per ml (0.5%) (*Rx*)	*Betoptic* (Alcon)
Suspension: 2.8 mg (equiv. to 2.5 mg base) per ml (0.25%) (*Rx*)	*Betoptic S* (Alcon)
CARTEOLOL HCl	
Solution: 1% (*Rx*)	*Ocupress* (Otsuka America)
LEVOBUNOLOL HCL	
Solution: 0.25% and 0.5% (*Rx*)	Various, *AKBeta* (Akorn), *Betagan Liquifilm* (Allergan)
METIPRANOLOL HCl	
Solution: 0.3% (*Rx*)	*OptiPranolol* (Bausch & Lomb)
TIMOLOL MALEATE	
Solution: 0.25% and 0.5% (*Rx*)	Various, *Timoptic* (Merck), *Betimol* (Ciba Vision)
Gel: 0.25% and 0.5% (*Rx*)	*Timoptic-XE* (Merck)

Actions:

Pharmacology: The exact mechanism of ocular antihypertensive action is not established, but it appears to be a reduction of aqueous production. However, some studies show a slight increase in outflow facility with timolol and metipranolol.

Pharmacokinetics:

Pharmacokinetics of Ophthalmic β-Adrenergic Blocking Agents

Drug	β-receptor selectivity	Onset (min)	Maximum effect (hr)	Duration (hr)
Carteolol	β_1 and β_2	nd[1]	nd[1]	12
Betaxolol	β_1	30	2	12
Levobunolol	β_1 and β_2	< 60	2 to 6	12 to 24
Metipranolol	β_1 and β_2	≤ 30	≈ 2	12 to 24
Timolol	β_1 and β_2	30	1 to 2	12 to 24

[1] nd = No data

Indications:

Glaucoma: Lowering IOP in patients with chronic open-angle glaucoma.

Contraindications:

Bronchial asthma, a history of bronchial asthma or severe chronic obstructive pulmonary disease; sinus bradycardia; second-degree and third-degree AV block; overt cardiac failure; cardiogenic shock; hypersensitivity to any component of the products.

Warnings:

Systemic absorption: These agents may be absorbed systemically. The same adverse reactions found with systemic β-blockers may occur with topical use.

Cardiovascular: Timolol can decrease resting and maximal exercise heart rate even in healthy subjects.

Non-allergic bronchospasm patients or patients with a history of chronic bronchitis, emphysema, etc, should receive β-blockers with caution; they may block bronchodilation produced by catecholamine stimulation of β_2-receptors.

Diabetes mellitus: Administer with caution to patients subject to spontaneous hypoglycemia or to diabetic patients (especially labile diabetics). Beta-blocking agents may mask signs and symptoms of acute hypoglycemia.

Thyroid: Beta-adrenergic blocking agents may mask clinical signs of hyperthyroidism (eg, tachycardia).

Cerebrovascular insufficiency: Because of potential effects of β-blockers on blood pressure and pulse, use with caution in patients with cerebrovascular insufficiency.

Pregnancy: Category C.

Lactation: It is not known whether betaxolol, levobunolol or metipranolol are excreted in breast milk.

Children: Safety and efficacy for use in children have not been established.

Precautions:

Angle-closure glaucoma: The immediate objective is to reopen the angle, requiring constriction of the pupil with a miotic. These agents have little or no effect on the pupil.

Muscle weakness: Beta-blockade may potentiate muscle weakness consistent with certain myasthenic symptoms (eg, diplopia, ptosis, generalized weakness).

Long-term therapy: Diminished responsiveness to **betaxolol** and **timolol** after prolonged therapy has been reported. However, in long-term studies (2 and 3 years), no significant differences in mean IOP were observed after initial stabilization.

Drug Interactions:

Ophthalmic beta blockers may affect oral beta blockers, ophthalmic epinephrine, quinidine and verapamil.

Other drugs that may interact with systemic β-adrenergic blocking agents may also interact with ophthalmic agents.

Adverse Reactions:

Headache; depression; arrhythmia; syncope; heart block; cerebral vascular accident; cerebral ischemia; congestive heart failure; palpitation; nausea; hypersensitivity, including localized and generalized rash; bronchospasm; respiratory failure; eratitis; bleparoptosis; visual disturbances including refractive changes; diplopia; ptosis.

Systemic β-adrenergic blocker-associated reactions: Consider potential effects with ophthalmic use.

The following adverse reactions have occurred with each individual agent:

Carteolol:

Ophthalmic – Transient irritation, burning, tearing, conjunctival hyperemia, edema (≈ 25%).

Betaxolol:

Ophthalmic – Brief discomfort (> 25%); occasional tearing (5%).

Metipranolol:

Ophthalmic – Transient local discomfort; conjunctivitis; eyelid dermatitis; blepharitis; blurred vision; tearing; browache; abnormal vision; photophobia; edema.

Levobunolol:

Ophthalmic – Transient burning/stinging (25%); blepharoconjunctivitis (5%).

Timolol:

Ophthalmic – Ocular irritation including conjunctivitis; blepharitis; keratitis; blepharoptosis; decreased corneal sensitivity; visual disturbaces including refractive changes; diplopia; ptosis.

Administration and Dosage:

LEVOBUNOLOL HCl:

Usual dose – 1 drop in the affected eye(s) once or twice a day.

BETAXOLOL HCl:

Usual dose – Instill 1 to 2 drops twice daily.

METIPRANOLOL HCl:

Usual dose – One drop in the affected eye(s) twice a day. If the patient's IOP is not at a satisfactory level on this regimen, more frequent administration or a larger dose is not known to be of benefit.

CARTEOLOL HCl:

Usual dose – One drop in affected eye(s) twice daily. If the patient's IOP is not at a satisfactory level on this regimen, concomitant therapy can be instituted.

TIMOLOL MALEATE:

Solution –

Initial therapy: 1 drop of 0.25% twice daily. If clinical response is not adequate, change the dosage to 1 drop of 0.5% solution twice a day. If the IOP is maintained at satisfactory levels, change the dosage to 1 drop once a day.

Gel – Administer other ophthalmics at least 10 min before the gel. Dose is 1 drop (0.25% or 0.5%) once daily. Dosages > 1 drop of 0.5% have not been studied. Consider concomitant therapy if IOP is not at a satisfactory level.

MIOTICS, DIRECT-ACTING

ACETYLCHOLINE CHLORIDE, INTRAOCULAR	
Solution: 1:100 acetylcholine chloride when reconstituted (*Rx*)	*Miochol-E* (Ciba Vision)
CARBACHOL, INTRAOCULAR	
Solution: 0.01% (*Rx*)	*Miostat* (Alcon), *Carbastat* (Ciba Vision)
CARBACHOL, TOPICAL	
Solution: 0.75%, 1.5%, 2.25% and 3% (*Rx*)	*Isopto Carbachol* (Alcon), *Carboptic* (Optopics)
PILOCARPINE HCl	
Solution: 0.25%, 0.5%, 1%, 2%, 3%, 4%, 5%, 6%, 8% and 10% (*Rx*)	Various, *Pilocar* (Ciba Vision), *Isopto Carpine* (Alcon)
Gel: 4% (*Rx*)	*Pilopine HS* (Alcon)
PILOCARPINE NITRATE	
Solution: 1%, 2% and 4% (*Rx*)	*Pilagan* (Allergan)
PILOCARPINE OCULAR THERAPEUTIC SYSTEM	
Ocular Therapeutic System: Releases 20 or 40 mcg pilocarpine/hour for 1 week (*Rx*)	*Ocusert Pilo-20*, *Ocusert Pilo-40* (Alza)

Actions:

Pharmacology: The direct-acting miotics are parasympathomimetic (cholinergic) drugs which duplicate the muscarinic effects of acetylcholine. When applied topically, these drugs produce pupillary constriction, stimulate the ciliary muscles and increase aqueous humor outflow facility. With the increase in outflow facility, there is a decrease in intraocular pressure (IOP). Topical ophthalmic instillation of acetylcholine causes no discernible response as cholinesterase destroys the molecule more rapidly than it can penetrate the cornea; therefore, acetylcholine is only used intraocularly.

Pharmacokinetics:

Miosis Induction of Direct-Acting Miotics

Miotic	Onset	Peak	Duration
Acetylcholine, intraocular	seconds	—	10 min
Carbachol			
Intraocular	seconds	2 to 5 min	1 to 2 days
Topical	10 to 20 min	—	4 to 8 hours
Pilocarpine, topical	10 to 30 min	—	4 to 8 hours

Indications:

Carbachol, topical; pilocarpine:

Glaucoma – To decrease elevated IOP in glaucoma.

Acetylcholine; carbachol, intraocular:

Miosis – To induce miosis during surgery.

Contraindications:
Hypersensitivity to any component of the formulation; where constriction is undesirable (eg, acute iritis, acute or anterior uveitis, some forms of secondary glaucoma, pupillary block glaucoma, acute inflammatory disease of the anterior chamber).

Warnings:
Corneal abrasion: Use carbachol with caution in the presence of corneal abrasion to avoid excessive penetration.

Pregnancy: Category C (carbachol, pilocarpine).

Lactation: It is not known whether these drugs are excreted in breast milk.

Children: Safety and efficacy for use in children have not been established.

Precautions:
Systemic reactions: Caution is advised in patients with acute cardiac failure, bronchial asthma, peptic ulcer, hyperthyroidism, GI spasm, urinary tract obstruction, Parkinson's disease, recent MI, hypertension or hypotension.

Retinal detachment has been caused by miotics in susceptible individuals, in individuals with preexisting retinal disease or in those who are predisposed to retinal tears.

Miosis usually causes difficulty in dark adaptation. Advise patients to use caution while night driving or performing hazardous tasks in poor light.

Angle-closure: Although withdrawal of the peripheral iris from the anterior chamber angle by miosis may reduce the tendency for narrow-angle closure, miotics can occasionally precipoitate angle closure by increasing resistance to aqueous flow from posterior to anterior chamber.

Pilocarpine ocular system (Ocusert): Carefully consider and evaluate patients with acute infectious conjunctivitis or keratitis prior to use.

Adverse Reactions:
Acetylcholine:

Ophthalmic – Corneal edema; corneal clouding; corneal decompensation.

Systemic – Bradycardia; hypotension; flushing; breathing difficulties; sweating.

Carbachol:

Ophthalmic – Transient stinging and burning; corneal clouding; persistent bullous keratopathy; retinal detachment; transient ciliary and conjunctival injection; ciliary spasm with resultant temporary decrease of visual acuity.

Systemic – Headache; salivation; GI cramps; vomiting; diarrhea; asthma; syncope; cardiac arrhythmia; flushing; sweating; epigastric distress; tightness in bladder; hypotension; frequent urge to urinate.

Pilocarpine:

Ophthalmic – Transient stinging and burning; tearing; ciliary spasm; conjunctival vascular congestion; temporal, peri- or supra-orbital headache; superficial keratitis induced myopia; blurred vision; poor dark adaptation; reduced visual acuity in poor illumination in older individuals and in individuals with lens opacity.

Administration and Dosage:
ACETYLCHOLINE CHLORIDE, INTRAOCULAR:

Solution – 0.5 to 2 ml produces satisfactory miosis. Solution need not be flushed from the chamber after miosis occurs.

CARBACHOL, INTRAOCULAR: Bently instill no more than 0.5 ml into the anterior chamber before or after securing sutures. Miosis is usually maximal 2 to 5 minutes after application.

CARBACHOL, TOPICAL: Instill 2 drops into eye(s) up to 3 times daily.

PILOCARPINE:

Solution –

Initial: 1 or 2 drops 3 to 4 times daily. Individuals with heavily pigmented irides may require higher strengths.

Gel – Apply a 0.5 inch ribbon in the lower conjunctival sac of affected eye(s) once daily at bedtime.

PILOCARPINE NITRATE:

Glaucoma – 1 to 2 drops 2 to 4 times daily.

Emergency miosis – 1 to 2 drops of higher concentrations.

Reversal of mydriasis – Dosage and strength required are dependent on the cycloplegic used.

PILOCARPINE OCULAR THERAPEUTIC SYSTEM:

Initiation of therapy: It has been estimated that *Ocusert* 20 mcg is roughly equal to 0.5% or 1% drops and 40 mcg is roughly equal to 2% or 3% drops. Therapy may be started with the 20 mcg system, regardless of the strength of pilocarpine solution the patient previously required. Because of the patient's age, family history and disease status or progression, however, therapy may be started with the 40 mcg system.

If pressure is satisfactorily reduced with the 30 mcg system, the patient should continue its use, replacing each unit every 7 days. If IOP reduction greater than that achieved by 20 mcg is needed, transfer the patient to the 40 mcg system.

MIOTICS, CHOLINESTERASE INHIBITORS

DEMECARIUM BROMIDE

Solution: 0.125% and 0.25% (*Rx*) — *Humorsol* (Merck)

ECHOTHIOPHATE IODIDE

Powder for Reconstitution: 1.5 mg to make 0.03%, 3 mg to make 0.06%, 6.25 mg to make 0.125%, 12.5 mg to make 0.25% (*Rx*) — *Phospholine Iodide* (Wyeth-Ayerst)

PHYSOSTIGMINE (Eserine)

Ointment: 0.25% (as sulfate) (*Rx*) — *Eserine Sulfate* (Ciba Vision)

Actions:

Pharmacology: These indirect-acting agents inhibit the enzyme cholinesterase, potentiating the action of acetylcholine on the parasympathomimetic end organs. Topical application to the eye produces intense miosis and muscle contraction. Intraocular pressure (IOP) is reduced by a decreased resistance to aqueous outflow.

Cholinesterase-Inhibiting Miotics

Miotics	Miosis		IOP reduction		
	Onset (minutes)	Duration	Onset (hours)	Peak (hours)	Duration
Reversible					
Physostigmine	20 to 30	12 to 36 hrs	—	2 to 6	12 to 36 hrs
Demecarium	15 to 60	3 to 10 days	—	24	7 to 28 days
Irreversible					
Echothiophate	10 to 30	1 to 4 weeks	4 to 8	24	7 to 28 days

Indications:

Glaucoma: Therapy of open-angle glaucoma.

Contraindications:

Hypersensitivity to cholinesterase inhibitors or any component of the formulation;active uveal inflammation or any inflammatory disease of the iris or ciliary body; glaucoma associated with iridocyclitis.

Demecarium Pregnancy.

Echothiophate Most cases of angle-closure glaucoma (due to the possibility of increasing angle-block).

Warnings:

Myasthenia gravis: Because of possible additive adverse effects, administer demecarium and echothiophate only with extreme caution to patients with myasthenia gravis who are receiving systemic anticholinesterase therapy.

Surgery: In patients receiving cholinesterase inhibitors, administer succinylcholine with extreme caution before and during general anesthesia. Use prior to ophthalmic surgery only as a considered risk because of th possible occurrence of hyphema.

Pregnancy: Category X (demecarium).
Category C (physostigmine, echothiophate).

Lactation: It is not known whether these drugs are excreted in breast milk.

Children: The occurrence of iris cysts is more frequent in children. Exercise extreme caution in children receiving demecarium and isoflurophate who may require general anesthesia. Safety and efficacy for use of physostigmine have not been established.

Precautions:

Concomitant therapy: Cholinesterase inhibitors may be used in combination with adrenergic agents, β-blockers, carbonic anhydrase inhibitors or hyperosmotic agents.

Narrow angle glaucoma: Use with caution in patients with chronic angle-closure (narrow-angle) glaucoma or in patients with narrow angles, because of the possibility of producing pupillary block and increasing angle blockage. Temporarily discontinue if cardiac irregularities occur.

Special risk patients: Use caution in patients with marked vagotonia, bronchial asthma, spastic GI disturbances, peptic ulcer, pronounced bradycardia/hypotension, recent MI, epilepsy, parkinsonism and other disorders that may respond adversely to vagotonic effects.

Ophthalmic ointments may retard corneal healing.

Miosis usually causes difficulty in dark adaptation. Use caution while driving at night or performing hazardous tasks in poor light.

Gonioscopy: Use only when shorter-acting miotics have proven inadequate. Gonioscopy is recommended prior to use of medication.

Concomitant ocular conditions: When an intraocular inflammatory process is present, breakdown of the blood-aqueous barrier from anticholinesterase therapy requires abstention from, or cautious use of, these drugs. Use with great caution where there is a history of quiescent uveitis.

Systemic effects: Repeated administration may cause depression of the concentration of cholinesterase in the serum and erythrocytes, with resultant systemic effects.

Iris cysts: Iris cysts may form, enlarge and obscure vision (more frequent in children).

Drug Interactions:

Drugs that may interact with cholinesterase inhibitors include carbamate/organophosphate insecticides and pesticides, succinylcholine and systemic anticholinesterases.

Adverse Reactions:

Ophthalmic: Iris cysts; burning; lacrimation; lid muscle twitching; conjunctival and ciliary redness; browache; headache; activation of latent iritis or uveitis; induced myopia with visual blurring.

Systemic: Nausea; vomiting; abdominal cramps; diarrhea; urinary incontinence; fainting; sweating; salivation; difficulty in breathing; cardiac irregularities.

Administration and Dosage:

PHYSOSTIGMINE (ESERINE):

Ointment – Apply small quantity to lower fornix, up to 3 times daily.

DEMECARIUM BROMIDE:

Glaucoma –

Initial: Place 1 or 2 drops into eye(s).

Usual dose: 1 or 2 drops twice a week to 1 or 2 drops twice a day. The 0.125% strength used tice daily usually results in smooth control of the physiologic diurnal variation in IOP.

Strabismus –

Diagnosis: Instill 1 drop daily for 2 weeks, then 1 drop every 2 days for 2 to 3 weeks. If the eyes become straighter, an accomodative factor is demonstrated.

Therapy: In esotropia uncomplicated by amblyopia or anisometropia, instill not more than 1 drop at a time in both eyes every day for 2 to 3 weeks; too severe a degree of miosis may interfere with vision. Then reduce dosage to 1 drop every other day for 3 to 4 weeks and reevaluate the patient's status. Continue with a dosage of 1 drop every 2 days 1 drop twice a week. If improvement continues, reduce to 1 drop once a week and eventually to trial without medication.

ECHOTHIOPHATE IODIDE:

Glaucoma – Two doses per day are preferred to maintain as smooth a diurnal tension curve as possible, although 1 dose/day or every other day has been used with satisfactory results. Instill the daily dose or 1 of the 2 daily doses just before bedtime to avoid inconvenience due to miosis.

Early chronic simple glaucoma: Instill a 0.03% solution just before retiring and in the morning in cases not controlled with pilocarpine.

Advanced chronic simple glaucoma and glaucoma secondary to cataract surgery: Instill 0.03% solution twice daily, as above.

Accomodative esotropia –

Diagnosis: Instill 1 drop of 0.125% solution once a day into both eyes at bedtime for 2 or 3 weeks. If the esotropia is accommocative, a favorable response may begin within a few hours.

Treatment: After initial period of treatent for diagnostic purposes, reduce schedule to 0.125% every other day or 0.06% every day. The 0.03% strength has proven effective in some cases. The maximum recommended dose is 0.125% once a day, although more intensive therapy has been used for short periods.

DORZOLAMIDE HCl

Solution: 2% (*Rx*)	*Trusopt* (Merck)

Actions:

Pharmacology: Dorzolamide is a carbonic anhydrase inhibitor formulated for topical ophthalmic use.

Pharmacokinetics: When topically applied, dorzolamide reaches the systemic circulation. The drug is primarily excreted unchanged in the urine, and the metabolite is also excreted in urine.

Indications:

Elevated intraocular pressure (IOP): Treatment of elevated IOP in patients with ocular hypertension or open-angle glaucoma.

Contraindications:

Hypersensitivity to any component of this product.

Warnings:

Systemic effects: Dorzolamide is a sulfonamide and, although administered topically, is absorbed systemically. Therefore, the same types of adverse reactions attributable to sulfonamides may occur with topical administration of dorzolamide.

Renal function impairment: Dorzolamide has not been studied in patients with severe renal impairment (Ccr < 30 ml/min). However, because dorzolamide and its metabolite are excreted predominantly by the kidney, dorzolamide is not recommended in such patients.

Elderly: No overall differences in efficacy or safety were observed between these patients and younger patients.

Pregnancy: Category C.

Lactation: It is not known whether this drug is excreted in breast milk.

Children: Safety and efficacy in children have not been established.

Precautions:

Corneal endothelium effects: The effect of continued administration of dorzolamide on the corneal endothelium has not been fully evaluated.

Acute angle-closure glaucoma: The management of patients with acute angle-closure glaucoma requires therapeutic interventions in addition to ocular hypotensive agents. Dorzolamide has not been studied in patients with acute angle-closure glaucoma.

Ocular effects: Local ocular adverse effects, primarily conjunctivitis and lid reactions, were reported with chronic administration of dorzolamide.

Concomitant oral CA inhibitors: There is a potential for an additive effect on the known systemic effects of CA inhibition in patients receiving an oral CA inhibitor and dorzolamide. The concomitant administration of dorzolamide and oral CA inhibitors is not recommended.

Contact lenses: The preservative in dorzolamide solution, benzalkonium chloride, may be absorbed by soft contact lenses. Dorzolamide should not be administered while wearing soft contact lenses.

Drug Interactions:

Although acid-base and electrolyte disturbances were not reported in the clinical trials with dorzolamide, these disturbances have been reported with oral CA inhibitors and have, in some instances, resulted in drug interactions (eg, toxicity associated with high-dose salicylate therapy).

Adverse Reactions:

Adverse reactions occurring in ≥ 3% of patients include ocular burning, stinging or discomfort immediately following administration; bitter taste following administration; superficial punctate keratitis; signs and symptoms of ocular allergic reaction; blurred vision; tearing; dryness; photophobia.

Administration and Dosage:

Dosage: One drop in the affected eye(s) 3 times daily.

Concomitant therapy: If more than one ophthalmic drug is being used, administer the drugs at least 10 minutes apart.

LATANOPROST

Solution: 0.005% (50 mcg/ml) (*Rx*)	*Xalatan* (Pharmacia)

Actions:

Pharmacology: Latanoprost is a prostaglandin $F_{2\alpha}$ analog that is believed to reduce the intraocular pressure (IOP) by increasing the outflow of aqueous humor.

Pharmacokinetics:

Absorption – Latanoprost is absorbed through the cornea where the isopropyl ester prodrug is hydrolyzed by esterases to the biologically active acid. Peak concentration in the aqueous humor is reached ≈ 2 hours after topical administration.

Distribution – The distribution volume in humans is 0.16 L/kg.

Metabolism – The active acid of latanoprost reaching systemic circulation is primarily metabolized by the liver to the 1,2–dinor and 1,2,3,4–tetranor metabolites via fatty acid β-oxidation.

Excretion – The elimination of the acid of latanoprost from human plasma was rapid (half-life was 17 minutes) after both IV and topical administration. Systemic clearance is ≈ 7 ml/min/kg. Following hepatic β-oxidation, the metabolites are mainly eliminated via the kidneys. Approximately 88% to 98% of the administered dose is recovered in the urine after topical and IV dosing, respectively.

Indications:

Elevated intraocular pressure (IOP): For reduction of elevated IOP in patients with open-angle glaucoma and ocular hypertension who are intolerant of other IOP-lowering medications or insufficiently responsive to another IOP-lowering medication.

Contraindications:

Hypersensitivity to any component of this product.

Warnings:

Eye pigment changes: Latanoprost may gradually change eye color, increasing the amount of brown pigment in the iris by increasing the number of melanosomas (pigment granules) in melanocytes.

Pregnancy: Category C.

Lactation: It is not known whether this drug or its metabolites are excreted in breast milk.

Children: Safety and efficacy in children have not been established.

Precautions:

Cornea: Latanoprost is hydrolyzed in the cornea. The effect of continued administration of latanoprost on the corneal endothelium has not been fully evaluated.

Bacterial keratitis: There have been reports of bacterial keratitis associated with the use of multiple-dose containers of topical ophthalmic products. These containers had been inadvertently contaminated by patients who, in most cases, had a concurrent corneal disease or a disruption of the ocular epithelial surface.

Contact lenses: Do not administer latanoprost while wearing contact lenses.

Drug Interactions:

In vitro studies have shown that precipitation occurs when eye drops containing thimerosal are mixed with latanoprost. If such drugs are used, administer with an interval of at least 5 minutes between applications.

Adverse Reactions:

Local: The ocular adverse events and ocular signs and symptoms reported in 5% to 15% of the patients on latanoprost in a 6–month controlled trial were blurred vision, burning and stinging, conjunctival hyperemia, foreign body sensation, itching, increased pigmentation of the iris and punctate epithelial keratopathy. Also reported were dry eye, excessive tearing, eye pain, lid crusting, lid edema, lid erythema, lid discomfort/pain and photophobia (1% to 4%).

Systemic: The most common systemic adverse events seen with latanoprost were upper respiratory tract infection/cold/flu (4%).

Administration and Dosage:

The recommended dosage is one drop (1.5 mcg) in the affected eye(s) once daily in the evening. Do not exceed once-daily dosage because it has been shown that more frequent administration may decrease the IOP-lowering effect. Reduction of the IOP starts ≈ 3 to 4 hours after administration, and the maximum effect is reached after 8 to 12 hours.

Latanoprost may be used concomitantly with other topical ophthalmic drug products to lower IOP. If more than one topical ophthalmic drug is being used, administer the drugs at least 5 minutes apart.

Storage/Stability: Protect from light. Refrigerate unopened bottle at 2° to 8°C (36° to 46°F). Once opened, the container may be stored at room temperature up to 25°C (77°F) for 6 weeks.

CORTICOSTEROID

FLUOROMETHOLONE	
Suspension: 0.1% and 0.25% (*Rx*)	*Fluor-Op* (Ciba Vision), *FML Forte* (Allergan)
Suspension: 0.1% fluormetholone acetate (*Rx*)	*Flarex* (Alcon)
Ointment: 0.1% (*Rx*)	*FML S.O.P.* (Allergan)
MEDRYSONE	
Suspension: 1% (*Rx*)	*HMS* (Allergan)
PREDNISOLONE	
Suspension: 0.12%, 0.125%, 1% prednisolone acetate (*Rx*)	Various, *Econopred* (Alcon), *Pred Forte* (Allergan)
Solution: 0.125% and 1% prednisolone sodium phosphate (*Rx*)	Various, *AK-Pred* (Akorn), *Inflamase Mild* (Iolab)
DEXAMETHASONE	
Solution: 0.1% (*Rx*)	Various, *AK-Dex* (Akorn), *Decadron Phosphate* (Merck)
Suspension: 0.1% (*Rx*)	Various, *Maxidex* (Alcon)
Ointment: 0.05% (*Rx*)	Various, *AK-Dex* (Akorn), *Decadron Phosphate* (Merck)
RIMEXOLONE	
Suspension: 1% (*Rx*)	*Vexol* (Alcon)

Actions:

Pharmacology: Topical corticosteroids exert an anti-inflammatory action. Steroids inhibit inflammatory response to inciting agents of mechanical, chemical or immunological nature.

Indications:

Inflammatory conditions: Treatment of steroid responsive inflammatory conditions of the palpebral and bulbar conjunctiva, lid, cornea and anterior segment of the globe, such as: Allergic conjunctivitis; nonspecific superficial keratitis; superficial punctate keratitis; herpes zoster keratitis; iritis; cyclitis; and selected infective conjunctivitis when the inherent hazard of steroid use is accepted to obtain a diminution in edema and inflammation.

Corneal injury: Also used for corneal injury from chemical, radiation or thermal burns or penetration of foreign bodies.

Graft rejection: May use to suppress graft reaction after keratoplasty.

Contraindications:

Acute superficial herpes simplex keratitis; fungal diseases of ocular structures; vaccinia, varicella and most other viral diseases of the cornea and conjunctiva; ocular tuberculosis; hypersensitivity; after uncomplicated removal of a superficial corneal foreign body.

Medrysone is not for use in iritis and uveitis; its efficacy has not been demonstrated.

Warnings:

Moderate to severe inflammation: Use higher strengths for moderate to severe inflammations. In difficult cases of anterior segment eye disease, systemic therapy may be required. When deeper ocular structures are involved, use systemic therapy.

Ocular damage: Prolonged use may result in glaucoma, elevated IOP, optic nerve damage, defects in visual acuity and fields of vision, posterior subcapsular cataract formation or secondary ocular infections from pathogens liberated from ocular tissues.

Mustard gas keratitis or Sjogren's keratoconjunctivitis: Topical steroids not effective.

Infections: Acute, purulent, untreated eye infection may be masked or activity enhanced by steroids. Fungal infections of the cornea have been reported with long-term local steroid applications.

Pregnancy: Category C.

Lactation: It is not known whether topical steroids are excreted in breast milk.

Children: Safety and efficacy have not been established in children.

Adverse Reactions:

Glaucoma (elevated IOP) with optic nerve damage, loss of visual acuity and field defects; posterior subcapsular cataract formation; secondary ocular infection from pathogens, including herpes simplex liberated from ocular tissues; perforation of globe; blurred vision, discharge, discomfort, ocular pain, foreign body sensation, hyperemia, pruritus (rimexolone).

Systemic: Systemic side effects may occur with extensive use.

Administration and Dosage:

Suspensions and solutions: Instill 1 or 2 drops into the conjunctival sac every hour during the day and every 2 hours during the night. When a favorable response is observed, reduce dosage to 1 drop every 4 hours. Later, 1 drop 3 or 4 times daily may suffice to control symptoms. For postoperative inflammation, instill 1 to 2 drops 4 times daily beginning 24 hours after surgery; continue throughout the first 2 weeks of the postoperative period.

Ointments: Apply a thin coating in the lower conjunctival sac 3 or 4 times a day. When a favorable response is observed, reduce the number of daily applications to twice, and later to once a day as a maintenance dose if sufficient to control symptoms.

LODOXAMIDE TROMETHAMINE

Solution: 0.1% (*Rx*)	*Alomide* (Alcon)

Actions:

Pharmacology: Lodoxamide is a mast cell stabilizer that inhibits the in vivo Type I immediate hypersensitivity reaction. Although lodoxamide's precise mechanism of action is unknown, the drug may prevent calcium influx into mast cells upon antigen stimulation.

Pharmacokinetics: The disposition of lodoxamide was studied in six healthy adult volunteers receiving a 3 mg oral dose. Urinary excretion was the major route of elimination. The elimination half-life was 8.5 hours in urine. In a study in 12 healthy adult volunteers, topical administration of one drop in each eye 4 times per day for 10 days did not result in any measurable lodoxamide plasma levels at a detection limit of 2.5 ng/ml.

Indications:

Treatment of the ocular disorders referred to by the terms vernal keratoconjunctivitis, vernal conjunctivitis and vernal keratitis.

Contraindications:

Hypersensitivity to any component of this product.

Warnings:

For ophthalmic use only. Not for injection.

Contact lenses: As with all ophthalmic preparations containing benzalkonium chloride, instruct patients not to wear soft contact lenses during treatment with lodoxamide.

Pregnancy: *Category B.*

Lactation: It is not known whether lodoxamide is excreted in breast milk.

Children: Safety and efficacy in children < 2 years of age have not been established.

Precautions:

Burning/Stinging: Patients may experience a transient burning or stinging upon instillation of lodoxamide. Should these symptoms persist, advise patients to contact their physicians.

Adverse Reactions:

Adverse reactions occurring in ≥ 3% of patients include transient burning, stinging or discomfort upon instillation; ocular itching/pruritus; blurred vision; dry eye; tearing/discharge; hyperemia; crystalline deposits and foreign body sensation.

Administration and Dosage:

Adults and children > 2 years of age: 1 to 2 drops in each affected eye 4 times daily for up to 3 months.

LEVOCABASTINE HCl

Ophthalmic suspension: 0.05% (*Rx*)	*Livostin* (Iolab)

Actions:

Pharmacology: Levocabastine is a potent, selective histamine H_1-receptor antagonist for topical ophthalmic use. Antigen challenge studies performed 2 and 4 hours after initial drug instillation indicated activity was maintained for at least 2 hours.

Pharmacokinetics: After instillation in the eye, levocabastine is systemically absorbed. However, the amount of systemically absorbed levocabastine after therapeutic ocular doses is low.

Indications:

Allergic conjunctivitis: For the temporary relief of the signs and symptoms of seasonal allergic conjunctivitis.

Contraindications:

Hypersensitivity to any components of the product; while soft contact lenses are being worn.

Warnings:

For ophthalmic use only: Not for injection.

Pregnancy: Category C.

Lactation: Levocabastine is excreted in breast milk.

Children: Safety and efficacy in children < 12 years of age have not been established.

Adverse Reactions:

Adverse reactions occurring in ≥ 3 % of patients include: Mild, transient stinging and burning; headache; visual disturbances; dry mouth; fatigue; pharyngitis; eye pain/dryness; somnolence; red eyes; lacrimation/discharge; cough; nausea; rash/erythema; eyelid edema; dyspnea.

Administration and Dosage:

Shake well before using.

The usual dose is 1 drop instilled in affected eyes 4 times daily. Treatment may be continued for up to 2 weeks.

ANTIBIOTICS

CHLORAMPHENICOL	
Ointment: 10 mg/g (*Rx*)	Various, *Chloromycetin* (Parke-Davis), *Chloroptic S.O.P.* (Allergan)
Powder for solution: 25 mg/vial (*Rx*)	*Chlormycetin* (Parke-Davis)
Solution: 5 mg/ml (*Rx*)	Various, *Chloroptic* (Allergan), *AK-Chlor* (Akorn)
ERYTHROMYCIN	
Ointment: 5 mg/g (*Rx*)	Various, *Ilotycin* (Dista)
GENTAMICIN SULFATE	
Ointment: 3 mg/g (*Rx*)	Various, *Garamycin* (Schering), *Genoptic S.O.P.* (Allergan)
Solution: 3 mg/ml (*Rx*)	Various, *Garamycin* (Schering), *Genoptic* (Allergan)
TOBRAMYCIN	
Ointment: 3 mg/g (*Rx*)	Various, *Tobrex* (Alcon)
Solution: 0.3% (*Rx*)	Various, *AKTob* (Akorn), *Tobrex* (Alcon)
POLYMYXIN B SULFATE	
Powder for solution: 500,000 units (*Rx*)	*Polymyxin B Sulfate Sterile* (Roerig)

BACITRACIN	
Ointment: 500 units/g (*Rx*)	Various, *AK-Tracin* (Akorn)
CIPROFLOXACIN	
Solution: 3.5 mg/ml (equivalent to 3 mg base) (*Rx*)	*Ciloxan* (Alcon)
NORFLOXACIN	
Solution: 3 mg/ml (*Rx*)	*Chibroxin* (Merck)
OFLOXACIN	
Solution: 3 mg/ml (*Rx*)	*Ocuflox* (Allergan)

Indications:

Infections: Treatment of superficial ocular infections involving the conjunctiva or cornea (eg, conjunctivitis, keratitis, keratoconjunctivitis, corneal ulcers, blepharitis, blepharoconjunctivitis, acute meibomianitis and dacryocystitis) due to strains of microorganisms susceptible to antibiotics.

Tetracycline and erythromycin are also indicated for the prophylaxis of ophthalmia neonatorum due to Neisseria gonorrhoeae or *Chlamydia trachomatis*.

Chloramphenicol: Use chloramphenicol only in those serious infections for which less potentially dangerous drugs are ineffective or contraindicated (see Warnings).

Topical Ophthalmic Antibiotic Preparations

		Miscellaneous						Quinolones			Amino-glycosides			Tetra-cyclines			Sulfon-amides	
	Organism/Infection	Bacitracin	Gramicidin	Polymyxin B	Erythromycin	Chloramphenicol	Trimethoprim	Norfloxacin	Ciprofloxacin	Ofloxacin	Neomycin	Gentamicin	Tobramycin	Tetracycline	Chlortetracycline	Oxytetracycline	Sodium Sulfacetamide	Sulfisoxazole
Gram-Positive	Staphylococcus sp	✓	✓					✓	✓	✓		✓	✓					
	S aureus	✓	✓		✓	✓	✓	✓	✓	✓	✓	✓	✓	✓	✓		✓	
	Streptococcus sp	✓	✓			✓			✓	✓			✓	✓			✓	
	S pneumoniae	✓	✓		✓	✓	✓	✓	✓	✓		✓[1]	✓	✓	✓			
	α-hemolytic streptococci (viridans group)				✓													
	β-hemolytic streptococci	✓										✓[1]	✓					
	S pyogenes	✓			✓		✓		✓	✓		✓			✓			
	Corynebacterium sp	✓	✓		✓						✓	✓	✓					

Topical Ophthalmic Antibiotic Preparations

		Miscellaneous						Quinolones			Amino-glycosides			Tetra-cyclines			Sulfon-amides	
	Organism/Infection	Bacitracin	Gramicidin	Polymyxin B	Erythromycin	Chloramphenicol	Trimethoprim	Norfloxacin	Ciprofloxacin	Ofloxacin	Neomycin	Gentamicin	Tobramycin	Tetracycline	Chlortetracycline	Oxytetracycline	Sodium Sulfacetamide	Sulfisoxazole
Gram-Negative	Escherichia coli			✓		✓	✓	✓	✓	✓	✓	✓	✓	✓	✓	✓	✓	✓
	Haemophilus aegyptius					✓	✓	✓				✓	✓				✓	✓
	H ducreyi					✓			✓			✓	✓		✓	✓		
	H influenzae			✓	✓	✓	✓	✓	✓	✓	✓	✓	✓		✓	✓		
	Klebsiella sp					✓		✓	✓	✓	✓					✓		
	K pneumoniae			✓			✓	✓	✓	✓		✓	✓		✓			
	Neisseria sp	✓				✓			✓		✓	✓	✓	✓				
	N gonorrhoeae	✓			✓[2]			✓	✓	✓		✓		✓[2]	✓		✓	
	Proteus sp						✓	✓	✓	✓	✓	✓	✓					
	Acinetobacter calcoaceticus							✓	✓	✓		✓	✓					
	Enterobacter aerogenes			✓			✓	✓	✓		✓	✓	✓			✓		
	Enterobacter sp					✓		✓	✓	✓	✓	✓	✓					
	Serratia marcescens							✓	✓	✓		✓	✓					
	Moraxella sp					✓				✓		✓	✓					
	Chlamydia trachomatis				✓[2]				✓	✓				✓[3]	✓[3]		✓[4]	✓
	Pasteurella tularensis														✓	✓		
	Pseudomonas aeruginosa			✓		✓		✓	✓	✓		✓[1]	✓					
	Bartonella bacilliformis															✓		
	Bacteroides sp				✓									✓	✓	✓		
	Vibrio sp					✓		✓	✓			✓	✓			✓		
	Yersinia pestis														✓	✓		

[1] Increasing resistance has been seen.
[2] For prophylaxis.
[3] In conjunction with oral therapy
[4] Adjunct in systemic sulfonamide therapy.

Contraindications:

Hypersensitivity to any component of these products; epithelial herpes simplex keratitis (dendritic keratitis); vaccinia; varicella; mycobacterial infections of the eye; fungal diseases of the ocular structure; use of steroid combinations after uncomplicated removal of a corneal foreign body.

Warnings:

Sensitization from the topical use of an antibiotic may contraindicate the drug's later systemic use in serious infections.

Cross-sensitivity: Allergic cross-reactions may occur that could prevent future use of any or all of these antibiotics – Kanamycin, neomycin, paromomycin, streptomycin, and possibly, gentamicin.

Chloramphenicol – Hematopoietic toxicity has occurred occasionally with the systemic use of chloramphenicol and rarely with topical administration.

Pregnancy: Category B *(tobramycin)*, Category C *(gentamicin, ciprofloxacin, norfloxacin, ofloxacin)*.

Lactation: It is not known whether **ciprofloxacin, norfloxacin** or **ofloxacin** appears in breast milk following ophthalmic use. Exercise caution when administering **ciprofloxacin** to a nursing mother.

Children: **Tobramycin** is safe and effective in children. Safety and efficacy of **ciprofloxacin** in children < 12 years of age and **norfloxacin** and **ofloxacin** in infants < 1 year of age have not been established.

Precautions:

Superinfection: Do not use topical antibiotics in deep-seated ocular infections or in those that are likely to become systemic.

Systemic antibiotics – In all except very superficial infections, supplement the topical use of antibiotics with appropriate systemic medication.

Crystalline precipitate – A white crystalline precipitate located in the superficial portion of the corneal defect was observed in ≈ 17% of patients on **ciprofloxacin**.

Adverse Reactions:

Sensitivity reactions such as transient irritation, burning, stinging, itching, inflammation, angioneurotic edema, urticaria, vesicular and maculopapular dermatitis have occurred in some patients.

Chloramphenicol: Hematological events (including aplastic anemia) have been reported.

Ciprofloxacin: White crystalline precipitates; lid margin crusting; crystals/scales; foreign body sensation; itching; conjunctival hyperemia; bad taste in mouth; corneal staining; keratopathy/keratitis; allergic reactions; lid edema; tearing; photophobia; corneal infiltrates; nausea; decreased vision.

Norfloxacin: Conjunctival hyperemia; chemosis; photophobia; bitter taste in mouth.

Administration and Dosage:

Administration and dosage varies for the individual products. Refer to the individual manufacturer inserts.

NATAMYCIN

Suspension: 5% (*Rx*)	*Natacyn* (Alcon)

Actions:

Pharmacology: Natamycin, a tetraene polyene antibiotic, is derived from *Streptomyces natalensis*.

It possesses in vitro activity against a variety of yeast and filamentous fungi, including *Candida*, *Aspergillus*, *Cephalosporium*, *Fusarium* and *Penicillium*. The mechanism of action appears to be through binding of the molecule to the fungal cell membrane. The polyenesterol complex alters membrane permeability, depleting essential cellular constituents. Although activity against fungi is dose-related, natamycin is predominantly fungicidal.

Pharmacokinetics: Topical administration appears to produce effective concentrations within the corneal stroma, but not in intraocular fluid. Absorption from the GI tract is very poor. Systemic absorption should not occur after topical administration.

Indications:

Fungal blepharitis, conjunctivitis and keratitis caused by susceptible organisms. Natamycin is the initial drug of choice in Fusarium solani keratitis.

Contraindications:

Hypersensitivity to any component of the formulation.

Warnings:

Pregnancy: Safety for use during pregnancy has not been established.

Precautions:

For topical use only. Not for injection.

Fungal endophthalmitis: The effectiveness of topical natamycin as a single agent in fungal endophthalmitis has not been established.

Resistance: Failure of keratitis to improve following 7 to 10 days of administration suggests that the infection may be caused by a microorganism not susceptible to natamycin. Base continuation of therapy on clinical reevaluation and additional laboratory studies.

Toxicity: Adherence of the suspension to areas of epithelial ulceration or retention in the fornices occurs regularly. Should suspicion of drug toxicity occur, discontinue the drug.

Diagnosis/Monitoring: Determine initial and sustained therapy of fungal keratitis by the clinical diagnosis (laboratory diagnosis by smear and culture of corneal scrapings) and by response to the drug. Whenever possible, determine the in vitro activity of natamycin against the responsible fungus. Monitor tolerance to natamycin at least twice weekly.

Adverse Reactions:

One case of conjunctival chemosis and hyperemia, thought to be allergic in nature, was reported.

Administration and Dosage:

Fungal keratitis: Instill 1 drop into the conjunctival sac at 1 or 2 hour intervals. The frequency of application can usually be reduced to 1 drop 6 to 8 times daily after the first 3 to 4 days. Generally, continue therapy for 14 to 21 days, or until there is resolution of active fungal keratitis. In many cases, it may help to reduce the dosage gradually at 4 to 7 day intervals to ensure that the organism has been eliminated.

Fungal blepharitis and conjunctivitis: 4 to 6 daily applications may be sufficient.

ANTIVIRAL AGENTS

The topical ophthalmic antiviral preparations appear to interfere with viral reproduction by altering DNA synthesis. Idoxuridine, vidarabine and trifluridine are effective treatment for herpes simplex infections of the conjunctiva and cornea. Ganciclovir is indicated for use in immunocompromised patients with cytomegalovirus (CMV) retinitis and for prevention of CMV retinitis in transplant patients. Foscarnet is indicated for use only in AIDS patients with CMV retinitis.

Monographs for idoxuridine, vidarabine and trifluridine follow this introduction. Prescribing information for foscarnet and ganciclovir appear in the Antivirals section of the Anti-Infectives chapter.

Viral infection, especially epidemic keratoconjunctivitis (EKC), is more often associated with a follicular conjunctivitis, a serous conjunctival discharge and preuricular lymphadenopathy. The exceptionally contagious organism causing EKC is not susceptible to antiviral therapy at this time.

IDOXURIDINE (IDU)

Solution: 0.1% (*Rx*)	*Herplex* (Allergan)

Actions:

Pharmacology: Idoxuridine (IDU) blocks reproduction of herpes simplex virus by altering normal DNA synthesis.

In chemical structure, IDU closely approximates the configuration of thymidine, one of the four building blocks of DNA. As a result, IDU replaces thymidine in the enzymatic step of viral replication. The consequent production of faulty DNA results in a pseudostructure which cannot infect or destroy tissue.

Indications:

Herpes simplex keratitis treatment. Epithelial infections, characterized by the presence of a dendritic figure, respond better than stromal infections.

Contraindications:

Hypersensitivity to IDU or any component of the formulation.

Warnings:

Recurrences are common. IDU will often control the infection, but will have no effect on accumulated scarring, vascularization or resultant progressive loss of vision. Recurrence may be seen if medication is not continued for 5 to 7 days after the epithelial lesion is apparently healed.

Sensitization: IDU may be sensitizing; this is more common with dermal than with ocular use.

Corticosteroids can accelerate the spread of a viral infection and are usually contraindicated in herpes simplex epithelial infections.

Pregnancy: Category C.

Lactation: It is not known whether IDU is excreted in breast milk.

Children: Safety and efficacy in children have not been established.

Precautions:

Resistance: Some strains of herpes simplex appear to be resistant. If there is no lessening of fluorescein staining in 14 days, undertake another form of therapy.

Frequency/Duration: Do not exceed the recommended frequency and duration of administration.

Drug Interactions:

Drugs that may interact with idoxuridine include boric acid-containing solutions.

Adverse Reactions:

Adverse reactions may include: Irritation, pain, pruritus, inflammation or edema of the eyes or lids; allergic reactions; photophobia; corneal clouding; stippling and punctate defects in the corneal epithelium.

Administration and Dosage:

For optimal results, keep infected tissues saturated with IDU.

Examine patients at frequent intervals. In epithelial infections, improvement is usually seen within 7 to 8 days. If the patient continues to improve, continue therapy, usually ≤ 21 days.

Solution: Initially, place 1 drop into infected eye(s) every hour during the day and every 2 hours at night. Continue until definite improvement has taken place, as evidenced by loss of staining with fluorescein. Then reduce dosage to 1 drop every 2 hours during the day and every 4 hours at night. To minimize recurrences, continue therapy at this reduced dosage for 3 to 7 days after healing appears complete.

Alternate dosing schedule – Instill 1 drop every minute for 5 minutes. Repeat every 4 hours, day and night.

Concomitant therapy: In the management of herpes simplex with stromal lesions, corneal edema or iritis, topical corticosteroids may be used with IDU. Use such combined therapy for as long as the condition warrants. It is important to continue IDU therapy a few days after the steroid has been withdrawn.

Antibiotics may be used with IDU to control secondary infections, and **atropine** preparations may be employed adjunctively as indicated.

VIDARABINE (Adenine Arabinoside; Ara-A)

Ophthalmic Ointment: 3% vidarabine monohydrate (equivalent to 2.8% vidarabine) (*Rx*)	*Vira-A* (Parke-Davis)

Actions:

Pharmacology: The antiviral mechanism of action has not been established. Vidarabine appears to interfere with the early steps of viral DNA synthesis. It is rapidly deaminated to arabinosylhypoxanthine (Ara-Hx), the principal metabolite. Ara-Hx also possesses in vitro antiviral activity less than vidarabine's.

Pharmacokinetics:

Absorption – Systemic absorption is not expected to occur following ocular administration and swallowing lacrimal secretions.

Distribution – Because of its low solubility, trace amounts of both vidarabine and Ara-Hx can be detected in the aqueous humor only if there is an epithelial defect in the cornea. If the cornea is normal, only trace amounts of Ara-Hx can be recovered from the aqueous humor.

Indications:

Acute keratoconjunctivitis and recurrent epithelial keratitis due to herpes simplex virus types 1 and 2.

Superficial keratitis caused by herpes simplex virus which has not responded to topical idoxuridine, or when toxic or hypersensitivity reactions to idoxuridine have occurred.

Contraindications:

Hypersensitivity to vidarabine; sterile trophic ulcers.

Warnings:

Efficacy in other conditions: Vidarabine is not effective against RNA virus; adenoviral ocular infections; bacterial, fungal or chlamydial infections of the cornea; or trophic ulcers. Effectiveness against stromal keratitis and uveitis due to herpes simplex virus has not been established.

Corticosteroids alone are normally contraindicated in herpes simplex virus eye infections. If vidarabine is coadministered with topical corticosteroid therapy, consider corticosteroid-induced ocular side effects such as glaucoma or cataract formation and progression of bacterial or viral infection.

Temporary visual haze may be produced with vidarabine.

Pregnancy: Category C.

Lactation: It is not known whether vidarabine is excreted in breast milk.

Precautions:

Viral resistance to vidarabine has not been observed, although this possibility exists.

Adverse Reactions:

Adverse reactions may include: Lacrimation; foreign body sensation; conjunctival infection; burning; irritation; superficial punctate keratitis; pain; photophobia; punctal occlusion; sensitivity; uveitis; stromal edema; secondary glaucoma; trophic defects; corneal vascularization and hyphema.

Administration and Dosage:

Administer approximately 0.5 inch of ointment into the lower conjunctival sac(s) 5 times daily at 3 hour intervals.

If there are no signs of improvement after 7 days, or if complete reepithelialization has not occurred in 21 days, consider other forms of therapy. Some severe cases may require longer treatment.

After reepithelialization has occurred, treat for an additional 7 days at a reduced dosage to prevent recurrence.

Concomitant therapy: Topical antibiotics or topical steroids have been administered concurrently with vidarabine without an increase in adverse reactions, although their advantages and disadvantages must be considered.

TRIFLURIDINE (Trifluorothymidine)

Ophthalmic Solution: 1% (Rx)	*Viroptic* (Burroughs Wellcome)

Actions:

Pharmacology: A fluorinated pyrimidine nucleoside with in vitro and in vivo activity against herpes simplex virus types 1 and 2, and vaccinia virus. Some strains of adenovirus are also inhibited in vitro. Its antiviral mechanism of action is not completely known.

Pharmacokinetics:

Absorption – Intraocular penetration occurs after topical instillation. Decreased corneal integrity or stromal or uveal inflammation may enhance the penetration into the aqueous humor. Systemic absorption following therapeutic dosing appears negligible.

Indications:

Primary keratoconjunctivitis and recurrent epithelial keratitis due to herpes simplex virus types 1 and 2.

Epithelial keratitis that has not responded clinically to topical idoxuridine, or when ocular toxicity or hypersensitivity to idoxuridine has occurred. In a smaller number of patients resistant to topical vidarabine, trifluridine was also effective.

Contraindications:

Hypersensitivity reactions or chemical intolerance to trifluridine.

Warnings:

Efficacy in other conditions: The clinical efficacy in the treatment of stromal keratitis and uveitis due to herpes simplex or ophthalmic infections caused by vaccinia virus and adenovirus, or in the prophylaxis of herpes simplex virus keratoconjunctivitis and epithelial keratitis has not been established by well controlled clinical trials. Not effective against bacterial, fungal or chlamydial infections of the cornea or trophic lesions.

Dosage/Frequency: Do not exceed the recommended dosage or frequency of administration.

Pregnancy: Safety for use during pregnancy has not been established.

Lactation: Safety and efficacy have not been established.

Precautions:

Viral resistance, although documented in vitro, has not been reported following multiple exposure to trifluridine; this possibility may exist.

Adverse Reactions:

Adverse reactions may include: Mild, transient burning or stinging upon instillation; palpebral edema; superficial punctate keratopathy; epithelial keratopathy; hypersensitivity reaction; stromal edema; irritation; keratitis sicca; hyperemia and increased intraocular pressure.

Administration and Dosage:

Instill 1 drop onto the cornea of the affected eye(s) every 2 hours while awake for a maximum daily dosage of 9 drops until the corneal ulcer has completely reepithelialized. Following reepithelialization, treat for an additional 7 days with 1 drop every 4 hours while awake for a minimum daily dosage of 5 drops.

If there are no signs of improvement after 7 days, or if complete reepithelialization has not occurred after 14 days, consider other forms of therapy. Avoid continuous administration for periods exceeding 21 days because of potential ocular toxicity.

PILOCARPINE HCl

Tablets: 5 mg (*Rx*) — *Salagen* (MGI Pharma)

Actions:

Pharmacology: Pilocarpine is a cholinergic parasympathomimetic agent exerting a broad spectrum of pharmacologic effects with predominant muscarinic action. Pilocarpine can increase secretion by the exocrine glands, can stimulate intestinal tract smooth muscle (dose-related)and may increase Bronchial smooth muscle tone. The tone and motility of urinary tract, gallbladder, and biliary duct smooth muscle may be enhanced. Pilocarpine may have paradoxical effects on the cardiovascular system. The expected effect of a muscarinic agonist is vasodepression, but administration of pilocarpine may produce hypertension after a brief episode of hypotension. Bradycardia and tachycardia have both been reported with use of pilocarpine.

Pharmacokinetics: Following single 5 and 10 mg oral doses, unstimulated salivary flow was time-related with an onset at 20 minutes and a peak at 1 hour with a duration of 3 to 5 hours.

Following 2 days of 5 or 10 mg oral pilocarpine given at 8 am, noon and 6 pm, the mean elimination half-life was 0.76 and 1.35 hours for the 5 and 10 mg doses, respectively. T_{max} was 1.25 and 0.85 hours and C_{max} was 15 and 41 ng/ml, respectively. The AUC was 33 and 108 hr•ng/ml, respectively, following the last 6 hour dose.

When taken with a high fat meal, there was a decrease in the rate of absorption of pilocarpine. Mean T_{max} was 1.47 and 0.87 hours and mean C_{max} was 51.8 and 59.2 ng/ml for fed and fasted states, respectively.

Inactivation of pilocarpine is thought to occur at neuronal synapses and probably in plasma. Pilocarpine and its minimally active or inactive degradation products, including pilocarpic acid, are excreted in the urine.

Indications:

Xerostomia: Treatment of symptoms of xerostomia from salivary gland hypofunction caused by radiotherapy for cancer of the head and neck.

Contraindications:

Uncontrolled asthma; hypersensitivity to pilocarpine; when miosis is undesirable.

Warnings:

Cardiovascular disease: Patients with significant cardiovascular disease may be unable to compensate for transient changes in hemodynamics or rhythm induced by pilocarpine. Pulmonary edema has been reported as a complication of pilocarpine toxicity from high ocular doses given for acute angle-closure glaucoma. Administer pilocarpine with caution and under close medical supervision in patients with cardiovascular disease.

The dose-related cardiovascular effects of pilocarpine include hypotension, hypertension, bradycardia and tachycardia.

Ocular effects: Carefully examine the fundus prior to initiating therapy with pilocarpine. An association of ocular pilocarpine use and retinal detachment in patients with preexisting retinal disease has been reported. The systemic blood level that is associated with this finding is not known.

Ocular formulations of pilocarpine have caused visual blurring which may result in decreased visual acuity, especially at night and in patients with central lens changes, and impairment of depth perception. Advise caution while driving at night or performing hazardous activities in reduced lighting.

Pulmonary disease: Pilocarpine has been reported to increase airway resistance, bronchial smooth muscle tone and bronchial secretions. Administer with caution and under close medical supervision in patients with controlled asthma, chronic bronchitis or chronic obstructive pulmonary disease.

Elderly: Adverse events reported by those > 65 and those ≤ 65 years of age were comparable. Elderly women volunteers had a higher C_{max} and AUC than elderly men.

Pregnancy: Category C.

Lactation: It is not known whether this drug is excreted in breast milk.

Children: Safety and efficacy in children have not been established.

Precautions:

Toxicity: Toxicity is characterized by an exaggeration of parasympathomimetic effects which may include: Headache; visual disturbance; lacrimation; sweating; respiratory distress; GI spasm; nausea; vomiting; diarrhea; AV block; tachycardia; bradycardia; hypotension; hypertension; shock; mental confusion; cardiac arrhythmia; tremors.

Biliary tract: Administer with caution to patients with known or suspected cholelithiasis or biliary tract disease. Contractions of the gallbladder or biliary smooth muscle could precipitate complications including cholecystitis, cholangitis and biliary obstruction.

Renal colic: Pilocarpine may increase ureteral smooth muscle tone and could theoretically precipitate renal colic (or "ureteral reflux"), particularly in patients with nephrolithiasis.

Psychiatric disorder: Cholinergic agonists may have dose-related CNS effects. Consider this when treating patients with underlying cognitive or psychiatric disturbances.

Drug Interactions:

Drugs that may interact with pilocarpine include beta blockers and anticholinergics.

Drug/Food interactions. The rate of absorption of pilocarpine is decreased when taken with a high fat meal. Maximum concentration is decreased and time to reach maximum concentration is increased.

Adverse Reactions:

The most frequent adverse experiences associated with pilocarpine were a consequence of the expected pharmacologic effects. Adverse reactions occurring in ≥ 3% of patients include sweating, nausea, rhinitis, chills, flushing, urinary frequency, dizziness, asthenia, headache, dyspepsia, lacrimation, diarrhea, edema, abdominal pain, amblyopia, vomiting, pharyngitis and hypertension.

Administration and Dosage:

The recommended dose for the initiation of treatment is 5 mg 3 times/day. Titration up to 10 mg 3 times/day may be considered for patients who have not responded adequately and who can tolerate lower doses. The incidence of the most common adverse events increases with dose. Use the lowest dose that is tolerated and effective for maintenance.

TRETINOIN (trans-Retinoic Acid; Vitamin A Acid)

Cream: 0.025%, 0.05%, 0.1% (*Rx*) **Gel:** 0.025%, 0.01% (*Rx*) **Liquid:** 0.05% (*Rx*)	*Retin-A* (Ortho)

Actions:

Pharmacology: Although the exact mode of action of tretinoin is unknown, current evidence suggests that topical tretinoin decreases cohesiveness of follicular epithelial cells with decreased microcomedone formation. Additionally, tretinoin stimulates mitotic activity and increased turnover of follicular epithelial cells, causing extrusion of the comedones.

Indications:

Topical treatment of acne vulgaris.

Unlabeled uses: Tretinoin has been used to treat several different forms of skin cancer, and various dermatologic conditions including lamellar ichthyosis, mollusca contagiosa, verrucae plantaris, verrucae planae juveniles, ichthyosis vulgaris, bullous congenital ichthyosiform and pityriasis rubra pilaris.

Tretinoin appears to enhance the percutaneous absorption of topical minoxidil.

Tretinoin 0.025% to 0.1% appears to significantly improve photoaged skin, especially wrinkling and liver spots. Long-term consequences are unknown.

Contraindications:

Hypersensitivity to any component of the product.

Warnings:

For external use only: Keep tretinoin away from the eyes, mouth, angles of the nose and mucous membranes.

Irritation: Tretinoin may induce severe local erythema and peeling at the application site. If the degree of local irritation warrants, use medication less frequently, discontinue use temporarily or completely. Tretinoin may cause severe irritation to eczematous skin; use with caution in patients with this condition.

Pregnancy: Category C.

Lactation: It is not known whether this drug is excreted in breast milk.

Precautions:

Excessive application: Redness, peeling or discomfort may occur if medication is applied excessively, and results will not be improved.

Photosensitivity: It is advisable to "rest" a patient's skin until effects of keratolytic agents subside before beginning tretinoin. Minimize exposure to sunlight and sunlamps and advise patients with sunburn not to use tretinoin until fully recovered because of heightened susceptibility to sunlight as a result of use. Patients who undergo considerable sun exposure due to occupation and those with inherent sun sensitivity should exercise particular caution. Use sunscreen products and protective clothing over treated areas. Other weather extremes, such as wind and cold, also may be irritating.

Drug Interactions:

Drugs that may interact with tretinoin include sulfur, resorcinol, benzoyl peroxide and salicylic acid.

Adverse Reactions:

Adverse reactions may include excessively red, edematous, blistered or crusted skin; hyperpigmentation, hypopigmentation.

Administration and Dosage:

Apply once a day, before bedtime. Cover the entire affected area lightly. Thoroughly wash hands immediately after applying tretinoin.

Liquid: Apply with fingertip, gauze pad or cotton swab. Do not oversaturate gauze or cotton to the extent that liquid will run into unaffected areas.

Gel: Excessive application results in "pilling" of the gel, which minimizes the likelihood of overapplication by the patient.

Closely monitor alterations of vehicle, drug concentration or dose frequency. During the early weeks of therapy, an apparent exacerbation of inflammatory lesions may occur due to the action of the medication on deep, previously undetected lesions; this is not a reason to discontinue therapy.

Therapeutic results should be seen after 2 to 3 weeks, but may not be optimal until after 6 weeks. Once lesions have responded satisfactorily, maintain therapy with less frequent applications or other dosage forms.

Patients may use cosmetics, but thoroughly cleanse area to be treated before applying medication.

ISOTRETINOIN (13-cis-Retinoic Acid)

Capsules: 10, 20 and 40 mg (Rx) — *Accutane* (Roche)

Warning:

Women who are pregnant or who may become pregnant must not use isotretinoin. There is an extremely high risk that a deformed infant will result if pregnancy occurs while taking this drug in any amount even for short periods. Potentially all exposed fetuses can be affected.

Contraindicated in women of childbearing potential unless the patient meets all of the following conditions:

- has severe disfiguring cystic acne that is recalcitrant to standard therapies
- is reliable in understanding and carrying out instructions
- is capable of complying with the mandatory contraceptive measures
- has received both oral and written warnings of the hazards of taking isotretinoin during pregnancy and the risk of possible contraception failure and has acknowledged her understanding of these warnings in writing
- has had a negative *serum* pregnancy test within 2 weeks prior to beginning therapy. (It is also recommended that pregnancy testing and contraception counseling be repeated on a monthly basis.)
- will begin therapy only on the second or third day of the next normal menstrual period

Major human fetal abnormalities related to use of the drug have included hydrocephalus, microcephaly, external ear abnormalities (micropinna, small or absent external auditory canals), microphthalmia, facial dysmorphia, cleft palate, cardiovascular abnormalities, thymus gland abnormalities, parathyroid hormone deficiency and cerebellar malformation. There is also an increased risk of spontaneous abortion.

Effective contraception must be used for at least 1 month before beginning therapy, during therapy and for 1 month following discontinuation of therapy. It is recommended that two reliable forms of contraception be used simultaneously unless abstinence is the chosen method.

Actions:

Pharmacology: Isotretinoin is an isomer of retinoic acid, a metabolite of retinol (vitamin A). The exact mechanism of action is unknown. Clinical improvement in cystic acne patients is associated with reduction in sebum secretion. This temporary decrease is related to dose and treatment duration; it reflects a reduction in sebaceous gland size and inhibition of sebaceous gland differentiation. Isotretinoin and other retinoids may also prevent abnormal keratinization.

Sebum lipid production and composition is altered during isotretinoin therapy, but returns to pretreatment composition upon discontinuation, even though sebum production may not return to pretreatment levels.

Pharmacokinetics:

Absorption/Distribution – Oral bioavailability from oil-filled capsules is ≈ 23% to 25%. Plasma levels may be better maintained if the drug is taken with meals. After oral administration of 80 mg, peak plasma concentrations of 98 to 535 ng/ml (mean, 256 to 262 ng/ml) were measured at 2.9 to 3.2 hours. The minimum steady-state blood concentration of isotretinoin averaged 160 ± 19 ng/ml with 40 mg twice daily administration. The drug is 99.9% bound to plasma albumin. Maximum concentrations of 4-oxo-isotretinoin, the major metabolite, were 87 to 399 ng/ml, and were reached in 6 to 20 hours.

Metabolism/Excretion – The major metabolite in blood, 4-oxo-isotretinoin, generally exceeds the concentration of isotretinoin after 6 hours. Terminal elimination half-life of isotretinoin is 10 to 20 hours. Elimination half-life of 4-oxo-isotretinoin ranges from 17 to 50 hours (average, 25 hours).

Relatively equal amounts of radioactivity were recovered in the urine and feces with 65% to 83% of the dose recovered.

Indications:

Severe recalcitrant cystic acne: Adverse effects are significant; reserve treatment for patients unresponsive to conventional therapy, including systemic antibiotics. A single course has resulted in complete, prolonged remission in many patients. Patients may continue to improve while not receiving the drug.

Unlabeled uses: Isotretinoin has been used in the treatment of keratinization disorders such as keratosis follicularis (Darier-White disease), pityriasis rubra pilaris, lamellar ichthyosis, keratosis palmaris et plantaris congenital ichthyosiform erythroderma, rosacea, lichen planus, psoriasis and other ichthyotic conditions.

Success has been reported in the treatment of cutaneous T-cell lymphoma (mycosis fungoides) and leukoplakia.

High dose isotretinoin (2 mg/kg/day) has been used in the prevention of skin cancers in patients with xeroderma pigmentosum.

In patients who have been treated for squamous-cell carcinoma of the head and neck, high-dose isotretionoin (50 to 100 mg/m^2) appears to be effective in preventing second primary tumors.

Contraindications:

Pregnancy; hypersensitivity to parabens (used as preservatives in the formulation).

Warnings:

Pseudotumor cerebri (benign intracranial hypertension) has occurred with isotretinoin. Early signs and symptoms include papilledema, headache, nausea, vomiting and visual disturbances. Screen patients with these symptoms for papilledema; if present, discontinue drug immediately and consult a neurologist. **Minocycline** and **tetracycline** have been associated with pseudotumor cerebri or papilledema in isotretinoin patients.

Corneal opacities have appeared in patients receiving isotretinoin for acne and more frequently in patients on higher dosages for keratinization disorders. If visual difficulties occur, discontinue the drug and perform an ophthalmological examination. Corneal opacities have either completely resolved or were resolving at follow-up 6 to 7 weeks after discontinuation.

Decreased night vision has occurred during therapy. Because the onset in some patients was sudden, advise patients of this potential problem and warn them to be cautious when driving or operating any vehicle at night.

Inflammatory bowel disease (including regional ileitis) has been temporally associated with isotretinoin in patients with no history of intestinal disorders. Discontinue treatment immediately if abdominal pain, rectal bleeding or severe diarrhea occurs.

Hypertriglyceridemia occurs in ≈ 25% of patients; 15% develop a *decrease* in high density lipoproteins (HDL) and ≈ 7% show an increase in cholesterol. Obtain baseline values, then perform tests weekly or biweekly until lipid response is established (usually 4 weeks).

These effects are reversible generally within 8 weeks after cessation of therapy. Patients with increased tendency to develop hypertriglyceridemia include those with diabetes mellitus, obesity, increased alcohol intake and a familial history.

Musculoskeletal symptoms (including arthralgia) develop in ≈ 16% of patients. In general, these are mild to moderate and occasionally require discontinuation. They generally clear rapidly after discontinuing isotretinoin, and rarely persist.

In clinical trials of keratinization, a high prevalence of skeletal hyperostosis was noted with a mean dose of 2.24 mg/kg/day. Two children showed x–ray findings suggestive of premature closure of the epiphyses.

Minimal skeletal hyperostosis has been observed by x–ray in prospective studies of cystic acne patients treated with a single course of therapy at recommended doses.

Hepatotoxicity: Several cases of clinical hepatitis are possibly or probably related to isotretinoin therapy. Additionally, mild to moderate elevations of liver enzymes have been seen in ≈ 15% of patients, some of which normalized with dosage reduction or continued administration of the drug. If normalization does not readily occur, or if hepatitis is suspected, stop the drug and further investigate etiology.

Pregnancy: Category X.

Lactation: It is not known whether this drug is excreted in breast milk. Because of the potential for adverse effects, do not give to a nursing mother.

Children: One study showed X-ray findings suggestive of premature closure of the epiphyses in two children; another study suggested potential benefits in children 2 to 76 months of age with juvenile chronic myelogenous leukemia.

Precautions:

Healing response: As may be seen with healing cystic acne lesions, an occasional exaggerated healing response, manifested by exuberant granulation with crusting, has occurred.

Bleeding: Isotretinoin may increase fibrinolysis in patients with pre-existing bleeding disorders; tissue plasminogen activator productionmay also be stimulated.

Exacerbation of acne (transient) has occurred, generally during initial therapy period.

Contact lens tolerance may decrease.

Diabetes: Certain patients have experienced problems in the control of their blood sugar.

Blood donation: Due to isotretinoin's teratogenic potential, patients receiving the drug should not donate blood for transfusion for 30 days after discontinuing therapy.

Photosensitivity: Photosensitization (photoallergy or phototoxicity) may occur; caution patients to take protective measures (ie, sunscreens, protective clothing) against exposure to ultraviolet light or sunlight until tolerance is determined.

Drug Interactions:

Drugs that may interact with isotretinoin include vitamin A, tetracycline, minocycline and carbamazepine.

Drug/Food interactions: When taken with food or milk, the absorption of isotretinoin is increased.

Adverse Reactions:

Most adverse reactions are reversible upon discontinuation; however, some have persisted after cessation of therapy. Many are similar to those described in patients taking high doses of vitamin A.

Dermatologic: Cheilitis, usually dose-related (> 90%); dry skin, pruritus; skin fragility (up to 80%); facial skin desquamation, drying of mucous membranes (30%); petechiae (25%); nail brittleness (10%); rash (including erythema, seborrhea and eczema), thinning of hair which has rarely persisted (< 10%); peeling of palms and soles, skin infections, photosensitivity (5%).

GI: Dry mouth (up to 80%); nausea, vomiting, abdominal pain (20%); nonspecific GI symptoms (5%); anorexia (4%).

Ophthalmic: Conjunctivitis (40%).

CNS: Fatigue, headache (5%).

GU: White cells in urine (10% to 20%); proteinuria, microscopic or gross hematuria (< 10%); nonspecific urogenital findings (5%).

Musculoskeletal: Mild to moderate musculoskeletal symptoms which occasionally required drug discontinuation and rarely persisted after discontinuation (16%); skeletal hyperostosis; arthralgia, bone, joint and muscle pain and stiffness (16% to 17%).

Miscellaneous: Epistaxis, dry nose (up to 80%).

Lab test abnormalities: Elevated sedimentation rate (40%); reversible dose-related triglyceride elevation (25%; approximately 4% to 11% showed triglyceride elevation > 500 mg/dl); reversible mild to moderate decrease in HDL (16%); changes in serum lipids; decreased red blood cell parameters and white blood cell counts, elevated platelet counts, increased alkaline phosphatase, AST, ALT, GGTP and LDH (10% to 20%); reversible minimal elevation of cholesterol (7%); increased fasting blood sugar, hyperuricemia, thrombocytopenia, elevated CPK levels in patients who undergo vigorous physical activity (< 10%).

Administration and Dosage:

Individualize dosage. Adjust the dose according to side effects and disease response.

Recommended course of therapy: Initial dose is 0.5 to 1 mg/kg/day (range, 0.5 to 2 mg/kg/day) divided into 2 doses, for 15 to 20 weeks. Patients whose disease is very severe or is primarily manifest on the body may require up to the maximum recommended dose, 2 mg/kg/day. If the total cyst count decreases by > 70% prior to this time, the drug may be discontinued. After ≥ 2 months off therapy, and if warranted by persistent or recurring severe cystic acne, a second course of therapy may be initiated.

Doses as low as 0.05 mg/kg/day have been effective with minimal toxicity; however, relapses were more frequent.

CORTICOSTEROIDS, TOPICAL

Product	Trade Name (Manufacturer)
ACLOMETASONE DIPROPIONATE	
Ointment: 0.05% (*Rx*)	*Aclovate* (Glaxo)
Cream: 0.05% (*Rx*)	
AMCINONIDE	
Ointment: 0.01% (*Rx*)	*Cyclocort* (Fujisawa)
Cream: 0.1% (*Rx*)	
Lotion: 0.1% (*Rx*)	
AUGMENTED BETAMETHASONE DIPROPIONATE	
Cream: 0.05% (*Rx*)	*Diprolene* AF (Schering)
Ointment: 0.05% (*Rx*)	*Diprolene* (Schering)
Gel: 0.05% (*Rx*)	
Lotion: 0.05% (*Rx*)	
BETAMETHASONE BENZOATE	
Cream: 0.025% (*Rx*)	*Uticort* (Parke-Davis)
Lotion: 0.025% (*Rx*)	
Gel: 0.025% (*Rx*)	
BETAMETHASONE DIPROPIONATE	
Ointment: 0.05% (*Rx*)	Various, *Diprosone* (Schering), *Maxivate* (Westwood-Squibb)
Cream: 0.05% (*Rx*)	
Lotion: 0.05% (*Rx*)	
Aerosol: 0.1% (*Rx*)	
BETAMETHASONE VALERATE	
Ointment: 0.1% (*Rx*)	Various, *Betatrex* (Savage), *Valisone* (Schering)
Cream: 0.01%, 0.05%, 0.1% (*Rx*)	Various, *Valisone* (Schering)
Lotion: 0.1% (*Rx*)	Various, *Valisone* (Schering), *Betatrex* (Savage)
Powder for compounding (*Rx*)	*Betamethasone Valerate* (Paddock)
CLOBETASOL PROPIONATE	
Ointment: 0.05% (*Rx*)	Various, *Temovate* (Glaxo Wellcome)
Cream: 0.05% (*Rx*)	
Scalp application: 0.05% (*Rx*)	*Temovate* (Glaxo Wellcome)
Gel: 0.05% (*Rx*)	
CLOCORTOLONE PIVALATE	
Cream: 0.1% (*Rx*)	*Cloderm* (Hermal)
DESONIDE	
Ointment: 0.05% (*Rx*)	Various, *DesOwen* (Owen/Galderma), *Tridesilon* (Miles Inc)
Cream: 0.05% and 0.25% (*Rx*)	*DesOwen* (Owen/Galderma), *Tridesilon* (Miles Inc)
Lotion: 0.05% (*Rx*)	*DesOwen* (Owen/Galderma)
DESOXIMETASONE	
Ointment: 0.25% (*Rx*)	*Topicort* (Hoechst-Roussel)
Cream: 0.05% and 0.25% (*Rx*)	Various, *Topicort* (Hoechst-Roussel)
Gel: 0.05% (*Rx*)	*Topicort* (Hoechst-Roussel)
DEXAMETHASONE SODIUM PHOSPHATE	
Aerosol: 0.01% and 0.04% (*Rx*)	*Aeroseb-Dex* (Herbert)
DIFLORASONE DIACETATE	
Ointment: 0.05% (*Rx*)	*Florone* (Dermik), *Maxiflor* (Herbert), *Psorcon* (Dermik)
Cream: 0.05% (*Rx*)	
FLUOCINOLONE ACETONIDE	
Ointment: 0.025% (*Rx*)	Various, *Flurosyn* (Rugby), *Synalar* (Syntex)
Cream: 0.01%, 0.025%, 0.2% (*Rx*)	
Solution: 0.01% (*Rx*)	Various, *Synalar* (Syntex)
Shampoo: 0.01% (*Rx*)	*FS Shampoo* (Hill)
Oil: 0.01%(*Rx*)	*Derma-Smoothe/FS* (Hill)

FLUOCINONIDE	
Cream: 0.05% (*Rx*)	Various, *Fluonex* (ICN), *Lidex* (Syntex)
Ointment: 0.05% (*Rx*)	Various, *Lidex* (Syntex)
Solution: 0.05% (*Rx*)	
Gel: 0.05% (*Rx*)	
FLURANDRENOLIDE	
Ointment: 0.025% and 0.05% (*Rx*)	*Cordran* (Oclassen)
Cream: 0.025% and 0.05% (*Rx*)	*Cordran SP* (Oclassen)
Lotion: 0.05% (*Rx*)	Various, *Cordran* (Oclassen)
Tape: 4 mcg per square cm (*Rx*)	*Cordran* (Oclassen)
FLUTICASONE PROPIONATE	
Cream: 0.05% (*Rx*)	*Cutivate* (Glaxo Dermatology)
Ointment: 0.005% (*Rx*)	
HALCINONIDE	
Ointment: 0.1% (*Rx*)	*Halog* (Princeton)
Cream: 0.025% and 0.1% (*Rx*)	*Halog* (Princeton), *Halog-E* (Princeton)
Solution: 0.1% (*Rx*)	*Halog* (Princeton)
HALOBETASOL PROPIONATE	
Ointment: 0.05% (*Rx*)	*Ultravate* (Westwood-Squibb)
Cream: 0.05% (*Rx*)	
HYDROCORTISONE	
Ointment: 0.5%, 1%, 2.5% (*Rx and otc*)	Various, *Cortizone•5* (Thompson), *Cortizone•10* (Thompson), *Hytone* (Dermik)
Cream: 0.5%, 1%, 2.5% (*Rx and otc*)	Various, *Dermolate* (Schering-Plough), *Dermacort* (Solvay), *Procort* (Roberts)
Lotion: 0.25%, 0.5%, 1%, 2%, 2.5% (*Rx*)	Various, *Cetacort* (Owen/Galderma), *Ala-Scalp* (Del-Ray)
Liquid: 1% (*otc*)	*Scalpicin* (Combe), *T/Scalp* (Neutrogena)
Gel: 0.5% and 1% (*otc*)	*Extra Strength CortaGel* (Norstar)
Solution: 1% (*Rx*)	*Penecort* (Herbert), *Texacort* (GenDerm)
Aerosol/Pump Spray: 0.5% (*Rx and otc*)	*Aeroseb-HC* (Herbert), *Cortaid* (Upjohn)
Pump Spray: 1% (*otc*)	*Maximum Strength Cortaid* (Upjohn)
Stick, roll-on: 1% (*otc*)	*Maximum Strength Cortaid Faststick* (Upjohn)
HYDROCORTISONE ACETATE	
Ointment: 0.5% and 1% (*otc*)	*Lanacort-5* (Combe), *Maximum Strength Lanacort 10* (Combe), *Anusol HC-1* (Parke-Davis)
Cream: 0.5% and 1% (*Rx*)	*Cortaid with Aloe* (Upjohn), *U-Cort* (Thames)
HYDROCORTISONE BUTYRATE	
Solution: (*Rx*)	*Locoid* (Ferndale)
HYDROCORTISONE VALERATE	
Ointment: 0.2% (*Rx*)	*Westcort* (Westwood-Squibb)
Cream: 0.2% (*Rx*)	
MOMETASONE FUROATE	
Ointment: 0.1% (*Rx*)	*Elocon* (Schering)
Cream: 0.1%(*Rx*)	
Lotion: 0.1% (*Rx*)	
PREDNICARBATE	
Cream: 0.1% (*Rx*)	*Dermatop* (Hoechst-Roussel)
TRIAMCINOLONE ACETONIDE	
Ointment: 0.025%, 0.1%, 0.5% (*Rx*)	Various, *Kenalog* (Westwood-Squibb), *Aristocort* (Fujisawa)
Cream: 0.025%, 0.1%, 0.5% (*Rx*)	
Lotion: 0.025% and 0.1% (*Rx*)	Various, *Kenalog* (Westwood-Squibb)
Aerosol: (2 sec. spray) (*Rx*)	*Kenalog* (Westwood-Squibb)

Actions:

Pharmacology: The primary therapeutic effects of the topical corticosteroids are caused by their anti-inflammatory activity which is non-specific (eg, they act against most causes of inflammation including mechanical, chemical, microbiological and immunological).

Pharmacokinetics: The amount of corticosteroid absorbed from the skin depends on the intrinsic properties of the drug itself, the vehicle used, the duration of exposure and the surface area and condition of the skin to which it is applied. Occlusive dressings greatly enhance skin penetration and, therefore, increase drug absorption.

Vehicles – Ointments are more occlusive and are preferred for dry scaly lesions. Use creams on oozing lesions or in intertriginous areas where the occlusive effects of ointments may cause maceration and folliculitis.

Occlusive dressings – Occlusive dressings such as a plastic wrap increase skin penetration by tenfold by increasing the moisture content of the stratum corneum.

Relative potency – The relative potency of a product depends on several factors including the characteristics and concentration of the drug and the vehicle used.

Relative Potency of Selected Topical Corticosteroid Products

	Drug	Dosage Form	Strength
I.	***Very high potency***		
	Augmented betamethasone dipropionate	Ointment	0.05%
	Clobetasol propionate	Cream, Ointment	0.05%
	Diflorasone diacetate	Ointment	0.05%
	Halobetasol propionate	Cream, Ointment	0.05%
II.	***High potency***		
	Amcinonide	Cream, Lotion, Ointment	0.1%
	Augmented betamethasone dipropionate	Cream	0.05%
	Betamethasone dipropionate	Cream, Ointment	0.05%
	Betamethasone valerate	Ointment	0.1%
	Desoximetasone	Cream, Ointment	0.25%
		Gel	0.05%
	Diflorasone diacetate	Cream, Ointment (emollient base)	0.05%
	Fluocinolone acetonide	Cream	0.2%
	Fluocinonide	Cream, Ointment, Gel	0.05%
	Halcinonide	Cream, Ointment	0.1%
	Triamcinolone acetonide	Ointment	0.1%
III.	***Medium potency***		
	Betamethasone benzoate	Cream, Gel, Lotion	0.025%
	Betamethasone dipropionate	Lotion	0.05%
	Betamethasone valerate	Cream	0.1%
	Clocortolone pivalate	Cream	0.1%
	Desoximetasone	Cream	0.05%
	Fluocinolone acetonide	Cream, Ointment	0.025%
	Flurandrenolide	Cream, Ointment	0.025%
		Cream, Ointment, Lotion	0.05%
		Tape	4 mcg/cm^2
	Fluticasone propionate	Cream	0.05%
		Ointment	0.005%
	Hydrocortisone butyrate	Ointment, Solution	0.1%
	Hydrocortisone valerate	Cream, Ointment	0.2%
	Mometasone furoate	Cream, Ointment, Lotion	0.1%
	Triamcinolone acetonide	Cream, Ointment, Lotion	0.025%
		Cream, Ointment, Lotion	0.1%
		Cream, Ointment	0.5%
IV.	***Low potency***		
	Aclometasone dipropionate	Cream, Ointment	0.05%
	Desonide	Cream	0.05%
	Dexamethasone	Aerosol	0.01%
		Aerosol	0.04%
	Dexamethasone sodium phosphate	Cream	0.1%
	Fluocinolone acetonide	Cream, Solution	0.01%
	Hydrocortisone	Lotion	0.25%
		Cream, Ointment, Lotion, Aerosol	0.5%
		Cream, Ointment, Lotion, Solution	1%
		Cream, Ointment, Lotion	2.5%
	Hydrocortisone acetate	Cream, Ointment	0.5%
		Cream, Ointment	1%

Indications:

Pruritus:

Relief of inflammatory and pruritic manifestations of corticosteroid-responsive dermatoses.

Contact dermatitis, atopic dermatitis, nummular eczema, stasis eczema, asteatotic eczema, lichen planus, lichen simplex chronicus, insect and arthropod bite reactions, first- and second-degree localized burns and sunburns.

Alternative/Adjunctive treatment: Psoriasis, seborrheic dermatitis, severe diaper rash, disidrosis, nodular prurigo, chronic discoid lupus erythematosus, alopecia areata, lymphocytic infiltration of the skin, mycosis fungoides and familial benign pemphigus of Hailey-Hailey.

Possibly effective in the following conditions: Bullous pemphigoid, cutaneous mastocytosis, lichen sclerosus et atrophicus and vitiligo.

Nonprescription hydrocortisone preparations: Temporary relief of itching associated with minor skin irritations, inflammation and rashes due to eczema, insect bites, poison ivy, poison oak, poison sumac, soaps, detergents, cosmetics, jewelry, seborrheic dermatitis, psoriasis and external genital and anal itching.

Contraindications:

Hypersensitivity to any component; monotherapy in primary bacterial infections such as impetigo, paryonchia, erysipelas, cellulitis, angular cheilitis, erythrasma (clobetasol), treatment of rosacea, perioral dermatitis or acne; use on the face, groin or axilla (very high or high potency agents); ophthalmic use.

Warnings:

Pregnancy: Category C.

Lactation: It is not known whether topical corticosteroids could result in sufficient systemic absorption to produce detectable quantities in breast milk.

Children: Children may be more susceptible to topical corticosteroid-induced hypothalamic-pituitary-adrenal (HPA) axis suppression and Cushing's syndrome than adults because of a larger skin surface area to body weight ratio.

Precautions:

Systemic effects: Systemic absorption of topical corticosteroids has produced reversible HPA axis suppression, Cushing's syndrome, hyperglycemia and glycosuria.

As a general rule, little effect on the HPA axis will occur with use of a potent topical corticosteroid in amounts of < 50 g weekly for an adult and 15 g weekly for a small child, without occlusion. To cover the adult body one time requires 12 to 26 g.

Local irritation: If local irritation develops, discontinue use and institute appropriate therapy.

Skin atrophy is common and may be clinically significant in 3 to 4 weeks with potent preparations. Atrophy occurs most readily at sites where percutaneous absorption is high.

Psoriasis: Do not use topical corticosteroids as sole therapy in widespread plaque psoriasis.

Atrophic changes: Certain areas of the body, such as the face, groin and axillae, are more prone to atrophic changes than other areas of the body following treatment with corticosteroids.

Infections: Treating skin infections with topical corticosteroids can extensively worsen the infection.

For external use only: Avoid inhalation of aerosols, ingestion or contact with eyes.

Occlusive therapy: Discontinue the use of occlusive dressings if infection develops, and institute appropriate antimicrobial therapy.

Do not use occlusive dressings in augmented betamethasone dipropionate, betamethasone dipropionate, clobetasol, halobetasol propionate and **mometasone** treatment regimens.

Adverse Reactions:

Local: Burning; itching; irritation; erythema; dryness; folliculitis; hypertrichosis; pruritus; acneiform eruptions; hypopigmentation; perioral dermatitis; allergic contact dermatitis; numbness of fingers; stinging and cracking/tightening of skin; maceration of the skin; secondary infection; skin atrophy; striae; miliaria; telangiectasia. These may occur more frequently with occlusive dressings.

Administration and Dosage:

Usual dose: Apply sparingly to affected areas 2 to 4 times daily.

TRETINOIN

Cream: 0.05% (*Rx*)	*Renova* (Ortho)

Actions:

Pharmacology: The exact mechanism of action is unknown, although retinoids are believed to exert an effect on the growth and differentiation of various epithelial cells. When applied topically, however, there is no noted increase in desmosine, hydroxyproline or elastin mRNA in human skin. In addition, the role of the irritative nature of this product in bringing about its positive effects is not fully determined.

Pharmacokinetics: The transdermal absorption of tretinoin from various topical formulations ranged from 1% to 31% of applied dose, depending on whether it was applied to healthy skin or dermatatic skin.

Indications:

Dermatologic conditions: Adjunctive agent for use in the mitigation (palliation) of fine wrinkles, mottled hyperpigmentation and tactile roughness of facial skin in patients who do not achieve such palliation using comprehensive skin care and sun avoidance programs alone.

Topical tretinoin is also used as a treatment for acne vulgaris.

Contraindications:

Sensitivity reactions to any of the drug's components; discontinue if hypersensitivity to any ingredient is noted.

Warnings:

Mitigating effects: Tretinoin has shown no mitigating effects on significant signs of chronic sun exposure. Tretinoin does not eliminate wrinkles, repair sun damaged skin, reverse photoaging or restore a more youthful or younger dermal histologic pattern.

Many patients achieve a desired palliative effect on fine wrinkling, mottled hyperpigmentation and tactile roughness of facial skin with the use of comprehensive skin care and sun avoidance programs including sunscreens, protective clothing and emollient creams containing tretinoin.

Long-term use: There is evidence of atypical changes in melanocytes and keratinocytes and of increased dermal elastosis in some patients treated for > 48 weeks.

Photosensitivity: Because of heightened burning susceptibility, avoid or minimize exposure to sunlight (including sunlamps) during use of tretinoin. Warn patients to use sunscreens (minimum SPF of 15) and protective clothing when using tretinoin. Advise patients with sunburn not to use tretinoin until fully recovered. Patients who may have considerable sun exposure due to their occupations and those with inherent sensitivity to sunlight should exercise particular caution when using tretinoin.

Local reactions: Topical use may cause severe erythema, pruritus, burning, stinging and peeling at the site of application. In most patients, the dryness, peeling and redness recurred after the initial (24 weeks) decline. If the degree of local irritation warrants, direct patients to use less medication, decrease the frequency of application, discontinue use temporarily or discontinue use altogether.

Eczematous skin: Tretinoin has been reported to cause severe irritation on eczematous skin; use with utmost caution in patients with this condition.

Pregnancy: Category C.

Lactation: It is not known whether this drug is excreted in breast milk.

Children: Safety and efficacy in patients < 18 years of age have not been established.

Drug Interactions:

Topical preparations: Use caution with concomitant topical medications, medicated or abrasive soaps, shampoos, cleansers, cosmetics with a strong drying effect, products with high concentrations of alcohol, astringents, spices or lime, permanent wave solutions, electrolysis, hair depilatories or waxes, and products that may irritate the skin in patients being treated with tretinoin because they may increase irritation.

Photosensitizers: Do not use tretinoin if the patient is also taking drugs known to be photosensitizers (eg, thiazides, tetracyclines, fluoroquinolones, phenothiazines, sulfonamides) because of the possibility of augmented phototoxicity.

Adverse Reactions:

Adverse reactions include peeling; dry skin; burning; stinging; erythema; pruritus.

Administration and Dosage:

Apply tretinoin to the face once a day at bedtime, using only enough to cover the entire affected area lightly. Gently wash face with a mild soap, pat the skin dry, and wait 20 to 30 minutes before applying. Apply a pea-sized amount of cream to cover the entire face. Take caution to avoid contact with eyes, ears, nostrils and mouth.

Mitigation (palliation) of fine facial wrinkling, mottled hyperpigmentation and tactile roughness may occur gradually over the course of therapy. Up to 6 months of therapy may be required before the effects are seen. Most of the improvement noted with tretinoin is seen during the first 24 weeks of therapy. Thereafter, therapy primarily maintains the improvement noticed during the first 24 weeks.

CAPSAICIN

Cream: 0.025% and 0.075% in an emollient base (*otc*)	*Zostrix* (GenDerm), *Zostrix-HP* (GenDerm)
Cream: 0.025% (*otc*)	*Capzasin•P* (Thompson Medical)
Gel: 0.025% (*otc*)	*R-Gel* (Healthline Labs)
Lotion: 0.025% and 0.075% (*otc*)	*Capsin* (Fleming)
Roll-on: 0.075% (*otc*)	*No pain-HP* (Young Again Products)

Actions:

Pharmacology: Capsaicin is a natural chemical derived from plants of the solanaceae family. Although the precise mechanism of action is not fully understood, evidence suggests that the drug renders skin and joints insensitive to pain by depleting and preventing reaccumulation of substance P in peripheral sensory neurons. Substance P is thought to be the principle chemomediator of pain impulses from the periphery to the central nervous system.

Indications:

Temporary relief of pain from rheumatoid arthritis, osteoarthritis and relief of neuralgias such as the pain following shingles (herpes zoster) or painful diabetic neuropathy.

Unlabeled uses: Capsaicin is being investigated for use in other disorders including psoriasis, vitiligo and intractable pruritus, as well as postmastectomy and postamputation neuroma (phantom limb syndrome), vulvar vestibulitis, apocrine chromhidrosis and reflex sympathetic dystrophy.

Warnings:

For external use only. Avoid getting in eyes or on broken or irritated skin. Use care when handling contact lenses following application of capsaicin; irritation and burning may occur following lens insertion. Washing hands or using gloves or an applicator may alleviate this problem.

Bandage use: Do not bandage tightly.

Worsened condition: If condition worsens or if symptoms persist 14 to 28 days, discontinue use and consult physician.

Adverse Reactions:

Adverse reactions include burning; stinging; erythema; cough; respiratory irritation.

Administration and Dosage:

Adults and children ≥ 2 years of age: Apply to affected area not more than 3 or 4 times daily. May cause transient burning on application. This is observed more frequently when application schedules of < 3 or 4 times daily are used. If applied with the fingers, wash hands immediately after application.

PENCICLOVIR

Cream: 10 mg/kg (*Rx*)	*Denavir* (SmithKline Beecham)

Actions:

Pharmacology: Penciclovir is an antiviral agent active against herpes viruses. It has in vitro inhibitory activity against herpes simplex virus types 1 (HSV-1) and 2 (HSV-2).

Pharmacokinetics: Measurable penciclovir concentrations were not detected in plasma or urine of healthy male volunteers following single or repeat application of the 1% cream at a dose of 180 mg penciclovir daily (≈ 67 times the estimated usual clinical dose).

Indications:

Herpes labialis: For the treatment of recurrent herpes labialis (cold sores) in adults.

Contraindications:

Hypersensitivity to the product or any of its components.

Warnings:

Elderly: In patients ≥ 65 years of age, the adverse event profile was comparable with that observed in younger patients.

Pregnancy: Category B.

Lactation: There is no information on whether penciclovir is excreted in breast milk after topical administration.

Children: Safety and efficacy in pediatric patients have not been established.

Precautions:

Mucous membranes: Use penciclovir on herpes labialis on the lips and face only. Because no data are available, application to human mucous membranes is not recommended. Take particular care to avoid application in or near the eyes because it may cause irritation.

Immunocompromised patients: Penciclovir's effect in immunocompromised patients has not been established.

Adverse Reactions:

Adverse reactions occurring in ≥ 3% of patients included headache.

Administration and Dosage:

Apply penciclovir every 2 hours while awake for 4 days. Start treatment as early as possible (eg, during the prodrome or when lesions appear).

Chapter 11

ANTINEOPLASTICS

TAMOXIFEN CITRATE

Tablets: 10 and 20 mg (as citrate) (*Rx*)	Various, *Nolvadex* (Zeneca)

Actions:

Pharmacology: Tamoxifen is a nonsteroidal agent with potent antiestrogenic properties.

Pharmacokinetics: Tamoxifen is extensively metabolized after oral administration. Approximately 65% of an administered dose was excreted from the body over a period of 2 weeks with fecal excretion as the primary route of elimination.

After initiation of therapy, steady-state concentrations for tamoxifen are achieved in ≈4 weeks and steady-state concentrations for N-desmethyl tamoxifen are achieved in ≈ 8 weeks, suggesting a half-life of ≈14 days for this metabolite.

Indications:

Breast cancer:

Adjuvant therapy – For treatment of axillary node-negative breast cancer in women following total mastectomy or segmental mastectomy, axillary dissection and breast irradiation.

For treatment of node-positive breast cancer in postmenopausal women following total mastectomy or segmental mastectomy, axillary dissection, and breast irradiation.

Advanced disease therapy – Effective in the treatment of metastatic breast cancer in women and men. In premenopausal women with metastatic breast cancer, tamoxifen is an alternative to oophorectomy or ovarian irradiation. Estrogen receptor positive tumors are most likely to benefit.

Unlabeled uses: Tamoxifen has been used in the treatment of mastalgia and for decreasing the size and pain of gynecomastia. Studies are currently being considered for use of tamoxifen as chemosuppressive (preventive) therapy in women at high risk for primary breast cancer. Tamoxifen may also be useful in pancreatic and advanced/recurrent endometrial and heptocellular carcinoma.

Contraindications:

Hypersensitivity to the drug.

Warnings:

Visual disturbances, including corneal changes, cataracts and retinopathy, have occurred with tamoxifen use.

Hypercalcemia has occurred in some breast cancer patients with bone metastases within a few weeks of starting therapy with tamoxifen.

Hepatic effects: Tamoxifen has been associated with changes in liver enzyme levels and, on rare occasions, fatty liver, cholestasis, hepatitis and hepatic necrosis.

Pregnancy: Category D.

Lactation: It is not known whether this drug is excreted in breast milk.

Precautions:

Monitoring: Perform periodic complete blood counts, including platelet counts, and liver function tests.

Leukopenia/Thrombocytopenia: Use cautiously in patients with existing leukopenia or thrombocytopenia.

Hyperlipidemias have occurred infrequently.

Drug Interactions:

Drugs that may interact with tamoxifen include bromocriptine and anticoagulants.

Drug/Lab test interactions: T_4 elevations occurred in a few postmenopausal patients but were not accompanied by clinical hyperthyroidism. Variations in the karyopyknotic index on vaginal smears and various degrees of estrogen effect on Pap smears have been infrequently seen in postmenopausal patients.

Adverse Reactions:

Adverse reactions occuring in ≥ 3% of patients after 50year therapy include: Hot flashes, weight gain, fluid retention, vaginal discharge, nausea, irregular menses, weight loss, skin changes, increased BUN, diarrhea, increased AST and increased alkaline phosphatase.

Adverse reactions occurring in ≥ 3% of patients taking tamoxifen vs ovarian ablation include: Flushing, amenorrhea, altered menses, oligomenorrhea, bone pain, menstrual disorder, nausea, coughing, edema and fatigue.

Administration and Dosage:

10 or 20 mg twice daily (morning and evening).

Some studies have used dosages of 10 mg 2 or 3 times a day for 2 years, and 10 mg twice daily for 5 years. There was no indication that doses > 20 mg/day were more effective.

BLEOMYCIN SULFATE (BLM)

Powder for Injection: 15 units *(Rx)* — *Blenoxane* (Bristol-Myers Oncology)

Warning:

Pulmonary fibrosis is the most severe toxicity. It is most frequently seen as pneumonitis, which occasionally progresses to pulmonary fibrosis. Incidence is higher in elderly patients and in those receiving > 400 units total dose, but pulmonary toxicity has occurred in young patients and those treated with low doses.

A severe idiosyncratic reaction consisting of hypotension, mental confusion, fever, chills and wheezing has occurred in ≈ 1% of lymphoma patients.

Actions:

Pharmacology: Bleomycin sulfate is a mixture of cytotoxic glycopeptide antibiotics. The exact mechanism of action is unknown; however, the main mode of action appears to be inhibition of deoxyribonucleic acid (DNA) synthesis with lesser inhibition of ribonucleic acid (RNA) and protein synthesis. Bleomycin is cell cycle phase specific, with major effects in G_2 and M phases.

Pharmacokinetics:

Absorption/Distribution – Following IV administration, bleomycin has a rapid initial distribution half-life of 10 to 20 minutes. IM injection produces peak blood levels in 30 to 60 minutes that are ≈ ⅓ of those produced IV. Following intrapleural administration, bleomycin has a systemic absorption of ≈ 45%.

Metabolism/Excretion – 60% to 70% of an administered dose is recovered in the urine as active bleomycin. Only 20% to 40% of this amount is active drug. In patients with a creatinine clearance of > 35 ml/min, the plasma terminal elimination half-life is approximately 2 hours. At creatinine clearances of < 35 ml/min, the plasma terminal elimination half-life increases exponentially as the creatinine clearance decreases. Patients with moderately severe renal failure excreted < 20% of the dose in the urine.

Indications:

Palliative treatment in the following neoplasms as either a single agent or in combination with other chemotherapeutic agents:

Squamous cell carcinoma: Head and neck including mouth, tongue, tonsil, nasopharynx, oropharynx, sinus, palate, lip, buccal mucosa, gingiva, epiglottis, skin and larynx. Response is poorer in patients with head and neck cancer previously irradiated. Bleomycin is also indicated in carcinoma of the skin, penis, cervix and vulva.

Lymphomas: Hodgkin's, reticulum cell sarcoma and lymphosarcoma.

Testicular carcinoma: Embryonal cell, choriocarcinoma and teratocarcinoma.

Malignant pleural effusion: Effective as a sclerosing agent for malignant pleural effusion treatment and prevention of recurrent pleural effusion.

Contraindications:

Hypersensitivity or idiosyncrasy to bleomycin sulfate.

Warnings:

Renal or hepatic toxicity, beginning as a deterioration in renal or liver function tests, has occurred infrequently. These toxicities may occur at any time.

Pulmonary toxicities, the most serious side effect, occur in 10% of treated patients. In ≈ 1%, the drug-induced nonspecific pneumonitis progresses to pulmonary fibrosis and death. Although this is age- and dose-related, it is unpredictable. It is more common in patients > 70 years of age and in those receiving > 400 units total dose. When bleomycin is used in combination with other antineoplastic agents, pulmonary toxicities may occur at lower doses. Concomitant use of radiation therapy may also increase the incidence of pulmonary toxicity.

Identifying pulmonary toxicity is extremely difficult due to lack of specificity of the clinical syndrome. The earliest symptom is dyspnea; the earliest sign is fine rales.

Take chest X-rays every 1 to 2 weeks to monitor the onset of pulmonary toxicity. If changes are noted, discontinue treatment until it is determined if they are drug-related. Monitor the DL_{co} monthly; discontinue the drug when the DL_{co} falls below 30% to 35% of the pretreatment value. Maintain FIO_2 at concentrations approximating that of room air (25%) during surgery and the postoperative period and to carefully monitor fluid replacement, focusing more on colloid administration rather than crystalloid.

Renal function impairment: Bleomycin clearance may be reduced in patients with impaired renal function. Use with caution in patients with significant renal impairment.

Pregnancy: *Category D.*

Lactation: It is not known whether the drug is excreted in breast milk.

Children: Safety and efficacy have not been established.

Drug Interactions:

Drugs that may interact with bleomycin include digoxin (not capsules), granulocyte colony stimulating factors and phenytoin.

Adverse Reactions:

Adverse reactions may include erythema; rash; striae; vesiculation; hyperpigmentation; skin tenderness; hyperkeratosis; nail changes; alopecia; pruritus; stomatitis; skin toxicity; fever; chills; vomiting; anorexia; weight loss.

Administration and Dosage:

May administer IM, IV or SC. Administer IV solution over 10 minutes.

Because of the possibility of anaphylactoid reaction, treat lymphoma patients with ≤ 2 units for the first 2 doses. If no acute reaction occurs, follow the regular dosage schedule. The following schedule is recommended:

Squamous cell carcinoma, lymphosarcoma, non-Hodgkin's lymphoma, reticulum cell sarcoma, testicular carcinoma: 0.25 to 0.5 units/kg (10 to 20 units/m^2) IV, IM or SC once or twice/ week.

Hodgkin's disease: 0.25 to 0.5 units/kg (10 to 20 units/m^2) IV, IM or SC once or twice weekly. After a 50% response, administer a maintenance dose of 1 unit daily or 5 units weekly IV or IM. Improvement of Hodgkin's disease and testicular tumors is prompt (≤ 2 weeks). If no improvement is seen by this time, it is unlikely to occur. Squamous cell cancers respond more slowly, sometimes requiring 3 weeks before improvement is noted.

Malignant pleural effusion: 60 units administered as a single dose bolus intrapleural injection.

IV solution: Administer over 10 minutes.

PENTOSTATIN (2′-deoxycoformycin; DCF)

Powder for Injection: 10 mg/vial *(Rx)* — *Nipent* (Parke-Davis)

Warning:

The use of higher doses than those specified is not recommended. Dose-limiting severe renal, liver, pulmonary and CNS toxicities occurred in Phase I studies that used pentostatin at higher doses than recommended (20 to 50 mg/m^2 in divided doses over 5 days).

In a clinical investigation in patients with refractory chronic lymphocytic leukemia using pentostatin at the recommended dose in combination with fludarabine phosphate, four of six patients had severe or fatal pulmonary toxicity. The use of pentostatin in combination with fludarabine phosphate is not recommended.

Actions:

Pharmacology: Pentostatin is a potent transition state inhibitor of the enzyme adenosine deaminase (ADA).Pentostatin inhibition of ADA, particularly in the presence of adenosine or deoxyadenosine, leads to cytotoxicity due to elevated intracellular levels of dATP which can block DNA synthesis through inhibition of ribonucleotide reductase. Pentostatin can also inhibit RNA synthesis as well as cause increased DNA damage. However, the precise mechanism of pentostatin's antitumor effect in hairy cell leukemia is not known.

Pharmacokinetics: Following a single dose of 4 mg/m^2 pentostatin infused over 5 minutes, the distribution half-life was 11 minutes, the mean terminal half-life was 5.7 hours, the mean plasma clearance was 68 ml/min/m^2, and ≈ 90% of the dose was excreted in the urine as unchanged pentostatin or metabolites. The plasma protein binding of pentostatin is low, ≈ 4%.

Pentostatin half-life in patients with renal impairment (Ccr < 50 ml/min) was 18 hours, which was much longer than that observed in patients with normal renal function (Ccr > 60 ml/min), which was ≈ 6 hours.

Indications:

Single agent for adult patients with alpha-interferon-refractory hairy cell leukemia, defined as progressive disease after a minimum of 3 months of alpha-interferon treatment or no response after a minimum of 6 months of alpha-interferon.

Contraindications:

Hypersensitivity to pentostatin.

Warnings:

Myelosuppression: Patients with hairy cell leukemia may experience myelosuppression, primarily during the first few courses of treatment. Treat patients with infection only when the potential benefit justifies the potential risk to the patient. Attempt to control the infection before treatment is initiated or resumed.

Renal toxicity was observed at higher doses in early studies; however, in patients treated at the recommended dose, elevations in serum creatinine were usually minor and reversible.

Rashes, occasionally severe, were commonly reported and may worsen with continued treatment. Withholding of treatment may be required.

Pregnancy: Category D.

Lactation: It is not known whether pentostatin is excreted in breast milk. Decide whether to discontinue nursing or discontinue the drug, taking into account the importance of the drug to the mother.

Children: Safety and efficacy in children or adolescents have not been established.

Precautions:

Monitoring: Therapy with pentostatin requires regular patient observation and monitoring of hematologic parameters and blood chemistry values. If severe adverse reactions occur, withhold the drug and take appropriate corrective measures.

Prior to initiating therapy, assess renal function. Perform complete blood counts and serum creatinine before each dose and at other appropriate periods during therapy. Severe neutropenia has been observed following the early courses of treatment. If hematologic parameters do not improve with subsequent courses, evaluate patients for disease status, including a bone marrow examination. Perform periodic monitoring of the peripheral blood for hairy cells to assess the response to treatment.

In addition, bone marrow aspirates and biopsies may be required at 2 to 3 month intervals to assess the response to treatment.

CNS toxicity: Withhold or discontinue therapy in those with evidence of CNS toxicity.

Drug Interactions:

Drugs that may interact with pentostatin include allopurinol, fludarabine and vidarabine.

Adverse Reactions:

Adverse reactions occurring in ≥ 3% of patients include: Leukopenia; anemia; thrombocytopenia; ecchymosis; lymphadenopathy; petechia; nausea/vomiting; anorexia; diarrhea; constipation; flatulence; stomatitis; rash; skin disorder; eczema; dry skin; herpes simplex/zoster; maculopapular rash; vesiculobullous rash; pruritus; seborrhea; skin discoloration; sweating; fever; infection; fatigue; pain; allergic reaction; chills; death; sepsis; chest pain; abdominal pain; back pain; flu syndrome; asthenia; malaise; neoplasm; weight loss; peripheral edema; increased LDH; hepatic disorder/elevated liver function tests; cough; upper respiratory infection; lung disorder; bronchitis; dyspnea; epistaxis; lung edema; pneumonia; pharyngitis; rhinitis; sinusitis; GU disorder; hematuria; dysuria; increased BUN; increased creatinine; headache; anxiety; confusion; depression; dizziness; insomnia; nervousness; paresthesia; somnolence; abnormal thinking; myalgia; arthralgia; arrhythmia; abnormal ECG; thrombophlebitis; hemorrhage; abnormal vision; conjunctivitis; ear pain; eye pain.

Lab test abnormalities: Liver function test elevations occurred during treatment and were generally reversible.

Administration and Dosage:

Hydrate with 500 to 1000 ml of 5% Dextrose in 0.5 NaCl or equivalent before pentostatin administration. Administer an additional 500 ml of 5% Dextrose or equivalent after pentostatin is given.

Alpha-interferon-refractory hairy cell leukemia: 4 mg/m^2 every other week. Pentostatin may be administered IV by bolus injection or diluted in a larger volume and given over 20 to 30 minutes.

Higher doses are not recommended.

Duration/Response: Assess all patients receiving pentostatin at 6 months for response to treatment. If the patient has not achieved a complete or partial response, discontinue treatment.

If the patient has achieved a partial response, continue treatment in an effort to achieve a complete response. At any time that a complete response is achieved thereafter, two additional doses of pentostatin are recommended; then stop treatment. If the best response to treatment at the end of 12 months is a partial response, stop treatment with pentostatin.

Therapy/Dose discontinuation: Withholding or discontinuing individual doses may be needed when severe adverse reactions occur.

Patients who have elevated serum creatinine should have their dose withheld and a Ccr determined. There are insufficient data to recommend a starting or a subsequent dose for patients with impaired renal function (Ccr < 60 ml/min).

Renal function impairment: Treat patients only when potential benefit justifies potential risk. Two patients with impaired renal function (Ccr 50 to 60 ml/min) achieved complete response without unusual adverse events when treated with 2 mg/m^2.

Hematologic effects: No dosage reduction is recommended at the start of therapy in patients with anemia, neutropenia or thrombocytopenia. In addition, dosage reductions are not recommended during treatment in patients with anemia and thrombocytopenia if patients can be otherwise supported hematologically. Temporarily withhold pentostatin if the absolute neutrophil count falls below 200 cells/mm^3 during treatment in a patient who had an initial neutrophil count > 500 cells/mm^3; treatment may be resumed when the count returns to predose levels.

IDARUBICIN HCl

Powder for Injection (lyophilized): 5, 10 and 20 mg ***(Rx)*** *Idamycin* (Adria)

Warning:

Give idarubicin slowly into a freely flowing IV infusion. It must never be given IM or SC. Severe local tissue necrosis can occur if there is extravasation during administration. If signs or symptoms of extravasation occur, terminate the injection or infusion immediately and restart in another vein.

Idarubicin can cause myocardial toxicity leading to congestive heart failure. Cardiac toxicity is more common in patients who have received prior anthracyclines or who have pre-existing cardiac disease.

Severe myelosuppression occurs when idarubicin is used at therapeutic doses. Do not give to patients with pre-exisitng bone marrow suppression induced by previous drug therapy or radiotherapy unless the benefit warrants the risk.

The physician and institution must be capable of responding rapidly and completely to severe hemorrhagic conditions or overwhelming infection.

Reduce dosage in patients with impaired hepatic or renal function.

Actions:

Pharmacology: Idarubicin HCl is a synthetic antineoplastic anthracycline for IV use; it is a DNA-intercalating analog of daunorubicin which has an inhibitory effect on nucleic acid synthesis and interacts with the enzyme topoisomerase II. The compound has a high lipophilicity which results in an increased rate of cellular uptake compared with other anthracyclines.

Pharmacokinetics: Following IV administration to adult leukemia patients with normal renal and hepatic function, there is a rapid distributive phase with a very high volume of distribution presumably reflecting extensive tissue binding. The plasma clearance is twice the expected hepatic plasma flow indicating extensive extrahepatic metabolism. The drug is eliminated predominantly by biliary and to a lesser extent by renal excretion, mostly in the form of the primary active metabolite, 13-dihydroidarubicin (idarubicinol).

The estimated mean terminal half-life is ≈ 20 hours. The elimination of idarubicinol is considerably slower with an estimated mean terminal half-life that exceeds 45 hours.

The extent of drug and metabolite accumulation predicted in leukemia patients for days 2 and 3 of dosing is 1.7- and 2.3-fold, respectively, and suggests no change in kinetics following a 3 times daily regimen.

Peak cellular idarubicin concentrations are reached a few minutes after injection. Idarubicin and idarubicinol concentrations in nucleated blood and bone marrow cells are > 100 times the plasma concentrations. Idarubicin disappearance rates in plasma and cells were comparable with a terminal half-life of about 15 hours. The terminal half-life of idarubicinol in cells was about 72 hours.

The percentages of idarubicin and idarubicinol bound to human plasma proteins averaged 97% and 94%, respectively. The binding is concentration-independent.

Idarubicin studies in pediatric leukemia patients, at doses of 4.2 to 13.3 mg/m^2/day for 3 days, suggest dose-independent kinetics. There is no difference between the half-lives of the drug following 3 times daily or 3 times weekly administration.

Indications:

In combination with other approved antileukemic drugs for the treatment of acute myeloid leukemia (AML) in adults. This includes French-American-British (FAB) classifications M1 through M7.

Warnings:

Carcinogenesis: Idarubicin and related compounds have mutagenic and carcinogenic properties.

Pregnancy: Category D.

Lactation: It is not known whether this drug is excreted in breast milk. Because of the potential for serious adverse reactions in nursing infants, mothers should discontinue nursing prior to taking this drug.

Children: Safety and efficacy in children have not been established.

Precautions:

Monitoring: Therapy with idarubicin requires close observation of the patient and careful laboratory monitoring. Frequent complete blood counts and monitoring of hepatic and renal function tests are recommended.

Hyperuricemia secondary to rapid lysis of leukemic cells may be induced. Take appropriate measures to prevent hyperuricemia and to control any systemic infection before beginning therapy.

Administer slowly (over 10 to 15 minutes) into the tubing of a freely running IV infusion of 0.9% NaCl Injection, USP or 5% Dextrose Injection, USP. Attach the tubing to a butterfly needle or other suitable device and insert preferably into a large vein.

Adverse Reactions:

Adverse reactions occurring in ≥ 3% of patients include: Infection; nausea; vomiting; hair loss; abdominal cramps/diarrhea; hemmorage; mucositis; generalized rash; urticaria; bullous erythrodermatous rash of the palms and soles; hives at the injection site; mental status; fever; headache; severe hepatic function changes; seizure.

Administration and Dosage:

Induction therapy in adult patients with AML: 12 mg/m^2 daily for 3 days by slow (10 to 15 min) IV injection in combination with Ara-C, 100 mg/m^2 daily given by continuous infusion for 7 days or as a 25 mg/m^2 IV bolus followed by 200 mg/m^2 daily for 5 days by continuous infusion. In patients with unequivocal evidence of leukemia after the first induction course, a second course may be administered. Delay administration of the second course in patients who experience severe mucositis until recovery from this toxicity has occurred; a dose reduction of 25% is recommended. In patients with hepatic or renal impairment, consider a dose reduction of idarubicin. Do not administer if the bilirubin level is > 5 mg/dl.

DOXORUBICIN HCl (ADR)

Powder for Injection (lyophilized): 10, 20, 50, 100 and 150 mg *(Rx)*	*Rubex* (Bristol-Myers Oncology), *Adriamycin RDF* (Pharmacia), *Doxorubicin HCl* (Chiron)
Injection, aqueous: 2 mg/ml *(Rx)*	*Doxorubicin HCl* (Chiron)
Preservative Free Injection: 2 mg/ml *(Rx)*	*Adriamycin PFS* (Pharmacia)
Injection: 20 mg (lipid complex) *(Rx)*	*Doxil* (Sequus)

Warning:

Severe local tissue necrosis will result if extravasation occurs. Do not give IM or SC.

Serious irreversible myocardial toxicity with delayed congestive failure often unresponsive to supportive therapy may occur as total dosage approaches 550 mg/m^2. Myelosuppression requires careful monitoring.

Acute infusion-associated reactions (flushing, shortness of breath, facial swelling, headache, chills, back pain, tightness in the chest or throat and hypertension) have occurred in about 7% of patients treated with liposomal doxorubicin. In most patients, these reactions resolve over the course of several hours to a day once the infusion is terminated. In some patients, the reaction resolves by slowing the infusion rate.

Reduce dosage in patients with impaired hepatic function.

Severe myelosuppression may occur.

Actions:

Pharmacology: Doxorubicin is a cytotoxic anthracycline antibiotic. Its mechanism is related to its ability to bind to DNA and inhibit nucleic acid synthesis. Cell culture studies have shown rapid cell penetration, perinucleolar chromatin binding, rapid inhibition of mitotic activity and nucleic acid synthesis, mutagenesis and chromosomal aberrations.

Liposomal doxorubicin is encapsulated in long-circulating liposomes. Liposomes are microscopic vesicles composed of a phospholipid bilayer that are capable of encapsulating active drugs. The liposomes of liposomal doxorubicin are formualted with pegylation, to protect liposomes from detection by the mononuclear phagocyte system (MPS) and to increase blood circulation time.

The liposomes have a half-life of ≈ 55 hours in humans. They are stable in blood, and direct measurement of liposomal doxorubicin shows that at least 90% of the drug (the assay used cannot quantify < 5% to 10% free doxorubicin) remains liposome-encapsulated during circulation.

It is hypothesized that because of their small size (≈ 1000 nm) and persistence in the circulation to pegylated doxorubicin, liposomes are able to penetrate the altered and often compromised vasculature of tumors. This hypothesis is supported by studies using colloidal gold-containing liposomes, which can be visualized microscopically. Evidence of penetration of the liposomes from blood vessels and theri entry and accumulation in tumors have been seen in mice with C-26 colon carcinoma tumors and in transgenic mice with Kaposi's sarcoma-like lesions. Once the liposomes distribute to the tissue compartment, the encapsulated doxorubicin becomes available. The exact mechanism of release is not understood.

Liposomal encapsulation or incorporation in a lipid complex can substantially affect a drug's functional properties relative to those of the unencapsulated or nonlipid-assocaited drug. In addition, different liposomal or lipid-complexed products with a common activity ingredient may vary from one another in the chemical composition and physical form of the lipid component. Such differences may affect functional properties of these drug products.

Pharmacokinetics:

Absorption/Distribution –

Conventional doxorubicin undergoes rapid and extensive binding to tissue and plasma proteins after IV use. Does not cross blood-brain barrier.

Liposomal doxorubicin: In contrast to original doxorubicin, the steady-state volume of distribution of liposomal doxorubicin indicates that it is confined mostly to the vascular fluid volume. Plasma protein binding has not been determined.

Metabolism/Excretion –

Conventional doxorubicin: Plasma disappearance of doxorubicin follows a triphasic pattern with mean half-lives of 12 minutes, 3.3 hours and 29.6 hours. Doxorubicin is metabolized by carbonyl reduction to the active alcohol, doxorubicinol and inactive aglycones. Other inactive metabolites have been identified in urine and bile.

Liver function impairment, as reflected by elevated serum bilirubin, results in slower excretion and increased retention and accumulation of drug and metabolites in plasma and tissues. Other liver function abnormalities are not predictive. Urinary excretion accounts for ≈ 4% to 5% of the dose in 5 days. Biliary excretion is the major excretion route; 40% to 50% is recovered in bile or feces in 7 days.

Liposomal doxorubicin: Doxorubicinol, the major metabolite of doxorubicin, was detected at very low levels (range, 0.8 to 26.2 ng/ml) in the plasma of patients who received 10 or 20 mg/m^2 liposomal doxorubicin.

The plasma clearance of liposomal doxorubicin was slow, with a mean clearnace value of 0.041 L/hr/m^2 at a dose of 20 mg/m^2. This is in contrast to original doxorubicin.

Because of its slower clearance, the AUC of liposomal doxorubicin, primarily representing the circulation of liposome-encapsulated doxorubicin, is ≈ two to three orders of magnitude larger than the AUC for a similar dose of conventional doxorubicin as reported.

Indications:

Conventional doxorubicin: To produce regression in the following: Acute lymphoblastic leukemia, acute myeloblastic leukemia, Wilms' tumor, neuroblastoma, soft tissue and bone sarcomas, breast carcinoma, ovarian carcinoma, transitional cell bladder carcinoma, thyroid carcinoma, Hodgkin's and non-Hodgkin's lymphomas, bronchogenic carcinoma (the small cell histologic type is the most responsive) and gastric carcinoma.

Liposomal doxorubicin: Treatment of AIDS-related Kaposi's sarcoma in patients with disease that has progressed on prior combination chemotherapy or in patients who are intolerant to such therapy.

Contraindications:

Malignant melanoma, kidney carcinoma, large bowel carcinoma, brain tumors and metastases to the CNS are not significantly responsive to doxorubicin therapy.

Do not initiate therapy in patients with marked myelosuppression induced by previous treatment with other antitumor agents or by radiotherapy.

Conclusive data are not available on preexisting heart disease as a cofactor of increased risk of drug-induced cardiac toxicity. In such cases cardiac toxicity may occur at doses lower than recommended cumulative limit. Do not use doxorubicin in such cases.

A history of hypersensitivity reactions to conventional or liposomal doxorubicin or their components.

Patients who received previous treatment with complete cumulative doses of doxorubicin or daunorubicin.

Warnings:

Necrotizing colitis manifested by typhlitis (cecal inflammation), bloody stools and severe and sometimes fatal infections have occurred with doxorubicin given by IV push daily for 3 days combined with cytarabine continuous infusion daily for ≥ 7 days.

Cardiac toxicity must be given special attention. Although uncommon, acute left ventricular failure has occurred, particularly in patients who have received total dosage exceeding the recommended limit of 550 mg/m^2. The total dose of drug should also take into account any previous or concomitant therapy with other potentially cardiotoxic agents such as cyclophosphamide or daunorubicin. Cardiomyopathy or CHF may occur several weeks after drug discontinuation and is often unresponsive to medical or physical therapy.

Early diagnosis of drug-induced heart failure is essential for successful treatment with digitalis, diuretics, low salt diet and bed rest. Severe cardiac toxicity may occur precipitously without antecedent ECG changes. Perform a baseline ECG and prior to each dose or after 300 mg/m^2 cumulative dose. If test results indicate cardiac function change, carefully evaluate benefit of continued therapy against risk of producing irreversible cardiac damage. Preliminary evidence suggests cardiotoxicity may be reduced and total dosage safely increased by giving the drug on a weekly schedule or as a prolonged (48 to 96 hrs) continuous infusion.

The most definite test for anthracycline myocardial injury is endomyocardial biopsy. Other methods such as echocardiography or gated radionuclide scans have been used to monitor cardiac function during anthracycline therapy. If these test results indicate possible cardaic injury associated with doxorubicin or liposomal doxorubicin therapy, weigh the benefit of continued therapy against the risk of myocardial injury. Dexrazoxane, a cardioprotective agent, may be effective in preventing doxorubicin-induced cardiotoxicity (see individual monograph).

Infusion reactions appear to occur with the first infusion and do not appear to occur with later infusions if not present initially. In most patients, these reactions resolve over the course of several hours to a day once the infusion is terminated. In some patients, the reaction resolves by slowing the rate of infusion. Similar reactions have not been reported with conventional doxorubicin, and they presumably represent a reaction to liposomal doxorubicin or one of its surface components.

Many patients were able to tolerate further infusions without complications; however, six patients were terminated from therapy because of an infusion reaction to liposomal doxorubicin.

Palmar-plantar erythrodysesthesia – Among 705 patients with AIDS-related Kaposi's sarcoma treated with liposomal doxorubicin, 24 (3.4%) developed palmar-plantar skin eruptions characterized by swelling, pain, erythema and desquamation of the skin on the hands and feet. The syndrome was generally seen after ≥ 6 weeks of treatment but may occur earlier. The incidence of this reaction may be higher when liposomal doxorubicin is administered at doses that are higher or at intervals that are shorter than those recommended. In most patients, the reaction is mild and resolves in 1 to 2 weeks so that prolonged delay of therapy need not occur. The reaction can be severe and debilitating in some patients, however, and may require discontinuation of treatment.

Mucostitis may occur 5 to 10 days after administration, leading to ulceration, and represent a site of origin for severe infections. Incidence and severity of mucositis is greater with the 3 successive daily dosage regimen. Ulceration and necrosis of the colon, especially the cecum, may occur leading to bleeding or severe infections which can be fatal. This reaction has occurred in patients with acute non-lymphocytic leukemia treated with 3 days of doxorubicin plus cytarabine.

Carcinogenesis/Mutagenesis: Doxorubicin and related compounds have mutagenic and carcinogenic properties in experimental models.

Pregnancy: Category D.

Children: Children treated with doxorubicin during childhood are more likely to have abnormal cardiac function. Females may be at more risk.

Precautions:

Monitoring: Initial treatment requires close patient observation and extensive laboratory monitoring. Hospitalize patients at least during the first phase of treatment.

Hyperuricemia may be induced by doxorubicin secondary to rapid lysis of neoplastic cells. Monitor patient's blood uric acid level.

Urine discoloration: Doxorubicin imparts a red color to the urine for 1 to 2 days after administration.

Drug Interactions:

Doxorubicin may affect other antineoplastic agents (eg, cyclophosphamide, 6–mercaptopurine) and digoxin. Doxorubicin may be affected by barbiturates. Radiation-induced toxicities may be increased by doxorubicin.

Adverse Reactions:

Adverse reactions may include: Reversible complete alopecia; acute nausea and vomiting; mucositis (stomatitis and esophagitis) leading to ulceration; hyperpigmentation of nailbeds and dermal creases (primarily in children); onycholysis; recall of skin reaction due to prior radiotherapy; phlebosclerosis; facial flushing; severe cellulitis; erythematous streaking of veins; fever; chills; urticaria; anaphylaxis; lincomycin cross-sensitivity.

Acute infusion-associated reactions characterized by flushing, shortnesss of breath, facial swelling, headache, chills, back pain, tightness in the chest and throat and hypotension have occurred in ≈ 6.8% of patients treated with liposomal doxorubicin.

Administration and Dosage:

For IV use only.

Conventional doxorubicin::

Recommended dosage schedules: 60 to 75 mg/m^2, as a single IV injection administered at 21 day intervals. Give the lower dose to patients with inadequate marrow reserves due to old age, prior therapy or neoplastic marrow infiltration.

Alternative dose schedules: 30 mg/m^2 on each of 3 successive days, repeated every 4 weeks. Another alternative dose schedule is weekly doses of 20 mg/m^2 which may produce a lower incidence of CHF.

Dosage in patients with elevated bilirubin: Serum bilirubin 1.2 to 3 mg/dl, give 50% of normal dose; > 3 mg/dl, give 25% of normal dose.

Liposomal doxorubicin::

Recommended dosage schedule: Administer IV at a dose of 20 mg/m^2 (conventional doxorubicin equivalent) over 30 minutes, once every 3 weeks, for as long as the patient responds satisfactorily and tolerates treatment.

Do not administer as a bolus injection or an undiluted solution. Rapid infusion may increase the risk of infusion-related reactions.

Alternative dose schedules:

Liposomal Doxorubicin Dosing in Palmar-Plantar Erythrodysesthesia

Toxicity grade	Symptoms	Weeks since last dose	
		3	4
0	No Symptoms	Redose at 3-week interval	Redose at 3-week interval.
1	Mild erythema, swelling or desquamation not interfering with daily activities	Redose unless patient has experienced a previous grade 3 or 4 skin toxicity, in which case, wait an additional week.	Redose at 25% dose reduction; return to 3-week interval.
2	Erythema, desquamation or swelling interfering with, but not precluding, normal physical activities; small blisters or ulcerations < 2 cm in diameter	Wait an additional week.	Redose at 50% dose reduction; return to 3-week interval.
3	Blistering, ulceration or swelling interfering with walking or noraml daily activities; cannot wear regular clothing.	Wait an additional week.	Redose at 50% dose reduction; return to 3-week interval.
4	Diffuse or local process causing infectious complications, or a bedridden state or hospitalization	Wait an additional week.	Discontinue liposomal doxorubicin.

Liposomal Doxorubicin Dosing in Hematological Toxicity			
Grade	ANC (cells/mm³)	Platelets (cells/mm³)	Modification
1	1500-1900	75,000-150,000	None
2	1000- < 1500	50,000- < 75,000	None
3	500-999	25,000- < 50,000	Wait until ANC is ≥ 1,000 or platelets are ≥ 50,000 then redose at 25% dose reduction.
4	<500	< 25,000	Wait until ANC is ≥ 1,000 or platelets are ≥ 50,000 then redose at 50% dose reduction.

Liposomal Doxorubicin Dosing in Stomatitis		
Grade	Symptoms	Modification
1	Painless ulcers, erythema or mild soreness	None
2	Painful erythema, edema or ulcers, but can eat	Wait one week and if symptoms improve, redose at 100% dose.
3	Painful erythema, edema or ulcers, and cannot eat	Wait one week and if symptoms improve, redose at 25% dose reduction.
4	Requires parenteral or enteral support	Wait one week and if symptoms improve, redose at 50% dose reduction

Patients with impaired hepatic function: Limited clinical experience exists in treating hepatically impaired patients with liposomal doxorubicin. Therefore, based on experience with conventional doxorubicin, it is recommended that liposomal doxorubicin dosage be reduced if the bilirubin is elevated as follows: Serum bilirubin 1.2 to 3 mg/dl, give ½ normal dose, > 3 mg/dl, give ¼ normal dose.

IV infusion: Administer slowly into the tubing of a freely running IV infusion of NaCl Injection or 5% Dextrose Injection. Attach the tubing to a Butterfly needle inserted into a large vein. Avoid veins over joints or in extremities with compromised venous or lymphatic drainage. Rate depends on size of vein and dosage; however, do not administer in < 3 to 5 minutes. Local erythematous streaking along the vein as well as facial flushing may indicate too rapid administration.

DAUNORUBICIN CITRATE LIPOSOMAL

Injection: 2 mg/ml (equivalent to 50 mg daunorubicin base) *(Rx)* *DaunoXome* (NeXstar)

Actions:

Pharmacology: Daunorubicin is an anthracycline antibiotic with antineoplastic activity, which is originally obtained from *Streptomyces peucetius.*

Liposomal daunorubicin is a liposomal preparation of daunorubicin formulated to maximize the selectivity of daunorubicin for solid tumors in situ. In the circulation, the liposomal daunorubicin formulation helps to protect the entrapped daunorubicin from chemical and enzymatic degradation, minimizes protein binding and generally decreases uptake by normal (non-reticuloendothelial system) tissues. The specific mechanism by which liposomal daunorubicin is able to deliver daunorubicin to solid tumors in situ is not known. However, it is believed to be a function of increased permeability of the tumor neovasculature to some particles in the size range of liposomal daunorubicin. Once within the tumor environment, daunorubicin is released over time enabling it to exert its antineoplastic activity.

Pharmacokinetics:

Absorption/Distribution – Following IV injection, plasma clearance shows monoexponential decline. Plasma clearance is 17.3 ml/min, volume of distribution is 6.4 L, distribution half-life is 4.41 hrs, steady-state is 6.4 L and elimination half-life is 4.4 hrs. Daunorubicinol, the major active metabolite of daunorubicin, was detected at low levels in the plasma.

Indications:

Advanced HIV-associated Kaposi's sarcoma: First-line cytotoxic therapy for advanced HIV-associated Kaposi's sarcoma.

Contraindications:

Hypersensitivity reaction to previous doses or to any constituents of the product.

Warnings:

Myelosuppression: The primary toxicity of daunorubicin is myelosuppression, especially of the granulocytic series, which may be severe, with much less marked effects on the platelets and erythroid series.

Potential cardiac toxicity, particularly in patients who have received prior anthrocyclines or who have pre-existing cardiac disease, may occur. Although there is no reliable means of predicting CHF, cardiomyopathy induced by anthracyclines is usually associated with a decrease of left ventricular ejection fraction (LVEF). Certain ECG changes and a decrease in the systolic ejection fraction from pretreatment baseline may aid in recognizing those patients at greatest risk. Weigh the benefit of continued therapy against the risk.

Back pain, flushing and chest tightness has been reported in 13.8% of the patients. This generally occurs during the first 5 minutes of the infusion, subsides with interruption of the infusion and generally does not recur if the infusion is then resumed at a slower rate.

Extravasation at injection site: Conventional daunorubicin has been associated with local tissue necrosis at the site of drug extravasation. Although grade 3 to 4 injection site inflammation was reported in two patients treated with liposomal daunorubicin, no instances of local tissue necrosis were observed with extravasation.

Hepatic function impairment: Reduce dosage in patients with impaired hepatic function.

Elderly: Safety and efficacy in the elderly have not been established.

Pregnancy: *Category D.*

Children: Safety and efficacy in children have not been established.

Precautions:

Monitoring: Observe patient closely and monitor chemical and laboratory tests extensively. Evaluate cardiac, renal and hepatic function prior to each course of treatment. Repeat blood counts prior to each dose and withhold if the absolute granulocyte count is < 750 cells/mm^3. Monitor serum uric acid levels.

Hyperuricemia may be induced secondary to rapid lysis of leukemic cells. As a precaution, administer allopurinol prior to initiating antileukemic therapy.

Infection: Control any systemic infections before beginning therapy.

Adverse Reactions:

Adverse reactions that may occur in ≥ 3% of patients include: Depression; dizziness; fatigue; headache; insomnia; malaise; neuropathy; abdominal pain; anorexia; constipation; diarrhea; nausea; stomatitis; vomiting; arthralgia; back pain; myalgia; rigors; cough; dyspnea; rhinitis; sinusitis; alopecia; pruritus; abnormal vision; allergic reactions; chest pain; edema; fever; sweating; tenesmus; neutropenia; opportunistic infections/illnesses; influenza-like symptoms.

Administration and Dosage:

Administer IV over 1 hour at a dose of 40 mg/m^2. Repeat every 2 weeks. Continue treatment until there is evidence of progressive disease (eg, based on best response acheived; new visceral sites of involvement or progression of visceral disease; development of 10 or more new, cutaneous lesions or a 25% increase in the number of lesions compared with baseline; a change in the character of ≥ 25% of all previously counted flat lesions to raised; increase in surface area of the indicator lesions) or until other complications of HIV disease preclude continuation of therapy.

Hepatic or renal function impairment: Reduce dosage.

Liposomal Daunorubicin Dosage in Hepatic or Renal Function Impairment		
Serum bilirubin	Serum creatinine	Recommended dose
1.2 to 3 mg/dl		¾ normal dose
> 3 mg/dl	> 3 mg/dl	½ normal dose

MITOXANTRONE HCl

Injection: 2 mg mitoxantrone base per ml *(Rx)* — *Novantrone* (Immunex)

> **Warning:**
> When used in doses indicated for the treatment of leukemia, severe myelosuppression will occur. Give particular care to assuring full hematologic recovery before undertaking consolidation therapy (if this treatment is used); monitor patients closely during this phase.

Actions:

Pharmacology: Mitoxantrone is a synthetic antineoplastic anthracenedione for IV use. Although its mechanism of action is not fully elucidated, mitoxantrone is a DNA-reactive agent. It has a cytocidal effect on both proliferating and nonproliferating cultured human cells, suggesting lack of cell cycle phase specificity.

Pharmacokinetics:

Absorption/Distribution – Pharmacokinetic studies in adults following a single IV administration have demonstrated multi-exponential plasma clearance. Distribution to tissues is rapid and extensive. The apparent steady-state volume of distribution exceeds 1000 L/m^2. Elimination is slow with an apparent mean terminal plasma half-life of 5.8 days (range, 2.3 to 13). Mitoxantrone is 78% bound to plasma proteins in the concentration range of 26 to 455 ng/ml.

Metabolism/Excretion – Excretion is via the renal and hepatobiliary systems. Only 6% to 11% of the dose is recovered in the urine within 5 days after administration. Of the material recovered in the urine, 65% is unchanged drug; the remaining 35% is comprised of two inactive metabolites and their glucuronide conjugates (mono- and dicarboxylic acid derivatives). Hepatobiliary elimination of drug appears to be of greater significance; 25% of the dose is recovered in the feces within 5 days of IV dosing.

Indications:

In combination with other approved drug(s) in the initial therapy of acute nonlymphocytic leukemia (ANLL) in adults. This includes myelogenous, promyelocytic, monocytic and erythroid acute leukemias.

Unlabeled uses: Mitoxantrone may be beneficial, alone or in combination with other agents, in the treatment of breast cancer and refractory lymphomas. Response rates for breast cancer have been as high as 40% when used as a single agent. For non-Hodgkin's lymphoma, a high-dose intermittent dosage schedule appears to be more effective than a lower-dose weekly schedule.

Contraindications:

Hypersensitivity to mitoxantrone.

Warnings:

Cardiac: Functional cardiac changes including CHF and decreases in left ventricular ejection fraction (LVEF) occur. Cardiac toxicity may be more common in patients with prior treatment with anthracyclines, prior mediastinal radiotherapy, or with preexisting cardiovascular disease. Such patients should have regular cardiac monitoring of LVEF from the initiation of therapy.

Hepatoxicity: Patients have developed transient elevations of AST and ALT following mitoxantrone administration (4 to 24 days after treatment).

Pregnancy: Category D.

Lactation: It is not known whether this drug is excreted in breast milk. Because of the potential for serious adverse reactions in infants, discontinue breastfeeding before starting treatment.

Children: Safety and efficacy for use in children have not been established.

Precautions:

Monitoring: Accompany therapy by close and frequent monitoring of hematologic and chemical laboratory parameters, as well as frequent patient observation. Serial complete blood counts and liver function tests are necessary for appropriate dose adjustments.

For IV use only: Safety for use by routes other than IV administration has not been established. Do not use intrathecally.

Hyperuricemia may occur as a result of rapid lysis of tumor cells. Monitor serum uric acid levels and institute hypouricemic therapy prior to initiation of antileukemic therapy.

Systemic infections: Treat concomitantly with or just before starting mitoxantrone.

Adverse Reactions:

The following adverse reactions occurred in patients treated with mitoxantrone plus cytosine arabinoside: CHF; arrhythmias; chest pai; asymptomatic decreases in LVEF; tachycardia; ECG changes; hypotension; GI bleeding; petechiae/ecchymosis; nausea/vomiting; diarrhea; abdominal pain; mucositis/stomatitis; jaundice; UTI; pneumonia; sepsis; fungal infections; cough; dyspnea; seizures; headache; conjunctivitis; renal failure; fever; alopecia; myelosuppression; urticaria; rashes. It is clear that the combination of mitoxantrone plus cytosine arabinoside was responsible for nausea and vomiting, alopecia, mucositis/stomatitis and myelosuppression.

Administration and Dosage:

Mitoxantrone solution must be diluted prior to use. If extravasation occurs, stop administration immediately and restart in another vein. Avoid contact with the skin, mucous membranes or eyes.

Combination initial therapy for ANLL in adults: For induction, 12 mg/m^2/day on days 1 to 3 given as an IV infusion, and 100 mg/m^2 of cytosine arabinoside for 7 days given as a continuous 24 hour infusion on days 1 to 7.

Most complete remissions will occur following the initial course of induction therapy. In the event of an incomplete antileukemic response, a second induction course may be given. Give mitoxantrone for 2 days and cytosine arabinoside for 5 days using the same daily dosage levels.

If severe or life-threatening nonhematologic toxicity is observed during the first induction course, withhold the second induction course until toxicity clears.

Consolidation therapy used in two large randomized multicenter trials consisted of mitoxantrone 12 mg/m^2 given by IV infusion daily for days 1 and 2, and cytosine arabinoside 100 mg/m^2 for 5 days given as a continuous 24 hour infusion on days 1 to 5. The first course was given ≈ 6 weeks after the final induction course, the second was generally administered 4 weeks after the first. Severe myelosuppression occurred.

MITOMYCIN (Mitomycin-C; MTC)

Powder for Injection: 5,20 and 40 mg *(Rx)* — *Mutamycin* (Bristol-Myers Oncology)

Warning:

Bone marrow suppression, notably thrombocytopenia and leukopenia, which may contribute to overwhelming infection in an already compromised patient, is the most common and severe toxic effect.

Hemolytic uremic syndrome, a serious syndrome of microangiopathic hemolytic anemia, thrombocytopenia and irreversible renal failure has occurred.

Actions:

Pharmacology: Mitomycin is an antibiotic with antitumor activity isolated from *Streptomyces caespitosus*. It selectively inhibits the synthesis of deoxyribonucleic acid (DNA). The guanine and cytosine content correlates with the degree of mitomycin-induced cross-linking. At high concentrations, cellular ribonucleic acid (RNA) and protein synthesis are also suppressed.

Pharmacokinetics:

Absorption/Distribution – IV mitomycin is rapidly cleared from the serum. Maximal serum concentrations were 2.4 mcg/ml after IV injection of 30 mg; 1.7 mcg/ml after 20 mg and 0.52 mcg/ml after 10 mg. Serum half-life after a 30 mg bolus injection is 17 minutes.

Metabolism/Excretion – Clearance is effected primarily by hepatic metabolism, but metabolism occurs in other tissues as well. Clearance rate is inversely proportional to maximal serum concentration due to saturation of degradative pathways. About 10% of a dose is excreted unchanged in urine. Because of saturable metabolic pathways, the percent excreted in urine increases with increasing dose.

Indications:

Therapy of disseminated adenocarcinoma of stomach or pancreas combined with other chemotherapeutic agents, and as palliative treatment when other modalities fail.

Unlabeled uses: Mitomycin has been given by the intravesical route for the management of superficial bladder cancer. Mitomycin as an ophthalmic solution appears beneficial as an adjunct to surgical excision in primary or recurrent pterygia.

Contraindications:

Primary therapy as a single agent; to replace surgery or radiotherapy; hypersensitivity or idiosyncratic reaction to mitomycin; patients with thrombocytopenia, coagulation disorder or an increase in bleeding tendency due to other causes.

Warnings:

Bone marrow suppression, particularly thrombocytopenia and leukopenia, occurring in 64% of patients, is the most serious toxicity and is cumulative. Perform the following during and for at least 8 weeks following therapy: Platelet count, WBC, differential and hemoglobin. A platelet count < 100,000/mm^3 or a WBC < 4,000/mm^3, or a progressive decline in either, is an indication to interrupt therapy. Observe patients frequently during and after therapy. Deaths have occurred due to septicemia as a result of leukopenia.

Extravasation at injection site can cause severe local tissue necrosis. Stop the injection immediately. For management, see the Antineoplastics Introduction.

Renal function impairment: Observe patients for evidence of renal toxicity. Do not give to patients with a serum creatinine > 1.7 mg/dl.

Pregnancy: Safety for use during pregnancy has not been established.

Precautions:

Adult respiratory distress syndrome: A few cases have occurred in patients receiving mitomycin in combination with other chemotherapy and maintained at FIO_2 concentrations > 50% perioperatively. Use only enough oxygen to provide adequate arterial saturation since oxygen itself is toxic to the lungs. Pay careful attention to fluid balance; avoid overhydration.

Drug Interactions:

Vinca alkaloids: Vinca alkaloids interact with mitomycin.

Adverse Reactions:

Adverse reactions may include thrombocytopenia; leukopenia; cellulitis at injection site; stomatitis; alopecia; delayed erythema or ulceration (see Antineoplastics Introduction for management); hemolytic uremic syndrome (microangiopathic hemolytic anemia, thrombocytopenia, irreversible renal failure, pulmonary edema, neurologic abnormalities, hypertension); fever; anorexia; nausea; vomiting; headache; blurred vision; confusion; drowsiness; syncope; fatigue; edema; thrombophlebits; hematemesis; diarrhea; pain.

Administration and Dosage:

Give IV only.

After hematological recovery (see dosage adjustment guide) from previous chemotherapy use 20 mg/m^2 IV as a single dose at 6 to 8 week intervals.

Because of cumulative myelosuppression, reevaluate patients after each course of therapy; reduce dose if patient experiences any toxicity. Doses > 20 mg/m^2 are not more effective, and are more toxic than lower doses. Do not repeat dosage until leukocyte count has returned to 4000/mm^3 and platelet count to 100,000/mm^3. If disease continues to progress after two courses, discontinue; chances of response are minimal. When used with other myelosuppressives, adjust dosage appropriately.

Dosage Adjustment for Mitomycin

Nadir after prior dose per mm^3		% of prior dose to be given
Leukocytes	Platelets	
> 4000	> 100,000	100
3000-3999	75,000-99,999	100
2000-2999	25,000-74,999	70
< 2000	< 25,000	50

DACTINOMYCIN (Actinomycin D; ACT)

Lyophilized Powder for Injection: 0.5 mg *(Rx)* *Cosmegen* (Merck)

Warning:

Dactinomycin is extremely corrosive to soft tissue. If extravasation occurs during IV use, severe damage to soft tissues will occur. In at least one instance, this has led to contracture of the arms.

Actions:

Pharmacology: Dactinomycin is the principal component of the mixture of actinomycins. Dactinomycin anchors into a purine-pyrimidine (DNA) base pair by intercalation, inhibiting messenger RNA synthesis. Although maximal cell-kill is noted in G_1 phase, the cytotoxic action is primarily cell cycle nonspecific. Actively proliferating cells are more sensitive.

Pharmacokinetics: Very little active drug can be detected in circulating blood 2 minutes after IV injection. It concentrates in nucleated cells and does not cross the blood-brain barrier. Dactinomycin is minimally metabolized. Plasma half-life is ≈ 36 hours.

Indications:

Wilms' tumor: Combinations with vincristine, radiotherapy and surgery.

Rhabdomyosarcoma: Combinations with vincristine, cyclophosphamide and doxorubicin.

Metastatic and nonmetastatic choriocarcinoma: Combination with methotrexate.

Nonseminomatous testicular carcinoma.

Ewing's sarcoma: Palliative treatment alone, with other antineoplastics or X-ray.

Nonmetastatic Ewing's – Cyclosphosphamide and radiotherapy.

Sarcoma botryoides: Palliative treatment alone, with other antineoplastics or radiotherapy.

Radiation therapy effects may be potentiated by dactinomycin; the converse also appears likely. Dactinomycin may be tried in radiosensitive tumors not responding to x-ray therapy. Objective improvement in tumor size and activity may be observed when lower, better tolerated doses of both types of therapy are employed.

Perfusion technique: Dactinomycin alone or with other antineoplastics has been given by the isolation-perfusion technique, either as palliative treatment or as an adjunct to tumor resection; some tumors resistant to chemotherapy and radiation therapy may respond. Neoplasms in which dactinomycin has been tried using this technique include various types of sarcoma, carcinoma and adenocarcinoma. This technique offers advantages, provided drug leakage into the general circulation is minimal. By this technique the drug is in continuous contact with the tumor for the duration of treatment. The dose may be increased well over that used by the systemic route, usually without added toxicity.

Contraindications:

If given at or about the time of infection with chicken pox or herpes zoster, a severe generalized disease may occur, which could result in death.

Warnings:

Radiation: With combined dactinomycin-radiation therapy, the normal skin, as well as the buccal and pharyngeal mucosa, show early erythema.

Increased incidence of GI toxicity and marrow suppression has occurred when dactinomycin was given with x-ray therapy. Use particular caution in the first 2 months after irradiation for the treatment of right-sided Wilms' tumor, since hepatomegaly and elevated AST levels have been noted.

Reports indicate an increased incidence of second primary tumors following treatment with radiation and dactinomycin.

Carcinogenesis/Mutagenesis: The International Agency on Research on Cancer has judged that dactinomycin is a positive carcinogen in animals.

Dactinomycin has been mutagenic in a number of test systems in vitro and in vivo including human fibroblasts and leukocytes, and HELA cells.

Pregnancy: Category C.

Lactation: It is not known whether this drug is excreted in breast milk. Because of the potential for serious adverse reactions in nursing infants decide whether to discontinue nursing or to discontinue the drug, taking into account the importance of the drug to the mother.

Children: Do not give to infants < 6 to 12 months of age because of greater frequency of toxic effects.

Precautions:

Anaphylactoid reactions may occur; reactions may involve any body tissue.

Nausea and vomiting caused by dactinomycin necessitates intermittent administration. If stomatitis, diarrhea or severe hematopoietic depression appear, discontinue use until the patient has recovered.

Renal, hepatic and bone marrow function: Many abnormalities have occurred.

This drug is highly toxic. Handle and administer both powder and solution with care. Avoid inhalation of dust or vapors and contact with skin or mucous membranes, especially those of the eyes. Should accidental eye contact occur, immediately institute copious irrigation with water, followed by prompt ophthalmologic consultation. Should accidental skin contact occur, immediately irrigate the affected part with copious amounts of water for at least 15 minutes.

Drug Interactions:

Drug/Lab test interactions: Dactinomycin may interfere with bioassay procedures for the determination of antibacterial drug levels.

Adverse Reactions:

Toxic effects usually do not become apparent until 2 to 4 days after a course of therapy and may not be maximal before 1 to 2 weeks. Adverse reactions are usually reversible with discontinuation of therapy. Adverse reactions may include cheilitis; dysphagia; esophagitis; ulcerative stomatitis; pharyngitis Anorexia; abdominal pain; diarrhea; GI ulceration; proctitis; liver toxicity (including ascites, hepatomegaly, hepatitis and liver function test abnormalities); anemia (including aplastic anemia); agranulocytosis; leukopenia; thrombocytopenia; pancytopenia; reticulopenia (perform platelet and white cell counts daily. If either count markedly decreases, withhold drug until marrow recovery occurs; this often takes up to 3 weeks); alopecia; skin eruptions; acne; flare-up of erythema; increased pigmentation of previously irradiated skin; malaise; fatigue; lethargy; fever; myalgia; hypocalcemia; death.

Perfusion technique complications may consist of hematopoietic depression, absorption of toxic products from massive destruction of neoplastic tissue, increased susceptibility to infection, impaired wound healing and superficial ulceration of the gastric mucosa. Other side effects may include edema of the extremity involved, damage to soft tissues of the perfused area and (potentially) venous thrombosis.

Administration and Dosage:

Toxic reactions are frequent and may limit the amount of drug that may be given. Severity of toxicity varies and is only partly dependent on dose. Administer the drug in short courses.

IV: Individualize dosage. Do not exceed 15 mcg/kg or 400 to 600 mcg/m^2 daily IV for 5 days. Calculate the dosage for obese or edematous patients on the basis of surface area in an effort to relate dosage to lean body mass.

Adults – 0.5 mg/day IV for a maximum of 5 days.

Children – 0.015 mg/kg/day IV for 5 days. Alternative schedule is a total dosage of 2.5 mg/m^{2}IV over 1 week.

In both adults and children, administer a second course after at least 3 weeks, provided all signs of toxicity have disappeared.

Isolation-perfusion technique: 0.05 mg/kg for lower extremity or pelvis; 0.035 mg/kg for upper extremity. Use lower doses in obese patients, or when previous therapy has been employed. Complications are related to amount of drug that escapes into systemic circulation.

Use "two-needle technique" if given directly into the vein without use of an infusion. Reconstitute and withdraw dose from vial with one sterile needle. Use another needle for direct injection into vein.

PLICAMYCIN (Mithramycin)

Powder for Injection: 2500 mcg *(Rx)*	*Mithracin* (Miles)

Warning:

Severe thrombocytopenia, hemorrhagic tendency and even death may result from use. Although severe toxicity is more apt to occur in patients with advanced disease or patients otherwise considered poor risks for therapy, serious toxicity may also occasionally occur in patients who are in relatively good condition.

Actions:

Pharmacology: The exact mechanism of tumor inhibition is unknown; the drug forms a complex with deoxyribonucleic acid (DNA) and inhibits cellular ribonucleic acid (RNA) and enzymatic RNA synthesis. The binding to DNA in the presence of Mg^{++} (or other divalent cations) is responsible for the inhibition of DNA-dependent or DNA-directed RNA synthesis. This presumably accounts for plicamycin's biological properties.

Pharmacokinetics: Plicamycin is rapidly cleared from blood within the first 2 hrs; excretion is also rapid. Of measured excretion, 67% occurs within 4 hrs, 75% within 8 and 90% in the first 24 hours after injection. Plicamycin crosses the blood-brain barrier; brain tissue concentration is low, but it persists longer than in other tissues.

Indications:

Malignant testicular tumors when surgery or radiation is impossible.

Hypercalcemia and hypercalciuria in symptomatic patients (NOT responsive to conventional treatment) associated with advanced neoplasms.

Contraindications:

Thrombocytopenia, thrombocytopathy, coagulation disorders or increased susceptibility to bleeding due to other causes; bone marrow function impairment; pregnancy.

Warnings:

Hemorrhagic syndrome, the most important form of toxicity, usually begins with epistaxis. It can start with hematemesis which may progress to more widespread GI hemorrhage or to a more generalized bleeding tendency. It is most likely due to abnormalities in multiple clotting factors and is dose-related.

Renal function impairment: Use extreme caution. Monitor renal function carefully before, during and after treatment.

Pregnancy: Category X. Contraceptive measures are recommended during treatment.

Lactation: It is not known whether plicamycin is excreted in breast milk. Because of the potential for serious adverse reactions in nursing infants, discontinue nursing or the drug, taking into account the importance of the drug to the mother.

Precautions:

Monitoring: Obtain platelet count, prothrombin and bleeding times frequently during therapy and for several days following the last dose. Discontinue therapy if thrombocytopenia or a significant prolongation of prothrombin or bleeding times occurs.

Electrolyte imbalance (especially hypocalcemia, hypokalemia and hypophosphatemia): Correct with appropriate therapy prior to treatment. Calcium supplements are sometimes needed during plicamycin therapy.

Extravasation may cause local irritation and cellulitis at injection sites. Should thrombophlebitis or perivascular cellulitis occur, terminate infusion and reinstitute at another site. For management, see Antineoplastics Introduction.

Adverse Reactions:

Adverse reactions may include GI symptoms (anorexia, nausea, vomiting, diarrhea and stomatitis); fever; drowsiness; weakness; lethargy; malaise; headache; depression; phlebitis; facial flushing; skin rash; hepatotoxicity (mild, reversible); lab test abnormalities including increased AST, ALT, lactic dehydrogenase, alkaline phosphatase, serum bilirubin, ornithine carbamyl transferase, isocitric dehydrogenase, bromsulphalein retention, increased BUN and serum creatinine; proteinuria.

Administration and Dosage:

Base dose on body weight. Use ideal weight if patient has abnormal fluid retention.

Testicular tumors: 25 to 30 mcg/kg/day for 8 to 10 days unless significant side effects or toxicity occurs. Do not use > 10 daily doses. Do not exceed 30 mcg/kg/day.

In responsive tumors, some degree of regression is usually evident within 3 or 4 weeks following the initial course of therapy. If tumor masses remain unchanged, additional courses at monthly intervals are warranted.

When significant tumor regression is obtained, give additional courses of therapy at monthly intervals until complete regression is obtained or until definite tumor progression or new tumor masses occur, in spite of continued therapy.

Hypercalcemia and hypercalciuria (associated with advanced malignancy): 25 mcg/kg/day for 3 or 4 days. If desired degree of reversal is not achieved with initial course of therapy, repeat at intervals of ≥ 1 week to achieve desired result or to maintain serum and urinary calcium excretion at normal levels. It may be possible to maintain normal calcium balance with single, weekly doses or with 2 or 3 doses per week.

Administer IV only. Infuse slowly IV over 4 to 6 hrs. Avoid rapid direct IV injection; it may cause a higher incidence and greater severity of GI side effects.

PODOPHYLLOTOXIN DERIVATIVES

ETOPOSIDE (VP-16-213)	
Capsules: 50 mg *(Rx)*	*VePesid* (Bristol-Myers Oncology)
Injection: 20 mg/ml *(Rx)*	Various, *VePesid* (Bristol-Myers Oncology), *Toposar* (Pharmacia)
TENIPOSIDE (VM-26)	
Injection: 50 mg (10 mg/ml) *(Rx)*	*Vumon* (Bristol-Myers Oncology)

Warning:

Severe myelosuppression with resulting infection or bleeding may occur.

Hypersensitivity reactions, including anaphylaxis-like symptoms, may occur with initial dosing or at repeated exposure to teniposide. Epinephrine, with or without corticosteroids and antihistamines, has been used to alleviate symptoms.

Actions:

Pharmacology: These drugs are semisynthetic derivatives of podophyllotoxin.

Etoposide – Its main effect appears to be at the G_2 portion of the cell cycle. The predominant macromolecular effect appears to be DNA synthesis inhibition.

Teniposide is a phase-specific cytotoxic drug, acting in the late S or early G_2 phase of the cell cycle, thus preventing cells from entering mitosis. The mechanism of action appears to be related to the inhibition of type II topoisomerase activity since teniposide does not intercalate into DNA or bind strongly to DNA.

Pharmacokinetics:

Various Pharmacokinetic Parameters for Etoposide and Teniposide		
Parameter	Etoposide	Teniposide
Total body clearance (ml/min)	33-48	10.3
Terminal half-life (hrs)	4-11	5
Volume of distribution (L)	18-29	3-11 (children) 8-44 (adults)
Protein binding (%)	97	> 99
Elimination	Renal (35%) and nonrenal (ie, mostly metabolism, ≤ 6% bile)	Renal (44%) and fecal (≤ 10%)
Excreted unchanged in urine (%)	< 50	4-12

Etoposide –

Absorption/Distribution: The mean oral bioavailability is approximately 50% (range, 25% to 75%). There is no evidence of a first-pass effect for etoposide. On IV administration, the disposition of etoposide is a biphasic process with a distribution half-life of about 1.5 hours.

The pharmacokinetic characteristics of teniposide differ from those of etoposide. Teniposide is more extensively bound to plasma proteins and its cellular uptake is greater. Teniposide also has a lower systemic clearance, a longer elimination half-life and is excreted in the urine as parent drug to a lesser extent than etoposide.

Indications:

Etoposide:

Refractory testicular tumors in combination with other chemotherapeutic agents in patients who have received surgery, chemotherapy and radiotherapy. Adequate data on the use of oral etoposide are not available.

Small cell lung cancer in combination with other agents as first line treatment.

Teniposide: In combination with other approved anticancer agents for induction therapy in patients with refractory childhood acute lymphoblastic leukemia (ALL). Available under a Treatment IND since 1988 for relapsed or refractory ALL.

Unlabeled uses:

Etoposide has been used alone or in combination in acute nonlymphocytic leukemias (monocytic), Hodgkin's disease, non-Hodgkin's lymphomas, Kaposi's sarcoma and neuroblastoma.

Contraindications:

Hypersensitivity to etoposide, teniposide or Cremophor EL (polyoxyethylated castor oil, present in the teniposide preparation).

Warnings:

Myelosuppression: Observe patients for myelosuppression during and after therapy. Dose-limiting bone marrow suppression is the most significant toxicity.

Perform platelet count, hemoglobin, white blood cell count and differential at the start of therapy and prior to each subsequent dose. A platelet count < 50,000/mm^3 or an absolute neutrophil count < 500/mm^3 is an indication to withhold further therapy until the blood counts have sufficiently recovered.

Anaphylaxis may occur (etoposide, 0.7% to 2%; teniposide, ≈ 5%). The reactions usually respond to cessation of infusion and institution of appropriate therapy.

This reaction may occur with the first dose of teniposide and may be life threatening if not treated promptly. Patients who have experienced prior hypersensitivity reactions to teniposide are at risk for recurrence of symptoms and should only be retreated if the antileukemic benefit already demonstrated clearly outweighs the risk of a probable hypersensitivity reaction for that patient. When a decision is made to retreat a patient, pretreat with corticosteroids and antihistamines and carefully observe during and after the infusion.

Monitoring: In addition to hematologic tests, carefully monitor renal and hepatic function tests prior to and during therapy.

Hypotension: Administer by slow IV infusion (30 to 60 minutes or longer) since hypotension may occur with rapid IV injection.

Benzyl alcohol: Teniposide contains benzyl alcohol, which has been associated with a fatal "gasping" syndrome in premature infants.

CNS depression: Acute CNS depression and hypotension have occurred in patients receiving investigational infusions of high-dose teniposide who were pretreated with antiemetic drugs.

Hepatic function impairment: Exercise caution if teniposide is administered to patients with hepatic dysfunction. In children, elevated serum ALT levels are associated with reduced drug total body clearance of etoposide.

Carcinogenesis: These agents are possible carcinogens. Mutagenic and genotoxic potential has been established in mammalian cells.

Pregnancy: Category D. Contraceptive measures are recommended during treatment.

Lactation: It is not known whether this drug is excreted in breast milk. Because of the potential for serious adverse reactions in nursing infants, decide whether to discontinue nursing or the drug, accounting for the importance of the drug to the mother.

Children: Safety and efficacy for use of etoposide in children have not been established. Teniposide is indicated for use in children.

Drug Interactions:

Warfarin may be affected by etoposide. Drugs that may affect teniposide include sodium salicylate, sulfamethizole and tolbutamide. Methotrexate may be affected by teniposide.

Adverse Reactions:

Most adverse reactions are reversible if detected early. If severe reactions occur, reduce or discontinue dosage and institute corrective measures. Reinstitute therapy with caution, consider further need for the drug and be alert to recurrence of toxicity.

Adverse reactions occurring with etoposide in ≥ 3% of patients include: Myelosuppression, leukopenia, thrombocytopenia, anemia, nausea/vomiting, anorexia, diarrhea, atomatitis and alopecia.

Adverse reactions occurring with teniposide in ≥ 3%of patients include: Myelosuppression, leukopenia, neutropenia, thrombocytopenia, anemia, mucositis, nausea/vomiting, diarrhea, alopecia, rash, hypersensitivity/anaphylactic reactions, fever, infection and bleeding.

Administration and Dosage:

Handling:: Skin reactions may occur with accidental exposure. Use gloves. If solution contacts the skin or mucosa, immediately wash the area throughly with soap and water.

Etoposide (VP-16–213):: Modify the dosage, by either route, to account for the myelosuppressive effects of other drugs in combination, the effects of prior x-ray therapy or chemotherapy which may have compromised bone marrow reserve.

Administer solution over 30 to 60 minutes or longer. Do not give by rapid IV injection.

Testicular cancer –

Parental: Usual dose is 50 to 100 mg/m^2/day on days 1 to 5 to 100 mg/m^2/day on days 1, 3 and 5.

Small cell lung cancer –

Parental: 35 mg/m^2/day for 4 days to 50 mg/m^2/day for 5 days. Courses are repeated at 3 to 4 week intervals after recovery from toxicity.

Oral: 2 times the IV dose rounded to the nearest 50 mg.

Teniposide (VM-26):: Must be diluted prior to administration. Teniposide must be administered as an IV infusion. Take care to ensure that the IV catheter or needle is in the proper position and functional prior to infusion. Improper administration may result in extravasation causing local tissue necrosis or thrombophlebitis. In some instances, occlusion of cental venous access devices has occurred during 24–hour infusion at a concentration of 0.1 to 0.2 mg/ml. Frequent observation during these infusions is necessary to minimze the risk.

Administer over 30 to 60 minutes or longer. Do not give by rapid IV injection. Hypotension has been reportrd following rapid IV administration.

Hepatic/Renal function impairment – Adequate data in patients with hepatic or renal insufficiency are lacking, but dose adjustments may be necessary for patients with significant renal or hepatic impairment.

Down's syndrome patients – Reduce initial dosing; give the first course at half the usual dose.

VINORELBINE TARTRATE

Injection: 10 mg/ml *(Rx)*	*Navelbine* (Glaxo Wellcome)

Warning:

This product is for IV use only. Intrathecal administration of other vinca alkaloids has resulted in death.

Severe granulocytopenia resulting in increased susceptibility to infection may occur. Granulocyte counts should be ≥ 1000 cells/mm^3 prior to the administration of vinorelbine. Adjust dosage according to complete blood counts with differentials obtained on the day of treatment.

Improper administration of vinorelbine may result in extravasation causing local tissue necrosis or thrombophlebitis.

Actions:

Pharmacology: Vinorelbine is a semi-synthetic vinca alkaloid with antitumor activity that interferes with microtubule assembly. The antitumor activity of vinorelbine is thought to be due primarily to inhibition of mitosis at metaphase through its interaction with tubulin. Like other vinca alkaloids, vinorelbine may also interfere with:

1) amino acid, cyclic AMP and glutathione metabolism, 2) calmodulin-dependent Ca^{++}-transport ATPase activity, 3) cellular respiration and 4) nucleic acid and lipid biosynthesis.

Pharmacokinetics: The terminal phase half-life averages 27.7 to 43.6 hours and the mean plasma clearance ranges from 0.97 to 1.26 L/hr/kg. Steady-state volume of distribution values range from 25.4 to 40.1 L/kg.

Vinorelbine demonstrated high binding to human platelets and lymphocytes. The binding to plasma constituents in cancer patients ranged from 79.6% to 91.2%.

Vinorelbine undergoes substantial hepatic elimination, with large amounts recovered in feces. One metabolite, deacetylvinorelbine, possesses antitumor activity.

Approximately 18% of an administered dose was recovered in urine and 46% in feces; 10.9% was excreted unchanged in the urine.

Indications:

Non-small cell lung cancer (NSCLC): Single agent or in combination with cisplatin for the first-line treatment of ambulatory patients with unresectable, advanced NSCLC. In patients with Stage IV NSCLC, vinorelbine is indicated as a single agent or in combination with cisplatin. In Stage III NSCLC, vinorelbine is indicated in combination with cisplatin.

Unlabeled uses:

Breast cancer – Response rates of [illegible] to [illegible] (single agent) and 40% to 74% (combination therapy).

Ovarian carcinoma (cisplatin-resistant) – Response rates of 16% (single agent) to 35% (combination therapy).

Hodgkin's disease – Response rates of 34% to 90%.

Contraindications:

Patients with pretreatment granulocyte counts < 1000 cells/mm^3.

Warnings:

Granulocytopenia: Frequently monitor patients treated with vinorelbine for myelosuppression both during and after therapy. Granulocytopenia is dose-limiting. Perform complete blood counts with differentials and review results prior to giving each dose. Do not administer to patients with granulocyte counts < 1000 cells/mm^3.

Mutagenesis/Fertility impairment: In vivo, vinorelbine affects chromosome number and possibly structure.

Elderly: Greater sensitivity of some older individuals cannot be ruled out.

Pregnancy: Category D.

Lactation: It is not known whether the drug is excreted in breast milk. Nursing should be discontinued in women who are receiving vinorelbine therapy.

Children: Safety and efficacy in children have not been established.

Precautions:

Bronchospasm: Acute shortness of breath and severe bronchospasm have been reported infrequently following the administration of vinorelbine and other vinca alkaloids, most commonly when the vinca alkaloid was used in combination with mitomycin.

Neurotoxicity: If moderate or severe neurotoxicity develops, discontinue vinorelbine.

Eye contact: Avoid contamination of the eye with concentrations of vinorelbine used clinically.

Skin contact: Skin reactions may occur with accidental exposure. The use of gloves is recommended.

Drug Interactions:

Drugs that may affect vinorelbine include cisplatin and mitomycin.

Adverse Reactions:

Adverse reactions occurring in ≥ 3% of patients include: Granulocytopenia; leukopenia; thrombocytopenia; anemia; bilirubin elevation; nausea; voiting; anorexia; stomatitis; constipation; diarrhea; asthenia; injection site reactions or pain; phlebitis;

peripheral neuropathy; dyspnea; alopecia; cheast pain; shortness of breath; fatigue; jaw pain; myalgia; arthralgia and rash.

Administration and Dosage:

The usual initial dose is 30 mg/m^2 administered weekly. The recommended method of administration is an IV injection over 6 to 10 minutes. Adjust the dosage according to hematologic toxicity or hepatic insufficiency, whichever results in the lower dose.

Hematologic toxicity: Granulocyte counts should be ≥ 1000 cells/mm^3 prior to the administration of vinorelbine. Base dosage adjustments on granulocyte counts obtained on the day of treatment as follows:

Vinorelbine Dose Adjustments Based on Granulocyte Counts	
Granulocytes (cells/mm^3) on days of treatment	Dose (mg/m^2)
≥ 1500	30
1000 to 1499	15
<1000	Do not administer. Repeat granulocyte count in 1 week. If 3 consecutive weekly doses are held because granulocyte count is < 1000 cells/mm^3, discontinue vinorelbine.
Note: For patients who, during treatment, have experienced fever or sepsis while granulocytopenic or had 2 consecutive weekly doses held due to granulocytopenia, subsequent doses of vinorelbine should be: 22.5 mg/m^2 for granulocytes ≥ 1500 cells/mm^3 11.25 mg/m^2 for granulocytes 1000 to 1499 cells/mm^3	

Renal function impairment: No dose adjustments are required for renal insufficiency.

Hepatic function impairment: Administer with caution to patients with hepatic insufficiency. In patients who develop hyperbilirubinemia during treatment with vinorelbine, adjust the dose for total bilirubin as follows.

Vinorelbine Dose Modification Based on Total Bilirubin	
Total bilirubin (mg/dl)	Dose (mg/m^2)
≤ 2	30
2.1 - 3	15
> 3	7.5

VINCRISTINE SULFATE (VCR; LCR)

Injection: 1 mg/ml *(Rx)* — Various, *Oncovin* (Lilly), *Vincasar PFS* (Adria)

Warning:

It is extremely important that the IV needle or catheter be properly positioned before injection. Leakage into surrounding tissue may cause considerable irritation.

This preparation is for IV use only. Intrathecal use usually results in death.

Actions:

Pharmacology: Vincristine sulfate is an alkaloid obtained from the periwinkle (Vinca rosea Linn). Mode of action is unknown. In vitro, it arrests mitotic division at metaphase. Antineoplastic effects are related to interference with intracellular tubulin function. It reversibly binds to microtubule and spindle proteins in the S phase.

Pharmacokinetics:

Absorption/Distribution – Within 15 to 30 minutes following IV administration, > 90% of the drug is distributed from blood into tissue where it remains tightly, but not irreversibly, bound.

Metabolism/Excretion – Initial, middle and terminal half-lives are 5 min, 2.3 hrs and 85 hrs, respectively; the range of the terminal half-life is 19 to 155 hrs. The liver is the major excretory organ; ≈ 80% of a dose appears in feces and 10% to 20% in urine.

Indications:

Acute leukemia.

Combination therapy in Hodgkin's disease, non-Hodgkin's malignant lymphomas, rhabdomyosarcoma, neuroblastoma and Wilms' tumor.

Unlabeled uses: Vincristine has been used in the treatment of idiopathic thrombocytopenic purpura, Kaposi's sarcoma, breast cancer and bladder cancer.

Contraindications:

Do not give to patients with demyelinating form of Charcot-Marie-Tooth syndrome.

Warnings:

Administer IV only; intrathecal administration is uniformly fatal.

Hypersensitivity, temporally related to vincristine therapy, has occurred.

Pregnancy: Category D.

Lactation: It is not known whether this drug is excreted in breast milk.

Precautions:

Monitoring: Dose-limiting clinical toxicity is manifested as neurotoxicity; clinical evaluation (history, physical examination) is necessary to detect need for dosage modification. Perform complete blood count before each dose. Acute serum uric acid elevation may occur during induction of remission in acute leukemia; thus determine such levels frequently during the first 3 to 4 treatment weeks or take appropriate measures to prevent uric acid nephropathy.

Acute uric acid nephropathy has occurred.

CNS leukemia has occurred in patients undergoing otherwise successful therapy with vincristine.

Leukopenia or complicating infection: In the presence of these conditions, administration of the next dose warrants careful consideration.

Neuromuscular disease: Pay particular attention to dosage and neurological side effects if administered to patients with preexisting neuromuscular disease or when other neurotoxic drugs are used.

Eye contamination should be avoided with concentrations used clinically. If accidental contamination occurs, severe irritation (or, if drug was delivered under pressure, even corneal ulceration) may result.

Pulmonary reactions: Acute shortness of breath and severe bronchospasm have followed administration of vinca alkaloids, most frequently when the drug was used with mitomycin-C.

Concomitant radiation therapy: Do not give to patients receiving radiation therapy through ports that include the liver.

Drug Interactions:

Drugs that may affect vincristine include L-asparginase and mitomycin-C. Drugs that may be affected by vincristine include digoxin and phenytoin.

Adverse Reactions:

Adverse reactions may include: Loss of deep-tendon reflexes; ataxia; footdrop; paralysis; cranial nerve manifestations; severe pain may occur in the jaw, pharynx, parotid gland, bones, back and limbs; myalgias; convulsions; oral ulceration; abdominal cramps; nausea; vomiting; diarrhea; constipation; anorexia; intestinal necrosis or perforation; serious bone marrow depression; anemia; leukopenia; thrombocytopenia; anaphylaxis; rash; edema; polyuria; dysuria; urinary retention; optic atrophy with blindness; transient cortical blindness; ptosis; diplopia; photophobia; acute shortness of breath; severe bronchospasm; hyper- or hypotension; weight loss; fever; alopecia; headache.

Administration and Dosage:

Cautiously calculate and administer dose; overdosage may be serious or fatal.

Administer IV only, at weekly intervals. Injection may be completed in about 1 minute.

Adults: 1.4 mg/m^2.

Children: 2 mg/m^2. For children weighing ≤ 10 kg or having a body surface area < 1 m^2, give 0.05 mg/kg once a week.

Hepatic function impairment: A 50% reduction in the dose is recommended for patients having a direct serum bilirubin value > 3 mg/dl.

VINBLASTINE SULFATE (VLB)

Powder for Injection: 10 mg *(Rx)*	Various, *Velban* (Lilly)
Injection: 1 mg/ml *(Rx)*	Various

Actions:

Pharmacology: Vinblastine sulfate, an alkaloid, interferes with metabolic pathways of amino acids leading from glutamic acid to the citric acid cycle and urea. Studies have demonstrated an antimitotic effect and various atypical mitotic figures. Vinblastine has an effect on cell energy production required for mitosis and interferes with nucleic acid synthesis. In vitro, the drug arrests growing cells in metaphase.

Pharmacokinetics:

Absorption/Distribution – Similar to vincristine, vinblastine undergoes rapid distribution and extensive tissue binding following IV injection. Approximately 80% is bound to serum proteins. Vinblastine also localizes in platelets and leukocyte fractions of whole blood.

Metabolism/Excretion – Vinblastine is partially metabolized to deacetyl vinblastine which is more active than the parent drug. The initial, middle and terminal half-lives are 3.7 minutes, 1.6 hours and 24.8 hours, respectively.

Vinblastine is metabolized in the liver and the major route of excretion may be through the biliary system.

Indications:

Palliative treatment of the following:

Frequently responsive malignancies: Generalized Hodgkin's disease (stages III and IV, Ann Arbor modification of Rye staging system), lymphocytic lymphoma; histiocytic lymphoma; mycosis fungoides (advanced stages); advanced testicular carcinoma; Kaposi's sarcoma and Letterer-Siwe disease (histiocytosis X).

Less frequently responsive malignancies: Choriocarcinoma resistant to other chemotherapy; breast cancer unresponsive to surgery and hormonal therapy.

Hodgkin's disease: Vinblastine used as a single agent; advanced Hodgkin's disease has also been successfully treated with multiple-drug regimens that included vinblastine.

Advanced testicular germinal-cell cancers (embryonal carcinoma, teratocarcinoma and choriocarcinoma) are sensitive to vinblastine alone, but better clinical results are achieved with combination therapy.

Contraindications:

Leukopenia.

Presence of bacterial infection; infections must be under control prior to initiating therapy.

Significant granulocytopenia unless it is a result of the disease being treated.

Warnings:

Hematologic effects: Leukopenia is expected; leukocyte count is an important guide to therapy. In general, the larger the dose, the more profound and longer lasting the leukopenia will be.

Recently impaired bone marrow by prior therapy with radiation or with other oncolytic drugs may show thrombocytopenia (< 200,000 platelets/mm^3).

When cachexia or ulcerated skin surface occur, a more profound leukopenic response may occur; avoid use in older persons suffering from these conditions.

Hepatic function impairment: Toxicity may be enhanced in the presence of hepatic insufficiency.

Fertility impairment: Aspermia has been reported. Amenorrhea has occurred in some patients treated with a combination of an alkylating agent, procarbazine, prednisone and vinblastine.

Pregnancy: *Category D.*

Lactation: It is not known whether this drug is excreted in breast milk.

Precautions:

Using small amounts of drug daily for long periods is not advised, even though the resulting total weekly dose may be similar to that recommended. Strict adherence to the recommended dosage schedule is very important.

Avoid eye contamination; severe irritation or corneal ulceration (if the drug was delivered under pressure) may result.

Pulmonary reactions have occurred following use of vinca alkaloids and occur most frequently when the vinca alkaloid is used with mitomycin-C.

Drug Interactions:

Drugs that may interact with vinblastine include mitomycin-C and phenytoin.

Adverse Reactions:

Incidence of adverse reactions is dose-related. Adverse reactions may include:Leukopenia (granulocytopenia); anemia; thrombocytopenia (myelosuppression); hypertension; myocardial infarction and cerebrovascular accidents (combination chemotherapy); nausea and vomiting; pharyngitis; vesiculation of the mouth; ileus; diarrhea; constipation; anorexia; abdominal pain; rectal bleeding; hemorrhagic enterocolitis; bleeding from an old peptic ulcer; numbness of digits; paresthesias; peripheral neuritis; mental depression; loss of deep tendon reflexes; headache; convulsions; alopecia; vesiculation of the skin; malaise; weakness; dizziness; pain in tumor site; bone and jaw pain.

Administration and Dosage:

For IV use only. It is anticipated that intrathecal use would be fatal, as with vincristine.

Do not administer drug more than once weekly. Initiate therapy for adults with a single IV dose of 3.7 mg/m^2 of body surface. Thereafter, measure WBC counts to determine patient's sensitivity. A 50% dose reduction is recommended for patients having a direct serum bilirubin value > 3 mg/dl.

Incremental Dosage Weekly Intervals		
	Adult Dose (mg/m^2)	Pediatric Dose (mg/m^2)
First dose	3.7	2.5
Second dose	5.5	3.75
Third dose	7.4	5
Fourth dose	9.25	6.25
Fifth dose	11.1	7.5

Use the same increments until a max. dose not exceeding 18.5 mg/m^2 for adults and 12.5 mg/m^2 for children is reached. Do not increase dose after WBC count is reduced to ≈ 3000 cells/mm^3. For most adults the weekly dosage range is 5.5 to 7.4 mg/m^2.

Maintenance therapy: When the dose produces the above degree of leukopenia, administer a dose one increment smaller at weekly intervals for maintenance. Even though 7 days have elapsed, do not give the next dose until the WBC count has returned to at least 4000/mm^3.

IV: Inject into either the tubing of a running IV infusion or directly into a vein over 1 minute.

INTERFERON ALFA-2a (rIFN-A; IFLrA)

Injection Solution: 3 million IU/ml, 6 million IU/ml, 9 million IU/0.9 ml, 36 million IU/ml *(Rx)*	*Roferon*-A (Roche)
Powder for Injection: 6 million IU/ml when reconstituted *(Rx)*	

Actions:

Pharmacology: Interferon alfa-2a is a sterile protein product manufactured by recombinant DNA technology that employs a genetically engineered *Escherichia coli*bacterium. Interferon alfa-2a is a highly purified protein containing 165 amino acids. The mechanism by which interferons exert antitumor activity is not clearly understood. However, direct antiproliferative action against tumor cells and modulation of the host immune response may play important roles.

Pharmacokinetics:

Absorption/Distribution – In helathy people, interferon alfa-2a exhibited an elimination half-life of 3.7 to 8.5 hours (mean, 5.1 hours), volume of distribution at steady state of 0.223 to 0.748 L/kg (mean, 0.4 L/kg) and a total body clearance of 2.14 to 3.62 ml/min/kg (mean, 2.79 ml/min/kg) after a 36 million IU (2.2 x 10^8 pg) IV infusion. After IM and SC administrations of 36 million IU, peak serum concentrations ranged from 1500 to 2580 pg/ml (mean, 2020 pg/ml) at a mean time to peak of 3.8 hours and from 1250 to 2320 pg/ml (mean, 1730 pg/ml) at a mean time to peak of 7.3 hours, respectively. Multiple IM doses resulted in accumulation of 2 to 4 times the single dose serum concentrations. The apparent fraction of the dose absorbed after IM injection was greater than 80%.

Metabolism/Excretion – Alfa interferons are filtered through the glomeruli and undergo rapid proteolytic degradation during tubular reabsorption, rendering a negligible reappearance of intact alpha interferon in the systemic circulation, suggesting near complete reabsorption of interferon alfa-2a catabolites. Liver metabolism and subsequent biliary excretion are minor pathways of elimination.

Indications:

Hairy cell leukemia: In select patients ≥ 18 years of age.

AIDS-related Kaposi's sarcoma: In select patients 18 years of age and older.

Chronic myelogenous leukemia (CML): In chronic phase, Philadelphia chromosome (Ph) positive CML patients who are minimally pretreated (within 1 year of diagnosis).

Unlabeled uses: Alpha interferons have been used for a variety of conditions. Clinical trials are in progress to further determine clinical efficacy, optimal dosage and length of treatment.

Interferon Alfa Unlabeled Uses		
Significant activity	*Limited activity*	*No activity*
	Neoplastic Diseases	
Bladder tumors (local use for superficial tumors) Carcinoid tumor Cutaneous T-cell lymphoma Essential thrombocythemia Non-Hodgkin's lymphoma (low-grade)	Acute leukemias Cervical carcinoma Chronic lymphocytic leukemia Hodgkin's disease Malignant gliomas Melanoma Multiple myeloma Mycosis fungoides/Sézary syndrome Nasopharyngeal carcinoma Osteosarcoma Ovarian carcinoma Renal carcinoma	Breast cancer Colorectal carcinoma Gastric carcinoma Lung carcinoma Pancreatic carcinoma Prostatic carcinoma Soft tissue carcinoma

Interferon Alfa Unlabeled Uses		
Significant activity	*Limited activity*	*No activity*
Viral Infections		Miscellaneous
Chronic non-A, non-B hepatitis Condyloma acuminatum Cutaneous warts Cytomegaloviruses Herpes keratoconjunctivitis	Herpes simplex Papillomaviruses Rhinoviruses Vaccinia virus Varicella zoster Viral hepatitis B[1]	Hemangiomas of infancy (life-threatening) Multiple sclerosis

[1] May be more effective following prednisone withdrawal (immunologic priming).

Contraindications:

Hypersensitivity to alpha interferon or any component of the product.

Warnings:

GI hemorrhage: Infrequently, severe or fatal GI hemorrhage has been reported in association with alfa interferon therapy.

Laboratory tests: Prior to initiation of therapy, perform tests to quantitate peripheral blood hemoglobin, platelets, granulocytes and hairy cells and bone marrow hairy cells. Monitor periodically (eg, monthly) during treatment to determine response to treatment. If a patient does not respond within 6 months, discontinue treatment. If a response occurs, continue treatment until no further improvement is observed and these laboratory parameters have been stable for about 3 months. It is not known whether continued treatment after that time is beneficial.

Exercise caution in the following: In patients with severe renal or hepatic disease, seizure disorders or compromised CNS function or myelosuppression.

Administer with caution to patients with cardiac disease or with any history of cardiac illness. Acute, self-limited toxicities (eg, fever, chills) frequently associated with interferon alfa administration may exacerbate preexisting cardiac conditions.

Exercise caution when administering to patients with myelosuppression.

CNS reactions have occurred in a number of patients and included decreased mental status, exaggerated CNS function and dizziness. Careful periodic neuropsychiatric monitoring of all patients is recommended.

Leukopenia and elevation of hepatic enzymes occurred frequently but were rarely dose-limiting. Thrombocytopenia occurred less frequently. Proteinuria and increased cells in urinary sediment were also seen infrequently.

Neutralizing antibodies were detected in ≈ 27% of all patients (3.4% for patients with hairy cell leukemia). No clinical sequelae have been documented.

Anemia: In CML patients, a severe or life-threatening anemia was seen in 15% of patients. A severe life-threatening leukopenia and thrombocytopenia were seen in up to 27% of patients. Changes were usually reversible when therapy was discontinued.

Renal/Hepatic function impairment: Transient increases in liver transaminases or alkaline phosphatase of any intensity were seen in up to 50% of patients during treatment with interferon alfa-2a. Only 5% of patients had a severe or life-threatening increase in AST.

Dose-limiting hepatic or renal toxicities are unusual.

Pregnancy: Category C.

Lactation: It is not known whether this drug is excreted in breast milk. Because of the potential for serious adverse reactions in nursing infants, decide whether to discontinue nursing or to discontinue the drug, taking into account the importance of the drug to the mother.

Children: Safety and efficacy in children < 18 years of age have not been established.

Precautions:

Monitoring: Prior to initiation of therapy, perform tests to quantitate peripheral blood hemoglobin, platelets, granulocytes, hairy cells and bone marrow hairy cells. Monitor periodically (eg, monthly) during treatment to determine response to treatment. If a patient does not respond within 6 months, discontinue treatment. If a response occurs, continue treatment until no further improvement is observed and these laboratory parameters have been stable for about 3 months. It is not known whether continued treatment after that time is beneficial.

Because responses of hairy cell leukemia are not generally observed for 1 to 3 months after initiation of treatment, very careful monitoring for severe depression of blood cell counts is warranted during the initial phase of treatment.

Those patients who have preexisting cardiac abnormalities or who are in advanced stages of cancer should have ECGs taken prior to and during the course of treatment.

Drug Interactions:

Drugs that may be affected by interferon alfa-2a include aminophylline, theophylline, neurotoxic, hematotoxic or cardiotoxic drugs, interleukin-2 and CNS drugs.

Adverse Reactions:

Most adverse reactions are reversible if detected early. If severe reactions occur, reduce dosage or discontinue the drug; take appropriate corrective measures according to physician's clinical judgment. Reinstitute therapy with caution; consider further need for the drug, and be alert to possible recurrence of toxicity.

Adverse reactions occurring in ≥ 3% of patients include: Fever; fatigue; myalgias; headache; chills; arthralgia; coughing; dyspnea; hypotension; edema; chest pain; anorexia; nausea; diarrhea; emesis; abdominal pain; dizziness; decreased mental status; depression; confusion; diaphoresis; paresthesias; numbness; lethargy; visual or sleep disturbances; partial alopecia; rash; dryness or inflammation of the oropharynx; dry skin or pruritus; weight loss; change in taste; reactivation of herpes labialis; transient impotence; night sweats; rhinorrhea; lab test abnormalities including leukopenia; neutropenia; thrombocytopenia; decreased hemoglobin; abnormal AST-alkaline phosphatase, LDH and BUN; hypocalcemia; elevated fasting serum glucose and elevated serum phosphorus and serum phosphorus and serum uric acid neutralizing antibodies.

Administration and Dosage:

Give SC or IM. Subcutaneous administration is suggested for, but not limited to, patients who are thrombocytopenic (platelet count < 50,000/mm^3) or who are at risk for bleeding.

Hairy cell leukemia:

Induction dose – 3 million IU daily for 16 to 24 weeks, SC or IM.

Maintenance dose – 3 million IU 3 times per week. Dosage reduction by one-half or withholding of individual doses may be needed when severe adverse reactions occur.

The use of doses higher than 3 million IU is not recommended.

Treat patients for ≈ 6 months before determining whether to continue therapy. Patients with hairy cell leukemia have been treated for up to 20 consecutive months. The optimal duration of treatment for this disease has not been determined.

AIDS-related Kaposi's sarcoma:

Induction dose – 36 million IU daily for 10 to 12 weeks, administered IM or SC.

Maintenance dose – 36 million IU, 3 times per week. Dose reductions by one-half or withholding of individual doses may be required when severe adverse reactions occur. An escalating schedule of 3, 9 and 18 million IU daily for 3 days followed by 36 million IU daily for the remainder of the 10 to 12 week induction period has also produced equivalent therapeutic benefit with some amelioration of the acute toxicity in some patients.

When disease stabilization or a response to treatment occurs, treatment should continue until there is no further evidence of tumor or until discontinuation is required because of a severe opportunistic infection or adverse effects. The optimal duration of treatment for this disease has not been determined.

If severe reactions occur, modify dosage (50% reduction) or temporarily discontinue therapy until the adverse reactions abate. The need for dosage reduction should take into account the effects of prior x-ray therapy or chemotherapy that may have compromised bone marrow reserve. Minimum effective doses have not been established.

CML:

Chronic phase Ph positive CML – Prior to initiation of therapy, make a diagnosis of Ph positive CML in chronic phase by the appropriate peripheral blood, bone marrow and other diagnostic testing. Regularly monitor hematologic parameters (eg, monthly). Because significant cytogenic changes are not readily apparent until after hematologic response has occurred, and usually not until several months of therapy have elapsed, cytogenic monitoring may be performed at less frequent intervals. Achievement of complete cytogenic response has been observed up to 2 years following the start of interferon alfa-2a treatment.

Induction dose – 9 million units daily administered SC or IM. Based on clinical exsperience, short-term tolerance may be improved by gradually increasing the dose of interferon alfa-2a over the first week of administration from 3 million IU daily for 3 days to 6 million IU daily for 3 days to the target dose of 9 million IU daily for the duration of the treatment period.

Maintenance – Optimal dose and duration of therapy have not been determined.

Even though the median time to achieve the complete hematologic response was 5 months in clinical studies, hematologic responses have been observed up to 18 months after starting treatment. Continue therapy until disease progression. If severe side effects occur, a treatment interruption or reduction in either the dose or the frequency of injections may be necessary to achieve the individual maximally tolerated dose.

Children – Limited data are available on the use of interferon alfa-2a in children with CML. In one report of 15 children with Ph positive, adult-type CML, doses between 2.5 to 5 million IU/m^2/day given IM were tolerated. In another study, severe adverse effects including death were noted in children with previously untreated, Ph negative juvenile CML, who received interferon doses of 30 million IU/m^2/day.

INTERFERON ALFA-2b (IFN-alpha 2; rIFN-α2; α-2-interferon)

Powder for Injection, lyophilized: 3, 5, 10, 18, 25 and 50 million IU/vial *(Rx)*	*Intron* A (Schering)
Solution for Injection: 10 million, 18 million and 25 million IU/vial (*Rx*)	*Intron* A (Schering)

Actions:

Pharmacology: Interferon alfa is a protein produced by recombinant DNA techniques. Interferons exert their cellular activities by binding to specific membrane receptors on the cell surface. Once bound to the cell membrane, interferon initiates a complex sequence of intracellular events that includes the induction of certain enzymes. This process, at least in part, may be responsible for the various cellular responses to interferon, including inhibition of virus replication in virus-infected cells, suppression of cell proliferation and such immunomodulating activities as enhancement of the phagocytic activity of macrophages and augmentation of the specific cytotoxicity of lymphocytes for target cells.

Pharmacokinetics: Mean serum concentrations following IM and SC injections were comparable. Elimination half-lives were approximately 2 to 3 hours. Serum concentrations were below the detection limit by 16 hours after the injections.

After IV use, serum concentrations peaked by the end of infusion, then declined at a slightly more rapid rate than after IM or SC administration, becoming undetectable 4 hours after infusion. Elimination half-life was ≈ 2 hours.

Interferon could not be detected in urine; the kidney may be the main site of interferon catabolism.

Indications:

Hairy cell leukemia: In select patients ≥ 18 years of age, both previously splenectomized and nonsplenectomized.

Malignant melanoma: Adjuvant to surgical treatment in patients ≥ 18 years with malignant melanoma who are free of disease but at high risk for systemic recurrence within 56 days of surgery.

Condylomata acuminata: Intralesional treatment of genital or venereal warts in patients who do not respond to other treatment modalities or whose lesions are more readily treatable by interferon alfa-2b.

AIDS-related Kaposi's sarcoma: In select patients ≥ 18 years of age.

Chronic hepatitis non-A, non-B/C: In patients ≥ 18 years of age with compensated liver disease and a history of blood or blood product exposure or are HCV antibody positive.

Chronic hepatitis B: In patients ≥ 18 years of age with compensated liver disease and HBV replication. Patients must be serum HBsAg positive for at least 6 months and have HBV replication (serum HBeAg positive) with elevated serum ALT.

Unlabeled uses: Alpha interferons have been used for a variety of conditions, a list of which follows.

Interferon Alfa Unlabeled Uses		
Significant activity	Limited activity	No activity
	Neoplastic Diseases	
Bladder tumors (local use for superficial tumors)	Acute leukemias	Breast cancer
Carcinoid tumor	Cervical carcinoma	Colorectal carcinoma
Chronic myelogenous leukemia	Chronic lymphocytic leukemia	Gastric carcinoma
Cutaneous T-cell lymphoma	Hodgkin's disease	Lung carcinoma
Essential thrombocythemia	Malignant gliomas	Pancreatic carcinoma
Non-Hodgkin's lymphoma (low-grade)	Melanoma	Prostatic carcinoma
	Multiple myeloma	Soft tissue carcinoma
	Nasopharyngeal carcinoma	
	Osteosarcoma	
	Ovarian carcinoma	
	Renal carcinoma	
Viral Infections		**Miscellaneous**
Cutaneous warts	Papillomaviruses	Multiple sclerosis
Cytomegaloviruses	Rhinoviruses	
Herpes keratoconjunctivitis	Vaccinia virus	
Herpes simplex	Varicella zoster	

Contraindications:

Hypersensitivity to interferon alfa-2b or any components of the product.

Warnings:

Hairy cell leukemia:

Monitoring – Before initiating therapy, perform tests to quantitate peripheral blood hemoglobin, platelets, granulocytes and hairy cells and bone marrow hairy cells. Monitor periodically to determine response.

Do not give IM to patients with platelet counts < 50,000/mm^3. Instead, give SC.

Cardiovascular adverse experiences such as significant hypotension, arrhythmia or tachycardia (≥ 150 beats/min), were observed in ≈ 3% of patients studied with various malignancies who were treated at doses higher than those for hairy cell leukemia. Hypotension may occur during use, or for up to 2 days post-therapy, and may require supportive therapy, including fluid replacement, to maintain intravascular volume. Closely monitor patients with recent MI or previous or current arrhythmic disorder.

CNS effects (eg, depression, confusion, other alterations of mental status) were seen in ≈ 2% of hairy cell leukemia patients. Overall incidence in a larger patient population with other malignancies treated with higher doses was 10%.

Condylomata acuminata:

Do not use 3, 5 and 25 million IU strengths intralesionally; the dilution would result in a hypertonic solution. Do not use 50 million IU strength for condylomata.

AIDS-related Kaposi's sarcoma:

Monitoring – Perform lesion measurements and blood counts prior to initiation of therapy; monitor periodically during treatment.

Rapidly progressive visceral disease – Do not use.

Chronic hepatitis – NANB/C:

Monitoring – Before treatment, establish and consider the following criteria: Bilirubin ≤ 2 mg/dl; albumin stable and within normal limits; prothrombin time (PT) < 3 seconds prolonged; WBC ≥ 3000/mm^3; platelets > 70,000/mm^3; serum creatinine normal or near normal. Evaluate CBC and platelet counts; repeat at weeks 1 and 2 after therapy initiation, monthly thereafter. Evaluate ALT levels after 2, 16 and 24 weeks.

Pre-existing psychiatric condition/history of severe psychiatric disorder – Do not treat; discontinue therapy in any patient developing severe depression.

Pre-existing thyroid abnormalities – Patients whose thyroid function cannot be maintained in the normal range by medication should not be treated.

Chronic hepatitis B:

Monitoring – Before treatment, establish and consider the following criteria: Bilirubin normal; albumin stable and within normal limits; PT < 3 seconds prolonged; WBC ≥ 4000/mm^3; platelets ≥ 100,000/mm^3. Evaluate CBC and platelet counts, then repeat at weeks 1, 2, 4, 8, 12 and 16. Evaluate liver function tests, including serum ALT, albumin and bilirubin at treatment weeks 1, 2, 4, 8, 12 and 16. Evaluate HBeAg, HBsAg and ALT at the end of therapy and 3 and 6 months post-therapy.

ALT increase – A transient increase in ALT ≥ 2 times baseline (flare) can occur, generally 8 to 12 weeks after therapy initiation, and is more frequent in responders. Continue therapy unless signs and symptoms of hepatic failure occur.

Chronic hepatitis NANB/C and B: Do not treat patients with decompensated liver disease, autoimmune hepatitis; history of autoimmune disease, or immunosuppressed transplant recipients. In these patients, worsening liver disease, including jaundice, hepatic encephalopathy, hepatic failure and death have occurred following therapy.

Moderate to severe adverse experiences may require modification of the patient's dosage regimen, or in some cases, termination of therapy.

Fever/"flu-like" symptoms: Because of fever and other "flu-like" symptoms associated with this drug, use cautiously in debilitating medical conditions, such as those with a history of cardiovascular disease, pulmonary disease or diabetes mellitus prone to ketoacidosis. Observe caution in coagulation disorders or severe myelosuppression.

Pulmonary infiltrates, pneumonitis and pneumonia, including fatality, have been observed rarely. Take chest X-rays of any patient developing fever, cough, dyspnea or other respiratory symptoms.

Retinal hemorrhages, cotton wool spots and retinal artery or vein obstruction have been observed rarely.

Hypersensitivity reactions have not been observed in patients receiving interferon alfa-2b.

Hepatic function impairment: Do not treat patients with decompensated liver disease, autoimmune hepatitis, history of autoimmune disease, or or immunocompromised transplant recipients. In these patients, worsening liver disease, including jaundice, hepatic encephalopathy, hepatic failure and death have occurred following therapy.

Disconrinue therapy for any patient developing signs and symptoms of liver failure.

Fertility impairment: Interferon may impair fertility.

Pregnancy: Category C.

Lactation: It is not known if this drug is excreted in breast milk.

Children: Safety and efficacy in children < 18 years of age have not been established.

Precautions:

Monitoring: In addition to tests normally required for monitoring patients, the following are recommended for all patients on interferon therapy, prior to beginning treatment and periodically thereafter: Standard hematologic tests with complete blood counts and differential, platelet counts, blood chemistries, electrolytes and liver function tests. Patients with preexisting cardiac abnormalities, or in advanced stages of cancer, should have ECGs taken before and during treatment. Refer also to the monitoring sections under Warnings for each indication.

Baseline chest X-rays are suggested; repeat if clinically indicated.

For malignant melanoma patients, monitor differential, WBC count and liver function tests weekly during the induction phase of therapy and monthly during the maintenance phase of therapy.

Photosensitivity may occur.

Drug Interactions:

Drugs that may be affected by inteferon alfa 2–b include aminophylline and zidovudine.

Adverse Reactions:

The most frequently reported reactions are flu-like symptoms, particularly fever, headache, chills, myalgia and fatigue. Other adverse reactions include dizziness; paresthesia; depression; anxiety; confusion; hypoesthesia; amnesia; impaired concentration; nervousness; irritability; somnolence; decreased libido; nausea; diarrhea; vomiting; anorexia; dyspnea; constipation; loose stools; abdominal pain; pharyngitis; nasal congestion; dyspnea; coughing; sinusitis; dry mouth/thirst; arthralgia; asthenia; rigors; back pain; muscle pain/weakness; rash; pruritus; dry skin; dermatitis; alopecia; moniliasis; edema/facial edema; chest pain; increased sweating; malaise; taste alteration; insomnia; weight loss; herpes simplex; gingivitis; lab test abnormalities including hemoglobin, WBC count, platelet count, serum creatinine, alkaline phosphatase, AST, ALT and granulocyte count.

Administration and Dosage:

Patients should be well hydrated, especially during the initial stages of treatment.

Hairy cell leukemia: 2 million IU/m^2, IM or SC 3 times/week.

Maintain this dosage regimen unless the disease progresses rapidly, or severe intolerance occurs.

The patient may self-administer at bedtime.

Malignant melanoma: 20 million IU/m^2 IV on 5 consecutive days/weeks for 4 weeks. Maintenance dosage is 10 million IU/m^2 SC 3 times/week for 48 weeks.

Perform regular laboratory testing to monitor abnormalities for the purpose of dose modification. If adverse reactions develop during interferon alfa-2b treatment, particularly if granulocytes decrease to < 500/mm^3 or ALT/AST rises to > 5 × upper limit of normal, temporarily discontinue treatment until adverse reactions abate.

Restart interferon alfa-2b at 50% of the previous dose. If intolerance persists or if granulocytes decrease to < 250/mm^3 or ALT/AST rises to > 10 × upper limit of normal, discontinue interferon alfa-2b therapy.

Maintain therapy for 1 year unless there is a progression of disease.

Condylomata acuminata: 1 million IU/lesion 3 times/wk for 3 weeks intralesionally. Use only 10 million IU vial since dilution of other strengths required for intralesional use results in a hypertonic solution. Do not reconstitute 10 million IU vial with > 1 ml diluent. Use tuberculin or similar syringe and 25 to 30 gauge needle. Do not go beneath lesion too deeply or inject too superficially. As many as 5 lesions can be treated at one time.

Maximum response usually occurs 4 to 8 weeks after therapy initiation. If results are not satisfactory after 12 to 16 weeks, a second course may be instituted.

Drug delivery: Direct the needle at the center of the base of the wart and at an angle almost parallel to the plane of the skin. This will deliver the interferon to the dermal core of the lesion, infiltrating the lesion and causing a small wheal.

AIDS-related Kaposi's sarcoma: 30 million IU/m^2 3 times a week administered SC or IM. Use only 50 million IU vial. Maintain the selected dosage regimen unless the disease progresses rapidly or severe intolerance occurs. When patients initiate therapy at 30 million IU/m^2 3 times a week, average dose tolerated at end of 12 weeks therapy is 110 million IU/week and 75 million IU/week at end of 24 weeks therapy.

Chronic hepatitis non-A, non-B/C: 3 million IU 3 times/week SC or IM. Normalization of ALT levels may occur in some patients as early as 2 weeks after treatment initiation; however, current experience suggests completing a 6 month course of therapy in responding patients. Patients who relapse may be retreated with the same dosage regimen to which they had previously responded.

Chronic hepatitis B: 30 to 35 million IU per week SC or IM, either as 5 million IU daily or 10 million IU 3 times a week for 16 weeks.

Decreased granulocyte or platelet counts – Use the following guidelines:

Interferon Alfa-2b Dose with Decreased Granulocyte or Platelet Counts		
Granulocyte count	Platelet count	Interferon alfa-2b dose
< 750/mm^3	< 50,000/mm^3	Reduce by 50%
< 500/mm^3	< 30,000/mm^3	Interrupt

When platelet or granulocyte counts return to normal or baseline values, reinstitute therapy at up to 100% of initial dose.

LEVAMISOLE HCl

Tablets: 50 mg levamisole base *(Rx)*	*Ergamisol* (Janssen)

Actions:

Pharmacology: Levamisole is an immunomodulator. The effects of levamisole on the immune system are complex. The drug appears to restore depressed immune function rather than to stimulate response to above normal levels. Besides its immunomodulatory function, levamisole also inhibits alkaline phosphatase and has cholinergic activity.

Pharmacokinetics: It appears that levamisole is rapidly absorbed from the GI tract. The plasma elimination half-life is between 3 to 4 hours. Levamisole 150 mg is extensively metabolized by the liver, and the metabolites are excreted mainly by the kidneys (70% over 3 days). The elimination half-life of metabolite excretion is 16 hours. Approximately 5% is excreted in the feces; < 5% is excreted unchanged in the urine and < 0.2% unchanged in the feces. Approximately 12% is recovered in urine as the glucuronide of p–hydroxy-levamisole.

Indications:

Only as adjuvant treatment in combination with fluorouracil after surgical resection in patients with Dukes' stage C colon cancer.

Contraindications:

Hypersensitivity to the drug or its components.

Warnings:

Agranulocytosis: Levamisole has been associated with agranulocytosis, sometimes fatal. Neutropenia is usually reversible following discontinuation of therapy.

Higher than recommended doses of levamisole may be associated with an increased incidence of agranulocytosis, so do not exceed the recommended dose.

The combination of levamisole and fluorouracil has been associated with frequent neutropenia, anemia and thrombocytopenia.

Pregnancy: Category C.

Lactation: It is not known whether levamisole is excreted in breast milk; it is excreted in cows' milk.

Children: Safety and efficacy of levamisole in children have not been established.

Precautions:

Monitoring: On the first day of therapy with levamisole and fluorouracil, perform a CBC with differential and platelets, electrolytes and liver function tests. Thereafter, perform a CBC with differential and platelets weekly prior to each fluorouracil treatment; perform electrolyte and liver function tests every 3 months for a total of 1 year.

Drug Interactions:

Drugs that may be affected by levamisole include alcohol and phenytoin.

Adverse Reactions:

Adverse reactions occurring in ≥ 3% of patients include leukopenia; thrombocytopenia; anemia; dermatitis; alopecia; fatigue; fever; rigors; nausea; diarrhea; stomatitis; vomiting; anorexia; abdominal pain; constipation; taste perversion; arthralgia; myalgia; dizziness; headache; paresthesia; somnolence; abnormal tearing; infection.

Administration and Dosage:

Treatment: Initiate levamisole no earlier than 7 and no later than 30 days post-surgery at a dose of 50 mg every 8 hours for 3 days repeated every 14 days for 1 year. Initiate fluorouracil therapy no earlier than 21 days and no later than 35 days after surgery providing the patient is out of the hospital, ambulatory, maintaining normal oral nutrition, has well healed wounds and is fully recovered from any postoperative complications. If levamisole has been initiated from 7 to 20 days after surgery, initiate fluorouracil therapy coincident with the second course of levamisole, ie, at 21 to 34 days. If levamisole is initiated from 21 to 30 days after surgery, initiate fluorouracil simultaneously with the first course of levamisole.

ALTRETAMINE (Hexamethylmelamine)

Capsules: 50 mg *(Rx)*	*Hexalen* (US Bioscience)

Warning:

Monitor peripheral blood counts at least monthly, prior to the initiation of each course of altretamine therapy and as clinically indicated.

Because of the possibility of altretamine-related neurotoxicity, perform neurologic examination regularly during administration.

Actions:

Pharmacology: Altretamine, formerly known as hexamethylmelamine, is a synthetic cytotoxic antineoplastic s–triazine derivative. The precise mechanism by which altretamine exerts its cytotoxic effect is unknown.

Pharmacokinetics: Altretamine is well absorbed following oral administration, but undergoes rapid and extensive demethylation in the liver, producing variations in altretamine plasma levels. The principal metabolites are pentamethylmelamine and tetramethylmelamine. After oral administration to 11 patients with advanced ovarian cancer in doses of 120 to 300 mg/m^2, peak plasma levels were reached between 0.5 and 3 hours, varying from 0.2 to 20.8 mg/L. Half-life of the β-phase of elimination ranged from 4.7 to 10.2 hours. Altretamine and metabolites show binding to plasma proteins. The free fractions of altretamine, pentamethylmelamine and tetramethylmelamine are 6%, 25% and 50%, respectively.

Following oral administration of 4 mg/kg, urinary recovery was 61% at 24 hours and 90% at 72 hours. Human urinary metabolites were N–demethylated homologues of altretamine with < 1% unmetabolized altretamine excreted at 24 hours.

Indications:

For use as a single agent in the palliative treatment of patients with persistent or recurrent ovarian cancer following first-line therapy with a cisplatin- or alkylating agent-based combination.

Contraindications:

Hypersensitivity to altretamine.

Pre-existing severe bone marrow depression or severe neurologic toxicity; however, altretamine has been administered safely to patients heavily pretreated with cisplatin or alkylating agents including patients with pre-existing cisplatin neuropathies. Careful monitoring of neurologic function in these patients is essential.

Warnings:

Neurotoxicity: Altretamine causes mild to moderate neurotoxicity. Peripheral neuropathy and CNS symptoms (eg, mood disorders, disorders of consciousness, ataxia, dizziness, vertigo) have occurred. Neurologic toxicity appears to be reversible when therapy is discontinued.

Hematologic: Altretamine causes mild to moderate dose-related myelosuppression. Monitor peripheral blood counts prior to the initiation of each course of therapy, monthly and as clinically indicated.

Pregnancy: Category D.

Lactation: It is not known whether altretamine is excreted in breast milk. It is recommended that breastfeeding be discontinued if the mother is treated with altretamine.

Children: Safety and efficacy in children have not been established.

Precautions:

Nausea and vomiting: With continuous high-dose daily altretamine, nausea and vomiting of gradual onset occur frequently. In most instances, these symptoms are controllable with antiemetics; at times, however, the severity requires dose reduction or, rarely, discontinuation of therapy.

Drug Interactions:

Drugs that may interact with altretamine include cimetidine and monoamine oxidase inhibitors.

Adverse Reactions:

Adverse reactions occurring in ≥ 3% of patients include nausea and vomiting; increased alkaline phosphatase; peripheral sensory neuropathy; leukopenia; thrombocytopenia; anemia; changes in serum creatinine and BUN.

Administration and Dosage:

Altretamine is administered orally. Calculate doses on the basis of body surface area.

Altretamine may be administered either for 14 or 21 consecutive days in a 28 day cycle at a dose of 260 $mg/m^2/day$. Give the total daily dose as 4 divided oral doses after meals and at bedtime.

Temporarily discontinue altretamine (for ≥ 14 days) and subsequently restart at 200 $mg/m^2/day$ for any of the following situations: GI intolerance unresponsive to symptomatic measures; WBC < 2000/mm^3 or granulocyte count < 1000/mm^3; platelet count < 75,000/mm^3; progressive neurotoxicity.

If neurologic symptoms fail to stabilize on the reduced dose schedule, discontinue altretamine indefinitely.

CLADRIBINE (2-chlorodeoxyadenosine; CdA)

Injection: 1 mg/ml *(Rx)*	*Leustatin* (Ortho Biotech)

Warning:

Anticipate suppression of bone marrow function. This is usually reversible and appears to be dose-dependent. High doses (4 to 9 times the recommended dose for hairy cell leukemia) in conjunction with cyclophosphamide and total body irradiation as preparation for bone marrow transplantation, have been associated with severe, irreversible, neurologic toxicity (paraparesis/quadriparesis) or acute renal insufficiency in 45% of patients treated for 7 to 14 days.

Actions:

Pharmacology: Cladribine is a synthetic antineoplastic agent for continuous IV infusion. The selective toxicity of cladribine towards certain normal and malignant lymphocyte and monocyte populations is based on the relative activities of deoxycytidine kinase, deoxynucleotidase and adenosine deaminase. It is postulated that cells with high deoxycytidine kinase and low deoxynucleotidase activities will be selectively killed by cladribine as toxic deoxynucleotides accumulate intracellularly. Cladribine can be distinguished from other chemotherapeutic agents affecting purine metabolism in that it is cytotoxic to both actively dividing and quiescent lymphocytes and monocytes, inhibiting both DNA synthesis and repair.

Pharmacokinetics: For patients with normal renal function, the mean terminal half-life was 5.4 hours. Mean value for clearance and steady-state volume of distribution were 978 ± 422 ml/hr/kg and 4.5± 2.8 L/kg, respectively. Cladribine is bound approximately 20% to plasma proteins.

Indications:

Hairy cell leukemia (HCL): Treatment of active HCL as defined by clinically significant anemia, neutropenia, thrombocytopenia or disease-related symptoms.

Unlabeled uses: Cladribine appears to be beneficial in the following conditions: Advanced cutaneous T-cell lymphomas; chronic lymphocytic leukemia; non-Hodgkins lymphomas; acute myeloid leukemia; autoimmune hemolytic anemia; mycosis fungoides or the Sezary syndrome.

Contraindications:

Hypersensitivity to the drug or any of its components.

Warnings:

Bone marrow suppression: Severe bone marrow suppression, including neutropenia, anemia and thrombocytopenia, has been commonly observed in patients treated with cladribine, especially at high doses.

Nephrotoxicity/Neurotoxicity: In a study using high-dose cladribine (4 to 9 times the recommended dose for HCL) as part of a bone marrow transplant conditioning regimen, which also included high-dose cyclophosphamide and total body irradiation, acute nephrotoxicity and delayed onset neurotoxicity were observed.

Fever 37.8°C (≥100°F) was associated with the use of cladribine in ≈ 66% of patients in the first month of therapy.

Renal function impairment: Development of acute renal insufficiency in some patients receiving high doses of cladribine has been described.

Mutagenesis: As expected for compounds in this class, the actions of cladribine yield DNA damage.

Pregnancy: Category D.

Lactation: It is not known whether this drug is excreted in breast milk.

Children: Safety and efficacy in children have not been established.

Precautions:

Monitoring: Cladribine is a potent antineoplastic agent with potentially significant toxic side effects. Closely observe patients undergoing therapy for signs of hematologic and non-hematologic toxicity. Periodic assessment of peripheral blood counts, particularly during the first 4 to 8 weeks post-treatment, is recommended to detect the development of anemia, neutropenia and thrombocytopenia and for early detection of any potential sequelae.

Adverse Reactions:

Adverse reactions occurring in ≥ 3% of patients include: Severe neutropenia; severe anemia; thrombocytopenia; CD4 count suppression; bone marrow hypocellularity; fever; chills; infection; fatigue; rash; headache; injection site reactions; asthenia; diaphoresis; malaise; trunk pain; decreased appetite; nausea; vomiting; diarrhea; constipation; abdominal pain; purpura; petechiae; epistaxis; dizziness; insomnia; edema; tachycardia; abnormal breath sounds; cough; abnormal chest sounds; shortness of breath; pruritus; pain; erythema; myalgia and arthralgia.

Administration and Dosage:

Usual dose: The recommended dose and schedule for active HCL is a single course given by continuous infusion for 7 consecutive days at a dose of 0.09 mg/kg/day. Deviations from this dosage regimen are not advised. Consider delaying or discontinuing the drug if neurotoxicity or renal toxicity occurs.

HYDROXYUREA

Capsules: 500 mg ***(Rx)***	*Hydrea* (Immunex)

Actions:

Pharmacology: The precise mechanism of cytotoxic action is unknown. Hydroxyurea causes an immediate inhibition of deoxyribonucleic acid (DNA) synthesis without interfering with the synthesis of ribonucleic acid (RNA) or protein. It may also inhibit the incorporation of thymidine into DNA.

Pharmacokinetics:

Absorption/Distribution – Hydroxyurea is readily absorbed from the GI tract, reaching peak serum concentrations within 2 hours; by 24 hours the serum concentration is essentially zero. Hydroxyurea readily crosses the blood-brain barrier with peak CSF levels at 3 hours.

Metabolism/Excretion – About 50% of an oral dose is degraded in the liver and excreted into the urine as urea and as respiratory carbon dioxide; the remainder is excreted intact in the urine. Approximately 80% may be recovered in the urine within 12 hours.

Indications:

Melanoma; resistant chronic myelocytic leukemia; recurrent, metastatic or inoperable carcinoma of the ovary.

Concomitant administration with irradiation therapy in the local control of primary squamous cell (epidermoid) carcinomas of the head and neck, excluding the lip.

Contraindications:

Marked bone marrow depression (leukopenia < 2500/mm^3 WBC or thrombocytopenia < 100,000/mm^3 platelets); severe anemia.

Warnings:

Erythema: Patients who have received prior irradiation therapy may have an exacerbation of post-irradiation erythema.

Bone marrow suppression may occur, and leukopenia is generally the first and most common manifestation. Thrombocytopenia and anemia occur less often, seldom without a preceding leukopenia. Correct severe anemia with whole blood replacement before initiating hydroxyurea therapy.

Erythrocytic abnormalities: Self-limiting megaloblastic erythropoiesis is often seen early in hydroxyurea therapy. Hydroxyurea may delay plasma iron clearance and reduce the rate of iron utilization by erythrocytes, but it does not alter the RBC survival time.

Elderly patients may be more sensitive to the effects of hydroxyurea and may require a lower dosage regimen.

Renal function impairment: Hydroxyurea is excreted by the kidneys; therefore, use with caution in patients with marked renal dysfunction.

Pregnancy: Drugs that affect DNA synthesis may be mutagenic. Do not use in women who are or who may become pregnant, unless the potential benefits outweigh the possible hazards. Contraceptive measures are recommended during therapy.

Children: Dosage regimens for children have not been established.

Precautions:

Monitoring: Therapy requires close supervision. Determine the complete status of the blood, including bone marrow examination if indicated, as well as renal and liver function prior to and during treatment.

Hematology – Monitor hemoglobin, total leukocyte counts and platelet counts at least once a week throughout therapy.

Drug Interactions:

Drug/Lab test interactions: **Serum uric acid, BUN** and **creatinine**levels may be increased by hydroxyurea.

Adverse Reactions:

Adverse reactions may include leukopenia; anemia; thrombocytopenia; fever; chills; malaise; elevation of hepatic enzymes; abnormal BSP retention; severe gastric distress; stomatitis; anorexia; nausea; vomiting; diarrhea; constipation; maculopapular rash; facial erythema; moderate drowsiness.

Administration and Dosage:

Base dosage on the patient's actual or ideal weight, whichever is less.

An adequate trial period to determine effectiveness is 6 weeks. When there is regression in tumor size or arrest in tumor growth, continue therapy indefinitely. Interrupt therapy if the WBC drops below 2500/mm^3 or the platelet count below 100,000/mm^3. In these cases, recheck counts after 3 days, and resume therapy when the counts rise significantly toward normal. Since the hematopoietic rebound is prompt, it is usually necessary to omit only a few doses. If prompt rebound has not occurred during combined hydroxyurea and irradiation therapy, irradiation may also be interrupted. However, this is rare.

Solid tumors: Patients on intermittent therapy rarely require complete discontinuation of therapy because of toxicity.

Intermittent therapy – 80 mg/kg as a single dose every third day.

Continuous therapy – 20 to 30 mg/kg as a single daily dose.

Concomitant irradiation therapy (carcinoma of head and neck): 80 mg/kg as a single dose every third day. Begin hydroxyurea at least 7 days before initiation of irradiation and continue during radiotherapy and indefinitely afterwards, provided the patient is adequately observed and exhibits no unusual or severe reactions. Administer maximum irradiation dose appropriate for the therapeutic situation; adjustment of irradiation dosage is not usually necessary with concomitant hydroxyurea.

Resistant chronic myelocytic leukemia: Continuous therapy (20 to 30 mg/kg as a single daily dose) is recommended.

BCG, INTRAVESICAL

Freeze-dried suspension for reconstitution *(Rx)*	*TICE BCG* (Organon), *TheraCys* (Connaught)

Actions:

Pharmacology: BCG is a freeze-dried suspension of an attenuated strain of *Mycobacterium bovis* (Bacillus Calmette and Guerin) used in the non-specific active therapy of carcinoma in situ of the urinary bladder. BCG live (*TheraCys*) is used only for carcinoma in situ of the urinary bladder; BCG Vaccine (*TICE BCG*) is also used for immunization against tuberculosis.

BCG promotes a local inflammatory reaction with histiocytic and leukocytic infiltration in the urinary bladder. The local inflammatory effects are associated with an apparent elimination or reduction of superficial cancerous lesions of the urinary bladder. The exact mechanism is unknown.

Indications:

Intravesical use in the treatment of primary and relapsed carcinoma in situ of the urinary bladder to eliminate residual tumor cells and to reduce the frequency of tumor recurrence (*TheraCys*); primary or secondary treatment in absence of invasive cancer for patients with medical contraindications to radical surgery (*TICE BCG*).

Treatment of carcinoma in situ with or without associated papillary tumors. Not indicated for the treatment of papillary tumors occurring alone.

Therapy for patients with carcinoma in situ of the bladder following failure to respond to other treatment regimens.

Contraindications:

Patients on immunosuppressive or corticosteroid therapy, with compromised immune systems, or asymptomatic carriers with a positive HIV serology due to the risk of overwhelming systemic mycobacterial sepsis.

Fever, unless the cause of the fever is determined and evaluated.

Urinary tract infection because administration may result in the risk of disseminated BCG infection or in an increased severity of bladder irritation.

TheraCys: As an immunizing agent for the prevention of tuberculosis.

TICE BCG: Positive Mantoux test, only if there is evidence of an active TB infection.

Warnings:

Tuberculosis prevention: Do not use *TheraCys* as an immunizing agent to prevent TB. These agents may cause TB sensitivity.

Cancer prevention: These agents are not vaccines for cancer prevention.

Urinary status monitoring: Since administration of intravesical BCG causes an inflammatory response in the bladder and has been associated with hematuria, urinary frequency, dysuria and bacterial urinary tract infection, careful monitoring of urinary status is required.

BCG infection, systemic: Death has occurred due to systemic BCG infection; closely monitor for symptoms of such infection. Withhold BCG upon any suspicion of systemic infection (eg, granulomatous hepatitis).

Antimicrobial therapy: Evaluate patients undergoing antimicrobial therapy for other infections to assess whether the therapy will obviate the effects of BCG actions.

Small bladder capacity: Consider increased risk of severity of local irritation when deciding to treat with these agents.

Hypersensitivity: Allergic reactions are possible in individuals sensitive to the product components.

Pregnancy: Category C.

Lactation: It is not known whether BCG is excreted in breast milk.

Children: Safety and efficacy for use in children have not been established.

Precautions:

Contains viable attenuated mycobacteria. Handle as infectious. Use aseptic technique.

Urine disinfection: Disinfect urine voided for 6 hours after instillation with an equal volume of 5% hypochlorite solution (undiluted household bleach) and allow to stand for 15 minutes before flushing.

Transurethral resection: Do not give intravesical BCG any sooner than 1 to 2 weeks following transurethral resection. Fatalities due to disseminated BCG infection have occurred with BCG use after traumatic catheterization.

Drug Interactions:

Bone marrow depressants, immunosuppressants or **radiation** may impair response to BCG or increase the risk of osteomyelitis or disseminated BCG infection.

Adverse Reactions:

Adverse reactions occurring in ≥ 3% of patients include dysuria; urinary frequency; hematuria; cystitis; urinary urgency; urinary tract infection; urinary incontinence; cramps/pain; decreased bladder capacity; nocturia; malaise/fatigue; fever; chills; anemia; nausea/vomiting; anorexia; renal toxicity; genital pain; myalgia/arthralgia/arthritis; diarhea; leukopenia.

Administration and Dosage:

Intravesical treatment and prophylaxis for carcinoma in situ of the urinary bladder:

TheraCys – Begin between 7 to 14 days after biopsy or transurethral resection. Give a dose of 3 vials intravesically under aseptic conditions once weekly for 6 weeks (induction therapy). Follow the induction therapy by one treatment given 3, 6, 12, 18 and 24 months after initial treatment.

TICE BCG – Allow 7 to 14 days to elapse after bladder biopsy or transurethral resection before administration. Patients should not drink fluids for 4 hours before treatment and should empty their bladder prior to administration. The dose consists of one amp suspended in 50 ml preservative free saline. A standard treatment schedule consists of one instillation per week for 6 weeks. This may be repeated once if tumor remission has not been achieved and if the clinical circumstances warrant. Thereafter, continue approximately monthly for at least 6 to 12 months.

ALDESLEUKIN (Interleukin-2; IL-2)

Powder for Injection, lyophilized: 22 x 10^6 IU per vial (18 million IU [1.1 mg] per ml when reconstituted) *(Rx)*	*Proleukin* (Chiron)

Warning:

Aldesleukin administration has been associated with capillary leak syndrome (CLS). CLS results in hypotension and reduced organ perfusion which may be severe and can result in death (see Warnings).

Restrict therapy to patients with normal cardiac and pulmonary functions as defined by thallium stress testing and formal pulmonary function testing. Use extreme caution in patients with normal thallium stress tests and pulmonary function tests who have a history of prior cardiac or pulmonary disease.

Hold aldesleukin administration in patients developing moderate to severe lethargy or somnolence; continued administration may result in coma.

Actions:

Pharmacology: Aldesleukin, a human recombinant interleukin-2 product, is a highly purified protein (lymphokine) produced by recombinant DNA technology using a genetically engineered *Eschericia coli* strain containing an analog of the human interleukin-2 gene. Administration produces multiple immunological effects in a dose-dependent manner. These effects include activation of cellular immunity with profound lymphocytosis, eosinophilia and thrombocytopenia, the production of cytokines (including tumor necrosis factor, IL-1 and gamma interferon) and inhibition of tumor growth. The exact mechanism by which aldesleukin mediates its antitumor activity is unknown.

Pharmacokinetics: The pharmacokinetic profile of aldesleukin is characterized by high plasma concentrations following a short IV infusion, rapid distribution to extravascular, extracellular space and elimination from the body by metabolism in the kidneys with little or no bioactive protein excreted in the urine. Approximately 30% of the dose initially distributes to the plasma.

Following the initial rapid organ distribution, the primary route of clearance of circulating aldesleukin is the kidney; it is cleared from the circulation by both glomerular filtration and peritubular extraction. The mean clearance rate in cancer patients is 268 ml/min.

Indications:

Metastatic renal cell carcinoma in adults (≥ 18 years of age).

Unlabeled uses: Aldesleukin is being investigated in the treatment of Kaposi's sarcoma in combination with zidovudine. Aldesleukin may be beneficial for metastatic melanoma; 20% to 30% response rates have been reported in combination with low-dose cyclophosphamide. Aldesleukin has been used with some success in the treatment of colorectal cancer and non-Hodgkin's lymphoma, often in combination with lymphokine activated killer (LAK) cells.

Contraindications:

Hypersensitivity to interleukin-2 or any component of the formulation; abnormal thallium stress test or pulmonary function tests; organ allografts.

Retreatment is contraindicated in patients who experienced the following toxicities while receiving an earlier course of therapy.

Warnings:

Capillary leak syndrome (CLS): Aldesleukin has been associated with CLS which begins immediately after treatment starts and results from extravasation of plasma proteins and fluid into the extravascular space and loss of vascular tone. This usually results in a concomitant drop in mean arterial blood pressure within 2 to 12 hours after the start of treatment and reduced organ perfusion which may be severe and can result in death. With continued therapy, clinically significant hypotension (systolic blood pressure < 90 mm Hg or a 20 mm Hg drop from baseline systolic pressure) and hypoperfusion will occur. In addition, extravasation will lead to edema and effusions. The CLS may be associated with cardiac arrhythmias (supraventricular and ventricular), angina, MI, respiratory insufficiency requiring intubation, GI bleeding or infarction, renal insufficiency and mental status changes.

Clinical evaluation: Because of the severe adverse events which generally accompany therapy at the recommended dosages, perform thorough clinical evaluation to exclude from treatment patients with significant cardiac, pulmonary, renal, hepatic or CNS impairment.

CNS metastases: Aldesleukin may exacerbate disease symptoms in patients with clinically unrecognized or untreated CNS metastases. In addition, exercise extreme caution in treating patients with a history of seizure disorder because aldesleukin may cause seizures.

Bacterial infections: Intensive treatment is associated with impaired neutrophil function (reduced chemotaxis) and with an increased risk of disseminated infection, including sepsis and bacterial endocarditis. Consequently, adequately treat preexisting bacterial infections prior to initiation of therapy.

Renal/Hepatic function impairment: Occurs during treatment. Use of concomitant medications known to be nephrotoxic or hepatotoxic may further increase toxicity to the kidney or liver.

Fertility impairment: It is recommended that this drug not be administered to fertile persons of either sex not practicing effective contraception.

Pregnancy: Category C.

Lactation: It is not known whether this drug is excreted in breast milk.

Children: Safety and efficacy in children < 18 years of age have not been established.

Precautions:

Monitoring: The following clinical evaluations are recommended for all patients prior to beginning treatment and then daily during drug administration: Standard hematologic tests, including CBC, differential and platelet counts; blood chemistries, including electrolytes, renal and hepatic function tests; chest x-rays.

All patients should have baseline pulmonary function tests with arterial blood gases. Screen all patients with a stress thallium study. Document normal ejection fraction and unimpaired wall motion.

Daily monitoring during therapy should include vital signs (temperature, pulse, blood pressure and respiration rate) and weight. In a patient with a decreased blood pressure, especially < 90 mm Hg, conduct constant cardiac monitoring for rhythm. If an abnormal complex or rhythm is seen, perform an ECG. Take vital signs in these hypotensive patients hourly and check CVP.

Cardiac function is assessed daily by clinical examination and assessment of vital signs.

Anemia/Thrombocytopenia may occur. Leukopenia and neutropenia may also occur.

Mental status changes including irritability, confusion or depression may occur and may be indicators of bacteremia or early bacterial sepsis.

Thyroid function impairment has occurred following treatment. This impairment of thyroid function may be a manifestation of autoimmunity; consequently, exercise extra caution when treating patients with known autoimmune disease.

Allograft rejection: Aldesleukin enhancement of cellular immune function may increase the risk of allograft rejection in transplant patients.

Drug Interactions:

Drugs that may affect aldesleukin include antihypertensives, corticosteroids, cardiotoxic agents (eg, doxorubicin), hepatotoxic agents (eg, methotrexate), myelotoxic agents (eg, cytotoxic chemotherapy) and nephrotoxic agents (eg, aminoglycosides). Aldesleukin may affect psychotropic agents.

Adverse Reactions:

Adverse reactions occurring in ≥ 3% of patients include hypotension; sinus tachycardia; arrhythmias; bradycardia; PVCs; premature atrial contractions; myocardial ischemia; pulmonary congestion; dyspnea; pulmonary edema; respiratory failure; tachypnea; pleural effusion; wheezing; jaundice; ascites; anemia; thrombocytopenia; leukopenia; coagulation disorders; leukocytosis; eosinophilia; lab test abnormalities including elevated bilirubin, BUN, serum creatinine, transaminase, alkaline phosphatase, hypomagnesemia, acidosos, hypocalcemia, hypophophatemia, hypo- or hyperkalemia, hyperuricemia, hypoalbuminemia, hypoproteinemia, hyponatremia, alkalosis; nausea and vomiting; diarrhea; stomatitis, anorexia; GI bleeding; dyspepsia; constipation; mental status changes; dizziness; sensory dysfunction; special sensory disorders; syncope; oliguria/anuria; proteinuria; hematuria; dysuria; pruritus; erythema; rash; dry skin; exfoliative dermatitis; purpura/petechiae; arthralgia; myalgia; fever/chills; pain; fatigue/weakness/malaise; edema; infection; weight gain/loss; headache; conjunctivitis; injection site reactions.

Administration and Dosage:

Metastatic renal cell carcinoma in adults: Each course of treatment consists of two 5 day treatment cycles separated by a rest period: 600,000 IU/kg (0.037 mg/kg) administered every 8 hours by a 15 minute IV infusion for a total of 14 doses. Following 9 days of rest, repeat the schedule for another 14 doses, for a maximum of 28 doses per course.

Retreatment: Evaluate patients for response approximately 4 weeks after completion of a course of therapy and again immediately prior to the scheduled start of the next treatment course. Additional courses of treatment may be given to patients only if there is some tumor shrinkage following the last course and retreatment is not contraindicated. Separate each treatment course by a rest period of at least 7 weeks from the date of hospital discharge. Tumors have continued to regress up to 12 months following the initiation of therapy.

Dose modification: Accomplish dose modification for toxicity by holding or interrupting a dose rather than reducing the dose to be given.

PACLITAXEL

Injection: 30 mg/5 ml *(Rx)* — *Taxol* (Bristol-Myers Squibb)

Warning:

Severe hypersensitivity reactions characterized by dyspnea and hypotension requiring treatment, angioedema and generalized urticaria have occurred in 2% of patients. Pretreat patients receiving paclitaxel with corticosteroids, diphenhydramine and H_2 antagonists to prevent these reactions. Patients who experience severe hypersensitivity reactions to paclitaxel should not be rechallenged with the drug.

Do not give paclitaxel therapy to patients with baseline neutrophil counts of < 1500 cells/mm^3. In order to monitor the occurrence of bone marrow suppression, primarily neutropenia, which may be severe and result in infection, perform frequent peripheral blood cell counts on all patients receiving paclitaxel.

Actions:

Pharmacology: Paclitaxel is a natural product with antitumor activity. It is a novel antimicrotubule agent that promotes the assembly of microtubules from tubulin dimers and stabilizes microtubules by preventing depolymerization. This stability results in the inhibition of the normal dynamic reorganization of the microtubule network that is essential for vital interphase and mitotic cellular functions.

Pharmacokinetics: Following 1 and 6 hour infusions at dosing levels of 15 to 275 mg/m^2, mean terminal half-life ranges from 5.3 to 17.4 hours, mean values for total body clearance range from 5.8 to 16.3 L/hr/m^2, and the mean steady-state volume of distribution ranges from 42 to 162 L/m^2, indicating extensive extravascular distribution or tissue binding of paclitaxel. Mean values for total body clearance range from 14.2 to 17.2 L/hr/m^2 following 24 hour infusions of 200 to 275 mg/m^2. The drug is 89% to 98% protein bound.

The disposition of paclitaxel has not been fully elucidated. After IV administration of 15 to 275 mg/m^2 doses as 1, 6 and 24 hour infusions, mean values for cumulative urinary recovery of unchanged drug range from 1.3% to 12.6% of the dose, indicating extensive non-renal clearance.

Indications:

Metastatic carcinoma of the ovary: Treatment after failure of first-line or subsequent chemotherapy.

Unlabeled uses: Paclitaxel, alone or in combination with other chemotherapy agents, is being investigated for use in the following conditions: Advanced head and neck cancer; previously untreated extensive-stage small-cell lung cancer; adenocarcinoma of the upper GI tract; hormone-refractory prostate cancer; advanced non-small-cell lung cancer; metastatic breast cancer; leukemias. Further study is needed.

Contraindications:

Hypersensitivity reactions to paclitaxel or other drugs formulated in *Cremophor EL* (polyoxyethylated castor oil); baseline neutropenia of < 1500 cells/mm^3.

Warnings:

Bone marrow suppression (primarily neutropenia) is dose-dependent and is the major dose-limiting toxicity. Do not administer to patients with baseline neutrophil counts of < 1500 cells/mm^3.

Cardiac effects: Severe conduction abnormalities have been documented in two (< 1%) patients during therapy.

Hypersensitivity: Do not use in patients with a history of severe hypersensitivity reactions to products containing *Cremophor EL*. Minor symptoms such as flushing, skin reactions, dyspnea, hypotension or tachycardia do not require interruption of therapy.

Hepatic function impairment: Exercise caution when administering to patients with severe hepatic impairment.

Pregnancy: Category D.

Lactation: It is not known whether the drug is excreted in breast milk. Discontinue nursing when receiving paclitaxel therapy.

Children: Safety and efficacy of paclitaxel in children have not been established.

Precautions:

Cardiovascular: Hypotension and bradycardia have been observed during paclitaxel administration, but generally do not require treatment.

CNS: Although the occurrence of peripheral neuropathy is frequent, the development of severe symptomatology is unusual and requires a dose reduction of 20% for all subsequent courses of paclitaxel.

Drug Interactions:

Ketoconazole and cisplatin may affect paclitaxel.

Adverse Reactions:

Adverse reactions occurring in ≥ 3% of patients include neutropenia; leukopenia; thrombocytopenia; anemia; fever; infections including urinary tract, upper respiratory tract and sepsis; bleeding; packed cell transfusions; hypersensitivity reactions including flushing, rash and dyspnea; bradycardia and hypotension during infusion; abnormal ECG; peripheral neuropathy; myalgia/arthralgia; nausea and vomiting; diarrhea; mucositis; alopecia; bilirubin elevations; alkaline phosphatase elevations; AST elevations.

Administration and Dosage:

Premedicate all patients prior to administration in order to prevent severe hypersensitivity reactions. Such premedication may consist of oral dexamethasone 20 mg administered approximately 12 and 6 hours before paclitaxel, diphenhydramine (or its equivalent) 50 mg IV 30 to 60 minutes prior to paclitaxel, and cimetidine (300 mg) or ranitidine (50 mg) IV 30 to 60 minutes before paclitaxel.

Dosage: A dose of 135 mg/m^2 administered IV over 24 hours every 3 weeks is effective in patients with metastatic carcinoma of the ovary after failure of first-line or subsequent chemotherapy. Larger doses, with or without filgrastim, have so far produced responses similar to 135 mg/m^2. Do not repeat courses of paclitaxel until the neutrophil count is at least 1500 cells/mm^3 and the platelet count is at least 100,000 cells/mm^3. Reduce dosage by 20% for subsequent courses in patients who experience severe neutropenia (neutrophils < 500 cells/mm^3 for ≥ 1 week) or severe peripheral neuropathy during therapy. The incidence and severity of neurotoxicity and hematologic toxicity increase with dose, especially > 190 mg/m^2.

DOCETAXEL

Injection: 20 and 80 mg (*Rx*) *Taxotere* (Rhone-Poulenc Rorer)

Warning:

The incidence of treatment-related mortality associated with docetaxel is increased in patients with abnormal liver function and in patients receiving higher doses.

Docetaxel should generally not be given to patients with bilirubin > upper limit of normal (ULN), or to patients with AST or ALT > 1.5 × ULN concomitant with alkaline phosphatase (AP) > 2.5 × ULN because of an increased risk for the development of grade 4 neutropenia, febrile neutropenia, infections, severe thrombocytopenia, severe stomatitis, severe skin toxicity and toxic death. Patients with isolated elevations of transaminases > 1.5 × ULN also had a higher rate of febrile neutropenia grade 4 but did not have an increased incidence of toxic death.

Do not give to patients with neutrophil counts of < 1500 cells/mm^3.

Severe hypersensitivity reactions characterized by hypotension or bronchospasm or generalized rash/erythema occurred in 0.9% of patients who received the recommended dexamethasone premedication. Docetaxel must not be given to patients who have a history of severe hypersensitivity reactions to docetaxel or to other drugs formulated with polysorbate 80.

Severe fluid retention occurred in 6% of patients despite use of a 5–day dexamethasone premedication regimen. It was characterized by one or more of the following events: Poorly tolerated peripheral edema, generalized edema, pleural effusion requiring urgent drainage, dyspnea at rest, cardiac tamponade or pronounced abdominal distention (caused by ascites).

Actions:

Pharmacology: Docetaxel, an antineoplastic agent belonging to the taxoid family, is prepared by semisynthesis beginning with a precursor extracted from the renewable needle biomass of the yew plant. Docetaxel binds to free tubulin and promotes the assembly of tubulin into stable microtubules while simultaneously inhibiting their disassembly. This leads to the production of microtubule bundles without normal function and to the stabilization of microtubules, which results in the inhibition of mitosis in cells. Docetaxel's binding to microtubules does not alter the number of protofilaments in the bound microtubules, a feature which differs from most spindle poisons currently in clinical use.

Pharmacokinetics: The area under the curve (AUC) was dose-proportional following doses of 70 to 115 mg/m^2 with infusion times of 1 to 2 hours. Docetaxel's pharmacokinetic profile is consistent with a three-compartment pharmacokinetic model, with half-lives for the α, β and γ phases of 4 minutes, 36 minutes and 11.1 hours, respectively. Mean values for total body clearance and steady-state volume of distribution were 21 L/hr/m^2 and 113 L, respectively.

Docetaxel is eliminated in both the urine and the feces following oxidative metabolism of the tert-butyl ester group, but fecal excretion was the main elimination route. About 80% of the docetaxel recovered in the feces is excreted during the first 48 hours as one major and three minor metabolites with very small amounts (< 8%) of unchanged drug. Docetaxel is ≈ 94% protein bound, mainly to α_1—acid glycoprotein, albumin and lipoproteins.

Indications:

Breast cancer: For the treatment of patients with locally advanced or metastatic breast cancer who have progressed during anthracycline-based therapy or have relapsed during anthracycline-based adjuvant therapy.

Contraindications:

History of severe hypersensitivity reactions to docetaxel or to other drugs formulated with polysorbate 80; neutrophil counts of < 1500 cells/mm^3.

Warnings:

Toxic deaths: Docetaxel administered at 100 mg/m^2 was associated with deaths considered possibly or probably related to treatment in 2.4% of patients with normal liver function and in 11% of patients with abnormal liver function (AST or ALT > 1.5 × ULN together with AP < 2.5 × ULN). Sepsis accounted for the majority of the deaths.

Fluid retention: Premedicate patients with oral corticosteroids such as dexamethasone 16 mg/day for 5 days starting 1 day prior to docetaxel to reduce the severity of fluid retention and hypersensitivity reactions (see Warning Box).

Neutropenia: Neutropenia (< 2000 neutrophils/mm^3) occurs in virtually all patients given 60 to 100 mg/m^2 of docetaxel and grade 4 neutropenia (< 500 cells/mm^3) occurs in nearly all patients given 100 mg/m^2 and in 75% to 80% of patients given 60 to 75 mg/m^2. Frequent monitoring of blood counts is, therefore, essential so that dose can be adjusted. Do not administer to patients with neutrophils < 1500 cells/mm^3.

Cutaneous reactions: Reversible cutaneous reactions characterized by a rash including localized eruptions, mainly on the feet or hands, but also on the arms, face or thorax, usually associated with pruritus, have been observed. Eruptions generally occurred within 1 week after infusion, recovered before the next infusion and were not disabling.

Hypersensitivity: Observe patients closely for hypersensitivity reactions. Hypersensitivity reactions may occur within a few minutes following initiation of a docetaxel infusion.

Hepatic function impairment: Three breast cancer patients with severe liver impairment (bilirubin > 1.7 × ULN) developed fatal GI bleeding associated with severe drug-induced thrombocytopenia (see Warning Box).

Pregnancy: *Category D.*

Lactation: It is not known whether docetaxel is excreted in breast milk. Because of the potential for serious adverse reactions in nursing infants from docetaxel, discontinue nursing prior to taking the drug.

Children: Safety and efficacy in children < 16 years of age have not been established.

Precautions:

Monitoring: To monitor the occurrence of myelotoxicity, it is recommended that frequent peripheral blood cell counts be performed on all patients (see Warnings).

Obtain bilirubin, AST or ALT and alkaline phosphatase values prior to each cycle of docetaxel therapy.

Neurologic: Severe neurosensory symptoms (paresthesia, dysesthesia, pain) were observed among 7% of patients with anthracycline-resistant breast cancer. When these occur, dosage must be adjusted. If symptoms persist, discontinue treatment.

Asthenia: Severe asthenia has been reported in 11.1% of the patients but has led to treatment discontinuation in only 2.6%. It was reported in 23% of patients with anthracycline-resistant breast cancer and 5.5% of cycles received. Fatigue and weakness may last from a few days to several weeks and may be associated with deterioration of performance status in patients with progressive disease.

Drug Interactions:

Metabolism of docetaxel may be modified by concomitant administration of compounds that induce, inhibit or are metabolized by cytochrome P450 3A4, such as cyclosporine, terfenadine, ketoconazole, erythromycin and troleandomycin.

Adverse Reactions:

Adverse reactions that may occur in ≥ 5% of patients include: Neutropenia, leukopenia, thrombocytopenia, anemia, nausea, diarrhea, vomiting, stomatitis, myalgia, arthralgia, cutaneous reactions, nail changes, infection, fever, hypersensitivity reactions, fluid retention, neurosensory reactions, neuromotor reactions, alopecia, asthenia and infusion site reactions.

Administration and Dosage:

Recommended dose: 60 to 100 mg/m^2 administered IV over 1 hour every 3 weeks.

Premedication regimen: Premedicate patients with oral corticosteroids (see Warnings).

Dosage adjustment during treatment: Patients who are dosed initially at 100 mg/m^2 and who experience either febrile neutropenia, neutrophils < 500 cels/mm^3 for > 1 week, severe or cumulative cutaneous reactions or severe peripheral neuropathy during docetaxel therapy should have the dosage adjusted from 100 to 75 mg/m^2. If the patient continues to experience these reactions, either decrease the dosage from 75 to 55 mg/m^2 or discontinue treatment. Patients who are dosed at 60 mg/m^2 and do not experience these symptoms may tolerate higher doses.

PROCARBAZINE HCl (N-Methylhydrazine; MIH)

Capsules: 50 mg *(Rx)*	*Matulane* (Roche)

Actions:

Pharmacology: The mode of cytotoxic action is not clear; procarbazine may inhibit protein, ribonucleic acid (RNA) and deoxyribonucleic acid (DNA) synthesis. Procarbazine may inhibit transmethylation of methyl groups of methionine into t-RNA. In addition, procarbazine may directly damage DNA.

Pharmacokinetics:

Absorption/Distribution – Procarbazine is rapidly and completely absorbed from the GI tract and quickly equilibrates between plasma and cerebrospinal fluid (CSF). Peak CSF levels occur in 30 to 90 minutes. Following oral administration, maximum peak plasma concentrations occur within 60 minutes.

Metabolism/Excretion – The drug is metabolized in the liver to cytotoxic products. The major portion of drug is excreted in the urine as N-isopropylterephthalamic acid (≈ 70% within 24 hours following oral and IV administration). Less than 5% is excreted in urine unchanged. After IV injection, the plasma half-life is ≈ 10 minutes.

Indications:

Hodgkin's disease: In combination with other antineoplastics for treatment of Stage III and IV Hodgkin's disease. Use procarbazine as part of the MOPP (nitrogen mustard, vincristine, procarbazine, prednisone) regimen. It has also been used as part of the ChIVPP (chlorambucol, vinblastine, procarbazine, prednisone) regimen.

Contraindications:

Hypersensitivity to procarbazine. Inadequate marrow reserve demonstrated by bone marrow aspiration; consider in any patient with leukopenia, thrombocytopenia or anemia.

Warnings:

Toxicity common to many hydrazine derivatives is hemolysis and the appearance of Heinz-Ehrlich inclusion bodies in erythrocytes.

Discontinue if any of the following occurs: CNS signs or symptoms; leukopenia (WBC < 4000/mm^3); thrombocytopenia (platelets < 100,000 mm^3); hypersensitivity reaction; stomatitis (the first small ulceration or persistent spot soreness); diarrhea; hemorrhage or bleeding tendencies.

Resume therapy after side effects clear; adjust to a lower dosage schedule.

Renal/Hepatic function impairment: Undue toxicity may occur if used in patients with known impairment of renal or hepatic function.

Fertility impairment: Azoospermia and antifertility effects associated with procarbazine coadministered with other antineoplastics for treating Hodgkin's disease have occurred in human clinical studies.

Pregnancy: Category D. Contraceptive measures are recommended during therapy for both men and women.

Lactation: It is not known whether procarbazine is excreted in human milk. Mothers should not nurse while receiving this drug.

Children: Close clinical monitoring is mandatory. Toxicity, evidenced by tremors, convulsions and coma, has occurred.

Precautions:

Monitoring: Obtain baseline laboratory data prior to initiation of therapy. Monitor hemoglobin, hematocrit, WBC, differential, reticulocytes and platelets at least every 3 or 4 days. Bone marrow depression often occurs 2 to 8 weeks after the start of treatment. If leukopenia occurs, hospitalization may be needed to prevent systemic infection.

Evaluate hepatic and renal function prior to initiation of therapy.

Repeat urinalysis, transaminase, alkaline phosphatase and BUN at least weekly.

Use after radiation or other chemotherapy is known to have marrow depressant activity. Wait 1 month or longer before starting procarbazine. Interval length may also be determined by evidence of bone marrow recovery based on successive bone marrow studies.

Drug Interactions:

Drugs that may be affected by procarbazine include digitalis glycosides, levodopa, narcotics, sympathomimetics and tricyclic antidepressants.

Drugs that may affect procarbazine include alcohol.

Drug/Food interactions: Foods with high tyramine content may interact with procarbazine (eg, wine, yogurt, ripe cheese and bananas).

Adverse Reactions:

Adverse reactions may include leukopenia; anemia; thrombocytopenia; nausea; vomiting; anorexia; stomatitis; dysphagia; abdominal pain; diarrhea; constipation; pancytopenia; eosinophilia; hemolytic anemia; bleeding tendencies; hypotension; tachycardia; syncope; hematuria; urinary frequency; nocturia; dermatitis; pruritus; rash; urticaria; herpes; hyperpigmentation; flushing; alopecia; jaundice; paresthesias and neuropathies; headache; dizziness; depression; apprehension; nervousness; insomnia; nightmares; hallucinations; fatigue; drowsiness; tremors; coma; confusion; convulsions; retinal hemorrhage; nystagmus; photophobia; diplopia; inability to focus; papilledema; myalgia/arthralgia; hepatic dysfunction; pyrexia; diaphoresis; chills; intercurrent infections; pleural effusion; edema; cough; pneumonitis, photosensitivity; fainting; allergic reactions; hearing loss; slurred speech.

Administration and Dosage:

Base dosages on the patient's actual weight. Use estimated lean body mass (dry weight) if patient is obese or if there has been a spurious weight gain due to edema, ascites or other forms of abnormal fluid retention.

The following doses are for use of procarbazine as a single agent. When used in combination with other anticancer drugs, appropriately reduce procarbazine dosage (eg, in the MOPP regimen, the procarbazine dose is 100 mg/m^2 daily for 14 days).

Adults: To minimize nausea and vomiting, give single or divided doses of 2 to 4 mg/kg/day for the first week. Maintain daily dosage at 4 to 6 mg/kg/day until the WBC falls below 4,000/mm^3 or the platelets fall below 100,000/mm^3, or until maximum response is obtained. Upon evidence of hematologic toxicity, discontinue the drug until there has been satisfactory recovery. Resume treatment at 1 to 2 mg/kg/day. When maximum response is obtained, maintain the dose at 1 to 2 mg/kg/day.

Children: Close clinical monitoring is mandatory. Individualize dosage. This dosage schedule is a guideline only: 50 mg/m^2 daily for the first week. Maintain daily dosage at 100 mg/m^2 until leukopenia or thrombocytopenia occurs or maximum response is obtained. Upon evidence of hematologic toxicity, discontinue drug until there has been satisfactory response. When maximum response is attained, maintain the dose at 50 mg/m^2/day.

DACARBAZINE (DTIC; Imidazole Carboxamide)

Injection: 100 mg/10 ml vial, 100 and 200 mg/20 ml vial, 200 mg/30 ml vial, 500 mg/50 ml vial *(Rx)* — Various, *DTIC-Dome* (Miles Pharm)

Warning:

Hemopoietic depression is the most common toxicity.

Hepatic necrosis has been reported.

Actions:

Pharmacology: The exact mechanism of action is unknown. There is some evidence for activity via three mechanisms: Alkylation through an activated carbonium ion; inhibition of DNA synthesis by acting as a purine analog; and interaction with sulfhydryl groups in proteins. Both deoxyribonucleic acid (DNA) and ribonucleic acid (RNA) synthesis are inhibited.

Pharmacokinetics:

Absorption/Distribution – After IV administration of dacarbazine, volume of distribution exceeds total body water content suggesting tissue localization, probably in the liver.

Metabolism/Excretion – Plasma disappearance is biphasic with an initial half-life of 19 minutes and a terminal half-life of 5 hours. In renal and hepatic dysfunction, half-lives increase to 55 minutes and 7.2 hours.

An average of 40% of dacarbazine is excreted unchanged in the urine in 6 hours. Dacarbazine is subject to renal tubular secretion rather than glomerular filtration. Besides unchanged dacarbazine, 5-aminoimidazole-4 carboxamide (AIC) is a major metabolite in the urine.

Indications:

Metastatic malignant melanoma.

Second-line therapy in Hodgkin's disease in combination with other agents.

Unlabeled uses: In combiantion with cyclophosphamide and vincristine for malignant pheochromocytoma; coadministration with tamoxifen for metastatic malignant melanoma (more effective than dacarbazine alone).

Contraindications:

Hypersensitivity to dacarbazine.

Warnings:

Hemopoietic depression is the most common toxicity and involves primarily the leukocytes and platelets, although anemia sometimes occurs. Leukopenia and thrombocytopenia may be severe enough to cause death. Possible bone marrow depression requires careful monitoring of WBC, RBC and platelet levels. Hemopoietic toxicity may warrant temporary suspension or cessation of therapy.

Hepatotoxicity, accompanied by hepatic vein thrombosis and hepatocellular necrosis resulting in death, has been reported in approximately 0.01% of patients treated. This toxicity has been observed mostly when dacarbazine was coadministered with other antineoplastics, but it has also been reported with dacarbazine alone.

Anaphylaxis can occur following the administration of dacarbazine.

Pregnancy: Category C.

Lactation: It is not known if this drug is excreted in breast milk.

Precautions:

Hospitalization is not always necessary, but adequate lab facilities must be available.

Photosensitivity: Photosensitization (photoallergy or phototoxicity) may occur.

Adverse Reactions:

Adverse reactions may include anorexia; nausea; vomiting; flu-like syndrome; fever; myalgia; malaise; facial flushing; facial paresthesia; alopecia.

Anorexia, nausea and vomiting occur in over 90% of patients with the initial few doses. The vomiting lasts 1 to 12 hours and is incompletely and unpredictably palliated with phenobarbital or prochloperazine.

Administration and Dosage:

Administer IV only. Extravasation of the drug subcutaneously during IV administration may result in tissue damage and severe pain.

Malignant melanoma: 2 to 4.5 mg/kg/day IV for 10 days. Repeat at 4 week intervals.

Alternatively, administer 250 mg/m^2/day IV for 5 days. Repeat every 3 weeks.

Hodgkin's disease: 150 mg/m^2/day for 5 days, in combination with other effective drugs. Repeat every 4 weeks.

Alternatively, administer 375 mg/m^2 on day 1, in combination with other effective drugs; repeat every 15 days.

GEMCITABINE HCl

Powder, lyophilized: 20 mg/ml (*Rx*)	*Gemzar* (Lilly)

Actions:

Pharmacology: Gemcitabine is a nucleoside analog that exhibits antitumor activity through cell phase specificity, primarily killing cells undergoing DNA synthesis (S-phase), and also blocking the progression of cells through the G1/S-phase boundary. Gemcitabine is metabolized intracellulary by nucleoside kinases to the active diphosphate (dFdCDP) and triphosphate (dFdCTP) nucleosides. The cytotoxic effect of gemcitabine is attributed to a combination of two actions of the diphosphate and the triphosphate nucleosides, which leads to inhibition of DNA synthesis.

Pharmacokinetics: Volume of distribution of gemcitabine is significantly influenced by duration of infusion and gender. Clearance is affected by age and gender.

Gemcitabine Clearance and Half-Life for the "Typical" Patient

Age	Clearance Men (L/hr/m^2)	Clearance Women (L/hr/m^2)	Half-Life[1] Men (min)	Half-Life[1] Women (min)
29	92.2	69.4	42	49
45	75.7	57	48	57
65	55.1	41.5	61	73
79	40.7	30.7	79	94

[1] Half-life for patients receiving a short infusion (< 70 min).

The volume of distribution was increased with infusion length. Volume of distribution of gemcitabine was 50 L/m^2 following infusions lasting < 70 minutes, indicating that gemcitabine, after short infusions, is not extensively distributed into tissues. For long infusions, the volume of distribution rose to 370 L/m^2, reflecting slow equilibration of gemcitabine within the tissue compartment.

The maximum plasma concentrations of dFdU (inactive metabolite) were achieved up to 30 minutes after discontinuation of the infusions and the metabolites is excreted in urine without undergoing further biotransformation. The metabolite did not accumulate with weekly dosing, but its elimination is dependent on renal excretion, and could accumulate with decreased renal function.

Indications:

Adenocarcinoma of the pancreas: First-line treatment for patients with locally advanced (nonresectable Stage II or Stage III) or metastatic (Stage IV) adenocarcinoma of the pancreas. Gemcitabine is indicated for patients previously treated with 5–FU.

Contraindications:

Known hypersensitivity to the drug.

Warnings:

Infusion: Prolongation of the infusion time beyond 60 minutes and more frequent than weekly dosing have been shown to increase toxicity.

Myelosuppression: Gemcitabine can suppress bone marrow function as manifested by leukopenia, thrombocytopenia and anemia, and myelosuppression is usually the dose-limiting toxicity.

Fever: The overal incidence of fever was 41%. Fever was frequently associated with other flu-like symptoms and was usually mild and clinically manageable.

Rash: Rash was reported in 30% of patients. The rash was typically a macular or finely granular maculopapular pruritic eruption of mild to moderate severity involving the trunk and extremities. Pruritis was reported for 13% of patients.

Renal/Hepatic function impairment: Use gemcitabine with caution in patients with pre-existing renal impairment or hepatic insufficiency.

Elderly: Gemcitabine clearance is affected by age. There is no evidence, however, that usuaual dose adjustments are necessary in patients > 65 years of age. Grade 3/4 thrombocytopenia was more common in the elderly.

Gender – Older women were more likely not to proceed to a subsequent cycle and to experience grade 3/4 neutropenia and thrombocytopenia.

Pregnancy: Category D.

Lactation: It is not known whether gemcitabine or its metabolites are excreted in breast milk

Children: Safety and efficacy in pediatric patients have not been established.

Precautions:

Monitoring: Monitor patients receiving gemcitabine prior to each dose with a complete blood count (CBC), including differential and platelet count. Consider suspension or modification of therapy when marrow suppression is detected.

Hepatic and renal – Perform laboratory evaluation of renal and hepatic function prior to initiation of therapy and periodically thereafter.

Adverse Reactions:

Adverse reactions include: Anemia, leukopenia, neutropenia, thrombocytopenia, increased ALT and AST, increased alkaline phosphatase, increased bilirubin, proteinuria, hematuria, increased BUN, increased creatinine, nausea and vomiting, pain, fever, rash, dyspnea, constipation, diarrhea, hemorrhage, infection, alopecia, stomatitis, somnolence, peripheral edema, "flu syndrome," and paresthesia.

Administration and Dosage:

IV use only. Gemcitabine may be administered on an outpatient basis.

Adults: Administered IV at a dose of 1000 mg/m^2 over 30 minutes once weekly for up to 7 weeks (or until toxicity necessitates reducing or holding a dose), followed by a week of rest from treatment. Subsequent cycles should consist of infusions once weekly for 3 consecutive weeks out of every 4 weeks.

Gemcitabine Dosage Reduction Guidelines

Absolute granulocyte count ($\times 10^6$/L)		Platelet count ($\times 10^6$/L)	% of full dose
≥ 1000	and	≥ 100,000	100
500 to 999	or	50,000 to 99,000	75
< 500	or	< 50,000	hold

Patients who complete an entire 7–week initial cycle of gemcitabine therapy or a subsequent 3–week cycle at a dose of 1000 mg/m^2 may have the dose for subsequent cycles increased by 25% (to 1250 mg/m^2), provided that the absolute granulocyte count (AGC) and platelet nadirs exceed 1500 × 10^6/L and 100,000 × 10^6/L, respectively, and if nonhematologic toxicity has not been greater than World Health Organization Grade 1. If patients tolerate the subsequent course at a dose of 1250 mg/m^2, the dose for the next cycle can be increased to 1500 mg/m^2, provided again that the AGC and platelet nadirs exceed $1500 \times 10^6/L$ and $100{,}000 \times 10^6/L$, respectively, and again, if nonhematologic toxicity has not been greater than WHO Grade 1.

MITOTANE (o, p′-DDD)

Tablets: 500 mg *(Rx)* *Lysodren* (Bristol-Myers Oncology)

Warning:
Discontinue temporarily following shock or severe trauma since the prime action of mitotane is adrenal suppression. Administer exogenous steroids in such circumstances, since the depressed adrenal may not immediately start to function.

Actions:

Pharmacology: Mitotane is an adrenal cytotoxic agent, although it can cause adrenal inhibition without cellular destruction. The primary action is upon the adrenal cortex. The production of adrenal steroids is reduced. The biochemical mechanism of action is unknown. Data suggest that the drug modifies the peripheral metabolism of steroids and directly suppresses the adrenal cortex.

Pharmacokinetics:

Absorption/Distribution – Approximately 40% of oral mitotane is absorbed; it can be found in all body tissues but is primarily stored in fat. Blood levels detectable for up to 10 weeks after discontinuation of therapy may be related to a slow persistent release of drug from lipid storage sites. Blood levels do not appear to correlate with therapeutic or toxic effects.

Metabolism/Excretion – Approximately 10% to 25% of the drug is excreted in the urine as an unidentified water soluble metabolite. A variable amount of metabolite (1% to 17%) is excreted in the bile and the balance is apparently stored in tissues. Up to 60% is excreted unchanged in the stool. Following discontinuation of the drug, plasma terminal half-life has ranged from 18 to 159 days.

Indications:
Treatment of inoperable adrenal cortical carcinoma (functional and nonfunctional).

Contraindications:
Hypersensitivity to mitotane.

Warnings:
Surgically remove all possible tumor tissue from large metastatic masses before administration to minimize the possibility of infarction and hemorrhage in the tumor due to a rapid, cytotoxic effect of the drug.

Long-term therapy: Continuous administration of high doses may lead to brain damage and impairment of function.

Hepatic function impairment: Administer with care to patients with liver disease other than metastatic lesions of the adrenal cortex. Interference with mitotane metabolism may occur, causing drug accumulation.

Pregnancy: Category C. Contraceptive measures are recommended during therapy.

Lactation: It is not known whether this drug is excreted in breast milk.

Precautions:

Adrenal insufficiency may develop; consider adrenal steroid replacement in these patients.

Hazardous tasks: May produce sedation, lethargy, vertigo or other CNS side effects; observe caution while driving or performing other tasks requiring alertness.

Drug Interactions:
Drugs that may interct with mitotane include corticosteroids, warfarin and other drugs susceptible to the influence of hepatic enzyme reduction.

Drug/Lab test interactions: Protein-bound iodine (PBI) levels and urinary 17-hydroxycorticosteroids may be decreased by mitotane.

Adverse Reactions:

Adverse reactions occurring in ≥ 3% of patients include anorexia; nausea; vomiting; diarrhea; depression; lethargy; somnolence; dizziness; vertigo; skin rashes.

Administration and Dosage:

Start at 2 to 6 g/day in divided doses, 3 or 4 times daily. Increase dose incrementally to 9 to 10 g per day. If severe side effects appear, reduce to the maximum tolerated dose. If the patient can tolerate higher doses, and if improved clinical response appears possible, increase the dose until adverse reactions interfere. Maximum tolerated dose varies from 2 to 16 g/day (usually 9 to 10 g). The highest doses used in studies were 18 to 19 g/day.

Continue treatment as long as clinical benefits are observed (ie, maintenance of clinical status or slowing of growth of metastatic lesions). If no clinical benefits are observed after 3 months at the maximum tolerated dose, consider the case a clinical failure. However, 10% of the patients who showed a measurable response required more than 3 months at the maximum tolerated dose.

Chapter 12
MISCELLANEOUS DRUGS

ANTIDOTES

Drug	Trade Name (Distributor)	Toxic/Overdosed Substance
Dimercaprol (BAL)	*BAL In Oil* (H, W & D)	Arsenic, gold, mercury, lead
Deferoxamine Mesylate	*Desferal Mesylate* (Ciba)	Iron
Edetate Calcium Disodium	*Calcium Disodium Versenate* (Riker)	Lead
Sodium Thiosulfate		Arsenic, cyanide
Narcotic Antagonists Naloxone	 *Narcan* (DuPont)	Opioids
Physostigmine Salicylate	*Antilirium* (Forest Pharm.)	Anticholinergics (including tricyclic antidepressants) Diazepam, Morphine (CNS depression)
Pralidoxime Cl	*Protopam* (Ayerst)	Organophosphates; Anticholinesterases
Digoxin Immune Fab	*Digibind* (Glaxo Wellcome)	Digoxin
Methylene Blue	(Various)	Cyanide
Other agents used additionally as antidotes		
Leucovorin Calcium	*Wellcovorin* (Glaxo-Wellcome) *Leucovorin Calcium* (Lederle)	Folic acid antagonists (eg, methotrexate)
Hydroxocobalamin	(Various)	Cyanide poisoning from nitro prusside
Vitamin K	(Various)	Oral anticoagulants
Protamine Sulfate	(Various)	Heparin
Glucagon	(Lilly)	Insulin-induced hypoglycemia
Edetate Disodium	(Various)	Hypercalcemia Digitalis toxicity
Acetylcysteine	*Mucomyst* (Bristol-Myers) *Mucosol* (Dey Labs)	Acetaminophen
Atropine	(Various)	Cholinergic agents: Organophosphates, carbamates, pilocarpine, physostigmine or isofluorophate
Amyl nitrite, Na Nitrite, Na Thiosulfate	*Cyanide antidote kit* (Lilly)	Cyanide
Anticholinesterases Pyridostigmine Br Neostigmine Edrophonium Cl	 *Mestinon* (Roche) *Regonol* (Organon) *Prostigmin* (Roche) *Tensilon* (Roche)	Anticholinergics, Nondepolarizing muscle relaxants
Nonspecific therapy of overdoses include:		
Osmotic diuretics		Nonspecific, supportive therapies of overdoses. See also General Management Guidelines
Cathartics		
Peritoneal Dialysis Solutions		
Emetics Apomorphine Syrup of Ipecac Activated Charcoal	 (Lilly) (Various) (Various)	
Urinary Alkalinizers		
Urinary Acidifiers		

NALMEFENE HCl

Injection: 1 mg/ml (*Rx*)	*Revex* (Ohmeda)

Actions:

Pharmacology: Nalmefene, an opioid antagonist, is a 6-methylene analog of naltrexone. Nalmefene prevents or reverses the effects of opioids, including respiratory depression, sedation and hypotension. Nalmefene has no opioid agonist activity; it does not produce respiratory depression, psychotomimetic effects or pupillary constriction, and no pharmacological activity was observed when it was administered in the absence of opioid agonists. Nalmefene can produce acute withdrawal symptoms in individuals who are opioid-dependent.

Pharmacokinetics:

Absorption – Nalmefene is completely bioavailable following IM or SC administration. Nalmefene will be administered primarily as an IV bolus, however, it can be given IM or SC if venous access cannot be established. While the time to maximum plasma concentration was 2.3 hours following IM and 1.5 hours following SC administrations, therapeutic plasma concentrations are likely to be reached within 5 to 15 minutes after a 1 mg dose in an emergency.

Distribution – Following a 1 mg parenteral dose, nalmefene was rapidly distributed. A 1 mg dose blocked > 80% of brain opioid receptors within 5 minutes after administration. The apparent volumes of distribution centrally and at steady state are 3.9 and 8.6 L/kg, respectively. Over a concentration range of 0.1 to 2 mcg/ml, 45% is bound to plasma proteins.

Metabolism – Nalmefene is metabolized by the liver, primarily by glucuronide conjugation, and excreted in the urine; < 5% is excreted in the urine unchanged, and 17% is excreted in the feces.

Excretion – After IV administration of 1 mg to healthy males, plasma concentrations declined biexponentially with a redistribution and a terminal elimination half-life of 41 ± 34 minutes and 10.8 ± 5.2 hours, respectively. The systemic clearance of nalmefene is 0.8 L/hr/kg and the renal clearance is 0.08 L/hr/kg.

Indications:

Reversal of opioid effects: Complete or partial reversal of opioid drug effects, including respiratory depression, induced by either natural or synthetic opioids.

Opioid overdose: Management of known or suspected opioid overdose.

Contraindications:

Hypersensitivity to the product.

Warnings:

Emergency use: Nalmefene is not the primary treatment for ventilatory failure. In most emergency settings, treatment with nalmefene should follow, not precede, the establishment of a patent airway, ventilatory assistance, administration of oxygen and establishment of circulatory access.

Respiratory depression: Accidental overdose with long acting opioids (eg, methadone, levomethadyl) may result in prolonged respiratory depression. Observe patients until there is no reasonable risk of recurrent respiratory depression. While nalmefene has a longer duration of action than naloxone in fully reversing doses, be aware that a recurrence of respiratory depression is possible, even after an apparently initial response to nalmefene treatment.

Renal function impairment: There was a statistically significant 27% decrease in plasma clearance of nalmefene in the end-stage renal disease (ESRD) population during interdialysis (0.57 L/hr/kg) and a 25% decreased plasma clearance in the ESRD population during intradialysis (0.59 L/hr/kg) compared to controls (0.79 L/hr/kg). The elimination half-life was prolonged in ESRD patients from 10.2 (controls) to 26.1 hr.

Hepatic function impairment: Subjects with hepatic disease had a 28.3% decrease in plasma clearance of nalmefene compared to controls (0.56 vs 0.78 L/hr/kg, respectively).

Elimination half-life increased from 10.2 to 11.9 hours in the hepatically impaired. No dosage adjustment is recommended since nalmefene will be administered as an acute course of therapy.

Elderly: Dose proportionality was observed in nalmefene AUC following 0.5 to 2 mg IV administration to elderly male subjects. There was an apparent age-related decrease in the central volume of distribution that resulted in a greater initial nalmefene concentration in the elderly group. While initial plasma concentrations were transiently higher in the elderly, it would not be anticipated that this population would require dosing adjustment.

Pregnancy: Category B.

Lactation: Exercise caution when nalmefene is administered to a nursing woman.

Children: Safety and efficacy have not been established. Only use nalmefene in the resuscitation of the newborn when the expected benefits outweigh the risks.

Precautions:

Cardiovascular risks: Although nalmefene has been used safely in patients with preexisting cardiac disease, use all drugs of this class with caution in patients at high cardiovascular risk or who have received potentially cardiotoxic drugs.

Risk of precipitated withdrawal: Nalmefene is known to produce acute withdrawal symptoms and, therefore, should be used with extreme caution in patients with known physical dependence on opioids or following surgery involving high uses of opioids.

Incomplete reversal of buprenorphine: In animals, nalmefene doses up to 10 mg/kg (437 times the maximum recommended human dose) produced incomplete reversal of buprenorphine-induced analgesia. Hence, nalmefene may not completely reverse buprenorphine-induced respiratory depression.

Drug Interactions:

Flumazenil: Both flumazenil and nalmefene can induce seizures in animals. Remain aware of the potential risk of seizures from agents in these classes.

Adverse Reactions:

Adverse reactions occurring in ≥ 3% of patients include nausea; vomiting; tachycardia; hypertension; postoperative pain; fever; dizziness.

Administration and Dosage:

Administration: Titrate nalmefene to reverse the undesired effects of opioids. Once adequate reversal has been established, additional administration is not required and may actually be harmful due to unwanted reversal of analgesia or precipitated withdrawal.

Duration of action: The duration of action of nalmefene is as long as most opioid analgesics. The apparent duration of action will vary, however, depending on the half-life and plasma concentration of the narcotic being reversed, the presence or absence of other drugs affecting the brain or muscles of respiration and the dose of nalmefene administered. Partially reversing doses of nalmefene (1 mcg/kg) lose their effect as the drug is redistributed through the body, and the effects of these low doses may not last more than 30 to 60 minutes in the presence of persistent opioid effects. Fully reversing doses (1 mg/70 kg) last many hours, but may complicate the management of patients who are in pain, at high cardiovascular risk or who are physically dependent on opioids.

The recommended doses represent a compromise between a desirable controlled reversal and the need for prompt response and adequate duration of action. Using higher dosages or shorter intervals between incremental doses may increase the incidence and severity of symptoms related to acute withdrawal such as nausea, vomiting, elevated blood pressure and anxiety.

Patients tolerant to or physically dependent on opioids: Nalmefene may cause acute withdrawal symptoms in individuals who have some degree of tolerance to and dependence on opioids. Closely observe these patients for symptoms of withdrawal following administration of the initial and subsequent injections of nalmefene. Administer subsequent doses with intervals of at least 2 to 5 minutes between doses to allow the full effect of each incremental dose of nalmefene to be reached.

Reversal of postoperative opioid depression: Use 100 mcg/ml dosage strength (blue label); refer to the following table for initial doses. The goal of treatment with nalmefene in the postoperative setting is to achieve reversal of excessive opioid effects without inducing a complete reversal and acute pain. This is best accomplished with an initial dose of 0.25 mcg/kg followed by 0.25 mcg/kg incremental doses at 2 to 5 minute intervals, stopping as soon as the desired degree of opioid reversal is obtained. A cumulative total dose > 1 mcg/kg does not provide additional therapeutic effect.

Nalmefene Dosage for Reversal of Postoperative Opioid Depression

Body weight (kg)	Amount of nalmefene 100 mcg/ml solution (ml)
50	0.125
60	0.15
70	0.175
80	0.2
90	0.225
100	0.25

Cardiovascular risk patients: In cases where the patient is known to be at increased cardiovascular risk, it may be desirable to dilute nalmefene 1:1 with saline or sterile water and use smaller initial and incremental doses of 0.1 mcg/kg.

Management of known/suspected opioid overdose: Use 1 mg/ml dosage strength (green label). The recommended initial dose of nalmefene for nonopioid dependent patients is 0.5 mg/70 kg. If needed, this may be followed by a second dose of 1 mg/70 kg, 2 to 5 minutes later. If a total dose of 1.5 mg/70 kg has been administered without clinical response, additional nalmefene is unlikely to have an effect.

If there is a reasonable suspicion of opioid dependency, initially administer a challenge dose of 0.1 mg/70 kg. If there is no evidence of withdrawal in 2 minutes, follow the recommended dosing.

Repeated dosing: Nalmefene is the longest acting of the currently available parenteral opioid antagonists. If recurrence of respiratory depression does occur, the dose should again be titrated to clinical effect using incremental doses to avoid overreversal.

Hepatic and renal disease: Hepatic disease and renal failure substantially reduce the clearance of nalmefene. For single episodes of opioid antagonism, adjustment of nalmefene dosage is not required. However, in patients with renal failure, slowly administer the incremental doses (over 60 seconds).

Loss of IV access: Should IV access be lost or not readily obtainable, a single dose of nalmefene should be effective within 5 to 15 minutes after 1 mg IM or SC doses.

NALOXONE HCl

Injection: **0.4 and 1 mg/ml (*Rx*)** — Various, *Narcan* (DuPont Pharm.)
Neonatal Injection: **0.02 mg per ml (*Rx*)**

Actions:

Pharmacology: Naloxone, a pure narcotic antagonist, will precipitate abstinence syndrome in the presence of narcotic addiction. Since it is devoid of undesirable agonist properties, naloxone is preferred for reversal of narcotic-induced respiratory depression. Naloxone prevents or reverses opioid effects including respiratory depression, sedation, hypotension; it can reverse psychotomimetic and dysphoric effects of agonist-antagonists such as pentazocine.

Mechanism – The mechanism of action is not fully understood; evidence suggests that it antagonizes the opioid effects by competing for the same receptor sites.

Pharmacokinetics:

Distribution – After parenteral use, naloxone is rapidly distributed in the body. It is metabolized in the liver, primarily by glucuronide conjugation.

Excretion – Naloxone is excreted in the urine. The serum half-life in adults ranged from 30 to 81 minutes; in neonates, 3.1 ± 0.5 hours.

Onset, peak and duration: Onset of action of IV naloxone is generally apparent within 2 min; it is only slightly less rapid when given SC or IM. Duration of action of 1 to 4 hours depends upon dose and route. IM use produces a more prolonged effect than IV use.

Indications:

For the complete or partial reversal of narcotic depression, including respiratory depression, induced by opioids including natural and synthetic narcotics, propoxyphene, methadone, nalbuphine, butorphanol and pentazocine. Also indicated for the diagnosis of suspected acute opioid overdosage.

Unlabeled uses: Naloxone has been used to improve circulation in refractory shock. Naloxone has also been used for the reversal of alcoholic coma, dementia of the Alzheimer type and schizophrenia.

Contraindications:

Hypersensitivity to these agents.

Warnings:

Drug dependence: Administer cautiously to persons who are known or suspected to be physically dependent on opioids, including newborns of mothers with narcotic dependence. Reversal of narcotic effect will precipitate acute abstinence syndrome.

Repeat administration: The patient who has satisfactorily responded should be kept under continued surveillance. Administer repeated doses as necessary, since the duration of action of some narcotics may exceed that of the narcotic antagonist.

Respiratory depression: Not effective against respiratory depression due to nonopioid drugs.

Pregnancy: Category B.

Lactation: It is not known whether the drug is excreted in breast milk.

Precautions:

Other supportive therapy: Maintain a free airway and provide artificial ventilation, cardiac massage and vasopressor agents; employ when necessary to counteract acute narcotic overdosage.

Cardiovascular effects: Several instances of hypotension, hypertension, pulmonary edema and ventricular tachycardia and fibrillation have been reported in postoperative patients.

Adverse Reactions:

Abrupt reversal of narcotic depression may result in nausea, vomiting, sweating, tachycardia, increased blood pressure and tremulousness.

In postoperative patients, excessive dosage may result in excitement and significant reversal of analgesia, hypotension, hypertension, pulmonary edema and ventricular tachycardia and fibrillation.

Administration and Dosage:

Give IV, IM or SC. The most rapid onset of action is achieved with IV use, which is recommended in emergency situations.

Adults:

Narcotic overdose (known or suspected) – Initial dose is 0.4 to 2 mg IV; may repeat IV at 2 to 3 minute intervals. If no response is observed after 10 mg has been administered, question the diagnosis of narcotic-induced or partial narcotic-induced toxicity.

Postoperative narcotic depression (partial reversal) – Smaller doses are usually sufficient. Titrate dose according to the patient's response.

Initial dose: Inject in increments of 0.1 to 0.2 mg IV at 2 to 3 minute intervals to the desired degree of reversal.

Repeat dose: Repeat doses may be required within 1 or 2 hr intervals depending on the amount, type (ie, short- or long-acting) and time interval since last administration of narcotic. Supplemental IM doses have produced a longer lasting effect.

Children:

Narcotic overdose (known or suspected) – Initial dose is 0.01 mg/kg IV; give a subsequent dose of 0.1 mg/kg if needed. If an IV route is not available, may be given IM or SC in divided doses.

Postoperative narcotic depression – Follow the recommendations and cautions under adult administration guidelines. For initial reversal of respiratory depression, inject in increments of 0.005 to 0.01 mg IV at 2 to 3 minute intervals to desired degree of reversal.

Neonates:

Narcotic-induced depression – Initial dose is 0.01 mg/kg IV, IM or SC; may be repeated in accordance with adult administration guidelines.

NALTREXONE HCl

Tablets: 50 mg (*Rx*)	*ReVia* (DuPont)

Actions:

Pharmacology: Naltrexone, a pure opioid antagonist, markedly attenuates or completely reversibly blocks the subjective effects of IV opioids. In subjects physically dependent on opioids, naltrexone will precipitate withdrawal symptomatology.

Naltrexone blocks the effects of opioids by competitive binding at opioid receptors. This makes the blockade potentially surmountable.

Pharmacokinetics:

Absorption – Although well absorbed orally, naltrexone is subject to significant first-pass metabolism with oral bioavailability estimates ranging from 5% to 40%. Following oral administration, naltrexone undergoes rapid and nearly complete absorption with ≈ 96% of the dose absorbed from the GI tract. Peak plasma levels of both naltrexone and 6–β-naltrexol occur within 1 hour of dosing.

Distribution – The volume of distribution for naltrexone after IV administration is estimated to be 1350 L. In vitro, naltrexone is 21% bound to plasma proteins.

Metabolism/Excretion – The major metabolite of naltrexone is 6–β-naltrexol. The activity of naltrexone is believed to be due to both parent and the 6–β-naltrexol metabolite. The mean elimination half-life values for naltrexone and 6–β-naltrexol are 4 and 13 hours, respectively.

Renal elimination is primarily by glomerular filtration. Both parent drug and metabolites are excreted primarily by the kidney, however, urinary excretion of unchanged naltrexone accounts for < 2% of an oral dose and fecal excretion is a minor elimination pathway. The urinary excretion of unchanged and conjugated 6–β-naltrexone accounts for 43% of an oral dose. Naltrexone and its metabolites may undergo enterohepatic recycling.

Indications:

Narcotic addiction: Blockade of the effects of exogenously administered opioids.

Alcoholism: Treatment of alcohol dependence.

Unlabeled uses: Naltrexone has been used in eating disorders and in the treatment of post-concussional syndrome unresponsive to other treatments.

Contraindications:

Patients receiving opioid analgesics; opioid-dependent patients; patients in acute opioid withdrawal; failed naloxone challenge; positive urine screen for opioids; history of sensitivity to naltrexone; acute hepatitis or liver failure.

Warnings:

Hepatotoxicity: Naltrexone has the capacity to cause hepatocellular injury when given in excessive doses. It is contraindicated in acute hepatitis or liver failure, and its use in patients with active liver disease must be carefully considered in light of its hepatotoxic effects.

Warn patients of the risk of hepatic injury and advise them to stop naltrexone and seek medical attention if they experience symptoms of acute hepatitis.

Although no cases of hepatic failure have ever been reported, consider this as a possible risk of treatment.

Abstinence precipitation/syndrome: Unintended precipitation of abstinence or exacerbation of a preexisting subclinical abstinence syndrome may occur; therefore, patients should remain opioid-free for a minimum of 7 to 10 days before starting naltrexone.

Severe opioid withdrawal syndromes precipitated by accidental naltrexone ingestion have occurred in opioid-dependent individuals. Withdrawal symptoms usually appear within 5 minutes of ingestion and may last up to 48 hours.

Surmountable blockade: While naltrexone is a potent antagonist with a prolonged pharmacologic effect (24 to 72 hours), the blockade produced by naltrexone is surmountable. This poses a potential risk to individuals who attempt to overcome the blockade by self-administering large amounts of opioids. Any attempt by a patient to overcome the antagonism by taking opioids is very dangerous and may lead to fatal overdose.

Use with narcotics: Patients taking naltrexone may not benefit from opioid-containing medicines. Use a nonopioid-containing alternative, if available.

Pregnancy: Category C.

Lactation: It is not known if naltrexone is excreted in breast milk.

Children: Safety for use in children < 18 years of age has not been established.

Precautions:

Monitoring: A high index of suspicion for drug-related hepatic injury is critical if the occurrence of liver damage induced by naltrexone is to be detected at the earliest possible time.

Suicide: The risk of suicide is increased in patients with substance abuse with or without concomitant depression. This risk is not abated by treatment with naltrexone.

Drug Interactions:

Drugs that may be affected by naltrexone include opioid-containing products and thioridazine.

Adverse Reactions:

Adverse reactions associated with treatment of alcoholism include nausea, headache, dizziness, nervousness, fatigue, insomnia and vomiting.

Reactions associated with treatment of narcotic addiction include difficulty sleeping, anxiety, nervousness, headache, low energy, irritability, increased energy, dizziness, abdominal cramps/pain, nausea, vomiting, loss of appetite, diarrhea, constipation, joint/muscle pain, delayed ejaculation, decreased potency, skin rash, chills and increased thirst.

Administration and Dosage:

If there is any question of occult opioid dependence, perform a naloxone challenge test. Do not attempt treatment until naloxone challenge is negative.

Alcoholism: A dose of 50 mg once daily is recommended for most patients. An initial 25 mg dose, splitting the daily dose and adjusting the time of dosing have met with limited success.

Narcotic dependence: Initiate treatment using the following guidelines:

1. Do not attempt treatment until the patient has remained opioid-free for 7 to 10 days.

2. Administer a naloxone challenge test (see below). If signs of opioid withdrawal are still observed following challenge, do not treat with naltrexone. The naloxone challenge can be repeated in 24 hours.

3. Initiate treatment carefully, slowly increasing the dose. Administer 25 mg initially; observe patient for 1 hour. If no withdrawal signs occur, give the rest of the daily dose.

Maintenance treatment: Once the patient has been started on naltrexone, 50 mg every 24 hours will produce adequate clinical blockade of the actions of parenterally administered opioids. A flexible dosing regimen may be employed. Thus, patients may receive 50 mg every weekday with a 100 mg dose on Saturday, 100 mg every other day, or 150 mg every third day. Several studies have employed the following dosing regimen with success: 100 mg Monday, 100 mg Wednesday and 150 mg Friday.

FLUMAZENIL

Injection: 0.1 mg/ml (*Rx*)	*Romazicon* (Hoffman-La Roche)

Actions:

Pharmacology: Flumazenil antagonizes the actions of benzodiazepines on the CNS and competitively inhibits the activity at the benzodiazepine recognition site on the GABA/benzodiazepine receptor complex.

The duration and degree of reversal of benzodiazepine effects are related to the dose and plasma concentrations of flumazenil. The onset of reversal is usually evident within 1 to 2 minutes after the injection is completed. Within 3 minutes, 80% response will be reached, with the peak effect occurring at 6 to 10 minutes.

Pharmacokinetics: After IV administration, flumazenil has an initial distribution half-life of 7 to 15 minutes and a terminal half-life of 41 to 79 minutes. Peak concentrations of flumazenil are proportional to dose, with an apparent initial volume of distribution of 0.5 L/kg. After redistribution the apparent volume of distribution ranges from 0.77 to 1.6 L/kg. Protein binding is approximately 50%.

Flumazenil is a highly extracted drug. Clearance of flumazenil occurs primarily by hepatic metabolism and is dependent on hepatic blood flow. In healthy volunteers, total clearance ranges from 0.7 to 1.3 L/hr/kg, with < 1% of the administered dose eliminated unchanged in the urine. Elimination of drug is essentially complete within 72 hours, with 90% to 95% appearing in urine and 5% to 10% in the feces.

Indications:

Reversal of benzodiazepine sedation: For the complete or partial reversal of the sedative effects of benzodiazepines in cases where general anesthesia has been induced or maintained with benzodiazepines, where sedation has been produced with benzodiazepines for diagnostic and therapeutic procedures, and for the management of benzodiazepine overdose.

Contraindications:

Hypersensitivity to flumazenil or to benzodiazepines; benzodiazepine use for control of a potentially life-threatening condition; in patients who are showing signs of serious cyclic antidepressant overdose.

Warnings:

Seizures: The use of flumazenil has been associated with the occurrence of seizures. These are most frequent in patients who have been on benzodiazepines for long-term sedation or in overdose cases where patients are showing signs of serious cyclic antidepressant overdose. Individualize the dosage of flumazenil and be prepared to manage seizures.

Seizure risk: The reversal of benzodiazepine effects may be associated with the onset of seizures in certain high-risk populations.

Most convulsions associated with flumazenil administration require treatment and have been successfully managed with benzodiazepines, phenytoin or barbiturates.

Hypoventilation: Monitor patients who have received flumazenil for the reversal of benzodiazepine effects (after conscious sedation or general anesthesia) for resedation, respiratory depression or other residual benzodiazepine effects for an appropriate period (up to 120 minutes) based on the dose and duration of effect of the benzodiazepine employed, because flumazenil has not been established as an effective treatment for hypoventilation due to benzodiazepine administration.

Flumazenil may not fully reverse postoperative airway problems or ventilatory insufficiency induced by benzodiazepines. In addition, even if flumazenil is initially effective, such problems may recur because the effects of flumazenil wear off before the effects of many benzodiazepines.

Hepatic function impairment: Mean total clearance is decreased to 40% to 60% of normal in patients with moderate liver dysfunction and to 25% of normal in patients with severe liver dysfunction compared with age-matched healthy subjects. This results in a prolongation of the half-life from 0.8 hours in healthy subjects to 1.3 hours in patients with moderate hepatic impairment and 2.4 hours in severely impaired patients.

Pregnancy: Category C.

Labor and delivery – The use of flumazenil to reverse the effects of benzodiazepines used during labor and delivery is not recommended because the effects of the drug in the newborn are unknown.

Lactation: It is not known whether flumazenil is excreted in breast milk.

Children: Flumazenil is not recommended for use in children.

Precautions:

Monitoring: Monitor patients for resedation, respiratory depression or other persistent or recurrent agonist effects for an adequate period of time after administration of flumazenil.

Return of sedation: Resedation is least likely in cases where flumazenil is adminstered to reverse a low dose of a short-acting benzodiazepine. It is most likely in cases where a large single or cumulative dose of a benzodiazepine has been given in the course of a long procedure along with neuromuscular blocking agents and multiple anesthetic agents.

Intensive Care Unit (ICU): Use with caution in the ICU because of the increased risk of unrecognized benzodiazepine dependence in such settings.

Overdose situations: Flumazenil is intended as an adjunct to, not as a substitute for, proper management of airway, assisted breathing, circulatory access and support, internal decontamination by lavage and charcoal, and adequate clinical evaluation.

Head injury: Use with caution in patients with head injury as flumazenil may be capable of precipitating convulsions or altering cerebral blood flow in patients receiving benzodiazepines.

Neuromuscular blocking agents: Do not use flumazenil until the effects of neuromuscular blockade have been fully reversed.

Psychiatric patients: Flumazenil may provoke panic attacks in patients with a history of panic disorder.

Drug and alcohol dependent patients: Use with caution in patients with alcoholism and other drug dependencies due to the increased frequency of benzodiazepine tolerance and dependence observed in these patient populations.

Tolerance to benzodiazepines: Flumazenil may cause benzodiazepine withdrawal symptoms in individuals who have been taking benzodiazepines long enough to have some degree of tolerance. Slower titration rates of 0.1 mg/min and lower total doses may help reduce the frequency of emergent confusion and agitation.

Physical dependence on benzodiazepines: Flumazenil is known to precipitate withdrawal seizures in patients who are physically dependent on benzodiazepines, even if such dependence was established in a relatively few days of high-dose sedation in ICU environments. The risk of either seizures or resedation in such cases is high and patients have experienced seizures before regaining consciousness. Use flumazenil in such settings with extreme caution, because the use of flumazenil in this situation has not been studied and no information as to dose and rate of titration is available.

Pain on injection: To minimize the likelihood of pain or inflammation at the injection site, administer flumazenil through a freely flowing IV infusion into a large vein. Local irritation may occur following extravasation into perivascular tissues.

Respiratory disease: Appropriate ventilatory support is the primary treatment of patients with serious lung disease who experience serious respiratory depression due to benzodiazepines rather than the administration of flumazenil.

Ambulatory patients: Effects may wear off before a long-acting benzodiazepine is completely cleared from the body.

Mixed drug overdosage: Particular caution is necessary when using flumazenil in cases of mixed drug overdosage; toxic effects of other drugs taken in overdose (especially cyclic antidepressants) may emerge with reversal of the benzodiazepine effect by flumazenil.

Drug Interactions:

Drug/Food interactions: Ingestion of food during an IV infusion of flumazenil results in a 50% increase in flumazenil clearance, most likely due to the increased hepatic blood flow that accompanies a meal.

Adverse Reactions:

Adverse reactions may include death, convulsions, headache, injection site pain, increased sweating, fatigue, cutaneous vasodilation, nausea, vomiting, dizziness, agitation, dry mouth, tremors, palpitations, insomnia, dyspnea, hyperventilation, emotional lability, abnormal/blurred vision and paresthesia.

Administration and Dosage:

For IV use only. To minimize the likelihood of pain at the injection site, administer flumazenil through a freely running IV infusion into a large vein.

Individualization of dosage: In high-risk patients, it is important to administer the smallest amount of flumazenil that is effective. The 1 minute wait between individual doses in the dose-titration recommended for general clinical populations may be too short for high-risk patients because it takes 6 to 10 minutes for any single dose of flumazenil to reach full effects. Slow the rate of administration of flumazenil administered to high-risk patients.

Reversal of conscious sedation or in general anesthesia: The recommended initial dose is 0.2 mg (2 ml) administered IV over 15 seconds. If the desired level of consciousness is not obtained after waiting an additional 45 seconds, a further dose of 0.2 mg (2 ml) can be injected and repeated at 60 second intervals where necessary (up to a maximum of 4 additional times) to a maximum total dose of 1 mg (10 ml). Individualize the dose based on the patient's response, with most patients responding to doses of 0.6 to 1 mg.

In the event of resedation, repeated doses may be administered at 20 minute intervals as needed. For repeat treatment, administer no more than 1 mg (given as 0.2 mg/min) at any one time, and give no more than 3 mg in any one hour.

Suspected benzodiazepine overdose: The recommended initial dose is 0.2 mg (2 ml) administered IV over 30 seconds. If the desired level of consciousness is not obtained after waiting 30 seconds, a further dose of 0.3 mg (3 ml) can be administered over another 30 seconds. Further doses of 0.5 mg (5 ml) can be administered over 30 seconds at 1 minute intervals up to a cumulative dose of 3 mg.

Most patients with benzodiazepine overdose will respond to a cumulative dose of 1 to 3 mg, and doses beyond 3 mg do not reliably produce additional effects.

If a patient has not responded 5 minutes after receiving a cumulative dose of 5 mg, the major cause of sedation is likely not to be due to benzodiazepines, and additional flumazenil is likely to have no effect.

In the event of resedation, repeated doses may be given at 20 minute intervals if needed. For repeat treatment, give no more than 1 mg (given as 0.5 mg/min) at any one time and give no more than 3 mg in any one hour.

DIGOXIN IMMUNE FAB (Ovine)

Injection, lyophilized: 38 mg per vial (*Rx*)	*Digibind* (Glaxo Wellcome)

Actions:

Pharmacology: Digoxin immune fab (ovine) are antigen binding fragments (fab) derived from specific antidigoxin antibodies produced in sheep. Fab fragments bind molecules of digoxin, making them unavailable for binding at their site of action.

Pharmacokinetics: After IV injection in humans with normal renal function, the half-life appears to be 15 to 20 hours. Improvement in signs and symptoms of intoxication begins in less than half an hour.

The fab fragment-digoxin complex accumulates in the blood and is excreted by the kidneys.

Indications:

Digitalis intoxication: Treatment of potentially life-threatening digoxin intoxication. It has also been used successfully to treat life-threatening digitoxin overdose.

Warnings:

Hypersensitivity: Allergic reactions have not yet occurred, but consider the possibility of anaphylactic, hypersensitivity or febrile reactions. If an anaphylactoid reaction occurs, discontinue the drug infusion and initiate appropriate therapy. Have epinephrine 1:1000 immediately available. Refer to Management of Acute Hypersensitivity Reactions.

Patients allergic to ovine proteins are particularly at risk, as are individuals who have previously received antibodies or fab fragments raised in sheep.

Pregnancy: Category C.

Lactation: It is not known whether this drug is excreted in breast milk.

Children: This agent has been used successfully in infants with no apparent adverse sequelae. Digoxin immune fab is best used when ≥ 0.3 mg of digoxin/kg has been ingested, there is underlying heart disease or serum digoxin concentrations are ≥ 6.4 nmol/L.

Precautions:

Monitoring: Obtain serum concentrations before administration. Closely monitor the patient's temperature, blood pressure, ECG and potassium concentration during and after drug administration. The total serum digoxin concentration may rise precipitously following administration, but this will be almost entirely bound to the fab fragment. Fab fragments will interfere with digitalis immunoassay measurements.

Potassium – Monitor serum potassium concentration repeatedly, especially over the first several hours after the drug is given, and cautiously treat when necessary.

Withdrawal: Standard therapy for digitalis intoxication includes withdrawal of the drug and correction of factors that may contribute to toxicity such as electrolyte disturbances, hypoxia, acid-base disturbances and agents such as catecholamines.

Patients may deteriorate from withdrawal of digoxin. Additional support can be provided by use of IV inotropes or vasodilators. Do not use other types of digitalis glycosides or redigitalize until the fab fragments have been eliminated from the body; this may require several days.

Adverse Reactions:

Adverse reactions may include low cardiac output states; congestive heart failure; hypokalemia.

Administration and Dosage:

Administer IV over 15 to 30 minutes and infused through a 0.22 micron membrane filter. If cardiac arrest is imminent, give as a bolus injection.

Dosage varies according to the amount of digoxin to be neutralized. If, after several hours, toxicity has not reversed or appears to recur, readministration may be required. If a patient presents with digitalis toxicity from an acute ingestion, and neither a serum digitalis concentration nor an estimated ingestion amount is available, administer 20 vials (800 mg).

Dosage estimates: The dose need not be exactly equimolar. In general, a large dose has a faster onset but enhances the possibility of an allergic or febrile reaction.

Approximate Dose for Reversal of a Single Ingestion Digoxin Overdose

Number of Digoxin Tablets or Capsules Ingested*	Dose of digoxin immune fab (ovine)	
	mg	# of vials
25	340	10
50	760	20
75	1140	30
100	1520	40
150	2280	60
200	3040	80

* 0.25 mg tablets with 80% bioavailability or 0.2 mg *Lanoxicaps Capsules* (100% bioavailability).

Estimates of Fab Fragments From Serum Digoxin Concentration

Patient	Weight (kg)	Serum Digoxin Concentration (ng/ml)						
		1	2	4	8	12	16	20
Infants/Children (dose given in mg)	1	0.4 mg†:	1 mg†:	1.5 mg†:	3 mg	5 mg	6 mg	8 mg
	3	1 mg†:	2 mg†:	5 mg	9 mg	14 mg	18 mg	22 mg
	5	2 mg†:	4 mg	8 mg	15 mg	23 mg	30 mg	40 mg
	10	4 mg	8 mg	15 mg	30 mg	46 mg	61 mg	80 mg
	20	8 mg	15 mg	30 mg	61 mg	91 mg	122 mg	160 mg
Adults (dose given in vials [v])	40	0.5 v	1 v	2 v	3 v	5 v	2 v	8 v
	60	0.5 v	1 v	3 v	5 v	7 v	10 v	11 v
	70	1 v	2 v	3 v	6 v	8 v	11 v	13 v
	80	1 v	2 v	3 v	7 v	9 v	13 v	15 v
	100	1 v	2 v	4 v	8 v	11 v	16 v	19 v

† Dilution of reconstituted vial to 1 mg/ml may be desirable.

Chronic therapy:

Adults – Six vials (28 mg) usually is adequate to reverse most cases of toxicity. This dose can be used in patients who are in acute distress or for whom a serum digoxin or digitoxin concentration is not available.

Children – For those weighing ≤ 20 kg, a single vial usually should suffice.

SUCCIMER

Capsules: 100 mg (*Rx*)	*Chemet* (Bock)

Actions:

Pharmacology: Succimer is an orally active, heavy metal chelating agent; it forms water soluble chelates and, consequently, increases the urinary excretion of lead.

Toxicology – The kidney and the GI tract were the major target organs for succimer toxicity.

Pharmacokinetics: Absorption is rapid but variable, with peak blood levels between 1 and 2 hours. Approximately 49% of the dose was excreted: 39% in the feces, 9% in the urine and 1% as carbon dioxide from the lungs. The apparent elimination half-life was about 2 days.

Indications:

Treatment of lead poisoning in children with blood lead levels > 45 mcg/dl. Not indicated for prophylaxis of lead poisoning in a lead-containing environment; always accompany the use of succimer with identification and removal of the source of the lead exposure.

Unlabeled uses: Succimer may be beneficial in the treatment of other heavy metal poisonings (eg, mercury, arsenic).

Contraindications:

History of allergy to the drug.

Warnings:

Keep out of reach of children.

Not a substitute for effective abatement of lead exposure.

Pregnancy: Category C.

Lactation: It is not known whether this drug is excreted in breast milk. Discourage mothers requiring therapy from nursing their infants.

Children: There is no therapeutic experience with succimer in children < 1 year of age.

Precautions:

Carefully observe patients during treatment due to limited clinical experience with succimer.

Elevated blood lead levels and associated symptoms may return rapidly after discontinuation of succimer because of redistribution of lead from bone stores to soft tissues and blood. After therapy, monitor patients for rebound of blood lead levels by measuring the levels at least once weekly until stable. However, use the severity of lead intoxication (as measured by the initial blood lead level and the rate and degree of rebound of blood lead) as a guide for more frequent blood lead monitoring.

Renal function: Adequately hydrate all patients undergoing treatment. Exercise caution in using succimer therapy in patients with compromised renal function. Limited data suggest that succimer is dialyzable, but that the lead chelates are not.

Hepatic function: Transient mild elevations of serum transaminases have been observed in 6% to 10% of patients during the course of therapy. Monitor serum transaminases before the start of therapy and at least weekly during therapy. Closely monitor patients with a history of liver disease.

Repeated courses: Clinical experience is limited. The safety of uninterrupted dosing > 3 weeks has not been established and is not recommended.

Allergic reactions: The possibility of allergic or other mucocutaneous reactions to the drug must be borne in mind on readministration (as well as during initial courses). Monitor patients requiring repeated courses during each treatment course.

Drug Interactions:

Chelation therapy (eg, EDTA): Coadministration of succimer with other chelation therapy is not recommended.

Drug/Lab test interactions: Succimer may interfere with serum and urinary laboratory tests. In vitro, succimer caused false-positive results for ketones in urine using nitroprusside reagents such as Ketostix and falsely decreased measurements of serum uric acid and CPK.

Adverse Reactions:

Adverse reactions may include: Increases in serum transaminases; rash; nausea; vomiting; diarrhea; appetite loss; hemorrhoidal symptoms; loose stools; metallic taste in mouth; back/stomach/head/rib/flank pain; abdominal cramps; chills; fever; flu-like symptoms; heavy head; headache; moniliasis; elevated AST/ALT/alkaline phosphatase/serum cholesterol; drowsiness; dizziness; sensorimotor neuropathy; sleepiness; paresthesia; cloudy film in eye; ears plugged; otitis media; decreased urination; voiding difficulty; proteinuria increased.

Administration and Dosage:

Start dosage at 10 mg/kg or 350 mg/m^2 every 8 hours for 5 days; initiation of therapy at higher doses is not recommended. Reduce frequency of administration to 10 mg/kg or 350 mg/m^2 every 12 hours (two-thirds of initial daily dosage) for an additional 2 weeks of therapy. A course of treatment lasts 19 days. Repeated courses may be necessary if indicated by weekly monitoring of blood lead concentration. A minimum of 2 weeks between courses is recommended unless blood lead levels indicate the need for more prompt treatment.

Succimer Pediatric Dosing Chart

Weight			
lbs	kg	Dose (mg)[1]	Number of capsules[1]
18-35	8-15	100	1
36-55	16-23	200	2
56-75	24-34	300	3
76-100	35-44	400	4
> 100	> 45	500	5

[1] To be administered every 8 hours for 5 days, followed by dosing every 12 hours for 14 days.

Patients who have received EDTA with or without BAL may use succimer for subsequent treatment after an interval of 4 weeks. Data on the concomitant use of succimer with EDTA with or without BAL are not available, and such use is not recommended.

PENICILLAMINE

Capsules: 125 and 250 mg (*Rx*)	*Cuprimine* (MSD)
Tablets, titratable: 250 mg (*Rx*)	*Depen* (Wallace)

Actions:

Pharmacology:

Rheumatoid arthritis – The mechanism of action of penicillamine in rheumatoid arthritis is unknown. The onset of therapeutic response may not be seen for 2 or 3 months in those patients who respond.

Wilson's disease: Penicillamine is a chelating agent that removes excess copper in patients with Wilson's disease. Noticeable improvement may not occur for 1 to 3 months.

Poisoning: Penicillamine also forms soluble complexes with iron, mercury, lead and arsenic which are readily excreted by the kidneys. The drug may be used to treat poisoning by these metals.

Cystinuria: Penicillamine reduces excess cystine excretion in cystinuria. Penicillamine with conventional therapy decreases crystalluria and stone formation and may decrease the size of or dissolve existing stones. This is done, at least in part, by disulfide interchange between penicillamine and cystine, resulting in a substance more soluble than cystine and readily excreted.

Pharmacokinetics: It is well absorbed from the GI tract after oral administration (40% to 70%); peak plasma levels occur in 1 to 3 hours. Most (80%) of the plasma penicillamine is protein bound, primarily to albumin. Penicillamine is rapidly excreted in the urine; 50% is excreted in the feces. Metabolites may be detected in the urine for up to 3 months after stopping the drug. Half-life ranges are 1.7 to 3.2 hours.

Indications:

Rheumatoid arthritis.

Wilson's disease (hepatolenticular degeneration).

Cystinuria.

Unlabeled uses: The benefits of penicillamine's copper chelating and immunological effects have been investigated for use in the treatment of primary biliary cirrhosis.

Contraindications:

History of penicillamine-related aplastic anemia or agranulocytosis; rheumatoid arthritis patients with a history or other evidence of renal insufficiency; pregnancy; breastfeeding.

Warnings:

Fatalities: Penicillamine has been associated with fatalities due to aplastic anemia, agranulocytosis, thrombocytopenia, Goodpasture's syndrome and myasthenia gravis.

Hematologic: Leukopenia (2%) and thrombocytopenia (4%) have occurred. A reduction in WBC below 3500, neutrophils $< 2000/mm^3$, or monocytes $> 500/mm^3$ mandate permanent withdrawal of therapy.

Hepatotoxicity: Penicillamine has been associated with a mild elevation of hepatic enzymes that usually returns to normal even with continuation of the drug.

Autoimmune syndromes which may be caused by penicillamine include *polymyositis, diffuse alveolitis* and *dermatomyositis, Goodpasture's syndrome, myastheinc syndrome, pemphigus* and *obliterative bronchiolitis*

Pemphigoid-type reactions characterized by bullous lesions have required discontinuation of penicillamine and treatment with corticosteroids.

Lupus erythematosus: Certain patients will develop a positive antinuclear antibody (ANA) test and some may show a lupus erythematosus-like syndrome similar to other drug-induced lupus, but it is not associated with hypocomplementemia and may be present without nephropathy. A positive ANA test does not mandate drug discontinuance; however, a lupus erythematosus-like syndrome may develop later.

Sensitivity reactions: Once instituted for Wilson's disease or cystinuria, continue treatment with penicillamine on a daily basis. Interruptions for even a few days have been followed by sensitivity reactions after reinstitution of therapy.

Hypersensitivity: Allergic reactions occur in ≈ ⅓ of patients. They are more common at the start of treatment, and occur as generalized rashes or drug fever. Discontinue treatment and reinstitute at a low dosage such as 250 mg/day, with gradual increases. Administering prednisolone 20 mg/day for the first few weeks of penicillamine therapy reduces the severity of these reactions. Antihistamines may control pruritus.

Renal function impairment: Proteinuria and hematuria may develop and may be a warning sign of membranous glomerulopathy which can progress to a nephrotic syndrome.

Pregnancy: *Category D.*

Lactation: Safety has not been established.

Children: The efficacy of penicillamine in juvenile rheumatoid arthritis has not been established.

Precautions:

Monitoring: When indicated, monitor drug toxicity or efficacy through urinalysis. In rheumatoid arthritis patients, discontinue the drug if unexplained gross hematuria or persistent microscopic hematuria develops. Perform liver function tests and an annual x–ray for renal stones.

Monitor white and differential blood cell count, hemoglobin determination, and direct platelet count every 2 weeks for the first 6 months of penicillamine therapy and monthly thereafter.

Drug fever may appear in some patients, usually in the second to third week of therapy; it is sometimes accompanied by a macular cutaneous eruption.

Dermatologic – Skin rashes are the most frequent (44% to 50%) adverse reactions. Early rash occurs during the first few months of treatment and is more common.

A *late rash* is less commonly seen, usually after 6 months or more of treatment, and requires drug discontinuation. It usually appears on the trunk, is accompanied by intense pruritus, and is usually unresponsive to topical corticosteroids.

Pemphigoid rash, the most serious dermatologic reaction occurs most often after 6 to 9 months of penicillamine.

Oral ulcerations may develop which may have the appearance of aphthous stomatitis. Although rare, cheilosis, glossitis and gingivostomatitis have been reported.

Hypogeusia occurs in 25% to 33% of patients, except for a lesser incidence in Wilson's disease (4%).

Dietary supplementation: Because of their dietary restriction, give patients with Wilson's disease, cystinuria and rheumatoid arthritis whose nutrition is impaired 25 mg/day of pyridoxine during therapy, because penicillamine increases the requirement for this vitamin.

Iron deficiency may develop, especially in children and in menstruating women. This may be caused by diet. If necessary, give iron in short courses. A period of 2 hours should elapse between administration of penicillamine and iron, since orally administered iron reduces the effects of penicillamine.

Effects of penicillamine on collagen and elastin make it advisable to consider a reduction in dosage to 250 mg/day when surgery is contemplated.

Penicillamine may cause increased skin friability at sites subject to pressure or trauma, such as shoulders, elbows, knees, toes and buttocks.

Drug Interactions:

Drugs that may affect penicillamine include gold therapy, antimalarial or cytotoxic drugs, iron salts, antacids and food.

Drugs that may be affected by penicillamine include digoxin.

Adverse Reactions:

Penicillamine has a high incidence (over 50%) of untoward reactions, some of which are potentially fatal.

Adverse reactions that may occurin ≥ 3% of patients include: Anorexia; epigastric pain; nausea; vomiting; diarrhea; blunting/diminution/total loss of taste; taste perversion; thrombocytopenia; generalized pruritis; early and late rashes; proteinuria.

Administration and Dosage:

Give penicillamine on an empty stomach at least 1 hour before meals or 2 hours after meals and at least 1 hour apart from any other drug, food or milk.

Wilson's disease: Initial dosage is 1 g/day for children or adults. This may be increased, as indicated by the urinary copper analyses, but it is seldom necessary to exceed 2 g/day. In patients who cannot tolerate 1 g/day initially, initiating dosage with 250 mg/day and increasing gradually allows closer control of the drug. Give on an empty stomach in 4 divided doses, 30 minutes to 1 hour before meals and at bedtime (at least 2 hours after the evening meal).

Cystinuria:

Adult dosage – 2 g/day (range 1 to 4 g/day) in 4 divided doses.

Pediatric dosage – 30 mg/kg/day in 4 divided doses. If 4 equal doses are not feasible, give the larger portion at bedtime. Initiating dosage with 250 mg/day, and increasing gradually, allows closer control of the drug and may reduce the incidence of adverse reactions.

Patients should drink about a pint of fluid at bedtime and another pint once during the night when urine is more concentrated and more acid than during the day. The greater the fluid intake, the lower the dosage of penicillamine required.

Rheumatoid arthritis: Administer on an empty stomach at least 1 hour before meals and at least 1 hour apart from any other drug, food or milk.

Initial therapy: A single daily dose of 125 or 250 mg. Thereafter, increase dose at 1 to 3 month intervals by 125 or 250 mg/day as patient response and tolerance indicate. If satisfactory remission is achieved, continue the dose. If there is no improvement and if there are no signs of potentially serious toxicity after 2 to 3 months with doses of 500 to 750 mg/day, continue increases of 250 mg/day at 2 to 3 month intervals until satisfactory remission occurs or toxicity develops. If there is no discernible improvement after 3 to 4 months of treatment with 1 to 1.5 g/day, assume the patient will not respond and discontinue the drug.

Maintenance therapy: Many patients respond to 500 to 750 mg/day or less. In patients who respond but who evidence incomplete disease suppression after the first 6 to 9 months of treatment, increase daily dosage by 125 or 250 mg/day at 3 month intervals. Dosage above 1 g/day is unusual, but up to 1.5 g/day has been required.

Dosage frequency: Dosages ≤ 500 mg/day can be given as a single daily dose. Dosages > 500 mg/day should be administered in divided doses.

ALPROSTADIL (Prostaglandin E_1; PGE_1)

Lyophilized powder for injection: 6.15 mcg (5 mcg/ml), 11.9 mcg (10 mcg/ml) and 23.2 mcg (20 mcg/ml) (*Rx*)	*Caverject* (Upjohn)
Pellet: 125, 250, 500 or 1000 mcg (*Rx*)	*Muse* (Vivus)

Actions:

Pharmacology: Alprostadil induces erection by relaxation of trabecular smooth muscle and by dilation of cavernosal arteries.

Pharmacokinetics:

Distribution – Following intracavernosal injection, mean peripheral plasma concentrations at 30 and 60 minutes after injection were not significantly greater than baseline levels of endogenous alprostadil. Alprostadil is bound in plasma primarily to albumin (81% bound).

Intraurethral: Following intraurethral administration, alprostadil is absorbed from the urethral mucosa into the corpus spongosium. The half-life is short, varying between 30 seconds and 10 minutes.

Metabolism – Following IV administration, 60% to 90% of circulating alprostadil is metabolized in one pass through the lungs, primarily by beta- and omega-oxidation. The near-complete pulmonary first-pass metabolism of PGE_1 is the primary factor influencing the systemic pharmacokinetics of alprostadil and is a reason that peripheral venous plasma levels of PGE_1 are low or undetectable (< 2 pg/ml) following alprostadil administration. The enzyme catalyzing this process has been isolated from many tissues in the lower GU tract including the urethra, prostate and corpus cavernosum.

Excretion – The metabolites of alprostadil are excreted primarily by the kidney, with almost 90% of an administered IV dose excreted in urine within 24 hours post-dose. The remainder of the dose is excreted in the feces.

Indications:

Erectile dysfunction: Treatment of erectile dysfunction caused by neurogenic, vasculogenic, psychogenic or mixed etiology.

Intracavernosal alprostadil may be a useful adjunct to other diagnostic tests in the diagnosis of erectile dysfunction.

Unlabeled uses: Diagnostic peripheral arteriography (0.7 mcg/min for 10 min); treatment of atherosclerosis, gangrene and pain caused by peripheral vascular disease.

Contraindications:

Hypersensitivity to the drug; conditions that might predispose patients to priapism (eg, sickle cell anemia or trait, multiple myeloma, leukemia); patients with anatomical deformation of the penis; patients with penile implants (intracavernosal); use in women, children or newborns; use in men for whom sexual activity is inadvisable or contraindicated; for sexual intercourse with a pregnant woman unless the couple uses a condom barrier.

Warnings:

Priapism is known to occur following intracavernosal administration of vasoactive substances, including alprostadil. To minimize the chances of prolonged erection or priapism, titrate slowly to the lowest effective dose. Instruct the patient to seek immediate medical assistance for any erection that persists for > 6 hours. If priapism is not treated immediately, penile tissue damage and permanent loss of potency may result.

Penile fibrosis: Regular follow-up of patients, with careful examination of the penis, is strongly recommended to detect signs of penile fibrosis. Discontinue treatment in patients who develop penile angulation, cavernosal fibrosis or Peyronie's disease.

Penile pain after intracavernosal administration was reported. In the majority of the cases, penile pain was rated mild or moderate in intensity. Inject alprostadil slowly to decrease penile pain.

Hematoma/Ecchymosis: In most cases, hematoma/ecchymosis was judged to be a complication of a faulty injection technique.

Hemodynamic changes, manifested as decreases in blood pressure and increases in pulse rate, principally at doses > 20 mcg, were observed during clinical studies, and appeared to be dose-dependent.

Erectile dysfunction, causes: Diagnose and treat underlying treatable medical causes of erectile dysfunction prior to initiation of therapy.

Pulmonary disease: The pulmonary extraction of alprostadil following intravascular administration was reduced by 15% in patients with acute respiratory distress syndrome (ARDS).

Renal/Hepatic function impairment: Alterations in renal or hepatic function would not be expected to have a major influence on the pharmacokinetics of alprostadil.

Pregnancy: These products are not indicated for use in women. Do not use for sexual intercourse with a pregnant woman unless the couple uses a condom barrier.

Children: *Caverject* is not indicated for use in newborns or children. However, alprostadil (*Prostin VR Pediatric*) is used in newborns to maintain the patency of the ductus arteriosus in neonates with congenital heart defects.

Drug Interactions:

Drugs that may interact with alprostadil include anticoagulants, cyclosporine and vasoactive agents.

Adverse Reactions:

Adverse reactions occurring in ≥ 3% of patients receiving alprostadil by intracavernosal administration include penile pain, prolonged erection, penile fibrosis, hematoma, injection site hematoma, penis disorder and upper respiratory infection.

Adverse reactions in ≥ 3% of patients receiving alprostadil by intraurethral administration include penile pain, urethral pain, urethral burning, urethral bleeding/spotting, testicular pain, headache, dizziness, URI, flu syndrome, hypotension, pain and accidental injury.

Administration and Dosage:

Initial titration:

Erectile dysfunction of vasculogenic, psychogenic or mixed etiology – Initiate dosage titration at 2.5 mcg. If there is a partial response, the dose may be increased by 2.5 mcg to a dose of 5 mcg and then in increments of 5 to 10 mcg, depending on erectile response, until the dose that produces an erection suitable for intercourse and not exceeding a duration of 1 hour is reached. If there is no response to the initial 2.5 mcg dose, the second dose may be increased to 7.5 mcg, followed by increments of 5 to 10 mcg. If there is no response, then the next higher dose may be given within 1 hour. If there is a response, then there should be at least a 1-day interval before the next dose is given.

Erectile dysfunction of pure neurogenic etiology (spinal cord injury) Initiate dosage titration at 1.25 mcg. The dose may be increased by 1.25 mcg to a dose of 2.5 mcg, followed by an increment of 2.5 mcg to a dose of 5 mcg, and then in 5 mcg increments until the dose that produces an erection suitable for intercourse and not exceeding a duration of 1 hour is reached. If there is no response, then the next higher dose may be given within 1 hour. If there is a response, then there should be at least a 1-day interval before the next dose is given.

Maintenance therapy: The first injections of alprostadil must be done at the physician's office by medically trained personnel. Self-injection therapy by the patient can be started only after the patient is properly instructed and well-trained in the self-injection technique. The recommended frequency of injection is no more than 3 times weekly, with at least 24 hours between each dose.

Intraurethral: Administer as needed to acheive an erection. The onset of effect is within 5 to 10 minutes after administration. The duration of effect is ≈ 30 to 60 minutes. A medical professional should instruct each patient on proper technique for administering alprostadil prior to self-administration. The maximum frequency of use is no more than two systems per 24–hour period.

Initiation of therapy – Titrate dose under the supervision of a physician to test a patient's response to alprostadil, to demonstrate proper administration technique and to monitor for evidence of hypotension. Individually titrate patients to the lowest dose that is sufficient for sexual intercourse. If necessary, increase the dose (or decrease) on separate occasions in a stepwise manner until the patient achieves an erection that is sufficient for sexual intercourse.

DISULFIRAM

Tablets: 250 and 500 mg (*Rx*) Various, *Antabuse* (Wyeth-Ayerst)

Warning:

Never give to a patient in a state of alcohol intoxication, or without the patient's full knowledge. Instruct the patient's relatives accordingly.

Actions:

Pharmacology: Disulfiram produces an intolerance to alcohol which results in a highly unpleasant reaction when the patient under treatment ingests even small amounts of alcohol. Disulfiram blocks oxidation of alcohol at the acetaldehyde stage by inhibiting aldehyde dehydrogenase. Accumulation of acetaldehyde produces the disulfiram-alcohol reaction. This reaction persists as long as alcohol is being metabolized.

Pharmacokinetics: Disulfiram is rapidly absorbed from the GI tract and eliminated slowly from the body. About 12 hours are required for its full action. Disulfiram is metabolized to diethyldithiocarbamate, which is oxidized to carbon disulfide and diethylamine. Ingestion of alcohol may produce unpleasant symptoms for 1 to 2 weeks after the last dose of disulfiram.

Indications:

An aid in the management of selected chronic alcoholics who want to remain in a state of enforced sobriety.

Contraindications:

Severe myocardial disease or coronary occlusion; psychoses; hypersensitivity to disulfiram or to other thiuram derivatives used in pesticides and rubber vulcanization; patients receiving or who have recently received metronidazole, paraldehyde, alcohol, or alcohol-containing preparations.

Warnings:

Disulfiram-alcohol reaction: Disulfiram plus alcohol, even small amounts, produces flushing, throbbing in head and neck, throbbing headaches, respiratory difficulty, nausea, copious vomiting, sweating, thirst, chest pain, palpitations, dyspnea, hyperventilation, tachycardia, hypotension, syncope, marked uneasiness, weakness, vertigo, blurred vision and confusion. In severe reactions there may be respiratory depression, cardiovascular collapse, arrhythmias, myocardial infarction, acute congestive heart failure, unconsciousness, convulsions and death. The intensity of the reaction is proportional to the amounts of disulfiram and alcohol ingested.

Concomitant conditions: Because of the possibility of an accidental reaction, use with caution in patients with diabetes mellitus, hypothyroidism, epilepsy, cerebral damage, chronic and acute nephritis, hepatic cirrhosis or insufficiency.

Pregnancy: Category C.

Precautions:

Monitoring: Perform baseline and follow-up transaminase tests (10 to 14 days) to detect hepatic dysfunction resulting from therapy. Perform a CBC and SMA-12 test every 6 months.

Ethylene dibromide: Patients should not be exposed to ethylene dibromide or its vapors.

Drug Interactions:

Drugs that may interact with disulfiram include alcohol, benzodazepines, caffeine, hydantoins, isoniazid, metronidazole, tricyclic antidepressants and warfarin.

Adverse Reactions:

Adverse reactions may include: Peripheral neuropathy; polyneuritis; optic or retrobulbar neuritis (with impaired vision, color perceptions and blindness); drowsiness; headache; restlessness; occasional skin eruptions; acneiform eruptions; allergic dermatitis; metallic or garlic-like aftertaste; hepatotoxicity resembling viral or alcoholic hepatitis; multiple cases of both cholestatic and fulminant hepatitis; arthropathy; acetonemia; impotence.

Administration and Dosage:

Do NOT administer until the patient has abstained from alcohol for at least 12 hours.

Initial dosage schedule: Administer a maximum of 500 mg daily in a single dose for 1 to 2 weeks. If a sedative effect is experienced, take at bedtime or decrease dosage.

Maintenance regimen: The average maintenance dose is 250 mg daily (range, 125 to 500 mg), not to exceed 500 mg daily.

NICOTINE

NICOTINE TRANSDERMAL	
Transdermal System (*Rx*)	*Habitrol* (Basel Pharm.), *Nicoderm* (SmithKline-Beecham), *Nicotrol* (McNeil), *ProStep* (Lederle)
NICOTINE POLACRILEX	
Chewing gum: 2 mg (*otc*)	*Nicorette* (SK-Beecham)
4 mg nicotine (*otc*)	*Nicorette DS* (SK-Beecham)

Actions:

Pharmacology: Nicotine, the chief alkaloid in tobacco products, binds stereoselectively to acetylcholine receptors at the autonomic ganglia, in the adrenal medulla, at neuromuscular junctions and in the brain.

Pharmacokinetics:

Nicotine gum –

Absorption/Distribution: The nicotine is bound to an ion exchange resin and is released only during chewing; nicotine will not be released in significant amounts if the gum is swallowed. The blood level of nicotine will depend upon the vigor, rapidity and duration of chewing.

Metabolism/Excretion – Nicotine is metabolized mainly by the liver, and to a lesser extent, by the kidney and lung. The half-life of nicotine ranges from 1 to 2 hours. The primary metabolite of nicotine in plasma, cotinine, has a half-life of 15 to 20 hours and concentrations that exceed nicotine by 10-fold.

Nicotine transdermal system: All systems are labeled by the actual amount of nicotine absorbed by the patient. After application, plasma concentrations rise rapidly, then slowly decline until the system is removed, after which they decline more rapidly.

Following system removal, plasma nicotine concentrations decline in an exponential fashion with an apparent mean half-life of 3 to 4 hours, caused by continued absorption from the skin depot. Most nonsmoking patients will have nondetectable nicotine concentrations in 10 to 12 hours.

Indications:

As an aid to smoking cessation for the relief of nicotine withdrawal symptoms. Use as part of a comprehensive behavioral smoking-cessation program.

Contraindications:

Hypersensitivity to nicotine or any components of the transdermal system; nonsmokers; during the immediate postmyocardial infarction period; life-threatening arrhythmias; severe or worsening angina pectoris; active temporomandibular joint disease (nicotine polacrilex); pregnancy.

Warnings:

Cardiovascular: Specifically, screen and evaluate patients with coronary heart disease, serious cardiac arrhythmias or vasospastic diseases before nicotine is prescribed. There have been occasional reports of tachyarrhythmias associated with nicotine use; therefore, if an increase in cardiovascular symptoms occurs, discontinue the drug.

Endocrine: Because of the action of nicotine on the adrenal medulla, use with caution in patients with hyperthyroidism, pheochromocytoma or insulin-dependent diabetes.

Renal/Hepatic function impairment: Anticipate some influence of hepatic impairment on drug kinetics (reduced clearance). Only severe renal impairment should affect clearance of nicotine or its metabolites from circulation.

Elderly: Transdermal nicotine therapy appeared to be as effective in elderly patients > 60 years of age as in younger smokers. However, asthenia, various body aches and dizziness occurred slightly more often in elderly patients.

Pregnancy: Category X (nicotine polacrilex), *Category D* (transdermal nicotine). Nicotine is contraindicated in women who are or may become pregnant; advise patients to use contraceptive measures.

Lactation: Nicotine passes freely into breast milk and has the potential for serious adverse reactions in nursing infants.

Children: Safety and efficacy in children/adolescents who smoke are not evaluated. The amounts of nicotine that are tolerated by adult smokers can produce symptoms of poisoning and could prove fatal if the transdermal nicotine system is applied or ingested by children or pets.

Precautions:

Oral/GI: Use caution in patients with oral or pharyngeal inflammation and in those with history of esophagitis or peptic ulcer.

Skin disease: Systems are usually well tolerated by patients with normal skin, but may be irritating for patients with some skin disorders (atopic or eczematous dermatitis).

Allergic reactions: Caution patients with contact sensitization that a serious reaction could occur from exposure to other nicotine-containing products or smoking.

Dental problems might be exacerbated by chewing nicotine gum.

Drug abuse and dependence: Urge patients to stop smoking completely when initiating therapy. If patients smoke while using nicotine, they may experience adverse effects due to peak nicotine levels higher than those due to smoking alone.

To minimize risk of dependence, encourage patients to gradually withdraw or stop gum usage at 3 months, transdermal nicotine after 4 to 8 weeks. Chronic consumption is toxic and addicting.

Drug Interactions:

Smoking cessation, with or without nicotine substitutes, may alter response to concomitant medication in ex-smokers. Smoking may affect acetaminophen, caffeine, imipramine, oxazepam, pentazocine, propranolol, theophylline, catecholamines, cortisol, furosemide, glutethimide, insulin and propoxyphene.

Adverse Reactions:

Adverse reactions from nicotine polacrilex include: Traumatic injury to oral mucosa or teeth; jaw ache; eructation secondary to air swallowing; stomatitis; glossitis; gingivitis; pharyngitis; aphthous ulcers; changes in taste perception; nonspecific GI distress; nausea/vomiting; hiccoughs; edema; flushing; hypertension; palpitations; tachyarrhythmias; tachycardia; cardiac irritability; deaths; myocardial infarction; congestive heart failure; confusion; convulsions; depression; euphoria; numbness; paresthesia; syncope; tinnitus; weakness; erythema; itching; rash; urticaria; constipation; diarrhea; breathing difficulty; cough; hoarseness; sneezing; wheezing; dry mouth.

Reactions associated with transdermal nicotine include: Short-lived erythema; pruritus or burning at the application site; cutaneous hypersensitivity; asthenia; back pain; diarrhea; dyspepsia; constipation; nausea; headache; insomnia; abnormal dreams; nervousness; dizziness; increased cough; pharyngitis; rash; myalgia; arthralgia; taste perversion; dysmenorrhea.

Administration and Dosage:

Nicotine Transdermal:

Recommended Dosing Schedule of Transdermal Nicotine for Healthy Patients		
	Duration	
Dose	Per strength of patch	Entire course of therapy
Habitrol[1]		
21 mg/day	First 6 weeks	8 to 12 weeks
14 mg/day	Next 2 weeks[2]	
7 mg/day	Last 2 weeks[3]	
Nicoderm[1]		
21 mg/day	First 6 weeks	8 to 12 weeks
14 mg/day	Next 2 weeks[2]	
7 mg/day	Last 2 weeks	
Nicotrol		
15 mg/day	First 12 weeks	14 to 20 weeks
10 mg/day	Next 2 weeks[2]	
5 mg/day	Last 2 weeks	
ProStep[3]		
22 mg/day	4 to 8 weeks	6 to 12 weeks
11 mg/day[4]	2 to 4 weeks	

[1] Start with 14 mg/day for 6 weeks for patients who: Have cardiovascular disease; weigh < 100 lbs; smoke < ½ pack of cigarettes/day. Decrease dose to 7 mg/day for the final 2 to 4 weeks.
[2] Patients who have successfully abstained from smoking should have their dose reduced after each 2 to 4 weeks of treatment until the 7 mg/day dose (*Habitrol; Nicoderm*) or 5 mg/day dose (*Nicotrol*) has been used for 2 to 4 weeks.
[3] Start with 22 mg/day except for patients who weigh < 100 lbs; they may start with 11 mg/day with the dose increased as appropriate.
[4] Optional weaning dose.

Habitrol, Nicoderm, ProStep – After 24 hours, remove the used system and apply a new system to an alternate skin site. Skin sites should not be reused for at least a week. Caution patients not to continue to use the same system for > 24 hours.

Nicotrol – Each day apply a new system upon waking and remove at bedtime.

Nicotine Polacrilex: Increasing to the 4 mg dose may be considered for patients who fail to stop smoking with the 2 mg dose, or for those whose nicotine withdrawal symptoms remain so strong as to threaten relapse.

Recommended Nicotine Polacrilex Dosing Schedule for Healthy Patients			
Nicotine polacrililex	Cigarettes/day	Number of pieces to be used per day	Maximum pieces per day
4 mg	≥ 25	9 -12	20
2 mg	> 25	9 -12	30

Acidic beverages (eg, coffee, juices, wine, soft drinks) interfere with the buccal absorption before and during chewing of nicotine gum. Therefore, avoid eating and drinking for 15 minutes before and during chewing of nicotine gum.

Abstinence (quit) rates may be higher when patients chew nicotine gum on a fixed schedule (one piece every 1 to 2 hours) than when allowed to chew it as needed.

AZATHIOPRINE

Tablets: 50 mg (*Rx*)	*Imuran* (Glaxo Wellcome)
Injection: 100 mg (as sodium) per vial (*Rx*)	Various, *Imuran* (Glaxo Wellcome)

Warning:
Chronic immunosuppression with azathioprine increases the risk of neoplasia. Physicians using this drug should be familiar with this risk as well as with the mutagenic potential to both men and women and with possible hematologic toxicities.

Actions:

Pharmacology: Azathioprine, an imidazoyl derivative of 6–mercaptopurine (6–MP), has many biological effects similar to those of the parent compound.

Homograft survival – Although the use of azathioprine for inhibition of renal homograft rejection is well established, the mechanism(s) for this action are obscure.

Immunoinflammatory response – The severity of adjuvant arthritis is reduced by azathioprine. The mechanisms whereby it affects autoimmune diseases are not known.

Pharmacokinetics: Azathioprine is well absorbed following oral administration. Blood levels are of little value for therapy since the magnitude and duration of clinical effects correlate with thiopurine nucleotide levels in tissues rather than with plasma drug levels.

Indications:

Renal homotransplantation: As an adjunct for the prevention of rejection in renal homotransplantation.

Rheumatoid arthritis: Indicated only in adult patients meeting criteria for classic or definite rheumatoid arthritis as specified by the American Rheumatism Association. Restrict use to patients with severe, active and erosive disease not responsive to conventional management.

Unlabeled uses: Azathioprine has been used in the treatment of chronic ulcerative colitis; however, serious adverse effects may offset its limited value.

Azathioprine has been used for the treatment of generalized myasthenia gravis.

Azathioprine may be effective in controlling the progression of Behcet's syndrome, especially eye disease, the most serious manifestation.

Although controversial, low-dose azathioprine may be effective in treating Crohn's disease.

Contraindications:

Hypersensitivity to azathioprine; pregnancy in rheumatoid arthritis patients.

Warnings:

Hematologic effects: Severe leukopenia or thrombocytopenia, macrocytic anemia, severe bone marrow depression and selective erythrocyte aplasia may occur in patients on azathioprine. Hematologic toxicities are dose-related, may occur late in the course of therapy and may be more severe in renal transplant patients whose homograft is undergoing rejection. Perform complete blood counts, including platelet counts, weekly during the first month, twice monthly for the second and third months of treatment, then monthly or more frequently if dosage alterations or other therapy changes are necessary.

Infections: Serious infections are a constant hazard for patients on chronic immunosuppression, especially for homograft recipients. The incidence of infection in renal homotransplantation is 30 to 60 times that in rheumatoid arthritis. Fungal, viral, bacterial and protozoal infections may be fatal and should be treated vigorously.

GI toxicity: A GI hypersensitivity reaction characterized by severe nausea and vomiting has been reported. These symptoms may also be accompanied by diarrhea, rash, fever, malaise, myalgias, elevations in liver enzymes, and occasionally hypotension.

Hepatotoxicity with elevated serum alkaline phosphatase and bilirubin may occur primarily in allograft recipients. Periodically measure serum transaminases, alkaline phosphatase and bilirubin for early detection of hepatotoxicity.

Carcinogenesis/Mutagenesis/Fertility impairment: Azathioprine is carcinogenic in animals and may increase the patient's risk of neoplasia. Azathioprine is mutagenic in animals and humans.

Pregnancy: *Category D.*

Lactation: Use of azathioprine in nursing mothers is not recommended.

Children: Safety and efficacy in children have not been established. However, it has been used in children.

Drug Interactions:

Drugs that may affect azathioprine include ACE inhibitors, allopurinol and methotrexate.

Drugs that may be affected include anticoagulants, cyclosporine and nondepolarizing neuromuscular blockers.

Adverse Reactions:

The principal and potentially serious toxic effects are hematologic and GI. Adverse reactions may include leukopenia, infections and neoplasia.

Administration and Dosage:

Renal homotransplantation: Initial dose is usually 3 to 5 mg/kg/day, given as a single daily dose on the day of transplantation, and in a minority of cases, 1 to 3 days before transplantation. It is often initiated IV, with subsequent use of tablets (at the same dose level) after the postoperative period. Reserve IV administration for patients unable to tolerate oral medications. Maintenance levels are 1 to 3 mg/kg/day.

Children – An initial dose of 3 to 5 mg/kg/day IV or orally followed by a maintenance dose of 1 to 3 mg/kg/day has been recommended.

Rheumatoid arthritis: Initial dose is approximately 1 mg/kg (50 to 100 mg) given as a single dose or twice daily. The dose may be increased, beginning at 6 to 8 weeks and thereafter by steps at 4 week intervals, if there are no serious toxicities and if initial response is unsatisfactory. Use dose increments of 0.5 mg/kg/day, up to a maximum dose of 2.5 mg/kg/day.

Use the lowest effective dose for maintenance therapy; lower decrementally with changes of 0.5 mg/kg or approximately 25 mg/day every 4 weeks while other therapy is kept constant.

Renal function impairment: Relatively oliguric patients, especially those with tubular necrosis in the immediate postcadaveric transplant period, may have delayed clearance of azathioprine or its metabolites.

Use with allopurinol: Reduce dose of azathioprine to approximately 25% to 33% of the usual dose.

TACROLIMUS (FK506)

Capsules: 1 and 5 mg (*Rx*)	*Prograf* (Fujisawa)
Injection: 5 mg/ml (*Rx*)	

Warning:

Increased susceptibility to infection and the possible development of lymphoma may result from immunosuppression. Manage patients receiving the drug in facilities equipped and staffed with adequate laboratory and supportive medical resources.

Actions:

Pharmacology: Tacrolimus is a macrolide immunosuppressant. Tacrolimus prolongs the survival of the host and transplanted graft. Tacrolimus inhibits T-lymphocyte activation, although the exact mechanism of action is not known.

Pharmacokinetics:

Pharmacokinetic Parameters of Tacrolimus in Whole Blood After Oral Administration					
Population	Dose (mg/kg/12h)	C_{max} (ng/ml)	T_{max} (hr)	AUC (ng/ml•hr)	Absolute bioavailability
Liver transplant patients (n = 17)	0.15	68.5	2.3	519	21.8
Food	0.15	27.1	3.2	223	—
Fasting	0.15	52.4	1.5	290	—

The disposition of tacrolimus from whole blood was biphasic with a terminal elimination half-life of 11.7 hours in liver transplant patients.

Indications:

Organ (liver) rejection prophylaxis: Prophylaxis of organ rejection in patients receiving allogeneic liver transplants. It is recommended that tacrolimus be used concomitantly with adrenal corticosteroids.

Unlabeled uses: Tacrolimus is being investigated for kidney, bone marrow, cardiac, pancreas, pancreatic island cell and small bowel transplantation. It may be beneficial for the treatment of autoimmune disease and severe recalcitrant psoriasis.

Contraindications:

Hypersensitivity to tacrolimus; hypersensitivity to HCO-60 polyoxyl 60 hydrogenated castor oil (used in vehicle for injection).

Warnings:

Nephrotoxicity: Tacrolimus can cause nephrotoxicity, particularly when used in high doses. Nephrotoxicity has been noted in 33% to 40% of liver transplantation patients receiving the drug.

Hyperkalemia: Mild to severe hyperkalemia has been noted in liver transplant recipients treated with tacrolimus, which may require treatment.

Neurotoxicity, including tremor, headache and other changes in motor function, mental status and sensory function occurred in ≈ 55% of liver transplant recipients. Tremor and headache have been associated with high whole-blood concentrations of tacrolimus and may respond to dosage adjustment. Seizures have occurred in adult and pediatric patients. Coma and delirium also have been associated with high plasma concentrations of tacrolimus.

Lymphomas: As with other immunosuppressants, patients receiving tacrolimus are at increased risk of developing lymphomas and other malignancies, particularly of the skin.

Hypersensitivity: A few patients receiving the injection have experienced anaphylactic reactions. Although the exact cause of these reactions is not known, other drugs with castor oil derivatives in the formulation have been associated with anaphylaxis in a small percentage of patients.

Continuously observe patients receiving the injection for at least the first 30 minutes following the start of the infusion and at frequent intervals thereafter.

Renal/Hepatic function impairment: The use of tacrolimus in liver transplant recipients experiencing post-transplant hepatic impairment may be associated with increased risk of developing renal insufficiency related to high whole-blood levels of tacrolimus.

Carcinogenesis/Fertility impairment: An increased incidence of malignancy is a recognized complication of immunosuppression in recipients of organ transplants.

Pregnancy: Category C. The use of tacrolimus during pregnancy has been associated with neonatal hyperkalemia and renal dysfunction.

Lactation: Because tacrolimus is excreted in breast milk, avoid nursing.

Precautions:

Monitoring: Regularly assess serum creatinine and potassium. Perform routine monitoring of metabolic and hematologic systems as clinically warranted.

Hypertension is a common adverse effect of tacrolimus therapy. Mild or moderate hypertension is more frequently reported than severe hypertension.

Hyperglycemia was associated with the use of tacrolimus in 29% to 47% of liver transplant recipients, and may require treatment.

Drug Interactions:

Drugs that may affect tacrolimus include nephrotoxic agents (aminoglycosides, amphotericin B, cisplatin, cyclosporine), antifungals, bromocriptine, calcium channel blockers, cimetidine, clarithromycin, danazol, diltiazem, erythromycin, methylprednisolone, metoclopramide, carbamazepine, phenobarbital, phenytoin and rifamycins.

Drugs that may be affected include vaccines.

Because tacrolimus is metabolized mainly by the cytochrome P-450 IIIA enzyme systems, substances known to inhibit or induce these enzymes may affect the metabolism of tacrolimus with resultant increases or decreases in whole blood or plasma levels.

Drug/Food interactions: The presence of food reduced the absorption of tacrolimus (decrease in AUC and C_{max} and increase in T_{max}). The relative oral bioavailability (whole blood) was reduced by 27% compared to the fasting state.

Adverse Reactions:

The principal adverse reactions of tacrolimus are tremor, headache, diarrhea, hypertension, nausea and renal dysfunction. Other reactions may include insomnia, paresthesia, constipation, anorexia, vomiting, anemia, leukocytosis, thrombocytopenia, hyperglycemia, dyspnea, prutitus, rash, abndominal pain, fever, asthenia, back pain, ascites and peripheral edema, abnormal dreams, agitation, anxiety, confusion, convulsion, depression, dizziness, hallucinations, incoordination, nervousness, somnolence, thinking abnormal, abnormal vision, tinnitus, dyspepsia, flatulence, GI hemorrhage, GI perforation, hepatitis, increased appetite, jaundice, liver damage, oral moniliasis, chest pain, hypotension, tachycardia, hematuria, hyperlipemia, hyperphosphatemia, hyperuricemia, hypocalcemia, hypophosphatemia, hyponatremia, diabetes mellitus, coagulation disorder, ecchymosis, leukopenia, prothrombin decreased, abdomen enlarged, chills, peritonitis, photosensitivity reaction, arthralgia, generalized spasm, leg cramps, myalgia, asthma, bronchitis, cough increased, pulmonary edema, pharyngitis, rhinitis, sinusitis, voice alteration, alopecia, hirsutism, sweating.

Administration and Dosage:

Injection: For IV infusion only.

In patients unable to take the capsules, therapy may be initiated with the injection. Administer the initial dose no sooner than 6 hours after transplantation. The recommended starting dose is 0.05 to 0.1 mg/kg/day as a continuous IV infusion. Give adult patients doses at the lower end of the dosing range. Concomitant adrenal corticosteroid therapy is recommended early post-transplantation. Continue continuous IV infusion only until the patient can tolerate oral administration.

Oral: It is recommended that patients be converted from IV to oral therapy as soon as oral therapy can be tolerated. This usually occurs within 2 to 3 days. Give the first dose of oral therapy 8 to 12 hours after discontinuing the IV infusion. The recommended starting oral dose is 0.15 to 0.3 mg/kg/day administered in 2 divided daily doses every 12 hours. Administer the initial dose no sooner than 6 hours after transplantation. Give adult patients doses at the lower end of the dosing range.

Children (< 12 years): It is recommended that therapy be initiated in pediatric patients at the high end of the recommended adult IV and oral dosing ranges (0.1 mg/kg/day IV and 0.3 mg/kg/day oral).

Hepatic/Renal function impairment: Because of the potential for nephrotoxicity, give patients with renal or hepatic impairment doses at the lowest value of the recommended IV and oral dosing ranges.

Conversion from one immunosuppressive regimen to another: Do not use tacrolimus simultaneously with cyclosporine. Discontinue either agent at least 24 hours before initiating the other.

MYCOPHENOLATE MOFETIL

Capsules: 250 mg (*Rx*)	*CellCept* (Roche)

Warning:

Increased susceptibility to infection and the possible development of lymphoma may result from immunosuppression. Only physicians experienced in immunosuppressive therapy and management of renal transplant patients should use mycophenolate. Patients receiving the drug should be managed in facilities equipped and staffed with adequate laboratory and supportive medical resources. The physician responsible for maintenance therapy should have complete information requisite for the follow-up of the patient.

Actions:

Pharmacology: Mycophenolate is rapidly absorbed following oral administration and hydrolyzed to form MPA, which is the active metabolite. MPA is a potent, selective, uncompetitive and reversible inhibitor of inosine monophosphate dehydrogenase (IMPDH), and therefore inhibits the de novo pathway of guanosine nucleotide synthesis without incorporation into DNA.

Pharmacokinetics:

Absorption/Distribution – Following oral administration, mycophenolate undergoes rapid and extensive absorption and complete presystemic metabolism to MPA, the active metabolite.

Mean apparent volume of distribution of MPA in 12 healthy volunteers is ≈ 3.6 and 4 L/kg after IV and oral administration, respectively. MPA, at clinically relevant concentrations, is 97% bound to plasma albumin. MPAG is 82% bound to plasma albumin at MPAG concentration ranges normally seen in stable renal transplant patients; however, at higher MPAG concentrations (observed in patients with renal impairment or delayed graft function), the binding of MPA may be reduced as a result of competition between MPAG and MPA for protein binding.

Metabolism – In addition to MPA, other metabolites of the 2-hydroxyethyl- morpholino moiety are also recovered in the urine.

Excretion – Negligible amount of drug is excreted as MPA (< 1% of dose) in the urine. Oral administration resulted in complete recovery of the administered dose; 93% was recovered in the urine and 6% recovered in feces. Most (about 87%) of the administered dose is excreted in the urine as MPAG (phenolic glucuronide of MPA).

Mean Pharmacokinetic Parameters for MPA Following Mycophenolate				
Parameter	Dose	T_{max} (hr)	C_{max} (mcg/ml)	AUC (mcg•hr/ml)
Healthy volunteers (n = 129)	1 g	0.8	24.5	63.9 (n = 117)
Renal transplant patients				
Time after renal transplantation				
Early (< 40 days; n = 25)	1 g bid	1.31	8.16	27.3 [1]
Early (< 40 days; n = 27)	1.5 g bid	1.21	13.5	38.4 [1]
Late (> 3 months; n = 23)	1.5 g bid	0.9	24.1	65.3 [1]
Renal impairment (GFR, ml/min/ 1.73 m²)				
Healthy volunteers (GFR > 80; n = 6)	1 g	0.75	25.3	45 [2]
Mild renal impairment (GFR 50 to 80; n = 6)	1 g	0.75	26	59.9 [2]
Moderate renal impairment (GFR 25 to 49; n = 6)	1 g	0.75	19	52.9 [2]
Severe renal impairment (GFR < 25; n = 7)	1 g	1	16.3	78.6 [2]
Hepatic impairment				
Healthy volunteers (n = 6)	1 g	0.63	24.3	29 [3]
Alcoholic cirrhosis (n = 18)	1 g	0.85	22.4	29.8 [3]

[1] Interdosing interval $AUC_{0\ 12}$
[2] Interdosing interval $AUC_{0\ 96}$
[3] Interdosing interval $AUC_{0\ 48}$

Pediatrics:

Mean Pharmacokinetic Parameters for MPA Following Multiple Doses of Mycophenolate in Pediatric Renal Transplant Patients				
Age range	Dose	T_{max} (hr)	C_{max} (mcg/ml)	$AUC_{0\text{-}12}$ (mcg•hr/ml)
≥ 3 mo to < 6 yr (n = 4)	15 mg/kg bid	1.25	3.7	13.6
≥ 6 yr to < 12 yr (n = 4)	15 mg/kg bid	0.5	13.5	23.4
≥ 12 yr to 18 yr (n = 5)	15 mg/kg bid	0.5	13.2	30
≥ 12 yr to 18 yr (n = 7)	23 mg/kg bid	1.14	10.6	28.3

Indications:

Organ rejection: For the prophylaxis of organ rejection in patients receiving allogeneic renal transplants. Mycophenolate should be used concomitantly with cyclosporine and corticosteroids.

Contraindications:

Allergic reactions to mycophenolate have been observed; therefore, mycophenolate is contraindicated in patients with a hypersensitivity to the drug, mycophenolic acid or any component of the drug product.

Warnings:

Lymphomas/Malignancies: Patients receiving immunosuppressive regimens involving combinations of drugs, including mycophenolate, as part of an immunosuppressive regimen are at increased risk of developing lymphomas and other malignancies, particularly of the skin. Lymphoproliferative disease or lymphoma developed in ≈1% of patients in the controlled studies of prevention of rejection.

Neutropenia: Up to 2% of patients receiving mycophenolate developed severe neutropenia. Neutropenia has been observed most frequently in the period from 31 to 180 days post-transplant in patients treated for prevention of rejection.

Renal function impairment: Avoid mycophenolate doses > 1 g administered twice a day and carefully observe patients.

Pregnancy: Category C.

Lactation: It is not known whether this drug is excreted in human milk. Because of the potential for serious adverse reactions in nursing infants from mycophenolate, decide whether to discontinue nursing or to discontinue the drug, taking into account the importance of the drug to the mother.

Children: Safety and efficacy have not been established.

Precautions:

Monitoring: Perform complete blood counts weekly during the first month, twice monthly for the second and third months of treatment, then monthly through the first year.

GI hemorrhage: GI tract hemorrhage has been observed in ≈ 3% of patients treated with mycophenolate. GI tract perforations have rarely been observed.

Delayed graft function: In patients with delayed graft function post-transplant, mean MPA AUC was comparable, but MPAG AUC was two- to threefold higher, compared to that seen in post-transplant patients without delayed graft function. No dose adjustment is recommended for these patients, however, they should be carefully observed.

Drug Interactions:

Drugs that alter the GI flora: may interact with mycophenolate by disrupting enterohepatic recirculation. Interference of MPAG hydrolysis may lead to less MPA available for absorption.

Drugs that may be affected by mycophenolate include acyclovir, phenytoin and theophylline.

Drugs that may affect mycophenolate include acyclovir, ganciclovir, antacids, azathioprine, cholestyramine, probenecid and salicylates.

Drug/Food interactions: Food (27 g fat, 650 calories) had no effect on the extent of absorption (MPA AUC) of mycophenolate when administered at doses of 1.5 g twice daily to renal transplant patients. However, MPA C_{max} was decreased by 40% in the presence of food.

Adverse Reactions:

The principal adverse reactions associated with mycophenolate include diarrhea, leukopenia, sepsis and vomiting, and there is evidence of a higher frequency of certain types of infections.

Adverse reactions occurring in ≥ 3% of patients include: Pain; abdominal pain; fever; headache; infection; sepsis; asthenia; chest pain; back pain; hypertension; anemia; leukopenia; thrombocytopenia; hypochromic anemia; leukocytosis; urinary tract infection; hematuria; kidney tubular necrosis; urinary tract disorder; peripheral edema; hypercholesterolemia; hypophosphatemia; edema; hypokalemia; hyperkalemia; diarrhea; constipation; nausea; dyspepsia; vomiting; oral moniliasis; infection; dyspnea; cough increased; pharyngitis; bronchitis; pneumonia; acne; rash; tremor; insomnia; dizziness.

Patients receiving mycophenolate 2 g/day had an overall better safety profile than did patients receiving 3 g/day. Sepsis, which was generally CMV viremia, was slightly more common in patients treated with mycophenolate; diarrhea was most clearly increased in patients receiving mycophenolate.

The incidence of malignancies among the 1483 patients enrolled in controlled trials for the prevention of rejection who were followed for ≥ 1 year was similar to the incidence reported in the literature for renal allograft recipients. There was a slight increase in the incidence of lymphoproliferative disease in the mycophenolate treatment groups compared to the placebo and azathioprine groups.

Malignancies Observed with Mycophenolate in Prevention of Renal Rejection Trials (%)				
Malignancy	Mycophenolate 2 g/day (n = 501)	Mycophenolate 3 g/day (n = 490)	Placebo (n = 166)	Azathioprine 1 to 2 mg/kg/day or 100 to 150 mg/day (n = 326)
Lymphoma/Lymphoproliferative disease	0.6	1	0	0.3
Nonmelanoma skin carcinoma	4	1.6	0	2.4
Other malignancy	0.8	1.4	1.8	1.8

Incidence of Opportunistic Infections in Prevention of Renal Rejection with Mycophenolate (%) [1]				
Infection	Mycophenolate 2 g/day	Mycophenolate 3 g/day	Azathioprine 1 to 2 mg/kg/day or 100 to 150 mg/day	Placebo
Herpes simplex	15.2-16.7	12.5-20	19	6
CMV				
Viremia/Syndrome	13.4-15.2	12.4-15	13.8	13.3
Tissue invasive disease	3.6-8.3	7.5-11.5	6.1	2.4
Herpes zoster	6-6.7	6.9-7.6	5.8	2.4
Candida				
Fungemia/disseminated	0.6	0.6	0.3	0
Tissue invasive	0.6	0.6	0.3	0
Aspergillus/Mucor invasive disease	0.3	0.9	0.3	
Pneumocystis carinii	0.3	0	1.2	2.4

[1] Data pooled from three separate studies.

Other adverse reactions occurring in ≥ 3% of patients include: Albuminuria; dysuria; hydronephrosis; impotence; pain; pyelonephritis; urinary frequency; urinary tract disorder; angina pectoris; atrial fibrillation; cardiovascular disorder; hypotension; palpitation; peripheral vascular disorder; postural hypotension; tachycardia; thrombosis; vasodilatation; anorexia; esophagitis; flatulence; gastritis; gastroenteritis; GI hemorrhage; GI moniliasis; gingivitis; gum hyperplasia; hepatitis; ileus; infection; mouth ulceration; rectal disorder; asthma; lung disorder; lung edema; pleural effusion; rhinitis; sinusitis; alopecia; fungal dermatitis; hirsutism; pruritus; benign skin neoplasm; skin disorder; skin hypertrophy; skin ulcer; sweating; anxiety; depression; hypertonia; paresthesia; somnolence; diabetes mellitus; parathyroid disorder; arthralgia; joint disorder; leg cramps; myalgia; myasthenia; amblyopia; cataract; conjunctivitis; abdomen enlarged; accidental injury, chills and fever; cyst; face edema; flu syndrome; hemorrhage; hernia; malaise; pelvic pain; ecchymosis; polycythemia; increased alkaline phosphatase, creatinine, gamma glutamyl transpeptidase, lactic dehydrogenase, AST and ALT; hypercalcemia; hyperlipemia; hyperuricemia; hypervolemia; hypocalcemia; hypoglycemia; hypoproteinemia; weight gain; dehydration; acidosis.

Administration and Dosage:

Give the initial dose of mycophenolate within 72 hours following transplantation. A dose of 1 g administered twice a day (daily dose of 2 g) is recommended for use in combination with corticosteroids and cyclosporine in renal transplant patients. Although a dose of 1.5 g administered twice daily (daily dose of 3 g) was used in clinical trials and was shown to be safe and effective, no efficacy advantage could be established. Patients receiving 2 g/day demonstrated an overall better safety profile than did patients receiving 3 g/day. It is recommended that mycophenolate be administered on an empty stomach.

Dosage adjustments: In patients with severe chronic renal impairment (GFR < 25 ml/min/1.73 m^2) outside of the immediate post-transplant period, avoid doses > 1 g administered twice a day; carefully observe these patients. No dose adjustments are needed in patients experiencing delayed graft function post-operatively.

CYCLOSPORINE (Cyclosporin A)

Capsules, soft gelatin: 25, 50 and 100 mg (*Rx*)	*Sandimmune* (Sandoz)
Capsules, soft gelatin for microemulsion: 25 and 100 mg (*Rx*)	*Neoral* (Sandoz)
Oral Solution: 100 mg/ml (*Rx*)	*Sandimmune* (Sandoz)
Oral solution for microemulsion: 100 mg/ml (*Rx*)	*Neoral* (Sandoz)
IV Solution: 50 mg/ml (*Rx*)	*Sandimmune* (Sandoz)

Warning:

Administer *Sandimmune* with adrenal corticosteroids but not with other immunosuppressants. Increased susceptibility to infection and the possible development of lymphoma may result from immunosuppression. Cyclosporine for microemulsion (*Neoral*) may be given with other immunosuppressants.

Sandimmune capsules and oral solution have decreased bioavailability compared with *Neoral*. *Sandimmune* and *Neoral* are not bioequivalent and cannot be used interchangeably without physician supervision.

Absorption during chronic *Sandimmune* use is erratic. Monitor blood levels at repeated intervals and make dose adjustments to avoid toxicity (high levels) or possible organ rejection (low absorption). This is of special importance in liver transplants. For a given trough concentration, cyclosporine exposure will be greater with *Neoral* than with *Sandimmune*. If a patient who is receiving exceptionally high doses of *Sandimmune* is converted to *Neoral*, use particular caution.

Actions:

Pharmacology: Cyclosporine is a cyclic polypeptide immunosuppressant consisting of 11 amino acids.

Pharmacokinetics:

Absorption – From the GI tract is incomplete and variable. Peak blood and plasma concentrations are achieved at about 3.5 hours. *Neoral* has increased bioavailability compared with *Sandimmune*. Factors which may affect bioavailability include: 1) Food that may delay and impair absorption, 2) enterohepatic recirculation, 3) radioimmunoassay (RIA) vs high pressure liquid chromatography (HPLC) assay (RIA cross-reacts w/metabolites), 4) whole blood vs plasma specimen.

Distribution – Largely outside the blood volume; ≈ 33% to 47% is in plasma, 4% to 9% in lymphocytes, 5% to 12% in granulocytes and 41% to 58% in erythrocytes. In plasma, ≈ 90% is bound to proteins, primarily lipoproteins.

Metabolism – Cyclosporine is metabolized by the cytochrome P–450 hepatic enzyme system. The disposition from blood is biphasic with a terminal half-life of ≈ 19 hours (*Sandimmune*) or 8.4 hours (*Neoral*).

Excretion – Primarily biliary. Only 6% of the dose is excreted in urine.

Indications:

Immunosuppression: Prophylaxis of organ rejection in kidney, liver and heart allogeneic transplants. *Sandimmune* is always to be taken in conjunction with adrenal corticosteroids; *Neoral* has been used in combination with azathioprine and corticosteroids. *Sandimmune* may also be used to treat chronic rejection in patients previously treated with other immunosuppressants. Because of the risk of anaphylaxis, reserve the injection for patients unable to take the capsule or oral solution.

Unlabeled uses: Cyclosporine has had limited but successful use in other procedures including pancreas, bone marrow and heart/lung transplantation.

The following conditions have been treated with cyclosporine; oral dosages have ranged from 1 to 10 mg/kg/day: Alopecia areata; aplastic anemia; atopic dermatitis; Behcet's disease; biliary cirrhosis; corneal transplantation or other diseases of the eye which have an autoimmune component (compounded into ophthalmic drops; cyclosporine currently has orphan drug status for ophthalmic use); Crohn's disease; dermatomyositis; Graves, ophthalmopathy; insulin-dependent diabetes mellitus; lichen planus (topical preparation); lupus nephritis; multiple sclerosis;

myasthenia gravis; nephrotic syndrome; pemphigus and pemphigoid; polymyositis; psoriatic arthritis; pulmonary sarcoidosis; pyoderma gangrenosum; rheumatiod arthritis; severe psoriasis; ulcerative colitis; uveitis.

Contraindications:

Hypersensitivity to cyclosporine, polyoxyethylated castor oil or any compnent of the products.

Warnings:

Nephrotoxicity: Based on Sandimmune oral solution experience,

Nephrotoxicity has been noted in 25%, 38% and 37% of renal, cardiac and liver transplantation cases, respectively. Mild nephrotoxicity was generally noted 2 to 3 months after transplant and consisted of an arrest in the fall of preoperative elevations of BUN and creatinine. These elevations were often responsive to dosage reductione. More overt nephrotoxocity was seen early after transplantation and was characterized by a rapidly rising BUN and creatinine. This form of nephrotoxicity is usually responsive to *Sandimmune* dosage reduction.

Hepatotoxicity has been noted in 4%, 7% and 4% of renal, cardiac and liver transplantation cases, respectively. This usually occurred during the first month of therapy when high doses were used, and consisted of elevated hepatic enzymes and bilirubin.

Glomerular capillary thrombosis, which may result in graft failure, occasionally develops.

Convulsions have occurred in adult and pediatric patients receiving cyclosporine, particularly in combination with high-dose methylprednisolone.

Bioequivalency: Sandimmune is not bioequivalent to *Neoral.*

CNS toxicity may include: Headache; flushing; confusion; seizures; ataxia; hallucinations; mania; depression; encephalopathy; sleep problems; blurred vision.

Lipids: In one study, cyclosporine significantly increased total cholesterol, LDL and apolipoprotein B levels.

Glucose metabolism: There are conflicting reports of the drug's effects on glucose metabolism.

Hypersensitivity: Anaphylactic reactions are rare ($\approx$ 1 in 1000) in patients on cyclosporine injection. Continuously observe patients on IV cyclosoprine for at least the first 30 minutes after start of infusion and frequently thereafter. If anaphylaxis occurs, stop infusion.

Renal function impairment: Requires close monitoring and possibly frequent dosage adjustment. In patients with persistent high elevations of BUN and creatinine who are unresponsive to dosage adjustments, consider switching to other immunosuppressive therapy.

Carcinogenesis: The risk of malignancies in cyclosporine recipients is higher than in the healthy population but similar to that in patients receiving other immunosuppressive therapies.

With cyclosporine, some patients have developed a lymphoproliferative disorder, which regresses when the drug is discontinued. Patients receiving cyclosporine are at increased risk for development of lymphomas and other malignancies, particularly those of the skin. The increased risk appears related to the intensity and duration of immunosuppression rather than to the use of specific agents.

Pregnancy: Category C.

Lactation: Avoid nursing; cyclosporine is excreted in breast milk.

Children: Patients as young as 6 months of age have received *Sandimmune* with no unusual adverse effects.

Precautions:

Monitoring:

Blood levels – Blood level monitoring of cyclosporine is a useful and essential component in patient management. While no fixed relationships have yet been established, blood concentration monitoring may assist in the clinical evaluation of rejection and toxicity, dose adjustments and the assessment of compliance.

Of major importance to blood level analysis is the type of assay used, the transplanted organ and other immunosuppressant agents being administered.

While several assays and assay matrices are available, there is a consensus that parent-compound-specific assays correlate best with clinical events. Of these, HPLC is the standard reference, but the monoclonal antibody RIAs and the monoclonal antibody FPIA offer sensitivity, reproducibility and convenience.

Repeatedly assess renal and liver functions by measurement of BUN, serum creatinine, serum bilirubin and liver enzymes.

Malabsorption: Patients with malabsorption may have difficulty achieving therapeutic levels with oral *Sandimmune* use.

Hypertension is a fairly common side effect. Mild or moderate hypertension, which may occur in ≈ 50% of patients following renal transplantation and in most cardiac transplant patients, is more frequently encountered than severe hypertension and the incidence decreases over time. Hypertension appears to be most severe in children.

Drug Interactions:

Monitoring of circulating cyclosporine levels and appropriate dosage adjustment are essential when drugs that affect hepatic microsomal enzymes, particularly the cytochrome P450 III-A enzymes, are used concomitantly.

Nephrotoxic drugs: Use with caution in patients receiving cyclosporine.

Drugs that may affect cyclosporine pharmacokinetics include carbamazepine, phenobarbital, phenytoin, rifampin, rifabutin, TMP-SMZ IV, diltiazem, erythromycin, fluconazole, ketoconazole, nicardipine, imipenem-cilistatin, methylprednisolone (high-dose), prednisolone, metoclopramide, amiodarone, danazol, methyltestosterone, nicardipine and probucol.

Drugs that may pharmacologically affect cyclosporine include aminoglycosides, amphotericin B, NSAIDs, TMP-SMZ, cimetidine, ketoconazole, melphalan, quinolones, ranitidine, vancomycin, methylprednisolone, azathioprine, corticosteroids, cyclophosphamide, verapamil, digoxin, nondepolarizing muscle relaxants, colchicine, vaccines, lovastatin, nifedipine and potassium-sparing diuretics.

Drug/Food interactions: Administration of food with *Neoral* decreases the AUC and C_{max} of cyclosporine. A high-fat meal consumed within 30 minutes of *Neoral* administration decreased the AUC by 13% and C_{max} by 33%. The effects of a low-fat meal were similar. In addition, do not take cyclosporine simultaneously with grapefruit juice unless specifically instructed to do so; trough cyclosporine concentrations may be increased.

Adverse Reactions:

Adverse reactions may include: Renal dysfunction; tremor; infectious complications; hirsutism; hypertension; gum hyperplasia; cramps; acne; convulsions; paresthesia.

Administration and Dosage:

Bioequivalency: Sandimmune capsules and oral solution have decreased bioavailability compared with *Neoral. Sandimmune* and *Neoral* are NOT bioequivalent and cannot be used interchangeably without physician supervision.

Adjunct therapy with adrenal corticosteroids is recommended.

Oral:

Initially – 15 mg/kg/day 4 to 12 hours prior to transplantation. There is a trend towards use of even lower initial doses for renal transplantation in the ranges of 10 to 14 mg/kg/day. Continue dose postoperatively for 1 to 2 weeks, then taper by 5% per week to a maintenance level of 5 to 10 mg/kg/day. Some centers successfully tapered the dose to as low as 4 mg/kg in selected renal transplant patients without an apparent rise in rejection rate.

Parenteral: For infusion only. Patients unable to take the oral solution or capsules preoperatively or postoperatively may be given the IV concentrate. Use the IV form at ⅓ the oral dose.

Initial dose – 5 to 6 mg/kg/day given 4 to 12 hours prior to transplantation as a single IV dose. Continue this daily single dose postoperatively until the patient can tolerate the oral doseforms. Switch patients to oral therapy as soon as possible after surgery.

Children: May use same dose and dosing regimen, but higher doses may be required.

Neoral:

Initial dose – The initial dose of *Neoral* can be given 4 to 12 hours prior to transplantation or postoperatively. In newly transplanted patients, the initial dose of *Neoral* is the same as the initial oral dose of *Sandimmune*. The mean doses were 9 mg/kg/day for heart transplant patients, 8 mg/kg/day for liver transplant patients and 7 mg/kg/day for heart transplant patients. Divide total daily dose into two equal daily doses.

Conversion from Sandimmune to Neoral – In transplanted patients who are considered for conversion to *Neoral* from *Sandimmune*, start *Neoral* with the same daily dose as was previously used with *Sandimmune* (1:1 dose conversion). Subsequently adjust *Neoral* to attain the pre-conversion cyclosporine blood trough concentration. Using the same trough concentration target range for *Neoral* as for *Sandimmune* results in greater cyclosporine exposure when *Neoral* is administered.

Poor Sandimmune absorption – Patients with lower than expected cyclosporine blood trough concentrations in relation to the oral dose of *Sandimmune* may have poor or inconsistent absorption. After conversion to *Neoral*, patients tend to have higher cyclosporine concentrations. Because of the increase in bioavailability following conversion to *Neoral*, the cyclosporine blood trough concentration may exceed the target range.

MUROMONAB-CD3

Injection: 5 mg per 5 ml (*Rx*) — *Orthoclone OKT3* (Ortho Biotech)

Warning:

Anaphylactic or anaphylactoid reactions may occur following administration of any dose or course of muromonab-CD3. Serious and occasionally life-threatening systemic, cardiovascular and CNS reactions have been reported. These have included: Pulmonary edema, especially in patients with volume overload; shock; cardiovascular collapse; cardiac or respiratory arrest; seizures; coma.

Actions:

Pharmacology: Muromonab-CD3 is a murine monoclonal antibody to the T3 (CD3) antigen of human T cells which functions as an immunosuppressant. The antibody is a biochemically purified IgG_{2a} immunoglobulin. It reverses graft rejection, probably by blocking the T cell function, which plays a major role in acute renal rejection.

Pharmacokinetics: Serum levels are measured with an enzyme-linked immunosorbent assay (ELISA). During treatment with 5 mg/day for 14 days, mean serum trough levels rose over the first 3 days and then averaged 0.9 mcg/ml on days 3 to 14. Circulating serum levels > 0.8 mcg/ml block the function of cytotoxic T cells in vitro and in vivo.

Indications:

Renal allograft rejection: Treatment of acute allograft rejection in renal transplant patients.

Cardiac/Hepatic allograft rejection: Treatment of steroid-resistant acute allograft rejection in cardiac and hepatic transplant patients.

Contraindications:

Hypersensitivity to this or any product of murine origin; anti-mouse antibody titers ≥ 1:1000; patients in fluid overload or uncompensated heart failure, as evidenced by chest x-ray or > 3% weight gain within the week prior to treatment; history of seizures or predisposition to seizures; pregnancy, breastfeeding.

Warnings:

Cytokine release syndrome (CRS): Temporally associated with the administration of the first few doses of muromonab-CD3 (particularly, the first two to three doses), most patients have developed CRS that has been attributed to the release of cytokines by activated lymphocytes or monocytes. This clinical syndrome has ranged from a more frequently reported mild, self-limited, "flu-like" illness to a less frequently reported severe, life-threatening shock-like reaction, which may include serious cardiovascular and CNS manifestations. The syndrome typically begins approximately 30 to 60 minutes after administration of a dose (but may occur later) and may persist for several hours. The frequency and severity of this symptom complex is usually greatest with the first dose.

Pulmonary edema – Severe pulmonary edema has occurred in patients who appeared to be euvolemic. The pathogenesis of pulmonary edema may involve all or some of the following: Volume overload; increased pulmonary vascular permeability; reduced left ventricular compliance/contractility.

Serum creatinine – During the first 1 to 3 days of therapy, some patients have experienced an acute and transient decline in the GFR and diminished urine output with a resulting increase in the level of serum creatinine.

Patients at risk for more serious complications of the CRS may include those with the following conditions: Unstable angina; recent MI or symptomatic ischemic heart disease; heart failure of any etiology; pulmonary edema of any etiology; any form of chronic obstructive pulmonary disease; intravascular volume overload or depletion of any etiology (eg, excessive dialysis, recent intensive diuresis, blood loss); cerebrovascular disease; patients with advanced symptomatic vascular disease or neuropathy; history of seizures; septic shock.

Fluid status – Prior to administration, assess the patient's volume (fluid) status carefully. It is imperative, especially prior to the first few doses, that there be no clinical evidence of volume overload or uncompensated heart failure, including a clear chest X-ray and weight restriction of ≤ 3% above the patient's minimum weight during the week prior to injection.

Prevention/Minimization – Manifestations of the CRS may be prevented or minimized by pretreatment with 8 mg/kg methylprednisolone, given 1 to 4 hours prior to administration of the first dose of muromonab-CD3 and by closely following recommendations for dosage and treatment duration.

Neuro-Psychiatric events: Seizures, encephalopathy, cerebral edema, aseptic meningitis and headaches have occurred during therapy with muromonab-CD3, even following the first dose, resulting in part from T cell activation and subsequent systemic release of cytokines.

Aseptic meningitis syndrome – The incidence of this syndrome was 6%. Fever, headache, meningismus and photophobia were the most commonly reported symptoms; a combination of these four symptoms occurred in 5% of patients.

Headache is frequently seen after any of the first few doses and may occur in any of the aforementioned neurologic syndromes or by itself.

Patients who may be at greater risk for CNS adverse experiences include: Known or suspected CNS disorders; cerebrovascular disease (small or large vessel); conditions having associated neurologic problems; underlying vascular diseases; concomitant medication that may, by itself, affect the CNS.

Infections: Muromonab-CD3 is usually added to immunosuppressive therapeutic regimens, thereby augmenting the degree of immunosuppression. This increase in the total burden of immunosuppression may alter the spectrum of infections observed and increase the risk, the severity and the potential gravity (morbidity) of infectious complications.

Neoplasia: As a result of depressed cell-mediated immunity, organ transplant patients have an increased risk of developing malignancies.

Hypersensitivity: Serious and occasionally fatal, immediate (usually within 10 minutes) hypersensitivity reactions have occurred. Manifestations of anaphylaxis may appear similar to manifestations of the CRS.

Pregnancy: Category C.

Lactation: It is not known whether muromonab-CD3 is excreted in breast milk.

Children: Safety and efficacy in children have not been established. Muromonab-CD3 has been used in infants/children, beginning with a dose of ≤ 5 mg.

Precautions:

Monitoring: Monitor the following tests prior to and during therapy:

- *Renal* – BUN, serum creatinine, etc;
- *Hepatic* – Transaminases, alkaline phosphatase, bilirubin;
- *Hematopoietic* – WBCs and differential, platelet count, etc;
- *Chest X-ray* within 24 hours before initiating treatment, which should be free of any evidence of heart failure or fluid overload.

Monitor one of the following immunologic tests during therapy:

- Plasma levels determined by an ELISA; (target levels should be ≥ 800 ng/ml); or
- Quantitative T lymphocyte surface phenotyping (CD3, CD4, CD8); target CD3 positive T cells < 25 cells/mm^3.

Testing for human-mouse antibody titers is strongly recommended; a titer ≥ 1:1000 is a contraindication for use.

Intravascular thrombosis: As with other immunosuppressive therapies, arterial or venous thromboses of allografts and other vascular beds have been reported.

Drug Interactions:

Drugs that may affect muromonab include other immunosuppressants (eg, azathioprine, corticosteroids, cyclosporine) and indomethacin.

Adverse Reactions:

Adverse ractions associated with CRS may include high (often spiking, up to 107°F) fever, chills/rigors, abdominal pain, malaise, muscle/joint aches and pains, dyspnea, shortness of breath, tachypnea, respiratory arrest/failure/distress, cardiovascular collapse, cardiac arrest, angina/MI, nausea, vomiting, chest pain/tightness, hemodynamic instability, heart failure, pulmonary edema, adult respiratory distress syndrome, hypoxemia, apnea, arrhythmias, diarrhea, tremor, bronchospasm/wheezing, headache, tachycardia, rigor and hypertension.

Other adverse events may include pancytopeina, aplastic anemia, neutropenia, leukopenia, thrombocytopenia, lymphopenia, leukocytosis, lymphademopathy, coagulation disturbances, hypotension/shock, heart failure, angina/MI, tachycardia, bradycardia, tachypnea/hyperventilation, abnormal chest sounds, pneumonia/pneumonitis, rash, urticaria, pruritus, erythema, flushing, diaphoresis, diarrhea, bowel infarction, arthralgia, arthritis, blindness, blurred vision diplopia, hearing loss, otitis media, tinnitus, vertigo, photophobia, conjunctivitis, nasal/ear stuffiness and anuria/oliguria.

Administration and Dosage:

Muromonab-CD3 is for IV use only.

Administer as an IV bolus in < 1 minute. Do not give by IV infusion or in conjunction with other drug solutions.

Renal allograft rejection, acute: 5 mg/day for 10 to 14 days. Begin treatment once acute renal rejection is diagnosed.

Cardiac/hepatic allograft rejection, steroid resistant: 5 mg/day for 10 to 14 days. Begin treatment when it is determined that a rejection has not been reversed by an adequate course of corticosteroid therapy.

APPENDIX

FDA PREGNANCY CATEGORIES

The rational use of any medication requires a risk versus benefit assessment. Among the myriad of risk factors which complicate this assessment, pregnancy is one of the most perplexing.

The FDA has established five categories to indicate the potential of a systemically absorbed drug for causing birth defects. The key differentiation among the categories rests upon the degree (reliability) of documentation and the risk vs benefit ratio. Pregnancy Category X is particularly notable in that if any data exist that may implicate a drug as a teratogen and the risk vs benefit ratio does not support use of the drug, the drug is contraindicated during pregnancy. These categories are summarized below:

FDA Pregnancy Categories

Pregnancy Category	Definition
A	Adequate studies in pregnant women have not demonstrated a risk to the fetus in the first trimester of pregnancy and there is no evidence of risk in later trimesters.
B	Animal studies have not demonstrated a risk to the fetus but there are no adequate studies in pregnant women ... or ... Animal studies have shown an adverse effect, but adequate studies in pregnant women have not demonstrated a risk to the fetus during the first trimester of pregnancy and there is no evidence of risk in later trimesters.
C	Animal studies have shown an adverse effect on the fetus but there are no adequate studies in humans; the benefits from the use of the drug in pregnant women may be acceptable despite its potential risks ... or ... There are no animal reproduction studies and no adequate studies in humans.
D	There is evidence of human fetal risk, but the potential benefits from the use of the drug in pregnant women may be acceptable despite its potential risks.
X	Studies in animals or humans demonstrate fetal abnormalities or adverse reaction reports indicate evidence of fetal risk. The risk of use in a pregnant woman clearly outweighs any possible benefit.

Regardless of the designated Pregnancy Category or presumed safety, no drug should be administered during pregnancy unless it is clearly needed and potential benefits outweigh potential hazards to the fetus.

CONTROLLED SUBSTANCES

The Controlled Substances Act of 1970 regulates the manufacturing, distribution and dispensing of drugs that have abuse potential. The Drug Enforcement Administration (DEA) within the US Department of Justice is the chief federal agency responsible for enforcement.

DEA Schedules: Drugs under jurisdiction of the Controlled Substances Act are divided into five schedules based on their potential for abuse and physical and psychological dependence. All controlled substances listed in *Drug Facts and Comparisons®* are identified by schedule as follows:

Schedule I *(c-I)*: High abuse potential and no accepted medical use (eg, heroin, marijuana, LSD).

Schedule II *(c-II)*: High abuse potential with severe dependence liability (eg, narcotics, amphetamines, dronabinol, some barbiturates).

Schedule III *(c-III)*: Less abuse potential than schedule II drugs and moderate dependence liability (eg, nonbarbiturate sedatives, nonamphetamine stimulants, limited amounts of certain narcotics).

Schedule IV *(c-IV)*: Less abuse potential than schedule III drugs and limited dependence liability (eg, some sedatives, antianxiety agents, nonnarcotic analgesics).

Schedule V *(c-V)*: Limited abuse potential. Primarily small amounts of narcotics (codeine) used as antitussives or antidiarrheals. Under federal law, limited quantities of certain *c-V* drugs may be purchased without a prescription directly from a pharmacist if allowed under state statutes. The purchaser must be at least 18 years of age and must furnish suitable identification. All such transactions must be recorded by the dispensing pharmacist.

Registration: Prescribing physicians and dispensing pharmacies must be registered with the DEA, PO Box 28083, Central Station, Washington, DC 20005.

Inventory: Separate records must be kept of purchases and dispensing of controlled substances. An inventory of controlled substances must be made every 2 years.

Prescriptions: Prescriptions for controlled substances must be written in ink and include: Date; name and address of the patient; name, address and DEA number of the physician. Oral prescriptions must be promptly committed to writing. Controlled substance prescriptions may not be dispensed or refilled more than 6 months after the date issued or be refilled more than five times. A written prescription signed by the physician is required for schedule II drugs. In case of emergency, oral prescriptions for schedule II substances may be filled; however, the physician must provide a signed prescription within 72 hours. Schedule II prescriptions cannot be refilled. A triplicate order form is necessary for the transfer of controlled substances in schedule II. Forms are available for the individual prescriber at no charge from the DEA.

State Laws: In many cases state laws are more restrictive than federal laws and therefore impose additional requirements (eg, triplicate prescription forms).

MANAGEMENT OF ACUTE HYPERSENSITIVITY REACTIONS

Type I hypersensitivity reactions (immediate hypersensitivity or anaphylaxis) are immunologic responses to a foreign antigen to which a patient has been previously sensitized. Anaphylact*oid* reactions are not immunologically mediated; however, symptoms and treatment are similar.

Signs and Symptoms

Acute hypersensitivity reactions typically begin within 1 to 30 minutes of exposure to the offending antigen. Tingling sensations and a generalized flush may proceed to a fullness in the throat, chest tightness or a "feeling of impending doom." Generalized urticaria and sweating are common. *Severe* reactions include life-threatening involvement of the airway and cardiovascular system.

Treatment:

Appropriate and immediate treatment is imperative. The following general measures are commonly employed:

Epinephrine 1:1000, 0.2 to 0.5 mg (0.2 to 0.5 ml) SC is the primary treatment. In children, administer 0.01 mg/kg or 0.1 mg. Doses may be repeated every 5 to 15 minutes if needed. A succession of small doses is more effective and less dangerous than a single large dose. Additionally, 0.1 mg may be introduced into an injection site where the offending drug was administered. If appropriate, the use of a tourniquet above the site of injection of the causative agent may slow its absorption and distribution. However, remove or loosen the tourniquet every 10 to 15 minutes to maintain circulation.

Epinephrine IV (generally indicated in the presence of hypotension) is often recommended in a 1:10,000 dilution, 0.3 to 0.5 mg over 5 minutes; repeat every 15 minutes, if necessary. In children, inject 0.1 to 0.2 mg or 0.01 mg/kg/dose over 5 minutes; repeat every 30 minutes.

A conservative IV epinephrine protocol includes 0.1 mg of a 1:100,000 dilution (0.1 mg of a 1:1000 dilution mixed in 10 ml normal saline) given over 5 to 10 minutes. If an IV infusion is necessary, administer at a rate of 1 to 4 mcg/min. In children, infuse 0.1 to 1.5 (maximum) mcg/kg/min.

Dilute epinephrine 1:10,000 may be administered through an endotracheal tube, if no other parenteral access is available, directly into the bronchial tree. It is rapidly absorbed there from the capillary bed of the lung.

Airway: Ensure a patent airway via endotracheal intubation or cricothyrotomy (ie, inferior laryngotomy, used prior to tracheotomy) and administer oxygen. Severe respiratory difficulty may respond to IV aminophylline or to other bronchodilators.

Hypotension: The patient should be recumbent with feet elevated. Depending upon the severity, consider the following measures:

- Establish a patent IV catheter in a suitable vein.
- Administer IV fluids (eg, normal saline, lactated Ringer's).
- Administer plasma expanders.

- Administer cardioactive agents (see group and individual monographs). Commonly recommended agents include dopamine, dobutamine, norepinephrine and phenylephrine.

Adjunctive therapy does not alter acute reactions, but may modify an ongoing or slow-onset process and shorten the course of the reaction.

- *Antihistamines: Diphenhydramine* – 50 to 100 mg IM or IV, continued orally at 5 mg/kg/day or 50 mg every 6 hours for 1 to 2 days. For children, give 5 mg/kg/day, maximum 300 mg per day.
  Chlorpheniramine – (adults, 10 to 20 mg; children, 5 to 10 mg) IM or slowly IV.
  Hydroxyzine – 10 to 25 mg orally or 25 to 50 mg IM 3 to 4 times daily.
- *Corticosteroids*, eg, hydrocortisone IV 100 to 1000 mg or equivalent, followed by 7 mg/kg/day IV or oral for 1 to 2 days. The role of corticosteroids is controversial.
- *H_2 antagonists: Cimetidine* – *Children*, 25 to 30 mg/kg/day IV in six divided doses; *adults*, 300 mg every 6 hours.
  Ranitidine – 50 mg IV over 3 to 5 minutes. May be of value in addition to H_1 antihistamines, although this opinion is not universally shared.

CALCULATIONS

To calculate milliequivalent weight: $\text{mEq} = \frac{\text{gram molecular weight/valence}}{1000}$

$\text{mEq} = \frac{\text{mg}}{\text{eq wt}}$ equivalent weight or eq wt = $\frac{\text{gram molecular weight}}{\text{valence}}$

Commonly used mEq weights			
Chloride	35.5 mg = 1 mEq	Magnesium	12 mg = 1 mEq
Sodium	23 mg = 1 mEq	Potassium	39 mg = 1 mEq
Calcium	20 mg = 1 mEq		

To convert temperature °C ↔ °F: $\frac{°C}{°F - 32} = \frac{5}{9}$ *or* $°C = \frac{5}{9}(°F - 32)$

$$°F = 32 + \frac{9}{5}\,°C$$

To calculate creatinine clearance (Ccr) from serum creatinine:

Male: $\text{Ccr} = \frac{\text{weight (kg)} \times (140 - \text{age})}{72 \times \text{serum creatinine (mg/dl)}}$ Female: Ccr = 0.85 × calculation for males

To calculate ideal body weight (kg):

Male = 50 kg + 2.3 kg (each inch > 5 ft) Female = 45.5 kg + 2.3 kg (each inch > 5 ft)

To calculate body surface area (BSA) in adults and children:

1) *Dubois method:*

$\text{SA (cm}^2) = \text{wt (kg)}^{0.425} \times \text{ht (cm)}^{0.725} \times 71.84$

$\text{SA (m}^2) = K \times \sqrt[3]{\text{wt}^2 \text{ (kg)}}$ (common K value 0.1 for toddlers, 0.103 for neonates)

2) *Simplified method:*

$\text{BSA (m}^2) = \sqrt{\frac{\text{ht (cm)} \times \text{wt (kg)}}{3600}}$

To approximate surface area (m^2) *of children from weight (kg):*

Weight range (kg)	≈ Surface area (m^2)
1 to 5	(0.05 x kg) + 0.05
6 to 10	(0.04 x kg) + 0.10
11 to 20	(0.03 x kg) + 0.20
21 to 40	(0.02 x kg) + 0.40

Suggested Weights for Adults	
Height*	Weight in pounds†
4'10"	91-119
4'11"	94-124
5'0"	97-128
5'1"	101-132
5'2"	104-137
5'3"	107-141
5'4"	111-146
5'5"	114-150
5'6"	118-155
5'7"	121-160
5'8"	125-164
5'9"	129-169
5'10"	132-174
5'11"	136-179
6'0"	140-184
6'1"	144-189
6'2"	148-195
6'3"	152-200
6'4"	156-205
6'5"	160-211
6'6"	164-216

* Without shoes. † Without clothes.

The higher weights in the ranges generally apply to people with more muscle and bone. Source: Nutrition and Your Health: Dietary Guidelines for Americans, 4th ed, 1995. US Department of Agriculture, US Department of Health and Human Services. At press time, these new guidelines had not been officially released. It is possible some changes to this chart will occur.

NORMAL LABORATORY VALUES

In the following tables, normal reference values for commonly requested laboratory tests are listed in traditional units and in SI units. The tables are a guideline only. Values are method dependent and "normal values" may vary between laboratories.

Blood, Plasma or Serum

Determination	Reference Value: Conventional Units	Reference Value: SI Units
Ammonia (NH_3)	10-80 µg/dl	5-50 µmol/L
Amylase	≤ 130 U/L	≤ 130 U/L
Antinuclear antibodies	negative at 1:10 dilution of serum	negative at 1:10 dilution of serum
Antithrombin III (AT III)	80%-120%	
Bilirubin: conjugated	≤ 0.2 mg/dl	≤ 4 µmol/L
total	0.1-1 mg/dl	2-18 µmol/L
Calcitonin	< 100 pg/ml	< 100 ng/L
Calcium: female < 50 years old	8.8-10 mg/dl	2.2-2.5 mmol/L
female > 50 years old	8.8-10.2 mg/dl	2.2-2.56 mmol/L
male	8.8-10.3 mg/dl	2.2-2.58 mmol/L
all populations	4.4-5.1 mEq/L	2.2-2.56 mmol/L
Carbon dioxide content	22-28 mEq/L	22-28 mmol/L
Carcinoembryonic antigen	< 3 ng/ml	< 3 µg/L
Chloride	95-105 mEq/L	95-105 mmol/L
Coagulation screen:		
Bleeding time	3-9.5 min	180-570 sec
Prothrombin time	< 2 sec from control	< 2 sec from control
Partial thromboplastin time (activated)	22-37 sec	22-37 sec
Protein C	58%-148%	
Protein S	58%-148%	
Copper, total	70-140 µg/dl	11-22 µmol/L
Corticotropin (ACTH)	20-100 pg/ml	4-22 pmol/L
Cortisol: 0800 hr	4-19 µg/dl	110-520 nmol/L
1800 hr	2-15 µg/dl	50-410 nmol/L
2400 hr	< 5 µg/dl	< 140 nmol/L
Creatine phosphokinase, total (CK, CPK)	≤ 150 U/L	≤ 150 U/L
Creatine kinase isoenzymes, MB fraction	> 5% in MI	> 0.05 fraction of 1
Creatinine	0.6-1.2 mg/dl	50-110 µmol/L
Fibrinogen (coagulation factor I)	150-350 mg/dl	1.5-3.5 g/L
Follicle stimulating hormone (FSH):		
female	2-15 mIU/ml	2-15 IU/L
peak production	20-50 mIU/ml	20-50 IU/L
male	1-10 mIU/ml	1-10 IU/L
Glucose, fasting	70-110 mg/dl	3.9-6.1 mmol/L
Haptoglobin	50-220 mg/dl	0.5-2.2 g/L
Hematologic tests:		
Hematocrit (Hct), female	33%-43%	0.33-0.43 fraction of 1
male	39%-49%	0.39-0.49 fraction of 1
Hemoglobin (Hb), female	11.5-15.5 g/dl	115-155 g/L
male	14-18 g/dl	140-180 g/L
Leukocyte count (WBC)	3200-9800/mm^3	3.2-9.8 x 10^9/L
Erythrocyte count (RBC), female	3.5-5 × 10^6/mm^3	3.5-5 x 10^{12}/L
male	4.3-5.9 × 10^6/mm^3	4.3-5.9 x 10^{12}/L
Mean corpuscular volume (MCV)	76-100 μm^3	76-100 fL

Blood, Plasma or Serum		
	Reference Value	
Determination	Conventional Units	SI Units
Mean corpuscular hemoglobin (MCH)	27-33 pg	27-33 pg
Mean corpuscular hemoglobin concentration (MCHC)	33-37 g/dl	330-370 g/L
Erythrocyte sedimentation rate (sedrate, ESR): female	≤ 30 mm/hr	≤ 30 mm/hr
male	≤ 20 mm/hr	≤ 20 mm/hr
Erythrocyte enzymes:		
Glucose-6-phosphate dehydrogenase (G6PD)	5-15 U/g Hb	5-15 U/g Hb
Pyruvate kinase	13-17 U/g Hb	13-17 U/g Hb
Ferritin	18-300 ng/ml	18-300 μg/L
Folic acid: normal	> 3.3 ng/ml	> 7.3 nmol/L
borderline	2.5-3.2 ng/ml	5.75-7.39 nmol/L
Platelet count	130-400 × $10^3/mm^3$	130-400 × 10^9/L
Vitamin B_{12}	200-1000 pg/ml	150-750 pmol/L
Iron: female	60-160 μg/dl	11-29 μmol/L
male	80-180 μ/dl	14-32 μmol/L
Iron binding capacity	250-460 μg/dl	45-82 μmol/L
Lactic acid (lactate)	0.5-2 mEq/L	0.5-2 mmol/L
Lactic dehydrogenase	50-150 U/L	50-150 U/L
Lead	≤ 60 μg/dl	≤ 2.9 μmol/L
Lipids:		
Lipids, total	400-850 mg/dl	4-8.5 g/L
Total cholesterol		
< 29 years old	< 200 mg/dl	< 5.2 mmol/L
30-39 years old	< 225 mg/dl	< 5.85 mmol/L
40-49 years old	< 245 mg/dl	> 6.35 mmol/L
> 50 years old	< 265 mg/dl	< 6.85 mmol/L
LDL	50-190 mg/dl	1.3-4.9 mmol/L
HDL: female	30-90 mg/dl	0.8-2.35 mmol/L
male	30-70 mg/dl	0.8-1.8 mmol/L
Triglycerides	< 460 mg/dl	< 1.8 g/L
Magnesium	1.6-2.4 mEq/L	0.8-1.2 mmol/L
Osmolality	280-300 mOsm/kg	280-300 mmol/kg
Oxygen saturation (arterial)	96%-100%	0.96-1 fraction of 1
PCO_2, arterial	35-45 mmHg	4.7-6 kPa
pH, arterial	7.35-7.45	7.35-7.45
PO_2, arterial: Breathing room air[1] On 100% O_2	75-100 mmHg > 500 mmHg	10-13.3 kPa
Phosphatase (acid), total:	≤ 3 King-Armstrong units/dl ≤ 3 Bodansky units/dl	≤ 5.5 U/L ≤ 16.1 U/L
Phosphatase (alkaline)[2]	30-120 U/L	30-120 U/L
Phosphorus, inorganic[3] (phosphate)	2.5-5 mg/dl	0.8-1.6 mmol/L
Potassium	3.5-5 mEq/L	3.5-5 mmol/L
Progesterone		
Follicular phase	< 2 ng/ml	< 6 nmol/L
Luteal phase	2-20 ng/ml	6-64 nmol/L
Prolactin	< 20 ng/ml	< 20 μg/L
Prostate specific antigen	0-4 ng/ml	

Blood, Plasma or Serum

Determination	Reference Value: Conventional Units	Reference Value: SI Units
Protein: Total	6-8 g/dl	60-80 g/L
Albumin	4-6 g/dl	40-60 g/L
Globulin	2.3-3.5 g/dl	23-35 g/L
Rheumatoid factor	< 80 IU/ml	< 80 kIU/L
Sodium	135-147 mEq/L	135-147 mmol/L
Testosterone: female	< 0.6 ng/ml	< 2 nmol/L
male	4-8 ng/ml	14-28 nmol/L
Thyroid Hormone Function Tests:		
Thyroid-stimulating hormone (TSH)	2-11 μU/ml	2-11 mU/L
Thyroxine-binding globulin capacity	12-28 μg/dl	150-360 nmol/L
Total triiodothyronine (T_3)	75-220 ng/dl	1.2-3.4 nmol/L
Total thyroxine by RIA (T_4)	4-11 μg/dl	51-142 nmol/L
T_3 resin uptake	25%-35%	0.25-0.35 fraction of 1
Transaminase, AST (aspartate aminotransferase, SGOT)	≤ 35 U/L	≤ 35 U/L
Transaminase, ALT (alanine aminotransferase, SGPT)	≤ 35 U/L	≤ 35 U/L
Urea nitrogen (BUN)	8-18 mg/dl	3-6.5 mmol/L
Uric acid	2-7 mg/dl	120-420 μmol/L
Vitamin A (retinol)	10-50 μg/dl	0.35-1.75 μmol/L
Zinc	75-120 μg/dl	11.5-18.5 μmol/L

[1] Age-dependent.
[2] Infants and adolescents up to 104 U/L.
[3] Infants in the first year up to 6 mg/dl.

Urine

Determination	Reference Value: Conventional Units	Reference Value: SI Units
Catecholamines: Epinephrine	< 10 μg/day	< 55 nmol/day
Norepinephrine	< 100 μg/day	< 590 nmol/day
Creatinine: female	14-22 mg/kg/24 hr	0.12-0.19 mmol/kg/day
male	20-26 mg/kg/24 hr	0.18-0.23 mmol/kg/day
Potassium (diet-dependent)	25-100 mEq/day	25-100 mmol/day
Protein, quantitative	< 150 mg/day	< 0.15 g/day

Steroids:	Age (yrs)	(mg/day) male	(mg/day) female	(μmol/day) male	(μmol/day) female
17-Ketosteroids	10	1-4	1-4	3-14	3-14
	20	6-21	4-16	21-73	14-56
	30	8-26	4-14	28-90	14-49
	50	5-18	3-9	17-62	10-31
	70	2-10	1-7	7-35	3-24
17-Hydroxycorticosteroids (as cortisol):					
female		2-8 mg/day		5-25 μmol/day	
male		3-10 mg/day		10-30 μmol/day	

Drug Levels†			
		Reference Value	
Drug Determination		Conventional Units	SI Units
Aminoglycosides (peak levels)	Amikacin	16-32 μg/ml	nd
	Gentamicin	4-8 μg/ml	nd
	Kanamycin	15-40 μg/ml	nd
	Netilmicin	6-10 μg/ml	nd
	Streptomycin	20-30 μg/ml	nd
	Tobramycin	4-8 μg/ml	nd
Antiarrhythmics	Amiodarone	0.5-2.5 μg/ml	nd
	Bretylium	0.5-1.5 μg/ml	nd
	Digitoxin	9-25 μg/L	11.8-32.8 nmol/L
	Digoxin	0.5-2.2 ng/ml	0.6-2.8 nmol/L
	Disopyramide	2-8 μg/ml	6-18 μmol/L
	Flecainide	0.2-1 μg/ml	nd
	Lidocaine	1.5-6 μg/ml	4.5-21.5 μmol/L
	Mexiletine	0.5-2 μg/ml	nd
	Procainamide	4-8 μg/ml	17-34 μmol/ml
	Propranolol	50-200 ng/ml	190-770 nmol/L
	Quinidine	2-6 μg/ml	4.6-9.2 μmol/L
	Tocainide	4-10 μg/ml	nd
	Verapamil	0.08-0.3 μg/ml	nd
Anti-convulsants	Carbamazepine	4-12 μg/ml	17-51 μmol/L
	Phenobarbital	15-40 μg/ml	65-172 μmol/L
	Phenytoin	10-20 μg/ml	40-80 μmol/L
	Primidone	5-12 μg/ml	25-46 μmol/L
	Valproic acid	50-100 μg/ml	350-700 μmol/L
Antidepressants	Amitriptyline	110-250 ng/ml	nd
	Amoxapine	200-500 ng/ml	nd
	Bupropion	25-100 ng/ml	nd
	Clomipramine	80-100 ng/ml	nd
	Desipramine	125-300 ng/ml	nd
	Doxepin	100-200 ng/ml	nd
	Imipramine	200-350 ng/ml	nd
	Maprotiline	200-300 ng/ml	nd
	Nortriptyline	50-150 ng/ml	nd
	Protriptyline	100-200 ng/ml	nd
	Trazodone	800-1600 ng/ml	nd
Antipsychotics	Chlorpromazine	30-500 ng/ml	nd
	Fluphenazine	0.13-2.8 ng/ml	nd
	Haloperidol	5-20 ng/ml	nd
	Perphenazine	0.8-1.2 ng/ml	nd
	Thiothixene	2-57 ng/ml	nd
Miscellaneous	Amantadine	300 ng/ml	nd
	Amrinone	3.7 μg/ml	nd
	Chloramphenicol	10-20 μg/ml	31-62 μmol/L
	Cyclosporine[1]	250-800 ng/ml (whole blood, RIA)	nd
		50-300 ng/ml (plasma, RIA)	nd
	Ethanol[2]	0 mg/dl	0 mmol/L
	Hydralazine	100 ng/ml	nd
	Lithium	0.5-1.5 mEq/L	0.5-1.5 mmol/L
	Salicylate	100-200 mg/L	724-1448 μmol/L
	Sulfonamide	5-15 mg/dl	nd
	Terbutaline	0.5-4.1 ng/ml	nd
	Theophylline	10-20 μg/ml	55-110 μmol/L
	Vancomycin (peak)	30-40 ng/ml	nd

† The values given are generally accepted as desirable for achieving therapeutic effect without toxicity for most patients. However, exceptions are not uncommon.

[1] 24 hour trough values. [2] Toxic: 50-100 mg/dl (10.9-21.7 mmol/L). nd – No data available.

STANDARD ABBREVIATIONS

ac before meals
bid twice daily
°C degrees Celsius
bpm beats per minute
Ca calcium
Cal Calorie (kilocalorie)
Ccr creatinine clearance
CDC Centers for Disease Control and Prevention
CHF congestive heart failure
Cl chloride
CNS central nervous system
CPK creatine phosphokinase
CSF cerebrospinal fluid
cu cubic
Cu copper
dl deciliter (100 ml)
DNA Deoxyribonucleic acid
ECG or EKG electrocardiogram
EEG electroencephalogram
F fluoride
°F degrees Fahrenheit
FA folic acid
FDA Food and Drug Administration
Fe iron
g gram
G-6-PD glucose-6-phosphate dehydrogenase
gal gallon
GI gastrointestinal
GU genitourinary
h or hr hour
hs at bedtime
I iodine
IM intramuscular
IU international units
IV intravenous
K potassium
kg kilogram
L liter
lb pound
m meter
m^2 square meter
mcg microgram
mCi millicurie
mEq milliequivalent
mg milligram
Mg magnesium
MIC minimum inhibitory concentration
min minute
ml milliliter
mm millimeter
mm^3 cubic millimeter
Mn manganese
Mo molybdenum
mOsm milliosmole
MRI Magnetic resonance imaging
Na sodium
NF National Formulary
ng nanogram
otc over the counter (nonprescription)
oz ounce
P phosphorus
pc after meals
po by mouth
ppm parts per million
prn as needed
pt pint
qid four times daily
qt quart
RDA Recommended Dietary Allowance
RNA ribonucleic acid
Rx prescription only
SC subcutaneous
Se selenium
t½ half-life
tid three times daily
tbsp tablespoon
tsp teaspoon
U unit
UD unit dose package
USP United States Pharmacopeia
V_d Volume of distribution
WHO World Health Organization
Zn zinc

GENERAL MANAGEMENT OF ACUTE OVERDOSAGE

Rapid intervention is essential to minimize morbidity and mortality in an acute toxic ingestion. Institute measures to prevent absorption and hasten elimination as soon as possible; however, symptomatic and supportive care takes precedence over other therapy. It is assumed that basic life support measures, ie, cardiopulmonary resuscitation (CPR), have been instituted. The discussion below outlines procedures used in the management of acute overdosage of orally ingested systemic drugs.

Advanced Life Support Measures:

Adequate Airway must be established and maintained, generally via oropharyngeal or endotracheal airways, cricothyrotomy or tracheostomy.

Ventilation may then be performed via mouth-to-mouth insufflation, hand-operated bag (ambu bag) or a mechanical ventilator.

Circulation must be maintained.

- *Hypotension:* If hypotension/hypoperfusion occurs, place the patient in shock position (head lowered, feet elevated); specific therapy may include:

  Establish IV access and initiate IV fluids (eg, normal [0.9%] saline, 0.45% saline, Ringer's lactate, dextrose solutions). A maintenance flow rate is generally 100 to 200 ml/hour; individualize as necessary.

  Plasma, plasma protein fractions, whole blood or plasma expanders may be required.

  Severe hypotension may require judicious use of cardiovascular active agents. The most commonly recommended agents are dopamine, dobutamine and norepinephrine.
- *Arrhythmia* treatment is dictated by the offending drug.
- *Hypertension*, sometimes severe, may occur.

Seizures: Simple isolated seizures may require only observation and supportive care. Repetitive seizures or status epilepticus require therapy. Diazepam IV or phenytoin are generally the agents of choice; phenobarbital may also be considered.

Reduction of Drug Absorption:

Gastric emptying is generally recommended as soon as possible; however, this is generally not very effective unless employed within the first 1 to 2 hours after ingestion. Syrup of ipecac and gastric lavage are the two most commonly employed methods.

- *Syrup of ipecac* is the method of choice outside the hospital, but administer only on the advice of a qualified health-care professional.
- *Gastric lavage* is indicated in the comatose patient and for those in whom syrup of ipecac fails to produce emesis. Airway protection via endotracheal intubation is appropriate for the patient without a gag reflex. Position the patient on his left side and use a large bore tube. Instill warm water or saline 37° C (98.6° F), 100 to 300 ml per wash for adults; 10 ml/kg to a maximum of 250 ml for children, until lavage solution returns clear. Instill the fluid over 1 to 2 minutes, leave in place about 1 minute and drain over 3 to 4 minutes.

Adsorption, using activated charcoal after completion of emesis or lavage, is indicated for virtually all significant toxic ingestions. It adsorbs a wide variety of toxins and there are no contraindications. However, it adsorbs many orally administered antidotes as well, so space dosage properly.

Catharsis is sometimes recommended, generally using a saline or osmotic cathartic (eg, magnesium sulfate or citrate or sorbitol) to promote passage of the toxin through the GI tract.

Whole bowel irrigation (WBI) utilizes rapid administration of large volumes of lavage solutions, such as PEG. It may be most useful for removal of iron tablets and cocaine-containing condoms or balloons.

Elimination of Absorbed Drug:

Interruption of enterohepatic circulation by "gastric dialysis" uses scheduled doses of activated charcoal for 1 to 2 days. Gastric dialysis not only interrupts the enterohepatic cycle of some drugs, but also creates an osmotic gradient, drawing drug from the plasma back into the gastrointestinal lumen where it is bound by the charcoal and excreted in the feces.

Diuresis may be effective.

- *Forced diuresis* is occasionally useful. The most common agents employed are furosemide and osmotic diuretics.
- *Alkaline diuresis* is appropriate for certain compounds (eg, phenobarbital, salicylates) and is usually accomplished by the administration of IV sodium bicarbonate.
- *Acid diuresis* may be indicated (eg, in overdose with amphetamines, fenfluramine, quinine) but use with caution in patients with renal or liver disease. It is usually accomplished with oral or IV ascorbic acid or ammonium chloride.

Dialysis is indicated in a minority of severe overdose cases. Drug factors that alter dialysis effectiveness include volume of distribution, drug compartmentalization, protein binding and lipid/water solubility.

- *Peritoneal dialysis* and *hemodialysis* have been the most common methods used. *Charcoal or resin hemoperfusion* is a relatively new procedure with promising clinical potential (eg, with theophylline).

Poison Control Center:

Consultation with a regional poison control center is highly recommended.

COMMON ABBREVIATIONS

Word	Abbreviation	Meaning
ana	āā, aa	of each
ante cibum	a.c.	before meals or food
ad	ad	to, up to
aurio dextra	a.d.	right ear
ad libitum	ad lib	at pleasure
aurio laeva	a.l.	left ear
ante meridiem	A.M.	morning
aqua	aq	water
aqua destilata	aq.dest.	distilled water
aurio sinister	a.s.	left ear
aures ultrae	a.u.	each ear
bis in die	b.i.d.	twice daily
bowel movement	b.m.	bowel movement
blood pressure	b.p.	blood pressure
cong	c.	a gallon
cum	c̄	with
capsula	caps	capsule
	cc	cubic centimeter
compositus	comp	compound
dies	d	day
dilue	dil	dilute
dispensa	disp	dispense
divide	div	divide
dentur tales doses	d.t.d.	give of such a dose
elixir	el	elixir
	e.m.p.	as directed
et	et	and
	ex aq	in water
fac, fiat, fiant	f., ft.	make, let be made
Food and Drug Administration	FDA	Food and Drug Administration
gramma	Gm., g	gram
granum	gr	grain
gutta	gtt	a drop
hora	h	hour
hora somni	h.s., hor. som.	at bedtime
	i.m., I.M.	intramuscular
	i.v.	intravenous
liquor	liq	a liquor, solution
	mcg	microgram
	mg	milligram
	ml	milliliter
misce	M.	mix
quantum sufficiat	q.s.	a sufficient quantity
	q.s. ad	a sufficient quantity to make
semis	s̄s̄., ss	one-half
United States Adopted Names	USAN	official adopted names
United States Pharmacopeia	U.S.P.	United States Pharmacopeia
while awake	w.a.	while awake

COMMON SYSTEMS OF WEIGHT AND MEASURE*

METRIC SYSTEM

Metric Weight

1 microgram†	μg (mcg)	=	0.000,001	g
1 milligram	mg	=	0.001	g
1 centrigram	cg	=	0.01	g
1 decigram	dg	=	0.1	g
1 gram	g	=	1.0	g
1 dekagram	Dg	=	10.0	g
1 hectogram	Hg	=	100.0	g
1 kilogram	Kg	=	1000.0	g

Metric Liquid Measure

1 microliter	μl	=	0.000,001	L
1 milliliter	ml	=	0.001	L
1 Centiliter	cl	=	0.01	L
1 deciliter	dl	=	0.1	L
1 liter	L	=	1.0	L
1 dekaliter	Dl	=	10.0	L
1 hectoliter	Hl	=	100.0	L
1 kiloliter	Kl	=	1000.0	L

APOTHECARY SYSTEM

Apothecary Weight

1 grain‡	gr	=	1 gr		
1 scruple	+	=	20 gr		
1 dram	/	=	60 gr	=	3+
1 ounce	0	=	480 gr	=	8/
1 pound	G	=	5760 gr	=	120

Apothecary Liquid Measure

1 minim	.	=	1.		
1 fluidram	f/	=	60.		
1 fluidounce	f0	–	480.	=	8 f/
1 pint	pt	=	7680.	=	16 f0
1 quart	qt	=	15630.	=	32 f0
1 gallon	gal	=	61440.	=	8 pt0

AVOIRDUPOIS SYSTEM

Avoirdupois Weight

1 ounce	=	1 oz	=	437.5 grains (gr)		
1 pound	=	1 lb	=	16 ounces (oz)	=	7000 grains (gr)

* The listing of common systems of weight and measure is included to aid the practitioner in calculating dosages.

† Note: The abbreviation μg or mcg is used for microgram in pharmacy rather than gamma (γ) as in biology.

‡ Note: The grain in each of the above systems has the same value, and thus serves as a basis for the interconversion of the other units.

INDEX

A

B

D

E

F

G

H

I

J

K

L

M

N

O

P

Q

R

S

T

U

V

W

X

Z